Pancreatic Cancer

Daniel D. Von Hoff, MD
Professor of Medicine, Molecular and Cellular Biology and Pathology

Director, Arizona Health Sciences Center's Cancer and Therapeutics Program
University of Arizona

Director, Translational Drug Development Division
Translational Genomics Research Institute (TGen)
Phoenix, AZ

Douglas B. Evans, MD
Hamill Foundation
Distinguished Professor of Surgery
The University of Texas M. D. Anderson Cancer Center, Houston, TX

Ralph H. Hruban, MD
Professor of Pathology and Oncology
The Sol Goldman Pancreatic Cancer Research Center
The Johns Hopkins Medical Institutions, Baltimore, MD

JONES AND BARTLETT PUBLISHERS
Sudbury, Massachusetts
BOSTON TORONTO LONDON SINGAPORE

World Headquarters
Jones and Bartlett Publishers
40 Tall Pine Drive
Sudbury, MA 01776
978-443-5000
info@jbpub.com
www.jbpub.com

Jones and Bartlett
Publishers Canada
2406 Nikanna Road
Mississauga, ON L5C
2W6
CANADA

Jones and Bartlett
Publishers International
Barb House, Barb Mews
London W6 7PA
UK

Jones and Bartlett's books and products are available through most bookstores and online booksellers. To contact Jones and Bartlett Publishers directly, call 800-832-0034, fax 978-443-8000, or visit our website www.jbpub.com.

Substantial discounts on bulk quantities of Jones and Bartlett's publications are available to corporations, professional associations, and other qualified organizations. For details and specific discount information, contact the special sales department at Jones and Bartlett via the above contact information or send an email to specialsales@jbpub.com.

Library of Congress Cataloging-in-Publication Data

Pancreatic cancer / [edited] by Daniel D. Von Hoff, Douglas B. Evans, Ralph H. Hruban.– 1st ed.
p. ; cm.
Includes bibliographical references and index.
ISBN 0-7637-2178-6
1. Pancreas--Cancer.
[DNLM: 1. Pancreatic Neoplasms–therapy. 2. Pancreatic Neoplasms--diagnosis. WI 810 P18815 2005] I. Von Hoff, Daniel D. II. Evans, Douglas B. (Douglas Brian), 1956- III. Hruban, Ralph H.
RC280.P25P342 2005
616.99'437--dc22
2004013095

Production Credits
Chief Executive Officer: Clayton Jones
Chief Operating Officer: Don W. Jones, Jr.
President, Jones and Bartlett Higher Education: Robert Holland
V.P., Design and Production: Anne Spencer
V.P., Manufacturing and Inventory Control: Therese Bräuer
Executive Publisher: Christopher Davis
Production Director: Amy Rose
Marketing Manager: Matthew Payne
Editorial Assistant: Kathy Richardson
Production Assistant: Caroline Senay
Production Assistant: Kate Hennessy
Text Design: Anne Spencer
Cover Design: Ko Design Studio
Composition: Graphic World
Illustrations and Technical Art: Graphic World
Printing and Binding: Courier Kendallville
Cover Printing: Courier Kendallville and Courier Westford

Printed in the United States of America
09 08 07 06 05 10 9 8 7 6 5 4 3 2 1

The Editors dedicate this book to the people who lost their lives battling pancreatic cancer and to those who have survived the disease with the hope that knowledge and hard work will defeat it.

Daniel D. Von Hoff, MD
Douglas B. Evans, MD
Ralph H. Hruban, MD

Contents

Pancreatic cancer is now the fourth leading cause of cancer death in the United States, and mortality almost equals incidence. Because of progress against other types of cancer, it is very likely that the number of deaths from pancreatic cancer each year will surpass the number of deaths from other more common cancers, such as breast cancer. In addition to the sheer mortality from the disease, pancreatic cancer causes significant morbidity for patients, including pain, severe fatigue, weight loss, and cachexia. Pancreatic cancer also does the worst thing a disease can do—it robs those affected of all hope. It is clear that more needs to be done to treat and prevent this disease.

Based on new molecular findings, there is reason to believe that pancreatic cancer has a unique genetic profile that may be vulnerable to attack. One way to help galvanize that attack is to have a reference source of our current knowledge of pancreatic cancer, both basic and clinical, so that individuals from different disciplines can use this resource as both a stepping stone for treating patients who already have the disease and as a foundation for the discovery of new ways to treat or prevent pancreatic cancer. Therefore, the purpose of *Pancreatic Cancer* is to serve as a knowledge base for those who want to make a difference for patients both now and in the future.

A wonderful group of 115 individual investigators from seven countries has contributed their expertise, time, and considerable energy to put this knowledge base together. We sincerely hope that this information will be an important foundation for the prevention and treatment of pancreatic cancer and will serve to further stimulate the growing body of clinicians and investigators who work to improve the outcome of patients with this disease.

Daniel D. Von Hoff, MD
Douglas B. Evans, MD
Ralph H. Hruban, MD

THE LUSTGARTEN FOUNDATION FOR PANCREATIC CANCER RESEARCH

www.lustgarten.org

The Board of Directors of The Lustgarten Foundation for Pancreatic Cancer Research applauds the efforts of Drs. Daniel Von Hoff, Douglas Evans, and Ralph Hruban for helping to bring much-needed attention to a disease that too often goes unnoticed. We are proud to join with such outstanding leaders in the fight against pancreatic cancer.

The Lustgarten Foundation is pleased to encourage the distribution of this comprehensive resource by Jones and Bartlett Publishers. We believe that *Pancreatic Cancer* will prove a significant stepping stone in the advancement of education among members of the scientific and medical communities. Thank you all for your incredible dedication to this important work.

The editors are especially grateful to the following people, whose incredible enthusiasm and hard work contributed to this book.

We want to thank Chris Davis, Executive Publisher, Medicine, of Jones and Bartlett Publishers, who saw how great a problem pancreatic cancer is and enthusiastically agreed to take on the challenge of a definitive textbook in the area. The editors are very grateful for his vision and leadership on the project. Kathy Richardson, Editorial Assistant, Medicine; Amy Rose, Production Manager; and Caroline Senay, Production Assistant, of Jones and Bartlett Publishers worked so hard on the compilation of the contributions and the copyediting of the manuscripts.

We are very appreciative of those who have dedicated special time to this book, including: Kathleen D. Wagner at The University of Texas M. D. Anderson Cancer Center, who coordinated the development of all color illustrations, Dante Trusty and Norman Barker at The Johns Hopkins Medical Institutions for their invaluable assistance with specimen photography and microscopic photography expertise respectively, and Dr. Haiyong Han at the Arizona Cancer Center for some of the photo contributions for the text cover. In addition, we are grateful to our assistants Mrs. Susan K. Hogue of The University of Texas M. D. Anderson Cancer Center, Mrs. Sandra Markowitz at The Johns Hopkins Medical Institutions, and Ms. Elva Apodaca and Ms. Angela Wakeham of the Arizona Cancer Center for their hard work, dedication, and professionalism they devoted to this project.

We are very grateful to our colleagues, who contributed their perspectives, their expertise, and their time to this text. Without their devotion, this book would not exist.

Daniel D. Von Hoff, MD
Douglas B. Evans, MD
Ralph H. Hruban, MD

A Special Thank You

We gratefully acknowledge the generous support of the Heriette Pickelner Fund for Pancreatic Cancer Research at The University of Texas M. D. Anderson Cancer Center, which made possible the color figures throughout the text. We are fortunate to have Heriette's family provide the following brief insight into this wonderfully talented woman whose legacy lives on in the battle against pancreatic cancer.

We could not believe it when the doctors told Heriette she had pancreatic cancer. She was too young, too healthy. At first, the tumor did not look like cancer, but it was. We hoped that it was caught early enough or that a particular treatment would work—that was not to be. When Heriette learned she had pancreatic cancer, the doctors told her that her life expectancy may be as short as six months. Instead, she fought this disease for two and a half years. She was an ideal patient, baking treats for the staff at M. D. Anderson and cooking dinner for her doctors (and even telling them that if they want more, they need to keep her alive). She educated herself as much as she could about her illness, was an active researcher on the Internet, and often talked to other patients. When she realized the lethality of pancreatic cancer, she decided to do something about it and established a research fund in the hope that she could, in some small way, help find a cure for pancreatic cancer. She knew that her fund would not be able to help her, but she had the faith and vision that it would help others. She believed no one should have to go through the occasional painful treatments, the dashed hopes, and the agony of loss that accompany cancer treatment. Heriette loved her family and was more worried about them than she was about herself. In the end, she was not afraid of death; instead she felt guilty that she was leaving her husband, sons, parents, sister, and nieces. The reality of it, though, was that we were all very proud of her; by the time she succumbed to the cancer, she had unknowingly taught us so much about being strong, staying positive, always having hope, and never, ever, giving up.

We have every expectation that a young doctor will read this textbook and take an interest in fighting pancreatic cancer. Maybe an experienced physician will learn something new and help identify pancreatic cancer in its early stages; hopefully, saving someone's life. And maybe, just maybe, this textbook will lead to finding a cure. That is why Heriette created her research fund. The Pickelner Fund for Pancreatic Cancer Research is dedicated to the blessed memory of Heriette Pickelner, a loving woman of valor and dignity.

Bob, Aaron, and Daniel Pickelner
Marcee, Dan, Samantha, and Monica Lundeen
Milton and Eleanor Gaman

Eddie K. Abdalla, MD
Assistant Professor of Surgery
The University of Texas M. D. Anderson Cancer Center, Houston, TX

Ross A. Abrams, MD
Chairman, Department of Radiation Oncology
Rush University Medical Center, Chicago, IL

N. Volkan Adsay, MD
Associate Professor
The Karmanos Cancer Institute and Wayne State University, Harper Hospital, Detroit, MI

Jorge Albores-Saavedra, MD
Professor of Pathology
Director, Division of Anatomic Pathology
Louisiana State University Health Sciences Center, Shreveport, LA

Syed Z. Ali, MD
Associate Professor of Pathology
The Sol Goldman Pancreatic Cancer Research Center
The Johns Hopkins Medical Institutions, Baltimore, MD

Nabeel Bardeesy, PhD
Instructor, Harvard Medical School
Dana-Farber Cancer Institute, Boston, MA

Peter J. Biggs, PhD
Associate Professor of Radiation Oncology
Harvard Medical School
Massachusetts General Hospital, Boston, MA

John D. Birkmeyer, MD
G.D. Zuidema Professor of Surgery,
University of Michigan, Ann Arbor, MI

Michael Bouvet, MD
Associate Professor of Surgery
University of California, San Diego, CA

Kieran Brune, BS
Department of Pathology
The Sol Goldman Pancreatic Cancer Research Center
The Johns Hopkins Medical Institutions, Baltimore, MD

Mark P. Callery, MD
Associate Professor of Surgery
Harvard Medical School
Chief, Division of General Surgery
Beth Israel Deaconess Medical Center, Boston, MA

Kenneth J. Chang, MD
Associate Professor of Medicine, University of California
Executive Director, H. H. Chao Comprehensive Digestive Disease Center, Irvine, CA

Chusilp Charnsangavej, MD
Robert D. Moreton Distinguished Chair in Diagnostic Imaging
Professor of Radiology and Associate Deputy Division Head for Research
The University of Texas M. D. Anderson Cancer Center, Houston, TX

Haesun Choi, MD
Associate Professor of Radiology
The University of Texas M. D. Anderson Cancer Center, Houston, TX

John D. Christein, MD
Fellow, Advanced GI Surgery
Mayo Clinic, Rochester, MN

Yun Shin Chun, MD
Resident in Surgery
Mayo Clinic College of Medicine, Rochester, MN

Bryan M. Clary, MD
Assistant Professor of Surgery
Duke University Medical Center, Durham, NC

Kevin C. Conlon, MD, MBA
Professor & Chair of Surgery
Trinity College Dublin,
The Adelaide & Meath Hospital incorporating the National Children's Hospital, Dublin, Ireland

Christopher H. Crane, MD
Associate Professor of Radiation Oncology
The University of Texas M. D. Anderson Cancer Center, Houston, TX

David T. Curiel, MD, PhD
Professor and Director
Gene Therapy Center, University of Alabama at Birmingham, Birmingham, AL

Michael J. Demeure, MD
Professor of Surgery
University of Arizona, Tucson, AZ

Benedict M. Devereaux, MBBS
Consultant Gastroenterologist
Royal Brisbane and Women's Hospital, Brisbane, Australia

Gerard M. Doherty, MD
N.W. Thompson Professor of Surgery
University of Michigan, Ann Arbor, MI

Lee M. Ellis, MD
Professor of Surgery and Cancer Biology
The University of Texas M. D. Anderson Cancer Center, Houston, TX

Ahmed Elsayem, MD
Assistant Professor
The University of Texas M. D. Anderson Cancer Center, Houston, TX

Richard A. Erickson, MD
Professor of Medicine
Texas A&M University System Health Science Center
Director, Division of Gastroenterology, Scott & White Clinic and Hospital, Temple, TX

Douglas B. Evans, MD
Professor of Surgery
The University of Texas M. D. Anderson Cancer Center, Houston, TX

Bingliang Fang, PhD
Associate Professor
The University of Texas M. D. Anderson Cancer Center, Houston, TX

Silvana C. Faria, MD
Associate Professor of Radiology
The University of Texas M. D. Anderson Cancer Center, Houston, TX

Michael B. Farnell, MD
Professor of Surgery
Chair, Division of Gastroenterologic and General Surgery
Mayo Medical School, Rochester, MN

Olivera J. Finn, PhD
Professor of Immunology
University of Pittsburgh School of Medicine, Pittsburgh, PA

Marsha L. Frazier, PhD
Associate Professor
The University of Texas M. D. Anderson Cancer Center, Houston, TX

Carlos Frenández-del Castillo, MD
Associate Professor of Surgery
Harvard Medical School
Massachusetts General Hospital, Boston, MA

Scott F. Gallagher, MD
Assistant Professor of Surgery
University of South Florida College of Medicine, Tampa General Hospital, Tampa, FL

Michael C. Garofalo, MD
Assistant Professor of Radiation Oncology
University of Maryland Medical Center, Baltimore, MD

Michael G. Goggins, MD
Associate Professor of Pathology, Medicine, Oncology
The Sol Goldman Pancreatic Cancer Research Center
The Johns Hopkins Medical Institutions, Baltimore, MD

Sanjay Gupta, MD
Assistant Professor
The University of Texas M. D. Anderson Cancer Center, Houston, TX

Ralph H. Hruban, MD
Professor of Pathology and Oncology
The Sol Goldman Pancreatic Cancer Research Center
The Johns Hopkins Medical Institutions, Baltimore, MD

Kelly K. Hunt, MD
Professor of Surgery
The University of Texas M. D. Anderson Cancer Center, Houston, TX

Christine A. Iacobuzio-Donahue, MD, PhD
Assistant Professor of Pathology and Oncology
The Sol Goldman Pancreatic Cancer Research Center
The Johns Hopkins Medical Institutions, Baltimore, MD

Elizabeth M. Jaffe, MD
Professor of Oncology
The Sol Goldman Pancreatic Cancer Research Center
Sidney Kimmel Comprehensive Cancer Center
The Johns Hopkins Medical Institutions, Baltimore, MD

Li Jiao, MD
Fellow, Department of Gastrointestinal Medical
The University of Texas M. D. Anderson Cancer Center, Houston, TX

Eric Jonasch, MD
Assistant Professor of Medicine
The University of Texas M. D. Anderson Cancer Center, Houston, TX

Matthew H. Katz, MD
Senior Resident in Surgery
University of California, San Diego, CA

Michael L. Kendrick, MD
Assistant Professor of Surgery
Mayo Clinic College of Medicine, Rochester, MN

Scott E. Kern, MD
Professor of Oncology
The Sol Goldman Pancreatic Cancer Research Center
Sidney Kimmel Comprehensive Cancer Center
The Johns Hopkins Medical Institutions, Baltimore, MD

Alison Klein, PhD
Assistant Professor of Oncology
The Sol Goldman Pancreatic Cancer Research Center
Sidney Kimmel Comprehensive Cancer Center
The John Hopkins Medical Institutions, Baltimore, MD

David S. Klimstra, MD
Attending Pathologist
Memorial Sloan-Kettering Cancer Center, New York, NY

Andrew H. Ko, MD
Assistant Clinical Professor of Medicine
UCSF Comprehensive Cancer Center, San Francisco, CA

Jason A. Konner, MD
Clinical Assistant Attending
Memorial Sloan-Kettering Cancer Center, New York, NY

Maria A. Kouvaraki, MD, PhD
Fellow
The Department of Surgical Oncology, Section of Endocrine Tumor Surgery
The University of Texas M. D. Anderson Cancer Center, Houston, TX

Young Kwok, MD
Assistant Professor of Radiation Oncology
University of Maryland Medical Center, Baltimore, MD

Daniel A. Laheru, MD
Assistant Professor of Oncology
The Sol Goldman Pancreatic Cancer Research Center
Sidney Kimmel Comprehensive Cancer Center
The Johns Hopkins Medical Institutions, Baltimore, MD

Laura A. Lambert, MD
Fellow, Department of Surgical Oncology
The University of Texas M. D. Anderson Cancer Center, Houston, TX

Gregory Y. Lauwers, MD
Associate Professor of Pathology, Harvard Medical School
Director, Gastrointestinal Pathology Service, Massachusetts General Hospital, Boston, MA

Steven D. Leach, MD
The Paul K. Neumann Professor in Pancreatic Cancer
The Sol Goldman Pancreatic Cancer Research Center
The Johns Hopkins Medical Institutions, Baltimore, MD

Jeffrey E. Lee, MD
Professor of Surgery
The University of Texas M. D. Anderson Cancer Center, Houston, TX

Jonathan J. Lewis, MD, PhD
Chairman and CEO
ZIOPHARM, Inc., New York, NY

Donghui Li, PhD
Associate Professor of Medicine
The University of Texas M. D. Anderson Cancer Center, Houston, TX

John W. Lin, MD
Fellow, Department of Surgery
The Sol Goldman Pancreatic Cancer Research Center
The Johns Hopkins Medical Institutions, Baltimore, MD

Daniel S. Longnecker, MD
Professor of Pathology
Dartmouth Medical School, Hanover, NH

Evelyne M. Loyer, MD
Associate Professor of Radiology
The University of Texas M. D. Anderson Cancer Center, Houston, TX

Stephen McRae, MD
Assistant Professor of Radiology
The University of Texas M. D. Anderson Cancer Center, Houston, TX

Mari Mino, MD
Instructor in Pathology, Harvard Medical School
Assistant Pathologist, Massachusetts General Hospital, Boston, MA

Abdool R. Moossa, MD
Professor of Surgery
University of California, San Diego, CA

Michel M. Murr, MD
Associate Professor of Surgery
University of South Florida College of Medicine, Tampa General Hospital, Tampa, FL

G. Johan A. Offerhaus, MD, PhD
Professor of Pathology
Academic Medical Center, University of Amsterdam, The Netherlands

Eileen M. O'Reilly, MD
Assistant Professor of Medicine
Assistant Attending Physician
Memorial Sloan-Kettering Cancer Center, New York, NY

Theodore N. Pappas, MD
Professor of Surgery
Duke University Medical Center

John V. Pearson, BS
Translational Genomics Research Institute (TGen), Phoenix, AZ

Gloria M. Petersen, PhD
Professor of Epidemiology
Mayo Clinic College of Medicine, Rochester, MN

Vincent J. Picozzi, Jr., MD
Hematologist/Oncologist
Virginia Mason Medical Center, Seattle, WA

Peter W. T. Pisters, MD
Professor of Surgery
The University of Texas M. D. Anderson Cancer Center, Houston, TX

Scott Plevy, MD
Associate Professor of Medicine and Immunology
University of Pittsburgh School of Medicine, Pittsburgh, PA

Miquel Porta, MD, PhD
Professor and Head, Clinical & Molecular Epidemiology of Cancer Unit
Institut Municipal d'Investigació Mèdica
Universitat Autònoma de Barcelona, Spain

Chandrajit P. Raut, MD
Instructor, Harvard Medical School
Associate Surgeon, Brigham and Women's Hospital, Boston, MA

Suresh K. Reddy, MD
Associate Professor
The University of Texas M. D. Anderson Cancer Center, Houston, TX

William F. Regine, MD
Professor and Chairman of Radiation Oncology
University of Maryland Medical Center, Baltimore, MD

Taylor S. Riall, MD
Instructor, Department of Surgery
The Sol Goldman Pancreatic Cancer Research Center
The Johns Hopkins Medical Institutions, Baltimore, MD

Marcel Rozencweig, MD
Sr. VP, Drug Development
GPC Biotech, Princeton, NJ

Eric P. Sandgren, VMD, PhD
Associate Professor of Pathobiological Sciences
School of Veterinary Medicine, University of Wisconsin-Madison, Madison, WI

Michael G. Sarr, MD
James C. Masson Professor of Surgery
Mayo Clinic College of Medicine, Rochester, MN

Charles R. Scoggins, MD
Assistant Professor of Surgery, Division of Surgical Oncology
University of Louisville, Louisville, KY

Suzanne E. Shapiro, MS
The Department of Surgical Oncology, Section of Endocrine Tumor Surgery
The University of Texas M. D. Anderson Cancer Center, Houston, TX

Saima Sharif, MD
Fellow, Department of Medicine
University of Pittsburgh and University of Pittsburgh Cancer Institute, Pittsburgh, PA

Diane M. Simeone, MD
Associate Professor of Surgery
University of Michigan Medical Center, Ann Arbor, MI

Carmen C. Solorzano, MD
Assistant Professor of Surgery
University of Miami/Jackson Memorial Medical Center and The Sylvester Cancer Center, Miami, FL

Gregg A. Staerkel, MD
Professor of Pathology
The University of Texas M. D. Anderson Cancer Center, Houston, TX

Janio Szklaruk, MD
Associate Professor of Radiology
The University of Texas M. D. Anderson Cancer Center, Houston; TX

Rudranath Talukdar, MD
Research Associate, Molecular and Cellular Oncology
The University of Texas M. D. Anderson Cancer Center, Houston, TX

Eric P. Tamm, MD
Assistant Professor of Radiology
The University of Texas M. D. Anderson Cancer Center, Houston, TX

Margaret A. Tempero, MD
Professor of Medicine and Chief
Deputy Director, Director of Clinical Sciences
UCSF Comprehensive Cancer Center, San Francisco, CA

Sarah P. Thayer, MD, PhD
Assistant Professor of Surgery
Harvard Medical School
Massachusetts General Hospital, Boston, MA

Geoffrey B. Thompson, MD
Professor of Surgery, Mayo Medical School
Mayo Clinic, Rochester, MN

Michael J. Tisdale, PhD
Pharmaceutical Sciences Research Institute, Aston University, Birmingham, England

Jeffrey M. Trent, PhD
President and Scientific Director
Translational Genomics Research Institute (TGen), Phoenix, AZ

Olga N. Tucker, MD
Senior (Specialist) Registrar in Surgery
The Adelaide & Meath Hospital incorporating the National Children's Hospital, Dublin, Ireland

Douglas S. Tyler, MD
Professor of Surgery
Duke University Medical Center, Durham, NC

Michiel S. van der Heijden, MD
Fellow, Department of Pathology
The Sol Goldman Pancreatic Cancer Research Center
The Johns Hopkins Medical Institutions, Baltimore, MD

Susanne van Eeden, MD
Assistant Professor of Pathology
Academic Medical Center, University of Amsterdam, The Netherlands

Chandu Vemuri, MD
Resident in Surgery
University of Michigan, Ann Arbor, MI

Charles M. Vollmer, Jr., MD
Visiting Assistant Professor of Surgery
Harvard Medical School
Beth Israel Deaconess Medical Center, Boston, MA

Daniel D. Von Hoff, MD
Professor of Medicine, Molecular and Cellular Biology and Pathology

Director, Arizona Health Sciences Center's Cancer and Therapeutics Program
University of Arizona

Director Translational Drug Development Division
Translational Genomics Research Institute (TGen)
Phoenix, AZ

Michael J. Wallace, MD
Associate Professor of Radiology
The University of Texas M. D. Anderson Cancer Center, Houston, TX

Kay Washington, MD, PhD
Professor of Pathology
Vanderbilt University Medical Center, Nashville, TN

David Whitaker, MBBS
Gastroenterology Registrar
Royal Brisbane and Women's Hospital, Brisbane Australia

David C. Whitcomb, MD, PhD
Professor of Medicine, Cell Biology & Physiology, and Human Genetics Chief
Division of Gastroenterology, Hepatology and Nutrition
University of Pittsburgh and University of Pittsburgh Medical Center, Pittsburgh, PA

Rebekah R. White, MD
Chief Resident in Surgery
Duke University Medical Center, Durham, NC

Christopher G. Willett, MD
Professor and Chair of Radiation Oncology
Duke University Medical Center, Durham, NC

Robert A. Wolff, MD
Associate Professor of Medicine
Department of Gastrointestinal Medical Oncology
The University of Texas M. D. Anderson Cancer Center, Houston, TX

Masato Yamamoto, MD, PhD
Research Assistant Professor
Gene Therapy Center, University of Alabama at Birmingham, Birmingham, AL

James C. Yao, MD
Associate Professor of Medicine
The University of Texas M. D. Anderson Cancer Center, Houston, TX

Tina W. F. Yen, MD
Assistant Professor of Surgery
Medical College of Wisconsin, Milwaukee, WI

Charles J. Yeo, MD
The John L. Cameron Professor of Surgery
The Sol Goldman Pancreatic Cancer Research Center
The Johns Hopkins Medical Institutions, Baltimore, MD

Emmanuel E. Zervos, MD
Assistant Professor of Surgery
University of South Florida College of Medicine, Tampa General Hospital, Tampa, FL

SECTION 1

Anatomy

CHAPTER

1

Gross and Microscopic Anatomy of the Pancreas

Mary Kay Washington, MD, PhD

Gross Anatomy

Anatomic Location

The pancreas, a yellow-tan lobulated organ, lies in a relatively inaccessible retroperitoneal location in the posterior abdomen, anterior to the aorta. The anterior surface of the pancreas is covered with peritoneum; other surfaces are encased in a poorly defined capsule of fibrous tissue. In adults, the pancreas weighs roughly 100 g in men, and 85 g in women. A wide variation in dimensions is seen in the adult, with the pancreas measuring from 15–25 cm in length, 1.4–4 cm from anterior to posterior surfaces, and 3–9 cm in height.[1]

The pancreas is regionally divided into the head, neck, body, and tail, with most of the pancreatic parenchyma (60%–70%) lying in the head and uncinate process. The head inserts into the "C" loop of duodenum (Fig. 1.1). The uncinate process, an extension of the head of the pancreas, curves behind the superior mesenteric artery and vein; these vessels may produce an indentation in the uncinate process known as the *vascular groove* or *pancreatic notch*. The border between the head and the body of the pancreas is designated the *neck*, and the neck is defined as that portion of the pancreas anterior to the superior mesenteric vein and the beginning of the portal vein. Most of the pancreatic body lies behind the gastric antrum, with the pancreatic tail extending to the hilum of the spleen. The distinction between the pancreatic body and tail is poorly defined.

The Pancreatic Ductal System

The main pancreatic duct (the duct of Wirsung) begins in the tail of the pancreas and runs along the posterior surface of the body of the gland to drain into the second portion of the duodenum at the major papilla, the ampulla of Vater. The average diameter of the main pancreatic duct is 3 mm.[1] Smaller ducts join the main duct in a "herringbone" pattern. The accessory pancreatic duct (the duct of Santorini) empties into the minor papilla, or it ends blindly in 20% of cases. The minor papilla usually empties into the duodenum several centimeters proximal (cephalad) to the major papilla. As is discussed in greater detail in Chapter 5, the embryonic dorsal and ventral pancreatic ducts usually fuse, with the short portion of the dorsal duct near the duodenum becoming the accessory duct. Failure of the two embryonic ducts to fuse results in the draining of the bulk of the pancreatic secretions through the diminutive minor papilla. This condition, known as *pancreas divisum*, is found in roughly 10% of the population.

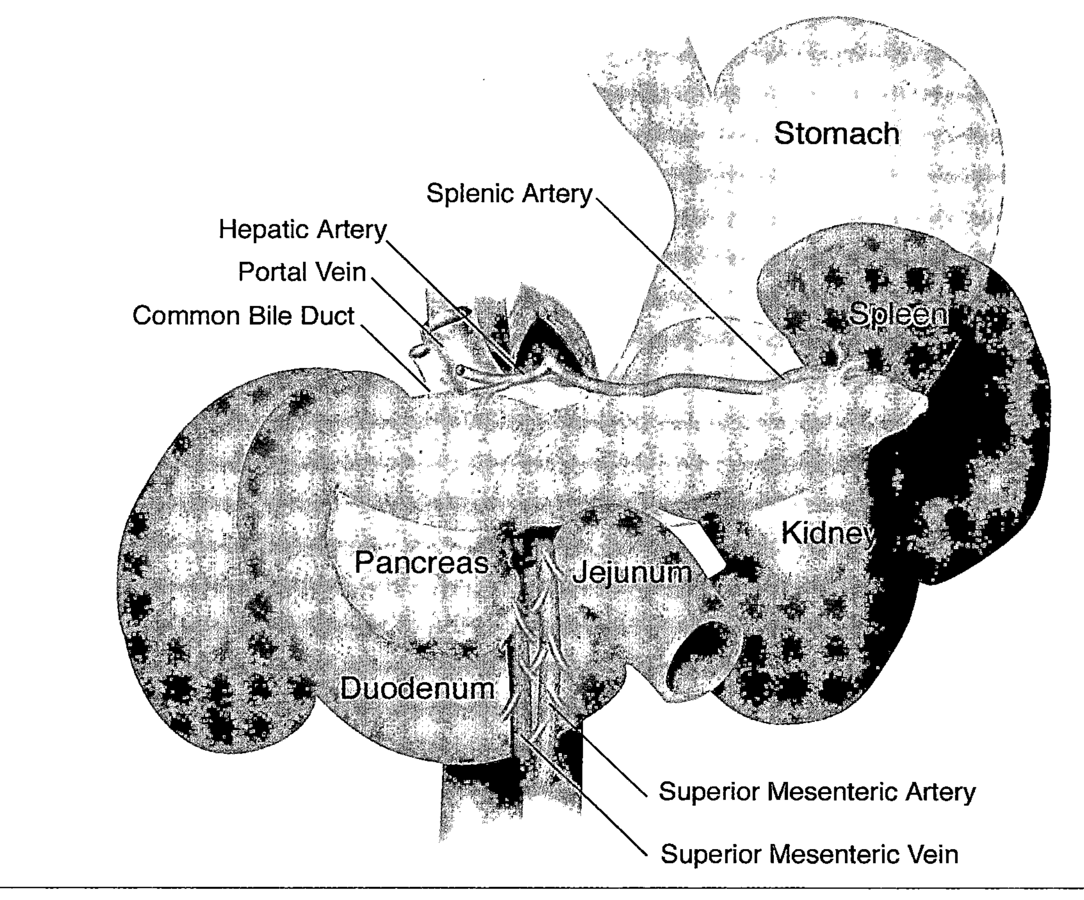

Figure 1.1
Relationship of the pancreas to intra-abdominal organs and major vessels.

The major papilla (papilla of Vater), the confluence of the common bile duct and the main pancreatic duct, is subject to anatomic variations. The common bile duct and the pancreatic duct may open separately or may form a common channel 1–12 mm long. This common channel, found in roughly two thirds of the population,[2] is referred to as the ampulla of Vater. The ducts usually join near the orifice without forming a true dilated ampulla; the pancreatic duct enters the ampulla caudal or slightly lateral to the common bile duct. The sphincter of Oddi, the intrinsic smooth muscle of the vaterian system, regulates the flow of bile and has a complex and variable arrangement of muscle fibers. The minor papilla is located approximately 2 cm proximal to the major papilla.

Blood Supply and Lymphatic Drainage

The major veins and arteries supplying the pancreas course posterior to the main pancreatic duct. Although the origin and distribution of blood vessels supplying the pancreas are subject to considerable variation,[3-8] the following general statements apply in most cases. The celiac trunk, through two of its three major branches (the splenic artery and the common hepatic artery), and the superior mesenteric artery constitute the main blood supply to the pancreas. The gastroduodenal branch of the common hepatic artery, with its anterior and posterior superior pancreaticoduodenal artery branches, is an important source of blood for the head of the pancreas. As many as nine branches of the splenic artery supply the body (supplied by the arteria pancreatica magna) and tail (supplied by the arteria cauda pancreatica) of the pancreas. Branches of the inferior pancreaticoduodenal artery, itself a branch of the superior mesenteric artery, form anastomoses with the anterior and posterior superior pancreaticoduodenal arteries to supply the pancreas and duodenum. Intrinsic blood supply to the pancreas is well developed, with branches of larger vessels supplying interlobular arteries; in general, a single intralobular artery supplies each pancreatic lobule. These arteries typically travel at the periphery of the lobules and are therefore normally separated from the pancreatic ducts by acinar tissue.

The venous drainage of the pancreas is through the superior mesenteric vein and splenic veins, which combine posterior to the pancreas to form the hepatic portal vein. Veins correspond to relative arteries and follow the same general course.

The lymphatic drainage of the pancreas is a matter of considerable interest, given its importance in pancreatic cancer. Small lymphatic vessels, small channels lined by a single layer of endothelial cells, are inconspicuous in routine microscopic sections of the pancreas; these are found within the acini and drain into larger vessels in the interlobular fibrous tissue. These intralobular lymphatics are rather sparse, and most lymphatic vessels lie in the interlobular septa.[9] Lymphatic vessels have a close relationship with acini but are not as closely associated with islets of Langerhans. Larger interlobular lymphatics emerge on the surface of the pancreas and travel with blood vessels toward peripancreatic lymph nodes. Lymph from more superficial lymph nodes, which constitute a ring around the pancreas, drains into deeper nodes, such as preaortic lymph nodes, and ultimately into the thoracic duct. The periaortic lymph nodes may also receive lymph directly from the pancreas.[9] Peripancreatic lymph nodes are abundant, with up to 240 nodes per specimen in some autopsy studies.[10] Regional peripancreatic lymph nodes for cancer staging purposes may be grouped into lymph nodes found along the course of the hepatic artery, the celiac axis, the splenic artery, and the pyloric and splenic regions.[11]

Nerve Supply

The pancreas is innervated by intrinsic and extrinsic neural systems. The extrinsic components, which belong to the parasympathetic and sympathetic systems, may be functionally classified as afferent and efferent nerves. Anatomically, the major components of the extrinsic system are the anterior and posterior branches of the vagus nerve and the splanchnic nerve trunks. The intrinsic neural component is composed of intrapancreatic ganglia scattered throughout the pancreatic parenchyma. In addition to acetylcholine and norepinephrine, a large number of neurotransmitters and neuromodulators have been identified, such as peptidergic neurotransmitters, including vasoactive intestinal polypeptide, neuropeptide Y, and gastrin-releasing peptide. Peptidergic innervation may involve both intrinsic and extrinsic components, and specific peptides are localized to different innervation targets. For instance, localization of substance P/tachykinins, neuropeptide K, and calcitonin gene-related polypeptide around pancreatic vasculature suggests a role in the regulation of pancreatic blood flow.[12]

The extrinsic nerve supply to the pancreas is through efferent fibers of the parasympathetic and sympathetic systems. The parasympathetic supply, which stimulates pancreatic secretion, is via the vagus nerve through the celiac plexus; parasympathetic nerve fibers form a network in the adventitia of blood vessels, and nerves enter the pancreas with arterial branches to end in intrinsic ganglia. Fibers from the intrinsic ganglia course throughout the pancreatic substance to end close to parenchymal cells.

The sympathetic nerve supply to the pancreas is involved in regulating pancreatic blood flow. Fibers from nerve cell bodies in the intermediolateral cell column of the thoracic spinal cord pass through the sympathetic chain ganglia and descend in the greater splanchnic nerve to end in the celiac ganglia. Postganglionic fibers travel in company with parasympathetic fibers to enter the pancreas.

Thin, unmyelinated visceral afferent fibers travel with both the sympathetic and the parasympathetic nervous supply to the pancreas. Those traveling with parasympathetic fibers terminate in the nucleus tractus solitarius. Those traveling with the sympathetic supply traverse the celiac plexus and ascend though greater splanchnic nerves. The cell bodies for this pathway are located in dorsal root ganglia at the thoracic level. It is generally agreed that these fibers are the pathway for pain into the central nervous system from the pancreas.

Microscopic Anatomy

The pancreas is classified as a compound exocrine-endocrine gland; on low-magnification microscopic examination, scattered islets are seen embedded within the acinar tissue of the exocrine pancreas (Fig. 1.2). By volume, the exocrine portion of the pancreas represents up to 84% of total pancreatic volume, with the duct system representing 2%–4% and the endocrine portion constituting about 2%.[1] The organizational unit of the exocrine pancreas is the lobule. The pancreatic lobule consists of a heterogeneous arrangement of acini separated by delicate incomplete stromal septa containing vessels, lymphatics, nerves, and interlobular ducts. The connective tissue within normal lobular units is sparse; a variable amount of connective tissue and fat is present in interlobular areas.

Although classically represented as spherical, grape-like clusters, acini may be spherical, elongated or cylindrical, or irregular. The three-dimensional anatomy of the acinar/ductal system is more complex than previously appreciated and may constitute a tubular-like glandular arrangement[13] rather than a grouping of simple acinar structures. Pancreatic secretions may pass through a complex pathway before reaching ducts.

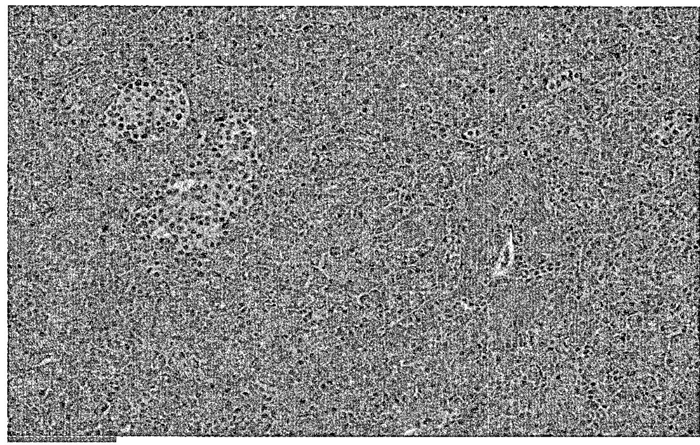

Figure 1.2
The pancreas is a compound exocrine/endocrine organ. Most of the parenchyma consists of acini, with scattered islets of Langerhans. An interlobular duct is present in this field. Hematoxylin and eosin, original magnification ×100.

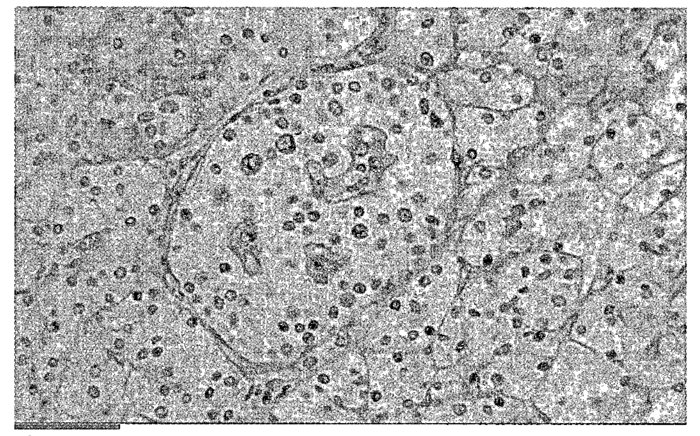

Figure 1.4
The acini rest on a basement membrane containing collagen type IV, shown here. Capillaries are highlighted in the islet of Langerhans. Indirect immunoperoxidase stain, collagen type IV, original magnification ×400.

Acinar Cells

The major cell type in the pancreas is the acinar cell, the fundamental exocrine secretory cell of the pancreas.[14] The acinar cell produces enzymatically inert proenzymes that are activated in the duodenal lumen. By light microscopy, the acinar cell is a large pyramidal cell with a basally located round nucleus (Fig. 1.3). The basal aspect has a basal lamina composed of type IV collagen (Fig. 1.4), laminin, and fibronectin. The small apex opens to the acinar lumen, where the luminal surface of the cell is lined by numerous microvilli. The basal cytoplasm of the acinar cell is strongly basophilic because of abundant rough endoplasmic reticulum; the apical cytoplasm is more eosinophilic and is filled with refractile periodic acid–Schiff positive zymogen granules, which contain the storage forms of the digestive enzymes synthesized and secreted by the acinar cells. Occasionally, clear cytoplasmic vacuoles are present. The acinar cells are held together by junctional complexes, of which the tight junction is the most important. Tight junctions are located near the apical surface, where they help to confine proteolytic secretions to the lumen. Acinar cells label with antibodies to the pancreatic exocrine enzymes trypsin, chymotrypsin, lipase, amylase, and elastase. Acinar cells also typically label with the anticytokeratin clone CAM5.2 (Fig. 1.5) and are weakly positive or negative with AE1/AE3 and with antibodies against cytokeratins 7 and 20 (Table 1.1).

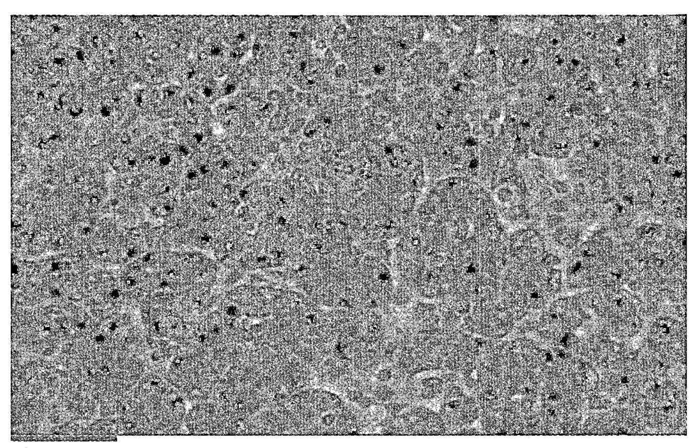

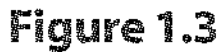

Figure 1.3
The acinar cells of the pancreas have polarized cytoplasm, with apical eosinophilia due to numerous zymogen granules. Pale-staining centroacinar cells and intercalated ducts are distributed among the acini. Hematoxylin and eosin, original magnification ×400.

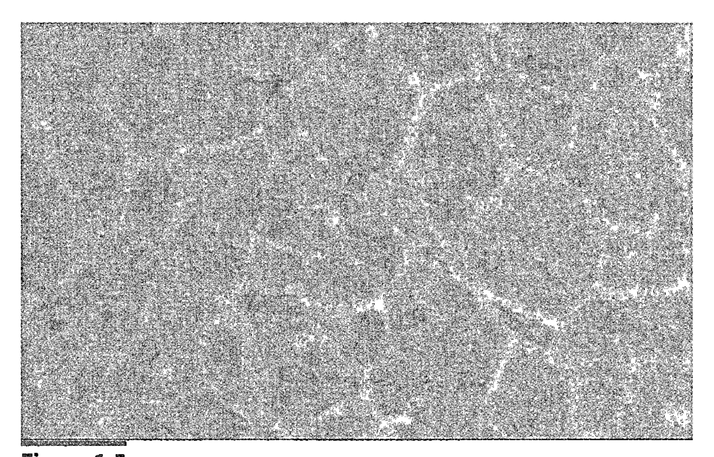

Figure 1.5
Acinar cells are positive for cytokeratin CAM5.2 but negative for cytokeratins 7 and 20. Indirect immunoperoxidase, cytokeratin CAM5.2, original magnification ×400.

Table 1.1 Immunohistochemical Markers of Normal Pancreatic Cells

Pancreatic Cell Type	Immunohistochemical Markers	Other Comments
Acinar	CAM5.2, trypsin, chymotrypsin, lipase, amylase, elastase	Butyrate esterase +; CK7 −; CK20−
Duct	CAM5.2, AE1/AE3, epithelial membrane antigen, cystic fibrosis transmembrane receptor, CK7+, CK19+	CK7+, CK19+
Endocrine	Chromogranin, neuron specific enolase, synaptophysin	Specific products: insulin, glucagon, somatostatin, pancreatic polypeptide, serotonin
Stellate	Alpha smooth muscle actin (activated state)	

Abbreviation: CK, cytokeratin.

Ultrastructural features The acinar cell has the ultrastructural features of a classic protein-producing and -secreting cell. The basal cytoplasm contains abundant rough endoplasmic reticulum, occupying up to 20% of the cell volume.[13] The Golgi apparatus is prominent, and vacuoles containing digestive enzyme precursors form at the condensing face of the Golgi apparatus. These vacuoles coalesce as the glycoproteins within them are condensed, forming the zymogen granules, which store the exocrine enzymes until they are secreted. Zymogen granules are membrane bound, measure up to 1.5 μm in diameter, and are closely packed in the apical cytoplasm; microtubules and actin filaments are associated with the granule membranes and may be involved in movement of the granules to the cell surface,[13] where they are discharged to the lumen by exocytosis.

Table 1.2 Mucin Expression in Normal Pancreas

Apomucin Type	Expression in Normal Pancreas (reference)
MUC1	Ductal epithelial cells; some acini[18]
MUC2	Negative[18]
MUC3	Negative[18]
MUC4	Negative[16]
MUC5	Negative[18]
MUC6	Negative[17]

Ductal System

The pancreatic ductal system starts with centroacinar cells, small cells embedded within acini, and proceeds through progressively larger ducts, termed *intercalated*, *intralobular*, *interlobular*, and *major ducts* in increasing order of size. The ductal system, in addition to serving as a conduit for pancreatic exocrine secretions, also modifies the composition of pancreatic juice by secreting sodium chloride, water, and bicarbonate. This buffering of pancreatic juice stabilizes the exocrine proenzymes.[15] Ductal cells in normal pancreas are negative by immunohistochemical studies for expression of apomucins MUC2, MUC3, MUC4, MUC5, and MUC6 but do express MUC1[16-18] (Table 1.2).

The centroacinar cell constitutes the beginnings of the intercalated duct draining the acinus and is located within the acinus, near its center (Fig. 1.3). The centroacinar cell is smaller than the acinar cell and is a relatively nondescript round-to-elongated cell with pale cytoplasm and an elongated nucleus. The pallor of the cytoplasm, relative to acinar cells, is due to the absence of zymogen granules and the paucity of other organelles. Some centroacinar cells display more granular and eosinophilic cytoplasm because of larger numbers of mitochondria.

The smallest unit of the ductal system is the intercalated duct, starting in the acinus (Fig. 1.6). The cells of the intercalated ducts are flattened, low, cuboidal cells, similar to centroacinar cells. The transition from isolated centroacinar cells to the intercalated duct is imperceptible, with the main difference between ductular cells and centroacinar cells being the central location of centroacinar cells within the acinus. Intercalated duct cells typically contain a small number of microvilli on the luminal surface. Solitary modified cilia (kinocilia) project from the luminal surface.[13]

The intralobular ducts are formed by confluence of intercalated ducts; the smallest intralobular ducts are smaller than an acinus. The larger intralobular ducts have minimal accumulation of apical mucin on special stains, such as alcian blue and periodic acid–Schiff. Although these ducts represent the major area for localization of

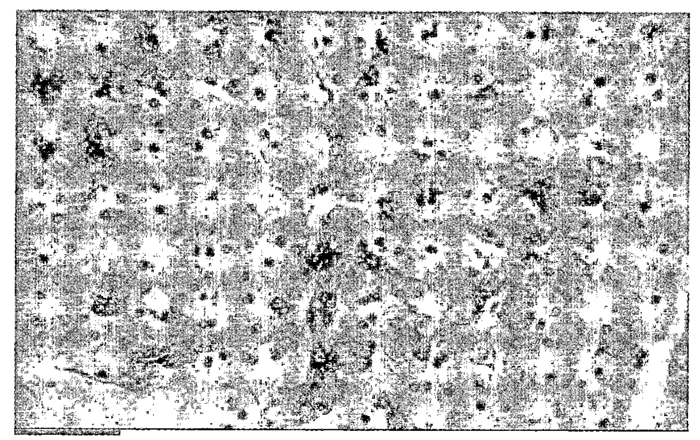

Figure 1.6
Intercalated ducts and centroacinar cells are highlighted with AE1/AE3. Indirect immunoperoxidase, AE1/AE3, original magnification ×400.

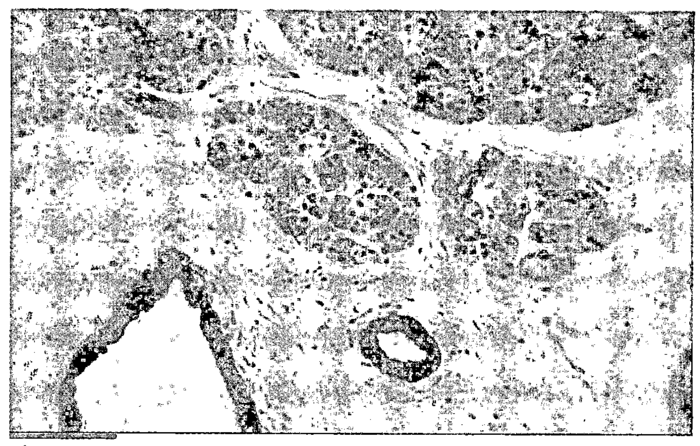

Figure 1.8
Like intercalated and intralobular ducts, interlobular ducts label with AE1/AE3. Indirect immunoperoxidase, AE1/AE3, original magnification ×200.

carbonic anhydrase, some isozymes of carbonic anhydrase may also be found in acinar cells.[15]

The interlobular ducts are invested by a layer of collagen (Fig. 1.7) and are lined by medium-to-tall columnar cells with some accumulation of mucin, mostly neutral and sialomucins, with some sulfomucins. As duct size increases, the amount of sulfomucin decreases, whereas sialomucins increase. A progressive increase in the height of the epithelial cell and the mucin content occurs with increasing duct size. The cystic fibrosis transmembrane conductance regulator is a duct cell marker and is present in interlobular ducts but not in acinar cells.[19]

The major ducts are surrounded by a variable cuff of collagen and are lined by a single layer of tall columnar cells; occasional goblet cells are found. A few endocrine cells; mostly glucagons and pancreatic polypeptide (PP)-producing cells, are found among the columnar duct epithelial cells; these endocrine cells are inconspicuous on routinely stained slides but are easily identified through immunolabeling for neuroendocrine markers. The gel-forming mucus secreted by the columnar cells acts as a defensive barrier to injury by the digestive enzymes. Ductal epithelial cells exhibit multiple short microvilli on their luminal surface. Immunolabeling reveals that the pancreatic duct cells are positive for keratins CAM5.2 and AE1/AE3 (Fig. 1.8). They normally express epithelial membrane antigen but not carcinoembryonic antigen.

As the main pancreatic duct enters the ampulla of Vater, the mucosal lining is thrown into broad papillary folds, or "valvules" (Fig. 1.9). The stroma contains

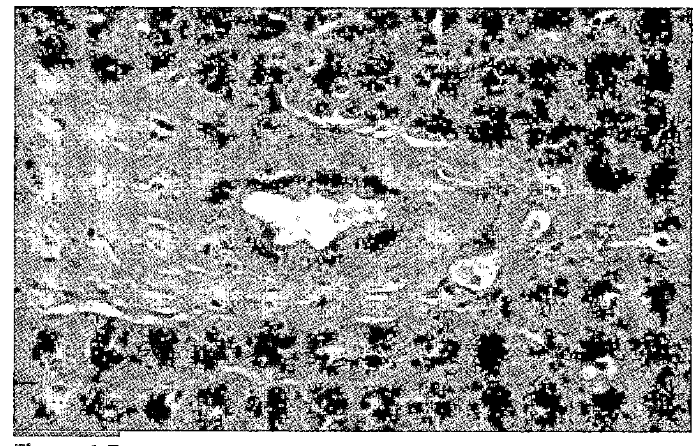

Figure 1.7
Interlobular ducts are surrounded by a cuff of fibrous stroma of variable thickness. Hematoxylin and eosin, original magnification ×400.

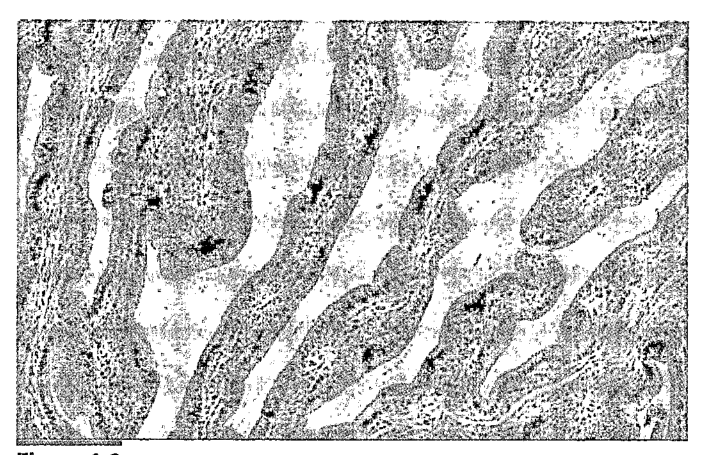

Figure 1.9
The mucosa of the ampulla of Vater and of the distal portion of the main pancreatic duct is thrown into papillary fronds. Hematoxylin and eosin, original magnification ×400.

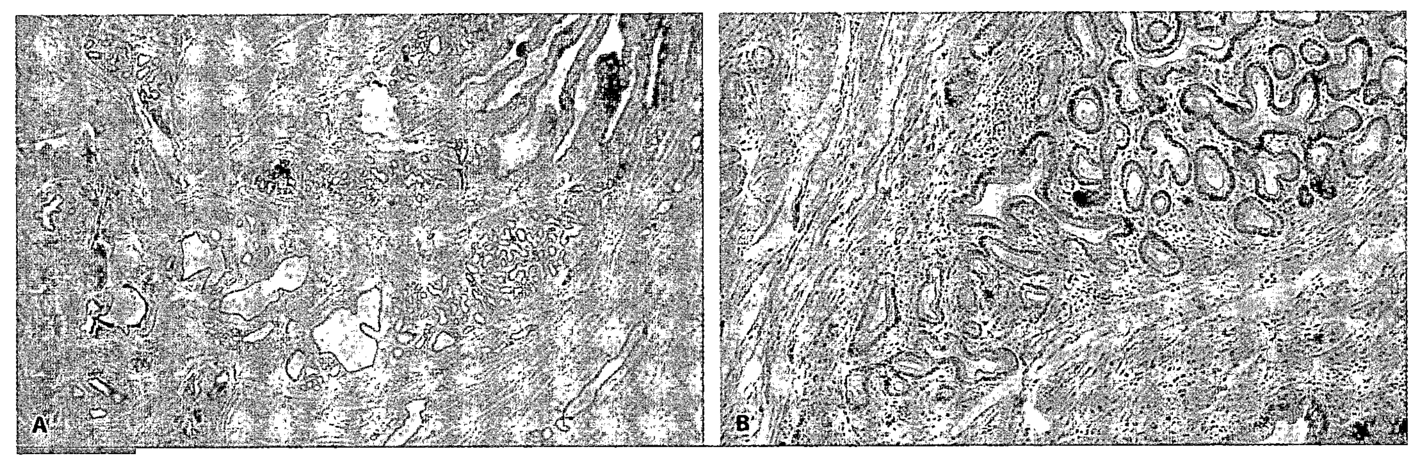

Figure 1.10
Mucin-secreting glands are present in the fibromuscular stroma of the ampulla of Vater. Recognition of the clustered architecture of these glands can help avoid confusion with infiltrating carcinoma. **(A)** Hematoxylin and eosin, original magnification ×200. **(B)** Hematoxylin and eosin, original magnification ×400.

abundant collagen and elastic fibers. Glandular outpouchings are commonly found in the fibrous tissue surrounding the duct and the ampulla (Fig. 1.10). The epithelial lining is identical to that of the common bile duct, and the epithelial cells contain sulfated acid mucin. Various metaplastic changes, such as pyloric metaplasia, are common findings. The presence of smooth muscle bundles, those of the sphincter choledochus, in the wall of the duct, further contributes to the complex microanatomy of this structure (Fig. 1.10A). A transition from ductal epithelium to intestinal epithelium is seen at the orifice of the ampulla (Fig. 1.11).

Stroma

The pancreatic stroma consists of fibrous tissue with variable amounts of adipose tissue separating lobules and surrounding the pancreas. Intralobular fat may not be uniformly distributed throughout the organ but is sometimes less prominent in PP-rich areas of the posterior head.[20] Within the stroma are nerve fibers and intrinsic ganglia of parasympathetic system. Pacinian corpuscles are occasionally reported.[21]

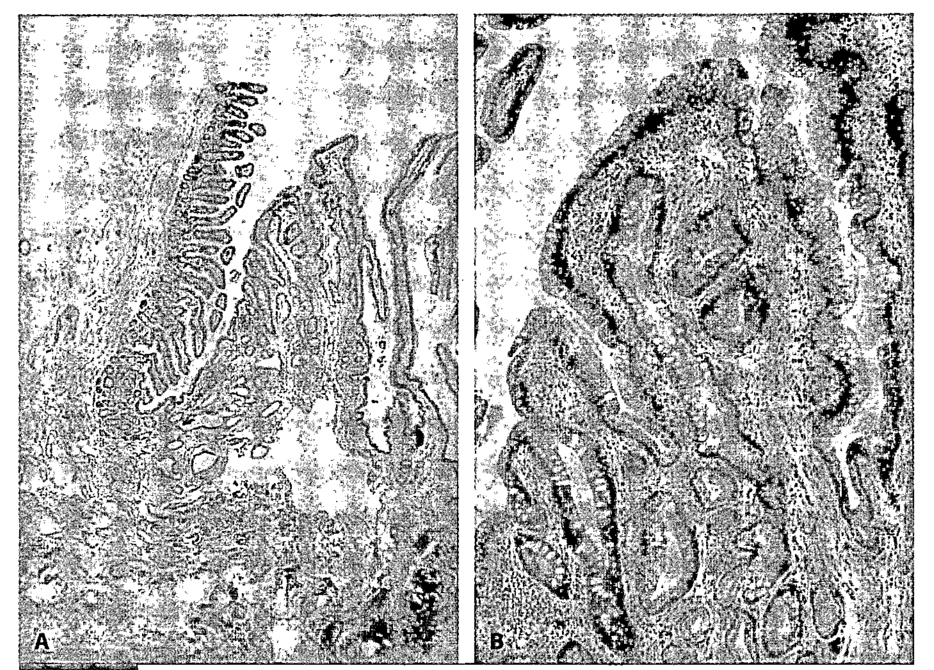

Figure 1.11
Transition from ductal epithelium to small bowel mucosa occurs at the junction of the ampulla with the duodenum. **(A)** Hematoxylin and eosin, original magnification × 40. **(B)** Hematoxylin and eosin, original magnification ×200.

Pancreatic stellate cells, retinoid-containing fat storage cells located in the interlobular and interacinar stroma, have been implicated in pancreatic fibrosis.[22] These cells are probably pericytes and are similar in many ways to hepatic stellate cells. Stellate cells are inconspicuous in normal pancreas but are found in increased numbers in chronic pancreatitis. On activation, these cells assume a myofibroblastic phenotype with increased collagen synthesis, primarily collagen type I, and increased numbers of pancreatic stellate cells are found in areas of fibrosis. Activated pancreatic stellate cells may be visualized by immunohistochemistry by staining with antibodies directed against alpha smooth muscle actin[22] (Fig. 1.12). Ac-

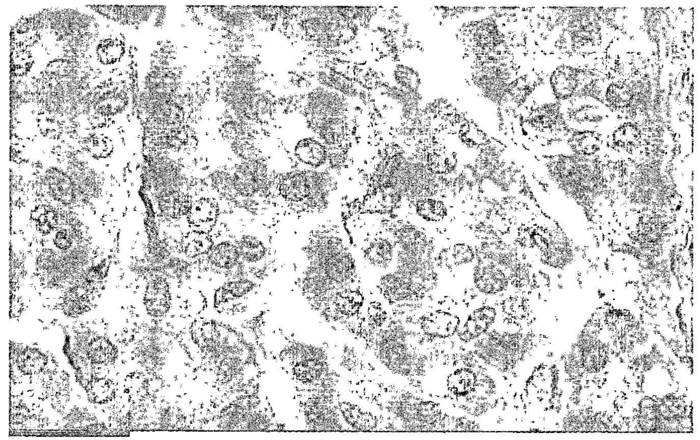

Figure 1.12
Activated pancreatic stellate cells express alpha smooth muscle actin. Stellate cell bodies and long cytoplasmic processes in close approximation to acinar cells are present in the interlobular stroma. Indirect immunoperoxidase, alpha smooth muscle actin, original magnification ×1000.

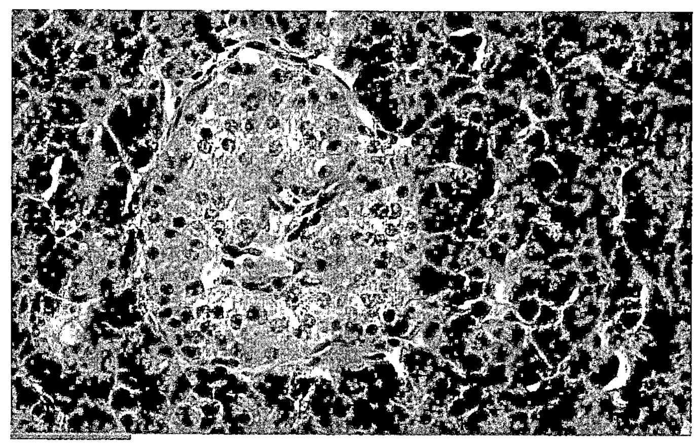

Figure 1.13
Islets of Langerhans are pale staining and sharply demarcated from surrounding acinar tissue. The endocrine cells are arranged in short cords. The central microvasculature is visible in this example. Hematoxylin and eosin, original magnification ×400.

tivating factors include proinflammatory cytokines, such as transforming growth factor-β and platelet-derived growth factor.

Endocrine Pancreas

Up to 90% of pancreatic endocrine cells are contained within the islets of Langerhans (Figs. 1.2 and 1.13); the remainder are dispersed among acini as single cells or located in or near ducts. The islets of Langerhans constitute roughly 1%–2% of adult pancreas but account for a larger proportion (15%) in the newborn, due in part to underdevelopment of the exocrine pancreas. Most islets in the human adult pancreas measure 75–225 μm (mean size, 140 μm)[1] in greatest dimension and contain approximately 1000 cells. Distribution of islets may not be uniform within the pancreas, although conflicting reports may be cited. Association of islets with ducts is normal in both adults and infants. While they are embedded in inconspicuous reticulin and collagen fibers, islets lack a true capsule.

The islets constitute a compact collection of endocrine cells arranged in clusters and cords and intermingled with a dense network of capillaries. Each islet is penetrated by one to five short arterioles, and a disproportionate amount of blood flow to the pancreas, roughly 20%, is directed to the islets. The capillaries of the islets are lined by layers of endocrine cells in direct contact with vessels, and most endocrine cells are in direct contact with blood vessels, either by cytoplasmic processes or by direct apposition. The capillaries of the islet resemble a glomerulus and are fenestrated, unlike capillaries in the exocrine pancreas. Blood leaving the islet capillary plexus flows into a second capillary plexus in the acinus, a circulatory arrangement referred to as the *insuloacinar portal system*.

Islet cells are roughly cuboidal, with pale eosinophilic cytoplasm that stains more lightly than acinar cells. Nuclei are round with finely stippled chromatin typical of endocrine cells. Nuclear variability is common, generally in insulin cells, and diploid, tetraploid, and octoploid nuclei are common. Islet cells label with antibodies against neuron-specific enolase, chromogranin A, and synaptophysin. They are in general keratin negative but may show faint labeling with CAM5.2.

The islets in posterior part of the head and the uncinate process, which originate from ventral pancreatic anlage, are irregular, arranged in distinct trabeculae, and are rich in PP (Fig. 1.14). These islets are larger than typical compact islets and may measure up to 400–500 μm in greatest dimension.[1]

The topographical distribution of various types of endocrine cells within islets is not random. Insulin-producing cells (B cells or β cells) constitute 60%–70% of the islet cell population and are mostly found in islet cores (Fig. 1.15). Insulin-producing cells are more numerous in adults than in infants. Glucagon-producing cells (A cells or α cells) constitute 15%–20% of total endocrine cells; they lie at the periphery of the islet (Fig. 1.16) and are arranged along capillaries in the interior (15%–20% of cells). These cells are smaller, more elongated, and darker staining than insulin-producing cells but cannot be reliably differentiated from other endocrine cell types on hematoxylin and eosin staining. Glucagon-producing cells are sparse in the PP-rich islets of the pancreatic head and uncinate process. Somatostatin-producing cells have no particular location within the islet (Fig. 1.17). These cells constitute a larger proportion of endocrine cells in children than in adults (5%–10%). PP-producing cells are

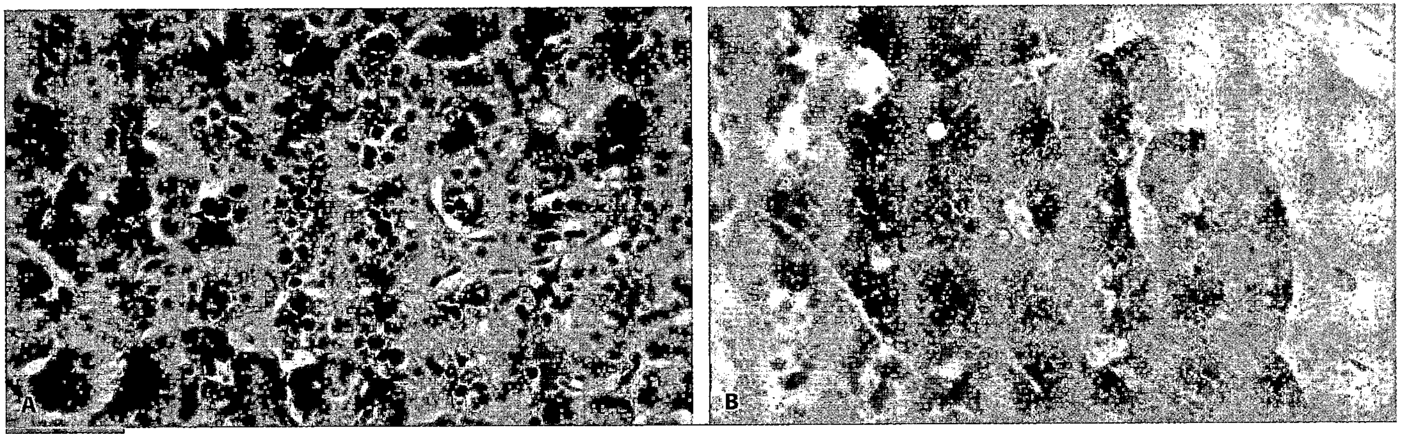

Figure 1.14
Large irregular islets with prominent trabecular architecture, located in the posterior head, contain large numbers of pancreatic polypeptide-producing cells. **(A)** Hematoxylin and eosin, original magnification ×400 **(B)** Indirect immunoperoxidase, pancreatic polypeptide, original magnification ×400.

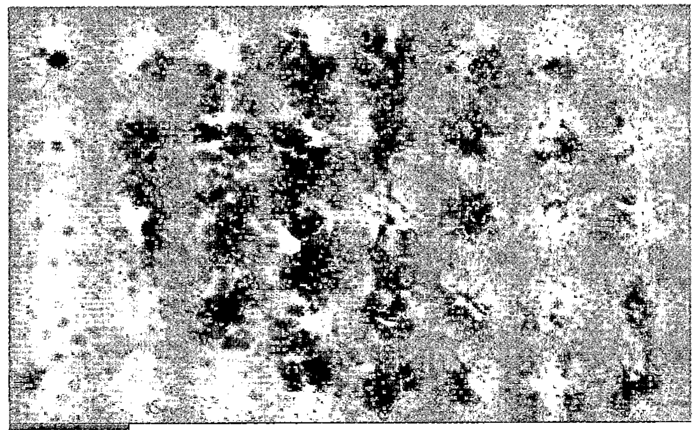

Figure 1.15
Insulin-producing cells (B cells) constitute a large percentage of islet cells, and are widely distributed throughout the islet, with some concentration within the core. Indirect immunoperoxidase, insulin, original magnification ×400.

rare in compact islets but when present are found mostly at the periphery. These cells often found among acinar cells and along small ducts. They constitute up to 70% of the irregular islets of the uncinate process and posterior pancreatic head but only 2%–5% of regular islets. Other, rarer types of endocrine cells may be found within the pancreas. Rare serotonin cells are found along the large ducts.

Innervation of pancreatic islets is by both sympathetic and parasympathetic nerve fibers running alongside blood vessels. Peptidergic fibers originating from the ganglia of the intrinsic autonomic nervous system serve as neuroregulators involved in local control of endocrine function.[12]

On ultrastructural examination, islet cells are joined by tight and gap junctions. Their secretory granules are membrane bound and electron dense; granule morphology varies with secretory product.

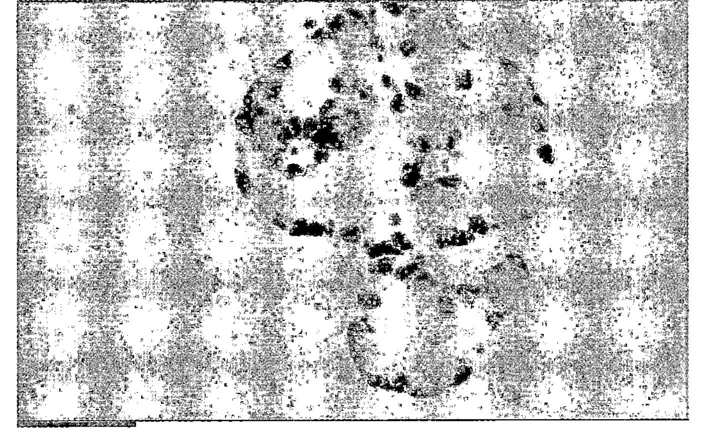

Figure 1.16
Glucagon-producing cells (A cells) constitute roughly 20% of islet cells, and are located at the periphery. Indirect immunoperoxidase, glucagon, original magnification ×400.

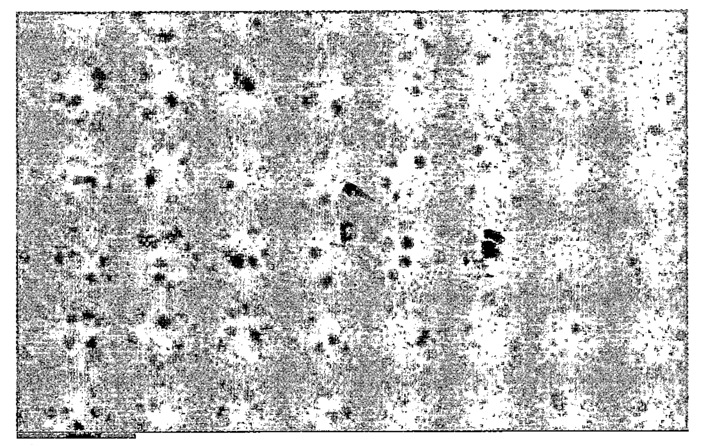

Figure 1.17
Somatostatin-producing cells are sparse within the islets, and are irregularly distributed. Indirect immunoperoxidase, glucagon, original magnification ×400.

References

1. Solcia E, Capella C, Klöppel G. *Tumors of the Pancreas*. 3rd series, ed. Washington, DC: Armed Forces Institute of Pathology; 1997.
2. Di Magno E, Shorter R, Taylor W, Go V. Relationships between pancreaticobiliary ductal anatomy and pancreatic ductal and parenchymal histology. *Cancer.* 1982;49:361–368.
3. Bertelli E, Di Gregorio F, Bertelli L, Civeli L, Mosca S. The arterial blood supply of the pancreas: a review. III. The inferior pancreaticoduodenal artery. An anatomical review and a radiological study. *Surg Radiol Anat.* 1996;18:67–74.
4. Bertelli E, Di Gregorio F, Bertelli L, Civeli L, Mosca S. The arterial blood supply of the pancreas: a review. II. The posterior superior pancreaticoduodenal artery. An anatomical and a radiological study. *Surg Radiol Anat.* 1996;18:1–9.
5. Bertelli E, Di Gregorio F, Bertelli L, Orazioli D, Bastianini A. The arterial blood supply of the pancreas: a review. IV. The anterior inferior and posterior pancreaticoduodenal aa., and minor sources of blood supply for the head of the pancreas. An anatomical review and a radiological study. *Surg Radiol Anat.* 1997;19:203–212.
6. Bertelli E, Di Gregorio F, Mosca S, Bastianini A. The arterial blood supply of the pancreas: a review. V. The dorsal pancreatic artery. An anatomic review and a radiological study. *Surg Radiol Anat.* 1998;20:445–452.
7. Ibukuro K. Vascular anatomy of the pancreas and clinical applications. *Int J Gastroint Cancer.* 2001;30:87–104.
8. Murakami G, Hirata K, Takamuro T, Mukaiya M, Hata F, Kitagawa S. Vascular anatomy of the pancreaticoduodenal region: a review. *J Hepatobiliary Pancreat Surg.* 1999;6:55–68.
9. O'Morchoe CC. Lymphatic system of the pancreas. *Microsc Res Tech.* 1997;37:456–477.
10. Nagai H, Kuroda A, Morioka Y. Lymphatic and local spread of T1 and T2 pancreatic cancer. *Ann Surg.* 1986;204:65–71.
11. American Joint Commission on Cancer. Exocrine pancreas. In: Greene FL, Page DL, Fleming ID et al, eds. *AJCC Cancer Staging Manual.* 6th ed. New York: Springer; 2002:157–164.
12. Salvioli B, Bovara M, Barbara G, et al. Neurology and neuropathology of the pancreatic innervation. *J Pancreas.* [electronic resource] 2002;3:26–33.
13. Motta PM, Macchiarelli G, Nottola SA, Correr S. Histology of the exocrine pancreas. *Microsc Res Tech.* 1997;37:384–398.
14. Klimstra DS. Pancreas. In: Sternberg SS, ed. *Histology for Pathologists.* 2nd ed. Philadelphia: Lippincott-Raven Publishers; 1997:613–647.
15. Nishimori I, Fujuikawa-Adachi K, Onishi S, Hollingsworth MA. Carbonic anhydrase in human pancreas: hypotheses for the pathophysiological roles of CA isozymes. *Ann NY Acad Sci.* 1999;880:5–16.
16. Andrianifahanana M, Moniaux N, Schmied BM, et al. Mucin (MUC) gene expression in human pancreatic adenocarcinoma and chronic pancreatitis: a potential role of MUC4 as a tumor marker of diagnostic significance. *Clin Cancer Res.* 2001;7:4033–4040.
17. Harris A. The duct cell in cystic fibrosis. *Ann NY Acad Sci.* 1999;880:17–30.
18. Terada T, Ohta T, Sasaki M, Nakanuma Y, Kim YS. Expression of MUC apomucins in normal pancreas and pancreatic tumours. *J Pathol.* 1996;180:160–165.
19. Marino C, Matovcik L, Gorelick F, Cohn J. Localization of the cystic fibrosis transmembrane conductance regulator in pancreas. *J Clin Invest.* 1988;88:712–716.
20. Orci L, Mallaisse-Legae F, Baetens D, Perrelet A. Pancreatic polypeptide-rich regions in human pancreas. *Lancet.* 1978;2:1200–1201.
21. Standop J, Ulrich A, Schneider MB, Andren-Sandberg A, Pour PM. Pacinian corpuscle in the human pancreas. *Pancreas.* 2001;23:36–39.
22. Bachem MG, Schneider E, Gross H, et al. Identification, culture, and characterization of pancreatic stellate cells in rats and humans. *Gastroenterology.* 1998;115:421–432.

2

Exocrine Pancreas

Biology

Exocrine Pancreas—Diagnosis and Staging

CHAPTER 2

Pathology of the Exocrine Pancreas

Ralph H. Hruban, MD
Syed Z. Ali, MD

Neoplasms of the pancreas can be broadly divided into neoplasms with predominantly endocrine differentiation and neoplasms with predominantly exocrine differentiation. The pathology of endocrine neoplasms is discussed by Dr. Klimstra in Chapter 41. Neoplasms of the exocrine pancreas can be further subdivided into solid neoplasms and cystic neoplasms. The pathology of cystic neoplasms is covered by Dr. Adsay in Chapter 51. This chapter focuses on the pathology of three solid neoplasms of the exocrine pancreas–infiltrating ductal adenocarcinoma and its variants, acinar cell carcinoma, and pancreatoblastoma (Table 2.1). We also discuss pancreatic intraepithelial neoplasia (PanIN), the noninvasive precursor to infiltrating ductal adenocarcinoma.

Infiltrating ductal adenocarcinoma is by far the most common malignant neoplasm of the pancreas, and, unfortunately, infiltrating ductal adenocarcinoma is also the most deadly. In 2004 it is estimated that ~ 30,000 Americans will be diagnosed with infiltrating ductal adenocarcinoma of the pancreas, and ~ 30,000 will die of it.[1] The prognosis for patients with other pancreatic neoplasms, particularly the cystic neoplasms, is usually significantly better than it is for ductal adenocarcinomas, and the most appropriate therapy varies dramatically, depending on tumor type. It is therefore critical that neoplasms of the pancreas are correctly classified pathologically.

Infiltrating Ductal Adenocarcinoma

Infiltrating ductal adenocarcinoma is an invasive gland-forming malignant epithelial neoplasm.[2] By definition, these carcinomas at least focally show glandular or ductal differentiation, and they do not have a predominant component of one of the other more specific variants of pancreatic cancer, such as a dominant component with acinar differentiation. Characteristically, infiltrating ductal adenocarcinomas induce an intense host desmoplastic stromal reaction.[3] It is this desmoplastic reaction that gives adenocarcinomas of the pancreas their firm consistency.

Most infiltrating ductal adenocarcinomas arise in the head of the gland (65%), but adenocarcinomas can also arise in the body of the gland or in the tail, or they can even diffusely involve the entire length of the pancreas.[2] Approximately 80% of these carcinomas are unresectable at the time of diagnosis because they have either invaded into adjacent organs or large vessels or because they have metastasized to more distant organs, including the liver and lung.[2,4]

Grossly, infiltrating ductal adenocarcinomas form poorly defined firm white-yellow masses (Fig. 2.1).[2] Some can grow quite large and show central necrosis or cystic change, whereas others are so small as to be grossly imperceptible. Microscopically infiltrating duct carcinomas, by definition, at least focally show glandular or ductal differentiation.[2] Gland formation is characterized by a cuboidal-to-columnar epithelium with polarized nuclei and central lumen formation (Fig. 2.2). In addition, almost all of these carcinomas induce an intense nonneoplastic desmoplastic reaction. This desmoplastic reaction is composed of myofibroblasts, dense collagen, and a mixture of inflammatory cells, including lymphocytes and plasma cells. The neoplastic mass also often contains trapped nonneoplastic pancreatic parenchyma, including islets of Langerhans and residual acini.[3]

The neoplastic cells of *well-differentiated* infiltrating ductal adenocarcinomas are relatively uniform, they form well-defined glands, and they show only mild nuclear and architectural pleomorphism.[2] The gland formation in *moderately differentiated* infiltrating ductal adenocarcinomas is, by contrast, not as well defined. The neoplastic glands frequently have incomplete lumina, and they may show cribriforming. In addition, there is greater nuclear pleomorphism and more numerous mitoses (Fig. 2.2). *Poorly differentiated* infiltrating ductal adenocarcinomas, as one would expect, do not form well-defined glands. Instead, the neoplastic cells show dramatic nuclear pleomorphism and grow in sheets or as individual cells (Fig. 2.3). Numerous mitotic figures, some of which are bizarre, may be seen. In these instances, it may be necessary to perform special stains for mucin to demonstrate glandular differentiation. Whatever the degree of differentiation, the feature that best distinguishes infiltrating ductal adenocarcinomas from benign glands in the pancreas is that infiltrating ductal adenocarcinomas grow haphazardly. This haphazard growth can often be appreciated at low magnification. Benign glands have an orderly, predictable, branching growth pattern, whereas there is no order to the growth of infiltrating carcinomas.

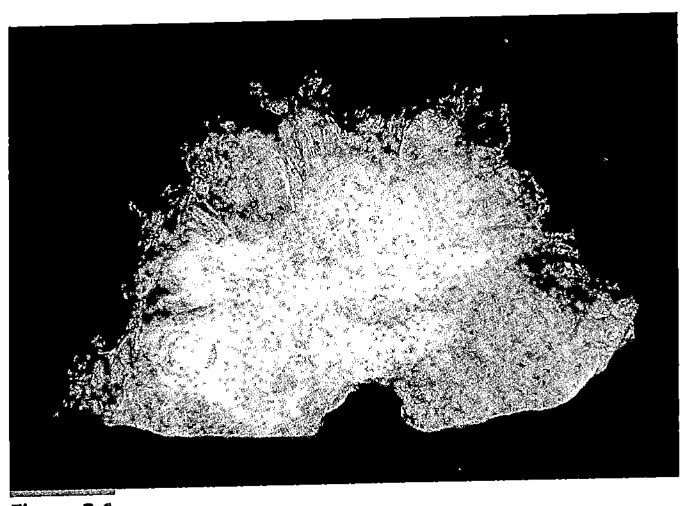

Figure 2.1
Cross-section of an infiltrating adenocarcinoma of the pancreas. The carcinoma is white-yellow and poorly defined. The black at the periphery is India ink placed to help evaluate the surgical margins.

In addition to a haphazard growth pattern, most infiltrating ductal adenocarcinomas, even the resectable ones, show perineural, vascular, and lymphatic invasion (Figs. 2.4 and 2.5). Perineural invasion is important because it is a significant pathway by which infiltrating ductal adenocarcinomas extend beyond the pancreas. Perineural invasion within the pancreas is associated with perineural invasion outside of the gland and into

Table 2.1 Solid Exocrine Neoplasms of the Pancreas

	Age in Years	Direction of Differentiation	Immunolabeling	5-Year Survival Rate
Ductal adenocarcinoma	Most 60–80	Infiltrating glands with an intense desmoplastic reaction	Cytokeratins 7, 8, 13, 18 and 19, MUC1, MUC3, MUC4, MUC5, CEA	4%
Acinar cell carcinoma	Mean, 58	Pancreatic exocrine enzymes, including trypsin, chymotrypsin, and lipase	Trypsin, chymotrypsin, lipase	6%
Pancreatoblastoma	Mean age, 2.5 in children, 40 in adults	Multiple, including acinar. Distinctive squamoid nests	Trypsin, chymotrypsin, lipase. Often chromogranin, synaptophysin	55%

Abbreviation: CEA, carcinoembryonic antigen.

retroperitoneal soft tissues. Involvement of the retroperitoneal soft tissues is one of the reasons that surgical resections of infiltrating ductal adenocarcinomas often fail. Similarly, lymphatic invasion is important because it is associated with spread beyond the gland and metastasis to lymph nodes. Venous invasion is relatively unusual in most cancer types, but it is seen in adenocarcinomas of the pancreas, and when it occurs, it often has an unusual morphology, with the neoplastic epithelium lining the lumen of the vessel.

Infiltrating ductal adenocarcinomas can metastasize to almost any organ in the body. The most frequent sites of metastases include the liver, lungs, skin, peritoneum, and adrenals.[2] Metastases to the liver need to be distinguished from benign bile duct proliferations, including bile duct hamartomas and bile duct adenomas.[5-7] Bile duct hamartomas are usually multiple, contain bile, and are lined by a flattened epithelium that lacks atypia (Fig. 2.6). Bile duct adenomas are usually single, do not contain bile, and are lined by a low cuboidal epithelium without atypia (Fig. 2.7). In contrast, most metastases to the liver show significant nuclear and architectural atypia, as well as an infiltrative pattern of growth. Metastases are also often multiple and can measure >1 cm. The current (sixth edition) American Joint Committee on Cancer staging for pancreatic exocrine neoplasms is shown in Table 2.2.

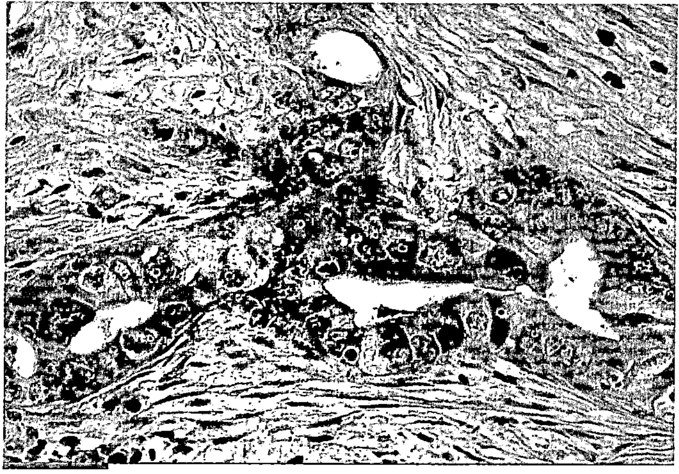

Figure 2.2
Infiltrating adenocarcinoma. Note the gland formation, the pleomorphism, and the numerous mitoses.

The intraoperative frozen section diagnosis is an essential tool for guiding the surgeon.[8,9] Sections can be used to determine the nature of a mass in the pancreas and the extent of the pathology. Frozen sections of the pancreas are, however, extremely difficult to interpret. In fact, some well-differentiated infiltrating carcinomas appear better differentiated than benign reactive glands. Criteria useful in distinguishing between benign and neoplastic glands include (1) incomplete gland lumina, (2) haphazard arrangement of the glands, (3) variation in nuclear size by more than 4 to 1 in a single gland (the so-called 4 to 1 rule), (4) perineural invasion (Fig. 2.4), (5) lymphatic invasion (Fig. 2.5), (6) mitoses (Fig. 2.2), particularly atypical mitoses, and (7) necrotic luminal debris.[8,9] Most importantly, frozen section diagnoses require open communication between the surgeon and the pathologist. A well-differentiated gland without atypia may signify carcinoma if the biopsy was taken from outside the parenchyma of the pancreas, whereas the same finding may be nonspecific if the biopsy specimen was taken from the pancreatic parenchyma.

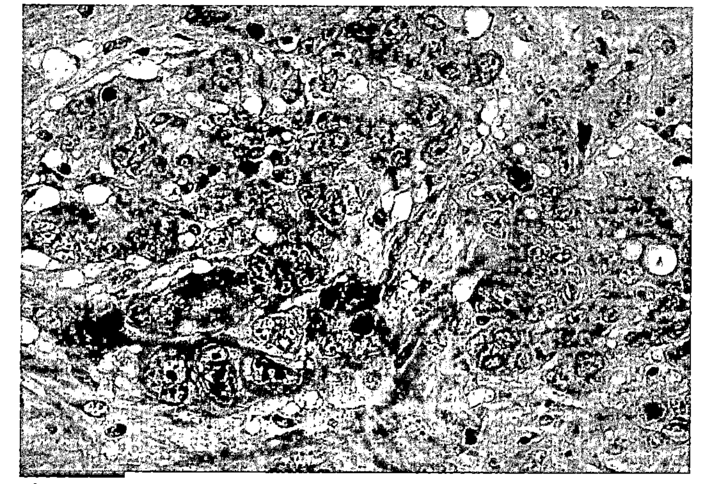

Figure 2.3
Infiltrating poorly differentiated adenocarcinoma.

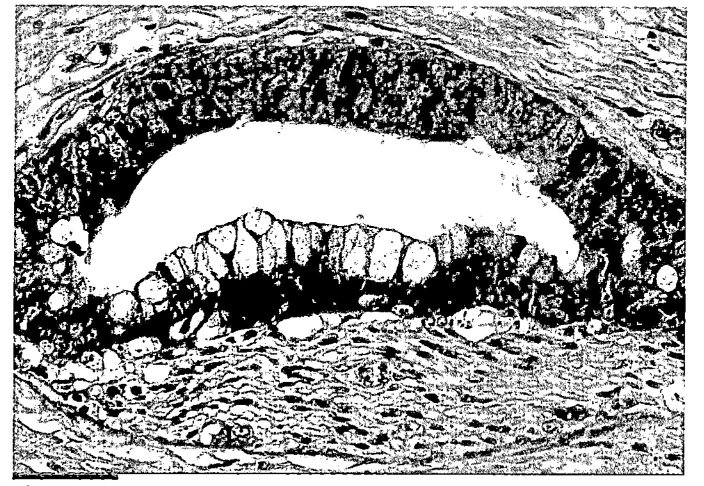

Figure 2.4
Perineural invasion in an infiltrating adenocarcinoma.

A growing number of fine needle aspiration (FNA) biopsies are being performed on pancreatic lesions. Cytomorphologic features of an infiltrating ductal adenocarcinoma include cellular smears with fragments and single malignant cells. The cellularity is highly variable and dependent on the technique of the aspirator and the degree of desmoplasia present in the invasive carcinoma. In general, FNA of well-differentiated adenocarcinoma reveals predominantly cohesive tissue fragments with a flat monolayered appearance, which is often deceptively bland. In contrast to nonneoplastic ductal epithelium, the cancerous cells display distinct nuclear enlargement,

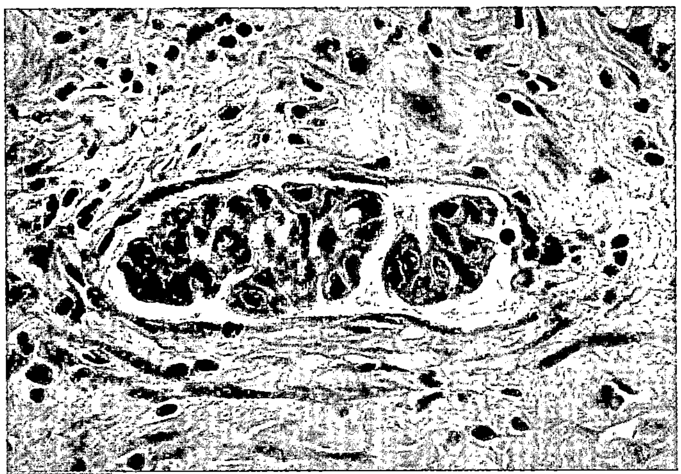

Figure 2.5
Lymphatic invasion.

Table 2.2 Tumor, Node, Metastasis Classification

Primary Tumor (T)

TX Primary tumor cannot be assessed
T0 No evidence of primary tumor
Tis Carcinoma *in situ*
T1 Tumor limited to the pancreas, 2 cm or less in greatest dimension
T2 Tumor limited to the pancreas, more than 2 cm in greatest dimension
T3 Tumor extends beyond the pancreas but without involvement of the celiac axis or the superior mesenteric artery
T4 Tumor involves the celiac axis or the superior mesenteric artery (unresectable primary tumor)

Regional Lymph Nodes (N)

NX Regional lymph nodes cannot be assessed
N0 No regional lymph node metastasis
N1 Regional lymph node metastasis

Distant Metastasis

MX Distant metastasis cannot be assessed
M0 No distant metastasis
M1 Distant metastasis

Stage Grouping

Stage 0	Tis	N0	M0
Stage IA	T1	N0	M0
Stage IB	T2	N0	M0
Stage IIA	T3	N0	M0
Stage IIB	T1	N1	M0
	T2	N1	M0
	T3	N1	M0
Stage III	T4	Any N	M0
Stage IV	Any T	Any N	M1

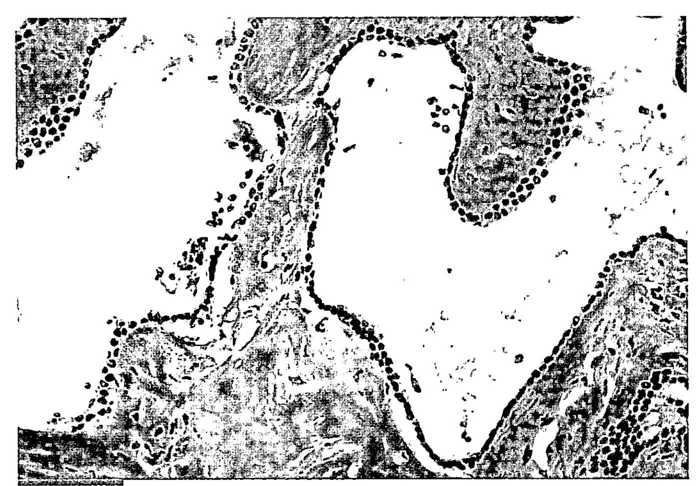

Figure 2.6
Bile duct hamartoma in the liver. These lesions can be multiple and contain bile.

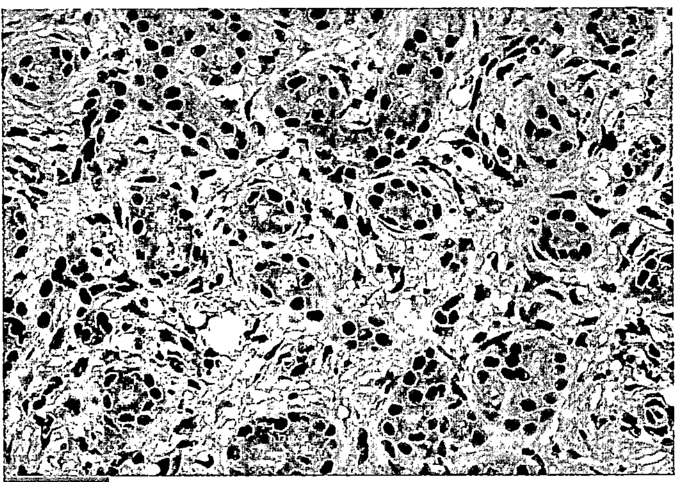

Figure 2.7
Bile duct adenoma in the liver.

pleomorphism, and frequent mitoses (Fig. 2.8). As a result of the high nuclear/cytoplasmic ratio, the tumor fragments show prominent nuclear crowding and overlap, and they lose the fine "honeycomb" arrangement of normal ductal epithelium. Also noticeable are irregularities in the nuclear membrane and chromatin distribution in the cells. Another helpful finding is the absence of pancreatic acinar epithelium (the more abundant type of epithelium in normal pancreatic aspirates), resulting in the presence of only ductal-type epithelium. Mucin may be present in the form of extracellular material and less often as intracytoplasmic vacuoles.

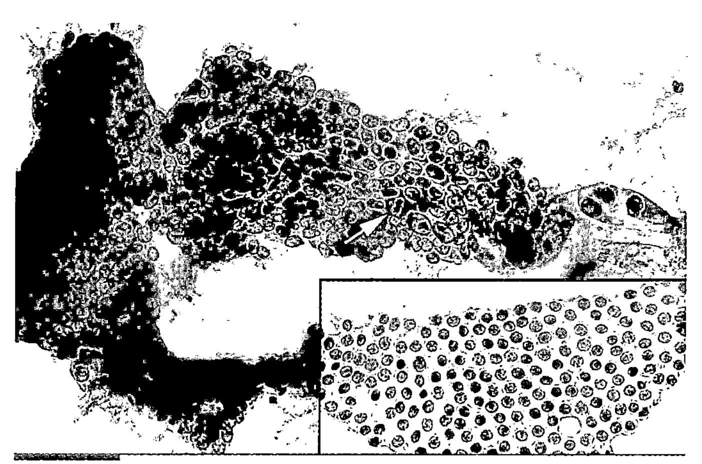

Figure 2.8
Well-differentiated ductal adenocarcinoma. Fine-needle aspiration (FNA): a crowded fragment of malignant cells. Note nuclear enlargement and pleomorphism. A mitotic figure is noted in the center of the field (*arrow*). The inset shows normal ductal epithelium for comparison. Papanicolaou stain, ×400.

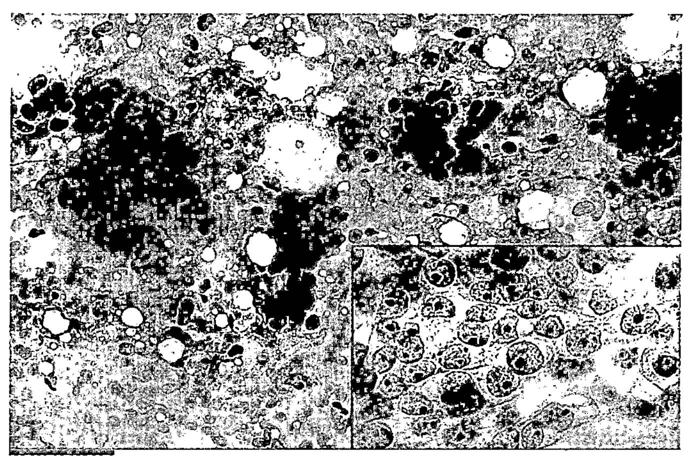

Figure 2.9
Poorly differentiated ductal adenocarcinoma. Fine-needle aspiration (FNA): note cellular discohesiveness, marked pleomorphism, and prominent nucleoli. Papanicolaou and Diff-Quik stain, ×400.

Poorly differentiated adenocarcinomas cytomorphologically display clearly malignant features, and the FNA diagnosis rarely poses a challenge. Although tissue fragments are still present, the size of these fragments is often smaller, with a more three-dimensional appearance. Single discohesive cells are observed scattered in the slide background. In contrast to more well-differentiated neoplasms, poorly differentiated carcinomas tend to have marked nuclear enlargement, coarser nuclear chromatin, and more prominent nucleoli (Fig. 2.9). Karyorrhectic nuclei, as well as frequent cellular necrosis, are additional findings. Another characteristic of these neoplasms is the presence of either focal or prominent "squamous cell" change characterized by presence of syncytial cellular aggregates or single neoplastic cells with dark nuclei and thick, "hard" cytoplasm. Keratinized cells may be observed as well.

Various special stains can help in the interpretation of difficult biopsies. The mucicarmine and periodic acid–Schiff stains can be used to confirm the production of mucin. Immunohistochemical labeling can also be used to establish the direction of differentiation of a neoplasm. Most infiltrating ductal adenocarcinomas express cytokeratins 7, 8, 13, 18, and 19.[2] By contrast, most colorectal cancers express cytokeratin 20, but not cytokeratin 7. The pattern of mucin antigen expression can also be helpful. Most infiltrating ductal adenocarcinomas of the pancreas express MUC1, MUC3, MUC4, and MUC5AC, but not MUC2.[10-12] This pattern of labeling contrasts with that seen in mucinous cystic neoplasms and intraductal papillary mucinous neoplasms of the pancreas, both of which express MUC2 but not MUC1.[11] Other helpful immunostains include immunolabeling for the *DPC4* gene product dpc4, and carcinoembryonic antigen (CEA). Expression of dpc4 is intact in benign processes of the pancreas but is completely lost because of genetic inactivation of the *DPC4* gene in 55% of infiltrating ductal carcinomas (Fig. 2.10).[13] Conversely, CEA is expressed in most infiltrating ductal carcinomas but not in most benign processes.[14] Finally, markers specific for other lines of differentiation are usually not expressed in ductal adenocarcinomas. Infiltrating ductal adenocarcinomas either do not express or at most only focally express markers of acinar differentiation (trypsin, chymotrypsin, and lipase), nor do they express markers of endocrine differentiation (chromogranin and synaptophysin). The significant expression of one of these markers in a neoplasm with ductal differentiation suggests a mixed carcinoma, either a mixed ductal-acinar or a mixed ductal-endocrine carcinoma.[15]

A growing body of evidence suggests that many infiltrating ductal adenocarcinomas of the pancreas arise from noninvasive epithelial precursor lesions. These lesions are critical because their detection and treatment provide the opportunity to prevent the development of an invasive adenocarcinoma. Epithelial precursors in the pancreas include noninvasive intraductal papillary mucinous neoplasms (IPMNs), noninvasive mucinous cystic neoplasms, and proliferations in the small pancreatic ducts, called *pancreatic intraepithelial neoplasias* (PanINs).[16,17] IPMNs and mucinous cystic neoplasms are discussed in detail in Chapter 51.

PanINs have been recognized for close to a century,[18] but three recently developed lines of evidence have firmly established that some PanINs progress to infiltrating adenocarcinoma.[19] First, morphologic studies have demonstrated that PanINs are more common in pancreata with an invasive ductal adenocarcinoma than they are in pancreata without cancer.[20] Second, there have been a handful of case reports of patients with histologically documented PanINs who years later develop an infiltrating adenocarcinoma of the pancreas.[21,22] Third, and perhaps most importantly, a large body of molecular genetic work has shown that PanINs harbor many of the same genetic alterations in cancer-associated genes as are present in infiltrating ductal adenocarcinomas.[17,21-24] The proportion of PanINs that progress and the time frame at which PanINs progress have not been established. Nonetheless, just as the recognition and treatment of adenomas of the colon can reduce colon cancer mortality, so, too, does the recognition and treatment of PanINs have the potential of reducing pancreatic cancer mortality.

A major advance in the study of PanINs has been the establishment of internationally accepted morphologic standards for the classification of varying histologic grades of PanINs.[16] PanIN-1A is the term used to designate flat epithelial proliferations without architectural or cytologic atypia (Fig. 2.11A). PanIN-1B also lacks atypia, but in contrast to PanIN-1A, the epithelial cells form intraluminal papillae (Fig. 2.11B). The intraductal proliferations in PanIN-2 show moderate nuclear and architectural atypia (Fig. 2.11C). The nuclear abnormalities in PanIN-2 include a mild loss of polarity, crowding of the nuclei, enlarged nuclei, nuclear pseudostratification, and nuclear hyperchromasia. Mitoses are only rarely seen and when present are located basally. PanIN-3 lesions are characterized by the presence of significant architectural and cytological atypia (Fig. 2.11D). Architecturally, these lesions are usually papillary, and small clusters of cells can be seen budding off into the ductal lumina. In some cases, luminal necrosis is present. The nuclei in PanIN-3 are enlarged and overlapping and show a loss of orientation such that they are no longer oriented perpendicular to the basement membrane. Nucleoli can be prominent, and mitoses, some of which may be luminal or atypical, can be found. Additional examples of each grade of PanIN can be found on the web (http://pathology.jhu.edu/PANCREAS_PANIN).

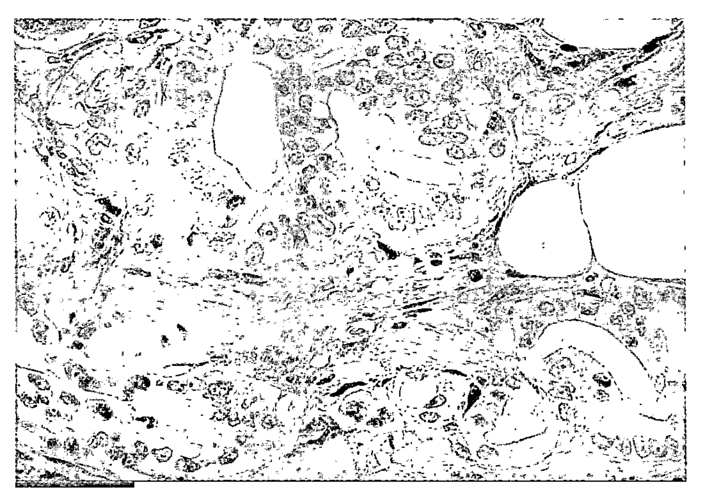

Figure 2.10
Loss of dpc4 expression in an infiltrating ductal adenocarcinoma.

The histologic categorization of PanINs is helpful because it has been used to show that genetic alterations are more common in high-grade PanINs (PanIN-3) than they are in PanINs without atypia (PanINs-1A and -1B).[21] For example, although activating point mutations in codon 12 of the *KRAS2* oncogene can be found in PanINs-1A and -1B, inactivation of the *TP53*, *DPC4*, and *BRCA2* tumor suppressor genes is limited to PanIN-3 and infiltrating carcinoma.[17,21-24] Most importantly, the appreciation that histologically distinct noninvasive precursors to invasive ductal adenocarcinoma exist provides a foundation for the detailed study of precursor lesions in the pancreas and should lead to the eventual development of tests for the early detection of pancreatic neoplasia and to the development strategies for the chemoprevention of invasive pancreatic cancer.

PanINs are distinguished from IPMNs (Chapter 51) primarily on the basis of size.[16] Most PanINs are <5 mm, and most IPMNs are ≥ 1 cm. Rarely, however, PanINs are larger than 5 mm, and rarely, IPMNs can involve ducts smaller than 1 cm.[25] In these cases, serial sections can be used to determine whether the lesion in question is in direct continuity with a larger lesion that meets diagnostic criteria for an IPMN. Similarly, radiologic images, if available, may help establish the presence or absence of a larger

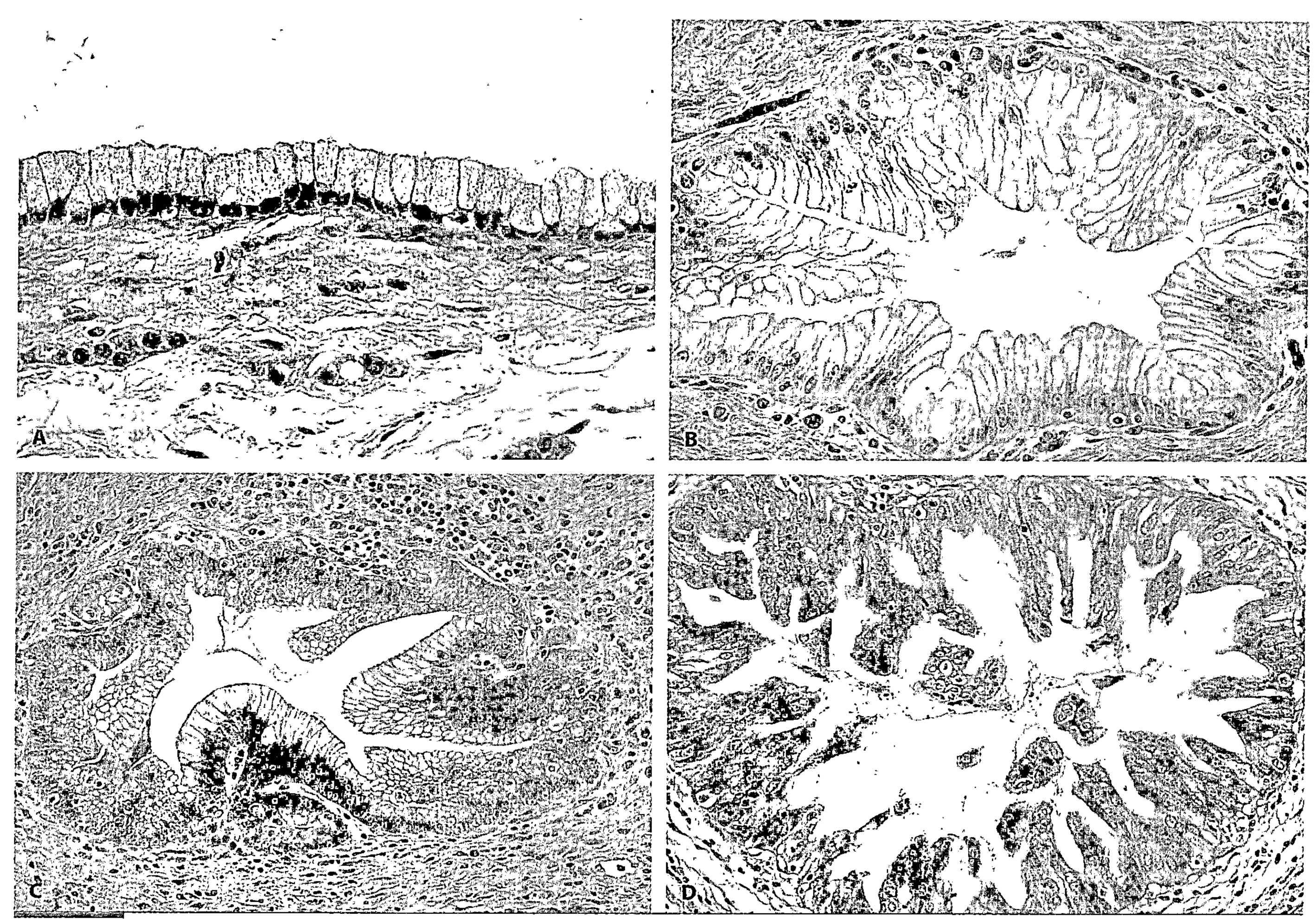

Figure 2.11
Pancreatic intraepithelial neoplasia (PanIN). **(A)** PanIN-1A; **(B)** PanIN-1B; **(C)** PanIN-2; **(D)** PanIN-3.

IPMN. In addition, the papillae in PanINs usually are not as tall and complex as those in IPMNs, whereas abundant luminal mucin production is a feature of IPMNs. MUC2 expression is a specific, but relatively insensitive, marker of an IPMN.[11]

The differential diagnosis for infiltrating ductal adenocarcinoma includes chronic pancreatitis, other tumors of the exocrine pancreas, and endocrine neoplasms of the pancreas. Chronic pancreatitis should be at the top of the differential diagnosis because the treatment of chronic pancreatitis differs so dramatically from that of adenocarcinoma. Several features of chronic pancreatitis can mimic ductal adenocarcinoma. The residual epithelial cells in chronic pancreatitis can show significant reactive atypia, and the stroma can be very fibrotic, mimicking a desmoplastic reaction to a neoplasm. However, the ducts in chronic pancreatitis retain a predictable branching pattern. By contrast, the glands in ductal adenocarcinomas grow in a haphazard, unpredictable fashion. For example, in the normal pancreas, the ducts and arteries are physically separated by nonneoplastic pancreatic parenchyma. The ducts are present in the center of the pancreatic lobules, and the arteries run in the periphery of the lobules. Ductal adenocarcinomas can violate this organization, and neoplastic glands can be seen immediately adjacent to arteries. Growth outside of the pancreas and perineural, vascular, and lymphatic permeation are also manifestations of the infiltrative growth pattern of ductal adenocarcinoma.

Lymphoplasmacytic sclerosing pancreatitis is a recently recognized form of pancreatitis that can clinically and grossly mimic infiltrating ductal adenocarcinoma.[26] Patients with lymphoplasmacytic sclerosing pancreatitis often have elevated serum immunoglobulin G4 levels.[27] Lymphoplasmacytic sclerosing pancreatitis can form a mass lesion and can produce obstructive jaundice. The light microscopic appearance of lymphoplasmacytic sclerosing pancreatitis is, however, very distinct from that of infiltrating adenocarcinoma. Lymphoplasmacytic sclerosing pancreatitis is characterized by an intense mixed inflammatory cell infiltrate composed primarily of lymphocytes and plasma cells. This infiltrate is centered around the pancreatic ducts and ductules, and a prominent venulitis is often present. The histologic changes of invasive carcinoma, including a haphazard arrangement of the glands and significant cytologic and architectural atypia, are not seen. The separation of lymphoplasmacytic sclerosing pancreatitis from pancreatic cancer is critical because some patients with lymphoplasmacytic sclerosing pancreatitis respond to steroid therapy and do not require surgery.[27]

Acinar cell carcinoma and *pancreatoblastoma* should also be included in the differential diagnosis of infiltrating ductal adenocarcinomas. Both acinar cell carcinoma and pancreatoblastoma show acinar differentiation, including cells polarized around small lumina, granular cytoplasm, and basally oriented nuclei.[28,29] These cells often have single prominent nucleoli. Pancreatoblastomas also have focal "squamoid islands." In difficult cases, immunohistochemical labeling for exocrine markers, including trypsin, chymotrypsin, and lipase, can be used to establish acinar differentiation.

Several variants of infiltrating ductal adenocarcinoma should be noted. The *undifferentiated carcinoma with osteoclast-like giant cells* is a distinctive neoplasm characterized by atypical mononuclear cells admixed with large multinucleated osteoclast-like giant cells (Fig. 2.12).[30] The nuclei in the multinucleated giant cells are uniform, and some giant cells can be seen phagocytizing adjacent cells and debris. In addition, in situ and invasive adenocarcinomas, including mucinous cystic neoplasms and PanINs, are often present. For years, it was not clear whether undifferentiated carcinomas with osteoclast-like giant cells were epithelial or mesenchymal neoplasms, but genetic analyses of carefully microdissected tumors has shown that the infiltrating mononuclear cells are most consistent with neoplastic cells arising from epithelial precursors, whereas the osteoclast-like giant cells are reactive nonneoplastic cells.[30] Although it was originally believed that undifferentiated carcinomas with osteoclast-like giant cells had a better prognosis than infiltrating ductal adenocarcinomas, these neoplasms are, in fact, fully malignant, with an average survival of only ~ 12 months.

The *anaplastic carcinoma*, as the name suggests, is an extremely poorly differentiated variant of ductal adenocarcinoma characterized by dramatic pleomorphism. Large atypical cells and bizarre mitotic figures are often present. These carcinomas are extremely aggressive and confer a median survival of less than a few months.

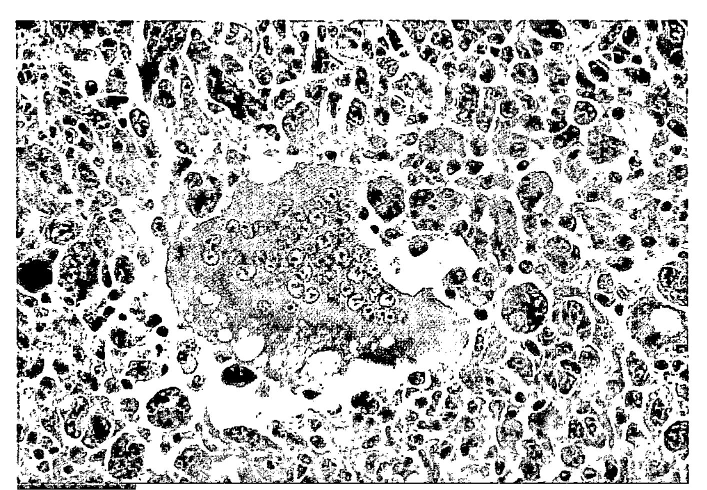

Figure 2.12
Undifferentiated carcinoma with osteoclast-like giant cells.

The *adenosquamous carcinoma* is a malignant epithelial neoplasm that shows both squamous and glandular differentiation.[31] The squamous component can predominate, but a careful examination of multiple sections from these neoplasms almost always reveals at least focal glandular differentiation. Pure squamous carcinomas of the pancreas are rare, and the finding of a pure squamous carcinoma should raise the possibility of a metastasis to the pancreas.

The *medullary carcinoma* of the pancreas is a poorly differentiated carcinoma with a syncytial pattern of growth, pushing borders, and an associated intense lymphocytic infiltrate (Fig. 2.13).[32,33] These carcinomas frequently show microsatellite instability at the molecular level, and inactivation of the *hMLH1* gene either by hypermethylation or biallelic genetic mutations.[32,33] Medullary carcinomas are important to recognize because patients with medullary carcinomas are more likely to have a family history of cancer, and some have hereditary nonpolyposis colorectal cancer syndrome.[32,33] Medullary carcinomas of the pancreas are therefore one of the first tumor types of the pancreas with a known link between a tumor morphology and a specific set of genetic alterations.

The *mucinous noncystic carcinoma* is also known as colloid carcinoma.[34,35] These gland-forming epithelial neoplasms produce copious quantities of extracellular mucin, such that the neoplastic cells are embedded in large pools of mucin. Carcinomas in which at least 80% of the neoplasm shows this pattern of growth

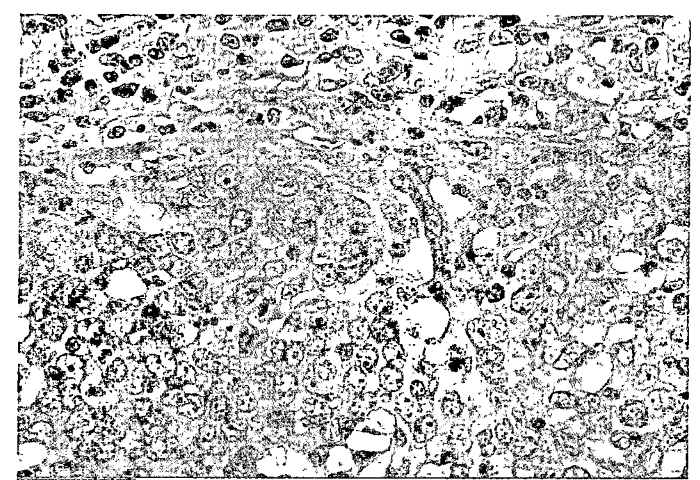

Figure 2.13
Medullary carcinoma of the pancreas. Note the poor differentiation, syncytial growth pattern, and pushing borders.

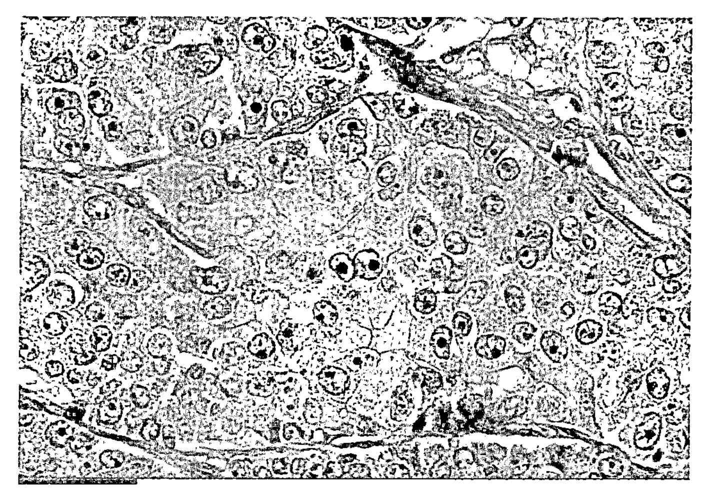

Figure 2.14
Acinar cell carcinoma. Note the granular cytoplasm and the single prominent nucleoli.

appear to have a better prognosis than infiltrating ductal adenocarcinomas. Of note, most mucinous noncystic carcinomas of the pancreas arise in association with an IPMN (see Chapter 51).[35]

The *signet ring cell carcinoma* of the pancreas is extremely rare.[36] This is a malignant mucin-producing epithelial neoplasm in which the neoplastic cells are not cohesive and, as the name suggests, form individual signet ring cells. Carcinomas with signet ring differentiation more commonly arise in the stomach and the breast (lobular carcinoma). Metastases from these other organs should be ruled out before a diagnosis of a signet ring cell carcinoma primary to the pancreas is established.

Acinar Cell Carcinoma

Acinar cell carcinomas are malignant epithelial neoplasms with exocrine enzyme production.[2,29] This enzyme production can be demonstrated immunohistochemically or ultrastructurally. Acinar cell carcinomas are rare, accounting for <2% of pancreatic malignancies. The average age at diagnosis is ~60 years, and acinar cell carcinomas are more common in men than they are in women.[2,29] Up to 15% of the patients experience a dramatic clinical syndrome caused by lipase release into the circulation. These patients have peripheral eosinophilia, polyarthralgias, and metastatic fat necrosis.[37]

Acinar cell carcinomas can arise in any portion of the pancreas. They are usually very large (average size, 10 cm) and usually well-circumscribed.[2,29] On cut section, acinar cell carcinomas are white to tan to red, and soft and fleshy. These carcinomas tend to be soft and fleshy because, in contrast to infiltrating ductal adenocarcinomas, they are usually cellular neoplasms with only minimal fibrous stroma. By light microscopy, the neoplastic cells usually grow as solid sheets, but they at least focally form acini.[2,29] The acini formed by the neoplastic cells are small glandular structures with minute lumina, similar to nonneoplastic acini. The nuclei in these acinar structures are basally located and the cytoplasm granular (Fig. 2.14). Nuclear pleomorphism is usually not dramatic, but prominent single nucleoli are a characteristic feature of acinar cell carcinomas. Single prominent nucleoli can be a very helpful clue to the diagnosis for acinar cell carcinomas that grow as solid sheets with minimal acini formation.

FNA of acinar cell carcinoma produces cellular smears with abundance of only one cell type, that is, pancreatic acinar epithelium. Ductal or islet epithelium is conspicuously absent. The latter feature assumes a significant diagnostic importance in well-differentiated acinar cell carcinomas, a situation in which the cytologic distinction from normal acinar epithelium can be extremely difficult. In general, acinar cell carcinomas cytologically show cells in small or large sheets often arranged as acini, short cords, or more often as irregular solid nests. The neoplastic cells lack the distinct compact and lobular architecture of the normal pancreatic acini. In contrast to ductal adenocarcinoma, the nuclei are eccentrically placed in the cytoplasm and often display one or two prominent nucleoli. The cytoplasm is distinctly granular and usually appears metachromatic on staining. Less often, because of the paucity of zymogen granules, the cytoplasm assumes a clearer or more vacuolated appearance. In addition, as a result of cytoplasmic disintegration, numerous naked nuclei, resembling lymphocytes can be observed in the slide background. Mitosis and necrosis are rarely observed.

Immunohistochemical labeling is often needed to establish the diagnosis of an acinar cell carcinoma. The most useful markers to establish exocrine enzyme production are trypsin, chymotrypsin, and lipase.[2,29] Of interest, many acinar cell carcinomas also focally express endocrine markers, such as chromogranin. The presence of a minor endocrine component should not lead to the erroneous diagnosis of a well-differentiated neuroendocrine neoplasm in a neoplasm with otherwise extensive acinar differentiation. The diagnosis of a mixed acinar-endocrine carcinoma should be established if the endocrine component makes up >25% of the neoplasm.[15]

Of note, in contrast to most ductal adenocarcinomas, which express cytokeratin 7 and 19, most acinar cell carcinomas do not express cytokeratin 7, 19, or 20.[2,29] Epithelial membrane antigen is expressed in about half of acinar cell carcinomas.

Although largely supplanted by immunohistochemical labeling, electron microscopy can be used to demonstrate pancreatic exocrine differentiation in these neoplasms. Acinar cell carcinomas contain numerous zymogen granules. Zymogen granules are homogeneously electron dense 125- to 1000-nm granules with a closely applied limiting membrane.

The differential diagnosis for acinar cell carcinomas includes ductal adenocarcinoma, pancreatic endocrine neoplasms, and pancreatoblastoma.[2,29] Although both acinar cell carcinomas and pancreatic endocrine neoplasms can grow in solid sheets, pancreatic endocrine neoplasms usually have a more abundant hyalinized stroma, and the neoplastic cells tend to form nests and ribbons. Pancreatic endocrine neoplasms also have central, not basal, nuclei and a salt and pepper chromatin pattern. Pancreatic endocrine neoplasms lack the single prominent nucleolus that is so characteristic of acinar cell carcinomas. Immunohistochemical labeling can be used in difficult cases. Chromogranin and synaptophysin strongly and diffusely label pancreatic endocrine neoplasms, whereas immunolabeling for trypsin and chymotrypsin is negative.

Pancreatoblastomas, by definition, show significant acinar differentiation, and pancreatoblastomas can therefore mimic acinar carcinomas.[28] Although there is overlap, most pancreatoblastomas occur in children, and most acinar cell carcinomas, in adults. The presence of squamoid nests in pancreatoblastomas distinguishes them from acinar cell carcinomas.

Pancreatoblastoma

Pancreatoblastomas are malignant epithelial neoplasms with both acinar differentiation and squamoid nests.[2,28,38] In addition, many pancreatoblastomas show endocrine, ductal, and even mesenchymal differentiation. Most pancreatoblastomas arise in children, but up to a third arise in adults.[2,28] Pancreatoblastomas are slightly more common in males than in females, and they are more common in Asians than in Caucasians. Some patients have elevated α-fetoprotein levels, and when they are elevated, α-fetoprotein levels can be used to monitor response to therapy.[39,40] Pancreatoblastomas have been reported in infants with the Beckwith-Weidemann syndrome, and most pancreatoblastomas show loss of chromosome 11p, a genetic finding common to other infantile embryonal neoplasms, including hepatoblastomas.[38] A case of a pancreatoblastoma arising in a patient with familial adenomatous polyposis has recently been published.[38]

Pancreatoblastomas involve the head and the body/tail of the gland with equal frequencies.[2,28] As is true for acinar cell carcinomas, pancreatoblastomas tend to be large (mean ~ 10 cm), well-circumscribed, and at least partially encapsulated.[28] On cut section, most are soft and fleshy, but some are firm and fibrous, depending on the proportion of fibrous connective tissue in the neoplasm. Pancreatoblastomas are usually off-white to tan, and the larger cases can show central necrosis.

Multiple directions of differentiation can be seen by light microscopy.[28] All pancreatoblastomas show acinar differentiation and squamoid nests (Fig. 2.15). These squamoid nests appear as rounded islands of flattened eosinophilic cells scattered amongst the other neoplastic cells. In addition, endocrine differentiation, ductal differentiation, and mesenchymal differentiation can be present. Cells with endocrine differentiation appear as round cells with centrally placed nuclei. The ductal cells form well-defined larger lumina, and mesenchymal differentiation can range from spindle-shaped cells to frank bone and cartilage formation.

Immunohistochemical stains can be used to confirm the multiple directions of differentiation in these neoplasms.[2,28] As expected, the cells with acinar differentiation label with antibodies to trypsin, chymotrypsin, and lipase, the endocrine cells with chromogranin and synaptophysin, and the ductal cells with cytokeratin 7 and 19. The labeling of the squamoid nests is more variable.

On FNA, pancreatoblastomas display an abundance of neoplastic cells. These cells usually form tight

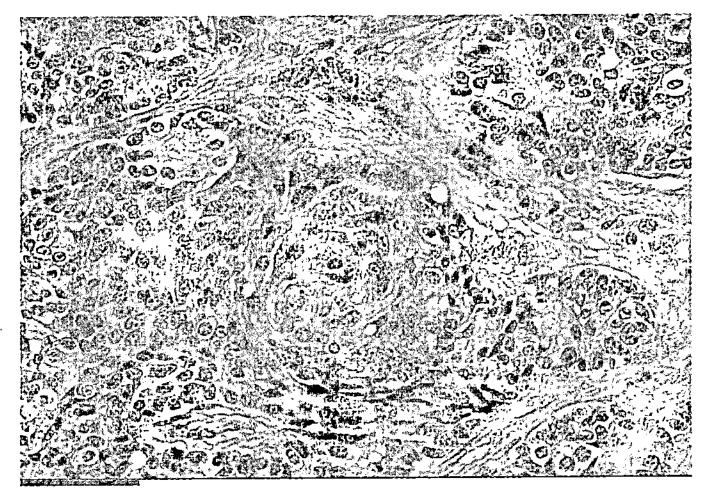

Figure 2.15
Pancreatoblastoma. Note the prominent squamoid nest arising in the setting of acinar differentiation.

cohesive fragments and, less often, single cells. The neoplastic cells show small to intermediate-sized primitive-appearing nuclei, which are usually extremely hyperchromatic. The cytoplasm is scant, giving the cells a high nuclear/cytoplasmic ratio. The neoplasm may contain oval, cuboidal to spindle-shaped cells. Mesenchymal tissue fragments as well as cells in acinar-type arrangements are also seen. Mitoses are frequent. A predominant architecture of single discohesive cells may be apparent in some cases. Traversing fine capillary vessels may be observed within the nests of neoplastic cells. As one might expect, squamoid corpuscles and acinar differentiation have also been described on FNA.

Acinar cell carcinoma is the main neoplasm to consider in the differential diagnosis of pancreatoblastoma.[2,28] Although pancreatoblastomas tend to occur in children, and acinar cell carcinomas more often occur in adults, there is considerable overlap, and age cannot be used as the sole criterion to distinguish between these two entities. Both neoplasms can also show acinar and endocrine differentiation. The feature that distinguishes between these two entities is therefore the squamoid nests in pancreatoblastomas.

Fine-Needle Aspiration

FNA cytology has proven useful in distinguishing the various neoplastic processes discussed earlier. Despite the difficult anatomic location of the pancreas within the abdomen, virtually any segment of the gland is approachable by FNA. Most commonly, a percutaneous transabdominal route is used, guided by real-time ultrasound study or computed tomographic imaging. A transgastric or transduodenal endoscopic ultrasound approach may also be used to sample pancreatic lesions. In these cases, the possibility of intestinal contamination of the sample must be considered in the interpretation of the cytology.

The primary indication for an FNA is a mass lesion suspected to be neoplastic. In addition, FNAs are also routinely used in cystic lesions, as well as in suspected cases of chronic pancreatitis, which cannot be adequately diagnosed on the basis of clinical and radiologic findings. FNA is considered a safe technique with a high rate of diagnostic accuracy. Complications are rare (one series reported less than 1%)[41] and include vasovagal reactions, hemorrhagic or necrotizing pancreatitis, pancreatic fistula, infectious necrosis, and tumor seeding of the needle tract. If the procedure is performed via endoscopic route with ultrasound guidance, additional complications of acute pancreatitis and aspiration pneumonia have been reported.[42,43]

The diagnostic profile of FNA for pancreatic pathology has been well studied.[43,44] An overall sensitivity of 90% and a specificity approaching 100% have been documented in various studies with an efficiency of 90%. Another series found FNA to have a positive predictive value of 100% and a negative predictive value of 80%.[45] Comparison of the diagnostic accuracy of FNA with that of tissue core biopsy shows an accuracy of 91% versus 56%, respectively.[46] For the endoscopic route with ultrasound guidance, the sensitivity, specificity, and accuracy for diagnosis of pancreatic carcinoma have been reported to be 91%, 100%, and 92%, respectively.[47] The latter technique is particularly well-suited for cystic pancreatic lesions because it can provide highly detailed imaging without interference by bowel or air. The endoscopic route with ultrasound guidance is also considered highly accurate for sampling small functioning neuroendocrine neoplasms not evident on computed tomography and for identifying patients with multiple lesions.[48] FNA of cystic lesions provides an excellent means to obtain cyst fluid for chemical analysis, a test that is often helpful in distinguishing nonneoplastic from neoplastic cysts. A high carbohydrate antigen of 19.9, a low CEA level, and high amylase levels in cyst fluid are indicative of mucinous tumors, serous cystadenomas, and pseudocysts, respectively.[49] A cytologic sample not only furnishes an accurate morphologic diagnosis but also helps with various ancillary studies (flow cytometry) and molecular genetics evaluation. For example, it has been suggested that the finding of mutant *KRAS2* genes in an FNA sample supports the diagnosis of pancreatic cancer.[50]

A potential pitfall for a false-positive cancer diagnosis is overinterpretation of normal epithelium (both pancreatic and extrapancreatic, e.g., gastrointestinal) when they are present in an FNA sample. One recent study found that such misinterpretations were relatively common (10%) in the pancreas.[51] Other diagnostically problematic areas include chronic pancreatitis with reactive epithelial atypia, well-differentiated carcinomas, mucinous cystic neoplasms, and occasionally neuroendocrine neoplasms. Despite this, pancreatic FNA is considered the first-line diagnostic modality in patients with pancreatic disease. It allows a safe, rapid, accurate, and cost-effective alternative to conventional tissue biopsies or exploratory laparotomy.

Conclusion

Our understanding of the pathology of pancreatic cancer has grown significantly in the past decade. Histologic precursors to invasive carcinoma have been defined, and studies of these precursors have led to the development of a progression model in which noninvasive PanINs accumulate genetic abnormalities and progress to an invasive and eventually metastatic carcinoma. Studies of invasive carcinoma have led to the recognition of new subtypes of pancreatic cancer, such as the medullary carcinoma, with specific genetic alterations. One can easily imagine that the application of modern molecular diagnostic techniques to FNAs will improve our ability to make accurate diagnoses on ever-smaller biopsy specimens, thereby sparing patients more invasive diagnostic procedures.

References

1. Jemal A, Thomas A, Murray T, Thun M. Cancer statistics, 2002. *CA: Cancer J Clin.* 2002;52:23-47.
2. Solcia E, Capella C, Klöppel G. *Atlas of Tumor Pathology: Tumors of the Pancreas.* 3rd series ed. Washington, DC: Armed Forces Institute of Pathology; 1997.
3. Iacobuzio-Donahue CA, Ryu B, Hruban RH, Kern SE. Exploring the host desmoplastic response to pancreatic carcinoma: gene expression of stromal and neoplastic cells at the site of primary invasion. *Am J Pathol.* 2002;160:91–99.
4. Niederhuber JE, Brennan MF, Menck HR. The National Cancer Data Base Report on Pancreatic Cancer. *Cancer.* 1995;76:1671–1677.
5. Hruban RH, Sturm PDJ, Slebos RJC, et al. Can K-*ras* codon 12 mutations be used to distinguish benign bile duct proliferations from metastases in the liver? A molecular analysis of 101 liver lesions from 93 patients. *Am J Pathol.* 1997;151:943–949.
6. Allaire GS, Rabin L, Ishak KG, Sesterhenn IA. Bile duct adenoma: a study of 152 cases. *Am J Surg Pathol.* 1988;12: 708–715.
7. Salo J, Bru C, Vilella A, et al. Bile duct hamartomas presenting as multiple focal lesions on hepatic ultrasonography. *Am J Gastroenterol.* 1992;87:221–223.
8. Hyland C, Kheir SM, Kashlan MB. Frozen section diagnosis of pancreatic carcinoma: a prospective study of 64 biopsies. *Am J Surg Pathol.* 1981;5:179–191.
9. Cioc AM, Ellison EC, Proca DM, Lucas JG, Frankel WL. Frozen section diagnosis of pancreatic lesions. *Arch Pathol Lab Med.* 2002;126:1169–1173.
10. Monges GM, Mathoulin-Portier MP, Acres RB, et al. Differential MUC1 expression in normal and neoplastic human pancreatic tissue: an immunohistochemical study of 60 samples. *Am J Clin Pathol.* 1999;112:635–640.
11. Adsay NV, Merati K, Andea A, et al. The dichotomy in the preinvasive neoplasia to invasive carcinoma sequence in the pancreas: differential expression of MUC1 and MUC2 supports the existence of two separate pathways of carcinogenesis. *Mod Pathol.* 2002;15:1087–1095.
12. Andrianifahanana M, Moniaux N, Schmied BM, et al. Mucin (MUC) gene expression in human pancreatic adenocarcinoma and chronic pancreatitis: a potential role of MUC4 as a tumor marker of diagnostic significance. *Clin Cancer Res.* 2001;7:4033–4040.
13. Wilentz RE, Su GH, Dai JL, et al. Immunohistochemical labeling for Dpc4 mirrors genetic status in pancreatic adenocarcinomas: a new marker of DPC4 inactivation. *Am J Pathol.* 2000;156:37–43.
14. Shimizu M, SaitohY, Ohyanagi H, Itoh H. Immunohistochemical staining of pancreatic cancer with CA19-9, KM01, unabsorbed CEA, and absorbed CEA. *Arch Pathol Lab Med.* 1990;114:195–200.
15. Klimstra DS, Rosai J, Heffess CS. Mixed acinar-endocrine carcinomas of the pancreas. *Am J Surg Pathol.* 1994; 18:765–778.
16. Hruban RH, Adsay NV, Albores-Saavedra J, et al. Pancreatic intraepithelial neoplasia (PanIN): a new nomenclature and classification system for pancreatic duct lesions. *Am J Surg Pathol.* 2001;25:579–586.
17. Hruban RH, Wilentz RE, Kern SE. Genetic progression in the pancreatic ducts. *Am J Pathol.* 2000;156:1821–1825.
18. Hulst SPL. Zur Kenntnis Der Genese Des Adenokarzinoms Und Karzinoms Des Pankreas. *Virchows Arch* (B) 1905;180:288–316.
19. Hruban RH, Goggins M, Parsons JL, Kern SE. Progression model for pancreatic cancer. *Clin Cancer Res.* 2000;6: 2969–2972.
20. Cubilla AL, Fitzgerald PJ. Morphological lesions associated with human primary invasive nonendocrine pancreas cancer. *Cancer Res.* 1976;36:2690–2698.
21. Goggins M, Hruban RH, Kern SE. *BRCA2* is inactivated late in the development of pancreatic intraepithelial neo-

plasia: evidence and implications. *Am J Pathol.* 2000;156: 1767–1771.
22. Wilentz RE, Geradts J, Maynard R, et al. Inactivation of the *P16 (INK4A)* tumor-suppressor gene in pancreatic duct lesions: loss of intranuclear expression. *Cancer Res.* 1998; 58:4740–4744.
23. Wilentz RE, Iacobuzio-Donahue CA, Argani P, et al. Loss of expression of Dpc4 in pancreatic intraepithelial neoplasia: evidence that *DPC4* inactivation occurs late in neoplastic progression. *Cancer Res.* 2000;60:2002–2006.
24. Moskaluk CA, Hruban RH, Kern SE. *P16* and *K-ras* gene mutations in the intraductal precursors of human pancreatic adenocarcinoma. *Cancer Res.* 1997;57:2140–2143.
25. Takaori K. Dilemma in classifications of possible precursors of pancreatic cancer involving the main pancreatic duct: PanIN or IPMN? *J Gastroenterol.* 2003;38:311–313.
26. Abraham SC, Wilentz RE, Yeo CJ, et al. Pancreaticoduodenectomy (Whipple resections) in patients without malignancy: are they all "chronic pancreatitis"? *Am J Surg Pathol.* 2003;27:110–120.
27. Hamano H, Kawa S, Horiuchi A, et al. High serum IgG4 concentrations in patients with sclerosing pancreatitis. *N Engl J Med.* 2001;344:732–738.
28. Klimstra DS, Wenig BM, Adair CF, Heffess CS. Pancreatoblastoma: a clinicopathologic study and review of the literature. *Am J Surg Pathol.* 1995;19:1371–1389.
29. Klimstra DS, Heffess CS, Oertel JE, Rosai J. Acinar cell carcinoma of the pancreas: a clinicopathologic study of 28 cases. *Am J Surg Pathol.* 1992;16:815–837.
30. Westra WH, Sturm PJ, Drillenburg P, et al. K-*ras* oncogene mutations in osteoclast-like giant-cell tumors of the pancreas and liver: genetic evidence to support origin from the duct epithelium. *Am J Surg Pathol.* 1998;22:1247–1254.
31. Ishikawa O, Matsui Y, Aoki I, et al. Adenosquamous carcinoma of the pancreas: a clinicopathologic study and report of three cases. *Cancer.* 1980;46:1192–1196.
32. Goggins M, Offerhaus GJA, Hilgers W, et al. Pancreatic adenocarcinomas with DNA replication errors (RER+) are associated with wild-type K-*ras* and characteristic histopathology: poor differentiation, a syncytial growth pattern, and pushing borders suggest RER+. *Am J Pathol.* 1998;152:1501–1507.
33. Wilentz RE, Goggins M, Redston M, et al. Genetic, immunohistochemical, and clinical features of medullary carcinomas of the pancreas: a newly described and characterized entity. *Am J Pathol.* 2000;156:1641–1651.
34. Adsay NV, Pierson C, Sarkar F, et al. Colloid (mucinous noncystic) carcinoma of the pancreas. *Am J Surg Pathol.* 2001;25:26–42.
35. Seidel G, Zahurak M, Iacobuzio-Donahue CA, et al. Almost all infiltrating colloid carcinomas of the pancreas and periampullary region arise from in situ papillary neoplasms: a study of 39 cases. *Am J Surg Pathol.* 2002;26:56–63.
36. Tracey KJ, O'Brien MJ, Williams LF, et al. Signet ring carcinoma of the pancreas, a rare variant with very high CEA values: immunohistologic comparison with adenocarcinoma. *Dig Dis Sci.* 1984;29:573–576.
37. van Klaveren RJ, de Mulder PHM, Boerbooms MT, et al. Pancreatic carcinoma with polyarthritis, fat necrosis, and high serum lipase and trypsin activity. *Gut.* 1990;31: 953–955.
38. Abraham SC, Wu TT, Klimstra DS, Finn L, Hruban RH. Distinctive molecular genetic alterations in sporadic and familial adenomatous polyposis-associated pancreatoblastomas: frequent alterations in the APC/β-catenin pathway and chromosome 11p. *Am J Pathol.* 2001;159:1619–1627.
39. Morohoshi T, Sagawa F, Mitsuya T. Pancreatoblastoma with marked elevation of serum alpha-fetoprotein. *Virchows Arch A Pathol Anat Histol.* 1990;416:265–270.
40. Iseki M, Suzuki T, Koizumi Y, et al. Alpha-fetoprotein-producing pancreatoblastoma. A case report. *Cancer.* 1986; 57:1833–1835.
41. Alpern GA, Dekker A. Fine needle aspiration cytology of the pancreas: an analysis of its use in 52 patients. *Acta Cytol.* 1985;29:873–878.
42. O'Toole D, Palazzo L, Arotcarena R, et al. Assessment of complications of EUS-guided fine needle aspiration. *Gastrointest Endosc.* 2001;53:470–474.
43. Teplick SK, Haskin PH, Kline TS, Sammon JK, Laffey PA. Percutaneous pancreaticobiliary biopsies in 173 patients using primarily ultrasound or fluoroscopic guidance. *Cardiovasc Intervent Radiol.* 1988;11:26–28.
44. David O, Green L, Reddy V, et al. Pancreatic masses: a multi-institutional study of 364 fine needle aspiration biopsies with histopathologic correlation. *Diagn Cytopathol.* 1998;19:423–427.
45. Al-Kaisi N, Siegler EE. Fine needle aspiration cytology of the pancreas. *Acta Cytol.* 1989;33:145–152.
46. Keighley MR, Moore J, Thompson H. The place of fine needle aspiration cytology for the intraoperative diagnosis of pancreatic malignancy. *Ann R Coll Surg Engl.* 1984;66: 405–408.
47. Raut CP, Grau AM, Staerkel GA, et al. Diagnostic accuracy of endoscopic ultrasound-guided fine needle aspiration in patients with presumed pancreatic cancer. *J Gastrointest Surg.* 2003;7:118–126.
48. Gines A, Vazquez-Sequeiros E, Soria MT, Clain JE, Wiersema MJ. Usefulness of EUS-guided fine needle aspiration (EUS-FNA) in the diagnosis of functioning neuroendocrine tumors. *Gastrointest Endosc.* 2002;56:291–296.
49. Hammel P, Levy P, Voitot H, et al. Preoperative cyst fluid analysis is useful for the differential diagnosis of cystic lesions of the pancreas. *Gastroenterology.* 1995;108: 1230–1235.
50. Evans DB, Frazier ML, Charnsangavej C, Katz RL, Larry L, Abbruzzese JL. Molecular diagnosis of exocrine pancreatic cancer using a percutaneous technique. *Ann Surg Oncol.* 1996;3:241–246.
51. Young NA, Mody DR, Davey DD. Misinterpretation of normal cellular elements in fine needle aspiration biopsy specimens. *Arch Pathol Lab Med.* 2002;126:670–675.

COMMENTARY

G. Johan A. Offerhaus, MD, PhD
Susanne van Eeden, MD

A Poem About the Pancreas[1]
Even if you open up a practice
on Harley Street
no patient will come in with complaints
about his pancreas:
"I think it's my pancreas, Doc!"
—unless he's a fellow professional
also educated
out of his natural mind; few patients
will be alarmed by the word—how unlike
"the heart"
a word that means "the biscuit"
to the best of us.

Years from now
when you trundle in
thin and yellow, depressed,
for abdominal films,
you too will have forgotten
your pancreas; and the news "It's cancer
of the pancreas" will hit
like an old family secret you knew all along;
"I'm sorry, but it's cancer
of the sweetbread!"
"Not the sweetbread!"—"Yes,
and, with proper medical management
early surgery
and a very rigid diet,
you can look forward to at least
another three months"; when the pancreas goes
it goes.

Those among us who are diabetic
whom the pancreas torments
by degrees
cannot describe that Familiar; even a poet
is at a loss for a metaphor;
nothing short of a surgical exploration
will unearth
the thick spongy worm
buried deep in the viscera
silent behind its curtain of peritoneum;
—with a head, a body,
and a tail,
using the man's face.

The aforementioned poetry summarized the highlights of the lecture on pancreatic pathology given by Dr. Boittnot, Professor of Pathology and past Co-Director of the Department of Pathology of The Johns Hopkins Medical Institutions, during the pathology course for medical students in the 1980s. Among the audience were residents and fellows, such as Ralph Hruban and Scott Kern, who taught the lab sessions to the students after the lectures. They must have embraced Boitnott's message by deciding to devote their professional lives to altering the dismal outlook of patients with pancreatic cancer. In the 1990s, the pancreatic cancer research group at Johns Hopkins was established by Drs. Hruban and Kern, and it was fertilized by the pancreata removed by the surgeons at Hopkins. It has grown ever since. Many of the authors of the different chapters in this book are (or were) members of the Hopkins group that covers all aspects of pancreatic cancer research. The architecture of the group is analogous to the Bowel Tumor Working Group at Hopkins, and its research efforts have proved to be as successful. Our knowledge and understanding of pancreatic cancer tumorigenesis have increased dramatically, and the poetry of pancreatic cancer may have to be rewritten in the future. At the same time, one has to admit that in practice, translation of these insights into patient benefits is still limited. For the great majority of patients, the bottom line of Dr Boitnott's lecture still counts: when the pancreas goes, it goes!

In Chapter 2, Drs. Hruban and Ali carefully describe and nicely illustrate the histopathology and cytopathology of the different forms of pancreatic cancer and their differential diagnoses. Obviously, we as pathologists are asked by our surgeons or gastroenterologists to delineate the specific types of cancer and provide degrees of differentiation in the pathology report because different forms may behave somewhat differently. However, by far the most important information is the extent of the disease because only this will ultimately determine whether or not cure is a serious option. Small cancers, less than 2 cm, that are restricted to the pancreas, without vascular or perineural invasion and without spread to the lymph nodes, may be cured when radically resected,[2] but we all know that these are the exceptions in our daily practice. Early detection is the only thing that may change this fact, and at the present time, it can be considered as a sine qua non to improve the prognosis of pancreatic cancer. Importantly, the pathologist may also play a role in the early detection of pancreatic cancer, and some of the ingredients that may be of help are mentioned in this chapter.

With regard to the different forms of pancreatic cancer, the medullary type, which was originally described at Hopkins, is important to recognize, even though it is rare. It may not only have a significantly better prognosis but it can also be due to an inherited mismatch repair defect, and the pathologist should raise this possibility.[3] Surveillance could then potentially lead to the early detection of other cancers in family members. Pancreatoblastoma is generally not listed among the extraintestinal cancers for which familial adenomatous polyposis patients carry an increased risk,[4] and its association with familial adenomatous polyposis still needs to be determined. Pancreatoblastoma falls outside the usually differential diagnosis for pancreatic cancer and is typically a tumor of the younger ages (rarely above 50 years of age), whereas conventional ductal pancreatic cancers are only rarely present in those younger than 50.[5]

In recent years, it has become evident that infiltrating ductal carcinomas of the pancreas are preceded by noninvasive precursor stages. Once we are capable of reliably diagnosing these so-called pancreatic intraepithelial neoplasia (PanIN) lesions, they will provide a realistic time window of early detection before invasive growth takes place. Largely because of the research of the Hopkins group, these consecutive precursor stages are now relatively well defined phenotypically and genotypically, and a tumor progression model analogous to the adenoma carcinoma sequence in the colorectum currently exists for the pancreas.[6] It is clear that access to the pancreas is much more difficult than access to the colorectum. In addition, the prevalence of the precursors in the general population compared with, for example, colorectal adenomas, does not justify large-scale screening of the general population. However, an increased number of high-risk groups for pancreatic cancer are being identified in which screening is a consideration.[7] It is therefore most likely that pathologists will be faced with these precursor lesions more often in the near future and will be paying attention to properly classifying PanINs.

Although in accordance with the international guidelines, a tripartite classification needs to be followed in grading the PanIN lesions, it would not be surprising if low-grade versus high-grade (intraepithelial neoplasia) becomes the standard, similar to other parts of the digestive tract.[8] To some extent, this is already indicated in the text of this chapter when the comparison of the genetic profile of PanINs-1 with the high-grade lesions is discussed. Not only does this correspond with other compartments of the digestive tract but it also makes sense because this dual partition will guide practical implications. The differential diagnosis between PanIN and intraductal papillary mucinous neoplasm (IPMN) is important and can be difficult. MUC2 immunostaining is mentioned as a specific marker, but because we have also rarely seen positivity in PanINs, this immunolabeling pattern needs to be interpreted with caution.

In this chapter, fine needle aspiration (FNA) is presented as the method of choice to reach a firm cytologic diagnosis before surgery. Preferences may vary among institutions, depending on the clinical setting and the experience of the investigators. The figures for sensitivity and specificity are therefore not always easily translatable to one's own institution, and comparison of performance characteristics between different diagnostic modalities can be difficult. Because of the problem of obtaining an accurate preoperative tissue diagnosis, surgery is regularly performed without a firm diagnosis. Comparable to other experienced institutions, such as ours, almost one tenth of the pancreatectomies performed at Johns Hopkins for suspected cancer have no neoplasm in the definitive surgical specimen. In fact, review of such cancer-negative specimens over the years has led to the recent recognition of entities such as lymphoplasmacytic sclerosing pancreatitis that may clinically mimic infiltrating ductal carcinoma. Our experience with FNA is also favorable. In the case of cystic lesions or neuroendocrine tumors, FNA can be performed at endoscopy and under ultrasound guidance. FNA is then often successful. Invasive growth in cystic neoplasms cannot be reliably diagnosed on cytology. Another approach used in our institution, and not mentioned in this chapter, is brush cytology obtained during endoscopic retrograde cholangiopancreatography (ERCP). It is the method of choice in the case of a potentially malignant stenosis of the distal common bile duct. It may well be that, in the future, brush cytology will appear the most attractive modality when we are asked to provide accurate diagnoses of PanIN grades in patients who participate in surveillance programs. Shed cells can be studied by light microscopy, but in addition, ancillary molecular studies may contribute to the distinction between low- and high-grade PanINs.[9,10] Sampling error may be less of a problem than when FNA is applied.

Finally, as far as the cytology is concerned, another methodology worth mentioning is the fresh cytologic touch preparation. It provides whole cells, which are of value not only for accurate diagnosis but also for molecular studies, such as in situ hybridization, that assess gains or losses of certain specific genetic regions in the DNA. Molecular profiling of solid tumors is rapidly evolving, and so in the near future, our clinicians may be more interested in the presence or absence of certain specific molecular profiles than in the grade of differentiation or cancer type in order to fine tune their treatment and therapeutic options.

In summary, because this field is changing so rapidly, this chapter and book will have to be updated regularly in the years to come and presumably by many of the same authors. It is predicted that the emphasis in the pathology of ductal pancreatic cancer will change from the advanced to the early stages, from the phenotype to the genotype, and from autopsy and surgical resection specimens to preoperative techniques. Given this rapidly moving field of pancreatic cancer research, this chapter is in good hands.

References

1. Charach R. Poetry. *N Engl J Med.* 1979;301:508.
2. Cameron JL, Crist DW, Sizmann JV, et al. Factors influencing survival after pancreaticoduodenectomy for pancreatic cancer. *Am J Surg.* 1991;161:120–125.

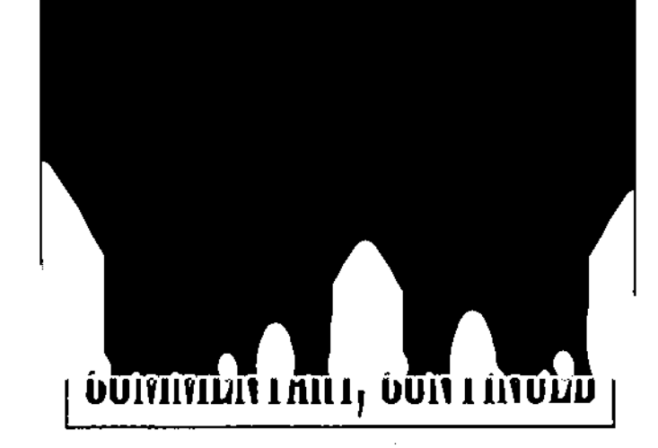

3. Goggins M, Offerhaus GJA, Higers W, et al. Pancreatic adenocarcinomas with DNA replication errors (RER+) are associated with wild-type K-*ras* and characteristic histopathology *Am J Pathol.* 1998;152:1501–1507.
4. Giardiello FM, Offerhaus GJA. Phenotype and cancer risk of various polyposis syndromes. *Eur J Cancer.* 1995;31:1085–1087.
5. Klimstra DS, Wenig BM, Adair CF, Heffess CS. Pancreatoblastoma: a clinicopathological study and review of the literature. *Am J Surg Pathol.* 1995;19:1371–1389.
6. Hruban HR, Wilentz RE, Goggins M, Offerhaus GJA, Yeo CJ, Kern SE. Pathology of incipient pancreatic cancer. *Ann Oncol.* 1999;10:9–11.
7. Vos tot Nederveen Capel WH, Offerhaus GJA, Puijenbroek M, et al. Pancreatic carcinoma in carriers of a specific 19bp deletion of *CDKN2A/p16 (p16-Leiden). Clin Cancer Res.* 2003;9:3598–3605.
8. Offerhaus GJA, Correa P, van Eeden S, et al. Report of an Amsterdam working group on Barrett Esophagus. *Virchows Arch.* 2003;443:602–608.
9. Sturm PDJ, Rauws EAJ, Hruban RH, et al. The clinical value of analysis of K-*ras* codon 12 and endobiliary brush cytology for the diagnosis of extrahepatic distal bile duct stenosis. *Clin Cancer Res.* 1999;5:629–635.
10. Tascilar M, Sturm PDJ, Caspers E, et al. Diagnostic p53 immunostaining of endobiliary brush cytology. *Cancer.* 1999;87:306–311.

CHAPTER 3

Molecular Genetic Alterations in Cancer-Associated Genes

Michiel S. van der Heijden, MD
Scott E. Kern, MD

Pancreatic cancer is fundamentally a genetic disease. This view is supported by the recurrent pattern of genetic changes associated with the transformation of normal pancreatic ductal cells into one of the deadliest forms of cancer (Table 3.1). Each of the key genetic alterations contributes to neoplastic progression by providing the developing neoplastic cells with a selective growth advantage over their neighboring cells. This leads to the serial outgrowth of naturally selected clonal populations of neoplastic cells, and these neoplastic cells can slowly evolve from a noninvasive precursor lesion (pancreatic intraepithelial neoplasia [PanIN]) to an invasive and eventually metastatic carcinoma.

The growth advantage provided by certain genetic changes also implies a pattern of mutually exclusive genetic mutations. That is, a second genetic change in a mutated pathway does not usually result in an additional growth advantage; multiple changes in the same pathway are therefore usually not encountered. The view that pancreatic cancer is fundamentally a genetic disease is also supported by the occurrence of multiple pancreatic cancers in families with a germline genetic alteration in a cancer-associated gene. The genetics of familial pancreatic cancer are discussed in Chapter 9; this chapter focuses on the genetics of sporadic pancreatic ductal adenocarcinoma.

The mutational analysis of pancreatic cancer is made extremely difficult by the fact that most often, only a minority of the cells constituting a pancreatic tumor are neoplastic cells. Pancreatic cancers characteristically induce an intense desmoplastic reaction composed of fibroblasts, inflammatory cells, and vessels. These nonneoplastic cells contain vast amounts of normal DNA that can mask the subtle changes in the neoplastic cells. To enrich for neoplastic cells, cell culture or the technique of *xenografting* is used: surgically resected pieces of tumor are transplanted into immunodeficient nude mice, where the population of neoplastic cells expands to form a xenograft—tumors with a very high percentage of malignant cells and few human nonneoplastic cells (Fig. 3.1).[1] Using this approach, the mutational changes in pancreatic cancer have been well studied, and pancreatic cancer has emerged as one of the genetically best-understood forms of cancer. Most of the mutational data originate in studies of xenografts and cell lines, subsequently confirmed in primary carcinomas. Metastatic carcinomas have not been studied molecularly to any significant extent. A routine distinction should be made between conventional ductal adenocarcinoma and a less common, histologically and genetically distinct, variant growing in a medullary pattern.[2,3] This distinction is clarified in this chapter.

Table 3.1 Summary of Genetic Alterations in Pancreatic Cancer

Gene	Locus	Function	Frequency (%)
Caretaker genes			
BRCA2	13q	DNA repair	7%
FANCC, FANCG	9q, 9p	DNA repair	<5%
Oncogenes			
Kras2	12	Signal transduction	85%–95%
CCNE	19q	G_1/S cell cycle transition	NA
Tumor-suppressor genes			
p16	9p	G_1/S cell cycle arrest	98%
p53	17p	Cell cycle arrest, apoptosis	50%–75%
MADH4	18q	TGF-β/activin pathway	55%
LKB1/STK11	19p	Serine/threonine kinase	5%
TGF-β, activin receptors		TGF-β/activin pathway	5%
BAX	19q	Apoptosis	<5%
FBXW7	4q	G_1 cell cycle transition	<5%

Abbreviation: TGF-β, transforming growth factor β.

Genetic Instability and Caretaker Genes

Pancreatic cancer is caused by a sequence of genetic changes, distributed in time over many years. Evidence is accumulating that genetic instability, leading to a higher frequency of mutations affecting oncogenes and tumor-suppressor genes, is an early event in the development of pancreatic cancer.[4-6] Although the mechanisms underlying this instability are still only starting to be understood, important progress has been achieved in recent years.

Most pancreatic cancers (> 90%) are aneuploid: they contain losses and gains of large portions of chromosomes or whole chromosomes, translocations, and rearrangements, leading to a grossly abnormal karyotype, reflecting an underlying chromosomal instability (CIN). A detailed assessment of allelic loss in pancreatic cancer xenografts has been made by Iacobuzio-Donahue et al.,[7] using 386 microsatellite markers (markers for loss of heterozygosity [LOH]) in 93 pancreaticobiliary carcinomas. The most frequent sites of allelic loss (> 60% of carcinomas) were loci of known tumor-suppressor genes: 9p (*p16/CDKN2A*), 17p (*TP53*), and 18q (*DPC4/MADH4*), but moderately frequent losses (40%–60%) were also seen at 1p, 3p, 6q, 8p, 17q, 18p, 21q, and 22q, loci not known at present to harbor a tumor-suppressor gene. The average loss was 15% of all tested markers per carcinoma. Interestingly, a significant difference in loss of heterozygosity was found between smokers and nonsmokers, with carcinomas from smokers displaying more LOH, a difference also noted in lung cancer.[8] A detailed study of chromosomal arms 17p and 18q in PanINs has indicated that loss of one allele of a tumor-suppressor gene is frequently the first "hit," followed by an intragenic mutation in the second copy of the targeted gene.[9]

A minority of pancreatic cancers has microsatellite instability (MIN): their chromosome numbers are usually normal, but these cancers have a more subtle defect at the nucleotide level. As is discussed later in greater detail, several specific genetic alterations have been implicated as potential causes of this genetic instability in pancreatic cancer.

Telomeres

Defective telomeres may be the major cause of the chromosomal instability observed in many cancers and in the vast majority of pancreatic cancers. Telomeres are present at the end of chromosomes and consist of specific repeated DNA sequences in association with telomere-binding proteins. Among other functions, telomeres protect chromosomes from self-perpetuating breakage-fusion-bridge cycles: fusion of chromosomal ends, followed by breakage and generation of highly recombinogenic free DNA ends, a phenomenon first described in 1941 by Barbara McClintock[10] and later identified in human tumors.[11] Chromosome fusions preferentially involve the chromosomes with the shortest telomeres, as shown by Hemann et al.[12] by digital karyotyping of splenocytes in genetically defined mice. Telomeres and their chromosome-protective functions can be maintained by the enzyme telomerase; however, most somatic human cells do not express this enzyme. A lack of telomerase leads to the progressive shortening of telomeres, which when proceeding beyond a critical limit leads to cellular senescence. However, cells that escape senescence, perhaps because of the failure of a key regulatory gene for the cell division cycle, would enjoy a tremendous growth advantage relative to the arrested cells that surround them.[13] Without telomere caps, unprotected chromosome ends may result in chromosomal fusion, creating fused chromosomes with two centromeres. At the next mitosis, these cells may form *anaphase bridges* in which the two centromeres of this unusual chromosome are pulled to opposite spindle poles, forming an irregular, long chromosome spanning between the two centromeres (a bridge). These bridges may subsequently break, leading to daughter cells with highly recombinogenic chromosome ends and a series of breakage-fusion-bridge cycles, or they may result in cytokinetic failure, with the formation of binucleated cells with supernumerary chromosomes. Thus, telomere dysfunction can lead to both structural and numerical instability of chromosomes.

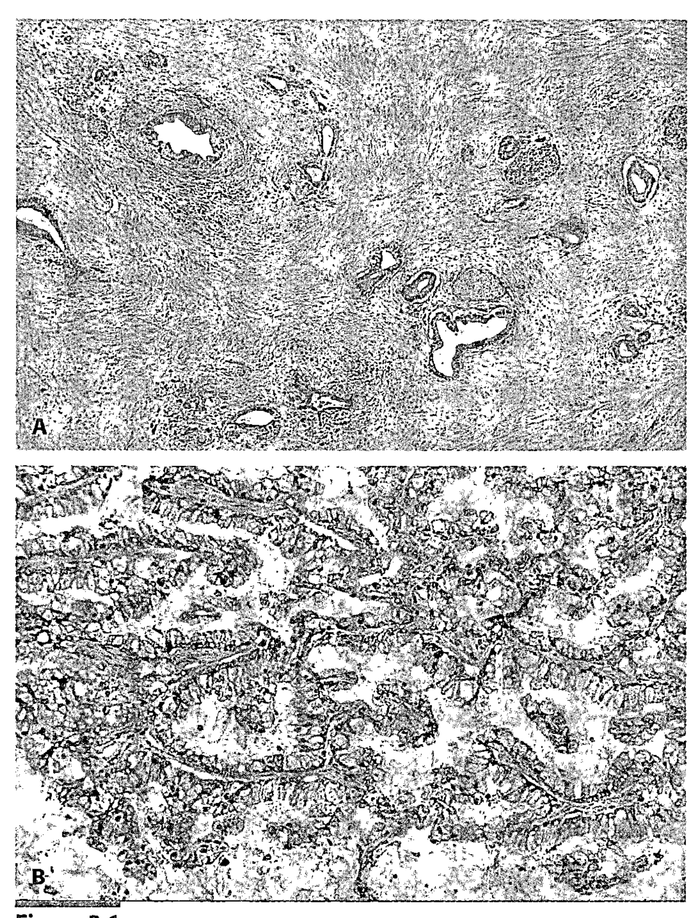

Figure 3.1
Xenografting. **(A)** Primary ductal pancreatic adenocarcinoma **(B)** Pancreatic adenocarcinoma xenograft.

Chromosomal instability provides a tumor with the genetic diversity to overcome certain barriers in carcinogenesis. However, ultimately, chromosomal instability might prove detrimental to tumor growth, which may explain why neoplasms seem to acquire mechanisms to elongate their telomeres at later stages in the development of a malignancy, often through the reactivation of the enzyme telomerase.

An elegant fluorescence in situ hybridization assay to detect intact telomeres in archival tissue sections has been developed recently by Meeker et al.[14] Van Heek et al.[15] used this protocol to show that telomeres were shortened in 79 (96%) of 82 PanINs (Fig. 3.2), perhaps accounting for the early chromosomal instability seen in the development of pancreatic cancer. A reduction in telomere intensity was even seen in 91% of PanIN-1a, the earliest putative precursor lesion in the pancreatic cancer progression model.[15]

Fanconi/Brca2 Pathway

Germline mutations in the *BRCA2* gene are present in a significant percentage of patients with familial breast, ovarian, young-onset prostate, and pancreatic cancer.[16-19] Germline mutations in the *BRCA2* gene may also play a significant role in apparently sporadic pancreatic cancers. The cloning of the *BRCA2* gene was greatly aided by the identification of a homozygous deletion in a sporadic pancreatic cancer, and germline mutations in the *BRCA2* gene are found in about 7% of sporadic pancreatic cancer.[17] The Brca2 protein is thought to play a role in DNA repair through homologous recombination, a process by which DNA damage, in particular DNA-interstrand crosslinks, can be repaired by use of the sister chromatid or the homologous chromosome.[20]

Other members of the Brca2 pathway may also play an important role in the development of pancreatic cancer. In 2002, Howlett et al.[21] found that biallelic mutations in the *BRCA2* gene are responsible for a subset of Fanconi anemia cases. Fanconi anemia is a hereditary cancer susceptibility disorder, with the occurrence of hematologic abnormalities or acute myelogenous leukemia at an early age, usually leading to death before the age of 20. Patients who survive into adulthood often develop solid tumors, especially squamous cell carcinomas of the head and neck or the anogenital region.[22] After the discovery of these mutations of the *BRCA2* gene in Fanconi anemia, other Fanconi genes were surveyed in pancreatic cancer. In an initial study of 22 pancreatic xenografts

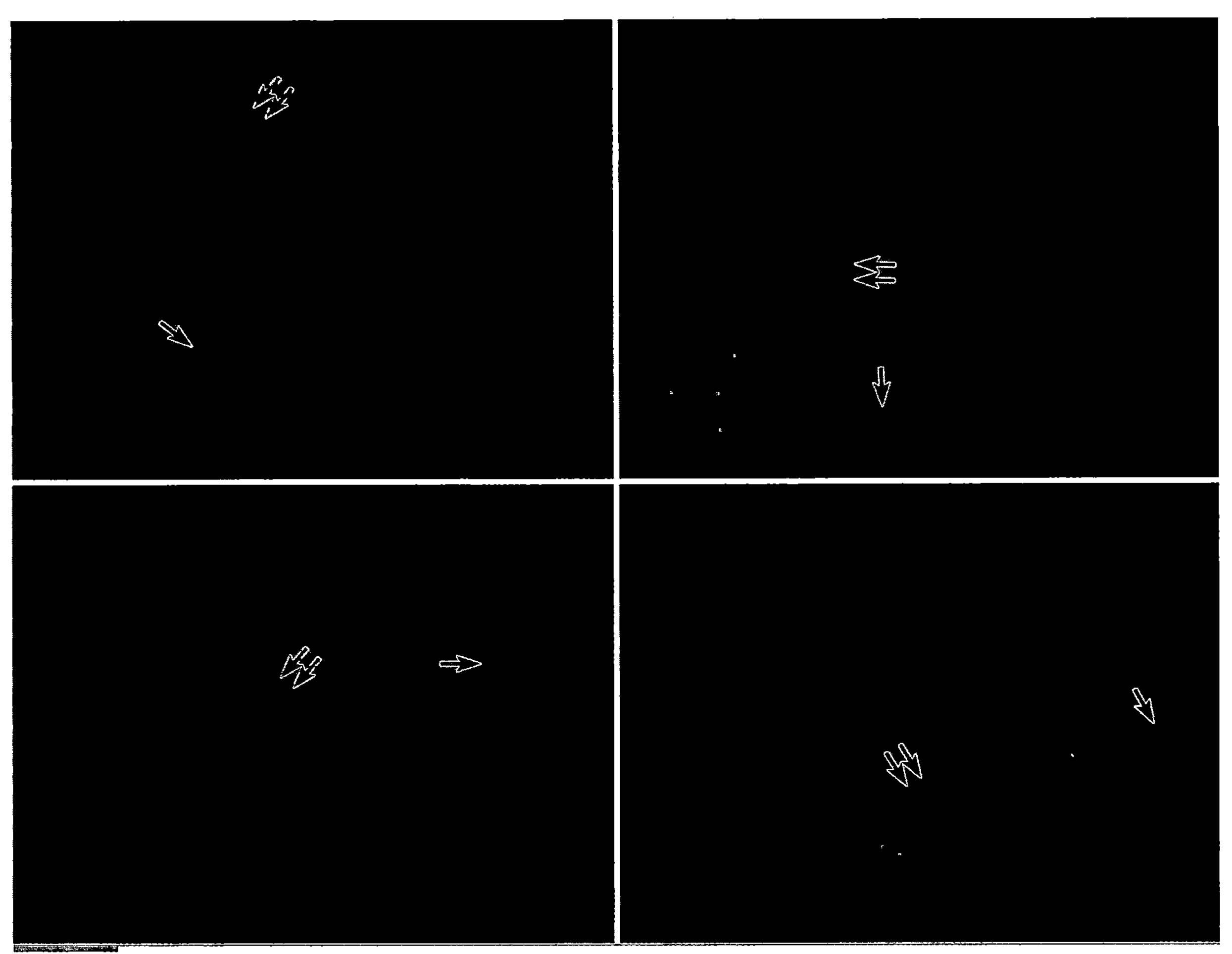

Figure 3.2
Telomere length in pancreatic intraepithelial neoplasia (PanIN) lesions adjacent to pancreatic adenocarcinoma. Telomeres are labeled red; DNA is counterstained with DAPI (blue). **(A)** Weak telomeric signals in the nuclei of low-grade PanIN (PanIN-1a) (*double arrows*); intense labeling in adjacent nuclei of normal epithelium (*arrows*). **(B)** Low-grade PanIN-1b. **(C)** Sharp transition between high-grade PanIN-3 and normal epithelium. **(D)** Weak telomeric signal in cancerized ducts (carcinoma growing into normal ducts, *double arrows*); interspersed bright signals are lymphocytes (*arrow*). (From reference [15]; with permission).

and 11 cell lines, two convincing mutations were found: a germline nonsense mutation in the *FANCG* gene in a cell line and a somatic frameshift mutation in the *FANCC* gene in a xenograft, both accompanied by loss of the second allele.[23] In addition, several missense mutations were found, of which the functional significance remains undetermined. The Fanconi genes *FANCA*, *FANCC*, *FANCE*, *FANCF*, *FANCG*, and *FANCL* form a nuclear complex that is necessary for the monoubiquitination of Fancd2, the central protein in this pathway.[24-26] A defect in monoubiquitination, which can be detected by a Western blot, indicates that one of the upstream *FANC* genes is defective. A total of 21 pancreatic cancer cell lines (including the already sequenced 11 cell lines) were recently screened using Fancd2 monoubiquitination as a functional assay (Fig. 3.3).[27] In this screen, another pancreatic cancer cell line was found to be defective in the Fanconi pathway, which led to the discovery of a large homozygous deletion of the *FANCC* gene in this cell. Large numbers of carcinomas have not been screened yet, but the frequency of mutations in the *FANCC* and *FANCG* genes is expected to be at least 3%.

Cells with inactivating mutations in the Fanconi genes (including *BRCA2*) have an increased in vitro sensitivity to mitomycin and other DNA-interstrand crosslinking agents. Patients with "sporadic" pancreatic cancers defective in this pathway are not themselves hypersensitive to these agents. Therefore, the occurrence of Fanconi-defective carcinomas in Fanconi-proficient hosts could provide a very useful therapeutic window for the treatment of these patients with DNA-interstrand crosslinking agents, such as mitomycin and cisplatin. Why mutations in the

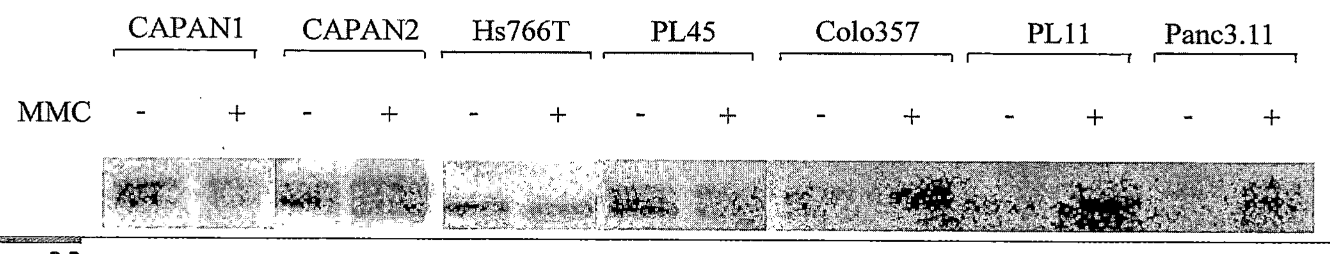

Figure 3.3
Screen for Fanconi anemia gene defects by Fancd2 monoubiquitination assay. The Fanconi proteins Fanca, Fancc, Fance, Fancf, Fancg, and Fancl assemble in a nuclear complex that is necessary for the monoubiquitination of Fancd2. The lower band on a Fancd2 immunoblot indicates the nonubiquitinated isoform; the upper band indicates the monoubiquitinated isoform. If any of the Fanconi genes other than *BRCA2* (as in CAPAN1 cells) is defective, only a single band is visible, as seen in the cell lines Hs766T (*FANCQ*) and PL11 (*FANCC*).

Fanconi/Brca2 pathway are selected for during tumorigenesis is not yet clear. An obvious suggestion would be that defects in this pathway could lead to the initiation of genetic instability.[28] However, genetic instability can be assumed to be present before the abrogation of members of the Fanconi/Brca2 pathway because the inactivation of the *BRCA2*, *FANCC*, or *FANCG* genes is always due in part to the deletion of one of the alleles. Also, the loss of the second allele in carriers of a *BRCA2* germline mutation occurs late in carcinogenesis.[29] Possibly, defects in the Fanconi/Brca2 pathway lead to a form of genetic instability that is needed to help a neoplasm overcome certain genetic barriers. As noted by Swift in 1971,[30] rare recessive syndromes, such as Fanconi anemia, may be of great value in understanding the origin of clinically common and important neoplasms.

Mitotic Checkpoints

In 1998, Cahill et al.[31] showed that all colorectal cancers displaying CIN, but not those demonstrating MIN, are defective in the mitotic checkpoint normally observed after treatment with mitotic spindle-disrupting agents. In some of these carcinomas, mutations were found in the *BUB1* gene in combination with a wild-type second allele. When these mutants were transfected into MIN tumors, the same type of mitotic checkpoint defect was found, even though the wild-type allele was still present, indicating that these mutations have a dominant negative effect. A survey of pancreatic cancer cell lines for these checkpoint abnormalities was conducted by Hempen et al.[32] In contrast to MIN cancer cells, the CIN-pancreatic cancer cell lines did not display a distinct mitotic block after treatment with a mitotic spindle-disrupting agent. In one of these cell lines, two missense mutations were found in a single allele in exon 8 of the *BUB1* gene, possibly accounting, at least in this cell line, for the observed mitotic checkpoint defect. The occurrence of dominant negative mutations in these checkpoint genes could contribute to aneuploidy and is in accordance with the genetically dominant nature of CIN.[33]

Mismatch Repair

Most human tumors, including pancreatic adenocarcinomas, have CIN, producing complex karyotypes with significant alterations in chromosomal copy numbers (aneuploidy).[34,35] However, some carcinomas have an almost diploid (normal) chromosome number. These cancers have a more subtle genetic instability: they have defects in mismatch repair, resulting in elevated rates of sequence mutations and very high rates of mutations in *microsatellites*: simple repetitive sequences, hence the term *microsatellite instability*. Defects in mismatch repair in cancer were initially reported in colorectal cancer.[36-38] Hereditary nonpolyposis colorectal cancer syndrome is caused by germline mutations in one of the mismatch repair genes (including *MSH2* and *MLH1*). Proteins encoded by these genes repair single-base-pair changes and small insertions and deletions. Cancers mutated in these genes accumulate changes of coding and noncoding regions of the genome.

Microsatellite instability is found in approximately 4% of pancreatic cancers,[1,2,39] and pancreatic cancer has been reported in some hereditary nonpolyposis colorectal cancer kindreds.[40,41] Pancreatic cancers with microsatellite instability are associated with a medullary histopathology: poor differentiation, a syncytial growth pattern, and pushing borders.[2,3] A medullary histology is always seen in MIN cancers, although half or more medullary tumors do not have MIN. Genetically, they are *KRAS2* wild-type and commonly contain mutations in the *TGFBRII*, *ACVR2* and *BRAF* genes, all in contrast with the usual findings in microsatellite stable pancreatic cancer. Recently, a diagnostic tool was developed by Montgomery et al.[42] that uses the appearance of anaphase bridges as a distinguishing sign between CIN and MIN tumors. In a study consisting of sarcomas and colorectal and pancreatic tumors, all chromosomally stable tumors (MIN tumors) lacked anaphase bridges, whereas anaphase bridges were found in most CIN sarcomas and carcinomas.

Oncogenes

Oncogenes encode for proteins that when mutationally activated, contribute to neoplastic progression.

KRAS2

The *KRAS2* gene encodes for a G (guanosine triphosphate–binding) protein that is involved in the transduction of signals from growth factor receptors and other signaling inputs. The Kras2 protein can be constitutively activated by point mutations in codons 12, 13, or 61 of the *KRAS2* gene. These point mutations impair the guanosine triphosphatase activity of the Kras2 protein. The *KRAS2* gene is mutated in more than 90% of pancreatic cancers, usually by a mutation in codon 12, the highest rate of mutations for the *KRAS2* gene in any type of cancer.[43] Studies in PanINs show the *KRAS2* gene to be mutated early in the development of pancreatic cancer, although the prevalence of *KRAS2* gene mutations rises in more advanced lesions.[44,45] There are a few reports of *KRAS2* gene amplification,[46,47] although whether these serve the same tumorigenic role as classic missense *KRAS2* gene mutations remains undetermined.

BRAF

The *BRAF* gene encodes a serine/threonine kinase located immediately downstream from Kras2 in the Ras signaling pathway, and the *BRAF* gene is a mutational target in several cancers, including melanomas (66%) and colorectal cancer (10%).[48] Mutations in the *KRAS2* and *BRAF* genes seem to be, in large part, mutually exclusive: in a study by Rajagopalan et al.,[49] mutations of *KRAS2* and *BRAF* were analyzed in 330 colorectal tumors. The *BRAF* gene was mutated in 32 (10%) of the carcinomas, and the *KRAS2* gene in 169 (51%); none of these carcinomas contained mutations in both genes. Furthermore, the prevalence of *BRAF* gene mutations is much higher in mismatch repair–deficient cancers (31%) than in mismatch repair–proficient cancers (7%). In a study by Calhoun et al.,[50] nine *KRAS2* wild-type pancreatic cancers were screened for mutations in the *BRAF* gene; three of these carcinomas (33%) harbored a somatic missense mutation, V599E, previously shown to stimulate the kinase activity of Braf[48]; two of these three carcinomas had a mismatch repair defect. Among 74 *KRAS2*-mutant cancers, no mutations in the *BRAF* gene were identified. These observances confirm that neoplasms seem to select for only one mutation in this pathway and that there seems to be nearly a requirement for *KRAS2*-related signal activation in the development of pancreatic cancer.

Cyclin E

Cyclin E is a known proto-oncogene, overexpressed in several different types of cancer, and the protein product of cyclin E functions as a cell cycle regulator. *Cyclin E* is targeted for degradation by the ubiquitin ligase Fbxw7 (Ago, Cdc4).[51,52] Using microarrays and immunohistochemical labeling, Calhoun et al.[50] determined that 6% of pancreatic adenocarcinomas overexpress cyclin E. The authors also reported low-level amplification and ectopic copies of *CCNE* (coding for cyclin E) in separate cell lines, as well as a somatic missense mutation in the *FBXW7* gene (H460R) in a xenografted pancreatic cancer. *FBXW7* functions as a tumor-suppressor gene, with the second allele inactivated by loss of heterozygosity. This biallelic mutation of the *FBXW7* gene was accompanied by strong nuclear immunopositivity for cyclin E, indicating an impaired degradation.

Other Amplified Regions

Amplification of genomic regions besides *CCNE* may occur occasionally. Amplified regions include the *AKT2* gene within an amplicon on chromosome 19q and the *MYB* gene on 6q, involving about 10%–20% of cases studied,[53-55] although the functional targets of these amplicons are not fully explored.

Tumor-Suppressor Genes

Tumor-suppressor genes are genes that when inactivated contribute to neoplastic progression. Tumor-suppressor genes usually code for proteins that have a direct or indirect role in governing the cell cycle or apoptosis, roles that restrict the expansion of cell populations. They can be inactivated by a combination of mutations, methylation, or the complete loss of one (LOH) or both (homozygous deletion) alleles.

p16/CDKN2A

Normal cells can progress through the G_1 phase of the cell cycle only if they can functionally inactivate the Rb protein by phosphorylation (reviewed in Sherr[56]). Rb is phosphorylated by a complex of cyclin D and cyclin-dependent kinases (Cdk4 and Cdk6). p16 inhibits promotion of the cell cycle by competing with cyclin D in binding to Cdk4 and Cdk6, preventing the phosphorylation (inactivation) of Rb. The hyperphosphorylation of Rb releases transcription factors that promote the G_1/S transition. Therefore, the p16/Rb pathway can be abrogated by alteration of p16, Rb, Cdk4/Cdk6, or cyclin D.

The *p16/CDKN2A* gene is located on 9p, a site of frequent allelic loss in pancreatic cancer, and is mutated in a variety of cancer types. Caldas et al. demonstrated homozygous deletions of *p16/CDKN2A* in 40% of pancreatic cancers and inactivating mutations of the gene in another 40% of pancreatic cancers by an intragenic mutation coupled with loss of the second allele[39]. In addition, Schutte et al. demonstrated that the *p16/CDKN2A* gene is inactivated by hypermethylation of its promoter in almost all of the remaining pancreatic cancers[57]. Inactivation of Rb is reported in a small number of pancreatic cancers: Huang et al. found loss of immunohistochemical staining for Rb in three of 30 pancreatic cancers.[58] A truncating mutation was found in one of these cancers, and a missense mutation was found on genomic sequencing in another of these three cancers. Thus, the p16/Rb pathway is inactivated in virtually all pancreatic cancers, leading to an inappropriate progression through the G_1 phase of the cell cycle.

TP53

p53, encoded by the *TP53* gene, is a nuclear DNA-binding protein that has an important role in the G_1/S cell cycle checkpoint, the maintenance of the G_2/M arrest, and the induction of apoptosis. The inactivation of the *TP53* gene results in the loss of important restraints on the initiation of replication and the loss of the induction of cell death. The *TP53* tumor-suppressor gene is located on the short arm of chromosome 17 (17p); this locus shows frequent loss of heterozygosity in pancreatic cancer.[1] The remaining *TP53* allele, when sequenced, harbors missense mutations or small frameshift mutations in 50%–75% of pancreatic cancers.[59-61] Thus, the *TP53* gene is inactivated in 50%–75% of pancreatic cancers.

TGF-*β*/Activin Pathway

The transforming growth factor type *β* (TGF-*β*) pathway is a tumor-suppressive signaling pathway activated by the binding of TGF-*β* ligands to cell surface receptors, and the subsequent phosphorylation, complexation, and nuclear localization of Smad proteins. This and related pathways can also be activated by the binding of related ligands, such as activin and bone morphogenic proteins.

The long arm of chromosome 18 (18q) is a site of frequent allelic loss in pancreatic cancer: almost 90% of pancreatic cancers have loss of heterozygosity at this locus. This led Hahn et al. [62,63] to search for a tumor-suppressor gene on 18q. While screening a panel of pancreatic xenografts, they found a region located at 18q21.1 to be homozygously deleted in a number of the carcinomas; they designated this region DPC4 (deleted in pancreatic cancer). Subsequently, several intragenic mutations were found in a gene located in this region, in xenografts without a homozygous deletion, but with LOH. This gene, *DPC4/MADH4/SMAD4*, encodes Madh4, a mediator of the TGF-*β* pathway, and is inactivated somatically in 55% of pancreatic cancers. In 35% of cancers, *MADH4* is inactivated by a homozygous deletion; in 20% by an intragenic mutation in combination with loss of the other allele. The prevalence of *MADH4* mutations in pancreatic cancer is much higher than that in other types of cancer. For example, *MADH4* is inactivated in 15% or less of breast and colorectal cancers.

The immunohistochemical labeling of Madh4 directly mirrors *MADH4* gene status. This has been shown for both homozygous deletions and truncating mutations of the *MADH4* gene[64] and, more recently, for most inactivating intragenic mutations: these mutant proteins are not stable and/or translated into proteins.[65] Immunohistochemical labeling for the Madh4 protein has been used to investigate the expression of Madh4 in PanINs by Wilentz et al.[66] Madh4 was expressed in all histologically low-grade lesions (PanIN-1 and -2), whereas Madh4 protein expression was lost in 31% of high-grade lesions (PanIN-3).

Multiple receptors, including TGF-*β* receptor type I (Tgfbr1/ALK5), TGF-*β* receptor type II (Tgfbr2), and the activin receptors type IB (Acvr1b/ALK4) and II (Acvr2), exert their effect through Madh4. In 1998, Goggins et al.[67] studied the genes *TGFBR1* and *TGFBR2* for inactivating mutations. One of 97 pancreatic and one of 12 biliary adenocarcinomas harbored a homozygous deletion of the *TGFBR1* gene. In addition, somatic alterations in the *TGFBR2* gene were identified in four out of 97 pancreatic adenocarcinomas. Three of these four mutations were homozygous frameshift mutations in a poly(A) tract, in pancreatic cancers with a mismatch repair defect. In a study by Hempen et al.,[68] mutations in the *ACVR2* gene were found in three mismatch repair defective pancreatic cancers; all of these three mutations were frameshift alterations in a poly(A) tract of the *ACVR2* gene, occurring in tumors that also harbored mutations in the *TGFBR2* gene. The occurrence of mutations in either gene in MIN carcinomas occurred at a higher rate than expected in a mathematical model, based on the prevalence of random alterations in short mononucleotide tracts in these carcinomas. In addition, a CIN pancreatic cancer was found with a frameshift mutation in the *ACVR2* gene combined with LOH of the second allele, establishing *ACVR2* as a tumor-suppressor gene targeted in pancreatic cancer.

In 2001, Su et al.[69] described a homozygous deletion and a 5-bp frameshift deletion in the activin receptor type 1B (*ACVR1B/ALK4*) gene in two pancreatic xenografts. *ACVR1B/ALK4* codes for an activin-receptor that signals through Madh4. The two pancreatic cancer xenografts with mutations in the *ACVR1B/ALK4* gene both had inactivating mutations in *MADH4*, creating an apparent contradiction with regard to the thesis that only one member of a linear cell pathway will be mutated in a cancer. However, these findings readily fit a more complex model of a branched signaling pathway in which, at an early stage, *MADH4* gene mutations would be detrimental to a developing neoplasm, whereas mutations of TGF-β and activin receptors, with only a partial inactivation of Madh4-mediated signaling, would provide the tumor with a selective advantage. In a later stage, when the cancer cells harbor new defects in cell cycle checkpoints and other regulatory systems, an inactivation of the *MADH4* gene would no longer be detrimental, but instead would be advantageous. This theory could explain the stepwise inactivation of members of a branched pathway tumor-suppressive system, like the TGF-β/activin pathway, and the empiric findings that *MADH4* loss in the pancreas appears restricted to late-stage PanINs and cancers.

Other Tumor-Suppressor Genes

Mutations in the *LKB1/STK11* gene are the cause of the autosomal-dominant inherited Peutz-Jeghers syndrome, characterized by mucocutaneous melanin macules and nonneoplastic gastrointestinal hamartomas (see Chapter 9).[70,71] In addition, patients with Peutz-Jeghers syndrome have an elevated risk of cancer: the average age at which cancer is diagnosed ranges from 38 to 50 years. The risk of death from gastrointestinal cancer is 13- to 30-fold greater than the risk in the general population; Giardiello et al.[72] found a relative risk of 132 for pancreatic cancer in Peutz-Jeghers patients. In a study by Su et al.,[73] the *LKB1/STK11* gene, encoding a serine/threonine kinase, was found to be homozygously deleted or to harbor a frameshift mutation accompanied by LOH in 4%–6% of 127 sporadic pancreatic and biliary adenocarcinomas. In addition, the wild-type allele in a patient with Peutz-Jeghers syndrome was found to be lost in a pancreatic cancer. The finding of inactivation of the *LKB1/STK11* gene in both familial and sporadic cases establishes the *LKB1/STK11* gene as a tumor-suppressive gene along the lines of the classical Nicholls/Knudson model.[74,75]

Many other tumor-suppressor genes that are targeted at low frequency in pancreatic cancer deserve mentioning. Intragenic mutations and homozygous deletions of the *MKK4* gene (mitogen-activated protein kinase 4) are seen in a small percentage of pancreatic cancers.[76] The *MKK4* gene codes for a component of a stress-activated protein kinase cascade and has roles in apoptosis and growth control. Frameshift mutations in the *BAX* gene, a mediator of apoptosis, have been reported in mismatch repair defective tumors at a rate higher than predicted based on the occurrence of random frameshifts in microsatellites.[68,77] The *EP300* gene codes for p300—a histone acetyltransferase that regulates transcription through chromatin remodeling. A truncating mutation in a pancreatic cancer cell line has been reported by Gayther et al.[78]; no larger studies of this gene in pancreatic cancer have been reported.

Conclusion

Through the study of pancreatic cancer precursor lesions, PanINs, a model for the progression of pancreatic ductal epithelium from noninvasive dysplastic intraepithelial lesions to an invasive cancer is emerging (Fig. 3.4).[79,80] The earliest recognizable and prevalent genetic defect is the shortening of telomeres. This defect could plausibly cause

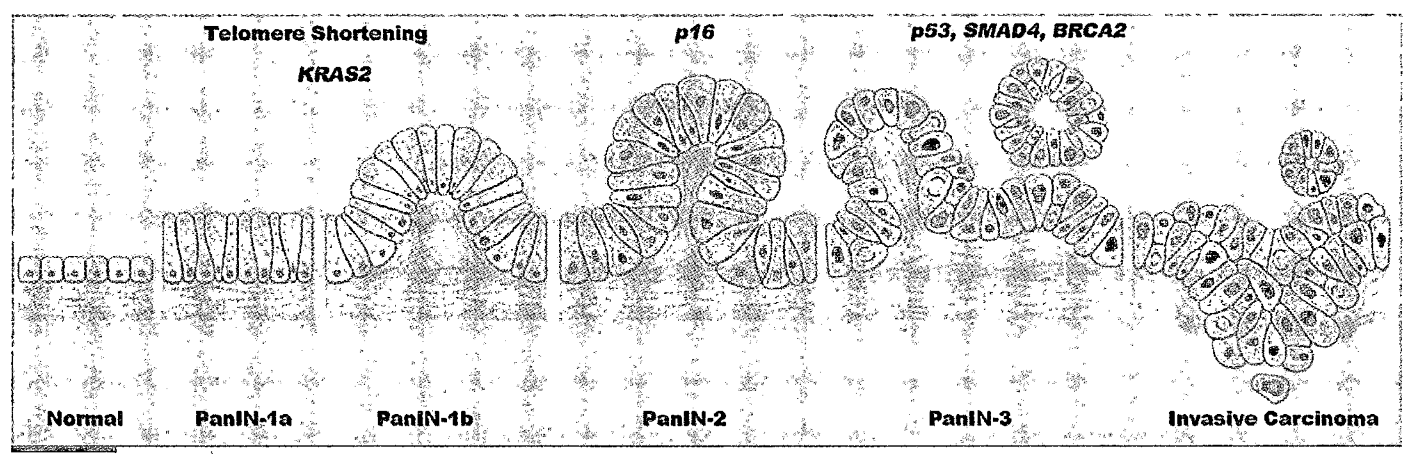

Figure 3.4
Progression model for pancreatic cancer. Specific genetic alterations accumulate during the progression from histologically normal epithelium to high-grade pancreatic intraepithelial neoplasia (PanIN) (*left to right*). (From Ref [80]; with permission).

CIN, leading to losses and gains of chromosomal arms; loss of heterozygosity of chromosome 9p (the location of *p16*) is seen in 13% of histologically low-grade duct lesions and in 90% of high-grade duct lesions.[1,59] All histologically high-grade PanIN lesions exhibit LOH at more than one chromosomal locus.[59] Activating mutations in the *KRAS2* gene can also occur early in this model, although the prevalence rises further down the road toward an invasive malignancy, suggesting that *KRAS2* gene mutations are not necessarily the first change (gatekeeper) needed for the development of ductal neoplasia. Alterations in the *p16* gene occur slightly later than *KRAS2* gene mutations, and the prevalence of loss of this gene also appears to rise with increasing grades of PanIN.[81,82] In this genetic progression model of pancreatic cancer, inactivation of the *DPC4*, *TP53*, and *BRCA2* genes seem to be relatively late events.[79]

The past decade has brought tremendous progress in understanding of the genetic causes of pancreatic cancer. However, it is unlikely that all genetic changes have been found as yet, as was demonstrated by recent discoveries of mutations in the *BRAF*, *FBXW7*, and Fanconi genes. Many genes still need to be investigated. The high mortality rate and paucity of therapeutic options for pancreatic cancer highlight the need to apply this extensive genetic knowledge to patient care. One such example would be the rational treatment of pancreatic cancers with defects in the Fanconi/Brca2 pathway with DNA-interstrand crosslinking agents, such as mitomycin and cisplatin, an approach that is currently being explored experimentally.

References

1. Hahn SA, Seymour AB, Hoque AT, et al. Allelotype of pancreatic adenocarcinoma using xenograft enrichment. *Cancer Res*. 1995;55:4670–4675.
2. Goggins M, Offerhaus GJ, Hilgers W, et al. Pancreatic adenocarcinomas with DNA replication errors (RER+) are associated with wild-type K-*ras* and characteristic histopathology: poor differentiation, a syncytial growth pattern, and pushing borders suggest RER+. *Am J Pathol*. 1998;152:1501–1507.
3. Wilentz RE, Goggins M, Redston M, et al. Genetic, immunohistochemical, and clinical features of medullary carcinoma of the pancreas: a newly described and characterized entity. *Am J Pathol*. 2000;156:1641–1651.
4. Rajagopalan H, Nowak MA, Vogelstein B, Lengauer C. The significance of unstable chromosomes in colorectal cancer. *Nat Rev Cancer*. 2003;3:695–701.
5. Nowak MA, Komarova NL, Sengupta A, et al. The role of chromosomal instability in tumor initiation. *Proc Natl Acad Sci USA*. 2002;99:16226–16231.
6. Cahill DP, Kinzler KW, Vogelstein B, Lengauer C. Genetic instability and Darwinian selection in tumours. *Trends Cell Biol*. 1999;9:M57–M60.
7. Iacobuzio-Donahue CA, Van der Heijden MS, Baumgartner MR, et al. Large scale allelotype of pancreaticobiliary carcinoma provides quantitative estimates of genome-wide allelic loss. *Cancer Res*. 2004;64:871–875.
8. Yoshino I, Fukuyama S, Kameyama T, et al. Detection of loss of heterozygosity by high-resolution fluorescent system in non-small cell lung cancer: association of loss of heterozygosity with smoking and tumor progression. *Chest*. 2003;123:545–550.
9. Lüttges J, Galehdari H, Brocker V, et al. Allelic loss is often the first hit in the biallelic inactivation of the *p53* and *DPC4* genes during pancreatic carcinogenesis. *Am J Pathol*. 2001;158:1677–1683.
10. McClintock B. The stability of broken ends of chromosomes in Zea mays. *Genetics*. 1941;26:234–282.
11. Gisselsson D, Pettersson L, Hoglund M, et al. Chromosomal breakage-fusion-bridge events cause genetic intratumor heterogeneity. *Proc Natl Acad Sci USA*. 2000;97:5357–5362.
12. Hemann MT, Strong MA, Hao LY, Greider CW. The shortest telomere, not average telomere length, is critical for cell viability and chromosome stability. *Cell*. 2001;107:67–77.
13. Hopkin K, Edwards P, Harris A, Klausner R, Peters G, Selby P, Stanley M., Cancer:1313–1362. In: Albert B, Johnson A, Lewis J, Raff M, Roberts K, Walter P (ed.) *Molecular Biology of the Cell*. 4th ed. New York: Garland Science; 2002:1313–1362.
14. Meeker AK, Gage WR, Hicks JL, et al. Telomere length assessment in human archival tissues: combined telomere fluorescence in situ hybridization and immunostaining. *Am J Pathol*. 2002;160:1259–1268.
15. van Heek NT, Meeker AK, Kern SE, et al. Telomere shortening is nearly universal in pancreatic intraepithelial neoplasia. *Am J Pathol*. 2002;161:1541–1547.
16. Edwards SM, Kote-Jarai Z, Meitz J, et al. Two percent of men with early-onset prostate cancer harbor germline mutations in the *BRCA2* gene. *Am J Hum Genet*. 2003;72:1–12.
17. Goggins M, Schutte M, Lu J, et al. Germline *BRCA2* gene mutations in patients with apparently sporadic pancreatic carcinomas. *Cancer Res*. 1996;56:5360–5364.
18. Murphy KM, Brune KA, Griffin C, et al. Evaluation of candidate genes *MAP2K4, MADH4, ACVR1B,* and *BRCA2* in familial pancreatic cancer: deleterious BRCA2 mutations in 17%. *Cancer Res*.2002;62:3789–3793.
19. Wooster R, Bignell G, Lancaster J, et al. Identification of the breast cancer susceptibility gene *BRCA2*. *Nature*. 1995;378:789–792.
20. van Gent DC, Hoeijmakers JH, Kanaar R. Chromosomal stability and the DNA double-stranded break connection. *Nat Rev Genet*.2001;2:196–206.
21. Howlett, NG, Taniguchi T, Olson S, et al. Biallelic inactivation of BRCA2 in Fanconi anemia. *Science*. 2002;297:606–609.
22. Kutler DI, Singh B, Satagopan J, et al. A 20-year perspective on the International Fanconi Anemia Registry (IFAR). *Blood*. 2003;101:1249–1256.
23. van der Heijden MS, Yeo CJ, Hruban RH, Kern SE. Fanconi anemia gene mutations in young-onset pancreatic cancer. *Cancer Res*. 2003;63:2585–2588.

24. Meetei AR, de Winter JP, Medhurst AL, et al. A novel ubiquitin ligase is deficient in Fanconi anemia. *Nat Genet.* 2003;35:165–170.
25. D'Andrea AD, Grompe M. The Fanconi anaemia/BRCA pathway. *Nat Rev Cancer.* 2003;3:23–34.
26. Joenje H, Patel KJ. The emerging genetic and molecular basis of Fanconi anaemia. *Nat Rev Genet.* 2001;2:446–457.
27. Van der Heijden MS, Brody JR, Gallmeier E, et al. Functional defects in the Fanconi anemia pathway in pancreatic cancer cells. *Am J Pathol.* 2004;165:651–657.
28. D'Andrea AD. The Fanconi road to cancer. *Genes Dev.* 2003;31:31.
29. Goggins M, Hruban RH, Kern SE. *BRCA2* is inactivated late in the development of pancreatic intraepithelial neoplasia: evidence and implications. *Am J Pathol.* 2000;156:1767–1771.
30. Swift M. Fanconi's anaemia in the genetics of neoplasia. *Nature.* 1971;230:370–373.
31. Cahill DP, Lengauer C, Yu J, et al. Mutations of mitotic checkpoint genes in human cancers. *Nature.* 1998;392:300–303.
32. Hempen PM, Kurpad H, Calhoun ES, Abraham S, Kern SE. A double missense variation of the *BUB1* gene and a defective mitotic spindle checkpoint in the pancreatic cancer cell line Hs766T. *Hum Mutat.* 2003;21:445.
33. Lengauer C, Kinzler KW, Vogelstein B. Genetic instability in colorectal cancers. *Nature.* 1997;386:623–627.
34. Griffin CA, Hruban RH, Long PP, Morsberger LA, Douna-Issa F, Yeo CJ. Chromosome abnormalities in pancreatic adenocarcinoma. *Genes Chromosomes Cancer.* 1994;9:93–100.
35. Bardi G, Johansson B, Pandis N, et al. Karyotypic abnormalities in tumours of the pancreas. *Br J Cancer.* 1993;67:1106–1112.
36. Thibodeau SN, Bren G, Schaid D. Microsatellite instability in cancer of the proximal colon. *Science.* 1993;260:816–819.
37. Ionov Y, Peinado MA, Malkhosyan S, Shibata D, Perucho M. Ubiquitous somatic mutations in simple repeated sequences reveal a new mechanism for colonic carcinogenesis. *Nature.* 1993;363:558–561.
38. Aaltonen LA, Peltomaki P, Leach FS, et al. Clues to the pathogenesis of familial colorectal cancer. *Science.* 1993;260:812–816.
39. Caldas C, Hahn SA, da Costa LT, et al. Frequent somatic mutations and homozygous deletions of the *p16* (MTS1) gene in pancreatic adenocarcinoma. *Nat Genet.* 1994;8:27–32.
40. Lynch HT, Voorhees GJ, Lanspa SJ, McGreevy PS, Lynch JF. Pancreatic carcinoma and hereditary nonpolyposis colorectal cancer: a family study. *Br J Cancer.* 1985;52:271–273.
41. Lynch HT, Smyrk T, Kern SE, et al. Familial pancreatic cancer: a review. *Semin Oncol.* 1996;23:251–275.
42. Montgomery E, Wilentz RE, Argani P, et al. Analysis of anaphase figures in routine histologic sections distinguishes chromosomally unstable from chromosomally stable malignancies. *Cancer Biol Ther.* 2003;2:248–252.
43. Almoguera C, Shibata D, Forrester K, Martin J, Arnheim N, Perucho M. Most human carcinomas of the exocrine pancreas contain mutant *c-K-ras* genes. *Cell.* 1988;53:549–554.
44. Caldas C, Hahn SA, Hruban RH, Redston MS, Yeo CJ, Kern SE. Detection of *K-ras* mutations in the stool of patients with pancreatic adenocarcinoma and pancreatic ductal hyperplasia. *Cancer Res.* 1994;54:3568–3573.
45. DiGiuseppe JA, Hruban RH, Offerhaus GJ, et al. Detection of *K-ras* mutations in mucinous pancreatic duct hyperplasia from a patient with a family history of pancreatic carcinoma. *Am J Pathol.* 1994;144:889–895.
46. Heidenblad M, Jonson T, Mahlamaki EH, Gorunova L, Karhu R, Johansson B, Hoglund M. Detailed genomic mapping and expression analyses of *12p* amplifications in pancreatic carcinomas reveal a 3.5-Mb target region for amplification. *Genes Chromosomes Cancer.* 2002;34:211–223.
47. Yamada H, Sakamoto H, Taira M, et al. Amplifications of both c-*K-ras* with a point mutation and c-myc in a primary pancreatic cancer and its metastatic tumors in lymph nodes. *Jpn J Cancer Res.* 1986;77:370–375.
48. Davies H, Bignell GR, Cox C, et al. Mutations of the *BRAF* gene in human cancer. *Nature.* 2002;417:949–954.
49. Rajagopalan H, Bardelli A, Lengauer C, Kinzler KW, Vogelstein B, Velculescu VE. Tumorigenesis: RAF/RAS oncogenes and mismatch-repair status. *Nature.* 2002;418:934.
50. Calhoun ES, Jones JB, Ashfaq R, et al. *BRAF* and *FBXW7* (CDC4, FBW7, AGO, SEL10) mutations in distinct subsets of pancreatic cancer: potential therapeutic targets. *Am J Pathol.* 2003;163:1255–1260.
51. Moberg KH, Bell DW, Wahrer DC, Haber DA, Hariharan IK. Archipelago regulates cyclin E levels in *Drosophila* and is mutated in human cancer cell lines. *Nature.* 2001;413:311–316.
52. Strohmaier H, Spruck CH, Kaiser P, Won KA, Sangfelt O, Reed SI. Human F-box protein hCdc4 targets cyclin E for proteolysis and is mutated in a breast cancer cell line. *Nature.* 2001;413:316–322.
53. Wallrapp C, Muller-Pillasch F, Solinas-Toldo S, et al. Characterization of a high copy number amplification at 6q24 in pancreatic cancer identifies *c-myb* as a candidate oncogene. *Cancer Res.* 1997;57:3135–3139.
54. Cheng JQ, Ruggeri B, Klein WM, et al. Amplification of *AKT2* in human pancreatic cells and inhibition of *AKT2* expression and tumorigenicity by antisense RNA. *Proc Natl Acad Sci USA.* 1996;93:3636–3641.
55. Miwa W, Yasuda J, Murakami Y, et al. Isolation of DNA sequences amplified at chromosome 19q13.1-q13.2 including the AKT2 locus in human pancreatic cancer. *Biochem Biophys Res Commun.* 1996;225:968–974.
56. Sherr CJ. Cancer cell cycles. *Science.* 1996;274:1672–1677.
57. Schutte M, Hruban RH, Geradts J, et al. Abrogation of the Rb/p16 tumor-suppressive pathway in virtually all pancreatic carcinomas. *Cancer Res.* 1997;57:3126–3130.
58. Huang L, Lang D, Geradts J, et al. Molecular and immunochemical analyses of RB1 and cyclin D1 in human ductal pancreatic carcinomas and cell lines. *Mol Carcinog.* 1996;15:85–95.
59. Yamano M, Fujii H, Takagaki T, Kadowaki N, Watanabe H, Shirai T. Genetic progression and divergence in pancreatic carcinoma. *Am J Pathol.* 2000;156:2123–2133.

60. Rozenblum E, Schutte M, Goggins M, et al. Tumor-suppressive pathways in pancreatic carcinoma. *Cancer Res.* 1997;57:1731–1734.
61. Pellegata NS, Sessa F, Renault B, et al. *K-ras* and *p53* gene mutations in pancreatic cancer: ductal and nonductal tumors progress through different genetic lesions. *Cancer Res.* 1994;54:1556–1560.
62. Hahn SA, Hoque AT, Moskaluk CA, et al. Homozygous deletion map at 18q21.1 in pancreatic cancer. *Cancer Res.* 1996;56:490–494.
63. Hahn SA, Schutte M, Hoque AT, et al. *DPC4*, a candidate tumor-suppressor gene at human chromosome 18q21.1. *Science.* 1996;271:350–353.
64. Wilentz RE, Su GH, Dai JL, et al. Immunohistochemical labeling for dpc4 mirrors genetic status in pancreatic adenocarcinomas: a new marker of *DPC4* inactivation. *Am J Pathol.* 2000;156:37–43.
65. Iacobuzio-Donahue CA, Song J, Parmiagiani G, Murphy K, Hruban RH, Kern SE. Missense mutations of *MADH4*: characterization of the mutational hotspot and functional consequences in human tumors. *Clin Cancer Res.* 2004;10:1597–1604.
66. Wilentz RE, Iacobuzio-Donahue CA, Argani P, et al. Loss of expression of Dpc4 in pancreatic intraepithelial neoplasia: evidence that *DPC4* inactivation occurs late in neoplastic progression. *Cancer Res.* 2000;60:2002–2006.
67. Goggins M, Shekher M, Turnacioglu K, Yeo CJ, Hruban RH, Kern SE. Genetic alterations of the transforming growth factor beta receptor genes in pancreatic and biliary adenocarcinomas. *Cancer Res.* 1998;58:5329–5332.
68. Hempen PM, Zhang L, Bansal RK, et al. Evidence of selection for clones having genetic inactivation of the activin A type II receptor (*ACVR2*) gene in gastrointestinal cancers. *Cancer Res.* 2003;63:994–999.
69. Su GH, Bansal R, Murphy KM, et al. *ACVR1B* (ALK4, activin receptor type 1B) gene mutations in pancreatic carcinoma. *Proc Natl Acad Sci.* 2001;98:3254–3257.
70. Hemminki A, Tomlinson I, Markie D, et al. Localization of a susceptibility locus for Peutz-Jeghers syndrome to *19p* using comparative genomic hybridization and targeted linkage analysis. *Nat Genet.* 1997;15:87–90.
71. Hemminki A, Markie D, Tomlinson I, et al. A serine/threonine kinase gene defective in Peutz-Jeghers syndrome. *Nature.* 1998;391:184–187.
72. Giardiello FM, Brensinger JD, Tersmette AC, et al. Very high risk of cancer in familial Peutz-Jeghers syndrome. *Gastroenterology.* 2000;119:1447–1453.
73. Su GH, Hruban RH, Bansal RK, et al. Germline and somatic mutations of the *STK11/LKB1* Peutz-Jeghers gene in pancreatic and biliary cancers. *Am J Pathol.* 1999; 154:1835–1840.
74. Knudson AG. Mutation and human cancer. *Adv Cancer Res.* 1973;17:317–352.
75. Nicholls EM. Somatic variation and multiple neurofibromatosis. *Hum Hered.* 1969;19:473–479.
76. Su GH, Hilgers W, Shekher MC, et al. Alterations in pancreatic, biliary, and breast carcinomas support MKK4 as a genetically targeted tumor-suppressor gene. *Cancer Res.* 1998;58:2339–2342.
77. Yamamoto H, Itoh F, Nakamura H, et al. Genetic and clinical features of human pancreatic ductal adenocarcinomas with widespread microsatellite instability. *Cancer Res.* 2001;61:3139–3144.
78. Gayther SA, Batley SJ, Linger L, et al. Mutations truncating the *EP300* acetylase in human cancers. *Nat Genet.* 2000;24:300–303.
79. Hruban RH, Wilentz RE, Kern SE. Genetic progression in the pancreatic ducts. *Am J Pathol.* 2000;156:1821–1825.
80. Hruban RH, Wilentz RE.:939–953. In: Kumar V, Fausto N, Abbas A. (ed.) *Robbins and Cotran Pathologic Basis of Disease.* 7th ed. Philadelphia, PA: W.B. Saunders Press; 2004.
81. Moskaluk CA, Hruban RH, Kern SE. *p16* and *K-ras* gene mutations in the intraductal precursors of human pancreatic adenocarcinoma. *Cancer Res.* 1997;57:2140-2143.
82. Geradts J, Hruban RH, Schutte M, Kern SE, Maynard R. Immunohistochemical P16 INK4a analysis of archival tumors with deletion, hypermethylation, or mutation of the *CDKN2/MTS1* gene: a comparison of four commercial antibodies. *Appl Immunohistochem Mol Morphol.* 2000;8:71–79.

CHAPTER

4

Molecular Signaling Pathways in Pancreatic Cancer

Nabeel Bardeesy, PhD

Molecular genetic studies have identified a mutational profile of pancreatic adenocarcinoma that is highly distinct among malignancies. This profile has helped to establish a genetic progression model that can guide studies aimed at a detailed understanding of the molecular signaling pathway alterations that lead to cancer genesis and progression. Elucidation of these processes will be critical for improvements in the diagnosis and treatment of this lethal disease.

Pancreatic adenocarcinoma is an invariably lethal condition—extensive clinical trials with cytotoxic therapies have had little effect on patient survival to date. It is well-recognized that improved understanding of pancreatic cancer biology will be necessary in achieving clinical advances.[1] An important challenge is in elucidating the biochemical basis for the distinguishing pathologic features of this cancer such as malignant progression from precursor lesions in the pancreatic ducts, marked stromal proliferation (desmoplasia), extreme aneuploidy, invasive growth, chemoresistance and age-dependent exponential increases in incidence (Fig. 4.1).[2] The discovery of a signature mutational profile of this cancer has provided a foundation for studies of the mechanisms regulating oncogenesis.[3] However, the identification of the specific signaling pathways that mediate disease pathogenesis—and the determination of the biologic consequences of their activation—remain areas of active investigation. Definitive solution of these questions should enable optimal selection of targets for effective therapies and improved diagnostics. Currently, direct experimental approaches are being employed to more fully dissect the components of these pathways and to demonstrate rigorously their causal pathogenic roles and specific biologic effects. Here we review current models of the molecular pathogenesis of pancreatic adenocarcinoma and address the oncogenic significance of these biochemical pathway alterations by considering experimental evidence from animal models and cell culture systems.

Genetic Progression of Pancreatic Adenocarcinoma

Pancreatic adenocarcinomas display a characteristic profile of genetic lesions, consisting of mutations in *CDKN2A*, *KRAS*, *SMAD4/DPC4* and *TP53* in a high proportion of tumors and less frequent mutations in *LKB1*, *BRCA2*, *MKK4*, and *ACVR1B*[3] (see Chapter 3 and Table 3.1). Ongoing studies have been directed at determining the biologic roles of these gene mutations, and in particular in relating these alterations to the processes of cancer initiation and progression. With respect to initiation, the existence of precursor lesions of pancreatic adenocarcinoma has been the subject of considerable debate although recent histopathologic and molecular studies have converged to establish a convincing model of the genetic and histologic progression of the disease.[4] The physical contiguity of pancreatic intraepithelial neoplasia (PanIN) lesions with malignant tumors has led to the hypothesis that these lesions represent incipient pancreatic adenocarcinoma (see Chapter 2).[5] PanINs show graded histologic abnormalities and increasing cytogenetic aberrations consistent with neoplastic progression.[6-9] Furthermore, the development of adenocarcinomas in patients previously documented to have PanIN has supported a PanIN-to-adenocarcinoma sequence.[10,11] At the molecular level, this progression model is further substantiated by the observation of common *INK4A* mutations in adjacent PanINs

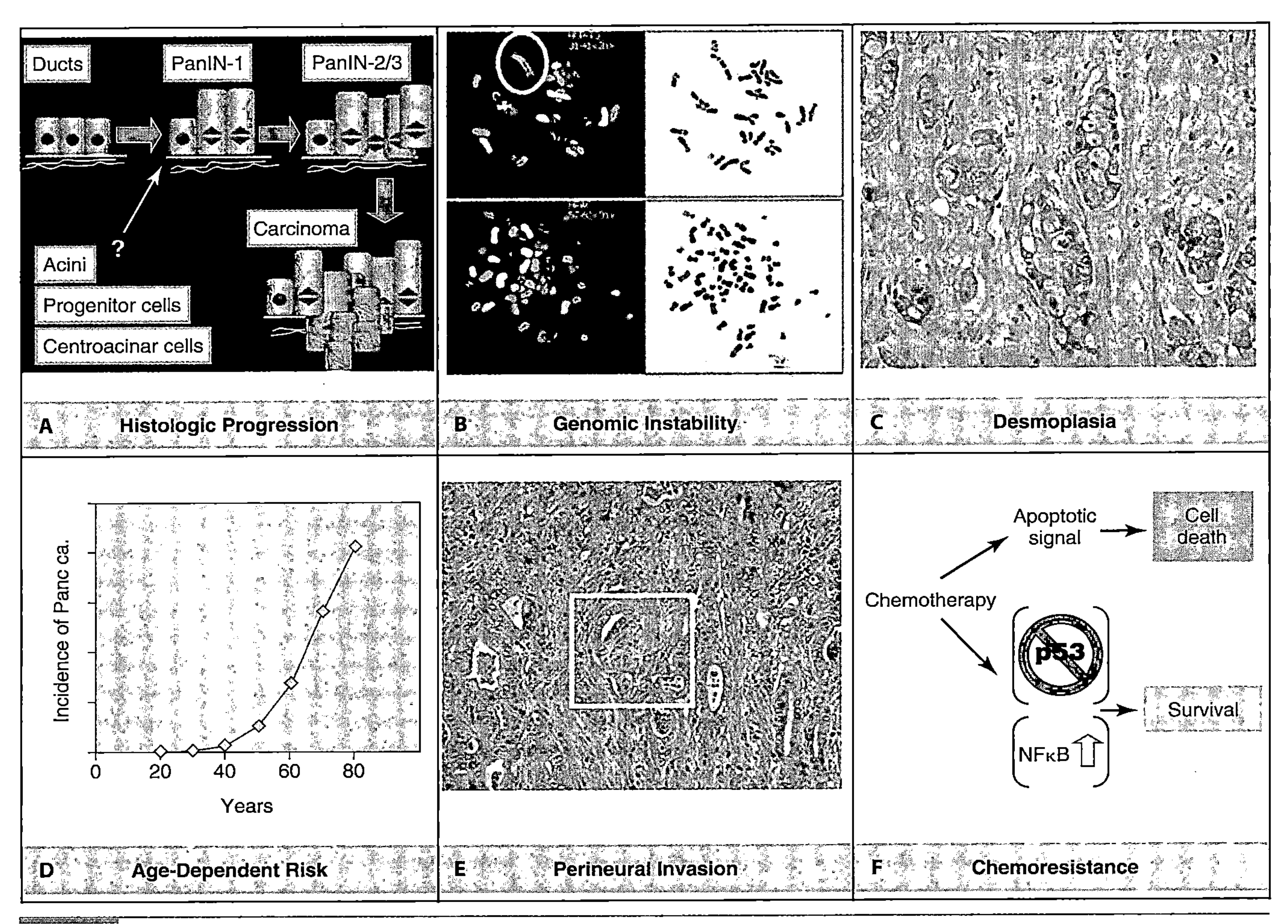

Figure 4.1
Characteristic phenotypes of pancreatic adenocarcinoma. **(A)** Histologic progression. Pancreatic adenocarcinomas are thought to arise from a series of premalignant ductal lesions known as pancreatic intraepithelial neoplasms (PanINs). Specific genetic lesions and gene expression changes have been correlated with different PanIN grades. It is important to determine the mechanistic role of these alterations in the pathogenic process. **(B)** Genomic instability. These tumors are markedly aneuploidy and show extensive chromosomal rearrangement consistent with ongoing genomic instability. The importance of genomic instability in disease pathogenesis and the biochemical basis for this phenotype are incompletely understood. **(C)** Desmoplasia. Extensive proliferation of stromal fibroblasts and deposition of extracellular matrix proteins—known as desmoplasia—is a hallmark of pancreatic adenocarcinoma. The signaling pathways contributing to desmoplasia and the impact of this process on tumorigenesis are under investigation. **(D)** Age-dependent risk. As with many epithelial cancers, pancreatic adenocarcinoma displays an age-dependent exponential rise in incidence. Several models have been proposed to account for this behavior. **(E)** Perineural invasion. This malignancy is characterized by tissue invasion—including invasion of the nerves—and metastasis, even at modest tumor burdens. **(F)** Chemoresistance. These tumors respond very poorly to existing therapies. Improved treatment will require an understanding of the biochemical basis for this chemoresistance.

and adenocarcinomas in a limited number of patients.[6] The progression model allows the correlation of specific molecular alterations with histopathogical changes, thereby providing a framework for detailed studies of the biologic effects of these lesions.

KRAS and Its Downstream Effectors

KRAS Activating *KRAS* gene mutations are present in virtually all pancreatic adenocarcinomas, a mutation rate that is uncommonly high among cancers.[6,12] *KRAS* encodes a small GTPase that, in its active, GTP-bound form, engages a broad series of cellular pathways relating to proliferation, survival, migration, metabolism and many other processes (Figs. 4.2 and 4.3).[13] Numerous signals, such as stimulated growth factor receptors, transduce their downstream effects through RAS guanine exchange factors (RAS-GEFs) that activate the RAS family proteins, K-, H- and NRAS (Fig. 4.2A). Conversely negative regulatory pathways induce RAS GTPase activating proteins (RAS GAPs) that attenuate RAS signaling. Oncogenic *KRAS* mutations—at codons 12, 13, and 61—encode constitutively active KRAS forms, obviating the need for upstream inducing signals and rendering the protein insensitive to inhibition (Fig. 4.2B). Activated KRAS engages multiple effector pathways, notably the RAF-mitogen activated protein kinase (MAPK), phosphoinositide-3-kinase (PI3K) and RalGDS pathways (Fig. 4.3). The elucidation of the critical KRAS effectors mediating pancreatic adenocarcinoma pathogenesis and the specific biologic processes provoked by KRAS signaling remain highly significant challenges in understanding the progression of this disease and in enabling the selection of effective drug targets.

The existing evidence points to a role of *KRAS* mutations in the initiation of pancreatic adenocarcinoma pathogenesis. *KRAS* activation is the earliest genetic alteration detected in PanIN progression—observed in about 25% of PanIN-1A lesions and increasing in frequency in higher grade PanINs.[6,14-20] These earliest lesions show cytologic abnormalities such as alterations in

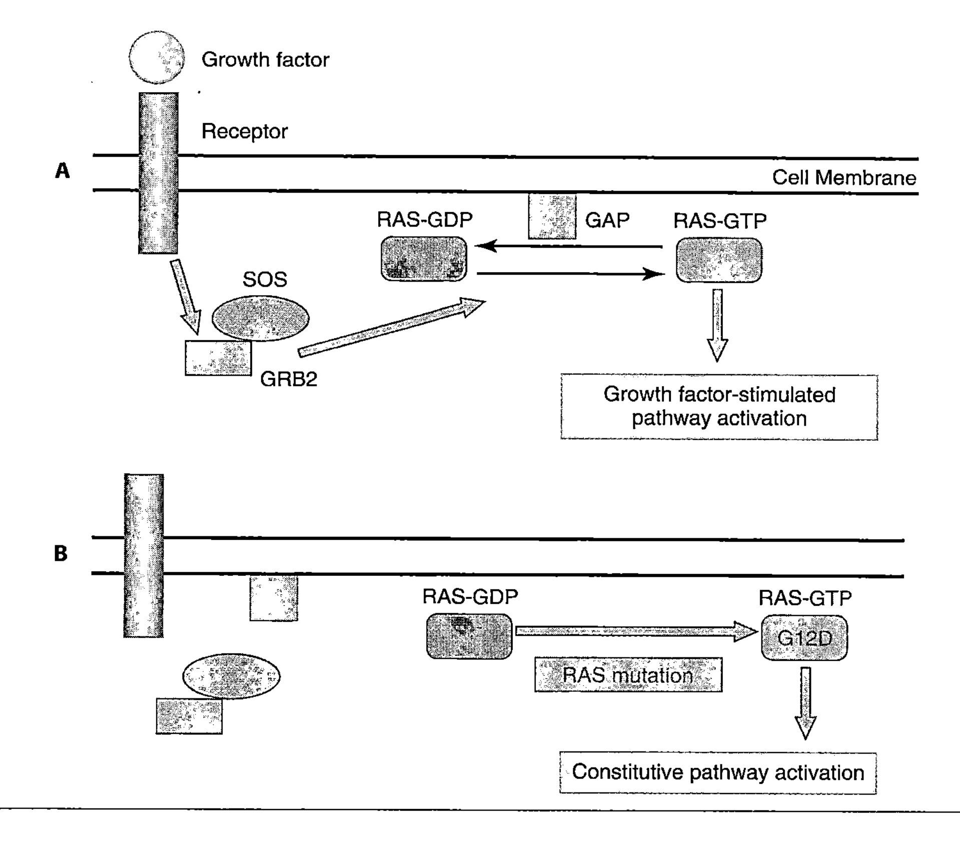

Figure 4.2
Activation of RAS family proteins. **(A)** Receptor-mediated activation. The binding of numerous growth factors to their receptors results in the recruitment of GRB2 and SOS and the conversion of RAS to its active guanosine triphosphate (GTP)-bound form. Activated RAS proteins engage numerous downstream signaling pathways. RAS guanosine triphosphatase (GTPase)–activating proteins (RAS GAPs) antagonize RAS activity by promoting GTP hydrolysis. **(B)** Oncogenic RAS mutations. Specific mutations cause RAS proteins to remain in a constitutively active GTP-bound state, eliminating the need for upstream signaling events and causing resistance to inhibition by RAS GAPs.

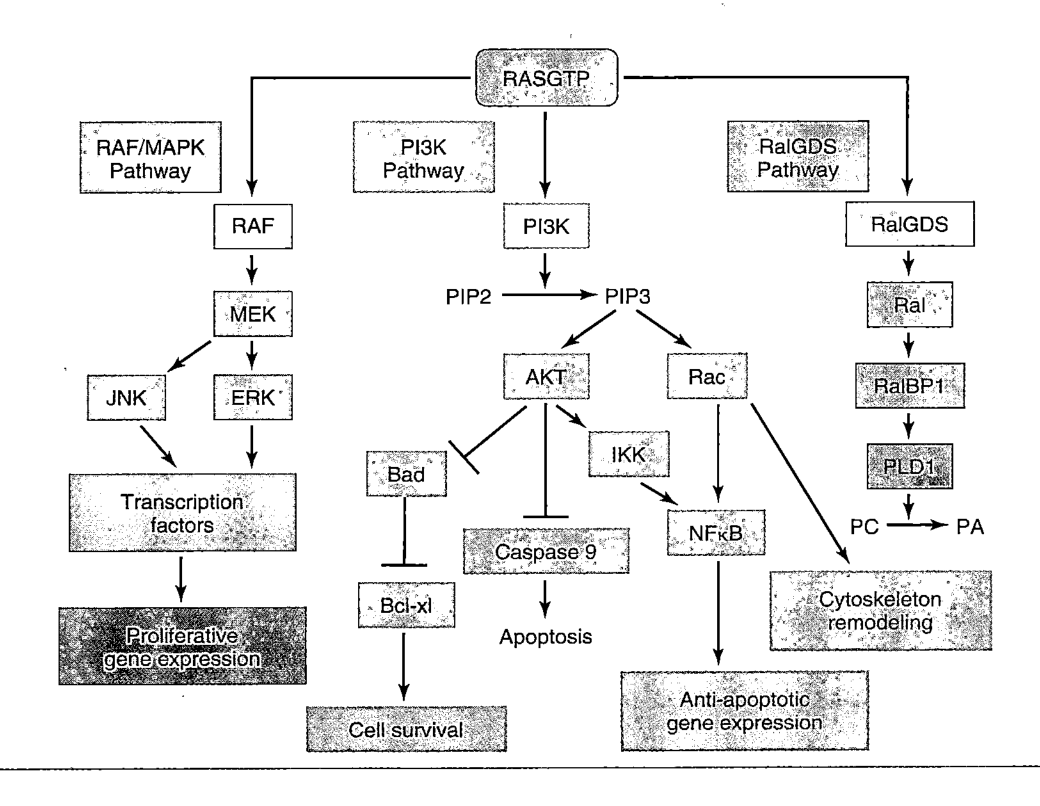

Figure 4.3
RAS signaling network. Activated RAS proteins engage multiple intersecting signaling pathways. The specific pathway modulations and the biologic outcomes of RAS activation vary, depending on cell type and cellular context. Note that in this simplified diagram, the induction of the three major signaling cascades through stimulation of RAF, phosphoinositide-3-kinase (PI3K), and Ral guanine nucleotide dissociation stimulator (RalGDS). PIP2, phosphatidylinositol-4,5-bisphosphate; PIP3, phosphotidylinositol-3,4,5 trisphophosphate; PC, phosphatidylcholine; PA, phosphatidic acid.

cell size, shape, and polarity and in expression of characteristic cellular differentiation markers.[21] The specific role of activated KRAS in producing these phenotypes is uncertain since it remains to be defined whether the earliest PanINs are clonal lesions. The proportion of cells within these lesions that harbor *KRAS* mutations needs to be established and it is important to determine whether the failure to detect KRAS alterations in a proportion of PanINs reflects the dispensability of this mutation in the onset of these first neoplastic stages or whether it is due to limitations in the detection methods. With respect to the later stages of malignancy, the detection of different KRAS mutations in separate neoplastic foci from the same pancreas suggests that while *KRAS* mutation is likely to be a critical event in the pathogenesis of this disease, other events are rate-limiting in the progression to invasive tumors.[6,18,19,22-24]

Mouse models have investigated the causal role of activated KRAS in the initiation of pancreatic ductal neoplasia (see Chapter 6). Based on studies of mouse strains in which an activated *Kras* allele (*Kras*^{G12D}) is expressed from its endogenous promoter—and hence at physiologic levels—in the pancreatic acinar, ductal and islet cells,[25,26] Kras activation appears to be an initiating step in pancreatic ductal neoplasia since these animals rapidly develop progressive lesions that closely resemble human PanINs. Pancreatic adenocarcinoma is very rarely observed in these mice in the absence of cooperating tumor suppressor mutations (see below). These results are consistent with a direct role of activated KRAS in the onset and progression of premalignant pancreatic ductal lesions and the insufficiency of this mutation for the development of advanced disease. It is notable that ductal, but not acinar or islet cell lesions, arise in these models indicating that endogenous levels of activated KRAS are incapable of transforming the nonductal compartment or that activated KRAS perturbs differentiation of other lineages towards a ductal phenotype.

In addition to a role in tumor initiation, it appears that KRAS activation is required for maintenance of the tumorigenic growth of established pancreatic adenocarcinomas since disruption of KRAS activity—via RNA interference, antisense RNA, or expression of dominant-negative KRAS^{N17}—attenuates the tumorigenicity of pancreatic adenocarcinoma cell lines.[27-29] Hence, KRAS activity seems to be required during all phases of pancreatic ductal tumorigenesis and thus activated KRAS, or its effectors, are likely to be appropriate targets for the prevention and therapy of this malignancy. It is notable, however, that the biochemical pathways induced by KRAS, and the resulting impact on cellular phenotypes, probably vary at different stages of tumorigenesis depending on the presence of other oncogenic mutations, on changes in intersecting signaling pathways, and on other alterations in the cellular context.[30-32] For example, phenotypes such enhanced proliferation and invasive growth—known to be associated with RAS activity—are restricted to the later stages of pancreatic neoplasia. Important future work is needed to resolve the context-dependent activities of KRAS and its signaling surrogates.

RAF-MAP kinase pathway The critical effectors of activated RAS proteins in promoting cancer have been the subject of considerable study (Fig. 4.3).[13] The high incidence of *BRAF* mutations and the mutually exclusive occurrence of *BRAF* and *RAS* mutations in human cancers suggest a primary role for the RAF-MAP kinase pathway in mediating the oncogenic effects of activated RAS,[33-36] although the RalGDS pathway may be central in some cancers.[37] There are suggestions that KRAS signaling plays a unique pathogenic role in pancreatic adenocarcinoma. The spectrum of *KRAS* mutations in pancreatic adenocarcinoma appears unusual among cancers; for example, the *KRAS*^{G12S} alteration, common in other malignancies and in early stage PanINs, is rare in pancreatic adenocarcinoma.[15,38] In addition, as noted above, *KRAS* mutations are more common in this cancer than in most other malignancies,[6,12] moreover—unlike other neoplasms with significant incidence of *RAS* mutations—*BRAF* mutations are rarely, if ever, observed (*BRAF* mutations do occur in a histologically and clinically distinct pancreatic tumor type, medullary carcinoma, that is associated with mismatch repair defects).[39] On the other hand, experimental studies using cell lines have suggested that there is a critical requirement for KRAS-dependent activation of RAF-MAP kinase for sustained tumorigenesis of established pancreatic adenocarcinomas since antisense inhibition of *kinase suppressor of ras-1 (KSR)*—a transducer of RAS signaling to RAF—strongly inhibits the tumorigenicity of xenografts, and expression of dominant-negative MAP kinase or MEKK inhibits colony formation *in vitro*.[29,40] Together, these findings indicate that RAF-MAP kinase pathway activation is necessary for the maintenance of established tumors while the progression of pancreatic adenocarcinoma likely requires KRAS functions beyond those induced by BRAF or by KRAS^{G12S}.

Epidermal growth factor receptor Autocrine signaling through the Epidermal Growth Factor Receptor (EGFR) family[41] is thought to be another important effector pathway of activated KRAS in pancreatic adenocarcinoma. Although EGF receptors are conventionally regarded as upstream activators of RAS proteins (Fig. 4.2A), they can also act as RAS signal transducers via RAS-induced autocrine activation of the EGFR family ligands (Fig. 4.4).[42,43] RAS transformation of several cell lineages requires the integrity of this autocrine loop and the resulting stimulation of PI3-kinase and other pathways.[43,44] Pancreatic adenocarcinomas show elevated expression of EGF receptors (EGFR, HER2/neu, and ERBB3) and their ligands (including transforming growth factor-α (TGF-α) and EGF) consistent with the presence of this autocrine loop.[45-53] EGFR, HER2, and TGF-α expression, induced in low grade PanINs, are among the first markers of pancreatic cancer progression, suggesting that autocrine EGFR family signaling may contribute to the earliest stages of pancreatic ductal neoplasia.[20,45,47,50] In line with a role of this signaling pathway in tumor initiation, *p53* mutant mice with transgenic expression of TGF-α in the acinar cells develop malignant pancreatic cancers with ductal features (see Chapter 6).[54] A related *p53* mutant, TGF-α transgenic model in which TGF-α expression becomes extinguished in premalignant lesions develops benign ductal tumors (serous cystadenomas)—rather than malignant tumors—suggesting that EGFR signaling is required for both initiation and progression of pancreatic ductal tumorigenesis.[55]

EGFR pathway is also likely to contribute to the maintenance of established tumors since disruption of EGFR signaling in human pancreatic adenocarcinoma cells—by expression of blocking antibodies or dominant-negative EGFR isoforms—inhibits growth *in vitro* and tumorigenesis in xenografts.[56-58] Attenuated EGFR signaling in xenografts results in apoptosis of the endothelial cells of the tumor vasculature, possibly involving loss of expression of angiogenic regulators such as vascular endothelial growth factor (VEGF).[58,59] The signal transducers and activators of transcription (STAT) factors—induced in pancreatic adenocarcinoma cells by EGFR/HER2 signaling through stimulation of the JAK serine-threonine kinase—may contribute to this VEGF induction.[60] (Fig. 4.4). Elevated STAT activity is detected in primary pancreatic adenocarcinomas and in cell lines, while disruption of this pathway in pancreatic adenocarcinoma cell lines, by expression of dominant negative STAT proteins, diminishes VEGF expression *in vitro* and blocks tumorigenic growth

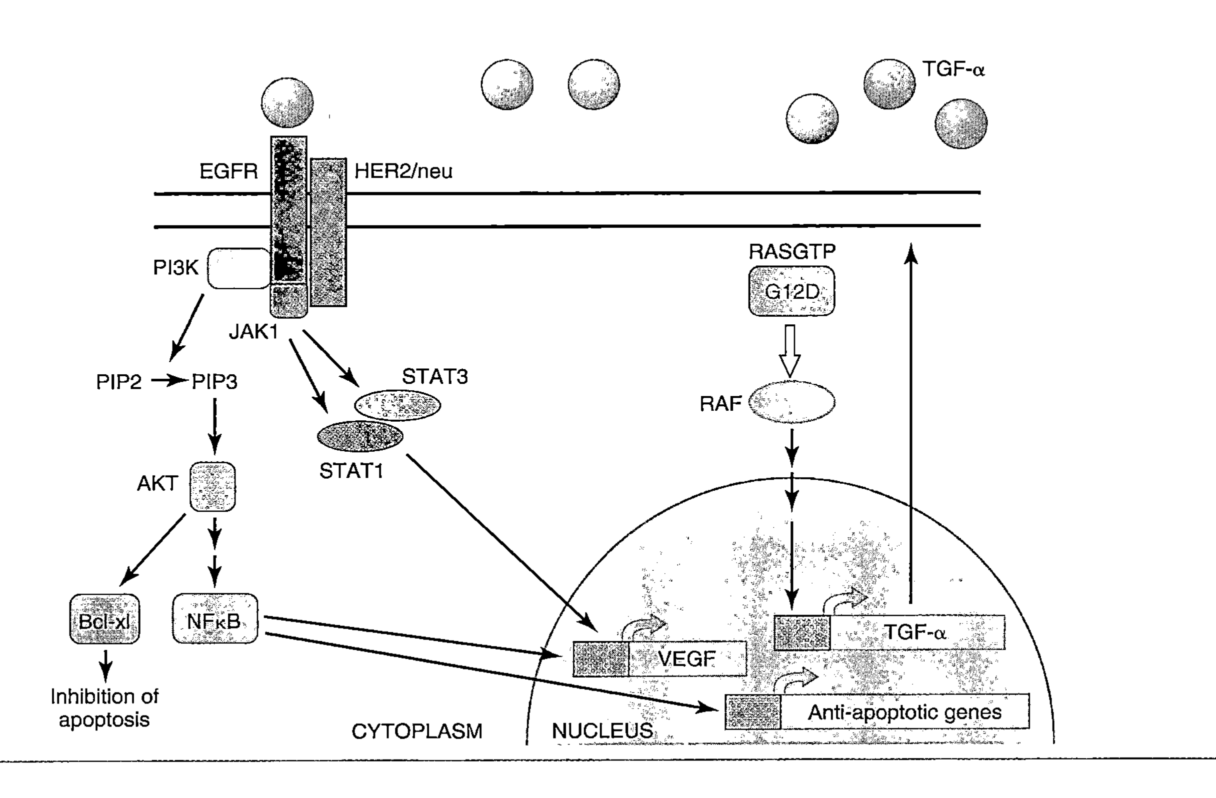

Figure 4.4
Autocrine epidermal growth factor receptor (EGFR) signaling. In pancreatic adenocarcinoma cells, activated KRAS alleles promote the expression of epidermal growth factor receptor (EGFR) family ligands, such as transforming growth factor-α (TGF-α). Because these cell lines also commonly express the EGF receptor (EGFR) and HER2/neu, there is a resulting autocrine signaling loop. Ligand activated EGFR—possibly by dimerization with HER2/neu—promotes cell survival and angiogenic programs through the activation of PI3K, JAK/STAT, and other pathways. These pathways are activated in primary pancreatic adenocarcinomas, suggesting that they may be important in oncogenesis and consequently may serve as suitable targets for therapeutics.

of xenografts.[60-62] Overall, the oncogenic effects of EGFR signaling in pancreatic adenocarcinoma are likely to be directed by numerous effectors (including PI3-kinase and NFκB, see below) and that regulate tumor angiogenesis as well as cell autonomous survival and proliferative processes. These observations support the use of therapies that target EGFR for both the treatment of pancreatic adenocarcinoma and possibly for chemoprevention in patients at risk for the malignancy. However, it should be noted that HER2 expression is reproducibly lost in highly advanced tumors which show undifferentiated histology.[50] This data should allow rational selection of patients most likely to benefit for anti-EGFR therapies.

Phosphoinositide-3-Kinase-AKT The PI3-kinase-AKT pathway is a key effector of RAS dependent transformation of many cell types and plays a role in cell survival, cell proliferation and other processes (Fig. 4.3).[63] AKT is constitutively active in primary pancreatic adenocarcinomas[64] and in xenografts[65] and disruption of the PI3-kinase-AKT pathway in cell lines, with chemical inhibitors or expression of dominant-negative AKT mutants, interferes with cell growth, survival, and response to chemotherapy.[66,67] The basis of PI3K-AKT activation in pancreatic adenocarcinoma is not clear: although RAS oncoproteins can activate the pathway directly, activation can also be achieved through KRAS-directed autocrine EGFR signaling (Fig. 4.4) or through the stimulation of other growth factor receptors such as the insulin-like growth factor-1 receptor (IGF-1R)[67,68] (see below for role of IGF-1R in pancreatic adenocarcinoma). Mutations in the PTEN (Phosphatase and tensin homolog) tumor suppressor, a negative regulator of PI3K, do not appear to contribute to AKT activation in this malignancy[69] although some tumors may have reduced PTEN expression levels.[70] In addition, chromosome 19 copy number increases spanning the *AKT* locus are detected in some pancreatic adenocarcinoma cell lines and primary tumors and correlate with high relative levels of AKT expression suggesting that gene copy increases may contribute to elevated AKT activity in some tumors.[71]

NFκB The nuclear factor κB (NFκB) transcription factor may be an important downstream mediator of KRAS signaling in pancreatic adenocarcinoma.[72] The dimeric NFκB complex controls the expression of a series of genes

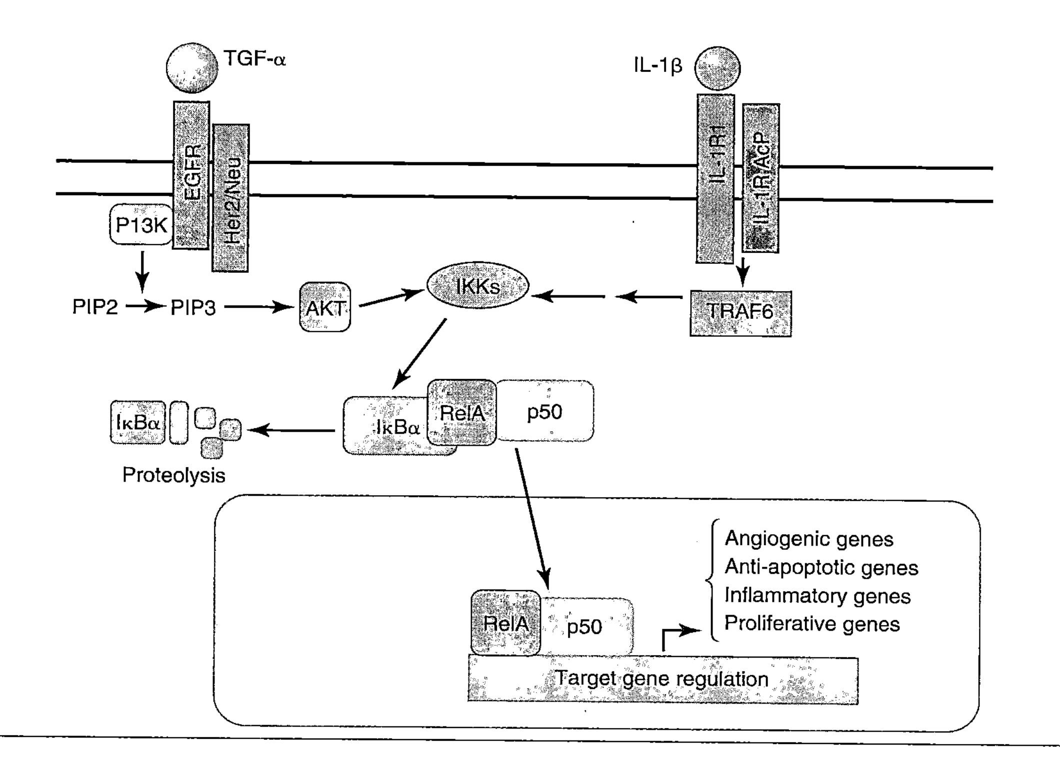

Figure 4.5

The NFκB signaling pathway. The heterodimeric NFκB transcription factor, composed of the p50 and p65 (RelA) subunits, is retained in an inactive cytoplasmic complex by binding to IκB family members. Numerous stimuli—including possibly epidermal growth factor receptor (EGFR) and interleukin-1β signaling in pancreatic adenocarcinoma—activate IκB kinases that promote the proteosomal degradation of IκB, resulting in the nuclear translocation and transcriptional activity of NFκB. The constitutive NFκB activity in pancreatic adenocarcinomas may contribute to such cell autonomous properties as tumor cell proliferation and survival as well as contributing to the angiogenic and inflammatory properties of this cancer.

that regulate the immune response, apoptosis, and many other processes (Fig. 4.5).[73] Normally sequestered in inactive form in the cytoplasm by binding to the IκB inhibitor, NFκB is activated and translocates to the nucleus following the phosphorylation and resulting proteosomal degradation of IκB.[74] This activation occurs in response to a variety of cell stresses through stimulation by pro-inflammatory cytokines, by growth factors, and by other regulators. Constitutive NFκB activity is observed in many cancers where it is thought to contribute to cell survival, angiogenesis, and invasion.[75] Most primary pancreatic cancers and cell lines, but not normal pancreatic specimens, show constitutive NFκB activity.[76] NFκB is likely to be an important effector of RAS oncoproteins in cancer since NFκB induction is required for RAS transformation of several cell types.[77,78] This induction may directly involve KRAS signaling since expression of dominant-negative *KRAS* alleles abrogates NFκB activity in pancreatic cancer cell lines.[76,79] This KRAS-dependent activation of NFκB requires MAP kinase-induced autocrine EGFR signaling and activation of the PI3K-AKT pathway[76,79,80]; an interleukin-1β autocrine loop may also contribute to NFκB activation.[81] The phenotypes mediated by NFκB activity are variable between different pancreatic adenocarcinoma cell lines: these include obligate roles in anchorage-independent cell survival and in anchorage-dependent cell survival *in vitro*, and requirements for tumorigenic growth or metastasis of orthotopic transplants.[79,82,83] These phenotypes appear to involve NFκB regulation of the apoptotic machinery and of VEGF, urokinase, and other pro-invasive or angiogenic factors.[79,82-84] The NFκB pathway may also contribute to the prominent chemoresistance of pancreatic adenocarcinomas.[85-87]

Feedback inhibition of KRAS signaling Specific genetic lesions are likely to be required to enable the full transformation potential of activated KRAS. One such alteration may be the loss of the wild-type allele of *KRAS*. Experimental studies have shown that wild-type *RAS* alleles can behave as tumor suppressors in cells with heterozygous activating *RAS* mutation, both *in vitro* and *in vivo*.[88,89] Loss of the wild type *KRAS* allele has been documented in some human pancreatic adenocarcinomas but not in adjacent PanINs suggesting that LOH is a late event in tumor progression,[16,22] although the functional significance of this lesion has not been determined. KRAS activity in pancreatic adenocarcinoma may also be enhanced by *KRAS* gene copy number increases as evidenced by the amplifications of chromosome 12p, the site of the *KRAS* locus, in a subset of primary tumors and derivative cell lines.[90-92] Tumors with these amplifications show coordinate increases in KRAS expression, a property likely to have functional significance since *in vitro* dosage increases of activated KRAS result in potentiated oncogenicity and induction of distinct signaling pathway.[93] A number of feedback loops regulate KRAS signaling and deregulation of some of these pathways may contribute to pancreatic adenocarcinoma progression. The dual specificity phosphatase-6 (DUSP-6), a negative regulator of the MAP kinase pathway, may be an example of such a loop; DUSP6 expression is induced in PanIN and is lost in some adenocarcinomas—coinciding with deletion of the locus.[94] Although numerous pathways are likely to impede the oncogenic potential of cells harboring activated *KRAS* alleles, the central regulator of this process appears to be the *INK4A/ARF* tumor suppressor locus, as discussed in the following section.

INK4A/ARF

Loss of function of the *INK4A* tumor-suppressor gene—by homozygous deletion, point mutation, or promoter hypermethylation—occurs in nearly all pancreatic adenocarcinomas and its pathogenetic relevance is underscored by the increased susceptibility in kindreds harboring germline *INK4A* mutations (see Chapters 3 and 9).[38,95,96] As is the case for the frequency of KRAS involvement, few cancers have a comparable incidence of *INK4A* loss.[97] *INK4A* encodes the cell cycle regulator, p16^{INK4A}, which restricts cell cycle progression by inhibiting cyclin-dependent kinase 4/6-mediated phosphorylation of the retinoblastoma (RB) family proteins (Fig. 4.6B).[98] Hypophosphorylated, hence functional, RB proteins arrest cells in the G1 phase of the cell cycle by binding to E2F transcription factors and preventing expression of genes required for G1 to S (DNA synthesis) phase cell cycle progression.

Approximately 40% of sporadic pancreatic adenocarcinomas display homozygous deletion of the *INK4A* locus,[99] suggesting that loss of the physically linked *ARF* tumor suppressor—encoded in an alternate reading frame and distinct first exon in the *INK4A/ARF* locus (Fig. 4.6A)[97]—may also contribute to the pathogenic process. The product of the *ARF* locus, p14^{ARF} (p19^{Arf} in mice) enhances p53 levels by blocking MDM2-mediated proteolysis and its loss attenuates p53 tumor-suppressor function (Fig. 4.6C).[100-103] It also appears that p14^{ARF} has p53-independent functions including the repression of ribosomal RNA synthesis, the inhibition of NFκB activity, and the targeting of E2F for degradation—suggesting that a number of other pathways are impaired by *INK4A/ARF* deletion.[104-106] Regarding the relative importance of either tumor suppressor at this locus, *INK4A* mutation seems to determine disease predisposition as there are both sporadic and germline mutations that specifically target *INK4A* yet spare *ARF*.[38,107-109] On the other hand, the loss of *ARF* in the tumors that have homozygous deletion of the locus,[38,110] and the high incidence of *p53* mutation in these tumors, may reflect an oncogenic role of *ARF* loss other than in p53 regulation (see below).

While *INK4A* mutations are associated with familial pancreatic adenocarcinoma, the risk of developing this cancer appears to be strongly modulated by environment or additional genetic factors; pancreatic adenocarcinoma is completely absent in some families while it occurs with high penetrance in others (see Chapter 9).[109,111,112] This variation is not due to the particular *INK4A* sequence alteration. The variable penetrance of pancreatic adenocarcinoma in association with germline *INK4A* mutations may suggest that *INK4A* plays a role in constraining malignant progression rather than in tumor initiation, a hypothesis supported by the observation that *INK4A/ARF* mutations occur subsequent to *KRAS* activation—in PanIN-2 and -3 lesions—in patients with sporadic malignancy.[6,113] These high-grade PanINs show nuclear abnormalities and have a significantly increased mitotic index compared to lower-grade lesions, features that are in accord with loss of the p16^{INK4A} (and p14^{ARF}) cell cycle regulatory function.

Genetic and biochemical interaction of *KRAS* and *INK4A/ARF* The loss of *INK4A* and activation of *KRAS* in virtually all pancreatic adenocarcinomas and the temporal order of these mutations fit well with models that implicate p16^{INK4A} in restraining the oncogenic activity of RAS proteins. These models arise from the observation that tumor types with activating *RAS* or *BRAF* mutations show a high concordance of *INK4A* loss and from *in vitro* and *in vivo* data showing that transformation by RAS oncogenes is facilitated by loss of *INK4A/ARF*.[12,33,38,97,114-118] It has been proposed that the mechanistic basis for the *in vivo* genetic interaction of activated *KRAS* and *INK4A/ARF* deficiency involves a feedback loop whereby activated RAS stimulates the MAP-kinase pathway leading directly to induction of p16^{INK4A} in human cells and subsequent growth arrest[114-117] (in rodent cells RAS-mediated arrest occurs via p19^{ARF} induction[119]). *In vivo*, *INK4A* normally

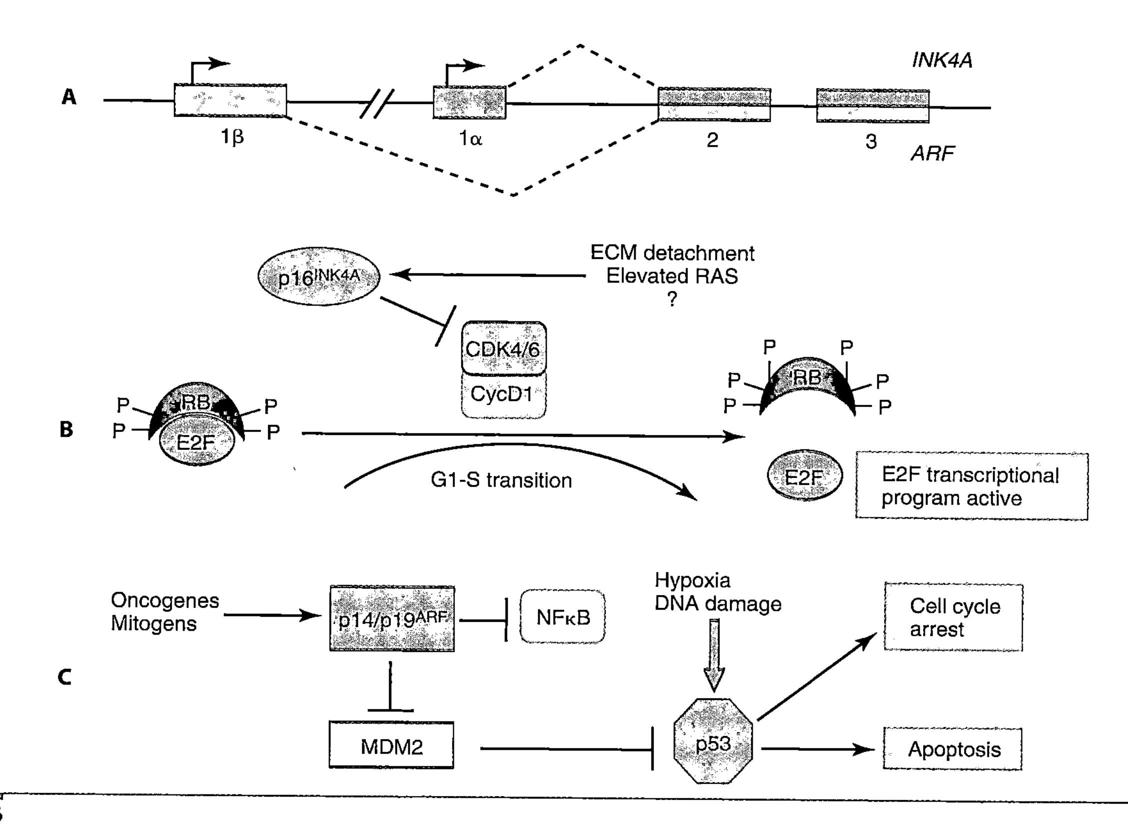

Figure 4.6

The *INK4A/RB* and *ARF/p53* pathways. **(A)** Structure of the *INK4A/ARF* tumor-suppressor locus. The *ARF* and *INK4A* genes are composed of distinct first exons (exons 1β and 1α, respectively) that splice into common exons 2 and 3. The resulting *ARF* and *INK4A* messenger RNAs utilize different translational reading frames, and thus the encoded proteins do not share any amino acid homology. **(B)** The *INK4A/RB* pathway. The RB family tumor-suppressor proteins binds to the E2F family transcription factors, thereby forming complexes that repress gene expression and maintain cells in the G1 phase of the cell cycle. Mitogenic stimuli induce cycle D/CDK4 complexes that phosphorylate RB, thereby releasing E2F that transactivates genes required for cycle progression. p16^{INK4A} prevents deregulated cell cycle progression by inactivating CDK4. The factors that induce *INK4A* expression in vivo are not fully established, although it is believed that cellular stresses, including extracellular matrix (ECM) detachment and aberrant mitogenic signals, contribute to this process. **(C)** The ARF/p53 pathway. *ARF* expression is thought to be induced after exposure to abnormal proliferative stimuli. p14^{ARF} (p19^{ARF} in mice) promotes p53 stabilization by interacting with MDM2 and inhibiting MDM2-directed proteolysis of p53. p19^{ARF} may also regulate other processes, such as interfering with NFκB transcriptional activity. Cellular stresses, such as DNA damage and hypoxia, induce p53 in an ARF-independent manner through the action of kinases that phosphorylate and inactivate the p53-binding ability of MDM2. p53 activation results in a gene expression program that either provokes G1 and G2 cell cycle arrest or apoptosis.

displays low levels and highly restricted patterns of expression but there is prominent *INK4A* induction in response to cellular stresses. *INK4A* expression is tightly controlled by both positive and negative regulators, modulated by such factors as integrin-extracellular matrix interactions[120,121] and mitogenic stimuli.[122,123] Although some *in vitro* studies have suggested that physiologic expression levels of activated KRAS may not normally induce *INK4A*,[93] it is tempting to speculate that the balance of these regulatory signals is altered in PanIN lesions enabling KRAS and other pathways to promote *INK4A* expression (Fig. 4.6B). The induction of *INK4A* may contribute to the low proliferation rate of early stage PanINs[9] and place selective pressure on the loss of *INK4A* during PanIN progression.

The genetic interactions of activated Kras and deletion of *Ink4a/Arf* have been studied in a mouse model.[25] As discussed above, Kras^{G12D} expression in the mouse pancreas produces PanINs that gradually develop into high-grade lesions but very rarely produce adenocarcinoma, while *Ink4a/Arf* deletion alone does not provoke a high susceptibility to pancreatic neoplasia (see also Chapter 6). Combined activation of Kras and *Ink4a/Arf* deficiency, however, results in the rapid onset of high-grade PanINs followed by the development of pancreatic adenocarcinomas. These observations are consistent with the PanIN-to-adenocarcinoma progression model and point to *Ink4a/Arf* loss as the critical regulator of the pathological transition to malignant disease. Rather than modulating the initiating stages of tumorigenesis in the pancreas, *Ink4a/Arf* deficiency has powerful synergy in promoting the advancement Kras^{G12D}-induced PanINs. The lack of progression of the murine PanINs in the presence of an intact *Ink4a/Arf* locus suggests that an efficient and potent p16^{Ink4a} and/or p19^{Arf}-mediated checkpoint impedes the malignant transformation of these initiated lesions.

Genomic Instability

The *p53* Tumor Suppressor Gene

The *TP53* tumor suppressor is mutated and shows loss of the wild-type allele in 50%–75% of pancreatic adenocarcinomas.[6] *TP53* encodes a transcription factor that is induced by a wide variety of cell-stress stimuli including DNA damage, oncogene expression, and hypoxia, and that activates programs for either G1 and G2 cell cycle arrest or apoptosis (Fig. 4.6C).[124] In contrast to the mutually exclusive relationship of *TP53* mutations and *ARF* loss in many tumor types, both of these lesions are present in a significant proportion of pancreatic adenocarcinomas, possibly reflecting an oncogenic role of *ARF* loss other than in p53 regulation and/or the specific role of p53 loss on the DNA damage response.[6] *TP53* mutations arise as late events in pancreatic neoplasia—occurring only in high-grade PanIN lesions and in adenocarcinomas—implying a role in malignant progression, including increased mitosis, nuclear abnormalities, chromosomal aberrations, and acquisition of an invasive phenotype.[8,20,125-128]

It is likely that p53 loss, and consequent disabling of the DNA checkpoint, contributes to the remarkable degree of chromosomal abnormalities that characterize this malignancy. The tumors are highly aneuploid, display numerous complex chromosomal rearrangements, and have intratumoral genomic heterogeneity, consistent with ongoing genomic instability during tumor progression.[7,92,129,130] In human carcinomas, the major genomic alterations are multiple complex chromosomal rearrangements, referred to as nonreciprocal translocations (NRTs). The processes leading to NRTs are thought to help drive the transformation process due to the fact that such rearrangements are invariably associated with regional amplification or deletion of the loci at the breakpoint.[131] Such a process results in rapid and widespread changes in gene ploidy throughout the genome, generating genetic diversity in a population of would-be cancer cells[132] and facilitating selection for cells bearing oncogenic changes. With respect to pancreatic adenocarcinoma, this hypothesis is supported by the existence of multiple recurrent chromosomal anomalies. In addition to the signature losses of chromosome 9p, 17p, and 18q, harboring the *INK4A/ARF*, *TP53*, and *SMAD4* loci, respectively, loss of 6q and 8p and gain of 5p, 8q, 12p, 19q, and 20q are commonly detected.[90,133-135] The pathogenic importance of this genetic instability is also suggested by genetic heterogeneity associated with pancreatic ductal neoplasia: different LOH patterns and *KRAS* mutations are detected in adjacent PanINs and invasive tumors, karyotypic analysis of primary tumor cells reveals the existence of multiple clones, and tumors frequently harbor multiple different mutant *KRAS* alleles.[6-8,18,19,22-24,129,130] Notably, adjacent neoplastic foci display similar genomic changes while more distant foci show increasingly divergent alterations.[7] These observations suggest that pancreatic adenocarcinomas arise from the clonal progression of one or more initiated PanINs that have acquired a mutator phenotype that enables acquisition of progression-associated genetic lesions. Such a mutator phenotype may also contribute to the profound chemoresistance of this malignancy.

Telomere Dynamics

Telomere attrition Loss of the chromosome capping structure, the telomere, is thought to contribute to the genomic instability of epithelial cancers. Most somatic cells lack telomerase, hence states of continuous cell division—such as epithelial renewal or response to proliferative stress—are accompanied by telomere erosion resulting in the generation of uncapped telomeres that are highly recombinogenic (Fig. 4.7).[136] The resulting chromosomal end-to-end fusions undergo breakage during anaphase creating new sites for recombination. These sequential breakage-fusion-bridge cycles produce chromosomal amplifications and deletions at the site of breakage and produce a high level of intratumoral heterogeneity.[131,137] *In vitro*, the survival of cells harboring critically short telomeres (crisis) and ongoing breakage-fusion-bridge events requires the inactivation of the p53-dependent DNA damage response.[138,139] The relevance of these processes to epithelial malignancies *in vivo* is provided by studies showing that combined p53 and telomerase deficiency in the mouse cooperate in the development of carcinomas in multiple tissues.[140] Together, these data have supported the hypothesis that continuous epithelial renewal results in age-dependent telomere erosion and attendant amplification/deletion, providing wholesale changes in gene ploidy that enable epithelial cells to reach a critical cancer threshold of mutations. These processes are likely to contribute to the remarkable age-dependent exponential increases in carcinoma incidence, such as the 80-fold increased risk of pancreatic adenocarcinoma at age 80 compared to age 40

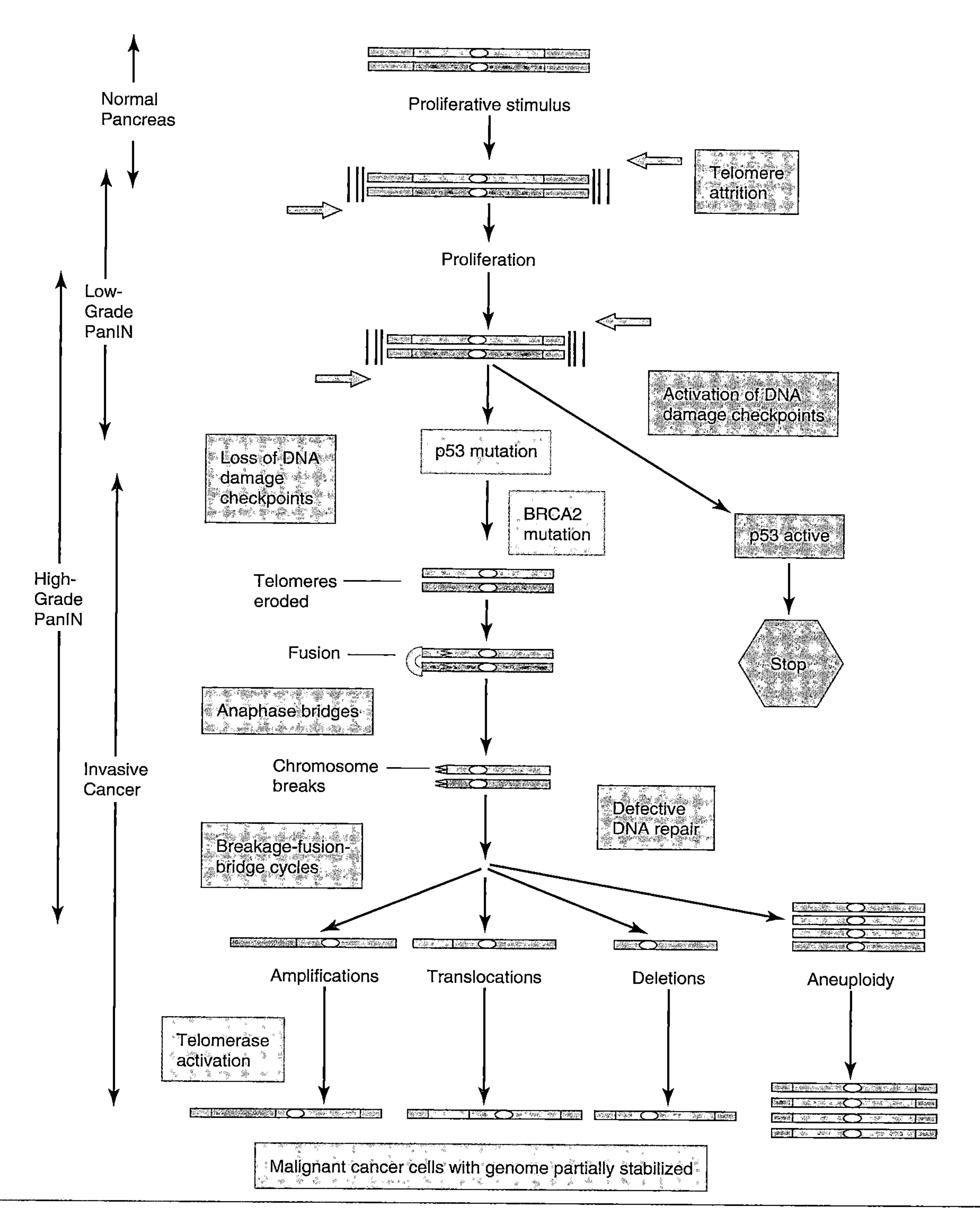

Figure 4.7
Telomere attrition and genomic instability in carcinoma progression. Most human somatic cells lack telomerase activity; hence telomere erosion occurs as these cells are induced to proliferate. Sustained proliferative stimuli, such as oncogenic mutations, lead to progressive telomere shortening that eventually activates *p53*-dependent DNA damage responses, resulting in growth arrest (highlighted in red to the right of the figure). Loss of checkpoint responses—such as by mutation of *TP53*—allows cells to continue proliferating, leading to critically shortened telomeres and telomere dysfunction (crisis). These critically shortened telomeres are highly recombinogenic and undergo chromosome breakage-fusion-bridge cycles that produce chromosomal amplifications, deletions, and translocations that contribute to tumor progression. *BRCA2* mutations also produce genomic instability by disabling the homologous recombination-based DNA repair pathway. Telomerase reactivation occurs at a late stage of tumorigenesis, stabilizing the genome and facilitating the immortal growth of the tumor cells.

(Fig. 4.1F).[141] We speculate that telomere attrition accompanying chronic epithelial cell turnover may play a particularly prominent role in the development of pancreatic adenocarcinomas in pancreatitis patients.[142]

A series of cytogenetic and molecular studies have provided strong evidence that telomere dynamics contributes to genomic instability in pancreatic adenocarcinoma (see Chapter 3). Specifically, *in situ* molecular analysis revealed shortened telomeres in PanIN-1 stage lesions, making telomere attrition the earliest known genetic alteration in the pathogenic process.[143] This comprehensive study corroborated conclusions of a previous report that revealed frequent absence of telomeres at chromosome ends and anaphase bridging in pancreatic adenocarcinoma cell lines indicative of persistent genomic instability associated with critically short telomeres.[144] These features were observed in cell lines derived from both low- and high-grade tumors suggesting that telomere dysfunction was an early step in the pathogenic process. Hence, although reactivation of telomerase is critical to the emergence of immortal cancer cells (see below), it appears to be a late event in pancreatic adenocarcinoma progression[145,146] and is preceded by a transient period of telomere shortening and dysfunction that is likely to contribute to carcinogenesis by leading to the formation of chromosomal rearrangements through breakage-fusion-bridge cycles. While low-grade PanINs have modest mitotic rates, there are prominent increases in cell proliferation in PanIN-3 lesions.[9] The increased cell turnover at this stage is likely to lead to critical telomere shortening of the already eroded telomeres and to activate DNA damage pathways, providing strong selective pressure for cells harboring *TP53* mutations.

Telomerase activation Telomerase activation is required for the immortalization and transformation of primary human cells *in vitro* and is a hallmark of carcinomas *in vivo*.[147] The induction of telomerase usually occurs late in tumorigenesis and is likely to produce a degree of genomic stabilization following the preceding, transient period of telomere attrition and ensuing oncogenic genomic rearrangements. Hence telomere regulation has a dual role in cancer: telomere dysfunction promotes initiation while telomere activation is necessary for malignant progression.[148,149] Telomerase activation detected up to 95% of pancreatic adenocarcinomas, and occurs relatively late in tumor progression,[145,146,150] perhaps at the transition from high-grade PanIN to carcinoma stages. There are numerous positive and negative regulators of telomerase expression and activity—including the Myc transcription factor (see following section) and the TGF-β pathway (see below)[151-153]—although the mechanism for telomerase activation in pancreatic adenocarcinoma has not been determined. The requirement for telomerase activity for the sustained proliferation of pancreatic adenocarcinoma cells suggests that targeting this process may be an appropriate therapeutic approach.[154,155]

Myc The Myc transcription factor is a potential inducer of telomerase and of ongoing genomic instability in pancreatic adenocarcinoma. Myc regulates the expression of a wide range of genes that are required for cell cycle progression and the overexpression of this gene results in cellular transformation *in vitro* and tumorigenesis *in vivo*.[156] The oncogenic effects are likely to involve a severe disruption of cell cycle control and attendant genomic instability.[157,158] The Myc transformation program is also thought to involve transcriptional activation of telomerase—an activity that is abrogated by the Myc co-repressor Mad1.[152,159,160] About 30% of primary pancreatic adenocarcinomas exhibit gains of chromosome 8q that produce increased copy numbers of the Myc gene, although the degree of amplification is usually modest.[92,133] Myc overexpression is also frequently seen in pancreatic adenocarcinomas and in some late-stage PanINs. Although functional data are lacking, it is reasonable to expect that aberrant Myc expression contributes to both telomerase activation as well as the ongoing chromosomal rearrangements associated with the progression of this malignancy.

The *BRCA2* Tumor Suppressor Gene

The *BRCA2* familial breast and ovarian tumor-suppressor gene is another regulator of genomic stability that has been implicated in pancreatic adenocarcinoma pathogenesis. *BRCA2* mutations do not appear to play a role in sporadic disease, but germline mutations are detected in up to 20% of pancreatic adenocarcinomas arising in a familial setting.[161-165] BRCA2 is required in the regulation of the homologous recombination pathway that mediates the repair of double-stranded DNA breaks.[166] In the context of a functional p53-dependent DNA damage checkpoint, the chromosomal abnormalities that arise due to BRCA2 dysfunction result in cell death. Hence the tumor promoting genomic instability caused by *BRCA2* loss requires previous inactivation of the p53 checkpoint. Correspondingly, loss of the wild-type *BRCA2* allele in patients with heterozygous germline mutations appears to be a late event in pancreatic adenocarcinoma progression, occurring between the PanIN-3 and adenocarcinoma stages.[19] Consistent with a role of BRCA2 in malignant progression rather than initiation, *BRCA2* mutation carriers do not have increased PanIN numbers and have a relatively low penetrance and late onset of pancreatic adenocarcinoma.[164,165]

Developmental Regulators and Pancreatic Adenocarcinoma

The processes of carcinogenesis and embryonic development have been long recognized to share many related features, including such phenotypes as rapid proliferation, cell renewal, and invasive growth (see Chapter 5).[167] Indeed molecular studies have revealed that developmental regulatory pathways are activated in an aberrant manner in cancer cells. These pathway alterations are likely to contribute to tumor initiation/progression through the inhibition of differentiation and expansion of progenitor/stem cell populations or to the disruptions in the de-differentiation of more committed lineages. Disturbances in a number of developmental signaling pathways appear to play unique roles in the pathogenesis of pancreatic adenocarcinoma.

TGF-β/SMAD4

Homozygous deletions of chromosome 18q, overlapping the *SMAD4/DPC4* gene, are present in about 30% of pancreatic adenocarcinomas.[168,169] The detection of intragenic point mutations—including nonsense and frameshift mutations—in another 15% of tumors is consistent with *SMAD4* being the pathogenic target of most of these deletions, although such intragenic lesions have been documented in only a limited number of primary tumor specimens. It is notable that the rate of *SMAD4* loss in pancreatic adenocarcinoma is significantly higher than in most other malignancies.[169] *SMAD4* encodes a transcription factor that is a central effector of the transforming growth factor-β (TGF-β) signaling pathway, an important regulator of embryonic pattern formation, cell differentiation, and a variety of processes relating to homeostasis—in particular wound healing, inflammation, and immune response (Fig. 4.8).[170] With respect to cellular growth control, the impact of TGF-β is highly dependent on the cell type and cell context. In numerous epithelial cell lines and in epithelial tissue *in vivo*,

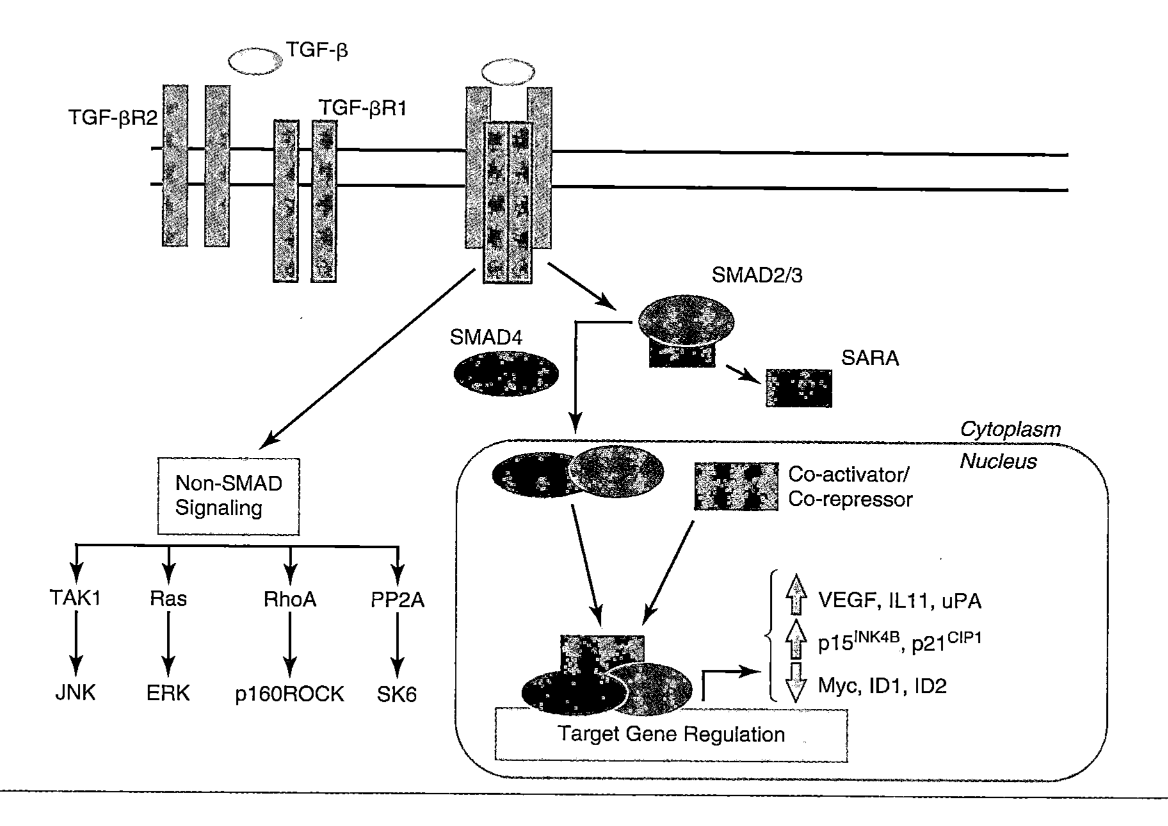

Figure 4.8
The transforming growth factor-β (TGF-β)/SMAD signaling pathway. TGF-β binds to the TGF-β type II receptor at the cell surface, promoting the recruitment and phosphorylation of the TGF-β type I receptor. The activated type I receptors activate the SMAD transcription factors by phosphorylating SMAD2 or 3, thereby releasing them from the SARA (SMAD anchor for receptor activation) cytoplasmic anchor proteins and enabling complex formation with SMAD4. These complexes translocate to the nucleus and modulate expression of specific target genes by associating with transcriptional co-activators and co-repressors.

TGF-β exerts a growth inhibitory program that involves modulation of expression of cell cycle regulators—such as induction of $p15^{INK4B}$ and $p27^{KIP1}$ and repression of c-Myc and ID family transcription factors—induction of apoptotic machinery and repression of telomerase.[152,153,171] Likewise, elevations in TGF-β signaling *in vivo* inhibit epithelial cancer initiation *in vivo* and lesions in this pathway promote intestinal, ovarian, and pancreatic tumorigenesis.[152,153,171] On the other hand TGF-β promotes the proliferation and transformation of fibroblasts, moreover, the epithelial-to-mesenchymal transition (EMT) in breast cancer and skin cancer—a process by which advanced carcinomas lose their differentiated features and acquire a highly aggressive, invasive phenotype—involves elevated activity of the TGF-β signaling pathway.[172-174] Therefore, in some carcinomas, the TGF-β signaling can have biphasic effects, inhibiting tumor initiation while promoting the high-grade advancement of established tumors (Fig. 4.9).[175]

SMAD4 loss is a late event in pancreatic adenocarcinoma pathogenesis, restricted to PanIN-3 lesions and invasive tumors, indicating a contribution to malignant progression,[8,176] however the specific tumorigenic impact of *SMAD4* mutation is ill-defined. The loss of *SMAD4* in pancreatic adenocarcinoma may have a primary role in modulating the interaction of the tumor with the microenvironment rather than in growth control of the tumor cells themselves since *SMAD4* restoration in some pancreatic cancer cell lines does not block cell growth *in vitro*, but it inhibits tumorigenesis in xenografts, an affect that appears to involve repression of angiogenesis and extracellular matrix remodeling.[177,178] On the other hand, stringent assays such as anchorage-independent growth, have revealed that *SMAD4* restoration (overexpression) is capable of mediating *in vitro* growth inhibition in some cell lines.[179] *SMAD4* deficiency does not appear to impart resistance to TGF-β–induced growth inhibition since the response of some pancreatic adenocarcinoma cell lines to this cytokine *in vitro* is not correlated with *SMAD4* status.[180-182] Rather, diminished expression of TGF-β type I receptor has been suggested to contribute to TGF-β resistance in some cell lines[183-185]; a number of genes implicated in TGF-β responsiveness in other cell types—including p53, $p15^{INK4B}$, Myc, and KRAS[186-188]—are also altered in pancreatic adenocarcinomas and consequently may regulate this phenotype. There appears to be a complex relationship between activated KRAS expression and TGF-β signaling. Activated KRAS may inhibit the expres-

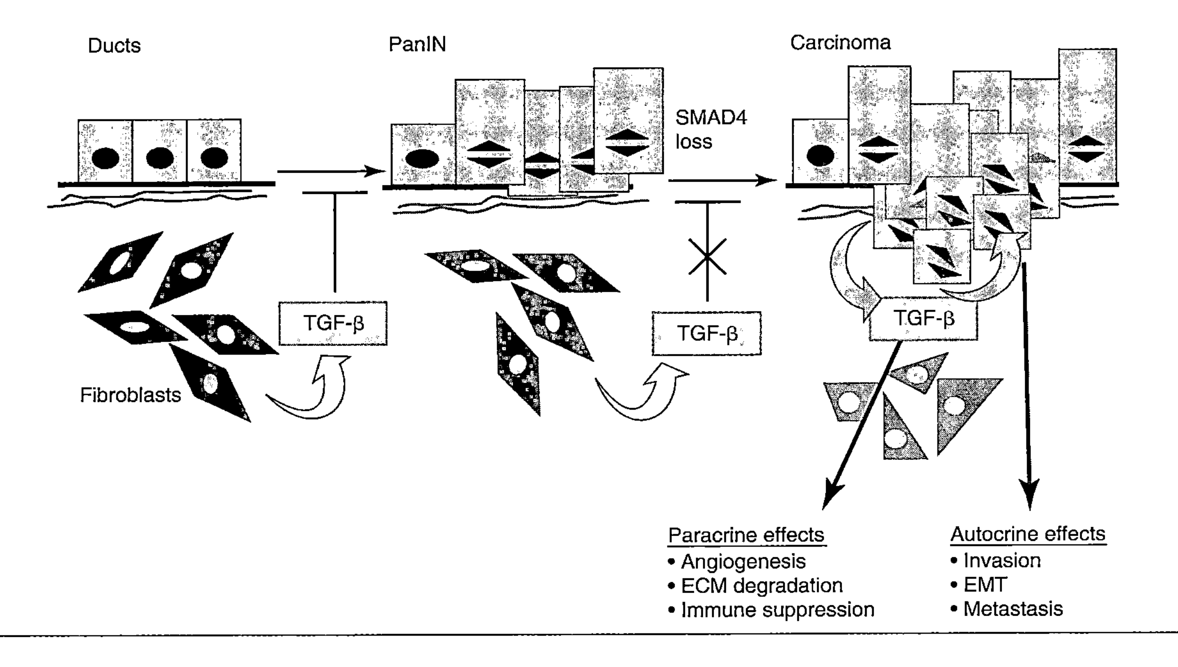

Figure 4.9
Stage-specific roles of transforming growth factor-β (TGF-β) signaling in carcinoma progression. TGF-β signaling is thought to play alternate roles in the initiation and progression of carcinomas. In experimental models, TGF-β inhibits epithelial tumor initiation stage by inducing cell cycle arrest or apoptosis while this cytokine stimulates the malignant progression of initiated lesions. In the pancreas, stromal-derived TGF-β may contribute to the maintenance of the pancreatic ductal epithelium in a quiescent state. *SMAD4 loss* or other lesions in TGF-β signaling, occurring in the later stages of pancreatic adenocarcinoma progression, are likely to attenuate the growth-inhibiting effects of TGF-β and promote malignant progression. Elevated TGF-β levels are detected in established pancreatic adenocarcinomas and may have stimulatory effects on tumorigenesis by both paracrine and autocrine signaling. The paracrine TGF-β signals may contribute to stromal alterations, such as angiogenesis, extracellular matrix (ECM) degradation, and immune suppression. The autocrine signals may encourage cell migration and epithelial-to-mesenchymal transitions (EMTs), leading to metastasis.

sion of TGF-β receptors in pancreatic adenocarcinoma cells providing a potential mechanism for TGF-β resistance.[189] On the other hand, in several cell types activated RAS and TGF-β produce cooperative effects on cellular phenotypes such as promoting migration and EMT indicating that RAS activation does not necessarily impair TGF-β function and rather, that RAS may inhibit the apoptotic effects of TGF-β while preserving other pro-invasive responses.[172,173,190]

In addition to the tumor–suppressor role of SMAD4 in pancreatic adenocarcinoma it appears that elevated TGF-β expression contributes to tumor progression. TGF-β1, TGF-β2 and TGF-β3 are all expressed at elevated levels in pancreatic adenocarcinoma cells relative to normal pancreas.[191] Secretion of the TGF-β ligands may help to promote the characteristic desmoplastic response of this malignancy as has been suggested from xenograft studies.[192] TGF-β signaling may also contribute to tumorigenesis in an autocrine manner since pancreatic adenocarcinomas also frequently overexpress the type II TGF-β receptor relative to normal pancreas.[193,194] The functionality of this autocrine signaling loop is suggested by the attenuated tumorigenicity and metastasis of xenografts subjected to the experimental blockade of TGF-β signaling by expression of soluble type II TGF-β receptor.[195,196] Furthermore, antibodies to TGF-β inhibit the invasion of pancreatic adenocarcinoma cell lines *in vitro* while exogenous addition of this cytokine enhanced invasion and promoted the epithelial-to-mesenchymal transition.[197,198] In line with this role of TGF-β in promoting advanced malignancy, overexpression of TGF-β2 or of the TGF-β receptors appear to correlate with shortened postoperative survival.[191,193,199]

In addition to these varied *in vitro* observations, opposing conclusions have been reached regarding the impact of *SMAD4* status on the prognosis of pancreatic adenocarcinoma; one study determined that patients expressing SMAD4 had significantly worse outcomes and did not benefit from surgery while another study indicated that SMAD4 expression predicted increased survival.[200,201] Overall, the complex response profiles to TGF-β suggest that TGF-β/SMAD4 signaling may have pleiotropic and context-dependent roles in pancreatic adenocarcinoma. These features add significant complexity in attempts to design therapeutic strategies directed against this pathway. Genetically-defined animal models may be of considerable value in resolving the oncogenic roles of TGF-β/SMAD4 in pancreatic adenocarcinoma.

A possible confounding factor in evaluating the pathogenic role of *SMAD4* loss is the possibility of an adjacent pancreatic adenocarcinoma tumor suppressor gene. This existence of such a locus is suggested by the detection of deletions at chromosome 18q in pancreatic adenocarcinoma cell lines that leave SMAD4 intact and by chromosome 18 transfer experiments in cell lines that result in growth inhibition *in vitro*, attenuated tumorigenesis of xenografts, and suppressed metastasis—effects occurring independent of the *SMAD4* status of the parental cells.[202-204] It will be important to identity definitively this putative adjacent pancreatic adenocarcinoma tumor suppressor locus.

Hedgehog

The mammalian Hedgehog family of secreted signaling proteins—comprised of Sonic, Indian, and Desert Hedgehog (Shh, Ihh, and Dhh, respectively)—regulates the growth and patterning of many organs during embryogenesis, while alterations that activate this pathway have been implicated in various cancers (see Chapter 5).[167] The Hedgehog pathway is under negative regulation by the Patched (PTC) tumor-suppressor protein that inactivates the Smoothed protein (Fig. 4.10). The Hedgehog ligands engage the PTC transmembrane protein, disrupting

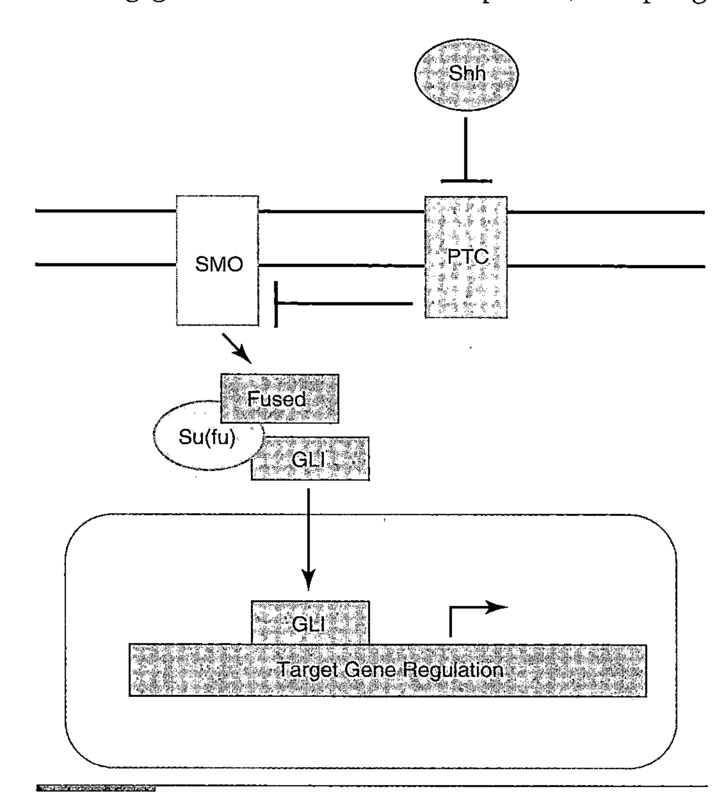

Figure 4.10
The Hedgehog signaling pathway. In the absence of ligand stimulation, the central regulator of the Hedgehog signaling pathway, the transcription factor GLI, is retained in the cytoplasm in a complex with fused and suppressor of fused (Su(fu)). The hedgehog signaling pathway is activated by the interaction of the Hedgehog family ligands—Sonic, Indian, and Desert Hedgehog (Shh, Ihh, and Dhh)—with the Patched (PTC) receptor. This interaction releases the inhibitory effects of PTC on Smoothened (SMO) and promotes the nuclear translocation and transcriptional activity of GLI, leading to expression of a series of proliferative and angiogenic target genes.

the inhibition of SMO and thereby enabling signal transduction to the GLI family of transcriptional regulators. Loss of *PTC*, activating mutations in *SMO* and overexpression of GLI and Hh proteins are associated with a variety of cancers.

Activation of the Hedgehog pathway has been implicated in both the initiation of pancreatic ductal neoplasia and in the maintenance of advanced cancers.[167] During embryogenesis, Shh is expressed throughout the developing gastrointestinal endoderm, with a notable exclusion from the developing pancreas.[205,206] Shh is also absent from the normal adult pancreas, but is activated in PanINs, exhibiting a graded increase in progressively later-stage lesions and carcinomas.[207,208] The Hedgehog pathway also appears to be activated in chronic pancreatitis in association with the development of tubular complexes that may be premalignant lesions in pancreatic neoplasia.[209] The functional importance of this pathway in the initiation of pancreatic ductal neoplasia is suggested by the demonstration that transgenic mice expressing Shh in the developing pancreas, under the control of the *Pdx1* promoter, display apparent transdifferentiation of acinar cells to tubular complexes.[208] Although an Shh-directed tubular metaplasia-PanIN sequence has not yet been demonstrated in the pathogenesis of human pancreatic adenocarcinoma, it is plausible that proliferative, dedifferentiated lesions produced by aberrant Shh activation may provide a suitable context for the development of oncogenic *KRAS* mutations and subsequent neoplastic transformation.

Beyond a potential role in tumor initiation, experimental studies have also pointed to a role of Shh in survival of established pancreatic adenocarcinomas. Specifically, attenuation of Shh signaling in human pancreatic adenocarcinoma cell lines—by exposure to cyclopamine, a chemical inhibitor of SMO—causes most cell lines to undergo apoptosis *in vitro* and to lose tumorigenicity in xenografts.[207,208] This requirement of Shh signaling for pancreatic adenocarcinoma maintenance appears to offer promising possibilities for new therapeutic approaches toward the disease. It will be important to identify the biochemical basis for Shh induction, to determine the relevance of Shh induction for tumorigenesis *in vivo*, and to identify the downstream mediators of such as Shh-directed tumorigenic initiation—and or maintenance—program.

Notch

The Notch signaling pathway is important in directing cell fate and cell proliferation during embryonic development, whereas aberrant activity of this pathway has been shown to contribute to cell transformation *in vitro* and to the development of human cancers (see also Chapter 5).[210] In mammals, this signaling pathway involves interaction of the membrane-bound Notch receptors (Notch 1-4) and Notch ligands (Delta-like and Jagged) on adjacent cells. Notch-ligand interactions induce the proteolysis of Notch and subsequent nuclear translocation of the Notch intracellular domain that transactivates a series of target genes following assembly into a multi-protein transcriptional activation complex (Fig. 4.11). During pancreatic development Notch signaling is necessary in restricting differentiation of pancreatic progenitor cells towards endocrine lineages thereby maintaining a sufficient population of undifferentiated precursors for exocrine development and organ size increases.[210,211] Notch and its ligands are expressed at low or undetectable levels in the normal adult pancreas, however there are prominent elevations in expression of these factors and an associated induction of transcriptional target genes such as *HES-1* in PanIN lesions and in pancreatic adenocarcinomas, consistent with activation of this pathway during malignant progression of this malignancy.[212] Although the role of Notch signaling in pancreatic adenocarcinoma pathogenesis remains to be established, experimental evidence has suggested that activation of this pathway may contribute to disease initiation, specifically through inducing the metaplastic conversion of acinar cells to ductular structures (tubular metaplasia),[212] a process associated with the pathogenesis of pancreatic tumors in some animal models.[54,55,213] Tubular metaplasia arises in the context of damage to the pancreas and resulting inflammation and can be generated experimentally by the ectopic expression of TGF-α in the acinar cells. *In vitro* experiments with explanted pancreatic acinar tissue have shown that TGF-α-induced acinar-ductal metaplasia proceeds through the direct activation of Notch signaling and that Notch activation is both necessary and sufficient for this process.[212] The ductal metaplastic phenotype is recapitulated in transgenic mice which have constitutive Notch activation in the pancreas.[214] Although tubular metaplasia has not yet been clearly implicated in human pancreatic adenocarcinoma development, the specific upregulation of Notch signaling in metaplastic ductal epithelium lesions and in PanINs may suggest a pathogenic link between these lesions. It will be important to investigate the role of Notch signaling in established tumors to determine whether targeting this pathway is a suitable therapeutic approach.

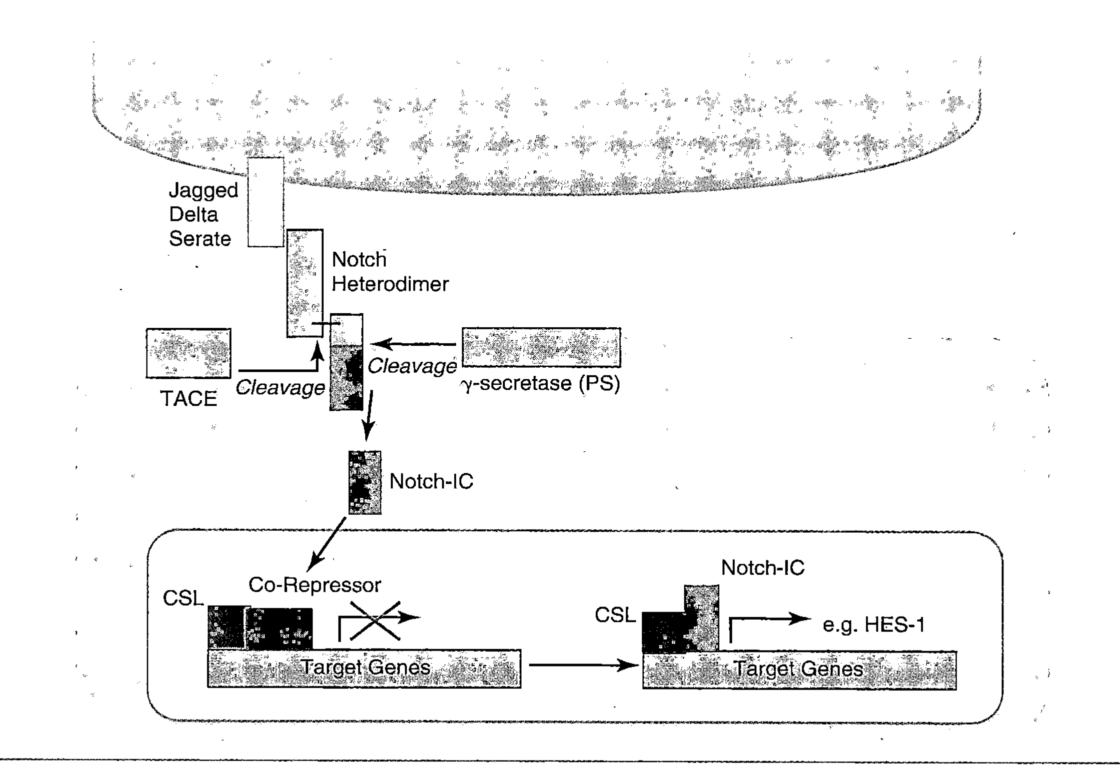

Figure 4.11
The Notch signaling pathway. The Notch transmembrane receptor is activated by binding to the ligands Jagged, Delta, or Serate on adjacent cells. This binding stimulates Notch proteolysis by tumor necrosis factor-α (TNF-α)–converting enzyme (TACE) and subsequently by γ-secretase and results in the release and nuclear translocation of the Notch intracellular domain (Notch-IC). Notch-IC activates gene transcription by interacting with CSL (also known as RBP-Jκ CBF1, Suppressor of Hairless, and Lag-1) and causing the release of a transcriptional co-repressor.

LKB1

Mutations in the *LKB1* tumor-suppressor gene are associated with the Peutz-Jeghers syndrome, a disorder consisting of pigmentation abnormalities, intestinal polyposis, and elevated cancer incidence (see Chapter 9).[215] The *LKB1* gene encodes a serine-threonine kinase that is required for mammalian embryogenesis and which has been implicated in the regulation of cell polarity and in cellular energy metabolism.[216-219] It has been reported that pancreatic cancers occur with elevated incidence in PJS patients and somatic *LKB1* mutations are detected in a small subset of sporadic pancreatic adenocarcinomas.[220,221] It remains to be established what is the relative incidence specifically of pancreatic adenocarcinoma in association with PJS since there is evidence that these patients are prone to other pancreatic tumor types including IPMN and cystadenomas. In the mouse, Lkb1 deficiency can produce pancreatic tubular metaplasia and subsequent cystadenoma development.[222] Study of the combined impact of Lkb1 deficiency and mutation in other pancreatic cancer genes in provoking malignant progression in the pancreas should help to more strongly establish a role of Lkb1 in the pathogenesis of pancreatic adenocarcinoma.

Growth Factors, Hormones, and Other Receptor-Mediated Pathways

Growth factor independence is a fundamental property of most cancers and often arises via the aberrant induction of receptors and ligands producing autocrine loops in the tumor cells. As discussed above, there is good evidence that the EGFR pathway is activated early in the pathogenesis of pancreatic adenocarcinoma and appears to be required for both tumor initiation as well as maintenance of established tumors. In addition a series of other receptor-mediated signaling pathways are thought to contribute to the tumorigenic process. Elucidating these pathways may be of particular importance from a therapeutic standpoint based on the promise of antibody-based treatments targeting receptors or ligands.

Insulin-Like Growth Factor Signaling

The insulin-like growth factor (IGF) signaling pathway regulates survival, invasion, and angiogenesis of many human cancers. Pancreatic adenocarcinomas show elevated expression of IGF-1 in both the tumor cells and the stroma and display aberrant activation of the IGF-1 receptor (IGF-1R) in tumor cells.[221-225] Analyses of pancreatic adenocarcinoma cell lines have suggested that PI3-K/AKT signaling may contribute to the elevated expression of IGF-1R.[226] *In vitro*, autocrine IGF-1 signaling promotes cell proliferation and growth factor independent survival.[68,223] Inhibition of the pathway by anti-IGF-1R antibodies or expression of a dominant negative form of IGF-1R inhibits the growth of xenografts and sensitizes cells to chemotherapy.[67,224,227] These processes apparently involve activation of both the MAP kinase and PI3K pathways.[68,224] Taken together, it appears that IGF-1 signaling contributes to tumorigenesis both by preventing tumor cell apoptosis and inducing tumor angiogenesis. The angiogenic phenotype may be mediated by stabilization of the hypoxia-inducible factor-1α (HIF-1α) and consequent transcriptional activation of vascular endothelial growth factor (VEGF).[224,228] Targeting IGF-1, IGF-1R, or the signaling surrogates of this pathway is a plausible therapeutic approach to treating pancreatic adenocarcinoma.

MET/HGF Signaling

The Met receptor tyrosine kinase and its ligand, hepatocyte growth factor (HGF)/scatter factor regulate cell motility, invasion, and proliferation and the deregulation of this signaling pathway contributes to the progression of several malignancies.[229] The Met receptor is expressed at low levels in the exocrine pancreas and shows marked upregulation in PanIN lesions and in pancreatic adenocarcinomas.[230-233] HGF is also induced during pancreatic adenocarcinoma progression—present in the epithelium of PanIN lesions and in the stromal cells of adenocarcinomas.[232,233] The induction of Met/HGF signaling in PanIN lesions—and in pancreatic regeneration models and in experimental and human pancreatitis[234-236]—may indicate a role of this pathway in tumor initiation. Experimental studies have also pointed to a role in the Met/HGF in the malignant growth of established tumors. HGF promotes motility of pancreatic adenocarcinoma cells *in vitro* and inhibition of this pathway through the administration of blocking antibodies or of the truncated HGF fragment, NK4, inhibits invasive growth and angiogenesis of xenografts.[232,237,238]

Fibroblast Growth Factors

Fibroblast growth factor (FGF) signaling[239] appears to contribute to mitogenesis and angiogenesis of pancreatic adenocarcinomas. Numerous FGF receptors including FGF receptor 1 (FGFR-1) and FGFR-2 and their ligands including FGF-1, FGF-2 (basic FGF), FGF-5 and FGF-7 (keratinocyte growth factor) are expressed by primary pancreatic adenocarcinomas as is glypican-1, a membrane heparin sulfate proteoglycan that facilitates FGF-FGFR interactions.[240-246] All of these factors are at elevated levels in the tumor cells although FGF-5 is also elevated in stromal fibroblasts and macrophages and FGF-7 and FGFR-2 are elevated in adjacent ductal and acinar cells consistent with roles of FGF signaling in the autocrine regulation of pancreatic cancer cell growth and in paracrine regulation of stromal responses and angiogenesis. FGF signaling may be necessary for pancreatic adenocarcinoma cell growth since the introduction of dominant-negative FGFR-1 mutants or antisense glypican-1 into pancreatic cancer cell lines inhibits growth *in vitro* and suppresses tumorigenesis of xenografts.[247-249] FGF signaling may also contribute to the desmoplasia of pancreatic adenocarcinomas since elevated FGF-2 levels are associated with this phenotype in primary tumors and in xenograft models.[192,250]

Vascular Endothelial Growth Factor

Although pancreatic adenocarcinomas are not markedly vascular, they do exhibit foci of endothelial cell proliferation consistent with an angiogenic phenotype.[251] While many of the factors discussed above—including EGF ligands, FGFs, HGF and TGF-β—are likely to contribute to angiogenesis, VEGF may play a particularly important role in this process (see also Chapter 39). This growth factor promotes endothelial cell proliferation and survival by binding to the VEGFR-1 and VEGFR-2 endothelial cell transmembrane receptors.[252] VEGF is overexpressed by pancreatic adenocarcinoma cells[253,254] whereas disruption of VEGF signaling—by expression of soluble VEGF receptors, by anti-VEGF antibodies, or by ribozymes—strongly suppresses the tumorigenicity of pancreatic cancer xenografts.[255-258] In addition to regulating tumor angiogenesis, it is possible that this signaling pathway also contributes to tumor cell growth in an autocrine manner since some pancreatic adenocarcinoma cells express VEGF receptors and proliferate in response to VEGF *in vitro*.[255,259] VEGF-C, a regulator of lymphoangiogenesis, is also overexpressed by pancreatic adenocarcinomas and may contribute to the lymph node metastasis of this malignancy.[260] Therapies directed against the VEGF pathway may be among the most promising emerging strategies for the treatment of pancreatic adenocarcinoma.

Nerve Growth Factors and Neurotransmitters

Pancreatic adenocarcinomas show a characteristic invasion of the pancreatic nerves, causing significant pain.[251] Numerous studies have investigated the link between the neurotrophic behavior of this cancer and the aberrant induction of neurotrophic (NT) or neuroendocrine hormone signaling. Specifically, the overexpression of NT family ligands—nerve growth factor (NGF) and NT-3—and the NGF receptor, TrkA are observed in these tumors.[261-264] There appears to be an association between NGF levels and both perineural invasion and pain suggesting that this signaling axis contributes to these phenotypes.[263] In addition, overexpression of NGF can promote growth and invasion of pancreatic cancer xenografts while the disruption of NGF signaling using small molecule inhibitors or antibodies impairs the tumorigenicity of xenografts.[265-267] The neurotransmitter receptor, neurokinin-1, is also overexpressed in pancreatic adenocarcinoma and in chronic pancreatitis and its activation is thought to both induce pain responses and to play a role in promoting inflammation.[268-270] Stimulation of neurokinin signaling by its ligand, substance P, promotes the growth *in vitro* of pancreatic adenocarcinoma cell lines. Neurotensin, another neurotransmitter that is overexpressed in pancreatic cancers also stimulates the proliferation of derivative cell lines.[271-273] It will be of considerable interest to determine the biologic roles of these neural signaling pathways in the pathogenesis of pancreatic adenocarcinoma *in vivo*. The targeting of these signaling pathways offers promise in the development of novel diagnostic, chemotherapeutic, and pain management approaches.

Cyclooxygenase and Lipoxygenase Metabolism

Cyclooxygenase (COX) and lipoxygenase (LOX) family enzymes regulate the metabolism of arachidonic acid into prostaglandins and other pro-inflammatory products.[274] The COX-2, 5-LOX, and 12-LOX isoforms of these enzymes have been implicated in tumorigenesis in which their metabolites activate a range of signaling pathways, leading to cancer cell proliferation, survival, invasion, and angiogenesis. Both COX-2 and 5-LOX are upregulated in the tumor cells of pancreatic adenocarcinomas and are associated with chronic pancreatitis.[275,276] COX-2 is expressed in PanINs and shows progressively increased expression in higher-grade lesions.[277] In addition to elevated 5-LOX expression, pancreatic adenocarcinoma cells show expression of receptors for metabolites of this pathway indicating that there is active autocrine signaling.[278] Pharmacologic inhibition of either COX-2 or 5-LOX suppresses proliferation and induces apoptosis of pancreatic adenocarcinoma cells *in vitro* and attenuates the growth of xenografts.[279-282] These pathways appear to be good targets for chemopreventative and chemotherapeutic intervention. It will be important to dissect the molecular mechanisms that induce COX-2 and 5-LOX in pancreatic adenocarcinoma and also to determine the specific downstream processes that become activated by the downstream signaling pathways.

Gastrointestinal Hormones

The deregulated expression of gastrointestinal hormones may contribute to the pathogenesis of pancreatic adenocarcinoma. For example, loss of expression of somatostatin receptors, and overexpression of gastrin and cholecystokinins and their receptors, have been linked to this malignancy in some, but not all studies.[283-286] Experiments *in vitro* and in animal models have indicated that there may be functional roles for these pathways in pancreatic adenocarcinoma cell growth[287-290]; however, the relevance of these pancreatic hormones to human pancreatic adenocarcinoma development *in vivo* is not well established.

Conclusion

Basic science investigations have uncovered numerous signaling pathways that become deregulated during the course of pancreatic adenocarcinoma progression. This information is vital in suggesting improved clinical approaches to this malignancy. Among the current challenges is the need to validate the requirement of sustained activity of these pathways for tumor cell survival in order to determine whether such pathways are appropriate therapeutic targets. It will also be important to more fully dissect these pathways to identify additional signaling components that may be more conducive to drug development. The identification of secreted biomarkers that are diagnostic for the activity of specific pathways will be critical for evaluating the efficacy of drugs targeting these pathways. For example, the modulation of the levels of a MAP kinase-regulated serum protein would provide a noninvasive gauge for whether anti-MAP kinase treatment is successfully reaching its target. Furthermore, the mechanisms of drug resistance of pancreatic adenocarcinomas will be important to determine. As discussed above, many agents show activity in pancreatic adenocarcinoma cell lines *in vitro* and in xenografts, however, the marked resistance of human pancreatic adenocarcinomas to existing therapeutic approaches and the plasticity conferred by the profound genomic instability of this malignancy make it likely the tumor cells will evolve to escape the cytotoxicity of many agents. Although targeted therapies have produced disappointing clinical outcomes to date, we can be optimistic that an improved understanding of the interaction of molecular signaling pathways in pancreatic adenocarcinoma biology—in conjunction with advances in drug development methods—will inform the design of rational and effective multiagent approaches towards this disease.

References

1. Kern S, Hruban R, Hollingsworth MA, et al. A white paper: the product of a pancreas cancer think tank. *Cancer Res.* 2001;61:4923–4932.
2. Bardeesy N, DePinho RA. Pancreatic cancer biology and genetics. *Nat Rev Cancer.* 2002;2:897–909.
3. Hansel DE, Kern SE, Hruban RH. Molecular pathogenesis of pancreatic cancer. *Annu Rev Genomics Hum Genet.* 2003;4:237–256.
4. Hruban RH, Wilentz RE, Kern SE. Genetic progression in the pancreatic ducts. *Am J Pathol.* 2000;156:1821–1825.
5. Cubilla AL, Fitzgerald PJ. Morphological lesions associated with human primary invasive nonendocrine pancreas cancer. *Cancer Res.* 1976;36:2690–2698.
6. Moskaluk CA, Hruban RH, Kern SE. p16 and K-ras gene mutations in the intraductal precursors of human pancreatic adenocarcinoma. *Cancer Res.* 1997;57:2140–2143.
7. Yamano M, Fujii H, Takagaki T, et al. Genetic progression and divergence in pancreatic carcinoma. *Am J Pathol.* 2000;156: 2123–2133.
8. Lüttges J, Galehdari H, Brocker V, et al. Allelic loss is often the first hit in the biallelic inactivation of the p53 and DPC4 genes during pancreatic carcinogenesis. *Am J Pathol.* 2001;158: 1677–1683.
9. Klein WM, Hruban RH, Klein-Szanto AJ, Wilentz RE. Direct correlation between proliferative activity and dysplasia in pancreatic intraepithelial neoplasia (PanIN): additional evidence for a recently proposed model of progression. *Mod Pathol.* 2002;15:441–447.
10. Brat DJ, Lillemoe KD, Yeo CJ, Warfield PB, Hruban RH. Progression of pancreatic intraductal neoplasias to infiltrating adenocarcinoma of the pancreas. *Am J Surg Pathol.* 1998;22: 163–169.
11. Brockie E, Anand A, Albores-Saavedra J. Progression of atypical ductal hyperplasia/carcinoma in situ of the pancreas to invasive adenocarcinoma. *Ann Diagn Pathol.* 1998;2:286–292.
12. Bos JL. ras oncogenes in human cancer: a review [published erratum appears in *Cancer Res.* 1990;50:1352]. *Cancer Res.* 1989;49:4682–4689.
13. Shields JM, Pruitt K, McFall A, Shaub A, Der CJ. Understanding Ras: "it ain't over 'til it's over." *Trends Cell Biol.* 2000;10:147–154.
14. Yanagisawa A, Ohtake K, Ohashi K, et al. Frequent c-Ki-ras oncogene activation in mucous cell hyperplasias of pancreas suffering from chronic inflammation. *Cancer Res.* 1993;53: 953–956.
15. Tada M, Ohashi M, Shiratori Y, et al. Analysis of K-ras gene mutation in hyperplastic duct cells of the pancreas without pancreatic disease. *Gastroenterology.* 1996;110:227–231.
16. Lüttges J, Schlehe B, Menke MA, Vogel I, Henne-Bruns D, Kloppel G. The K-ras mutation pattern in pancreatic ductal adenocarcinoma usually is identical to that in associated normal, hyperplastic, and metaplastic ductal epithelium. *Cancer.* 1999;85:1703–1710.
17. Terhune PG, Phifer DM, Tosteson TD, Longnecker DS. K-ras mutation in focal proliferative lesions of human pancreas. *Cancer Epidemiol Biomarkers Prev.* 1998;7:515–521.
18. DiGiuseppe JA, Hruban RH, Offerhaus GJ, et al. Detection of K-ras mutations in mucinous pancreatic duct hyperplasia from a patient with a family history of pancreatic carcinoma. *Am J Pathol.* 1994;144:889–895.
19. Goggins M, Hruban RH, Kern SE. BRCA2 is inactivated late in the development of pancreatic intraepithelial neoplasia: evidence and implications. *Am J Pathol.* 2000;156:1767–1771.
20. Apple SK, Hecht JR, Lewin DN, Jahromi SA, Grody WW, Nieberg RK. Immunohistochemical evaluation of K-ras, p53, and HER-2/neu expression in hyperplastic, dysplastic, and carcinomatous lesions of the pancreas: evidence for multistep carcinogenesis. *Hum Pathol.* 1999;30:123–129.
21. Hruban RH, Adsay NV, Albores-Saavedra J, et al. Pancreatic intraepithelial neoplasia: a new nomenclature and classification system for pancreatic duct lesions. *Am J Surg Pathol.* 2001;25:579–586.
22. Sugio K, Molberg K, Albores-Saavedra J, Virmani AK, Kishimoto Y, Gazdar AF. K-ras mutations and allelic loss at 5q and 18q in the development of human pancreatic cancers. *Int J Pancreatol.* 1997;21:205–217.
23. Lüttges J, Diederichs A, Menke MA, Vogel I, Kremer B, Kloppel G. Ductal lesions in patients with chronic pancreatitis show K-ras mutations in a frequency similar to that in the normal pancreas and lack nuclear immunoreactivity for p53. *Cancer.* 2000;88:2495–2504.
24. Laghi L, Orbetegli O, Bianchi P, et al. Common occurrence of multiple K-RAS mutations in pancreatic cancers with associated precursor lesions and in biliary cancers. *Oncogene.* 2002;21:4301–4306.
25. Aguirre AJ, Bardeesy N, Sinha M, et al. Activated Kras and Ink4a/Arf deficiency cooperate to produce metastatic pancreatic ductal adenocarcinoma. *Genes Dev.* 2003;17:3112–3126.
26. Hingorani SR, Petricoin EF, Maitra A, et al. Preinvasive and invasive ductal pancreatic cancer and its early detection in the mouse. *Cancer Cell.* 2003;4:437–445.
27. Brummelkamp TR, Bernards R, Agami R. Stable suppression of tumorigenicity by virus-mediated RNA interference. *Cancer Cell.* 2002;2:243–247.
28. Aoki K, Yoshida T, Sugimura T, Terada M. Liposome-mediated in vivo gene transfer of antisense K-ras construct inhibits pancreatic tumor dissemination in the murine peritoneal cavity. *Cancer Res.* 1995;55:3810–3816.
29. Hirano T, Shino Y, Saito T, et al. Dominant negative MEKK1 inhibits survival of pancreatic cancer cells. *Oncogene.* 2002;21:5923–5928.

30. Frame S, Balmain A. Integration of positive and negative growth signals during ras pathway activation in vivo. *Curr Opin Genet Dev.* 2000;10:106–113.
31. Ramaswamy S, Ross KN, Lander ES, Golub TR. A molecular signature of metastasis in primary solid tumors. *Nat Genet.* 2003;33:49–54.
32. Bernards R, Weinberg RA. A progression puzzle. *Nature.* 2002;418:823.
33. Davies H, Bignell GR, Cox C, et al. Mutations of the BRAF gene in human cancer. *Nature.* 2002;417:949–954.
34. Rajagopalan H, Bardelli A, Lengauer C, et al. Tumorigenesis: RAF/RAS oncogenes and mismatch-repair status. *Nature.* 2002;418:934.
35. Singer G, Oldt R 3rd, Cohen Y, et al. Mutations in BRAF and KRAS characterize the development of low-grade ovarian serous carcinoma. *J Natl Cancer Inst.* 2003;95:484–486.
36. Kimura ET, Nikiforova MN, Zhu Z, Knauf JA, Nikiforov YE, Fagin JA. High prevalence of BRAF mutations in thyroid cancer: genetic evidence for constitutive activation of the RET/PTC-RAS-BRAF signaling pathway in papillary thyroid carcinoma. *Cancer Res.* 2003;63:1454–1457.
37. Hamad NM, Elconin JH, KarnoubAE, et al. Distinct requirements for Ras oncogenesis in human versus mouse cells. *Genes Dev.* 2002;16:2045–2057.
38. Rozenblum E, Schutte M, Goggins M, et al. Tumor-suppressive pathways in pancreatic carcinoma. *Cancer Res.* 1997;57:1731–1734.
39. Calhoun ES, Jones JB, Ashfaq R, et al. BRAF and FBXW7 (CDC4, FBW7, AGO, SEL10) mutations in distinct subsets of pancreatic cancer: potential therapeutic targets. *Am J Pathol.* 2003;163:1255–1260.
40. Xing HR, Cordon-Cardo C, Deng X, et al. Pharmacologic inactivation of kinase suppressor of ras-1 abrogates Ras-mediated pancreatic cancer. *Nat Med.* 2003;9:1267–1268.
41. Olayioye MA, Neve RM, Lane HA, Hynes NE. The ErbB signaling network: receptor heterodimerization in development and cancer. *EMBO J.* 2000;19:3159–3167.
42. Schulze A, Lehmann K, Jefferies HB, McMahon M, Downward J. Analysis of the transcriptional program induced by Raf in epithelial cells. *Genes Dev.* 2001;15:981–994.
43. Sibilia M, Fleischmann A, Behrens A, et al. The EGF receptor provides an essential survival signal for SOS-dependent skin tumor development. *Cell.* 2000;102:211–220.
44. Oldham SM, Clark GJ, Gangarosa LM, Coffey RJ Jr, Der CJ. Activation of the Raf-1/MAP kinase cascade is not sufficient for Ras transformation of RIE-1 epithelial cells. *Proc Natl Acad Sci USA.* 1996;93:6924–6928.
45. Lemoine NR, Hughes CM, Barton CM, et al. The epidermal growth factor receptor in human pancreatic cancer. *J Pathol.* 1992;166:7–12.
46. Korc M, Chandrasekar B, Yamanaka Y, Friess H, Buchier M, Beger HG. Overexpression of the epidermal growth factor receptor in human pancreatic cancer is associated with concomitant increases in the levels of epidermal growth factor and transforming growth factor alpha. *J Clin Invest.* 1992;90:1352–1360.
47. Barton CM, Hall PA, Hughes CM, Gullick WJ, Lemoine NR. Transforming growth factor alpha and epidermal growth factor in human pancreatic cancer. *J Pathol.* 1991;163:111–116.
48. Friess H, Berberat P, Schilling M, Kunz J, Korc M, Buchler MW. Pancreatic cancer: the potential clinical relevance of alterations in growth factors and their receptors. *J Mol Med.* 1996;74:35–42.
49. Watanabe M, Nobuta A, Tanaka J, Asaka M. An effect of K-ras gene mutation on epidermal growth factor receptor signal transduction in PANC-1 pancreatic carcinoma cells. *Int J Cancer.* 1996;67:264–268.
50. Day JD, Digiuseppe JA, Yeo C, et al. Immunohistochemical evaluation of HER-2/neu expression in pancreatic adenocarcinoma and pancreatic intraepithelial neoplasms. *Hum Pathol.* 1996;27:119–124.
51. Friess H, Wang L, Zhu Z, et al. Growth factor receptors are differentially expressed in cancers of the papilla of vater and pancreas. *Ann Surg.* 1999;230:767–774;774–765.
52. Friess H, Yamanaka Y, Kobrin MS, Do DA, Buchler MW, Korc M. Enhanced erbB-3 expression in human pancreatic cancer correlates with tumor progression. *Clin Cancer Res.* 1995;1: 1413–1420.
53. Lemoine NR, Lobresco M, Leung H, et al. The erbB-3 gene in human pancreatic cancer. *J Pathol.* 1992;168:269–273.
54. Wagner M, Greten FR, Weber CK, et al. A murine tumor progression model for pancreatic cancer recapitulating the genetic alterations of the human disease. *Genes Dev.* 2001;15:286–293.
55. Bardeesy N, Morgan J, Sinha M, et al. Obligate roles for p16$^{(Ink4a)}$ and p19$^{(Arf)}$-p53 in the suppression of murine pancreatic neoplasia. *Mol Cell Biol.* 2002;22:635–643.
56. Wagner M, Cao T, Lopez ME, et al. Expression of a truncated EGF receptor is associated with inhibition of pancreatic cancer cell growth and enhanced sensitivity to cisplatinum. *Int J Cancer.* 1996;68:782–787.
57. Matsuda K, Idezawa T, You XJ, Kothari NH, Fan H, Korc M. Multiple mitogenic pathways in pancreatic cancer cells are blocked by a truncated epidermal growth factor receptor. *Cancer Res.* 2002;62:5611–5617.
58. Bruns CJ, Solorzano CC, Harbison MT, et al. Blockade of the epidermal growth factor receptor signaling by a novel tyrosine kinase inhibitor leads to apoptosis of endothelial cells and therapy of human pancreatic carcinoma. *Cancer Res.* 2000;60:2926–2935.
59. Baker CH, Kedar D, McCarty MF, et al. Blockade of epidermal growth factor receptor signaling on tumor cells and tumor-associated endothelial cells for therapy of human carcinomas. *Am J Pathol.* 2002;161:929–938.
60. DeArmond D, Brattain MG, Jessup JM, et al. Autocrine-mediated erbB-2 kinase activation of STAT3 is required for growth factor independence of pancreatic cancer cell lines. *Oncogene.* 2003;22:7781–7795.
61. Wei D, Le X, Zheng L, et al. Stat3 activation regulates the expression of vascular endothelial growth factor and human pancreatic cancer angiogenesis and metastasis. *Oncogene.* 2003;22:319–329.
62. Toyonaga T, Nakano K, Nagano M, et al. Blockade of constitutively activated Janus kinase/signal transducer and activator of transcription-3 pathway inhibits growth of human pancreatic cancer. *Cancer Lett.* 2003;201:107–116.
63. Vivanco I, Sawyers CL. The phosphatidylinositol-3-kinase/ AKT pathway in human cancer. *Nat Rev Cancer.* 2002;2: 489–501.

64. Semba S, Moriya T, Kimura W, Yamakawa M. Phosphorylated AKT/PKB controls cell growth and apoptosis in intraductal papillary-mucinous tumor and invasive ductal adenocarcinoma of the pancreas. *Pancreas.* 2003;26:250–257.
65. Bondar VM, Sweeney-Gotsch B, Andreeff M, Mills GB, McConkey DJ. Inhibition of the phosphatidylinositol 3-kinase-AKT pathway induces apoptosis in pancreatic carcinoma cells in vitro and in vivo. *Mol Cancer Ther.* 2002;1:989–997.
66. Ng SSW, Tsao MS, Chow S, Hedley DW. Inhibition of phosphatidylinosito–3-kinase enhances gemcitabine-induced apoptosis in human pancreatic cancer cells. *Cancer Res.* 2000;60:5451–5455.
67. Min Y, Adachi Y, Yamamoto H, et al. Genetic blockade of the insulin-like growth factor-1 receptor: a promising strategy for human pancreatic cancer. *Cancer Res.* 2003;63:6432–6441.
68. Nair PN, De Armond DT, Adamo ML, Strodel WE, Freeman JW. Aberrant expression and activation of insulin-like growth factor-1 receptor (IGF-1R) are mediated by an induction of IGF-1R promoter activity and stabilization of IGF-1R mRNA and contributes to growth factor independence and increased survival of the pancreatic cancer cell line MIA PaCa-2. *Oncogene.* 2001;20:8203–8214.
69. Okami K, Wu L, Riggins G, et al. Analysis of PTEN/MMAC1 alterations in aerodigestive tract tumors. *Cancer Res.* 1998;58:509–511.
70. Ebert MP, Fei G, Schandl L, et al. Reduced PTEN expression in the pancreas overexpressing transforming growth factor-β 1. *Br J Cancer.* 2002;86:257–262.
71. Cheng JQ, Ruggeri B, Klein WM, et al. Amplification of AKT2 in human pancreatic cells and inhibition of AKT2 expression and tumorigenicity by antisense RNA. *Proc Natl Acad Sci USA.* 1996;93:3636–3641.
72. Sclabas GM, Fujioka S, Schmidt C, Evans DB, Chiao PJ. NF-κB in pancreatic cancer. *Int J Gastrointest Cancer.* 2003;33:15–26.
73. Ghosh S, May MJ, Kopp EB. NF-κB and Rel proteins: evolutionarily conserved mediators of immune responses. *Annu Rev Immunol.* 1998;16:225–260.
74. Karin M, Ben-Neriah Y. Phosphorylation meets ubiquitination: the control of NF-[κ]B activity. *Annu Rev Immunol.* 2000;18:621–663.
75. Orlowski RZ, Baldwin AS Jr. NF-κB as a therapeutic target in cancer. *Trends Mol Med.* 2002;8:385–389.
76. Wang W, Abbruzzese JL, Evans DB, Larry L, Cleary KR, Chiao PJ. The nuclear factor-κ B RelA transcription factor is constitutively activated in human pancreatic adenocarcinoma cells. *Clin Cancer Res.* 1999;5:119–127.
77. Arsura M, Mercurio F, Oliver AL, Thorgeirsson SS, Sonenshein GE. Role of the IκB kinase complex in oncogenic Ras- and Raf-mediated transformation of rat liver epithelial cells. *Mol Cell Biol.* 2000;20:5381–5391.
78. Mayo MW, Wang CY, Cogswell PC, et al. Requirement of NF-κB activation to suppress p53-independent apoptosis induced by oncogenic Ras. *Science.* 1997;278:1812–1815.
79. Liptay S, Weber CK, Ludwig L, Wagner M, Adler G, Schmid RM. Mitogenic and antiapoptotic role of constitutive NF-κB/Rel activity in pancreatic cancer. *Int J Cancer.* 2003;105:735–746.
80. Sclabas GM, Fujioka S, Schmidt C, Fan Z, Evans DB, Chiao PJ. Restoring apoptosis in pancreatic cancer cells by targeting the nuclear factor-κB signaling pathway with the anti-epidermal growth factor antibody IMC-C225. *J Gastrointest Surg.* 2003;7:37–43; discussion 43.
81. Arlt A, Vorndamm J, Muerkoster S, et al. Autocrine production of interleukin 1β confers constitutive nuclear factor–κB activity and chemoresistance in pancreatic carcinoma cell lines. *Cancer Res.* 2002;62:910–916.
82. Fujioka S, Sclabas GM, Schmidt C, et al. Function of nuclear factor-κB in pancreatic cancer metastasis. *Clin Cancer Res.* 2003;9:346–354.
83. Fujioka S, Sclabas GM, Schmidt C, et al. Inhibition of constitutive NF-κ B activity by I κ B α M suppresses tumorigenesis. *Oncogene.* 2003;22:1365–1370.
84. Wang W, Abbruzzese JL, Evans DB, Chiao PJ. Overexpression of urokinase-type plasminogen activator in pancreatic adenocarcinoma is regulated by constitutively activated RelA. *Oncogene.* 1999;18:4554–4563.
85. Arlt A, Gehrz A, Muerkoster S, et al. Role of NF-kappaB and AKT/PI3K in the resistance of pancreatic carcinoma cell lines against gemcitabine-induced cell death. *Oncogene.* 2003;22: 3243–3251.
86. Dong QG, Sclabas GM, Fujioka S, et al. The function of multiple IkappaB: NF-κB complexes in the resistance of cancer cells to Taxol-induced apoptosis. *Oncogene.* 2002;21: 6510–6519.
87. Arlt A, Vorndamm J, Breitenbroich M, et al. Inhibition of NF-kappaB sensitizes human pancreatic carcinoma cells to apoptosis induced by etoposide (VP16) or doxorubicin. *Oncogene.* 2001;20:859–868.
88. Zhang Z, Wang Y, Vikis HG, et al. Wild-type Kras2 can inhibit lung carcinogenesis in mice. *Nat Genet.* 2001;29:25–33.
89. Finney RE, Bishop JM. Predisposition to neoplastic transformation caused by gene replacement of H-ras1. *Science.* 1993;260:1524–1527.
90. Heidenblad M, Jonson T, Mahlamaki EH, et al. Detailed genomic mapping and expression analyses of 12p amplifications in pancreatic carcinomas reveal a 3.5-Mb target region for amplification. *Genes Chromosomes Cancer.* 2002;34: 211–223.
91. Gisselsson D, Mandahl N, Palsson E, Gorunova L, Hoglund M. Locus-specific multifluor FISH analysis allows physical characterization of complex chromosome abnormalities in neoplasia. *Genes Chromosomes Cancer.* 2000;28:347–352.
92. Schleger C, Arens N, Zentgraf H, Bleyl U, Verbeke C. Identification of frequent chromosomal aberrations in ductal adenocarcinoma of the pancreas by comparative genomic hybridization (CGH). *J Pathol.* 2000;191:27–32.
93. Guerra C, Mijimolle N, Dhawahir A, et al. Tumor induction by an endogenous K-ras oncogene is highly dependent on cellular context. *Cancer Cell.* 2003;4:111–120.
94. Furukawa T, Sunamura M, Motoi F, Matsuno S, Horii A. Potential tumor suppressive pathway involving DUSP-6/MKP-3 in pancreatic cancer. *Am J Pathol.* 2003;162:1807–1815.
95. Goldstein AM, Fraser MC, Struewing JP, et al. Increased risk of pancreatic cancer in melanoma-prone kindreds with p16INK4 mutations. *N Engl J Med.* 1995;333: 970–974.

96. Whelan AJ, Bartsch D, Goodfellow PJ. Brief report: a familial syndrome of pancreatic cancer and melanoma with a mutation in the CDKN2 tumor-suppressor gene. *N Engl J Med.* 1995;333:975–977.
97. Ruas M, Peters G. The p16INK4a/CDKN2A tumor suppressor and its relatives. *Biochim Biophys Acta.* 1998;1378: F115–F177.
98. Lowe SW, Sherr CJ. Tumor suppression by INK4A-ARF: progress and puzzles. *Curr Opin Genet Dev.* 2003;13:77–83.
99. Quelle DE, Zindy F, Ashmun RA, Sherr CJ. Alternative reading frames of the INK4A tumor suppressor gene encode two unrelated proteins capable of inducing cell cycle arrest. *Cell.* 1995;83:993–1000.
100. Zindy F, Eischen CM, Randle DH, et al. Myc signaling via the ARF tumor suppressor regulates p53-dependent apoptosis and immortalization. *Genes Dev.* 1998;12:2424–2433.
101. Pomerantz J, Schreiber-Agus N, Liegeois NJ, et al. The Ink4a tumor-suppressor gene product, $p19^{ARF}$, interacts with MDM2 and neutralizes MDM2's inhibition of p53. *Cell.* 1998;92:713–723.
102. Stott FJ, Bates S, James MC, et al. The alternative product from the human CDKN2A locus, p14(ARF), participates in a regulatory feedback loop with p53 and MDM2. *EMBO J.* 1998;17:5001–5014.
103. Zhang Y, Xiong Y, Yarbrough WG. ARF promotes MDM2 degradation and stabilizes p53: ARF-INK4a locus deletion impairs both the Rb and p53 tumor-suppression pathways. *Cell.* 1998;92:725–734.
104. Martelli F, Hamilton T, Silver DP, et al. p19ARF targets certain E2F species for degradation. *Proc Natl Acad Sci USA.* 2001;98:4455–4460.
105. Rocha S, Campbell KJ, Perkins ND. p53- and Mdm2-independent repression of NF-κ B transactivation by the ARF tumor suppressor. *Mol Cell.* 2003;12:15–25.
106. Sugimoto M, Kuo ML, Roussel MF, Sherr CJ. Nucleolar Arf tumor suppressor inhibits ribosomal RNA processing. *Mol Cell.* 2003;11:415–424.
107. Liu L, Dilworth D, Gao L, et al. Mutation of the CDKN2A 5′ UTR creates an aberrant initiation codon and predisposes to melanoma. *Nat Genet.* 1999;21:128–132.
108. Lal G, Liu L, Hogg D, et al. Patients with both pancreatic adenocarcinoma and melanoma may harbor germline CDKN2A mutations. *Genes Chromosomes Cancer.* 2000;27: 358–361.
109. Lynch HT, Brand RE, Hogg D, et al. Phenotypic variation in eight extended CDKN2A germline mutation familial atypical multiple mole melanoma-pancreatic carcinoma-prone families: the familial atypical mole melanoma-pancreatic carcinoma syndrome. *Cancer.* 2002;94:84–96.
110. Geradts J, Wilentz RE, Roberts H. Immunohistochemical detection of the alternate INK4A-encoded tumor-suppressor protein p14(ARF) in archival human cancers and cell lines using commercial antibodies: correlation with p16(INK4a) expression. *Mod Pathol.* 2001;14: 1162–1168.
111. Borg A, Sandberg T, Nilsson K, et al. High frequency of multiple melanomas and breast and pancreas carcinomas in CDKN2A mutation-positive melanoma families. *J Natl Cancer Inst.* 2000;92:1260–1266.
112. Goldstein AM, Struewing JP, Chidambaram A, Fraser MC, Tucker MA. Genotype-phenotype relationships in US melanoma-prone families with CDKN2A and CDK4 mutations. *J Natl Cancer Inst.* 2000;92:1006–1010.
113. Wilentz RE, Geradts J, Maynard R, et al. Inactivation of the p16(INK4A) tumor-suppressor gene in pancreatic duct lesions: loss of intranuclear expression. *Cancer Res.* 1998;58:4740–4744.
114. Serrano M, Lin AW, McCurrach ME, Beach D, Lowe SW. Oncogenic ras provokes premature cell senescence associated with accumulation of p53 and p16INK4a. *Cell.* 1997;88:593–602.
115. Brookes S, Rowe J, Ruas M, et al. INK4a-deficient human diploid fibroblasts are resistant to RAS-induced senescence. *EMBO J.* 2002;21:2936–2945.
116. Drayton S, Rowe J, Jones R, et al. Tumor suppressor p16(INK4a) determines sensitivity of human cells to transformation by cooperating cellular oncogenes. *Cancer Cell.* 2003;4:301–310.
117. Zhu J, Woods D, McMahon M, Bishop JM. Senescence of human fibroblasts induced by oncogenic Raf. *Genes Dev.* 1998;12:2997–3007.
118. Chin L, Pomerantz J, Polsky D, et al. Cooperative effects of INK4a and ras in melanoma susceptibility in vivo. *Genes Dev.* 1997;11:2822–2834.
119. Kamijo T, Zindy F, Roussel MF, et al. Tumor suppression at the mouse INK4a locus mediated by the alternative reading frame product p19ARF. *Cell.* 1997;91:649–659.
120. Plath T, Detjen K, Welzel M, et al. A novel function for the tumor suppressor p16(INK4a): induction of anoikis via upregulation of the alpha(5)beta(1) fibronectin receptor. *J Cell Biol.* 2000;150:1467–1478.
121. Natarajan E, Saeb M, Crum CP, Woo SB, McKee PH, Rheinwald JG. Co-expression of p16(INK4A) and laminin 5 $\gamma 2$ by microinvasive and superficial squamous cell carcinomas in vivo and by migrating wound and senescent keratinocytes in culture. *Am J Pathol.* 2003;163:477–491.
122. Alani RM, Young AZ, Shifflett CB. Id1 regulation of cellular senescence through transcriptional repression of p16/Ink4a. *Proc Natl Acad Sci USA.* 2001;98:7812–7816.
123. Ohtani N, Zebedee Z, Huot TJ, et al. Opposing effects of Ets and Id proteins on p16INK4a expression during cellular senescence. *Nature.* 2001;409:1067–1070.
124. Vousden KH, Lu X. Live or let die: the cell's response to p53. *Nat Rev Cancer.* 2002;2:594–604.
125. Maitra A, Adsay NV, Argani P, et al. Multicomponent analysis of the pancreatic adenocarcinoma progression model using a pancreatic intraepithelial neoplasia tissue microarray. *Mod Pathol.* 2003;16:902–912.
126. Heinmoller E, Dietmaier W, Zirngibl H, et al. Molecular analysis of microdissected tumors and preneoplastic intraductal lesions in pancreatic carcinoma. *Am J Pathol.* 2000;157: 83–92.
127. DiGiuseppe JA, Hruban RH, Goodman SN, et al. Overexpression of p53 protein in adenocarcinoma of the pancreas. *Am J Clin Pathol.* 1994;101:684–688.
128. Boschman CR, Stryker S, Reddy JK, Rao MS. Expression of p53 protein in precursor lesions and adenocarcinoma of human pancreas. *Am J Pathol.* 1994;145:1291–1295.

129. Harada T, Okita K, Shiraishi K, Kusano N, Kondoh S, Sasaki K. Interglandular cytogenetic heterogeneity detected by comparative genomic hybridization in pancreatic cancer. *Cancer Res.* 2002;62:835–839.
130. Gorunova L, Hoglund M, Andren-Sandberg A, et al. Cytogenetic analysis of pancreatic carcinomas: intratumor heterogeneity and nonrandom pattern of chromosome aberrations. *Genes Chromosomes Cancer.* 1998;23:81–99.
131. Zhu C, Mills KD, Ferguson DO, et al. Unrepaired DNA breaks in p53-deficient cells lead to oncogenic gene amplification subsequent to translocations. *Cell.* 2002;109:811–821.
132. Albertson DG, Collins C, McCormick F, Gray JW. Chromosome aberrations in solid tumors. *Nat Genet.* 2003;34: 369–376.
133. Schleger C, Verbeke C, Hildenbrand R, Zentgraf H, Bleyl U. c-MYC activation in primary and metastatic ductal adenocarcinoma of the pancreas: incidence, mechanisms, and clinical significance. *Mod Pathol.* 2002;15:462–469.
134. Armengol G, Knuutila S, Lluis F, Capella G, Miro R, Caballin MR. DNA copy number changes and evaluation of MYC, IGF-1R, and FES amplification in xenografts of pancreatic adenocarcinoma. *Cancer Genet Cytogenet.* 2000;116:133–141.
135. Fukushige S, Waldman FM, Kimura M, et al. Frequent gain of copy number on the long arm of chromosome 20 in human pancreatic adenocarcinoma. *Genes Chromosomes Cancer.* 1997;19:161–169.
136. Maser RS, DePinho RA. Connecting chromosomes, crisis, and cancer. *Science.* 2002;297:565–569.
137. Gisselsson D, Pettersson L, Hoglund M, et al. Chromosomal breakage-fusion-bridge events cause genetic intratumor heterogeneity. *Proc Natl Acad Sci USA.* 2000;97:5357–5362.
138. Karlseder J, Broccoli D, Dai Y, Hardy S, de Lange T. p53- and ATM-dependent apoptosis induced by telomeres lacking TRF2. *Science.* 1999:283:1321–1325.
139. Chin L, Artandi SE, Shen Q, et al. p53 deficiency rescues the adverse effects of telomere loss and cooperates with telomere dysfunction to accelerate carcinogenesis. *Cell.* 1999;97: 527–538.
140. Artandi SE, Chang S, Lee SL, et al. Telomere dysfunction promotes non-reciprocal translocations and epithelial cancers in mice. *Nature.* 2000;406:641–645.
141. Anderson KE, Potter JD, Mack TM. Pancreatic cancer. In: Schottenfeld D, Fraumeni JJ, eds. *Cancer Epidemiology and Prevention.* New York: Oxford University Press; 1996:725–771.
142. Malka D, Hammel P, Maire F, et al. Risk of pancreatic adenocarcinoma in chronic pancreatitis. *Gut.* 2002;51:849–852.
143. van Heek NT, Meeker AK, Kern SE, et al. Telomere shortening is nearly universal in pancreatic intraepithelial neoplasia. *Am J Pathol.* 2002;161:1541–1547.
144. Gisselsson D, Jonson T, Petersen A. Telomere dysfunction triggers extensive DNA fragmentation and evolution of complex chromosome abnormalities in human malignant tumors. *Proc Natl Acad Sci USA.* 2001;98:12683–12688.
145. Suehara N, Mizumoto K, Muta T, et al. Telomerase elevation in pancreatic ductal carcinoma compared to nonmalignant pathological states. *Clin Cancer Res.* 1997;3:993–998.
146. Seki K, Suda T, Aoyagi Y, et al. Diagnosis of pancreatic adenocarcinoma by detection of human telomerase reverse transcriptase messenger RNA in pancreatic juice with sample qualification. *Clin Cancer Res.* 2001;7:1976–1981.
147. Hahn WC. Role of telomeres and telomerase in the pathogenesis of human cancer. *J Clin Oncol.* 2003;21:2034–2043.
148. Rudolph KL, Millard M, Bosenberg MW, DePinho RA. Telomere dysfunction and evolution of intestinal carcinoma in mice and humans. *Nat Genet.* 2001;28:155–159.
149. Hackett JA, Greider CW. Balancing instability: dual roles for telomerase and telomere dysfunction in tumorigenesis. *Oncogene.* 2002;21:619–626.
150. Buchler P, Conejo-Garcia JR, Lehmann G, et al. Real-time quantitative PCR of telomerase mRNA is useful for the differentiation of benign and malignant pancreatic disorders. *Pancreas.* 2001;22:331–340.
151. Cong YS, Wright WE, Shay JW. Human telomerase and its regulation. *Microbiol Mol Biol Rev.* 2002;66:407–425.
152. Lin SY, Elledge SJ. Multiple tumor suppressor pathways negatively regulate telomerase. *Cell.* 2003;113:881–889.
153. Yang H, Kyo S, Takatura M, Sun L. Autocrine transforming growth factor beta suppresses telomerase activity and transcription of human telomerase reverse transcriptase in human cancer cells. *Cell Growth Differ.* 2001;12: 119–127.
154. Shay JW, Wright WE. Telomerase: a target for cancer therapeutics. *Cancer Cell.* 2002;2:257–265.
155. Rha SY, Izbicka E, Lawrence R, et al. Effect of telomere and telomerase interactive agents on human tumor and normal cell lines. *Clin Cancer Res.* 2000;6:987–993.
156. Eisenman RN. Deconstructing MYC. *Genes Dev.* 2001;15: 2023–2030.
157. Felsher DW, Bishop JM. Transient excess of MYC activity can elicit genomic instability and tumorigenesis. *Proc Natl Acad Sci USA.* 1999;96:3940–3944.
158. Li Q, Dang CV. c-Myc overexpression uncouples DNA replication from mitosis. *Mol Cell Biol.* 1999;19:5339–5351.
159. Wu KJ, Grandori C, Amacker M, et al. Direct activation of TERT transcription by c-MYC. *Nat Genet.* 1999;21:220–224.
160. Wang J, Xie LY, Allan S, Beach D, Hannon GJ. Myc activates telomerase. *Genes Dev.* 1998;12:1769–1774.
161. Hahn SA, Greenhalf B, Ellis I, et al. BRCA2 germline mutations in familial pancreatic carcinoma. *J Natl Cancer Inst.* 2003;95:214–221.
162. Murphy KM, Brune KA, Griffin C, et al. Evaluation of candidate genes MAP2K4, MADH4, ACVR1B, and BRCA2 in familial pancreatic cancer: deleterious BRCA2 mutations in 17%. *Cancer Res.* 2002;62:3789–3793.
163. Lal G, Liu G, Schmocker B, et al. Inherited predisposition to pancreatic adenocarcinoma: role of family history and germ-line p16, BRCA1, and BRCA2 mutations. *Cancer Res.* 2000;60:409–416.
164. Goggins M, Schutte M, Lu J, et al. Germline BRCA2 gene mutations in patients with apparently sporadic pancreatic carcinomas. *Cancer Res.* 1996;56:5360–5364.
165. Ozcelik H, Schmocker B, Di Nicola N, et al. Germline BRCA2 6174delT mutations in Ashkenazi Jewish pancreatic cancer patients [letter]. *Nat Genet.* 1997;16:17–18.
166. Venkitaraman AR. Cancer susceptibility and the functions of BRCA1 and BRCA2. *Cell.* 2002;108:171–182.

167. Taipale J, Beachy PA. The Hedgehog and Wnt signalling pathways in cancer. *Nature*. 2001;411:349–354.
168. Hahn SA, Schutte M, Hoque AT, et al. DPC4, a candidate tumor-suppressor gene at human chromosome 18q21.1. *Science*. 1996;271:350–353.
169. Schutte M, Hruban RH, Hedrick L, et al. DPC4 gene in various tumor types. *Cancer Res*. 1996;56:2527–2530.
170. Massague J, Blain SW, Lo RS. TGF-β signaling in growth control, cancer, and heritable disorders. *Cell*. 2000;103: 295–309.
171. Siegel PM, Massague J. Cytostatic and apoptotic actions of TGF-β in homeostasis and cancer. *Nat Rev Cancer*. 2003;3: 807–820.
172. Oft M, Akhurst RJ, Balmain A. Metastasis is driven by sequential elevation of H-ras and Smad2 levels. *Nat Cell Biol*. 2002;4:487–494.
173. Janda E, Lehmann K, Killisch I, et al. Ras and TGF[β] cooperatively regulate epithelial cell plasticity and metastasis: dissection of Ras signaling pathways. *J Cell Biol*. 2002;156: 299–313.
174. Tang B, Vu M, Booker T, et al. TGF-β switches from tumor suppressor to prometastatic factor in a model of breast cancer progression. *J Clin Invest*. 2003;112:1116–1124.
175. Akhurst RJ, Derynck R. TGF-β signaling in cancer–a double-edged sword. *Trends Cell Biol*. 2001;11:S44–S51.
176. Wilentz RE, Iacobuzio-Donahue CA, Argani P, et al. Loss of expression of DPC4 in pancreatic intraepithelial neoplasia: evidence that DPC4 inactivation occurs late in neoplastic progression. *Cancer Res*. 2000;60:2002–2006.
177. Schwarte-Waldhoff I, Volpert OV, Bouck NP, et al. Smad4/DPC4-mediated tumor suppression through suppression of angiogenesis. *Proc Natl Acad Sci USA*. 2000;97: 9624–9629.
178. Duda DG, Sunamura M, Lefter LP, et al. Restoration of SMAD4 by gene therapy reverses the invasive phenotype in pancreatic adenocarcinoma cells. *Oncogene*. 2003;22:6857–6864.
179. Peng B, Fleming JB, Breslin T, et al. Suppression of tumorigenesis and induction of p15(ink4b) by Smad4/DPC4 in human pancreatic cancer cells. *Clin Cancer Res*. 2002;8: 3628–3638.
180. Dai JL, Schutte M, Bansal RK, Wilentz RE, Sugar AY, Kern SE. Transforming growth factor-beta responsiveness in DPC4/SMAD4-null cancer cells. *Mol Carcinog*. 1999;26:37–43.
181. Giehl K, Seidel B, Gierschik P, Adler G, Menke A. TGFbeta1 represses proliferation of pancreatic carcinoma cells which correlates with Smad4-independent inhibition of ERK activation. *Oncogene*. 2000;19:4531–4541.
182. Jonson T, Heidenblad M, Hakansson P, et al. Pancreatic carcinoma cell lines with SMAD4 inactivation show distinct expression responses to TGFβ1. *Genes Chromosomes Cancer*. 2003;36:340–352.
183. Nicolas FJ, Hill CS. Attenuation of the TGF-β-Smad signaling pathway in pancreatic tumor cells confers resistance to TGF-β-induced growth arrest. *Oncogene*. 2003;22: 3698–3711.
184. Baldwin RL, Friess H, Yokoyama M, et al. Attenuated ALK5 receptor expression in human pancreatic cancer: correlation with resistance to growth inhibition. *Int J Cancer*. 1996;67:283–288.
185. Wagner M, Kleeff J, Lopez ME, Bockman I, Massaque J, Korc M. Transfection of the type I TGF-β receptor restores TGF-beta responsiveness in pancreatic cancer. *Int J Cancer*. 1998;78:255–260.
186. Cordenonsi M, Dupont S, Maretto S, Insinga A, Imbriano C, Piccolo S. Links between tumor suppressors: p53 is required for TGF-β gene responses by cooperating with Smads. *Cell*. 2003;113:301–314.
187. Hannon GJ, Beach D. p15INK4B is a potential effector of TGF-β-induced cell cycle arrest. *Nature*. 1994;371: 257–261.
188. Staller P, Peukert K, Kiermaier A, et al. Repression of p15INK4b expression by Myc through association with Miz-1. *Nat Cell Biol*. 2001;3:392–399.
189. Alcock RA, Dey S, Chendil D, et al. Farnesyltransferase inhibitor (L-744,832) restores TGF-beta type II receptor expression and enhances radiation sensitivity in K-ras mutant pancreatic cancer cell line MIA PaCa-2. *Oncogene*. 2002;21:7883–7890.
190. Lehmann K, Janda E, Pierreux CE, et al. Raf induces TGFβ production while blocking its apoptotic but not invasive responses: a mechanism leading to increased malignancy in epithelial cells. *Genes Dev*. 2000;14:2610–2622.
191. Friess H, Yamanaka Y, Buchler M, et al. Enhanced expression of transforming growth factor β isoforms in pancreatic cancer correlates with decreased survival. *Gastroenterology*. 1993;105:1846–1856.
192. Lohr M, Schmidt C, Ringel J, et al. Transforming growth factor-beta1 induces desmoplasia in an experimental model of human pancreatic carcinoma. *Cancer Res*. 2001;61: 550–555.
193. Wagner M, Kleeff J, Friess H, Buchler MW, Korc M. Enhanced expression of the type II transforming growth factor-β receptor is associated with decreased survival in human pancreatic cancer. *Pancreas*. 1999;19:370–376.
194. Friess H, Yamanaka Y, Buchler M, et al. Enhanced expression of the type II transforming growth factor β receptor in human pancreatic cancer cells without alteration of type III receptor expression. *Cancer Res*. 1993;53:2704–2707.
195. Rowland-Goldsmith MA, Maruyama H, Matsuda K, et al. Soluble type II transforming growth factor-β receptor attenuates expression of metastasis-associated genes and suppresses pancreatic cancer cell metastasis. *Mol Cancer Ther*. 2002;1:161–167.
196. Rowland-Goldsmith MA, Maruyama H, Kusama T, Ralli S, Korc M. Soluble type II transforming growth factor-β(TGF-β) receptor inhibits TGF-beta signaling in COLO-357 pancreatic cancer cells in vitro and attenuates tumor formation. *Clin Cancer Res*. 2001;7:2931–2940.
197. Ellenrieder V, Hendler SF, Boeck W, et al. Transforming growth factor β1 treatment leads to an epithelial-mesenchymal transdifferentiation of pancreatic cancer cells requiring extracellular signal-regulated kinase 2 activation. *Cancer Res*. 2001;61:4222–4228.
198. Ellenrieder V, Hendler SF, Ruhland C, Boeck W, Adler G, Gress TM. TGF-β-induced invasiveness of pancreatic cancer cells is mediated by matrix metalloproteinase-2 and the urokinase plasminogen activator system. *Int J Cancer*. 2001;93:204–211.

199. Lu Z, Friess H, Graber HU, et al. Presence of two signaling TGF-β receptors in human pancreatic cancer correlates with advanced tumor stage. *Dig Dis Sci.* 1997;42:2054–2063.
200. Biankin AV, Morey AL, Lee CS, et al. DPC4/Smad4 expression and outcome in pancreatic ductal adenocarcinoma. *J Clin Oncol.* 2002;20:4531–4542.
201. Tascilar M, Skinner HG, Rosty C, et al. The SMAD4 protein and prognosis of pancreatic ductal adenocarcinoma. *Clin Cancer Res.* 2001;7:4115–4121.
202. Hilgers W, Song JJ, Haye M, et al. Homozygous deletions inactivate DCC, but not MADH4/DPC4/SMAD4, in a subset of pancreatic and biliary cancers. *Genes Chromosomes Cancer.* 2000;27:353–357.
203. Lefter LP, Sunamura M, Furukawa T, et al. Inserting chromosome 18 into pancreatic cancer cells switches them to a dormant metastatic phenotype. *Clin Cancer Res.* 2003;9: 5044–5052.
204. Lefter LP, Furukawa T, Sunamura M, et al. Suppression of the tumorigenic phenotype by chromosome 18 transfer into pancreatic cancer cell lines. *Genes Chromosomes Cancer.* 2002;34:234–242.
205. Hebrok M, Kim SK, Melton DA. Notochord repression of endodermal Sonic hedgehog permits pancreas development. *Genes Dev.* 1998;12:1705–1713.
206. Apelqvist A, Ahlgren U, Edlund H. Sonic hedgehog directs specialised mesoderm differentiation in the intestine and pancreas. *Curr Biol.* 1997;7:801–804.
207. Berman DM, Karhadkar SS, Maitra A, et al. Widespread requirement for Hedgehog ligand stimulation in growth of digestive tract tumours. *Nature.* 2003;425:846–851.
208. Thayer SP, Di Magliano MP, Heiser PW, et al. Hedgehog is an early and late mediator of pancreatic cancer tumorigenesis. *Nature.* 2003;425:851–856.
209. Kayed H, Kleeff J, Keleg S, Buchler MW, Friess H. Distribution of Indian hedgehog and its receptors patched and smoothened in human chronic pancreatitis. *J Endocrinol.* 2003;178:467–478.
210. Jensen J, Pedersen EE, Galante P, et al. Control of endodermal endocrine development by Hes-1. *Nat Genet.* 2000;24: 36–44.
211. Apelqvist A, Li H, Sommer L, et al. Notch signalling controls pancreatic cell differentiation. *Nature.* 1999;400:877–881.
212. Miyamoto Y, Maitra A, Ghosh B, et al. Notch mediates TGF α-induced changes in epithelial differentiation during pancreatic tumorigenesis. *Cancer Cell.* 2003;3:565–576.
213. Grippo PJ, Nowlin PS, Demeure MJ, Longnecker DS, Sandgren EP. Preinvasive pancreatic neoplasia of ductal phenotype induced by acinar cell targeting of mutant Kras in transgenic mice. *Cancer Res.* 2003;63:2016–2019.
214. Murtaugh LC, Stanger BZ, Kwan KM, Melton DA. Notch signaling controls multiple steps of pancreatic differentiation. *Proc Natl Acad Sci USA.* 2003;100:14920–14925.
215. Hemminki A. The molecular basis and clinical aspects of Peutz-Jeghers syndrome. *Cell Mol Life Sci.* 1999;55: 735–750.
216. Ossipova O, Bardeesy N, DePinho RA, Green JB. LKB1 (XEEK1) regulates Wnt signalling in vertebrate development. *Nat Cell Biol.* 2003;5:889–894.
217. Ylikorkala A, Rossi DJ, Korsisaari N, et al. Vascular abnormalities and deregulation of VEGF in Lkb1-deficient mice. *Science.* 2001;293:1323–1326.
218. Hawley SA, Boudeau J, Reid JL, et al. Complexes between the LKB1 tumor suppressor, STRADalpha/beta and MO25alpha/beta are upstream kinases in the AMP-activated protein kinase cascade. *J Biol.* 2003;2:28.
219. Martin SG, St Johnston D. A role for *Drosophila* LKB1 in anterior-posterior axis formation and epithelial polarity. *Nature.* 2003;421:379–384.
220. Giardiello FM, Brensinger JD, Tersmette AC, et al. Very high risk of cancer in familial Peutz-Jeghers syndrome. *Gastroenterology.* 2000;119:1447–1453.
221. Su GH, Hruban RH, Bansal RK, et al. Germline and somatic mutations of the STK11/LKB1 Peutz-Jeghers gene in pancreatic and biliary cancers. *Am J Pathol.* 1999;154: 1835–1840.
222. Bardeesy N, Sinha M, Hezel AF, et al. Loss of the Lkb1 tumour suppressor provokes intestinal polyposis but resistance to transformation. *Nature.* 2002;419:162–167.
223. Bergmann U, Funatomi H, Yokoyama M, Beger HG, Korc M. Insulin-like growth factor I overexpression in human pancreatic cancer: evidence for autocrine and paracrine roles. *Cancer Res.* 1995;55:2007–2011.
224. Stoeltzing O, Liu W, Reinmuth N, et al. Regulation of hypoxia-inducible factor-1α, vascular endothelial growth factor, and angiogenesis by an insulin-like growth factor-I receptor autocrine loop in human pancreatic cancer. *Am J Pathol.* 2003;163:1001–1011.
225. Ouban A, Muraca P, Yeatman T, Coppola D. Expression and distribution of insulin-like growth factor-1 receptor in human carcinomas. *Hum Pathol.* 2003;34:803–808.
226. Tanno S, Mitsuuchi Y, Altomare DA, Xiao GH, Testa JR. AKT activation up-regulates insulin-like growth factor I receptor expression and promotes invasiveness of human pancreatic cancer cells. *Cancer Res.* 2001;61:589–593.
227. Maloney EK, McLaughlin JL, Dagdigian NE, et al. An anti-insulin-like growth factor I receptor antibody that is a potent inhibitor of cancer cell proliferation. *Cancer Res.* 2003;63: 5073–5083.
228. Neid M, Datta K, Stephan S, Khanna I, Pal S, Shaw L, White M, Mukhopadhyay D. Role of insulin receptor substrates and protein kinase C-ζ in vascular permeability factor/vascular endothelial growth factor expression in pancreatic cancer cells. *J Biol Chem.* 2004;279: 3941–3948.
229. Danilkovitch-Miagkova A, Zbar B. Dysregulation of Met receptor tyrosine kinase activity in invasive tumors. *J Clin Invest.* 2002;109:863–867.
230. Di Renzo MF, Poulsom R, Olivero M, Comoglio PM, Lemoine NR. Expression of the Met/hepatocyte growth factor receptor in human pancreatic cancer. *Cancer Res.* 1995;55: 1129–1138.
231. Ebert M, Yokoyama M, Friess H, Buchler MW, Korc M. Coexpression of the c-met proto-oncogene and hepatocyte growth factor in human pancreatic cancer. *Cancer Res.* 1994;54:5775–5778.
232. Paciucci R, Vila MR, Adell T, et al. Activation of the urokinase plasminogen activator/urokinase plasminogen activa-

tor receptor system and redistribution of E-cadherin are associated with hepatocyte growth factor-induced motility of pancreas tumor cells overexpressing Met. *Am J Pathol.* 1998;153:201–212.
233. Furukawa T, Duguid WP, Kobari M, Matsuno S, Tsao MS. Hepatocyte growth factor and Met receptor expression in human pancreatic carcinogenesis. *Am J Pathol.* 1995;147: 889–895.
234. Otte JM, Kiehne K, Schmitz F, Folsch UR, Herzig KH. C-met protooncogene expression and its regulation by cytokines in the regenerating pancreas and in pancreatic cancer cells. *Scand J Gastroenterol.* 2000;35:90–95.
235. Menke A, Yamaguchi H, Giehl K, Adler G. Hepatocyte growth factor and fibroblast growth factor 2 are overexpressed after cerulein-induced acute pancreatitis. *Pancreas.* 1999;18: 28–33.
236. Ueda T, Takeyama Y, Hori Y, Nishikawa J, Yamamoto M, Saitoh Y. Hepatocyte growth factor in assessment of acute pancreatitis: comparison with C-reactive protein and interleukin-6. *J Gastroenterol.* 1997;32:63–70.
237. Saimura M, Nagai E, Mizumoto K, et al. Tumor suppression through angiogenesis inhibition by SUIT-2 pancreatic cancer cells genetically engineered to secrete NK4. *Clin Cancer Res.* 2002;8:3243–3249.
238. Tomioka D, Maehara N, Kuba K, et al. Inhibition of growth, invasion, and metastasis of human pancreatic carcinoma cells by NK4 in an orthotopic mouse model. *Cancer Res.* 2001;61:7518–7524.
239. Cross MJ, Claesson-Welsh L. FGF and VEGF function in angiogenesis: signalling pathways, biological responses and therapeutic inhibition. *Trends Pharmacol Sci.* 2001;22: 201–207.
240. Yamanaka Y, FriessH, Buchler M, et al. Overexpression of acidic and basic fibroblast growth factors in human pancreatic cancer correlates with advanced tumor stage. *Cancer Res.* 1993;53:5289–5296.
241. Kleeff J, Ishiwata T, Kumbasar A, et al. The cell-surface heparan sulfate proteoglycan glypican-1 regulates growth factor action in pancreatic carcinoma cells and is overexpressed in human pancreatic cancer. *J Clin Invest.* 1998;102: 1662–1673.
242. Ohta T, Yamamoto M, Numata M, et al. Expression of basic fibroblast growth factor and its receptor in human pancreatic carcinomas. *Br J Cancer.* 1995;72:824–831.
243. Kobrin MS, Yamanaka Y, Friess H, Lopez ME, Korc M. Aberrant expression of type I fibroblast growth factor receptor in human pancreatic adenocarcinomas. *Cancer Res.* 1993;53: 4741–4744.
244. Ishiwata T, Friess H, Buchler MW, Lopez ME, Korc M. Characterization of keratinocyte growth factor and receptor expression in human pancreatic cancer. *Am J Pathol.* 1998;153: 213–222.
245. Kornmann M, Ishiwata T, Beger HG, Korc M. Fibroblast growth factor-5 stimulates mitogenic signaling and is overexpressed in human pancreatic cancer: evidence for autocrine and paracrine actions. *Oncogene.* 1997;15: 1417–1424.
246. Kornmann M, Ishiwata T, Matsuda K, et al. IIIc isoform of fibroblast growth factor receptor 1 is overexpressed in human pancreatic cancer and enhances tumorigenicity of hamster ductal cells. *Gastroenterology.* 2002;123: 301–313.
247. Wagner M, Lopez ME, Cahn M, Korc M. Suppression of fibroblast growth factor receptor signaling inhibits pancreatic cancer growth in vitro and in vivo. *Gastroenterology.* 1998;114:798–807.
248. Ogawa T, Takayama K, Takakura N, Kitano S, Ueno H. Antitumor angiogenesis therapy using soluble receptors: enhanced inhibition of tumor growth when soluble fibroblast growth factor receptor-1 is used with soluble vascular endothelial growth factor receptor. *Cancer Gene Ther.* 2002;9:633–640.
249. Kleeff J, Wildi S, Kumbasar A, et al. Stable transfection of a glypican-1 antisense construct decreases tumorigenicity in PANC-1 pancreatic carcinoma cells. *Pancreas.* 1999;19: 281–288.
250. Kuniyasu H, Abbruzzese JL, Cleary KR, Fidler IJ. Induction of ductal and stromal hyperplasia by basic fibroblast growth factor produced by human pancreatic carcinoma. *Int J Oncol.* 2001;19:681–685.
251. Solcia E, Capella C, Kloppel G. *Tumors of the Pancreas.* Volume Fascicle 20. Washington, DC: Armed Forces Institute for Pathology; 1995.
252. Ferrara N, Gerber HP, LeCouter J. The biology of VEGF and its receptors. *Nat Med.* 2003;9:669–676.
253. Seo Y, Baba H, Fukuda T, Takashima M, Sugimachi K. High expression of vascular endothelial growth factor is associated with liver metastasis and a poor prognosis for patients with ductal pancreatic adenocarcinoma. *Cancer.* 2000;88: 2239–2245.
254. Itakura J, Ishiwata T, Friess H, et al. Enhanced expression of vascular endothelial growth factor in human pancreatic cancer correlates with local disease progression. *Clin Cancer Res.* 1997;3:1309–1316.
255. von Marschall Z, Cramer T, Hocker M, et al. De novo expression of vascular endothelial growth factor in human pancreatic cancer: evidence for an autocrine mitogenic loop. *Gastroenterology.* 2000;119:1358–1372.
256. Tokunaga T, Abe Y, Tsuchida T, et al. Ribozyme mediated cleavage of cell-associated isoform of vascular endothelial growth factor inhibits liver metastasis of a pancreatic cancer cell line. *Int J Oncol.* 2002;21:1027–1032.
257. Hotz HG, Hines OJ, Hotz B, et al. Evaluation of vascular endothelial growth factor blockade and matrix metalloproteinase inhibition as a combination therapy for experimental human pancreatic cancer. *J Gastrointest Surg.* 2003;7:220–227; discussion 227–228.
258. Hoshida T, Sunamura M, Duda DG, et al. Gene therapy for pancreatic cancer using an adenovirus vector encoding soluble flt-1 vascular endothelial growth factor receptor. *Pancreas.* 2002;25:111–121.
259. Itakura J, Ishiwata T, Shen B, Kornmann M, Korc M. Concomitant overexpression of vascular endothelial growth factor and its receptors in pancreatic cancer. *Int J Cancer.* 2000;85:27–34.
260. Tang RF, Itakura J, Aikawa T, et al. Overexpression of lymphangiogenic growth factor VEGF-C in human pancreatic cancer. *Pancreas.* 2001;22:285–292.

261. Miknyoczki SJ, Lang D, Huang L, Klein-Szanto AJ, Dionne CA, Ruggeri BA. Neurotrophins and Trk receptors in human pancreatic ductal adenocarcinoma: expression patterns and effects on in vitro invasive behavior. *Int J Cancer*. 1999;81:417–427.
262. Schneider MB, Standop J, Ulrich A, et al. Expression of nerve growth factors in pancreatic neural tissue and pancreatic cancer. *J Histochem Cytochem*. 2001;49:1205–1210.
263. Zhu Z, Friess H, diMola FF, et al. Nerve growth factor expression correlates with perineural invasion and pain in human pancreatic cancer. *J Clin Oncol*. 1999;17:2419–2428.
264. Ohta T, Numata M, Tsukioka Y. Neurotrophin-3 expression in human pancreatic cancers. *J Pathol*. 1997;181:405–412.
265. Miknyoczki SJ, Chang H, Klein-Szanto A, Dionne CA, Ruggeri BA. The Trk tyrosine kinase inhibitor CEP-701 (KT-5555) exhibits significant antitumor efficacy in preclinical xenograft models of human pancreatic ductal adenocarcinoma. *Clin Cancer Res*. 1999;5:2205–2212.
266. Zhu Z, Kleeff J, Kayed H, et al. Nerve growth factor and enhancement of proliferation, invasion, and tumorigenicity of pancreatic cancer cells. *Mol Carcinog*. 2002;35:138–147.
267. Miknyoczki SJ, Wan W, Chang H, et al. The neurotrophin-trk receptor axes are critical for the growth and progression of human prostatic carcinoma and pancreatic ductal adenocarcinoma xenografts in nude mice. *Clin Cancer Res*. 2002;8:1924–1931.
268. Friess H, Zhu Z, Liard V, et al. Neurokinin-1 receptor expression and its potential effects on tumor growth in human pancreatic cancer. *Lab Invest*. 2003;83:731–742.
269. Bhatia M, Saluja AK, Hofbauer B, et al. Role of substance P and the neurokinin 1 receptor in acute pancreatitis and pancreatitis-associated lung injury. *Proc Natl Acad Sci USA*. 1998;95:4760–4765.
270. Shrikhande SV, Friess H, di Mola FF, et al. NK-1 receptor gene expression is related to pain in chronic pancreatitis. *Pain*. 2001;91:209–217.
271. Reubi JC, Waser B, Friess H, Buchler M, Laissue J. Neurotensin receptors: a new marker for human ductal pancreatic adenocarcinoma. *Gut*. 1998;42:546–550.
272. Ishizuka J, Townsend CM Jr, Thompson JC. Neurotensin regulates growth of human pancreatic cancer. *Ann Surg*. 1993;217:439–445; discussion 446.
273. Guha S, Lunn JA, Santiskulvong C, Rozengurt E. Neurotensin stimulates protein kinase C-dependent mitogenic signaling in human pancreatic carcinoma cell line PANC-1. *Cancer Res*. 2003;63:2379–2387.
274. Funk CD. Prostaglandins and leukotrienes: advances in eicosanoid biology. *Science*. 2001;294:1871–1875.
275. Ding XZ, Hennig R, Adrian TE. Lipoxygenase and cyclooxygenase metabolism: new insights in treatment and chemoprevention of pancreatic cancer. *Mol Cancer*. 2003;2:10.
276. Koliopanos A, Friess H, Kleeff J, Roggo A, Zimmermann A, Buchler MW. Cyclooxygenase 2 expression in chronic pancreatitis: correlation with stage of the disease and diabetes mellitus. *Digestion*. 2001;64:240–247.
277. Maitra A, Ashfaq R, Gunn CR, et al. Cyclooxygenase 2 expression in pancreatic adenocarcinoma and pancreatic intraepithelial neoplasia: an immunohistochemical analysis with automated cellular imaging. *Am J Clin Pathol*. 2002;118: 194–201.
278. Hennig R, Ding XZ, Tong WG, et al. 5-lipoxygenase and leukotriene b(4) receptor are expressed in human pancreatic cancers but not in pancreatic ducts in normal tissue. *Am J Pathol*. 2002;161:421–428.
279. Molina MA, Sitja-Arnau M, Lemoine MG, Frazier ML, Sinicrope FA. Increased cyclooxygenase-2 expression in human pancreatic carcinomas and cell lines: growth inhibition by nonsteroidal anti-inflammatory drugs. *Cancer Res*. 1999;59: 4356–4362.
280. Yip-Schneider MT, Barnard DS, Billings SD, et al. Cyclooxygenase-2 expression in human pancreatic adenocarcinomas. *Carcinogenesis*. 2000;21:139–146.
281. Tong WG, Ding XZ, Witt RC, Adrian TE. Lipoxygenase inhibitors attenuate growth of human pancreatic cancer xenografts and induce apoptosis through the mitochondrial pathway. *Mol Cancer Ther*. 2002;1:929–935.
282. Ding XZ, Kuszynski CA, El-Metwally TH, Adrian TE. Lipoxygenase inhibition induced apoptosis, morphological changes, and carbonic anhydrase expression in human pancreatic cancer cells. *Biochem Biophys Res Commun*. 1999;266: 392–399.
283. Weinberg DS, Heyt GJ, Cavanagh M, Pitchon D, McGlynn KA, London WT. Cholecystokinin and gastrin levels are not elevated in human pancreatic adenocarcinoma. *Cancer Epidemiol Biomarkers Prev*. 2001;10:721–722.
284. Goetze JP, Nielsen FC, Burcharth F, Rehfeld JF. Closing the gastrin loop in pancreatic carcinoma: coexpression of gastrin and its receptor in solid human pancreatic adenocarcinoma. *Cancer*. 2000;88:2487–2494.
285. Caplin M, Savage K, Khan K, et al. Expression and processing of gastrin in pancreatic adenocarcinoma. *Br J Surg*. 2000;87:1035–1040.
286. Buscail L, Saint-Laurent N, Chastre E, et al. Loss of sst2 somatostatin receptor gene expression in human pancreatic and colorectal cancer. *Cancer Res*. 1996;56:1823–1827.
287. Reubi JC, Waser B, Gugger M, et al. Distribution of CCK1 and CCK2 receptors in normal and diseased human pancreatic tissue. *Gastroenterology*. 2003;125:98–106.
288. Povoski SP, Zhou W, Longnecker DS, Roebuck BD, Bell RH Jr. Stimulation of growth of azaserine-induced putative preneoplastic lesions in rat pancreas is mediated specifically by way of cholecystokinin-A receptors. *Cancer Res*. 1993;53: 3925–3929.
289. Delesque N, Buscail L, Esteve JP, et al. sst2 somatostatin receptor expression reverses tumorigenicity of human pancreatic cancer cells. *Cancer Res*. 1997;57:956–962.
290. Clerc P, Leung-Theung-Long S, Wang TC, et al. Expression of CCK2 receptors in the murine pancreas: proliferation, transdifferentiation of acinar cells, and neoplasia. *Gastroenterology*. 2002;122:428–437.

5

Pancreatic Development

John W. Lin, MD
Steven D. Leach, MD

The adult pancreas is a complex epithelial organ organized from comparatively simpler elements. Whether these elements are delineated functionally, as endocrine, exocrine and stromal cell types, or delineated structurally, as a branching ductal tree terminating in acini, interspersed with islets of Langerhans and mesenchymal elements, the genesis of such a complex organ requires a strictly choreographed developmental program. In developing pancreas, this program involves extensive interplay between soluble signals and nuclear transcription factors, culminating in normal regulation of growth and cytodifferentiation. Despite recent progress, our understanding of pancreatic organogenesis remains largely incomplete. Understanding its mechanistic framework will be an important advance in our ability to understand the organogenesis of other adult organs, given the likely conservation of mechanistic motifs within developing endoderm. In addition, such an understanding may enable both the isolation of a multipotent, self-renewing pancreatic precursor population and the transformation of these precursors to functional β cells; such an achievement will have clear applications in cell replacement therapy for diabetes mellitus.[1]

In addition, recent studies have suggested a novel paradigm in which common mechanisms may be operative in both pancreatic development and pancreatic cancer.[2,3] Among these, significant evidence has implicated inappropriately activated Notch[4] and Hedgehog[5,6] signaling pathways as characteristic features of early pancreatic cancer. In this review, we present a mechanistic framework of normal pancreatic development, providing a basis for understanding how aberrant regulation of these mechanisms may contribute to pancreatic carcinogenesis.

Morphogenetic Events in Pancreatic Development

Our understanding of the morphogenetic events in pancreatic development has required little modification since the classic descriptive works of Wessels and Cohen[7] and Pictet and Rutter.[8] Gastrulation of the mammalian embryo leads to formation of the three germ layers, ectoderm, mesoderm, and endoderm. Further maturation of body plan with cephalic and lateral in-folding leads to the formation of an endoderm-lined gut tube rostrally and caudally, with a floorless central portion in open communication with the yolk sac. The rostral and caudal borders of this central portion define the anterior and posterior intestinal portals, respectively, and these portals together divide the embryonic gut into its three domains: foregut, midgut, and hindgut.[9] Foregut endoderm ultimately gives rise to numerous epithelial organs, including thyroid, lung, liver, pancreas, esophagus, stomach, and duodenum. Despite similarities between pancreatic islet cells and neuroendocrine cells of neural crest origin, chick-quail chimera experiments have definitively demonstrated an endodermal origin for both exocrine and endocrine pancreas.[10,11]

The morphogenesis of the pancreas is similar across a variety of vertebrates, including amphibians,[12] reptiles,[13] chicks,[14] and mammals. The earliest recognizable pancreatic anlagen are the dorsal and ventral pancreatic buds. These begin as simple evaginations of cuboidal endoderm, which then elaborate further to produce a complex branching epithelial tree.[15] The dorsal pancreatic bud forms first, followed closely by the emergence of the ventral pancreatic buds. The ventral buds emerge as paired bilateral structures, although the right ventral bud regresses along with the right vitelline vein in mammals, resulting in a single ventral pancreatic bud at later embryonic stages.[16] Dorsal and ventral pancreatic buds fuse later in development, in concert with rotation of the gut. In humans, the duct of Wirsung (main pancreatic duct) results from fusion of the pancreatic duct of the ventral bud with the distal pancreatic duct of the dorsal bud; the proximal portion in the dorsal bud normally regresses but occasionally persists as an accessory duct of Santorini.[9]

After the establishment of the dorsal and ventral pancreatic buds is a period of remarkable growth and cytodifferentiation, a period that has been most thoroughly described in rodent animal models. In the mouse, the dorsal bud appears at E9.5 (embryonic days post coitum, with birth on day 19–20), and a single ventral bud appears at E10.5; these two fuse by E12.5. Cells immunoreactive for glucagon and bearing characteristic alpha granules on electron microscopic examination are evident in the early dorsal pancreatic epithelium.[8,17] A subpopulation of these early endocrine hormone–producing cells co-express more than one endocrine hormone, including insulin, but lineage tracing studies suggest that these early glucagon-positive cells contribute to adult α, but not β, cells.[18] In the mouse pancreas, the insulin and digestive zymogen content of the pancreatic buds exponentially increases at E13.5. Pictet and Rutter[8] referred to this period of cytodifferentiation as the "secondary transition." By E14.5, distinct acinar structures are visible, composed of polarized epithelial cells with characteristic apical zymogen granules. By E18.5, clusters of organized islets are also apparent.[8]

As previously suggested,[1,19] pancreatic morphogenesis can be conceptually divided into three phases: first, the specification and formation of dorsal and ventral pancreatic buds from foregut endoderm, followed by extensive branching morphogenesis of the epithelial tree, and completed with cytodifferentiation of endocrine and exocrine cell types. The mechanisms governing each of these three steps can be further grouped into two categories. The first category is that of transcriptional machinery, in which the orderly activation or repression of specific transcription factors is required for normal pancreatic organogenesis. The second category is composed of signaling pathways, in which local paracrine or cell–cell interactions regulate the transcriptional machinery of a target progenitor cell. A significant amount of recent work has involved the genetic dissection of both the transcriptional machinery and the signaling pathways involved in pancreatic development.

Specification and Early Development of Pancreatic Anlagen

Transcriptional Machinery

Modern understanding of the transcriptional regulation of pancreatic development began with the observation that targeted inactivation of *Pdx1* (pancreas duodenum homeobox 1), a ParaHox homeodomain transcription factor, leads to aborted pancreatic morphogenesis with sparing of most other aspects of embryogenesis.[20] Four transcription factors are currently known to be important for early development of the pancreatic anlagen, largely revealed by germline knockout phenotypes. Targeted inactivation of the homeobox gene *Hlxb9* results in dorsal pancreatic agenesis in mice. Ventral pancreatic bud development is unaffected, except for a moderate reduction in insulin-positive cells and a subtle alteration of islet architecture.[21,22] *Hlxb9* is expressed in two phases during murine pancreatic development: initial, transient expression in dorsal and ventral pancreatic anlagen, followed by later expression in differentiated insulin-positive cells. Transgenic misexpression of *Hlxb9* driven by a *Pdx1* promoter leads to a severe failure in pancreatic differentiation, including the adoption of intestine-like characteristics in pancreatic epithelium.[23]

The LIM homeodomain transcription factor *Isl1* is required for formation of dorsal pancreatic mesenchyme. *Isl1*$^{-/-}$ mice fail to develop dorsal pancreatic mesenchyme and subsequently fail to develop a dorsal pancreatic bud; in contrast, the ventral mesenchymal environment in

$Isl1^{-/-}$ mice appears unaffected, and development of ventral pancreatic bud epithelium is normal. The $Isl1^{-/-}$ defect is localized to mesenchyme, as $Isl1^{-/-}$ endoderm is competent to form a dorsal pancreatic bud if recombined with $Isl1^{+/+}$ dorsal mesenchyme.[24]

The homeobox gene *Pdx1* was initially isolated in several independent lines of investigation: in *Xenopus* as *XlHbox8*, a novel homeobox gene whose expression during development was restricted to a narrow band of foregut, including pancreatic anlagen,[25] and in rodents as IPF-1 (insulin promoter factor 1),[26] IDX-1 (islet/duodenum homeobox 1),[27] and STF-1 (somatostatin transcription factor 1),[28] reflecting the ability of *Pdx1* to transactivate expression of insulin and somatostatin promoters in mature β and δ cells. In situ hybridization demonstrates early expression of *Pdx1* transcripts in E8.5 foregut surrounding the pancreatic anlagen, as well as expression throughout dorsal and ventral pancreatic buds by E10.5[29] (Figs. 5.1A and 5.1B). *Pdx1* expression is extinguished as cytodifferentiation progresses and is largely restricted to mature β and δ cells in the adult pancreas.[30] Evidence from mice that have the bacterial *lacZ* reporter knocked into the endogenous *Pdx1* locus,[31] as well as formal lineage tracing utilizing Cre-loxP techniques,[32] have demonstrated that

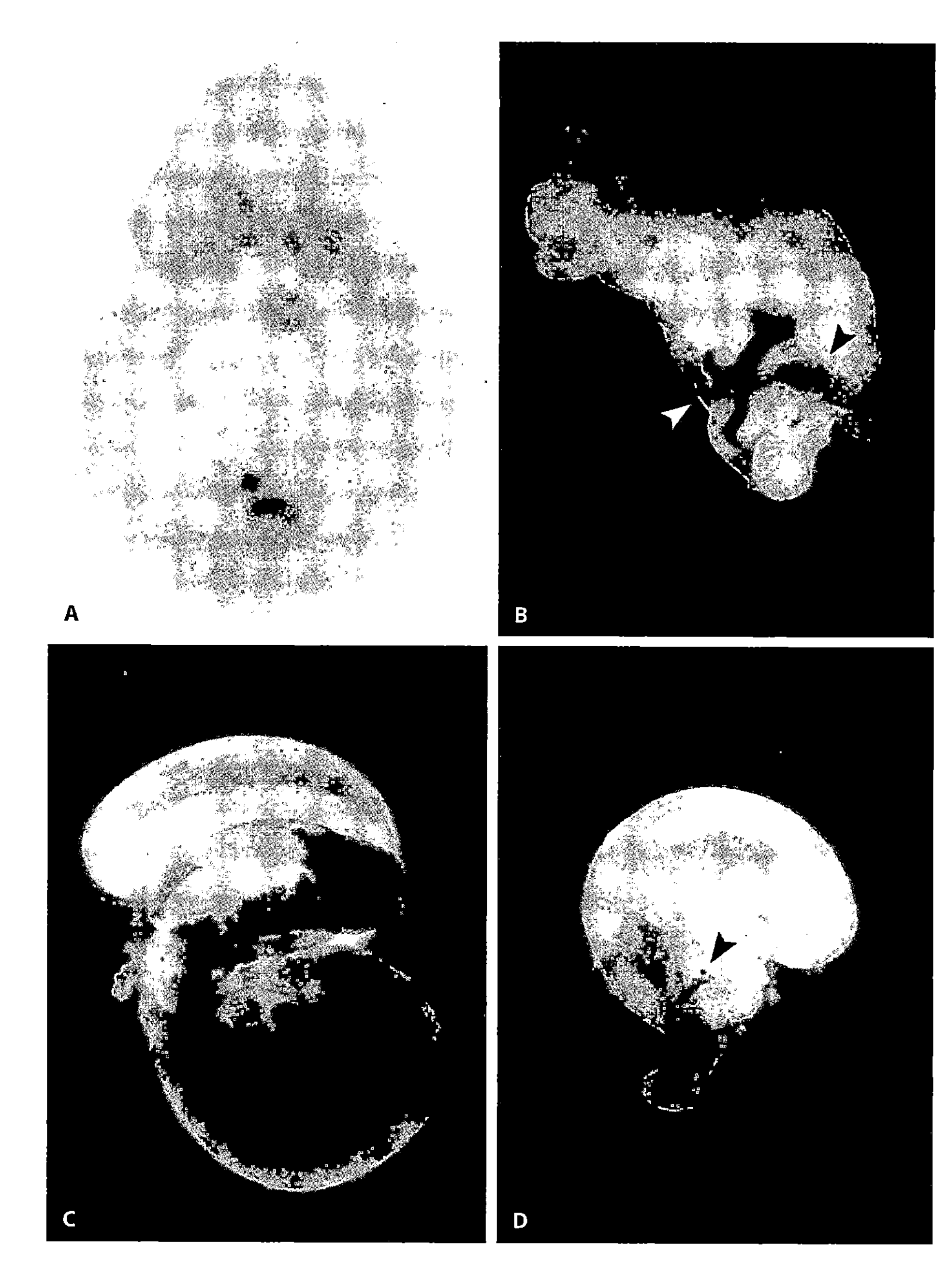

Figure 5.1
Pdx1 is expressed throughout developing pancreatic anlagen, and Pdx1 knockout mice have aborted pancreatic morphogenesis.[31] **(A)** and **(B)** Knock-in of lacZ into the endogenous Pdx1 locus and subsequent staining with X-Gal reveal normal domains of Pdx1 expression in Pdx1 lacZ/+ heterozygote embryos. **(A)** At E9.5, Pdx1 expression is found throughout nascent dorsal and ventral pancreatic buds. **(B)** At E11.5, expression persists throughout both dorsal and ventral buds (*arrowheads*), as well as in stomach, duodenum, and proximal hepatic diverticulum. **(C)** and **(D)** Comparison of X-Gal-stained Pdx1 lacZ/+ and Pdx1 lacZ/lacZ embryos at E16.5 reveals aborted pancreatic morphogenesis in Pdx1 knockouts. Pdx1 expression is seen throughout the dorsal and ventral pancreatic anlagen of Pdx1 lacZ/+ embryos at E16.5 **(C)** whereas E16.5 Pdx1 lacZ/lacZ mouse embryos, which lack PDX-1 protein, have a rudimentary pancreatic duct (*arrowhead*) and no pancreatic parenchyma **(D)**.

Pdx1-expressing cells contribute to adult stomach, duodenum, and distal bile duct, as well as to all acinar, endocrine, and ductal cells of the adult pancreas.

Targeted inactivation of *Pdx1* leads to aborted pancreatic morphogenesis.[20,33] *Pdx1*$^{-/-}$ mice do form a primitive pancreatic ductlike remnant as well as isolated clusters of differentiated glucagon-positive cells, but fail to form any acinar parenchyma or other endocrine cell types (Figs. 5.1C and 5.1D). Unlike *Isl1* knockouts, this effect is cell autonomous to endoderm; recombination of *Pdx1*$^{-/-}$ endoderm with wild-type mesenchyme fails to restore normal pancreatic development.[34] However, early hopes that *Pdx1* would be a master regulator of pancreatic development have yielded mixed results. Ectopic misexpression of *Pdx1* by in ovo electroporation of chick endoderm down-regulates several nonpancreatic transcription factors (e.g., *Hex*, *CdxA*) but fails to induce pancreatic bud formation or insulin production,[35] and misexpression of *Pdx1* in gastric and hindgut mesoderm (under control of the Hoxa4 promoter) failed to activate ectopic pancreas formation.[36] In contrast, adenoviral delivery of rat *Pdx1* driven by a cytomegalovirus (CMV) promoter to adult mouse liver results in endocrine hormone expression, persistent activation of endogenous *Pdx1*, and preserved glucostasis, despite ablation of pancreatic β cells by streptozotocin.[37,38] In addition, transgenic expression in *Xenopus* of a fusion protein combining a potent *VP16* transactivation domain with *Pdx1* results in expression of endocrine and exocrine markers within hepatic anlagen.[39] Therefore, overexpression of *Pdx1* in embryonic and mature liver is able to activate pancreas-specific gene expression, although neither experimental model is able to generate characteristic pancreatic structural elements, such as islets, acini, and ductal trees. Together, these results suggest that *Pdx1* is not required for the initial specification of pancreatic anlagen but plays a necessary role in subsequent morphogenesis and cytodifferentiation.

The class II basic helix-loop-helix (bHLH) transcription factor *Ptf1a-p48* is the exocrine pancreas-specific subunit of PTF1 (pancreas transcription factor 1), a heterotrimeric protein complex (PTF1a-P48, E47, REB) that is necessary and sufficient to transactivate expression of elastase, chymotrypsinogen, and several other acinar-specific digestive zymogens.[40] *Ptf1a-p48* is also expressed early in pancreatic development, within most cells of the nascent dorsal and ventral pancreatic buds. *Ptf1a-p48*$^{-/-}$ mice, like *Pdx1*$^{-/-}$ mice, fail to form a recognizable pancreas. *Ptf1a-p48*$^{-/-}$ mice are completely deficient in acinar cells. Although they do form differentiated endocrine hormone-producing cells, these endocrine cells are mislocated in isolated clusters along the remnant pancreatic mesentery and within the spleen, both of which are mesenchymal derivatives in close proximity to the dorsal pancreatic bud during development.[41] More recent work, employing genetically altered mice that have Cre recombinase knocked into the endogenous *Ptf1a-p48* locus, has demonstrated the expression of *Ptf1a-p48* during the ontogeny of all acinar and ductal cells, as well as most endocrine cells.[42] Interestingly, examination of *Ptf1a-p48*$^{Cre/Cre}$ mice revealed that cells that normally express *Ptf1a-p48* revert to an intestinal cell fate in the absence of PTF1a-P48 protein.[42] These results together suggest that *Ptf1a-p48*, like *Pdx1*, plays a necessary role in pancreatic development, determining pancreatic versus intestinal cell fates and controlling additional events subsequent to formation of the initial pancreatic bud. However, experiments involving ectopic overexpression of *Ptf1a-p48* remain to be conducted.

Signaling Pathways

In addition to the recognition of *Pdx1*, *Ptf1a-p48*, *Hlxb9*, and *Isl1* as important transcriptional regulators of early pancreatic development, modern experiments have uncovered important permissive and instructive roles for signaling molecules in early pancreatic development. Classic experiments have long suggested that soluble factors play an important role in pancreatic specification. In 1962, Golosow and Grobstein[43] reported that isolated E11.0 pancreatic buds failed to develop in vitro in the absence of mesenchyme; recombining these epithelial buds with mesenchyme—whether pancreatic or nonpancreatic—restored the ability of these in vitro cultured buds to develop a full complement of differentiated cell types. Furthermore, separation of the epithelial bud from the mesenchyme by a Millipore filter did not retard this trophic effect, suggesting that soluble growth factors were involved. In 1967, Wessels and Cohen[7] reported that early foregut endoderm (E8.0, 3–13 somites) was already competent to form pancreatic buds, if cultured in the presence of E11.0 pancreatic mesenchyme.[7] Attempts to purify a single "mesenchymal trophic factor" capable of driving pancreas development have been unsuccessful, reflecting the likely participation of multiple components.[44]

Hedgehog Signaling in Pancreatic Development

A significant body of evidence now implicates the soluble factor Sonic Hedgehog (*Shh*) and the Hedgehog signaling pathway in the specification of pancreatic anlagen. In the absence of ligand, the transmembrane Hedgehog receptor patched (*Ptc*) interacts with and inhibits the activity of another transmembrane protein, smoothened (*Smo*). Binding of a soluble Hedgehog ligand (Sonic, *Shh*, or Indian, *Ihh*) to *Ptc* results in derepression, and subsequent *Smo*-mediated activation of *Gli*, a nuclear transcription factor responsible for activation of Hedgehog-responsive target genes (Fig. 5.2).

Shh is widely expressed throughout intestinal epithelium at E9.5,[45] except in a sharply demarcated zone that marks the future dorsal and ventral pancreatic anlagen.[46] Mice ectopically misexpressing *Shh* in response to the *Pdx1* promoter fail to form a discrete pancreas but do bear exocrine zymogen and endocrine hormone-producing cells mislocated within intestinal-type epithelium.[46] Mice null for *Hhip*, a transmembrane protein that reduces Hedgehog signaling by binding and sequestering Hedgehog ligands, exhibit a similar but less dramatic phenotype.[47] Treatment of chick embryos with cyclopamine, an alkaloid inhibitor of *Shh* signaling, leads to pancreatic heterotopia throughout the foregut, consistent with an inhibitory influence of Hedgehog on pancreas specification during foregut development.[48]

Notochord, which is involved in dorsoventral patterning of neural floor plate through *Shh* signaling, appears to also regulate dorsal pancreatic bud patterning. Surgical removal of notochord in chick embryos results in failure of dorsal, but not ventral, pancreatic bud formation[49] as well as inappropriate expression of *Shh* in dorsal pancreatic anlage.[50] Ectopic grafting of notochord into chick embryos leads to down-regulation of *Shh* in adjacent intestinal endoderm.[50] The effect of notochord on *Shh* expression is reproducible by the soluble factors FGF2 (fibroblast growth factor 2) and activin-βB, a member of the TGF-β (transforming growth factor β) family.[50] Additional experiments in which foregut endoderm is co-cultured with isolated dorsal aortae have demonstrated a permissive role for signals from endothelium as well.[16] A series of in vivo chick-quail endoderm grafts have also suggested a potential instructive role of embryonic lateral plate mesoderm because peripancreatic lateral plate mesoderm is able to induce *Pdx1* expression in anterior, extrapancreatic endoderm; this effect is ablated by the activin antagonist follistatin and the BMP (bone morphogenetic protein) signaling pathway inhibitor noggin, suggesting that the TGF-β and BMP signaling pathways may mediate this instructive effect.[51]

In addition to patterning dorsal pancreas, *Shh* signaling also appears to regulate patterning of the ventral pancreatic bud. Unlike dorsal foregut endoderm, ventral pancreatic foregut endoderm from E8.0–8.5 embryos thrives in culture without a mesenchymal environment and adopts a pancreatic fate, as marked by *Pdx1* expression and *Shh* down-regulation. Culturing ventral pancreatic buds with FGF2 leads to down-regulation of *Pdx1* and expression of *Shh* and albumin, a marker of hepatic differentiation.[52] These results prompted a model in which ventral foregut endoderm is bipotential: *Shh* negative and pancreatic by default, converted to liver by mesenchymal signals. In contrast, dorsal foregut endoderm appears to be *Shh* positive and intestinal by default, converted to pancreas by signals from notochord and dorsal aorta.

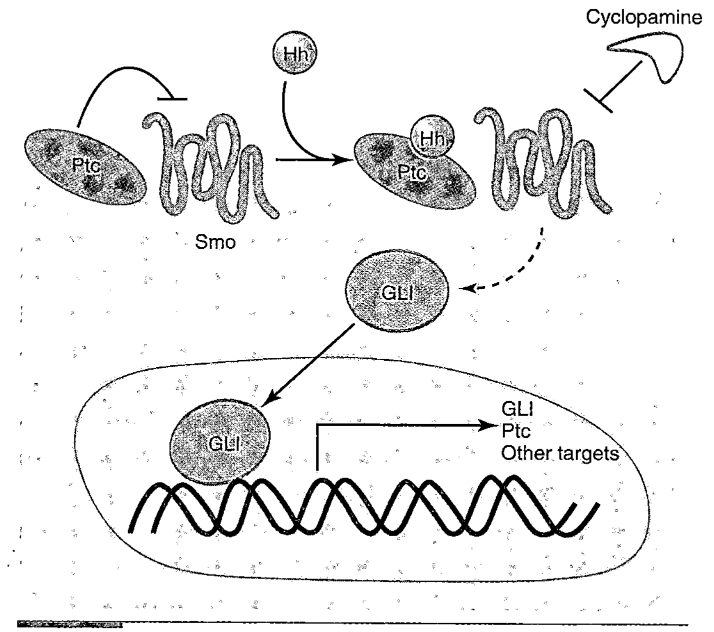

Figure 5.2
Hedgehog signaling pathway. In the absence of hedgehog ligand (*Hh*), the transmembrane protein Patched (*Ptc*) represses the seven-pass transmembrane protein Smoothened (*Smo*). The binding of hedgehog ligand leads to derepression of *Smo*, which is then able to activate the *Gli* family of nuclear transcription factors and induce expression of hedgehog target genes (e.g., *Gli*, *Ptc*). The steroidal alkaloid cyclopamine inhibits Hedgehog signal transduction through repression of *Smo*.

Endocrine and Exocrine Pancreatic Cytodifferentiation

Transcriptional Regulation of Endocrine Pancreatic Differentiation

Work over the past decade has identified numerous transcription factors necessary for normal endocrine differentiation. Neurogenin-3 (*ngn3*), a class II bHLH transcription factor, plays a unique role in the specification of endocrine precursors because targeted inactivation of *ngn3* leads to complete absence of all four differentiated endocrine cell types.[53] *ngn3* is expressed transiently in the pancreatic buds, with expression peaking at E15.5, coincident with the secondary transition of endocrine and exocrine cytodifferentiation. Expression is extinguished in adult pancreas, suggesting that *ngn3*-positive cells may represent an endocrine precursor population[54,55]; results of single-cell transcript analysis of developing pancreas support this view, with the onset of *ngn3* expression appearing to mark early commitment to an endocrine cell fate.[56] Overexpression of *ngn3* leads to an overabundance of differentiated endocrine cells in the pancreas, at the expense of exocrine cell types; these pancreata are hypomorphic, suggesting that *ngn3* overexpression may prematurely commit a precursor population to an endocrine cell fate, before normal proliferation and expansion of this precursor population can occur.[54,55]

Other transcription factors are also required for normal endocrine cytodifferentiation. The bHLH transcription factor *neuroD* (also known as BETA2, beta cell E-box transactivator-2) is inducible by *ngn3*[57] and enhances insulin promoter activity.[58] Targeted inactivation of *neuroD* leads to marked reduction of all endocrine cell types, but with preserved *ngn3* expression.[59] Knockout of the paired/homeodomain transcription factor *Pax4* leads to an absence of mature β and δ cells, with a preponderance of α cells and preservation of exocrine development, suggesting a role for *Pax4* as a switch favoring β/δ-cell fates over an α-cell fate.[60] Conversely, knockout of the related homeobox gene *Pax6* results in a pancreas with few or no α cells, in addition to significant reductions in β, δ, and PP cells.[61] *Nkx2.2*[62] and *Nkx6.1*[63] are members of the NK class of homeodomain proteins, both of which are broadly expressed in the early (E9.5/10.5) pancreatic bud and then progressively restricted to mature endocrine cells by E15.5. Knockout of either disrupts β-cell development, and analysis of double-knockout mice suggests that *Nkx6.1* lies downstream of *Nkx2.2*.[63]

Analysis of preserved endocrine cell types and preserved gene expression patterns in knockout phenotypes allows the epistatic ordering of these transcription factors into a preliminary, simplified cascade[58] (Fig. 5.3).

Transcriptional Regulation of Exocrine Pancreatic Differentiation

In contrast to the number of transcription factors known to be important in endocrine pancreatic differentiation, few elements of the exocrine pancreatic transcriptional machinery have been identified.[19] Single-cell transcript analysis has demonstrated co-expression of both *Nkx2.2* and *Nkx6.1* in putative exocrine pancreatic progenitors,[56] but the lack of a dramatic exocrine phenotype in respective knockouts[62,63] suggests that these NK class homeodomain transcription factors do not play a required role in exocrine cytodifferentiation.

Ptf1a-p48 is a class II bHLH transcription factor that, in the adult, is restricted to exocrine pancreas. Knockout mice have a dramatic exocrine phenotype, with a complete absence of differentiated acinar cells and only a rudimentary ductal remnant.[41] Endocrine cells of all four differentiated cell types persist in *Ptf1a-p48*$^{-/-}$ mice, but these are mislocated along the remnant pancreatic duct, along the pancreatic mesentery, and within the spleen. This knockout phenotype initially led to a model in which *Ptf1a-p48* is required for exocrine (but not endocrine) cytodifferentiation, with the endocrine phenotype resulting from lack of an exocrine parenchymal scaffolding for proper islet organization. However, subsequent lineage analysis of *Ptf1a-p48*$^{Cre/+}$ pancreata has implicated an additional direct role for *Ptf1a-p48* in the ontogeny of endocrine cell lineages.[42]

Mist1 is another recently identified class II bHLH transcription factor whose pancreatic expression is confined to acinar cells, although transcripts are also found in a variety of secretory extrapancreatic tissues, such as salivary acini, and serous cells of the stomach, prostate, and seminal vesicles.[64,65] In the embryonic pancreas, *Mist1* is detectable early (E10.5) in the dorsal pancreatic bud; at E14.0, when acinar structures are histologically distinct, *Mist1* expression is confined to acinar cells. *Mist1*$^{-/-}$ mice survive and at birth are reported to be grossly undistinguishable from control littermates. Examination of *Mist1*$^{-/-}$ mice later in life reveals defects in acinar cell organization and loss of acinar cell polarity; similar defects are also found in salivary and seminal vesicle epithelia.[66] The bHLH domain of *Mist1* is highly similar to that found in the recently characterized *Drosophila* transcription factor *dimmed*, which is required for amplified levels of secretory activity in *Drosophila* neuroendocrine cells.[67] Given the restriction of *Mist1* to secretory epithelial cell types in mammals, *dimmed* and *Mist1* may ultimately prove to be functional orthologs that both promote cellular machinery necessary to maintain a secretory cell type.

Signaling Pathways Regulating Endocrine and Exocrine Differentiation

Cre-loxP–based lineage tracing experiments suggest the existence of a multipotent pancreatic progenitor cell population that gives rise to the full complement of mature

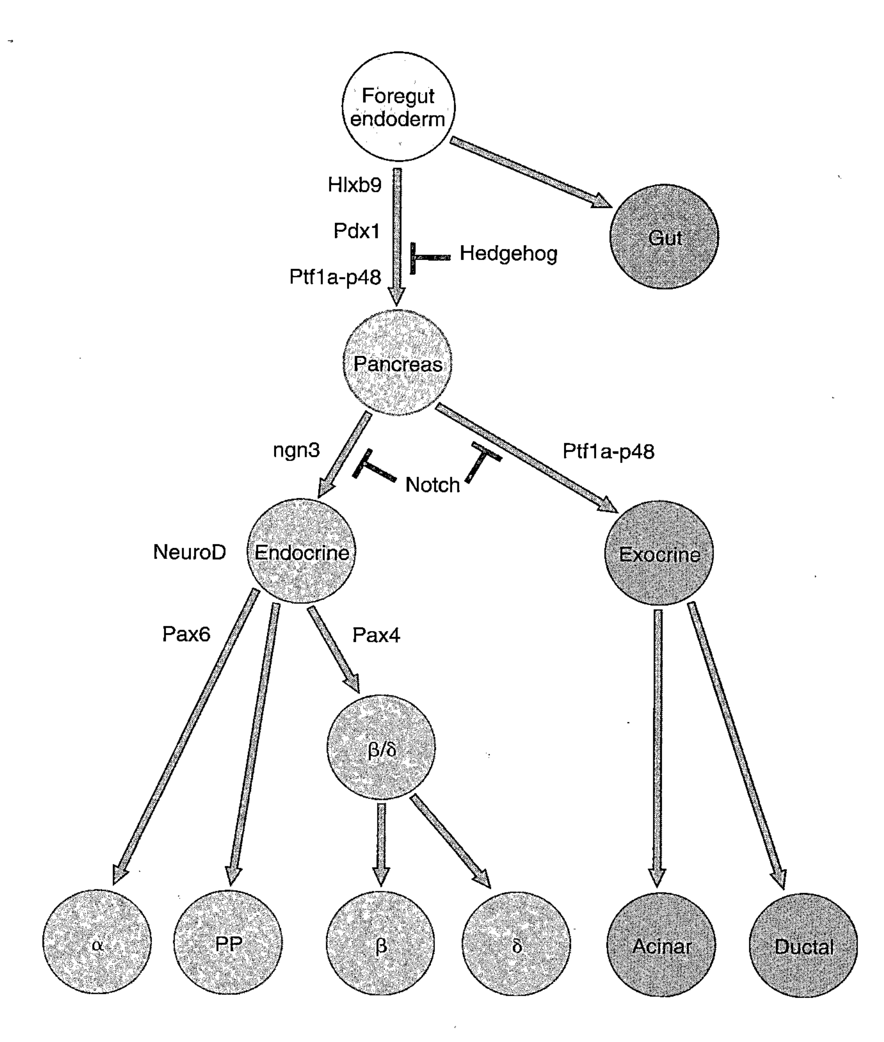

Figure 5.3
Schematic cascade of transcription factors in endocrine and exocrine pancreatic cytodifferentiation. Hlxb9, Pdx1, and Ptf1a-p48 are required for early formation of pancreatic anlage from foregut endoderm. The acquisition of ngn3 expression commits the precursor cell to an endocrine cell fate, marked by neuroD expression; Pax4 is required for β- and δ-cell differentiation, whereas Pax6 is required for α-cell differentiation. Active Hedgehog signaling appears to negatively regulate pancreas formation in foregut endoderm, diverting it toward an intestinal fate. Active Notch signaling appears to inhibit both endocrine and exocrine cytodifferentiation. PP, pancreatic polypeptide.

acinar, ductal, and endocrine lineages. Cells expressing the transcription factor *Pdx1* contribute to all differentiated epithelial cell types in the mature pancreas,[32] and cells expressing the transcription factor *Ptf1a-p48* contribute to all exocrine and most endocrine cell types.[42] Single-cell transcript analysis has also suggested the existence of a common precursor cell co-expressing *Pdx1*, *Ptf1a-p48*, *Nkx2.2*, and *Nkx6.1*. Precursor cells committed to an endocrine fate are marked by the acquisition of *ngn3* expression and loss of *Ptf1a-p48* expression, and cells committed to an exocrine fate are marked by the acquisition of *trypsin* and loss of *Nkx2.2* and *Nkx6.1*.[56] Accumulating evidence implicates several conserved signaling pathways in initiating (or preventing) cytodifferentiation within this multipotent pancreatic progenitor pool, as well as in altering the balance between endocrine and exocrine cell fates.

For example, members of the transforming growth factor-β (TGF-β) superfamily appear to affect the balance of endocrine and exocrine cytodifferentiation in in vitro models of pancreatic development. Treatment of cultured pancreatic buds with follistatin, an antagonist of activin and other members of the TGF-β superfamily, increases the ratio of acinar to endocrine cells.[68] Transgenic overexpression of a dominant negative TGF-β receptor leads to increased acinar cell mass and apoptosis.[69] Conversely, treatment of cultured pancreatic buds with TGF-β1 leads to an increased endocrine cell mass.[70]

E11.5 rat dorsal pancreatic buds cultured for 7 days in collagen gels fail to grow or develop exocrine differentiation in the absence of mesenchyme, but treatment with FGF1, FGF7, or FGF10 leads to marked growth and expansion of the exocrine, but not the endocrine, cell mass.[71] Treatment of naked E13.5 rat dorsal pancreatic buds cultured in collagen gels with epidermal growth factor (EGF) leads to a similar increase in epithelial cell mass, but with an apparent down-regulation of amylase, insulin, and glucagon expression. Withdrawal of EGF in these cultures is followed by the appearance of insulin expression throughout the enlarged bud.[72] Knockout mice lack-

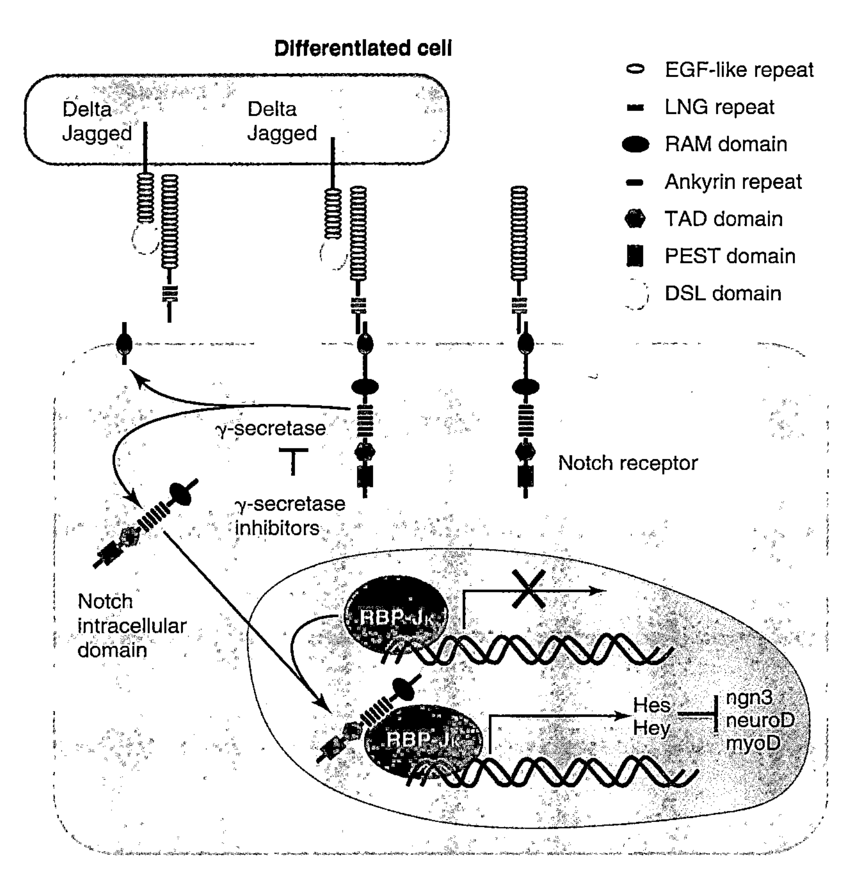

Figure 5.4
Notch signaling pathway in lateral inhibition. A differentiated cell expresses Notch ligands (e.g., Delta, Jagged) on its cell surface; these interact with Notch receptors on neighboring cells. This interaction leads to the γ-secretase–mediated release of the Notch intracellular domain (Notch ICD). This domain translocates to the nucleus and interacts with RBP-Jκ, converting it from a transcriptional repressor to a transcriptional activator. Notch target genes include the HES and HEY family of basic helix-loop-helix transcription factors, which generally act to maintain an undifferentiated, precursor state through repression of pro-cytodifferentiation genes, such as *ngn3*, *neuroD*, and *myoD*. Pharmacologic inhibition of Notch signaling can be induced by γ-secretase inhibitors, which prevent release of active Notch ICD. EGF, epidermal growth factor; LNG, Lin-12, Notch, Glp-1; TAD, transcriptional activator domain; PEST, proline-, glutamate-, serine-, threonine-rich domain; DSL, Delta, Serrate, Lag-2.

ing functional EGF receptors have a small pancreas with reduced endocrine cell mass; at birth, their pancreas lacks islets but has organized islet-like streaks of endocrine tissue along pancreatic ducts.[73] These results suggest that EGF receptor signaling may drive epithelial proliferation at the expense of epithelial differentiation. Mesenchymal-epithelial signaling mediated by a combination of EGF and FGF receptors and ligands may ultimately prove to illustrate Wessels and Cohen's elusive mesenchymal "trophic factor."[7]

Notch Signaling in Pancreatic Development

Several lines of evidence indicate that the Notch signaling pathway plays an important role in regulating pancreatic cytodifferentiation. The binding of cell-surface DSL (Delta, Serrate, Lag-2) ligands to Notch receptors on neighboring cells culminates in γ-secretase (presenilin-1)–mediated cleavage of the Notch receptor and liberation of the active intracellular domain.[74-76] This Notch intracellular domain translocates to the nucleus, where it interacts with RBP-Jκ (*Su(H)*, CBF-1), resulting in transactivation of Notch target genes, such as the HES (hairy enhancer of split) family of bHLH transcriptional repressors.[77] Notch effectors generally act to maintain cells in an undifferentiated, precursor state by further down-regulating pro-differentiation factors such as *achaete* and *scute* in *Drosophila* proneurons,[78] *myoD* in mammalian myoblasts,[79] and *ngn3* in mammalian islet cells.[80] Notch signaling also underlies the phenomenon of lateral inhibition seen in Drosophila neurogenesis, during which a committed neuron expresses DSL ligands and thus maintains its neighbors in an undifferentiated state[78] (Fig. 5.4).

Targeted inactivation of several Notch pathway components has been accomplished. Mice null for the Notch effector *Hes1* have a hypoplastic pancreas composed principally of endocrine cells, and largely devoid of exocrine parenchyma.[81] Knockout of the Notch ligand *Dll1* (delta-like ligand 1) leads to a similarly atrophic pancreas, consisting primarily of cells expressing endocrine lineage markers.[54] Knockout of RBP-Jκ leads to early embryonic death at E8.5–9.5, before pancreatic bud formation. Nevertheless, close examination of foregut endoderm at these stages reveals an increase in *ngn3*-positive cells, consistent with a pro-endocrine phenotype.[54] These results have been unified in a model in which active Notch signaling in a common precursor cell is required to prevent default endocrine cytodifferentiation. In the absence of Notch signaling, then, precocious endocrine differentiation occurs, resulting in a lack of exocrine cell types and pancreatic hypoplasia because cytodifferentiation occurs before proliferation of the undifferentiated precursor pool. However, recent work involving the transgenic overexpression of the active intracellular domain of *Notch1* by a *Pdx1* promoter has modified this view. In these mice, a paucity of both differentiated endocrine and exocrine cell types is observed, suggesting that active Notch signaling may act to reserve a population of precursor cells from either endocrine or exocrine differentiation, and that down-regulation of Notch is required for cytodifferentiation in either lineage.[82]

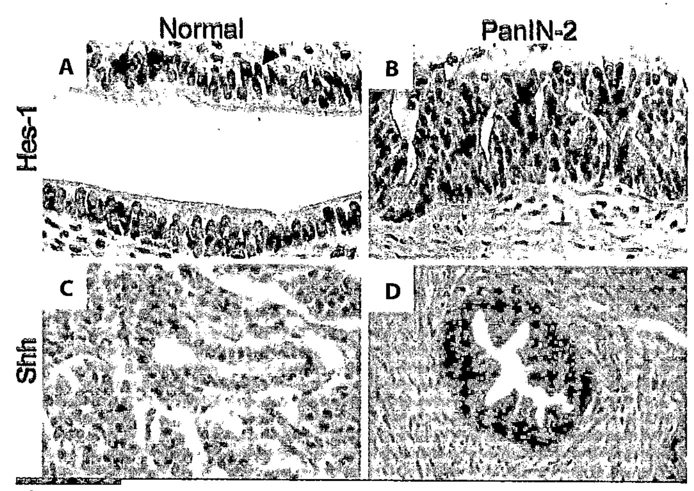

Figure 5.5
Notch and Hedgehog signaling pathways are inappropriately reactivated in early pancreatic cancer. The Notch effector HES-1 is detectable by immunohistochemistry in rare cells (*arrowhead*) of normal pancreatic ducts (**A**, 400×) but is detectable at high levels throughout PanIN-2 premalignant lesions (**B**, 400×). Similarly, Sonic hedgehog protein is absent in normal pancreatic ducts (**C**, 500×) but is expressed at moderate levels in PanIN-2 lesions (**D**, 250×). (Panels **A** and **B** adapted with permission from reference [4], and panels **C** and **D** adapted with permission from reference [6].)

Pancreatic Development and Pancreatic Cancer

Pathologic and molecular analysis of human pancreatic specimens has led to a stepwise progression model of human pancreatic carcinogenesis, analogous to the adenoma-carcinoma sequence described for colonic adenocarcinoma. In this model, the precursor lesion of pancreatic ductal adenocarcinoma is pancreatic intraepithelial neoplasia (PanIN), and several increasingly dysplastic grades of PanIN have been defined.[83] Molecular analysis of these lesions has revealed the stepwise accumulation of genetic defects, including mutations in *K-RAS*, *Smad4/DPC4*, and *TP53*.[84] In addition, recent evidence suggests that PanIN initiation may be related to changes in epithelial differentiation driven by signaling pathways that are normally active during foregut development.

The connection between pancreatic development and pancreatic cancer was first suggested by the observation that embryonic-like epithelium is expanded in early pancreatic cancer precursors.[2] Notably, human specimens of pancreatic ductal adenocarcinoma express a variety of cell-type markers, including those typically associated with acinar and ductal cells[85] as well as those associated with epithelial cells of the mature stomach, duodenum, and colon.[86] These expression patterns further support the concept that pancreatic carcinogenesis may be associated with the reacquisition of developmental pluripotency, acquired through a process of "de-differentiation."[3]

Murine PanIN-like lesions resulting from overexpression of the EGF ligand TGF-α are found to reactivate *Pdx1* and *Pax6*, transcriptional regulators normally extinguished in mature exocrine pancreas.[2] Notch pathway components are similarly extinguished in mature pancreatic ductal epithelium but are reactivated in specimens of human invasive pancreatic cancer and pancreatic intraepithelial neoplasia (PanIN)[4] (Figs. 5.5A and 5.5B). Using chip-based transcriptome comparisons and immunohistochemical analyses of human specimens, Miyamoto and colleagues[4] observed that multiple Notch pathway components were aberrantly up-regulated in PanIN and invasive pancreatic cancer. Notch receptors (*Notch1* through *Notch4*), ligands (*jag1*, *jag2*, *dlk1*), and target genes (*Hes1*, *Hes4*, *Hey1*, *HeyL*) were all up-regulated, suggesting the reactivation of a Notch signaling "module" in pancreatic cancer.[4] Further analysis demonstrated that Notch pathway activation is necessary and sufficient for in vitro TGF-α–induced transformation of isolated acinar cells to PanIN-like ductal lesions. Adenoviral delivery of activated Notch1 intracellular domain was able to induce acinar-to-ductal metaplasia in the absence of TGF-α, whereas addition of γ-secretase inhibitors (which interfere with endogenous Notch signaling) was able to ablate the metaplastic influence of TGF-α.[4] These results suggest that pancreatic neoplasia may be initiated by inappropriate reactivation of Notch signaling, a program normally active in embryonic, but not adult, pancreas.

In addition to reactivated Notch signaling, specimens of human pancreatic cancer also appear to be characterized by abnormal Hedgehog signaling. During mammalian pancreatic development, distinct mesenchymal signals from dorsal notochord or endothelium and ventral precardiac mesenchyme converge to extinguish sonic hedgehog (*Shh*) expression in pancreatic-fated endoderm. Similarly, no *Shh* expression is detectable in normal mature pancreas, including exocrine, endocrine, and ductal cell compartments. However, human PanIN lesions do express *Shh*, and at increasing levels with increasing grade of the lesion. PanIN-1 lesions express *Shh* and its receptor patched-1 (*Ptc1*) at low levels, whereas both PanIN-3 and invasive pancreatic cancer epithelia express these at moderate-to-high levels[6] (Figs. 5.5C and 5.5D). Up-regulation of Hedgehog pathway components is also found in many pancreatic cancer cell lines. As seen with Notch pathway components, Hedgehog receptors (*Ptc*), ligands (*Shh*, *Ihh*), and target genes (*Ptc*, *Gli*) are all up-regulated in a concerted manner.[5] Finally, *Ptc* transcript levels, a measure of Hedgehog pathway activity, were elevated in four of six human pancreatic cancers passaged as xenografts in nude mice.[5] Together, these results implicate up-regulation of Hedgehog signaling and Hedgehog pathway components in pancreatic cancers.

As with Notch pathway inhibition by γ-secretase inhibitors, endogenous Hedgehog signaling can be effectively ablated by the steroidal alkaloid cyclopamine. Treatment of human pancreatic cancer xenografts in nude mice with systemic cyclopamine led to a dramatic reduction of tumor mass in those four of six tumors that exhibited reactivated Hedgehog signaling (as assayed by *Ptc* transcripts)[5]; notably, growth of the other two of six tumors, with normal *Ptc* levels, was resistant to cyclopamine treatment. A similar, dose-dependent reduction in pancreatic cancer xenograft mass was also achieved by treatment with a neutralizing antibody, capable of binding Shh and Ihh ligands and preventing their interaction with the receptor *Ptc*.[5] Growth inhibition and increased apoptosis of pancreatic cancer cell lines are also seen after treatment with cyclopamine,[5,6] including dramatic reduction in tumor sizes of human pancreatic cancer cell lines transplanted into nude mice.[6] Finally, although transgenic misexpression of *Shh* by the *Pdx1* promoter typically converts pancreatic anlagen to an intestinal fate,[46] examination of pancreata that do form in these mice reveals numerous tubular complexes reminiscent of human PanIN.[6] Together, these results suggest that inappropriately active Hedgehog signaling is necessary for the maintenance, and potentially the induction, of human pancreatic cancer.

The paradigm of reactivated developmental pathways has also been observed in other models of epithelial cancer. In pulmonary epithelial development, Hedgehog signaling is transiently active in the embryonic period but is restricted in adult lungs to neuroendocrine progenitor cells. However, small-cell lung cancers have active Hedgehog signaling pathways, and inhibition by cyclopamine reduces the in vitro tumorigenicity of small-cell lung cancer cell lines.[87] Other work has implicated the wingless (Wnt) and Hedgehog signaling pathways in colon cancer and medulloblastoma,[88] and Notch activation appears capable of initiating malignant transformation in breast, lung, and myeloid precursors.[89] These observations in pancreatic and other epithelial cancers motivate the hypothesis that the earliest events in carcinogenesis may, in part, recapitulate regulatory programs that are normally active in development. The discovery of novel transcriptional regulators in pancreatic development may therefore affect our approach to tumor biology and may lead to novel strategies for chemotherapy, early detection, and chemoprevention.

References

1. Edlund H. Pancreatic organogenesis: developmental mechanisms and implications for therapy. *Nat Rev Genet.* 2002;3:524–532.
2. Song SY, Gannon M, Washington MK, et al. Expansion of Pdx1-expressing pancreatic epithelium and islet neogenesis in transgenic mice overexpressing transforming growth factor alpha. *Gastroenterology.* 1999;117:1416–1426.
3. Meszoely IM, Means AL, Scoggins CR, Leach SD. Developmental aspects of early pancreatic cancer. *Cancer J.* 2001;7:242–250.
4. Miyamoto Y, Maitra A, Ghosh B, et al. Notch mediates TGF alpha-induced changes in epithelial differentiation during pancreatic tumorigenesis. *Cancer Cell.* 2003;3:565–576.
5. Berman DM, Karhadkar SS, Maitra A, et al. Widespread requirement for Hedgehog ligand stimulation in growth of digestive tract tumours. *Nature.* 2003;425:846–851.
6. Thayer SP, Di Magliano MP, Heiser PW, et al. Hedgehog is an early and late mediator of pancreatic cancer tumorigenesis. *Nature.* 2003;425:851–856.
7. Wessels NK, Cohen JH. Early pancreas organogenesis: morphogenesis, tissue interactions, and mass effects. *Dev Biol.* 1967;15:237–270.
8. Pictet R, Rutter WJ. Development of the embryonic endocrine pancreas. In: Steiner DF, Frenkel N, eds. *Handbook of Physiology.* Vol Section 7, Volume 1. Washington, DC: Williams & Wilkins; 1972:25–66.
9. Carlson BM. *Human Embryology and Developmental Biology.* St. Louis, MO: Mosby; 1994.
10. Andrew A. An experimental investigation into the possible neural crest origin of pancreatic APUD (islet) cells. *J Embryol Exp Morphol.* 1976;35:577.

11. Fontaine J, Le Douarin NM. Analysis of endoderm formation in the avian blastoderm by the use of quail-chick chimaeras: the problem of the neuroectodermal origin of the cells of the APUD series. *J Embryol Exp Morphol.* 1977;41: 209–222.
12. Kelly OG, Melton DA. Development of the pancreas in *Xenopus laevis*. *Dev Dyn.* 2000;218:615–627.
13. Jackintell LA, Lance VA. Ontogeny and regional distribution of hormone-producing cells in the embryonic pancreas of Alligator mississippiensis. *Gen Comp Endocrinol.* 1994;94: 244–260.
14. Kim SK, Hebrok M, Melton DA. Pancreas development in the chick embryo. *Cold Spring Harb Symp Quant Biol.* 1997;62:377–383.
15. Slack JM. Developmental biology of the pancreas. *Development.* 1995;121:1569–1580.
16. Lammert E, Cleaver O, Melton D. Induction of pancreatic differentiation by signals from blood vessels. *Science.* 2001;294:564–567.
17. Herrera PL, Huarte J, Sanvito F, Meda P, Orci L, Vassalli JD. Embryogenesis of the murine endocrine pancreas: early expression of pancreatic polypeptide gene. *Development.* 1991;113:1257–1265.
18. Herrera PL. Adult insulin- and glucagon-producing cells differentiate from two independent cell lineages. *Development.* 2000;127:2317–2322.
19. Means AL, Leach SD. Lineage commitment and cellular differentiation in exocrine pancreas. *Pancreatology.* 2001;1: 587–596.
20. Jonsson J, Carlsson L, Edlund T, Edlund H. Insulin-promoter factor-1 is required for pancreas development in mice. *Nature.* 1994;371:606–609.
21. Harrison KA, Thaler J, Pfaff S, Gu H, Kehrl JH. Pancreas dorsal lobe agenesis and abnormal islets of Langerhans in Hlxb9-deficient mice. *Nat Genet.* 1999;23:71–75.
22. Li H, Arber S, Jessell TM, Edlund H. Selective agenesis of the dorsal pancreas in mice lacking homeobox gene Hlxb9. *Nat Genet.* 1999;23:67–70.
23. Li H, Edlund H. Persistent expression of Hlxb9 in the pancreatic epithelium impairs pancreatic development. *Dev Biol.* 2001;240:247i-253.
24. Ahlgren U, Pfaff S, Jessell TM, Edlund T, Edlund H. Independent requirement for ISL1 in the formation of the pancreatic mesenchyme and islet cells. *Nature.* 1997;385: 257–260.
25. Wright CV, Schnegelsberg P, De Robertis EM. XlHbox8: a novel homeoprotein restricted to a narrow band of endoderm. *Development.* 1988;104:787–794.
26. Ohlsson H, Karlsson K, Edlund T. IPF-1, a homeodomain-containing transactivator of the insulin gene. *EMBO J.* 1993;12:4251–4259.
27. Miller C, McGehee RE, Habener JF. IDX-1: a new homeodomain transcription factor expressed in rat pancreatic islets and duodenum that transactivates the somatostatin gene. *EMBO J.* 1994;13:1145–1156.
28. Leonard J, Peers B, Johnson T, Ferreri K, Lee S, Montminy MR. Characterization of somatostatin transactivating factor-1, a novel homeobox factor that stimulates somatostatin expression in pancreatic islet cells. *Mol Endocrinol.* 1993;7:1275–1283.
29. Guz Y, Montminy MR, Stein R, et al. Expression of murine STF-1, a putative insulin gene transcription factor, in β cells of pancreas, duodenal epithelium, and pancreatic exocrine and endocrine progenitors during ontogeny. *Development.* 1995;121:11–18.
30. Hui H, Perfetti R. Pancreas duodenum homeobox-1 regulates pancreas development during embryogenesis and islet cell function in adulthood. *Eur J Endocr.* 2002; 146:129–141.
31. Offield MF, Jetton JL, Labosky PA, et al. PDX-1 is required for pancreatic outgrowth and differentiation of the rostral duodenum. *Development.* 1996;122:983–995.
32. Gu G, Dubauskaite J, Melton DA. Direct evidence for the pancreatic lineage: NGN3+ cells are islet progenitors and are distinct from duct progenitors. *Development.* 2002;129:2447–2457.
33. Holland AM, Hale MA, Kagami H, Hammer RE, MacDonald RJ. Experimental control of pancreatic development and maintenance. *Proc Natl Acad Sci USA.* 2002; 99:12236-41.
34. Ahlgren U, Jonsson J, Edlund H. The morphogenesis of the pancreatic mesenchyme is uncoupled from that of the pancreatic epithelium in IPF1/PDX1-deficient mice. *Development.* 1996;122:1409–1416.
35. Grapin-Botton A, Majithia AR, Melton DA. Key events of pancreas formation are triggered in gut endoderm by ectopic expression of pancreatic regulatory genes. *Genes Dev.* 2001;15:444–454.
36. Heller RS, Stoffers DA, Hussain MA, Miller CP, Habener JF. Misexpression of the pancreatic homeodomain protein IDX-1 by the Hoxa-4 promoter associated with agenesis of the cecum. *Gastroenterology.* 1998;115:381–387.
37. Ber I, Shternhall K, Perl S, et al. Functional, persistent, and extended liver to pancreas transdifferentiation. *J Biol Chem.* 2003;278:31950–31957.
38. Ferber S, Halkin A, Cohen H, et al. Pancreatic and duodenal homeobox gene 1 induces expression of insulin genes in liver and ameliorates streptozotocin-induced hyperglycemia. *Nat Med.* 2000;6:568–572.
39. Horb ME, Shen C, Tosh D, Slack JM. Experimental conversion of liver to pancreas. *Curr Biol.* 2003;13:105–115.
40. Krapp A, Knofler M, Frutiger S, Hughes GJ, Hagenbuchle O, Wellauer PK. The p48 DNA-binding subunit of transcription factor PTF1 is a new exocrine pancreas-specific basic helix-loop-helix protein. *EMBO J.* 1996; 15:4317–4329.
41. Krapp A, Knöfler M, Ledermann B, et al. The bHLH protein PTF1-p48 is essential for the formation of the exocrine and the correct spatial organization of the endocrine pancreas. *Genes Dev.* 1998;12:3752–3763.
42. Kawaguchi Y, Cooper B, Gannon M, Ray M, MacDonald RJ, Wright CVE. The role of the transcriptional regulator PTF1-p48 in converting intestinal to pancreatic progenitors. *Nat Genet.* 2002;32:128–134.
43. Golosow N, Grobstein C. Epitheliomesenchymal interaction in pancreatic morphogenesis. *Dev Biol.* 1962;4:242–255.

44. Ronzio RA, Rutter WJ. Effects of a partially purified factor from chick embryos on macromolecular synthesis of embryonic pancreatic epithelia. *Dev Biol.* 1973;30:307–320.
45. Bitgood MJ, McMahon AP. Hedgehog and BMP genes are coexpressed at many diverse sites of cell-cell interaction in the mouse embryo. *Dev Biol.* 1995;172:126–138.
46. Apelqvist A, Ahlgren U, Edlund H. Sonic hedgehog directs specialised mesoderm differentiation in the intestine and pancreas. *Curr Biol.* 1997;7:801–804.
47. Kawahira H, Ma NH, Tzanakakis ES, McMahon AP, Chuang P, Hebrok M. Combined activities of hedgehog signaling inhibitors regulate pancreas development. *Development.* 2003;130:4871–4879.
48. Kim SK, Melton DA. Pancreas development is promoted by cyclopamine, a Hedgehog signaling inhibitor. *Proc Natl Acad Sci USA.* 1998;95:13036–13041.
49. Kim SK, Hebrok M, Melton DA. Notochord to endoderm signaling is required for pancreas development. *Development.* 1997;124:4243–4252.
50. Hebrok M, Kim SK, Melton DA. Notochord repression of endodermal Sonic hedgehog permits pancreas development. *Genes Dev.* 1998;12:1705–1713.
51. Kumar M, Jordan N, Melton D, Grapin-Botton A. Signals from lateral plate mesoderm instruct endoderm toward a pancreatic fate. *Dev Biol.* 2003;259:109–122.
52. Deutsch G, Jung J, Zheng M, Lora J, Zaret JS. A bipotential precursor population for pancreas and liver within the embryonic endoderm. *Development.* 2001;128:871–881.
53. Gradwohl O, Dierich A, LeMeur M, Guillemot F. Neurogenin3 is required for the development of the four endocrine cell lineages of the pancreas. *Proc Natl Acad Sci USA.* 2000;97:1607–1611.
54. Apelqvist A, Li H, Sommer L, et al. Notch signalling controls pancreatic cell differentiation. *Nature.* 1999;400:877–881.
55. Schwitzgebel VM, Scheel DW, Conners JR, et al. Expression of neurogenin3 reveals an islet cell precursor population in the pancreas. *Development.* 2000;127:3533–3542.
56. Chiang M, Melton DA. Single-cell transcript analysis of pancreas development. *Dev Cell.* 2003;4:383–393.
57. Huang HP, Liu M, El-Hodiri HM, Chu K, Jarnrich M, Tsai MJ. Regulation of the pancreatic islet-specific gene BETA2 (neuroD) by neurogenin 3. *Mol Cell Biol.* 2000;20:3292–3307.
58. Schwitzgebel VM. Programming of the pancreas. *Mol Cell Endocrinol.* 2001;185:99–108.
59. Naya FJ, Huang HP, Qiu Y, et al. Diabetes, defective pancreatic morphogenesis, and abnormal enteroendocrine differentiation in BETA2/neuroD-deficient mice. *Genes Dev.* 1997;11:2323–2324.
60. Sosa-Pineda B, Chowdhury K, Torres M, Oliver G, Gruss P. The Pax4 gene is essential for differentiation of insulin-producing beta cells in the mammalian pancreas. *Nature.* 1997;386:399–402.
61. St. Onge L, Sosa-Pineda B, Chowdhury K, Mansouri A, Gruss P. Pax6 is required for differentiation of glucagon-producing alpha-cells in mouse pancreas. *Nature.* 1997;387:406–409.
62. Sussel L, Kalamaras J, Hartigan-O'Connor DJ, et al. Mice lacking the homeodomain transcription factor Nkx2.2 have diabetes due to arrested differentiation of pancreatic beta cells. *Development.* 1998;125:2213–2221.
63. Sander M, Sussel L, Conners JR, et al. Homeobox gene Nkx6.1 lies downstream of Nkx2.2 in the major pathway of β-cell formation in the pancreas. *Development.* 2000;127:5533–5540.
64. Lemercier C, To RQ, Carrasco RA, Konieczny SF. The basic helix-loop-helix transcription factor Mist1 functions as a transcriptional repressor of MyoD. *EMBO J.* 1998;17:1412–1422.
65. Pin CL, Bonvissuto AC, Konieczny SF. Mist1 expression is a common link among serous exocrine cells exhibiting regulated exocytosis. *Anat Rec.* 2000;259:157–167.
66. Pin CL, Rukstalis JM, Johnson C, Konieczny SF. The bHLH transcription factor Mist1 is required to maintain exocrine pancreas cell organization and acinar cell identity. *J Cell Biol.* 2001;155:519–530.
67. Hewes RS, Park D, Gauthier SA, Schaefer AM, Taghert PH. The bHLH protein Dimmed controls neuroendocrine cell differentiation in *Drosophila*. *Development.* 2003;130:1771–1781.
68. Gittes GK, Galante PE, Hanahan D, Rutter WJ, Debas HT. Lineage-specific morphogenesis in the developing pancreas: role of mesenchymal factors. *Development.* 1996;122:439–447.
69. Bottinger EP, Jakubczak JL, Roberts ISD, et al. Expression of a dominant-negative mutant TGF-β type II receptor in transgenic mice reveals essential roles for TGF-β in regulation of growth and differentiation in the exocrine pancreas. *EMBO J.* 1997;16:2621–2633.
70. Sanvito F, Herrera PL, Huarte J, et al. TGF-β1 influences the relative development of the exocrine and endocrine pancreas in vitro. *Development.* 1994;120:3451–3462.
71. Miralles F, Czernichow P, Ozaki K, Itoh N, Scharfmann R. Signaling through fibroblast growth factor receptor 2b plays a key role in the development of the exocrine pancreas. *Proc Natl Acad Sci USA.* 1999;96:6267–6272.
72. Cras-Meneur C, Elghazi L, Czernichow P, Scharfmann R. Epidermal growth factor increases undifferentiated pancreatic embryonic cells in vitro: a balance between proliferation and differentiation. *Diabetes.* 2001;50:1571–1579.
73. Miettinen PJ, Huotari M, Koivisto T, et al. Impaired migration and delayed differentiation of pancreatic islet cells in mice lacking EGF-receptors. *Development.* 2000;127:2617–2627.
74. Mumm JS, Kopan R. Notch signaling: from the outside in. *Dev Biol.* 2000;228:151–165.
75. Fleming RJ. Structural conservation of Notch receptors and ligands. *Semin Cell Dev Biol.* 1998;9:599–607.
76. Baron M. An overview of the Notch signalling pathway. *Semin Cell Dev Biol.* 2003;14:113–119.
77. Beatus P, Lendahl U. Notch and neurogenesis. *J Neurosci Res.* 1998;54:125–136.
78. Fisher A, Caudy M. The function of hairy-related bHLH repressor proteins in cell fate decisions. *Bioessays.* 1998;20:298–306.

79. Kuroda K, Tani S, Tamura K, Minoguchi S, Kurooka H, Honjo T. Delta-induced Notch signaling mediated by RBP-J inhibits MyoD expression and myogenesis. *J Biol Chem.* 1999;274:7238–7244.
80. Lee JC, Smith SB, Watada H, et al. Regulation of the pancreatic pro-endocrine gene neurogenin3. *Diabetes.* 2001;50: 928–936.
81. Jensen J, Pedersen EE, Galante P, et al. Control of endodermal endocrine development by Hes-1. *Nat Genet.* 2000;24:36–44.
82. Hald J, Hjorth JP, German MS, Madsen OD, Serup P, Jensen J. Activated Notch1 prevents differentiation of pancreatic acinar cells and attenuate endocrine development. *Dev Biol.* 2003;260:426–437.
83. Hruban RH, Wilentz RE, Goggins M, Offerhaus GJ, Yeo CJ, Kern SE. Pathology of incipient pancreatic cancer. *Ann Oncol.* 1999;10[suppl. 4]:S9–S11.
84. Maitra A, Adsay NV, Argani P, et al. Multicomponent analysis of the pancreatic adenocarcinoma progression model using a pancreatic intraepithelial neoplasia tissue microarray. *Mod Pathol.* 2003;16:902–912.
85. Kim JH, Ho SB, Montgomery CK, Kim YS. Cell lineage markers in pancreatic cancer. *Cancer.* 1990;66:2134–2143.
86. Sessa F, Bonato M, Frigerio B, et al. Ductal cancers of the pancreas frequently express markers of gastrointestinal epithelial cells. *Gastroenterology.* 1990;98:1655–1665.
87. Watkins DN, Berman DM, Burkholder SG, Wang B, Beachy PA, Baylin SB. Hedgehog signalling within airway epithelial progenitors and in small-cell lung cancer. *Nature.* 2003;422:313–317.
88. Taipale J, Beachy PA. The hedgehog and Wnt signalling pathways in cancer. *Nature.* 2001;411:349–354.
89. Ball DW, Leach SD. Notch in malignancy. *Cancer Treat Res.* 2003;115:95–121.

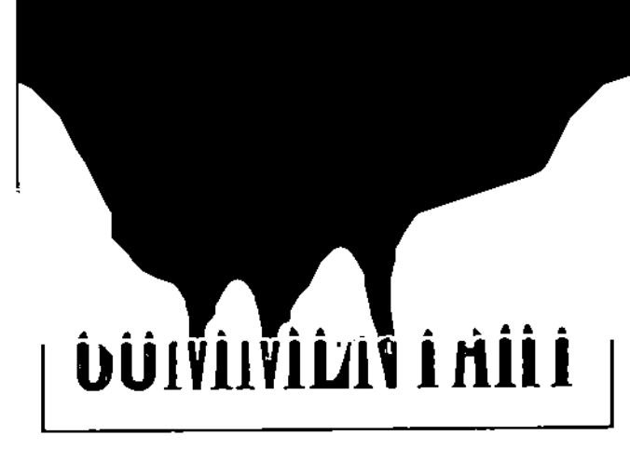

Sarah P. Thayer, MD, PhD

During development, the identity and patterning of the pancreas from the vertebrate foregut endoderm depends on the complex interactions of transcription factors and signal transduction pathways. Many of these factors are involved in decisions determining mechanisms that regulate self-renewal, differentiation, proliferation, and migration, which ultimately determine the fate of cells. It thus comes as no surprise that aberrant regulation of these developmental pathways has a critical role in the development of cancer. This chapter nicely summarizes our basic understanding of pancreatic development and how these genes and signaling pathways may contribute to pancreatic cancer, finally allowing us to make sense of old observations.

One unexplained observation mentioned by these authors is that ductal adenocarcinoma and its precursor lesions share many histologic features with the gastrointestinal epithelium. Infiltrating carcinoma of the pancreas appears to arise from histologically well-defined noninvasive precursor lesions, which have been termed PanINs (pancreatic intraepithelial neoplasias). Histologically, infiltrating ductal adenocarcinomas are composed of an atypical epithelium that recapitulates ductal structures, "tubular complexes" embedded in a dense reactive fibrosis.[1] In this progression, the normal cuboidal epithelium of the pancreatic ducts is replaced by an abnormal mucin-containing columnar epithelium that histologically resembles gastrointestinal epithelium. In humans, the pattern of mucin expression in the pancreatic epithelium can be a marker for neoplastic progression and malignant transformation.

PanIN and adenocarcinoma overexpress gastric mucins MUC1, MUC5AC, and MUC6, as well as a colonic mucin, MUC4, but not MUC2, an intestinal mucin.[2,3]

The abnormal epithelium of pancreatic cancer also frequently expresses other markers of gastrointestinal epithelial cells. Immunohistochemical staining has disclosed antigens normally found in gastric, colonic, and/or intestinal epithelial cells; these antigens included M1 and cathepsin E, markers of gastric surface-foveolar epithelial cells; pepsinogen II, a marker of gastroduodenal mucopeptic cells; CAR-5, a marker of colorectal epithelial cells; and M3SI, a marker of small-intestinal goblet cells.[4] Furthermore, this abnormal epithelium has even been found by ultrastructural analysis to have microvilli[5] and fine structural features characteristic of gastric foveolar cells, gastric mucopeptic cells, intestinal goblet cells, intestinal columnar cells, pancreatic duct epithelial cells, and cells with features of more than one cell type,[4] indicating that both precursor lesions (PanINs) and invasive adenocarcinoma of the pancreas may show gastric- and intestinal-type differentiation. Understanding pancreatic development has shed light on the molecular mechanisms that drive these metaplastic and atypical changes of the pancreatic epithelium.

PanIN lesions may represent a form of gastrointestinal metaplasia/neoplasia mediated by changes in Hh signaling. As described in Chapter 5, the Shh pathway plays a fundamental role in pancreatic development and appears to be an important and critical initiator of pancreatic cancer. Shh is expressed throughout the gut endoderm but is noticeably absent from the endoderm of the pancreatic bud.[6,7] Restriction of Shh in the endoderm is in fact critical for pancreatic development. In contrast, Shh exerts a significant inductive influence on the development of the gut, being important for morphogenesis and cytodifferentiation.[8,9] Here, Shh plays a pivotal and differentiative role, acting as a key switch between the fates of gastrointestinal and pancreatic cells. The fact that Shh, which is absent from the normal pancreas, is identified in human pancreatic cancer and its precursor lesions suggests that Shh may be responsible for these histologic changes that characterize pancreatic cancer by altering the developmental program. When Shh is misexpressed in Pdx-Shh mice, they form abnormal pancreata with features that histologically, immunohistochemically, and genetically resemble human pancreatic intraepithelial neoplastic lesions.[10] The epithelia of these mice, like those of human pancreatic adenocarcinoma, have an abnormal gastrointestinal-like organization of the epithelium and share histologic and immunohistochemical markers for gastrointestinal epithelial differentiation.

Shh may also play an important role in redirecting the mesenchyme of the pancreas in cancer. Human adenocarcinoma is characterized not only by abnormal epithelium but also by extensive desmoplastic reactions. Developmental studies have revealed that Shh misexpressed in the gut results in hyperplasia of gut-specific mesenchyme.[8,11] Similarly, misexpression of Shh in the developing pancreas of a mouse also results in the redirection of pancreatic mesenchyme into an intestinal mesenchyme.[12] Thus, Shh may play a critical and early role in the development of human pancreatic ductal malignancy via a gastrointestinal differentiation of both the epithelium and the mesenchyme.

Another long-standing observation is that cancer is by definition a disease of unregulated growth and self-renewal. Recently, the scientific community has identified similarities between stem cells and cancer cells, which suggest the existence of cancer stem cells—cells that possess indefinite potential for self-renewal and that drive tumorigenesis.[13] Perhaps one of the most striking similarities between stem cells and cancer cells/cancer stem cells is their capacity for indefinite self-renewal, their unlimited replicative potential, and their ability to give rise to cells that are phenotypically heterogeneous.[13-15] Therefore, stem cells and cancer cells may use similar pathways/mechanisms to regulate self-renewal. Understanding the normal developmental mechanisms that contribute to the regulation of normal stem cells may allow us to understand pancreatic cancer. Signaling pathways that are important in pancreatic development and that regulate stem cell renewal include Notch and Shh. Both of these pathways are aberrantly regulated in pancreatic cancer. The Notch and Shh pathways contribute to stem cell renewal in the retinal epithelium, in germline cells, and in the nervous and hematopoietic systems.[16-18] In the pancreas, Notch regulates differentiation of epithelial precursors, thereby preventing cellular differentiation, and appears to be important in maintaining a population of undifferentiated precursor cells.[19-21] Similarly, during development, Shh also inhibits terminal differentiation and maintains a high proliferative rate of precursor cells.[22] However, there is increasing evidence that suggests that these pathways also play a role in adult patterning and growth by regulating stem cell renewal in epithelia.[13,15,23] The Shh pathway, for example, now appears to play a role in the maintenance of gastric gland progenitor cells. Therefore, with the discovery that pancreatic neoplasia represents abnormal proliferative activity of cells capable of multipotential fates (gastric, intestinal, and colonic phenotypes), it is interesting to speculate that the misexpression of Shh and Notch may result in misspecification of cells toward a gastrointestinal stem cell-like fate.

The mechanisms by which these developmental genes act remain to be determined. Because pancreatic adenocarcinoma expresses different gastrointestinal markers, one mechanism that these authors suggest is the reacquisition, through a process of "dedifferentiation," of developmental pluripotency. However, some evidence suggests that stem cells themselves are targets of mutation.[13] In pancreatic cancer, however, as opposed to basal cell skin cancer, the mutations that activate the Shh pathway have yet to be identified; investigations suggest that activation of the Shh pathway may be initiated by ligand misexpression rather than by mutations.[24] Regardless of the mechanism—dedifferentiation, transdifferentiation, or an expansion of an already existent progenitor cell—what is clear is that developmental genes are being found to play an important role in altering the phenotype and proliferative potential of pancreatic cancer, allowing us to explain its malignant biologic behavior as well as its histology.

The search for the events underlying pancreatic development has led to a greater understanding of the molecular mechanisms that may govern and regulate the initiation, progression, and maintenance of pancreatic cancer, and that may one day lead to novel therapeutic and diagnostic approaches. Using developmental genes as targets for treatments has the potential advantage of allowing us to "turn off" not just one gene, but a host of genes that regulate growth and survival.

References

1. Wilentz RE, Hruban RH. Pathology of pancreatic cancer. In: Cameron JL, ed. *Pancreatic Cancer*. American Cancer Society Atlas of Clinical Oncology series. Hamilton, Ontario: BC Decker Inc.; 2001:37–66.
2. Kim GE, Bae HI, Park HU, et al. Aberrant expression of MUC5AC and MUC6 gastric mucins and sialyl Tn antigen in intraepithelial neoplasms of the pancreas. *Gastroenterology*. 2002;123:1052–1060.
3. Ringel J, Löhr M. The MUC gene family: their role in diagnosis and early detection of pancreatic cancer. *Mol Cancer*. 2003;2:9.
4. Sessa F, Bonato M, Frigerio B, et al. Ductal cancers of the pancreas frequently express markers of gastrointestinal epithelial cells. *Gastroenterology*. 1990;98:1655–1665.
5. Cubilla AL, Fitzgerald PJ. *Tumors of the Exocrine Pancreas*. 2nd edition. Washington DC: Armed Forces Institute of Pathology; 1984.
6. Ahlgren U, Jonsson J, Edlund H. The morphogenesis of the pancreatic mesenchyme is uncoupled from that of the pancreatic epithelium in IPF1/PDX1-deficient mice. *Development*. 1996;122:1409–1416.
7. Ahlgren U, Pfaff SL, Jessell TM, et al. Independent requirement for ISL1 in formation of pancreatic mesenchyme and islet cells. *Nature*. 1997;385:257–260.
8. Roberts DJ. Embryology of the gastrointestinal tract. In: Sanderson IR, Walker WA, eds. *Development of the Gastrointestinal Tract*. Hamilton, Ontario: BC Decker Inc.; 2000:1–12.
9. Fukuda K, Yasugi S. Versatile roles for sonic hedgehog in gut development. *J Gastroenterol*. 2002;37:239–246.
10. Thayer SP, Pasca di Magliano M, Heiser P, et al. Hedgehog is an early and late mediator of pancreatic cancer tumorigenesis. *Nature*. 2003;425:851–856.
11. Wicking C, Smyth I, Bale A. The hedgehog signaling pathway in tumorigenesis and development. *Oncogene*. 1999;18:7844–7851.
12. Apelqvist A, Ahlgren U, Edlund H. Sonic hedgehog directs specialized mesoderm differentiation in the intestine and pancreas. *Curr Biol*. 1997;7:801–804.
13. Reya T, Morrison SJ, Clarke MF, et al. Stem cells, cancer, and cancer stem cells. *Nature*. 2001;414:105–111.
14. Hanahan D, Weinberg RA. The hallmarks of cancer. *Cell*. 2000;100:57–70.
15. Taipale J, Beachy PA. The Hedgehog and Wnt signaling pathways in cancer. *Nature*. 2001;411:349–354.
16. Austin J, Kimble C. *glp-1* is required in the germ line for regulation of the decision between mitosis and meiosis in C. elegans. *Cell*. 1987;51:589–599.
17. Henrique D, Hirsinger E, Adam J, et al. Maintenance of neuroepithelial progenitor cells by Delta-Notch signaling in the embryonic chick retina. *Current Biol*. 1997;7:661–670.
18. Varnum-Finney B, Xu L, Brashem-Stein C, et al. Pluripotent cytokine-dependent, hematopoietic stem cells are immortalized by constitutive Notch1 signaling. *Nature Med*. 2000;6:1278–1281.
19. Apelqvist A, Li H, Sommer L, et al. Notch signaling controls pancreatic cell differentiation. *Nature*. 1999;400:877–881.

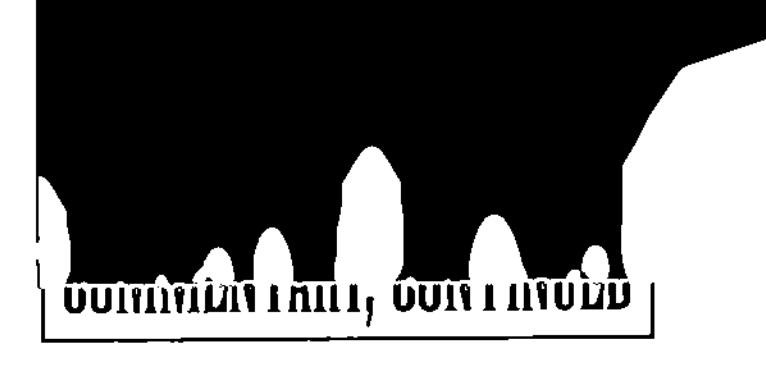

20. Jensen J, Heller RS, Funder-Nielsen T, et al. Independent development of pancreatic alpha- and beta-cells from neurogenin3-expressing precursors: a role for the notch pathway in repression of premature differentiation. *Diabetes*. 2000;49:163–176.
21. Murtaugh LC, Stanger BZ, Kwan KM, Melton DA. Notch signaling controls multiple steps of pancreatic differentiation. *Proc Natl Acad Sci USA*. 2003;100:14920–14925.
22. Wechsler-Reya R, Scott MP. The developmental biology of brain tumors. *Annu Rev Neurosci*. 2001;24:385–428.
23. van den Brink G, Hardwick JCH, Tytgat GNJ, et al. Sonic hedgehog regulates gastric gland morphogenesis in man and mouse. *Gastroenterology*. 2001;121:317–328.
24. Berman DM, Karhadkar SS, Maitra A, et al. Widespread requirement for Hedgehog ligand stimulation in growth of digestive tract tumours. *Nature*. 2003;425:846–851.

6

Mouse Models of Exocrine Pancreatic Cancer

Eric P. Sandgren, VMD, PhD

Many approaches are available for studying human disease, including the use of animals as surrogates for the human patient. Several species have been used to study pancreatic cancer, typically by evaluating the consequences of administering carcinogenic chemicals. This chapter addresses the current emphasis on the use of genetically manipulated mice to study exocrine pancreatic cancer. Changes in DNA constitute the molecular basis of cancer, and transgenic or gene-targeted mice let us select the specific gene changes and affected cell types that we wish to model. Thus, these techniques permit us to mimic, with variable precision, human cancer etiology in the mouse. Recent reviews have addressed selected aspects of both this subject and the role of other animal modeling approaches and should be consulted for additional background in this area.[1-6]

The Disease Is Human, So Why Study Mice? Model Validation

As outlined elsewhere in this book, exocrine pancreatic cancer is a devastating illness. Not only do we lack routinely effective treatments, but we also lack sufficient knowledge of the molecular, biochemical, and physiologic mechanisms that cause this disease. In view of the urgency to improve our understanding of human pancreatic cancer, why spend time and money re-creating this disease in mice? Animal models share one essential feature with their human counterparts: In both, disease develops in the natural context of a living organism, with its intact growth homeostatic mechanisms that must be evaded before disease can appear. However, we can precisely manipulate an animal's internal and external environments to an extent not possible in humans, which permits controlled studies of factors that influence disease onset, progression, or treatment. Finally, the DNA of mice can be altered almost at will, permitting unprecedented insight into gene–disease correlations. For these reasons, animals, more specifically mice, are used to explore the pathogenesis of many diseases that have a genetic component.

Unfortunately, the use of mouse models raises a potentially serious problem: the human–mouse mismatch. Mice are not people, and thus, how do we transfer our understanding of the disease in mice to the disease in humans? This issue is addressed by the process of "model validation," whereby we decide how closely the human and mouse diseases resemble one another. I believe there are three general criteria to consider during model validation: morphologic, molecular, and behavioral. These criteria are addressed later here.

Morphologic criteria must be established to determine whether human and mouse tumors have a similar appearance. For exocrine pancreas, we expect human adenocarcinomas to be modeled most closely by mouse lesions composed of duct-like cells, whereas acinar cell carcinomas are best modeled by lesions composed of acinar-like cells. Comparisons are made at the gross and microscopic (light and electron microscopic) levels and may consist of standard examination or may employ special histochemical stains, immunohistochemistry, and/or in situ hybridization to refine our characterization of lesion morphology. The histogenetic classification of neoplasia explicitly assumes that the cell type of origin is reflected by the cellular histotype in the neoplasm (although, as noted later, the pancreas may challenge this assumption). Therefore, we expect to favor the development of a morphologically valid model of pancreatic adenocarcinoma, for example, by targeting potentially carcinogenic DNA changes to pancreatic ductal epithelium.

Molecular evaluation also must be performed to address whether human and mouse tumors display the same molecular alterations. Human pancreatic neoplasms can be diverse with respect to DNA alterations, but several DNA changes are seen reproducibly in variable but high fractions of neoplastic cells: a mutation in the *K-RAS2* proto-oncogene and inactivation (via several mechanisms) of *TP53*, *p16*, and *SMAD4* tumor-suppressor genes.[7-9] Mouse tumors that display one or more of these changes are likely to serve as better models of the human disease than mouse tumors without these changes. We expect to favor the development of valid mouse models of the human disease by recreating these changes specifically in the pancreas.

Finally, behavioral criteria allow us to establish the similarities and differences between mouse and human tumor growth, invasiveness, metastasis, and effects on host. In one respect, these are the most important criteria because we are most interested in creating mouse cancer models that provide a prognosis and predict a response to therapy that mimics the human disease. There are no special steps that we can take to favor specifically the development of behaviorally valid models, other than directing relevant molecular changes to a relevant target cell(s), as outlined previously here. Rather, we must apply careful behavioral evaluation to each model that we create and then select the most valid models for subsequent study.

Methods to Manipulate Mouse DNA

Before describing past and current studies using genetically modified mice to study exocrine pancreatic carcinogenesis, the basic methods that let us perform these modifications are described.

Transgenic Mice

The first method for modifying mouse DNA involves the introduction of exogenous DNA into fertilized mouse ova, usually by microinjection, resulting in the production of transgenic mice.[10] In a typical microinjection experiment, 200 mouse ova are visualized microscopically one at a time; each has transgene DNA injected into one pronucleus, and then surviving eggs are surgically implanted into the oviduct of pseudopregnant recipient female mice. Viable ova will implant in the uterus and result in the birth of live mice, typically 20 to 40 of the 160 transferred. Of these, 5 to 10 founder mice will have incorporated one or more copies of the transgene into chromosomal DNA, and in a subset of the founders, the transgene may be expressed. Offspring of a single founder mouse constitute a transgenic line or lineage. Transgenes contain two parts: a gene regulatory element that activates transgene expression in specific cells and a coding sequence that mediates the production of a selected protein (Fig. 6.1).

Experiment design depends critically on the selection of these transgene genetic elements. The transgenic approach is used most often to model dominantly acting genetic changes, specifically oncogene mutation or overexpression. Thus, for example, to test the hypothesis that mutant *β-catenin* expression can induce cancer in pancreatic acinar cells, the acinar cell-specific elastase enhancer/promoter can be cloned upstream of DNA encoding a mutant *β-catenin* gene. When present in mice, this transgene will be expressed selectively in acinar cells, and the effects of mutant *β-catenin* in this cell type can be addressed systematically. Typically, two or more lineages expressing a particular transgene are evaluated in a study of this type because occasionally the site of transgene chro-

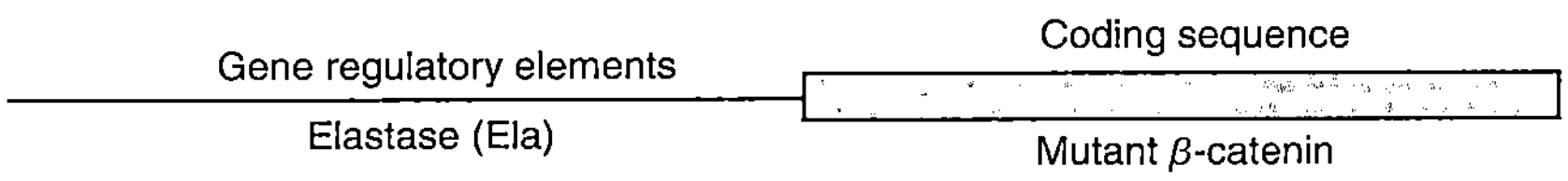

Gene regulatory elements | Coding sequence
Elastase (Ela) | Mutant β-catenin

Figure 6.1
Transgene structure. Typical transgenes include coding DNA from the gene of experimental interest and gene regulatory elements that direct the cell type specificity of transgene expression. This transgene, for example, would target expression of mutant β-catenin to pancreatic acinar cells.

mosomal integration can influence lesion development. Effects common to multiple lineages can be attributed specifically to transgene expression. A weakness of this approach is the lack of gene regulatory elements that exclusively target certain cell types, including pancreatic ductal epithelium. A second limitation is the inability to modulate transgene expression. The activity of most gene regulatory elements initiates during fetal development. The expression of transgenes using these regulatory elements also will initiate in the fetus and will remain present as long as the endogenous gene is expressed.

Gene Targeting

The second common method to modify the mouse genome, gene targeting, permits deletion or modification of selected regions of endogenous mouse DNA (Fig. 6.2).[10] This method requires an introduction of targeting vectors into mouse embryonic stem (ES) cells and selection and cloning of cells that have undergone homologous recombination between the vector and its endogenous target, transfer of modified cells into a recipient mouse blastocyst, and transfer of injected blastocysts into a recipient mouse uterus. Viable modified ES cells can participate in embryonic development, and offspring of some injected eggs are chimeric, composed of both blastocyst-derived and ES cell-derived cells. ES cell-derived germ cells can give rise to progeny carrying the targeted DNA modification. This approach is used most often to model recessively acting genetic changes. We can address the hypothesis that loss of a specific tumor suppressor gene activity contributes to carcinogenesis. For example, after a mating between two ES cell-derived mice heterozygous for a null mutation in the *TP53* gene, one fourth of the offspring will inherit two null alleles, and we can evaluate the effect of this gene defect on cancer development in pancreatic duct cells. A weakness of this approach is that the global loss of tumor-suppressor gene activity may be lethal during embryonic development, precluding evaluation of the role of that gene in cancer. Even if viable mice are born, multiple cell types may acquire an increased risk for cancer after tumor-suppressor gene loss so that the gene-null mouse becomes an effective model for only the type of neoplasm that develops first.

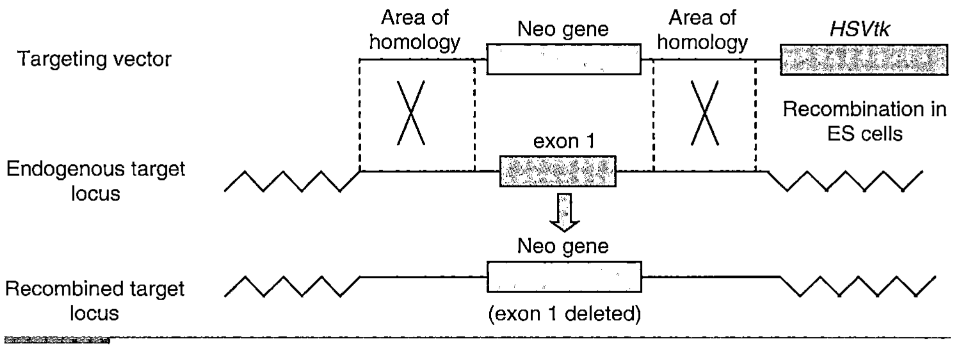

Figure 6.2
Gene targeting. Gene targeting requires the introduction of a targeting vector into ES cells. Targeting vectors recombine with homologous regions of chromosomal DNA in a small fraction of transfected ES cells, replacing endogenous DNA with part of the vector DNA. Correctly targeted cells must be identified, expanded, injected into blastocysts, and participate in recipient germ cell development in order to create gene-targeted mice. The *HSVtk* (herpes simplex virus thymidine kinase) gene is used for negative selection of ES cells into which the entire targeting vector has integrated nonhomologously.

Model Refinements: Transgene Inducibility and Cell-Specific Gene Knockouts

Two advances in experimental design have increased dramatically the utility of genetically modified mice for the study of disease. As noted earlier, both transgenic and gene targeting approaches have certain limitations. The timing of expression onset for most transgenes cannot be regulated, nor can we turn off transgene expression at a time of our choosing. These manipulations are important for several reasons. First, during spontaneous carcinogenesis, oncogene mutation or overexpression likely initiates postnatally, not in a fetal organ undergoing morphogenesis and differentiation. Second, engineered prenatal expression of certain oncogenes (e.g., mutant ras family members) induces developmental defects that include hyperplasia and altered differentiation,[11,12] and although interesting, these defects are not cancer.

Bujard and colleagues developed an inducible transgene system that can address these needs.[13-18] The system is based on the bacterial tetracycline (tet) operon (Fig. 6.3). The system employs two transgenes. The target transgene consists of the coding region for the gene under study preceded by a minimal promoter, which is incapable by itself of turning on transgene expression, and a multimerized tet operator sequence (tetO), which is a target for tet repressor protein binding. In most target transgenes, the tetO sequences are cloned upstream of the cytomegalovirus (CMV) minimal promoter. By itself, this transgene will not be expressed. The second transgene encodes a transactivator fusion protein, which combines the DNA binding domain of the tet repressor with the

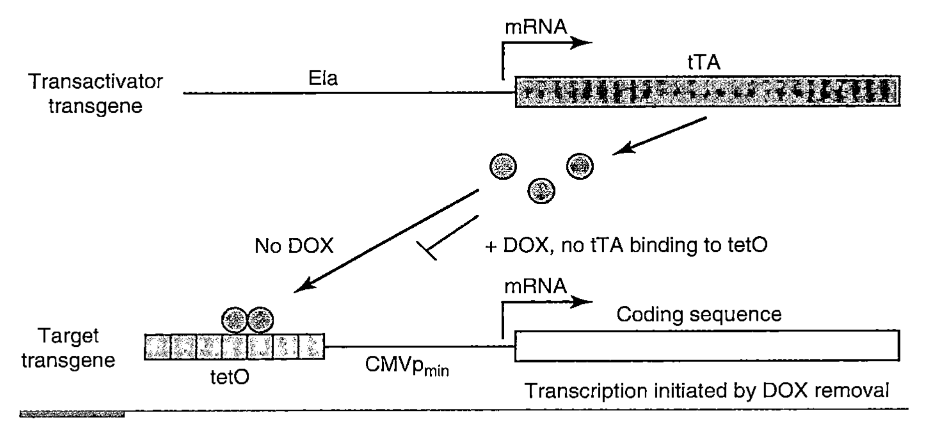

Figure 6.3
Tetracycline-inducible transgene expression. This system requires two transgenes. The first produces the tetracycline-transactivator protein (tTA), which binds to tet operator DNA (tetO) in the second (target) transgene. Once bound to tetO, the tTA protein interacts with other proteins bound to the CMV minimal promoter ($CMVp_{min}$), thereby mediating transcription of the target gene coding sequence. In the presence of DOX, tTA changes conformation so that it cannot bind to tetO. Without tTA binding, the tetO-$CMVp_{min}$ unit is not active. Cell-type specificity of this system is determined by the gene regulatory elements present in the tTA transgene.

transcriptional activation domain of the herpes viral protein VP16. The transactivator fusion protein binds to tetO in the absence of tetracycline. This brings the VP16 activation domain adjacent to the minimal promoter, creating a complete transcription unit capable of binding all necessary transcription factors. Transcription of the coding region ensues. Regulation of transgene expression makes use of the fact that tetracycline or an analogue, usually doxycycline (DOX), binds to the transactivator protein and changes its conformation so that it no longer binds tetO. The cell-type specificity of this system is controlled by the gene regulatory element selected to target transactivator expression. This system is called "DOX off." The converse system, in which several point mutations in the transactivator tet repressor domain create a protein that binds tetO in the presence of DOX, is called "DOX on." Thus, by regulating the DOX status of mice via feed or water, we can regulate the timing of transgene expression. Importantly, DOX passes to mice via placenta and milk, and thus, transgene expression can be regulated throughout life.

The second advance permits tissue-specific gene deletions, thereby avoiding disease associated with a loss of gene activity in some tissues during fetal development or in tissues that are not of primary interest to the investigator. This system uses the viral cre/lox elements (Fig. 6.4).[19-23] Lox sites are targets for the viral cre protein. When cre proteins bind to nearby direct repeats of the 34-bp lox element, they mediate deletion of DNA between the lox sites. Lox sites can be introduced into mouse DNA via homologous recombination in ES cells so that they flank an exon of a target gene. Mating can produce mice in which both alleles are "floxed" or flanked by lox. In the absence of cre protein, the gene remains normal. However, any cell into which cre has been introduced (via transgene expression, viral infection, or other means) will experience cre-mediated deletion of the target gene exon, thereby inactivating expression of that gene. A conceptually similar system employs the flp recombinase and its frt target sites.[24,25]

The inducible transgene and tissue-specific deletion methods can be combined to permit gene deletion at a specific stage of development or in the adult (Fig. 6.5).[26-28] Alone and together, these new approaches are allowing us to establish mouse models of disease that, at least with respect to molecular pathogenesis, more closely resemble their human counterparts.

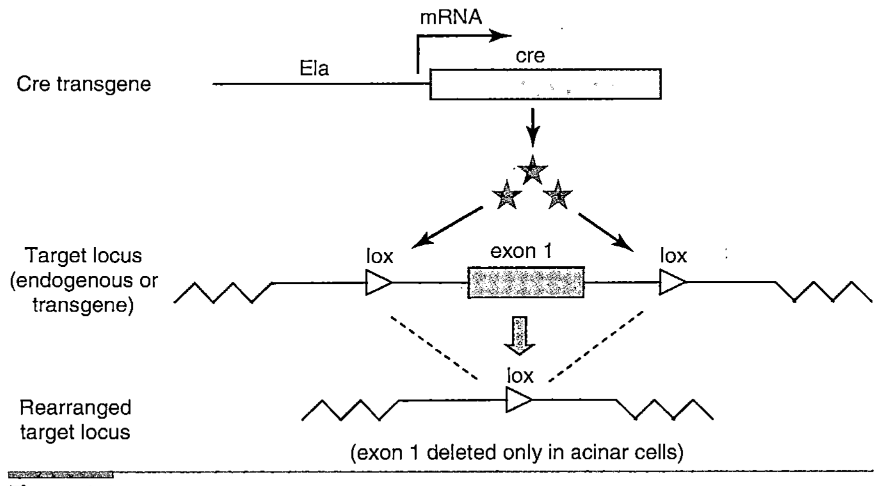

Figure 6.4
Cre-lox–mediated DNA deletion. The cre recombinase protein binds to nearby direct repeats of target lox sites and mediates deletion of intervening DNA. Typically, mice with a "floxed" (flanked by lox) target locus are generated by gene targeting in ES cells. Cell-type specificity of target deletion is determined by the method of cre delivery.

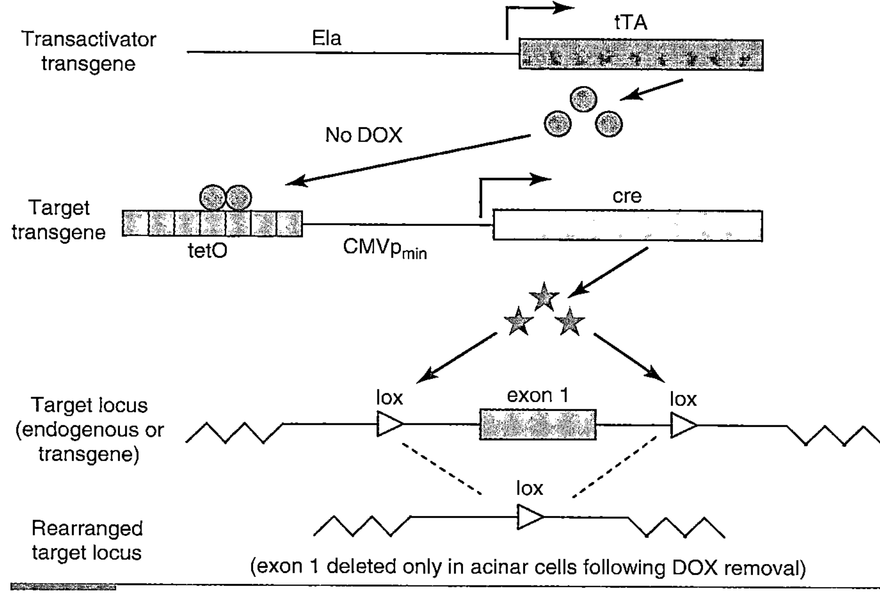

Figure 6.5
Inducible DNA deletion. This system represents a combination of the methods described in Figures 6.3 and 6.4 and permits cell type-specific and age-specific deletion of target DNA. Cell-type specificity of this system also is determined by the gene regulatory elements present in the tTA transgene.

The First Models

Single Genetic Changes

The first genetically manipulated models of exocrine pancreatic cancer, generated in the 1980s and 1990s, used cloned DNA fragments that were available at the time: the elastase (*Ela*) gene regulatory elements and coding regions for the oncogenes Simian Virus 40 Transforming Antigens (TAg), mutant *Hras*, *c-myc*, and transforming growth factor-α (*TGF-α*). The *Ela* enhancer/promoter region has been well characterized and is generally expressed specifically in pancreatic acinar cells.[29,30] TAg is a potent transforming oncogene in multiple mouse cell types and functions in part by binding to, thereby inactivating, the tumor-suppressor proteins p53 and pRb.[31] *Hras* mutations have not been identified in human pancreatic neoplasms, but mutant *H-ras* and *K-ras* activate similar downstream targets. Only recently have changes in the *c-myc* gene (generally amplification and/or overexpression) been linked to exocrine pancreatic cancer.[32-38] *TGF-α* is overexpressed in some primary pancreatic adenocarcinomas and cell lines derived from tumors.[39,40] Thus, for each of these oncogenes, there is a molecular relevance to human pancreatic cancer. However, for some, the link remains tenuous, and none represents the most commonly identified changes identified in the human disease.

As expected based on the targeting strategy, each transgene induced acinar-like lesions. Ela-TAg was generated first, and mice bearing this transgene displayed a reproducible spectrum of pancreatic lesion progression.[41-47] TAg alone was sufficient to induce acinar cell hyperplasia. Next, within this background of diffuse hyperplasia, focal lesions developed that generally were composed of small, basophilic cells and often displayed a loss of acinar architecture. These altered foci also displayed elevated mitotic indices and expanded by compressing surrounding parenchyma. Multifocal solid to acinar/glandular acinar cell carcinomas appeared with an incidence of 100% (Fig. 6.6A), but latency varied significantly depending on the transgenic lineage. The most rapid progression to carcinoma was 3 months, but mice in some lineages survived beyond a year. Metastasis occurred, but was infrequent (<10%). Interestingly, islet cell neoplasms developed in some mice of an Ela-TAg line that used a short form of the Ela gene regulatory element,[42] consistent with low-level expression from this promoter fragment in islet β-cells.

The series of publications describing Ela-TAg transgenic mice illustrated several important features of the use of transgenic animal models to study oncogene-induced pancreatic cancer. First, oncogene-associated carcinogenesis could be restricted to a chosen cell type by selection of the appropriate transgene targeting strategy. Second, within a transgenic lineage, single gene changes (in this example, acinar cell-directed expression of TAg) produce reproducible lesion pathogenesis. This finding was important because it indicated the utility of transgenic models to study the earliest changes during pancreatic cancer progression, a difficult task in humans because of the typically late stage of diagnosis. Third, despite the documented presence of TAg in all acinar cells in some lines of Ela-TAg mice, tumors were focal, indicating that other changes must occur in a subset of TAg-expressing acinar cells that permits them to develop into neoplasms. Fourth, the precise spectrum of lesions and lesion latency can vary considerably between different lineages of transgenic mice, representing the influence of

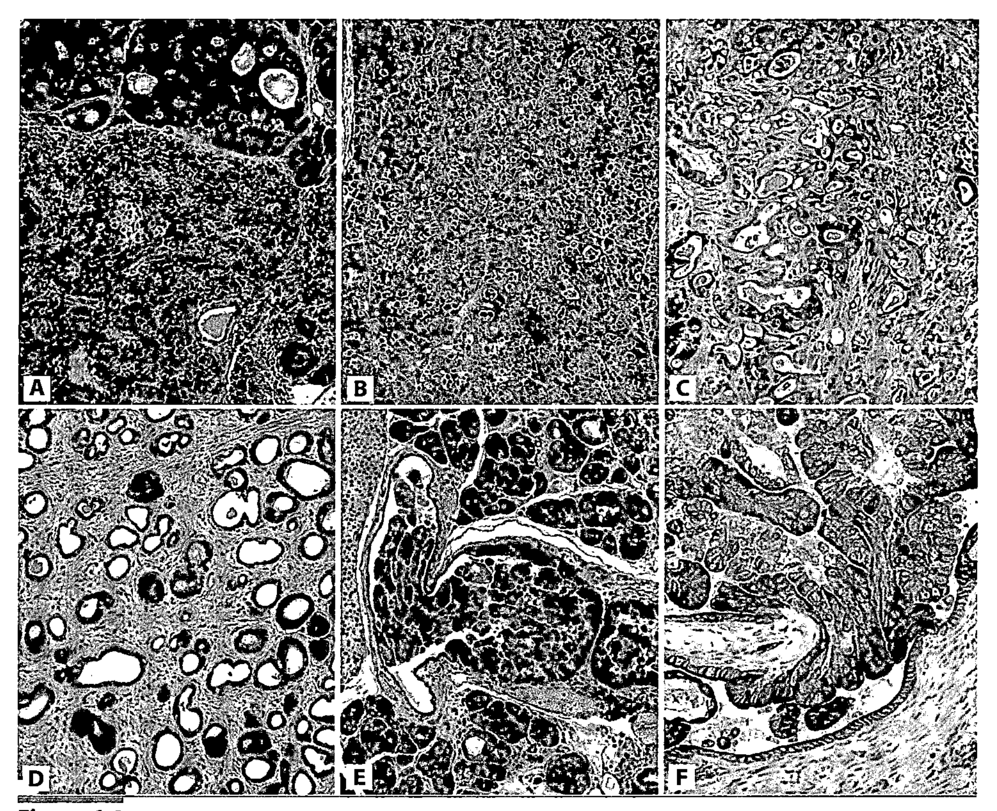

Figure 6.6
Microscopic appearance of mouse pancreatic lesions. **(A)** Adjacent acinar cell carcinomas in a 6-month-old Ela-TAg transgenic mouse. There are several normal-appearing acini in the extreme upper right of the photo. **(B)** Solid acinar cell carcinoma in a 5-month-old Ela-*c-myc* transgenic mouse. **(C)** Mixed acinar–ductal neoplasm in the same Ela-*c-myc* transgenic mouse, displaying multiple ductal structures, increased stroma, and a focus of inflammatory cells in the upper right of the photo. **(D)** Pancreas from a 12-month-old MT-TGF-α transgenic mouse displaying extensive fibrosis and multiple tubular complexes (lumen-containing structures derived from acini). Several normal-appearing acini are present in this section. **(E)** Neoplastic cells within and extending from the epithelium lining a ductal structure in pancreas from a 14-month-old Ela-*K-ras* transgenic mouse. There is no evidence of invasion. **(F)** Cytokeratin 19 protein (brown) in a noninvasive papillary-mucinous ductal carcinoma in situ. (A–E) Hematoxylin and eosin stain (original magnification, ×200). **(F)** Immunohistochemical stain (original magnification, ×400).

chromosomal site of transgene integration on characteristics of transgene expression. Finally, once characterized, transgenic mice are available to serve as subjects for additional molecular evaluation, permitting us both to identify genetic changes that correlate with lesion progression and to test whether other specific genetic changes can complement TAg expression to favor more rapid lesion onset or progression (see the next section).

Ela-mutant *H-ras* transgenic mice illustrated one of the limitations of the transgenic approach. Each of several mutations in *ras* genes encodes proteins with altered function, such that inactivation of ras signaling becomes ineffective. Most Ela-mutant *H-ras* founder mice were born with hyperplastic, poorly differentiated pancreata secondary to initiation of transgene expression in fetal pancreas.[11] This study demonstrated that mutant *H-ras* had a potent and disruptive effect on pancreatic development and growth. However, for this reason, the study could not identify the contribution of *H-ras* to pancreatic cancer in the adult mouse.

Ela-c-*myc* transgenic mice presented yet a third pattern of lesion morphogenesis.[48,49] During initial stages of lesion progression, Ela-c-*myc* transgenic mice resembled Ela-TAg mice. Overexpression of the transcription factor c-myc induced diffuse acinar hyperplasia and then multifocal solid masses of basophilic cells with a high mitotic index. Multiple acinar cell carcinomas (Fig. 6.6B) developed in each mouse between 3 and 12 months of age, with latency dependent on lineage. However, during latter stages of carcinogenesis, lesion morphology diverged between *c-myc* and TAg transgenic mice. Approximately 50% of all *c-myc*–induced carcinomas developed variable-sized areas of acinar-to-ductal metaplasia associated with increased stroma (Fig. 6.6C). The duct-like cells did not produce the acinar cell marker amylase but did express the duct cell marker cytokeratin 19 and often produced Alcian blue/periodic acid Schiff's-positive mucin. This model was intriguing because it suggested that a sequence of acinar-to-ductal metaplasia accompanied tumor progression in vivo.[48] Acinar-to-ductal metaplasia also has been identified in cultured human and animal pancreatic acinar cells, indicating plasticity in the differentiation state of this cell type.[50-58] The ductal component in Ela-*c-myc* tumors reproduced for the first time in mice one important morphologic feature of the disease in humans. Nevertheless, unlike human tumors, even ductal areas of the mixed neoplasms retained focal collections of amylase-positive acinar-like neoplastic cells with a high rate of cell replication.

Ela-*TGF-α* and metallothionein (MT)–*TGF-α* transgenic mice also developed unique lesions.[59-65] TGF-α is a ligand for the epidermal growth factor receptor and is synthesized as a transmembrane molecule, from which the active peptide is cleaved at the extracellular surface. When overexpressed specifically in pancreatic acinar cells via the Ela promoter or in acinar cells plus other epithelia via the MT promoter, TGF-α induced diffuse, progressive, moderate to severe pancreatic fibrosis (Fig. 6.6D). Importantly, fibrosis was not produced by overexpression of a cleavage-resistant form of TGF-α,[59] implicating secreted TGF-α in the effect. These findings identified a potent paracrine effect of this growth factor on pancreatic stroma. Accompanying this change was multifocal acinar-to-ductal metaplasia, in which single or adjacent groupings of acini became structurally reorganized to resemble ducts (Fig. 6.6D). This change, resulting in the development of "tubular complexes," is found also in response to certain forms of pancreatic injury. Metaplasia was accompanied by a loss of acinar cell markers (amylase) and acquisition of duct cell markers (CK19; occasional Alcian blue/periodic acid-Schiff positivity). Interestingly, metaplasia is inhibited when mice are deficient in matrix metalloproteinase-7 or Fas ligand.[64] With a very low incidence (<5%), the old Ela-*TGF-α* mice developed mixed exocrine pancreatic neoplasms (MT-*TGF-α* animals required euthanasia because of liver cancer at approximately 1 year of age).[59,63] In contrast, elastase-driven targeting of the epidermal growth factor ligand family member amphiregulin elicited intralobular duct and centroacinar cell proliferation, but not the development of tubular complexes or increased stroma, indicating a dramatic difference in the biological effects of these related molecules in vivo.[66]

Finally, elastase-driven targeting of the gastrin/cholecystokinin receptor in transgenic mice induced slight to moderate increases in pancreas weight and a 15% incidence of exocrine pancreatic neoplasms that were reported to have both acinar and ductal features.[67-69]

Collectively, the transgenic mouse models described previously here demonstrated that characteristic patterns of tissue change accompany the expression of individual oncogenes when they are targeted to pancreatic acinar cells, although the phenotypic changes can vary considerably when compared among different oncogenes. Of particular interest, c-myc and TGF-α induce acinar-to-ductal metaplasia, but in widely different contexts: c-myc within a neoplasm and TGF-α within non-neoplastic, fibrotic pancreas.

Combined Genetic Changes

Cancer is a multistage disease; therefore, subsequent studies were designed to examine whether selected genetic alterations could cooperate in mice to increase cancer multiplicity or reduce latency. As expected, interactions among factors were detected during lesion pathogenesis. As an example, I describe in detail the activity of TGF-α in the context of other genetic changes.

Recall that by itself TGF-α was only weakly oncogenic in pancreatic acinar cells. However, when expressed together with either TAg or *c-myc*, TGF-α dramatically reduced survival of bitransgenic mice relative to mice expressing either oncogene alone.[70] In fact, all TAg/TGF-α bitransgenic mice developed advanced pancreatic cancer and required euthanasia before the first Ela-TAg monotransgenic mouse reached this stage of disease: Survival curves did not overlap. TGF-α decreased the latency and increased the multiplicity of putative preneoplastic-altered pancreatic foci induced by TAg and dramatically increased the rate of growth of neoplasms induced by *c-myc*, suggesting that perhaps it could influence both early and late events in tumor progression. Metastasis, however, was not increased by TGF-α.

Schmid and colleagues examined the effect of the loss of one or both *TP53* alleles on TGF-α–induced pancreatic lesions.[63] Remarkably, Ela-TGF-α transgenic mice that carried gene targeting–induced null mutations in both *TP53* alleles (p53–/–) developed rapid-onset (within 4 months) invasive exocrine pancreatic neoplasms with 100% incidence. These neoplasms were morphologically complex. Many displayed areas of ductal differentiation

(CK19 expression), but like Ela-*c-myc* neoplasms, also displayed features of acinar cell carcinoma. Clearly, the p53 protein functions as a potent tumor suppressor in the context of TGF-α–induced mouse pancreatic neoplasia. Nevertheless, neoplasms remained focal, indicating that a lack of p53 and overexpression of TGF-α were not sufficient to induce cancer.

Heterozygous *TP53* null (p53 +/–) Ela-TGF-α mice displayed intermediate latency and incidence and were used by this group to identify molecular changes that could collaborate with TGF-α expression to favor tumor progression.[71] This study provides an outstanding example of the utility of careful molecular analysis of a mouse model of cancer. The authors reported several consistent molecular lesions in neoplasms. First, almost 90% of neoplasms lost the remaining normal *TP53* allele, rendering them p53 null, confirming the importance of *TP53* loss as a critical step in development of most of these tumors. Second, more than 50% of neoplasms displayed potential inactivation, typically via promoter methylation, of the cyclin-dependent kinase *cdkn2a* gene. Third, amplification or loss of genomic DNA was identified using comparative genomic hybridization, coupled with realtime polymerase chain reaction, to quantify the extent of selected amplifications. Comparative genomic hybridization permits detection of changes in chromosomal region copy number in tumors relative to the expected diploid copy number in normal tissues. By examining a large number of tumors (38 in this study), consistent changes in multiple tumors can be identified, and these are more likely to represent causative events during tumorigenesis. A fascinating pattern emerged, with chromosomal gains at proximal chromosome 11 (carrying the *Egfr* and *Rel* oncogenes), and either gains of distal chromosome 15, which carries the *c-myc* gene, or losses of distal chromosome 14, which carries the *Rb* tumor-suppressor gene. As the authors noted, a loss of *Rb* or overexpression of *c-myc* can facilitate passage through the G1/S phase arrest; they propose that one or the other DNA change may be an important event leading to tumor progression, although both are not necessary together. This report illustrates an effective molecular approach to supplement the pathobiologic data available from a mouse model. Discovering molecular changes that reproducibly complement lesion progression in mice identifies candidate genes that may be relevant to disease pathogenesis and, therefore, targets for therapy in humans.

Finally, Bardeesy et al.[72] examined the interaction between TGF-α overexpression and combined *TP53* and *p16/p19* heterozygous deficiencies in mouse pancreas. Like *TP53*, the *p16* tumor-suppressor gene is inactivated frequently in human pancreatic cancer. Although this combination of gene changes did not induce adenocarcinoma, it caused a high incidence of serous cystadenomas at a median age of approximately 10 months. These lesions morphologically resembled their human counterparts. Lesions also displayed inactivation of the remaining normal *p16* allele and a loss of the remaining *TP53* or *p19*.

Model Limitations

The models described previously here demonstrated the effectiveness of genetic manipulation to produce pancreatic cancer in mice. Nevertheless, when examined in the context of model validation, they exhibit certain limitations. First, lesion morphology does not reflect the dominant pattern of disease identified in human patients, ductal adenocarcinomas. Second, the effects of *K-ras* mutations on pancreatic cancer were not evaluated, yet *K-ras* is the most commonly identified target for mutational activation in the human disease. Third, lesion progression, especially the lack or low rate of metastasis, does not resemble human pancreatic cancer behavior. Thus, additional approaches incorporating the expression of mutant *K-ras* in mouse pancreas were necessary as a critical next step in model improvement.

Recent Models

Mutant *K-ras* Transgenic Mice

In 2003, several reports were published that significantly expanded and improved mouse models of exocrine pancreatic cancer. The first involved targeting of mutant *K-ras* to pancreas using transgenic mice. Brembeck et al.[73] used the cytokeratin 19 promoter to target mutant *K-ras* expression to simple epithelium in many organs, including pancreatic ductal epithelium. Focal inflammatory disease was observed in pancreas of these mice, but no preneoplastic lesions. Grippo et al.[12] used the Ela promoter to target mutant *K-ras* expression to acinar cells. In established lineages, they observed mild to moderate pancreatic atrophy and fibrosis, but most importantly, they also identified focal ductal lesions developing in older (>1 year of age) transgenic mice. Because it displays ductal lesions, the Ela-*K-ras* model is described in more detail.

Recall that targeting of mutant *H-ras* using the Ela promoter caused pancreatic hyperplasia and altered differentiation during fetal and early postnatal development.[11] Most Ela-mutant *K-ras* transgenic founder mice developed a similar condition.[12] However, two founders survived the postnatal period and were used to generate transgenic lines. In these lines, newborn mice displayed a relatively normal pancreatic phenotype with the exception of focal hyperplastic acini. Young adults developed diffuse pancreatic inflammation and exocrine atrophy, but this phenotype became less widespread as mice aged. Between 6 months and a year of age, focal areas of acinar dysplasia developed, in which focal cells within acini began to express the CK19 gene and mucin, both duct cell markers. After 1 year of age, approximately one half of the mice in one Ela-*K-ras* line displayed areas of noninvasive carcinoma in situ that in some cases resembled pancreatic intraepithelial neoplasia (PanIN) or papillary mucinous ductal carcinoma in situ (Fig. 6.6E and Fig. 6.6F), each a feature of pancreatic disease in humans. Cells in these lesions variably expressed CK19 and/or mucin.

Two aspects of this phenotype are of special note. First, at least some of these lesions develop via a process of acinar-to-ductal metaplasia: Primary ductal lesions have not been observed in these mice, and "intermediate" dysplastic structures, containing cells with both acinar and ductal features, are present. Unlike the metaplastic transition observed within tumors of Ela-*c-myc* transgenic mice, this transition occurs within non-neoplastic acinar epithelium. The generation of duct-like lesions from acinar precursor cells suggests that, at least in mice, acinar cells may serve as progenitors for ductal cancer in this organ. Second, mutant *K-ras* induced preinvasive lesions, but at least in the FVB/N strain background in which this model was developed, it did not induce progression beyond the preinvasive stage. This observation is consistent with suggestions that the *K-ras* mutation has a role in early exocrine pancreatic carcinogenesis but that additional genetic changes are required for development of more advanced disease.

Ela-*K-ras* mice also are being used to address mutant *K-ras*/tumor-suppressor gene loss interactions and the effect of strain background on lesion multiplicity (Sandgren et al., unpublished). Currently, expression of mutant *K-ras* cooperates with *TP53* loss to induce invasive and metastatic acinar cell carcinomas in young (less than 6 months of age) mice. Furthermore, one generation of backcrossing of FVB/N strain Ela-*K-ras* mice to some (although not all) other strains increases ductal lesion multiplicity in 14-month-old mice up to 20-fold. These preliminary findings illustrate the utility of Ela-*K-ras* mice to identify other genetic factors (tumor modifier loci) that may modulate mutant *K-ras*–induced pancreatic disease. The tetracycline-inducible transgene system also is being used to target mutant *H-ras* and mutant *K-ras* specifically to adult acinar cells, thereby avoiding any complications associated with mutant ras expression in developing pancreas (Sandgren et al., unpublished). Both mutant ras proteins induce pancreatic metaplastic lesions, but surprisingly, mutant *H-ras* appears more pathogenic in this system, despite the lack of *H-ras* mutations in human pancreatic cancer. These models, together with Ela-*K-ras* transgenic mice, should prove to be valuable tools to address the putative role of acinar cells in pancreatic ductal carcinogenesis.

More recently, several reports have taken additional steps to address *K-ras* mutations and pancreatic cancer (also reviewed in Leach[74]). These take advantage of a novel gene-targeting approach that allows expression of a mutant *K-ras* from its endogenous gene (Fig. 6.7). To accomplish this objective, mutant *K-ras*-encoding DNA preceded by a "floxed-stop" sequence was substituted for the endogenous *K-ras* coding region in ES cells, and these cells were used to generate mice. Before cre-mediated deletion of the transcriptional stop sequence, the targeted allele is silent (transcription from this allele stops before

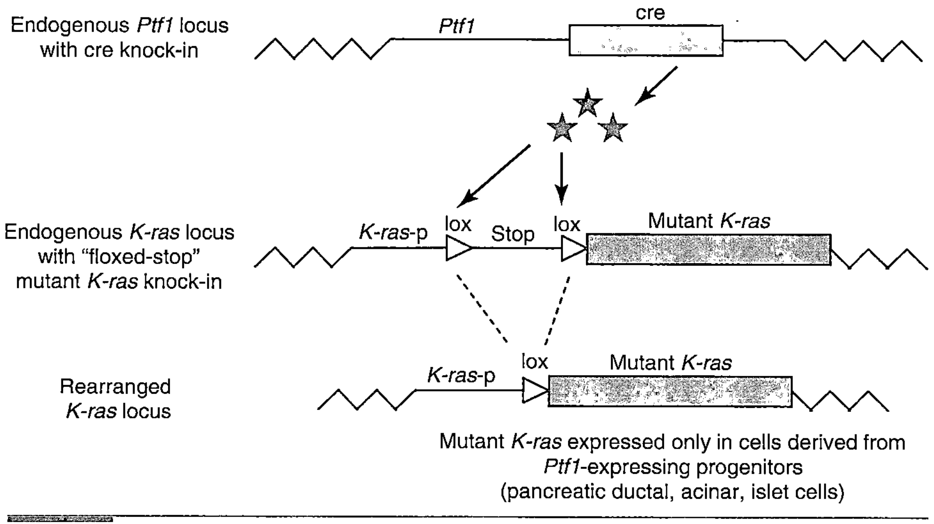

Figure 6.7
Activation of mutant *K-ras* expression in pancreatic epithelial cells. Cre protein is expressed from the endogenous *Ptf1* transcription factor gene promoter and mediates deletion of a transcriptional stop sequence upstream of a mutant *K-ras* coding sequence (Kras-p, endogenous *K-ras* gene promoter). This enables production of mutant *K-ras* from the endogenous *K-ras* locus. Both the *Ptf1* locus with a cre knock-in and the *K-ras* locus with a "floxed-stop" mutant *K-ras* knock-in were generated in ES cells via gene targeting.

it can progress to the coding region). The remaining normal allele produces wild-type *K-ras* mRNA and protein, and thus, these mice develop and grow normally. After cre-mediated stop sequence deletion, the targeted allele now permits transcription of an mRNA encoding mutant *K-ras*. This manipulation effectively recreates the genetic signature of the human disease: The mutation is present in the endogenous *K-ras* gene under transcriptional control of its own gene regulatory elements. Of course, the type of disease to develop depends critically on which cell types express cre and therefore activate expression of mutant *K-ras*.

Two cre-expressing mouse lines have been evaluated with this system. The first carried a cre transgene expressed from the *Pdx1* gene promoter. *Pdx1* encodes a transcription factor that is required for normal pancreatic development,[75,76] and it is expressed during fetal development in all pancreatic epithelial cell progenitors as well as some cells in the small intestine and stomach.[77] The second carried a cre "knock-in" at the *Ptf1* gene locus such that the coding sequence of one *Ptf1* allele was replaced by the coding sequence of cre. *Ptf1*, which also encodes a transcription factor, has a pattern of expression in the fetus that is restricted specifically to pancreatic epithelial cell precursors.[78,79] Mice carrying either of these cre-expressing systems plus the floxed-stop *K-ras* knock-in will activate mutant *K-ras* expression in multiple pancreatic cell types (and some extrapancreatic cells with Pdx1-cre), including ductal epithelial cells, beginning during fetal development. Hingorani et al.[80] described the effects of mutant *K-ras* expression using both cre systems. Aguirre et al.[81] described the effects of mutant *K-ras* expression plus cre-mediated loss of *p16/p19* (*Ink4a/Arf*) using Pdx1-cre. The results were fascinating.

First, with either cre mouse line, pancreatic lesions developed in adult mice that resembled PanINs. Lesions were not reported in the acinar or islet compartments, at least in young mice. As with Ela-*K-ras* lesions, most did not progress to the invasive stage, although Hingorani et al.[80] identified two mice that developed invasive and metastatic cancer at 6 and 8 months of age. Cells in PanIN lesions displayed CK19 and MUC-5 duct cell marker expression. PanINs also variably expressed or overexpressed *Hes1*, a marker of Notch signaling, cyclooxygenase-2 (*Cox-2*), involved in prostaglandin metabolism, and matrix metalloproteinase-7 (*MMP-7*). Each of these genes also is overexpressed in a subset of human PanINs. One adenocarcinoma displayed vascular and neural invasion and had spread to the liver, diaphragm, pleura, lung, lymph nodes, and adrenal cortex. As the authors noted, tumor behavior in this mouse is a close match to that displayed by the human disease. Finally, these authors performed serum proteomic analysis using the mass spectrometric method surface-enhanced laser desorption ionization time of flight. They compared differences in serum proteomic signatures between 39 mutant *K-ras*–expressing versus littermate control pancreases. Model parameters selected based on a pilot study allowed the authors to distinguish cases from control subjects in the experimental study set with a sensitivity of 90% and a specificity of 87%. This outcome represents a promising step in mouse model validation and suggests that we may be close to fulfilling the full promise of mouse pancreatic cancer models as surrogates for studying the human disease.

Aguirre et al.[81] carried the experimental design one step further, using the Pdx1-cre/floxed-stop *K-ras* model in combination with floxed alleles of the *Ink4a/Arf* (*p16/p19*) locus. In these mice, cre both activated mutant *K-ras* and deleted the *p16/p19* tumor-suppressor genes in pancreatic epithelial (and some other) cells. Between 7 and 11 weeks of age, all mutant *K-ras*–expressing plus *p16/p19* null mice developed invasive pancreatic adenocarcinomas that expressed ductal markers and occasionally metastasized to lymph nodes and liver. They also observed elevated expression of *Egfr* and *HER2/neu* in neoplasms. Again, these morphologic and molecular phenotypes resembled findings present in human patients.

Other Models

Several final studies to be discussed describe additional biologically and methodologically important models in the field of pancreatic cancer research. Miyamoto et al.[65] examined the notch signaling pathway in human and mouse pancreatic cancer. They demonstrated that expression of notch pathway components as well as downstream target genes is upregulated in pancreatic cancer precursor lesions in humans and mice and in invasive pancreatic cancer in humans. They further defined a requirement for Notch during TGF-α–induced acinar-to-ductal metaplasia in the mouse. The authors propose that notch pathway signaling secondary to augmented epidermal growth factor receptor activity promotes PanIN lesion formation in either metaplastic acinar or ductal epithelium.

Thayer et al.[82] identified abnormal hedgehog signaling in human pancreatic adenocarcinoma and precursor lesions and developed Pdx1-sonic hedgehog transgenic mice. By 3 weeks of age, the four mice examined displayed acinar to glandular transformation that resulted in pancreatic lesions somewhat resembling PanIN-1 and PanIN-

2. Remarkably, three of these pancreases overexpressed *HER-2/neu*, and two apparently displayed codon 12 *K-ras* mutations, each a molecular feature of human pancreatic cancer. These findings indicate that certain molecular features underlying lesion development and progression are shared among multiple carcinogenic pathways in pancreas.

Finally, Lewis et al.[83] established a model system that permits the introduction of transgenes into focal pancreatic epithelial cells. This system employs an elastase–TVA transgene. TVA is the receptor of avian leukosarcoma virus subgroup A. Two-day-old mice carrying this transgene express it in acinar but also other pancreatic epithelial cell types. When they are infected with appropriate viral vectors, the vectors bind to the cell surface receptor on pancreatic epithelial cells, are internalized, integrate into the DNA if the cell is replicating, and express vector open reading frames. Importantly, only scattered, focal cells within pancreas will be infected successfully, permitting identification of expressed gene effects in cells that are surrounded by otherwise normal cells. Using this approach, the authors introduced vectors expressing the polyoma virus middle T oncogene or the *c-myc* oncogene into *p16/p19* null mice. Polyoma virus middle T oncogene induced acinar and duct-like carcinomas in 70% of infected mice, whereas *c-myc* induced only endocrine tumors in 30% of infected mice (infected *p16/p19* wild-type mice displayed either no or only microscopic pancreatic lesions). Based on technical considerations and the microscopic and antigenic character of lesions, Lewis et al.[83] suggested that tumors originated from pancreatic progenitor cells, not mature pancreatic epithelium.

Conclusion

We have reached an exciting stage in pancreatic cancer model development. The use of mice permits precisely designed manipulation of pancreatic epithelial DNA in a living mammal. Recent designs finally incorporate mouse pancreas-specific targeting of the common molecular changes identified in human neoplasms, creating models of the human disease that are valid with respect to important molecular criteria. Several of these genetically manipulated mice also appear to provide valid models of lesion behavior, most importantly metastasis. Finally, multiple recent models display lesion morphology consistent with human pancreatic adenocarcinoma, although it appears that these duct-like lesions can arise from more than just ductal epithelium. There remains a critical need to correlate disease phenotype and biology with the specific pancreatic epithelial cell type and stage of development of that cell type into which molecular changes are introduced. The identification of a pancreatic cancer progenitor cell(s) (ductal, acinar, endocrine, stem) is an area of intense study.

Mice remain different from humans. However, by establishing a comprehensive understanding of the disease in the mouse, we can use what we already know about similarities and differences between mice and humans to guide our transfer of knowledge between species. In view of the recent progress in mouse modeling, the next several years hold the promise of producing tools that pancreatic cancer researchers can use to study molecular, biochemical, and physiologic mechanisms underlying pancreatic carcinogenesis, to identify modifier loci that influence disease risk, to correlate prognosis with specific molecular defects, to develop methods for early diagnosis, and to screen new therapies for effectiveness at multiple stages of disease.

Acknowledgments

The author thanks Allyson Holler for assistance with figures. Work in this area in the author's laboratory has been supported by the American Cancer Society and the National Cancer Institute, National Institutes of Health.

References

1. Hotz HG, Hines OJ, Foitzik T, Reber HA. Animal models of exocrine pancreatic cancer. *Int J Colorectal Dis*. 2000;15:136–143.
2. Standop J, Schneider MB, Ulrich A, et al. Experimental animal models in pancreatic carcinogenesis: lessons for human pancreatic cancer. *Dig Dis* 2001;19:24–31.
3. Bardeesy N, Sharpless NE, DePinho RA, et al. The genetics of pancreatic adenocarcinoma: a roadmap for a mouse model. *Semin Cancer Biol*. 2001;11:201–218.
4. Lowy AM, Clerc P, Saillan-Barreau C, et al. Transgenic models of pancreatic cancer. *Int J Gastrointest Cancer*. 2003;33:71–78.
5. Wei D, Xiong HQ, Abbruzzese JL, Xie K. Experimental animal models of pancreatic carcinogenesis and metastasis. *Int J Gastrointest Cancer*. 2003;33:43–60.
6. Heiser PW, Hebrok M. Development and cancer: lessons learned in the pancreas. *Cell Cycle*. 2004;3:270–272.
7. Hilgers W, Kern SE. Molecular genetic basis of pancreatic adenocarcinoma. *Genes Chromosomes Cancer*. 1999;26:1–12.
8. Hruban RH, Wilentz RE, Kern H. Genetic progression in the pancreatic ducts. *Am J Pathol*. 2000;156:1821–1825.
9. Sakorafas GH, Tsiotou AG, Tsiotos GG. Molecular biology of pancreatic cancer: oncogenes, tumour suppressor genes, growth factors, and their receptors from a clinical perspective. *Cancer Treat Rev*. 2000;26:29–52.
10. Nagy A, Gertsenstein M, Vintersten K, Behringer R. Manipulating the mouse embryo. *A Laboratory Manual*. 2003 Cold Spring Harbor Laboratory Press, Cold Spring Harbor, New York.

11. Quaife CJ, Pinkert CA, Ornitz DM, et al. Pancreatic neoplasia induced by ras expression in acinar cells of transgenic mice. *Cell.* 1987;48:1023–1034.
12. Grippo PJ, Nowlin PS, Demeure MJ, et al. Preinvasive pancreatic neoplasia of ductal phenotype induced by acinar cell targeting of mutant kras in transgenic mice. *Cancer Res.* 2003;63:2016–2019.
13. Gossen M, Bujard H. Tight control of gene expression in mammalian cells by tetracycline-responsive promoters. *Proc Natl Acad Sci USA.* 1992;89:5547–5551.
14. Gossen M, Freundlieb S, Bender G, et al. Transcriptional activation by tetracyclines in mammalian cells. *Science.* 1995;268:1766–1769.
15. Kistner A, Gossen M, Zimmermann F, et al. Doxycycline-mediated quantitative and tissue-specific control of gene expression in transgenic mice. *Proc Natl Acad Sci USA.* 1996;93:10933–10938.
16. Shockett PE, Schatz DG. Diverse strategies for tetracycline-regulated inducible gene expression. *Proc Natl Acad Sci USA.* 1996;93:5173–5176.
17. Forster K, Helbl V, Lederer T, et al. Tetracycline-inducible expression systems with reduced basal activity in mammalian cells. *Nucleic Acids Res.* 1999;27:708–710.
18. Blau HM, Rossi FM. Tet B or not tet B: advances in tetracycline-inducible gene expression. *Proc Natl Acad Sci USA.* 1999;96:797–799.
19. Kuhn R, Schwenk F, Aguet M, Rajewsky K. Inducible gene targeting in mice. *Science.* 1995;269:1427–1429.
20. Sauer B. Inducible gene targeting in mice using the Cre/lox system. *Methods.* 1998;14:381–392.
21. Muller U. Ten years of gene targeting: targeted mouse mutants, from vector design to phenotype analysis. *Mech Dev.* 1999;82:3–21.
22. Nagy A. Cre recombinase: the universal reagent for genome tailoring. *Genesis.* 2000;26:99–109.
23. Kwan KM. Conditional alleles in mice: practical considerations for tissue-specific knockouts. *Genesis.* 2002;32:49–62.
24. Farley FW, Soriano P, Steffen LS, Dymecki SM. Widespread recombinase expression using FLPeR (flipper) mice. *Genesis.* 2000;28:106–110.
25. Schaft J, Ashery-Padan R, van der Hoeven F, et al. Efficient FLP recombination in mouse ES cells and oocytes. *Genesis.* 2001;31:6–10.
26. St-Onge L, Furth PA, Gruss P. Temporal control of the Cre recombinase in transgenic mice by a tetracycline responsive promoter. *Nucleic Acids Res.* 1996;24:3875–3877.
27. Grieshammer U, Lewandoski M, Prevette D, et al. Muscle-specific cell ablation conditional upon Cre-mediated DNA recombination in transgenic mice leads to massive spinal and cranial motoneuron loss. *Dev Biol.* 1998;197:234–247.
28. Utomo AR, Nikitin AY, Lee WH. Temporal, spatial, and cell type-specific control of Cre-mediated DNA recombination in transgenic mice. *Nat Biotechnol.* 1999;17:1091–1096.
29. Ornitz DM, Palmiter RD, Hammer RE, et al. Specific expression of an elastase-human growth hormone fusion gene in pancreatic acinar cells of transgenic mice. *Nature.* 1985;313:600–602.
30. Hammer RE, Swift GH, Ornitz DM, et al. The rat elastase I regulatory element is an enhancer that directs correct cell specificity and developmental onset of expression in transgenic mice. *Mol Cell Biol.* 1987;7:2956–2967.
31. Ali SH, DeCaprio JA. Cellular transformation by SV40 large T antigen: interaction with host proteins. *Semin Cancer Biol.* 2001;11:15–23.
32. Mahlamaki EH, Hoglund M, Gorunova L, et al. Comparative genomic hybridization reveals frequent gains of 20q, 8q, 11q, 12p, and 17q, and losses of 18q, 9p, and 15q in pancreatic cancer. *Genes Chromosomes Cancer.* 1997;20:383–391.
33. Zojer N, Fiegl M, Mullauer L, et al. Chromosomal imbalances in primary and metastatic pancreatic carcinoma as detected by interphase cytogenetics: basic findings and clinical aspects. *Br J Cancer.* 1998;77:1337–1342.
34. Gorunova L, Hoglund M, Andren-Sandberg A, et al. Cytogenetic analysis of pancreatic carcinomas: intratumor heterogeneity and nonrandom pattern of chromosome aberrations. *Genes Chromosomes Cancer.* 1998;23:81–99.
35. Schleger C, Arens N, Zentgraf H, et al. Identification of frequent chromosomal aberrations in ductal adenocarcinoma of the pancreas by comparative genomic hybridization (CGH). *J Pathol.* 2000;191:27–32.
36. Armengol G, Knuutila S, Lluis F, et al. DNA copy number changes and evaluation of MYC, IGF1R, and FES amplification in xenografts of pancreatic adenocarcinoma. *Cancer Genet Cytogenet.* 2000;116:133–141.
37. Mahlamaki EH, Barlund M, Tanner M, et al. Frequent amplification of 8q24, 11q, 17q, and 20q-specific genes in pancreatic cancer. *Genes Chromosomes Cancer.* 2002;35:353–358.
38. Schleger C, Verbeke C, Hildenbrand R, et al. c-MYC activation in primary and metastatic ductal adenocarcinoma of the pancreas: incidence, mechanisms, and clinical significance. *Mod Pathol.* 2002;15:462–469.
39. Visser CJ, Bruggink AH, Korc M, et al. Overexpression of transforming growth factor-alpha and epidermal growth factor receptor, but not epidermal growth factor, in exocrine pancreatic tumours in hamsters. *Carcinogenesis.* 1996;17:779–785.
40. Friess H, Berberat P, Schilling M, et al. Pancreatic cancer: the potential clinical relevance of alterations in growth factors and their receptors. *J Mol Med.* 1996;74:35–42.
41. Ornitz DM, Hammer RE, Messing A, et al. Pancreatic neoplasia induced by SV40 T-antigen expression in acinar cells of transgenic mice. *Science.* 1987;238:188–193.
42. Bell RH Jr, Memoli VA, Longnecker DS. Hyperplasia and tumors of the islets of Langerhans in mice bearing an elastase I-SV40 T-antigen fusion gene. *Carcinogenesis.* 1990;11:1393–1398.
43. Longnecker DS, Kuhlmann ET, Freeman DH Jr, et al. Characterization of the elastase 1-simian virus 40 T-antigen mouse model of pancreatic carcinoma: effects of sex and diet. *Cancer Res.* 1990;50:7552–7554.
44. Bell RH, Brinck-Johnsen T, Longnecker DS, et al. Inhibitory effect of streptozotocin on tumor development in transgenic mice bearing an elastase I-SV40 T-antigen fusion gene. *Pancreas.* 1991;6:475–478.

45. Glasner S, Memoli V, Longnecker DS, et al. Characterization of the ELSV transgenic mouse model of pancreatic carcinoma: histologic type of large and small tumors. *Am J Pathol.* 1992;140:1237–1245.
46. Kuhlmann E, Terhune PG, Longnecker DS, Schaeffer BK. Evaluation of c-K-ras in pancreatic carcinomas from Ela-1, SV40E transgenic mice. *Carcinogenesis.* 1993;14:2649–2651.
47. Galvez JJ, Cardiff RD, Munn RJ, et al. Mouse models of human cancers (part 2). *Comp Med.* 2004;54:13–28.
48. Sandgren EP, Quaife CJ, Paulovich AG, et al. Pancreatic tumor pathogenesis reflects the causative genetic lesion. *Proc Natl Acad Sci USA.* 1991;88:93–97.
49. Schaeffer BK, Terhune PG, Longnecker DS. Pancreatic carcinomas of acinar and mixed acinar/ductal phenotypes in Ela-1-myc transgenic mice do not contain c-K-ras mutations. *Am J Pathol.* 1994;145:696–701.
50. De Lisle RC, Logsdon CD. Pancreatic acinar cells in culture: expression of acinar and ductal antigens in a growth-related manner. *Eur J Cell Biol.* 1990;51:64–75.
51. Hall PA, Lemoine NR. Rapid acinar to ductal transdifferentiation in cultured human exocrine pancreas. *J Pathol.* 1992;166:97–103.
52. Arias AE, Bendayan M. Differentiation of pancreatic acinar cells into duct-like cells in vitro. *Lab Invest.* 1993;69:518–530.
53. Pettengill OS, Faris RA, Bell RH Jr, et al. Derivation of duct-like cell lines from a transplantable acinar cell carcinoma of the rat pancreas. *Am J Pathol.* 1993;143:292–303.
54. Vila MR, Lloreta J, Real FX. Normal human pancreas cultures display functional ductal characteristics. *Lab Invest.* 1994;71:423–431.
55. Yuan S, Duguid WP, Agapitos D, et al. Phenotypic modulation of hamster acinar cells by culture in collagen matrix. *Exp Cell Res.* 1997;237:247–258.
56. Rooman I, Heremans Y, Heimberg H, Bouwens L. Modulation of rat pancreatic acinoductal transdifferentiation and expression of PDX-1 in vitro. *Diabetologia.* 2000;43:907–914.
57. Scarpelli DG, Rao MS, Reddy JK. Are acinar cells involved in the pathogenesis of ductal adenocarcinoma of the pancreas? *Cancer Cells.* 1991;3:275–277.
58. Schmid RM. Acinar-to-ductal metaplasia in pancreatic cancer development. *J Clin Invest.* 2002;109:1403–1404.
59. Sandgren EP, Luetteke NC, Palmiter RD, et al. Overexpression of TGF alpha in transgenic mice: induction of epithelial hyperplasia, pancreatic metaplasia, and carcinoma of the breast. *Cell.* 1990;61:1121–1135.
60. Jhappan C, Stahle C, Harkins RN, et al. TGF alpha overexpression in transgenic mice induces liver neoplasia and abnormal development of the mammary gland and pancreas. *Cell.* 1990;61:1137–1146.
61. Bockman DE, Merlino G. Cytological changes in the pancreas of transgenic mice overexpressing transforming growth factor alpha. *Gastroenterology.* 1992;103:1883–1892.
62. Song SY, Gannon M, Washington MK, et al. Expansion of Pdx1-expressing pancreatic epithelium and islet neogenesis in transgenic mice overexpressing transforming growth factor alpha. *Gastroenterology.* 1999;117:1416–1426.
63. Wagner M, Greten FR, Weber CK, et al. A murine tumor progression model for pancreatic cancer recapitulating the genetic alterations of the human disease. *Genes Dev.* 2001;15:286–293.
64. Crawford HC, Scoggins CR, Washington MK, et al. Matrix metalloproteinase-7 is expressed by pancreatic cancer precursors and regulates acinar-to-ductal metaplasia in exocrine pancreas. *J Clin Invest.* 2002;109:1437–1444.
65. Miyamoto Y, Maitra A, Ghosh B, et al. Notch mediates TGF alpha-induced changes in epithelial differentiation during pancreatic tumorigenesis. *Cancer Cell.* 2003;3:565–576.
66. Wagner M, Weber CK, Bressau F, et al. Transgenic overexpression of amphiregulin induces a mitogenic response selectively in pancreatic duct cells. *Gastroenterology.* 2002;122:1898–1912.
67. Yen TW, Sandgren EP, Liggitt HD, et al. The gastrin receptor promotes pancreatic growth in transgenic mice. *Pancreas.* 2002;24:121–129.
68. Clerc P, Saillan-Barreau C, Desbois C, et al. Transgenic mice expressing cholecystokinin 2 receptors in the pancreas. *Pharmacol Toxicol.* 2002;91:321–326.
69. Clerc P, Leung-Theung-Long S, Wang TC, et al. Expression of CCK2 receptors in the murine pancreas: proliferation, transdifferentiation of acinar cells, and neoplasia. *Gastroenterology.* 2002;122:428–437.
70. Sandgren EP, Luetteke NC, Qiu TH, et al. Transforming growth factor alpha dramatically enhances oncogene-induced carcinogenesis in transgenic mouse pancreas and liver. *Mol Cell Biol.* 1993;13:320–330.
71. Schreiner B, Baur DM, Fingerle AA, et al. Pattern of secondary genomic changes in pancreatic tumors of Tgf alpha/Trp53+/– transgenic mice. *Genes Chromosomes Cancer.* 2003;38:240–248.
72. Bardeesy N, Morgan J, Sinha M, et al. Obligate roles for p16(Ink4a) and p19(Arf)-p53 in the suppression of murine pancreatic neoplasia. *Mol Cell Biol.* 2002;22:635–643.
73. Brembeck FH, Schreiber FS, Deramaudt TB, et al. The mutant K-ras oncogene causes pancreatic periductal lymphocytic infiltration and gastric mucous neck cell hyperplasia in transgenic mice. *Cancer Res.* 2003;63:2005–2009.
74. Leach SD. Mouse models of pancreatic cancer: the fur is finally flying! *Cancer Cell.* 2004;5:7–11.
75. Ahlgren U, Jonsson J, Edlund H. The morphogenesis of the pancreatic mesenchyme is uncoupled from that of the pancreatic epithelium in IPF1/PDX1-deficient mice. *Development.* 1996;122:1409–1416.
76. Offield MF, Jetton TL, Labosky PA, et al. PDX-1 is required for pancreatic outgrowth and differentiation of the rostral duodenum. *Development.* 1996;122:983–995.
77. Gu G, Brown JR, Melton DA. Direct lineage tracing reveals the ontogeny of pancreatic cell fates during mouse embryogenesis. *Mech Dev.* 2003;120:35–43.
78. Krapp A, Knofler M, Ledermann B, et al. The bHLH protein PTF1-p48 is essential for the formation of the exocrine and the correct spatial organization of the endocrine pancreas. *Genes Dev.* 1998;12:3752–3763.
79. Kawaguchi Y, Cooper B, Gannon M, et al. The role of the transcriptional regulator Ptf1a in converting intestinal to pancreatic progenitors. *Nat Genet.* 2002;32:128–134.

80. Hingorani SR, Petricoin EF, Maitra A, et al. Preinvasive and invasive ductal pancreatic cancer and its early detection in the mouse. *Cancer Cell.* 2003;4:437–450.
81. Aguirre AJ, Bardeesy N, Sinha M, et al. Activated Kras and Ink4a/Arf deficiency cooperate to produce metastatic pancreatic ductal adenocarcinoma. *Genes Dev.* 2003;17:3112–3126.
82. Thayer SP, di Magliano MP, Heiser PW, et al. Hedgehog is an early and late mediator of pancreatic cancer tumorigenesis. *Nature.* 2003;425:851–856.
83. Lewis BC, Klimstra DS, Varmus HE. The c-myc and PyMT oncogenes induce different tumor types in a somatic mouse model for pancreatic cancer. *Genes Dev.* 2003;17:3127–3138.

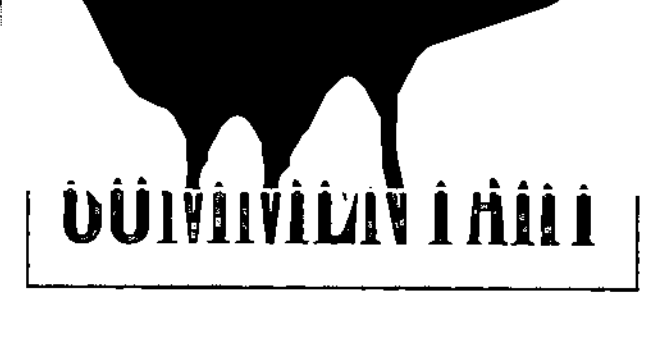

Daniel S. Longnecker, MD

Chapter 6 by Eric Sandgren provides a comprehensive review of genetically manipulated (transgenic) mouse models of exocrine pancreatic carcinoma. "Transgenic" has become the most frequently used generic designation for such models because of the way the field developed. Sandgren devoted part of the chapter to a description of methods used to introduce and manipulate genetic modifications in mice. Although early models were truly transgenic, not all of the mouse models discussed in Chapter 6 use transgene expression in the usual sense, explaining why "genetically manipulated" is a more accurate descriptive term. Both the promise and the limitations of the methods are highlighted.

Limitations include the fact that targeting is dependent on background knowledge of the relevant genes and their regulatory elements in the cells one wishes to target. The relevance to human disease is dependent on knowledge of the genetic basis of the disease that one wishes to mimic. Although the first transgenic models of pancreatic carcinoma were produced nearly two decades ago, this was before promoters were identified that allow targeting of pancreatic ductal epithelial cells and before our knowledge of the genetic basis of pancreatic cancer had progressed beyond the involvement of mutant *KRAS2*. As a result, we have several good models of acinar cell carcinoma in the mouse because of the early availability of the elastase-1 promoter, and we have learned something about acinar to ductal cell metaplasia in vivo. The latter observation sustains the possibility that duct-like carcinomas might arise from acinar cells in humans, although the current mainstream view is that ductal adenocarcinomas in the human pancreas arise from ductal cells.

As Sandgren stated, the dominant view in human oncology is that the cellular phenotype of the neoplasm reflects the cell of origin. However, there are notable exceptions in human pathology. Bronchogenic carcinomas often show squamous differentiation even though the cell of origin is pseudostratified columnar epithelium. Similarly, some squamous carcinomas of the uterine cervix are thought to arise from endocervical mucinous columnar epithelium that has undergone squamous metaplasia. Thus, the possibility that some presumably small fraction of human ductal adenocarcinomas arises from metaplastic acinar cells or from stem cells should remain an open question.

Modeling human pancreatic carcinoma is necessarily a complex challenge because of the wide variety of neoplasms that occur in the organ. The classification of pancreatic neoplasms by the World Health Organization[1] includes 10 histologic categories when one includes exocrine, neuroendocrine, mixed exocrine–endocrine tumors, pancreatoblastoma, and rare neoplasms of indeterminate type such as solid pseudopapillary tumors. Many of the major types have several subtypes, and several occur as both benign and malignant neoplasms (compare Chapters 2, 41, and 51).

The most common primary malignancy in the pancreas is ductal adenocarcinoma that, with closely related subtypes such as adenosquamous and anaplastic carcinoma, comprises approximately 90% of pancreatic exocrine neoplasms. It is the major focus for early diagnosis, treatment, and prevention in pancreatic neoplasia. It is therefore also the major focus for efforts to create animal models.

Premalignant lesions that progress to invasive ductal adenocarcinoma are now most frequently discussed using PanIN nomenclature in the context of the PanIN progression model (compare Chapter 2). PanIN denotes "pancreatic intraepithelial neoplasm" or "pancreatic intraepithelial neoplasia." PanINs are generally regarded as the precursor lesions for most ductal adenocarcinomas and their major subtypes. As is noted in Chapter 6, only the most recently reported transgenic models have yielded PanIN-like lesions and invasive carcinomas of ductal phenotype that are morphologically comparable to those found in humans. Sandgren cited a recent review by Steve Leach that provides a perceptive assessment of these new models (author's reference 74).

Recognition of intraductal papillary-mucinous neoplasms or tumors (IPMN or IPMT) during the past 25 years has provided additional insight into the genesis of pancreatic ductal adenocarcinomas. It is generally accepted that these neoplasms form an adenoma–carcinoma sequence and when invasion occurs the invasive component is most frequently a noncystic mucinous carcinoma (mucinous carcinoma, colloid carcinoma) but is nearly as often a ductal adenocarcinoma and is occasionally a cystadenocarcinoma.

Thus, it appears that there are at least two histogenetic pathways for the genesis of ductal adenocarcinomas in the human pancreas: the PanIN pathway and the IPMN progression pathway. The former is considered the major contributor and the latter an alternate minor pathway for genesis of a smaller fraction of these carcinomas. The IPMN pathway is considered a major and perhaps the only origin for noncystic mucinous carcinomas.

Mucinous cystic neoplasms (MCNs), which include adenoma, dysplastic noninvasive variants, and malignant variants, are sometimes cited as a third pathway for the origin of ductal adenocarcinomas. Because MCNs have not been consistently separated from IPMN in the past, the validity and importance of an MCN-based adenoma–carcinoma sequence as an origin for ductal adenocarcinomas are less clear.

To date, the IPMN pathway has not been modeled in genetically manipulated mice, although some lesions with IPMN-like appearance were noted in Sandgren's Ela-K-ras

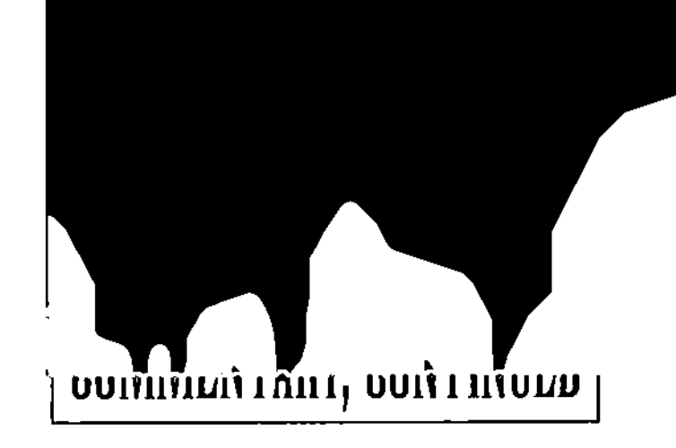

mouse lines. Because the latter lesions arise from a background of acinar-to-ductal metaplasia, this model seems an unlikely source for IPMN because in humans these neoplasms arise in the main pancreatic duct or its major branches. Development of a model for IPMN in genetically manipulated mice would likely provide useful insight into differences between the PanIN and IPMN pathways and would perhaps yield a model of noncystic mucinous carcinoma. A few carcinomas of the "noncystic mucinous" type have been observed in the N-nitrosobis(2-oxopropyl)amine (BOP)–induced hamster model of ductal adenocarcinoma that has been extensively characterized in the laboratories of Pour,[2] Scarpelli,[3] and Konishi et al.[4]

The development of the current group of mouse models has yielded some interesting but unanticipated results. One is the high incidence of islet cell neoplasms in one line of Ela-1-Tag transgenic mice—attributed by Sandgren to the use of a truncated elastase promoter. In these mice, the transgene is apparently expressed either in islet cells or in their precursor stem cells. Another surprise was the development of serous cystadenomas in mice that overexpressed transforming growth factor-α and lacked functional p16, p19, or p53. In humans, serous cystadenomas have been associated with loss of functional VHL tumor-suppressor gene.[5] Because of the justifiable major focus on creating models for ductal adenocarcinoma of the pancreas, it is likely that modeling of benign and rare pancreatic neoplasms will occur by accident rather than by design.

The introduction to Chapter 6 contains a discussion of model validation in which the author points out that morphology, molecular changes, and biological behavior should all be considered in evaluating the validity of each genetically manipulated mouse model of pancreatic carcinoma. The same approach may be applied to transplantation and chemically induced models. Models employing orthotopic implantation of human pancreatic carcinomas into the pancreas of nude mice[6] score well on this scale with two limitations. These are the inability to observe the early, premalignant stage of neoplastic development and the fact that the host is immunodeficient. The first of these makes the models unsuitable for studies of chemoprevention or early detection; the second limits their suitability for evaluation of experimental treatment. Both genetically manipulated mouse models and chemically induced models allow observation of early lesion development and yield carcinomas in immunocompetent hosts. The BOP-induced hamster model is the best characterized chemically-induced animal model of ductal adenocarcinoma in animals, and it scores fairly high in Sandgren's validation scheme. Experimental chemical carcinogenesis has also yielded several rat models of acinar cell carcinoma[7] (author's reference 1).

Overall, the models reviewed in Chapter 6 reflect remarkable progress in the methods of genetic manipulation in mice, in modeling human pancreatic neoplasms in mice, and in knowledge of the molecular basis of pancreatic ductal adenocarcinomas in humans.

References

1. Hamilton S, Aaltonen L, eds. *World Health Organization Classification of Tumours: Pathology and Genetics of Tumours of the Digestive System.* Lyon: IARC Press; 2000.
2. Fujii H, Egami H, Pour P, et al. Pancreatic ductal adenocarcinomas induced in Syrian hamsters by N-nitrosobis(2-oxopropyl)amine contain a c-Ki-ras oncogene with a point-mutated codon 12. *Mol Carcinog.* 1990;3:296–301.
3. Chang KW, Laconi S, Mangold KA, et al. Multiple genetic alterations in hamster pancreatic ductal adenocarcinomas. *Cancer Res.* 1995;55:2560–2568.
4. Konishi Y, Tsutsumi M, Tsujiuchi T. Mechanistic analysis of pancreatic ductal carcinogenesis in hamsters. *Pancreas.* 1998;16: 300–306.
5. Mohr V, Vortmeyer A, Zhuang Z, et al. Histopathology and molecular genetics of multiple cysts and microcystic (serous) adenomas of the pancreas in von Hippel-Lindau patients. *Am J Pathol.* 2000;157:1615–1621.
6. Hotz H, Reber H, Hotz B, et al. An orthotopic nude mouse model for evaluating pathophysiology and therapy of pancreatic cancer. *Pancreas.* 2003;26:e89–e98.
7. Longnecker DS. Experimental models of exocrine pancreatic tumors. In: Go VLW, et al., eds. *The Exocrine Pancreas: Biology, Pathobiology, and Diseases.* New York: Raven Press; 1993:551–564.

CHAPTER 7

Epidemiology

Donghui Li, PhD
Li Jiao, MD

Descriptive Epidemiology

Pancreatic cancer is a disease of developed countries.[1] In the United States, pancreatic cancer ranks ninth in cancer incidence and fourth in cancer-related mortality in both men and women.[2] The age-adjusted incidences are 9.8 and 12.6 per 100,000 person-years, respectively, for women and men of all races.[2] In 2003, about 30,700 Americans were projected to develop pancreatic cancer and 30,300 to die of this disease,[3] which accounts for 22% of gastrointestinal cancer–related deaths and 5% of all cancer-related deaths.[4] Pancreatic cancer is a rapidly fatal disease, with a death/incidence ratio of 0.99. The all-stage 5-year relative survival rate is less than 5%, the lowest among all types of cancer.[2]

The incidence of pancreatic cancer peaked in the 1970s after having steadily increased for at least 40 years.[5] Since then, there has been a slight and slow downward trend. During 1992–2000, the incidence went down slightly by 0.4% per year, but the mortality rate remained almost unchanged (annual percentage change, −0.1%).[2] The reduction in incidence during the 1980s and 1990s was entirely among men; the incidence among women actually showed a slight increase during the same period. The reason for the declining incidence is unclear, but a relationship with the declining smoking rate is postulated.

The most reliable and important predictor of pancreatic cancer incidence is age.[6,7] The age-specific incidence of pancreatic cancer in white American women and men increases continuously throughout life, even after the age of 85. About 80% of pancreatic cancer cases occur in people aged 60–80 years. Cases in people less than 40 years old are extremely rare; the risk of pancreatic cancer in people in the eighth decade of life is approximately 40 times that of those in the fourth decade of life. There is a higher age-adjusted incidence rate in men compared with women.[2] The male/female ratio of pancreatic cancer incidence in the general US population is about 1.3.

The incidence rate of pancreatic cancer in the US black population is considerably higher than in any other ethnic group.[2] The black population had an incidence of about 15.9 cases per 100,000 in 1996–2000, compared with about 10.8 cases per 100,000 in whites.[2] Black men also have the highest mortality rate, followed by black women and white men. Mortality rates among US blacks are higher than those among African blacks, suggesting that environmental factors are involved.[8] Hispanics and Asians tend to have lower pancreatic cancer incidence rates than non-Hispanic whites.

Table 7.1 Established and Suspected Risk Factors for Pancreatic Cancer

Factors	References
Established host etiologic factors	
Age	7
Male gender	2
Race (black>white)	2,8
Germline mutations	11–14
Hereditary pancreatitis	15
Family history of pancreatic cancer	9,10,16
Environmental factors	
Tobacco smoke	7,39–48
Suspected medical conditions	
Diabetes mellitus	17–22
Chronic pancreatitis	27–29,31,32
Gastrectomy or cholecystectomy	31,33,35,36,39
Helicobacter pylori infection	131,132
Dietary and lifestyle factors	
Fruit and vegetable intake	72–75
Saturated fat intake	74
Food preparation and cooking methods	87–90
Micronutrient deficiency	76,77,85,86
Alcohol intake	93-95,104
Coffee consumption	105
Obesity and physical activity	120–123
Carcinogen exposure	
Occupational exposures	106–110,117–119
Organochlorine compounds	111,112,127–129
Cadmium	130

Host Etiologic Factors

Hereditary Factors

Although hereditary genetic factors account for less than 10% of pancreatic cancer cases,[9-12] pancreatic cancer susceptibility has been linked to several germline gene mutations and familial cancer syndromes (Table 7.1). For example, carriers of the *BRCA2* and *p16* germline mutations have 10- and 20-fold increased risks, respectively, of developing pancreatic cancer.[13] Increased risk for the development of pancreatic cancer has been reported for patients with Peutz-Jeghers syndrome or hereditary nonpolyposis colorectal cancer; however, the degree of risk is difficult to estimate.[14] Patients with hereditary pancreatitis, an autosomal dominant syndrome characterized by the early onset of acute pancreatitis, have a four- to 16-fold higher risk of developing pancreatic cancer.[15] A family history of pancreatic cancer is associated with a 13-fold increased risk for this disease, and 7%–8% of patients with pancreatic cancer have such a history.[16]

Medical Conditions

Diabetes mellitus There has been long-standing evidence of an association between diabetes mellitus and pancreatic cancer, but whether these diseases are consequences of a common exposure or are causally connected remains unknown.[6,7,17] In some cases, diabetes appears to be a clinical manifestation of occult pancreatic cancer.[18] A meta-analysis of 20 epidemiologic studies published between 1975 and 1994 showed that pancreatic cancer occurred with increased frequency in patients with long-standing diabetes mellitus (more than 1 years' duration), with a pooled relative risk of 2.1 (95% confidence interval [CI] 1.6–2.8).[19] Later, two large cohort studies also showed that diabetes was positively associated with a risk of pancreatic cancer, and this association was only marginally lower when it was restricted to longer duration ($\geq$10 years).[20,21] More recently, Gapstur et al.[22] provided data showing that a higher postload plasma glucose level predicted elevated pancreatic cancer mortality. The US black population has higher incidence and mortality rates of diabetes mellitus than the white population. This is consistent with the higher incidence and mortality rates of pancreatic cancer among blacks.[23] Experimental studies attempting to prove a causal connection between diabetes and pancreatic cancer have been hampered by the lack of reliable animal models of type II diabetes. Some studies suggested that excess insulin or related growth factors stimulate pancreatic carcinogenesis.[24-26]

Chronic pancreatitis The hypothesis that chronic pancreatitis imparts a higher risk of pancreatic cancer has been examined in case-control studies, and there is evidence both for a positive association and for no association between the two conditions.[7,8,27-29] Chronic pancreatitis is most frequently associated with alcoholism, biliary tract diseases, or both. In two studies showing a positive association the risk of developing pancreatic cancer was increased only for those who developed pancreatitis less than 10 years before the cancer, suggesting that a common risk factor exists for both diseases or that some forms of pancreatitis are either predisposing conditions or early symptoms of the cancer.[30,31] Probably only 5%–6% of pancreatic cancer cases can be accounted for by preexisting chronic pancreatitis.[32]

Other medical conditions that have been associated with an increased risk of pancreatic cancer include those requiring gastrectomy or cholecystectomy.[6-8] Gastrectomy has been postulated to predispose an individual to pancreatic cancer through the enhanced formation of *N*-nitroso compounds.[33] There is evidence that duodenal ulcer patients treated with vagotomy and gastrojejunostomy have elevated gastric concentrations of nitrite and *N*-nitroso compounds.[34,35] Cholecystectomy may affect the risk of pancreatic cancer by increasing the circulating levels of cholecystokinin, a promoter of pancreatic carcinogenesis in rodents.[36]

Environmental Risk Factors

Smoking

The most prominent and consistent environmental risk factor for pancreatic cancer is cigarette smoking.[6-8] The relative risk of smokers versus that of nonsmokers is at least 1.5. The risk increases with the number of cigarettes smoked. The highest risk ratio, 10, existed in men who smoked more than 40 cigarettes daily.[37] The excess risk levels off 10–15 years after smoking cessation. Coughlin et al.[38] reported that smoking for 25 years or more was the strongest predictor of pancreatic cancer mortality. The positive association between smoking and pancreatic cancer has been demonstrated in at least eight prospective studies and in several case-control studies.[39-45] Hyperplastic changes in pancreatic duct cells, with atypical changes in their nuclei, have been observed in smokers at autopsy, and the extent of such changes seems to increase with the number of cigarettes smoked.[46] The risk of developing pancreatic cancer as a second malignancy may be higher in patients who already have a smoking-related malignancy, such as cancer of the lung, head and neck, or bladder.[47] Current estimates suggest that about 30% of pancreatic cancers may be attributable to cigarette smoking.[48] Smoking may account for the sex difference in the incidence of pancreatic cancer in the United States because there is no male/female difference in its incidence among nonsmokers.[8] Although black men have the highest incidence of pancreatic cancer, there is no evidence that blacks smoke more than whites. This suggests a role of other genetic or environmental risk factors.

Although cigarette smoking is considered to be a cause of pancreatic cancer, it is still uncertain which compounds in cigarettes are responsible for the disease. Some experimental evidence suggests a role of *N*-nitroso compounds and aromatic amines in pancreatic cancer. For example, *N*-nitroso compounds, which are present in cigarette smoke, can induce pancreatic cancer in animal models.[49] These compounds cause hyperplastic changes in the pancreatic ducts, which may be the precursor lesion to ductal adenocarcinoma. Pancreatic cancer has the highest frequency of *KRAS2* mutations among all human cancers,[50] and a higher frequency of *KRAS2* mutations has been associated with smoking and drinking alcohol.[51] Studies of the mutation spectra of the tumor-suppressor gene *TP53* have shown that specific endogenous or exogenous mutagens can produce characteristic patterns of DNA alterations in tumors—a "fingerprint" of exposure.[52] The spectra of *TP53* and *KRAS2* mutations in pancreatic adenocarcinoma are more similar to those of bladder cancer and colorectal cancer than to those of lung, head and neck, and esophageal cancers.[53] The predominant G-to-A transition observed in the former resembles that seen in animals exposed to aromatic amines or nitrosamines, whereas the G-to-T transversion observed implicates exposure to polycyclic aromatic hydrocarbon compounds. The association between *KRAS2* mutation and smoking status as well as the mutation spectrum support the hypothesis that exposure to carcinogens through cigarette smoking increases the frequency of gene mutations, which in turn contribute to pancreatic carcinogenesis, and that *N*-nitroso compounds and aromatic amines are the responsible tobacco carcinogens. In support of this hypothesis, tobacco-specific amines have been detected in human pancreatic juice,[54] smoking-related bulky DNA adducts have been detected in human pancreatic tissues,[55] and an aromatic amine-induced DNA adduct has been identified in human pancreatic tissues.[56]

How do tobacco carcinogens reach the pancreas? One proposed mechanism is the reflux of carcinogen-containing bile into the pancreatic duct.[57] However, the fact that Japanese men have the highest rates of cancer of the liver and biliary tract system in the world but fairly low rates of pancreatic cancer suggests that carcinogen-containing bile has different effects on these organs.[58] The pancreas may have some special tumor-promoting factors that allow mutated cells to gain a growth advantage and eventually develop into a tumor; alternatively, pancreatic duct cells may be able to metabolically activate carcinogens.[59] Because most carcinogens are converted into water-soluble noncarcinogenic compounds before being excreted in the bile, reconversion to an active form is necessary before such compounds would be carcinogenic in the pancreatic duct system. Evidence that carcinogen-activating enzymes are indeed present in human pancreatic tissues is available from several studies.[60-66]

What determines the organ specificity of smoking-related human cancers? Information on individual susceptibility to tobacco carcinogens and risk of pancreatic cancer is scarce. Three small case-control studies did not find any significant association between polymorphisms of several drug-metabolizing genes and the risk of pancreatic cancer.[67-69] Nevertheless, a recent large-scale population-based study demonstrated that the *GSTT1* null genotype was associated with a significantly higher risk of pancreatic cancer among smokers and that this effect was more evident among women than men.[70] Furthermore, the same study also demonstrated a significant role of a DNA repair gene, *XRCC1*, in this disease.[71] In a hospital-based study of 260 patients with pancreatic adenocarcinomas and 260 healthy control subjects, we have found a significant association between the *CYP1A2*1F* polymorphism and risk of pancreatic cancer (unpublished data, D. Li, et al., 2004). Similar to the observation for *GSTT1*, we observed a significant gene-environment interaction, especially among women. The odds ratios (ORs) of pancreatic cancer among ever-smokers with the variant allele were 3.4 (95% CI, 1.5–7.6) for women and 2.3 (95% CI, 1.1–4.6) for men compared with nonsmokers with the wild-type *CYP1A2*. CYP1A2 plays a critical role in the metabolic activation of tobacco carcinogens, such as tobacco-specific nitrosamines, aromatic amines, and heterocyclic amines. These data strongly support the hypothesis that individual variability in carcinogen metabolism and DNA repair is an important genetic determinant for the risk of smoking-related pancreatic cancer. Recent advances in the field of molecular epidemiology have offered new hopes of identifying high-risk individuals for the primary prevention of this lethal disease.

Nutritional Factors

The increased risk of pancreatic cancer in Western countries and the recent rise in its incidence in Japan are thought to be related to dietary factors.[72] Diet perhaps contributes to 30%–40% of pancreatic cancers, although epidemiologic findings linking diet to pancreatic cancer are limited and are not as consistent as those for smoking.[73,74] Recall bias and the influence of dietary changes after latent disease has developed undermine the validity of both case and proxy dietary information collection.[45] As a result, the consistency of results from studies that fail to collect dietary data from patients before the disease develops is compromised. Among the dietary studies that have been conducted, no single type of food source has been reported as an established risk factor.

Generally, the risk for pancreatic cancer seems to increase with the consumption of animal protein and fat and decrease with the consumption of vegetables and fruit. There is a positive correlation between the risk of pancreatic cancer and both per capita saturated fat and total saturated fat intake.[74] An international expert panel affiliated with the World Research Fund in association with the American Institute for Cancer Research concluded that fruits, vegetables, nonstarch polysaccharides, fiber, and vitamin C might decrease pancreatic cancer risk.[75] In studies to identify what components in fruits and vegetables are responsible for the protective effect, some micronutrients have been associated with a reduced risk of pancreatic cancer. For example, in a prospective study of 27,000 male Finnish smokers, dietary folate intake and serum folate and pyridoxine levels were inversely associated with pancreatic cancer risk.[76,77] Deficiencies in both folate and pyridoxine impair pancreatic exocrine function in rats.[78-82] This situation could theoretically lead to incomplete digestion of food, greater duodenal cholecystokinin release, and stimulation of pancreatic enzyme production, hypertrophy, and hyperplasia, thereby increasing the susceptibility of the pancreas to carcinogens. Furthermore, folate is an important nutrient involved in the methylation and synthesis of DNA. Imbalances in DNA methylation may affect chromosome stability and gene expression throughout carcinogenesis.[83,84] The association between folate status, DNA methylation, and risk of pancreatic cancer needs to be further explored.

Another dietary component that might be responsible for the protective effect of fruits and vegetables against pancreatic cancer is lycopene. Two studies have found that plasma levels of lycopene were significantly lower in patients with pancreatic cancer than in matched controls.[85,86] However, no study to date has analyzed lycopene intake and risk of pancreatic cancer. Lycopene may play a protective role in inflammation-related carcinogenesis.

Dietary Carcinogens

Pancreatic cancer risk is increased with high consumption of salt, smoked meats, dehydrated or fried foods, and refined sugars and is decreased with consumption of food containing no preservatives or additives, raw food, or food prepared by high-pressure cooking or in electric or microwave ovens.[87-89] Direct evidence linking specific dietary carcinogens to pancreatic cancer in humans is lacking. A recent study found a positive association between consumption of barbecued meat and risk of pancreatic cancer, which suggests a role of exposure to the food carcinogen heterocyclic aromatic amine (HCA) in pancreatic cancer.[90] This hypothesis is supported by evidence that HCA induces pancreatic tumors in experimental animals[91] and that the pancreas is highly susceptible to HCA-induced DNA damage.[92] In our ongoing case-control study, we have found a significant association between dietary intake of several HCA compounds and increased risk of pancreatic cancer[92]. Furthermore, we have detected a significantly higher level of HCA-induced DNA adducts in pancreatic tissue samples from patients with pancreatic cancer than in samples from controls without cancer. These findings strongly support the hypothesis that HCA exposure increases the risk for pancreatic cancer.

Alcohol and Coffee Consumption

A few studies have demonstrated an increased risk of pancreatic cancer in heavy drinkers of alcohol,[93-95] but more studies have revealed no significant association between alcohol consumption and pancreatic cancer.[96-103] Michaud et al.[104] analyzed data from both the Health Professionals Follow-Up Study and the Nurses Health Study and generated compelling evidence against a relationship between alcohol intake and pancreatic cancer risk. The pooled analysis of both cohorts revealed no association for either total alcohol intake or individual alcoholic beverages (wine, beer, or liquor). Alcohol consumption is often associated with cigarette smoking. Chronically high alcohol intake is generally agreed to contribute to increased risk of pancreatic cancer in cigarette smokers.[6-8]

The role of coffee consumption and risk of cancer has been controversial. In 1991, the International Agency for Research on Cancer concluded that there was a suggestive weak relationship between high levels of coffee consumption and pancreatic cancer.[105] However, bias and/or residual confounding (mostly cigarette smoking) may account for the association.[105]

Occupation

Excessively high rates of pancreatic cancer have been reported among workers in industries such as chemical manufacturing, coal and gas exploration, metal industries, leather tanning, textiles, aluminum milling, and transportation.[106-108] However, the available evidence is insufficient to identify any particular occupation as a certifiable cause of pancreatic cancer. Suggestive findings exist for people exposed to products of incomplete combustion,[109,110] certain pesticides,[111-113] and chemicals such as formaldehyde,[114] styrene,[115] and asbestos.[116] Nonspecific and inconsistent findings plague the studies that have been conducted to evaluate the excess risk of pancreatic cancer in industrial workers. Kauppinen et al.[117] specifically evaluated chemical and physical evidence from workers employed by the chemical, metallurgic, and aluminum industries. Using an exposure assessment strategy, these researchers found exposure to ionizing radiation (OR = 4.3), aromatic amines (OR = 1.9), acrylonitrile (OR = 2.1), pesticides (OR = 1.6), inorganic dusts (OR = 2.6), and organic solvents (OR = 2.0) to be associated with pancreatic cancer. Collins et al.[118] examined 14 studies using meta-analytic techniques to assess the association of formaldehyde exposure with pancreatic cancer across four different occupations: embalmers, pathologists, anatomists, and industrial workers. A small increase in pancreatic cancer risk was found but was limited to the first three of these occupations. Industrial workers with average and peak exposures to formaldehyde significantly higher than those of the other occupations examined had pancreatic cancer rates at expected levels of the general population. The finding of increased relative risk of pancreatic cancer among embalmers, pathologists, and anatomists is consistent across studies,[119] but the null findings among industrial workers who had the highest exposures suggest no relationship between pancreatic cancer and formaldehyde exposure. Findings regarding associations between pancreatic cancer and chlorinated hydrocarbon, hydrocarbon solvent, and polychlorinated biphenyls are still inconsistent and are currently under investigation.[119]

Other Possible Risk Factors

Obesity

Studies have shown that obesity and low levels of physical activity are etiologic factors in the development of pancreatic cancer in men and possibly in women.[120] Obesity also seems to contribute to the higher risk of pancreatic cancer in blacks than in whites in the United States.[121] The significant relationship between body mass index and caloric intake underscores the importance of energy balance in pancreatic carcinogenesis.[122] A recently published, large, prospective study of 900,000 individuals followed up for 16 years associated a high body mass index with a doubling of the risk of pancreatic cancer in both men and women.[123] Obesity is a known risk factor for diabetes, and obesity and diabetes may share some common mechanisms in contributing to cancer development. For example, elevated postload plasma glucose and high body mass index have been associated with impaired glucose tolerance, insulin resistance, and the resultant hyperinsulinemia.[124,125] Insulin has been shown to have a direct, dose-dependent, growth-promoting effect on pancreatic cancer cell lines in vitro.[23] Moreover, high concentrations of insulin are able to bind to and activate the insulin-like growth factor (IGF)-I) receptor and inactivate insulin-like growth factor–binding protein.[26]

As a consequence, the level of bioavailable insulin-like growth factor is increased, which could contribute to cancer development by stimulating cell proliferation. It has been estimated that the proportion of all deaths from cancer attributable to overweight and obesity in US adults 50 years of age or older may be as high as 14% in men and 20% in women.[123] More than 90,000 deaths per year from cancer might be avoided if the adult population could maintain a normal body weight. Because the prevalences of type II diabetes and obesity are steadily increasing, understanding the association between obesity, diabetes, and pancreatic cancer could have important implications for preventing this malignancy.

Organochlorine Compounds

Most epidemiologic studies on occupational or environmental exposure to organochlorine compounds and pancreatic cancer have found a weak association or no association. The most compelling evidence for a specific occupational exposure as a risk factor for pancreatic cancer comes from a case-control study of workers in a dichlorodiphenyltrichloroethane (DDT) manufacturing plant.[126] A seven-fold increased risk of pancreatic cancer was observed in workers whose average length of exposure to DDT was 47 months. In a population-based case-control study of pancreatic cancer in Michigan,[127] patients with pancreatic cancer were 10 times likelier to report having used ethylan than control subjects; however, actual exposure levels were not measured. A later study conducted in the San Francisco Bay area observed a higher serum concentration of 1,1,1-trichloro-2,2-bis(*p*-chlorophenyl)-ethane (p,p′-DDT), of its main metabolite and environmental degradation product, 1,1-dichloro-2,2-bis(*p*-chlorophenyl)-ethylene (p,p′-DDE), and of some polychlorinated biphenyls in patients with pancreatic cancer than in control subjects.[128] Furthermore, another study showed that patients with pancreatic cancer with mutations in the K-*ras* gene had higher concentrations of serum organochlorine compounds than control subjects without K-*ras* mutations.[129] A specific association was also found between serum concentration of DDE and DDT, and a G-to-T substitution was found at codon 12 of the *KRAS2* gene in pancreatic cancer.[129]

Cadmium

Schwartz and Reis[130] have proposed that various aspects of the epidemiology of pancreatic cancer might be explained by long-term exposure to cadmium, which accumulates in several human organs, including the pancreas. Substitution of cadmium for zinc was the proposed central mechanism underlying the carcinogenicity of cadmium. Risk factors for pancreatic cancer that was related to cadmium exposure include cigarette smoking and work in certain occupations or industries involving metal welding or soldering, pesticides, paints, or batteries. A meta-analysis of three cohorts with high exposure to cadmium showed an increased risk of pancreatic cancer (standardized mortality ratio = 166; 95% CI, 98–280; $P = 0.059$).[130]

Helicobacter Pylori

Two recent studies have shown a positive association between *Helicobacter pylori* infection and the risk of pancreatic cancer. In the first study, the *H. pylori* seroprevalence rates in 92 patients with pancreatic carcinoma and 92 matched control subjects were 65% and 45%, respectively ($P = 0.035$), which translate into an OR of 2.1 (95% CI, 1.1–4.1).[131] A later case-control study in 29,133 male Finnish smokers found that *H. pylori*–positive individuals had a 1.87-times greater risk of pancreatic cancer than *H. pylori*–negative individuals (95% CI, 1.05–3.34).[132] The exact role of *H. pylori* in pancreatic cancer has not been elucidated, but increased gastric/duodenal acidity and host inflammatory response associated with *H. pylori* colonization may contribute to pancreatic cancer development.[33]

Conclusion

The high mortality of pancreatic cancer and the scarcity of information on its etiology call for additional research. Epidemiologic studies have shown that the incidence and mortality of pancreatic cancer increased over several decades earlier in this century but have leveled off or slightly decreased in recent years. Incidence rates increase with age and are higher in men than in women and are higher in US blacks than in US whites. Both genetic and environmental factors may play significant roles in the etiology of pancreatic cancer. Exposure to carcinogens through cigarette smoking, diet, and occupational contact may increase the risk of pancreatic cancer. Other factors, such as nutrition and obesity, may also be important contributors to this disease. With advances in molecular biology and molecular epidemiology, we hope to develop new tools for identifying high-risk individuals. Understanding the etiologic and molecular events leading to the development of pancreatic carcinoma may provide a basis for developing effective strategies for the prevention, early diagnosis, and treatment of this disease.

References

1. International Agency for Research on Cancer. *Globocan 2000: Cancer Incidence, Mortality, and Prevalence Worldwide (2000 Estimates)*. http://www-dep.iarc.fr/globocan/globocan.html.
2. Ries LAG, Eisner MP, Kosary CL, et al., eds. *SEER Cancer Statistics Review, 1975-2000*. Bethesda, MD: National Cancer Institute, 2003. http://seer.cancer.gov/csr/1975_2000.
3. American Cancer Society. *Cancer Facts and Figures: 2003*. Atlanta: American Cancer Society, 2003.
4. Washaw A, Fernandez Del Castillo C. Pancreatic carcinoma. *N Engl J Med*. 1992;326:455–465.
5. Devesa SS, Blot WJ, Stone B, et al. Recent cancer trends in the United States. *J Natl Cancer Inst*. 1995;87:175–182.
6. Tominaga S, Kuroishi T. Epidemiology of pancreatic cancer. *Semin Surg Oncol*. 1998;15:3–7.
7. Anderson KE, Potter JD, Mack TM. Pancreatic cancer. In: Schottenfeld D and Fraumeni, JF Jr, editors. *Cancer Epidemiology and Prevention*. Oxford University Press, 1996;725–771.
8. Gold EB, Goldin SB. Epidemiology of and risk factors for pancreatic cancer. *Surg Oncol Clin North Am*. 1998;7:67–91.
9. Lynch HT, Smyrk T, Kern SE, et al. Familial pancreatic cancer: a review. *Semin Oncol*. 1996;23:251–275.
10. Lumadue JA, Griffin CA, Osman M, et al. Familial pancreatic cancer and the genetics of pancreatic cancer. *Surg Clin North Am*. 1995;75:845–855.
11. Hruban RH, Petersen GM, Ha PK, et al. Genetics of pancreatic cancer. *Surg Oncol Clin North Am*. 1998;7:1–23.
12. Lowenfels AB, Maisonneuve P. Pancreatic cancer: development of a unifying etiologic concept. *Ann NY Acad Sci*. 1999;880:191–200.
13. Goggins M, Schutte M, Lu J, et al. Germline *BRCA2* gene mutations in patients with apparently sporadic pancreatic carcinomas. *Cancer Res*. 1996;56:5360–5364.
14. Cowgill SM, Muscarella P. The genetics of pancreatic cancer. *Am J Surg*. 2003;186:279–286.
15. Whitcomb DC, Applebaum S, Martin SP. Hereditary pancreatitis and pancreatic carcinoma. *Ann NY Acad Sci*. 1999;880:201–209.
16. Tersmette AC, Petersen GM, Offerhaus GJ, et al. Increased risk of incident pancreatic cancer among first-degree relatives of patients with familial pancreatic cancer. *Clin Cancer Res*. 2001;7:738–744.
17. Noy A, Bilezikian JP. Clinical review 63. Diabetes and pancreatic cancer: clues to the early diagnosis of pancreatic malignancy. *J Clin Endocrinol Metab*. 1994;79:1223–1231.
18. Fisher WE. Diabetes: risk factor for the development of pancreatic cancer or manifestation of the disease? *World J Surg*. 2001;25:503–508.
19. Everhart J, Wright D. Diabetes mellitus as a risk factor for pancreatic cancer: a meta-analysis. *JAMA*. 1995;273:1605–1609.
20. Calle EE, Murphy TK, Rodriguez C, et al. Diabetes mellitus and pancreatic cancer mortality in a prospective cohort of United States adults. *Cancer Causes Control*. 1998;9:403–410.
21. Chow WH, Gridley G, Nyren O, et al. Risk of pancreatic cancer following diabetes mellitus: a nationwide cohort study in Sweden. *J Natl Cancer Inst*. 1995;87:930–931.
22. Gapstur SM, Gann PH, Lowe W, et al. Abnormal glucose metabolism and pancreatic cancer mortality. *JAMA*. 2000;283:2552–2558.
23. Cooper R, Liu K, Stamler J, et al. Prevalence of diabetes/hyperglycemia and associated cardiovascular risk factors in blacks and whites: Chicago Heart Association Detection Project in Industry. *Am Heart J*. 1984;108 (3 pt 2):827–833.
24. Fisher WE, Boros LG, Schirmer WJ. Insulin promotes pancreatic cancer: evidence for endocrine influence on exocrine pancreatic tumors. *J Surg Res*. 1996;63:310–313.
25. Korc M. Role of growth factors in pancreatic cancer. *Surg Oncol Clin North Am*. 1998;7:25–41.
26. Bergmann U, Funatomi H, Yokoyama M, et al. Insulin-like growth factor I overexpression in human pancreatic cancer: evidence for autocrine and paracrine roles. *Cancer Res*. 1995;55:2007–2011.
27. Lowenfels AB, Maisonneuve P, Gavallini G, et al. Pancreatitis and the risk of pancreatic cancer. *N Engl J Med*. 1993;28:1433–1437.
28. Ekbom A, McLaughlin JK, Nyren O, et al. Pancreatitis and pancreatic cancer: a population-based study. *J Natl Cancer Inst*. 1994;6:625–627.
29. Talamini G, Falconi M, Bassi C, et al. Incidence of cancer in the course of chronic pancreatitis. *Am J Gastroenterol*. 1999;4:1253–1260.
30. Ringborg U. Alcohol and risk of cancer. *Alcohol Clin Exp Res*. 1998;22[7 suppl]:323S–328S.
31. La Vecchia C, Negri E, D'Avanzo B, et al. Medical history, diet and pancreatic cancer. *Oncology*. 1990;47:463–466.
32. Bansal P, Sonnenberg A. Pancreatitis is a risk factor for pancreatic cancer. *Gastroenterology*. 1995;109:247–251.
33. Risch HA. Etiology of pancreatic cancer, with a hypothesis concerning the role of *N*-nitroso compounds and excess gastric acidity. *J Natl Cancer Inst*. 2003;95:948–960.
34. Schlag P, Böckler R, Ulrich H, et al. Are nitrite and *N*-nitroso compounds in gastric juice risk factors for carcinoma in the operated stomach? *Lancet*. 1980;1:727–729.
35. Watt PC, Sloan JM, Donaldson J, et al. Relation between gastric histology and gastric juice pH and nitrite and *N*-nitroso compound concentrations in the stomach after surgery for duodenal ulcer. *J Clin Pathol*. 1984; 37:511–515.
36. Howatson AG, Carter DC. Pancreatic carcinogenesis-enhancement by cholecystokinin in the hamster-nitrosamine model. *Br J Cancer*. 1985;51:107–114.
37. Ahlgren JD. Epidemiology and risk factors in pancreatic cancer. *Semin Oncol*. 1996;23:241–250.
38. Coughlin SS, Calle EE, Patel AV, et al. Predictors of pancreatic cancer mortality among a large cohort of United States adults. *Cancer Causes Control*. 2000;11:915–923.
39. Mack TM, Yu MC, Hanisch R, et al. Pancreas cancer and smoking, beverage consumption, and past medical history. *J Natl Cancer Inst*. 1986;76:49–60.
40. Silverman DT, Dunn JA, Hoover RN, et al. Cigarette smoking and pancreas cancer: a case-control study based on direct interview. *J Natl Cancer Inst*. 1994;86:1510–1516.

41. Muscat JE, Stellman SD, Hoffman D, et al. Smoking and pancreatic cancer in men and women. *Cancer Epidemiol Biomarkers Prev*. 1997;6:15–19.
42. Best EW. *A Canadian Study of Smoking and Health*. Ottawa: Department of National Health Welfare, 1996.
43. Floderus B, Cederlof R, Friberg L. Smoking and mortality: a 21-year follow-up based on the Swedish Twin Registry. *Int J Epidemiol*. 1988;17:332–340.
44. Doll R. Cancers weakly related to smoking. *Br Med Bull*. 1996;52:35–49.
45. Hammond EC. Smoking in relation to the death rates of one million men and women. *Natl Cancer Inst Monogr*. 1966;19:127–204.
46. Fraumeni JF. Cancers of the pancreas and bilary tract: epidemiological considerations. *Cancer Res*. 1975;35:3437–3446.
47. Neugut AI, Ahsan H, Robinson E. Pancreas cancer as second primary malignancy: a population-based study. *Cancer*. 1995;76:589–592.
48. Boyle P, Maisonneuve P, Bueno de Mesquita B, et al. Cigarette smoking and pancreatic cancer: a case control study for the search program of IARC. *Int J Cancer*. 1996;67:63–71.
49. Mizumoto K, Tsutsumi M, Denda A, et al. Rapid production of pancreatic carcinoma by initiation with *N*-nitroso-bis (2-oxopropyl)amine and repeated augmentation pressure in hamsters. *J Natl Cancer Inst*. 1988;80:1564–1567.
50. Almoguera C, Shibata D, Forrester K, et al. Most human carcinomas of the exocrine pancreas contain mutant c-K-*ras* genes. *Cell*. 1988;53:549–554.
51. Malats N, Porta M, Corominas JM, et al. K-*ras* mutations in exocrine pancreatic cancer: association with clinicopathological characteristics and with tobacco and alcohol consumption. *Int J Cancer*. 1997;70:661–667.
52. Hussain SP, Harris CC. Molecular epidemiology of human cancer: contribution of mutation spectra studies of tumor suppressor genes. *Cancer Res*. 1998;58:4023–4037.
53. Blanck HM, Tolbert PE, Hoppin JA. Patterns of genetic alterations in pancreatic cancer: a pooled analysis. *Environ Mol Mutagen*. 1999;33:111–122.
54. Prokopczyk B, Hoffmann D, Bologna M, et al. Identification of tobacco-derived compounds in human pancreatic juice. *Chem Res Toxicol*. 2002;15:677–685.
55. Thompson PA, Seyedi F, Lang NP, et al. Comparison of DNA adduct levels associated with exogenous and endogenous exposures in human pancreas in relation to metabolic genotype. *Mutat Res*. 1999;424:263–274.
56. Wynder El, Mabuchi K, Marruchi N, et al. Epidemiology of cancer of the pancreas. *J Natl Cancer Inst*. 1973;50:645–667.
57. Hirayama T. Smoking in relation to the death rates of 265,118 men and women in Japan: a report on five years of follow-up. Presented at the American Cancer Society's 14th Science Writers Seminar, Clearwater Beach, FL, 1972.
58. Morgan RG, Wormsley K. Progress report: cancer of the pancreas. *Gut*. 1977;18:580–592.
59. Harris CC, Autrup H, Stoner G, et al. Metabolism of benzo[a]pyrene and 7,12-dimethyl-benz[a]anthracene in cultured human bronchus and pancreatic duct. *Cancer Res*. 1977;37:3349–3355.
60. Foster JR, Idle JR, Hardwick JP, et al. Induction of drug-metabolizing enzymes in human pancreatic cancer and chronic pancreatitis. *J Pathol*. 1993;169:457–463.
61. Wacke R, Kirchner A, Prall F, et al. Up-regulation of cytochrome P450 1A2, 2C9, and 2E1 in chronic pancreatitis. *Pancreas*. 1998;16:521–528.
62. Chassagne P, Daujat M, Maurel P, et al. Cytochromes P-450 1A1 and 2E1 are present in human pancreas: evidence by molecular biology. *Gastroenterology*. 1995;108:A348.
63. Anderson KE, Hammons GJ, Kadlubar FK, et al. Metabolic activation of aromatic amines by human pancreas. *Carcinogenesis*. 1997;18:1085–1092.
64. Collier JD, Bennett MK, Hall A, et al. Expression of glutathione S-transferases in normal and malignant pancreas: an immunohistochemical study. *Gut*. 1994;35:266–269.
65. Ulrich AB, Standop J, Schmied BM, et al. Species differences in the distribution of drug-metabolizing enzymes in the pancreas. *Toxicol Pathol*. 2002;30:247–253.
66. Lee HC, Yoon YB, Kim CY. Association between genetic polymorphisms of the cytochromes P-450 (1A1, 2D6, and 2E1) and the susceptibility to pancreatic cancer. *Korean J Intern Med*. 1997;12:128–136.
67. Bartsch H, Malaveille C, Lowenfels AB, et al. Genetic polymorphism of N-acetyltransferases, glutathione S-transferase M1 and NAD(P)H:quinone oxidoreductase in relation to malignant and benign pancreatic disease risk. The International Pancreatic Disease Study Group. *Eur J Cancer Prev*. 1998;7:215–223.
68. Liu G, Ghadirian P, Vesprini D, et al. Polymorphisms in GSTM1, GSTT1 and CYP1A1 and risk of pancreatic adenocarcinoma. *Br J Cancer*. 2000;82:1646–1649.
69. Duell EJ, Holly EA, Bracci PM, et al. A population-based, case-control study of polymorphisms in carcinogen-metabolizing genes, smoking, and pancreatic adenocarcinoma risk. *J Natl Cancer Inst*. 2002;94:297–306.
70. Duell EJ, Wiencke JK, Cheng TJ, et al. Polymorphisms in the DNA repair genes XRCC1 and ERCC2 and biomarkers of DNA damage in human blood mononuclear cells. *Carcinogenesis*. 2000;21:965–971.
71. Hirayama T. Epidemiology of pancreatic cancer in Japan. *Jpn J Clin Oncol*. 1989;19:208–215.
72. Olsen GW, Mandel JS, Gibson RW, et al. Nutrients and pancreatic cancer: a population-based case-control study. *Cancer Causes Control*. 1991;2:291–297.
73. Lyon JL, Slattery ML, Mahoney AW, et al. Dietary intakes as a risk factor for cancer of the exocrine pancreas. *Cancer Epidemiol Biomarkers Prev*. 1993;2:513–518.
74. World Cancer Research Fund in association with American Institute for Cancer Research. *Food, Nutrition and the Prevention of Cancer: A Global Perspective*. Washington, DC: American Institute for Cancer Research; 1997.
75. Burney PG, Comstock GW, Morris JS. Serological precursors of cancer serum micronutrients and the subsequent risk of pancreatic cancer. *Am J Clin Nutr*. 1989;49:895–900.

76. Stolzenberg-Solomon RZ, Albanes D, Nieto FJ, et al. Pancreatic cancer risk and nutrition-related methyl-group availability indicators in male smokers. *J Natl Cancer Inst.* 1999;91:535–541.
77. Stolzenberg-Solomon RZ, Pietinen P, Taylor PR, et al. Prospective study of diet and pancreatic cancer in male smokers. *Am J Epidemiol.* 2002;155:783–792.
78. Balaghi M, Horne DW, Woodward SC, et al. Pancreatic one-carbon metabolism in early folate deficiency in rats. *Am J Clin Nutr.* 1993;58:198-203.
79. Balaghi M, Wagner C. Folate deficiency inhibits pancreatic amylase secretion in rats. *Am J Clin Nutr.* 1995;61:90–96.
80. Capdevila A, Decha-Umphai W, Song KH, et al. Pancreatic exocrine secretion is blocked by inhibitors of methylation. *Arch Biochem Biophys.* 1997;345:47–55.
81. Dubick MA, Gretz D, Majumdar AP. Overt vitamin B-6 deficiency affects rat pancreatic digestive enzyme and glutathionine reductase activities. *J Nutr.* 1995;125:20–25.
82. Singh M. Effect of vitamin B6 deficiency on pancreatic acinar cell function. *Life Sci.* 1980;26:715–724.
83. Chen RZ, Pettersson U, Beard C, et al. DNA hypomethylation leads to elevated mutation rates. *Nature.* 1998;395:89–93.
84. Baylin SB, Esteller M, Rountree MR, et al. Aberrant patterns of DNA methylation, chromatin formation and gene expression in cancer. *Hum Mol Genet.* 2001;10:687–692.
85. Burney PG, Comstock GW, Morris JS. Serologic precursors of cancer: serum micronutrients and the subsequent risk of pancreatic cancer. *Am J Clin Nutr.* 1989;49:895–900.
86. Comstock GW, Helzlsouer KJ, Bush TL. Prediagnostic serum levels of carotenoids and vitamin E as related to subsequent cancer in Washington County, Maryland. *Am J Clin Nutr.* 1991;53[suppl 1]:260S–264S.
87. Ghadirian P, Baillargeon J, Simard A, et al. Food habits and pancreatic cancer: a case-control study of the Francophone community in Montreal, Canada. *Cancer Epidemiol Biomarkers Prev.* 1995;4:895–899.
88. Knekt P, Steineck G, Jarvinen R, et al. Intake of fried meat and risk of cancer: a follow-up study in Finland. *Int J Cancer.* 1994;59:756–760.
89. Ohba S, Nishi M, Miyake H. Eating habits and pancreatic cancer. *Int J Pancreatol.* 1996;20:37–42.
90. Anderson KE, Sinha R, Kulldorff M, et al. Meat intake and cooking techniques: associations with pancreatic cancer. *Mutat Res.* 2002;506–507:225–231.
91. Yoshimoto M, Tsutsumi M, Iki K, et al. Carcinogenicity of heterocyclic amines for the pancreatic duct epithelium in hamsters. *Cancer Lett.* 1999;143:235–239.
92. Pfau W, Brockstedt U, Shirai T, et al. Pancreatic DNA adducts formed in vitro and in vivo by the food mutagens 2-amino-1-methyl-6-phenylimidazo[4,5-b]pyridine (PhIP) and 2-amino-3-methyl-9H-pyrido[2,3-b]indole (MeAalphaC). *Mutat Res.* 1997;378:13–22.
93. Durbec JP, Chevillotte G, Bidart JM, et al. Diet, alcohol, tobacco and risk of cancer of the pancreas: a case-control study. *Br J Cancer.* 1983;47:463–470.
94. Heuch I, Kvale G, Jacobsen BK, et al. Use of alcohol, tobacco and coffee, and risk of pancreatic cancer. *Br J Cancer.* 1983;48:637–643.
95. Silverman DT, Brown LM, Hoover RN, et al. Alcohol and pancreatic cancer in blacks and whites in the United States. *Cancer Res.* 1995;55:4899–4905.
96. Bouchardy C, Clavel F, La Vecchia C, et al. Alcohol, beer and cancer of the pancreas. *Int J Cancer.* 1990;45:842–846.
97. Bueno de Mesquita HB, Maisonneuve P, Moerman CJ, et al. Lifetime consumption of alcoholic beverage, tea, and coffee and exocrine carcinoma of the pancreas: a population-based case-control study in the Netherlands. *Int J Cancer.* 1992;50:514–522.
98. Clavel F, Benhamou E, Auquier A, et al. Coffee, alcohol, smoking and cancer of the pancreas: a case-control study. *Int J Cancer.* 1989;43:17–21.
99. Falk RT, Pickle LW, Fontham ET, et al. Life-style risk factors for pancreatic cancer in Louisiana: a case-control study. *Am J Epidemiol.* 1988;128:324–326.
100. Farrow DC, Davis S. Diet and the risk of pancreatic cancer in men. *Am J Epidemiol.* 1990;132:423–431.
101. Mizuno S, Watanabe S, Nakamura K, et al. A multi-institute case-control study on the risk factors of developing pancreatic cancer. *Jpn J Clin Oncol.* 1992;22:286–291.
102. Zatonski WA, Boyle P, Przewozniak K, et al. Cigarette smoking, alcohol, tea, and coffee consumption and pancreas cancer risk: a case-control study from Opole, Poland. *Int J Cancer.* 1993;53:601–607.
103. Longnecker MP, Enger SM. Epidemiologic data on alcoholic beverage consumption and risk of cancer. *Clin Chem Acta.* 1996;246:121–141.
104. Michaud DS, Giovannucci E, Willett WC, et al. Coffee and alcohol consumption and the risk of pancreatic cancer in two prospective United States cohorts. *Cancer Epidemiol Biomark Prev.* 2001;10;429–437.
105. International Agency for Research on Cancer. Coffee, tea, mate methylxanthines, and methylglyoxal. *IARC Monographs Evaluation of Carcinogenic Risks in Humans.* Lyon, France: IARC; 1991.
106. Norell S, Ahlbom A, Olin R, et al. Occupational factors and pancreatic cancer. *Br J Indust Med.* 1986;43:775–778.
107. Kauppinen T, Partanen T, Degerth R, et al. Pancreatic cancer and occupational exposures. *Epidemiology.* 1995;6:498–502.
108. Ji BT, Silverman DT, Dosemeci M, et al. Occupation and pancreatic cancer risk in Shanghai, China. *Am J Ind Med.* 1999;35:76–81.
109. Park RM, Mirer FE. A survey of mortality at two automotive engine manufacturing plants. *Am J Ind Med.* 1996;30:664–673.
110. Bardin JA, Eisen EA, Tolbert PE, et al. Mortality studies of machining fluid exposure in the automobile industry. V: a case-control study of pancreatic cancer. *Am J Ind Med.* 1997;32:240–247.
111. Garabrani DH, Held J, Langholz B, et al. DDT and related compounds and risk of pancreatic cancer. *J Natl Cancer Inst.* 1992;84:764–771.

112. Fryzek J, Garabrant DH, Harlow SD, et al. A case-control study of self-reported exposures to pesticides and pancreas cancer in southern Michigan. *Int J Cancer*. 1997;72:62–67.
113. Jaga K, Brosius D. Pesticide exposure: human cancers on the horizon. *Rev Environ Health*. 1999;14:39–50.
114. Kernan GJ, Ji BT, Dosemeci M, et al. Occupational risk factors for pancreatic cancer: a case-control study based on death certificates from 24 US states. *Am J Ind Med*. 1999;36:260–270.
115. Anttila A, Pukkala E, Riala R, et al. Cancer incidence among Finnish workers exposed to aromatic hydrocarbons. *Int Arch Occup Environ Health*. 1998;71:187–193.
116. Jarvholm B, Sanden A. Lung cancer and mesothelioma in the pleura and peritoneum among Swedish insulation workers. *Occup Environ Med*. 1998;55:766–770.
117. Kauppinen T, Partanen T, Degerth R. Pancreatic cancer and occupational exposures. *Epidemiology*. 1995;6498–6502.
118. Collins JJ, Esmen NA, Hall TA. A review and meta-analysis of formaldehyde exposure and pancreatic cancer. *Am J Ind Med*. 2001;39:336–345.
119. Ojajarvi IA, Partanen TJ, Ahlbom A, et al. Occupational exposures and pancreatic cancer: a meta-analysis. *Occup Environ Med*. 2000;57:316–324.
120. Hanley AJ, Johnson KC, Villeneuve PJ, et al. Canadian Cancer Registries Epidemiology Research Group. Physical activity, anthropometric factors and risk of pancreatic cancer: results from the Canadian Enhanced Cancer Surveillance System. *Int J Cancer*. 2001;94:140–147.
121. Carroll KK. Obesity as a risk factor for certain types of cancer. *Lipids*. 1998;33:1055–1059.
122. Silverman DT, Swanson CA, Gridley G, et al. Dietary and nutritional factors and pancreatic cancer: a case-control study based on direct interviews. *J Natl Cancer Inst*. 1998;90:1710–1719.
123. Calle EE, Rodriguez C, Walker-Thurmond K, et al. Overweight, obesity, and mortality from cancer in a prospectively studied cohort of US adults. *N Engl J Med*. 2003;348:1625–1638.
124. Smith GD, Egger M, Shipley MJ, et al. Post-challenge glucose concentration, impaired glucose tolerance, diabetes, and cancer mortality in men. *Am J Epidemiol*. 1992;136:1110–1114.
125. Gapstur SM, Gann PH, Lowe W, et al. Abnormal glucose metabolism and pancreatic cancer mortality. *JAMA*. 2003;283:2552–2558.
126. Garabrant DH, Held J, Langholz B, et al. DDT and related compounds and risk of pancreatic cancer. *J Natl Cancer Inst*. 1992;84:764–771.
127. Fryzek JP, Garabrant DH, Harlow SD, et al. A case-control study of self-reported exposures to pesticides and pancreas cancer in southeastern Michigan. *Int J Cancer*. 1997;72:62–67.
128. Hoppin JA, Tolbert PE, Holly EA, et al. Pancreatic cancer and serum organochlorine levels. *Cancer Epidemiol Biomarkers Prev*. 2000;9:199–205.
129. Porta M, Malats N, Jariod M, et al. Serum concentrations of organochlorine compounds and K-*ras* mutations in exocrine pancreatic cancer. PANKRAS II Study Group. *Lancet*. 1999;354:2125–2129.
130. Schwartz GG, Reis IM. Is cadmium a cause of human pancreatic cancer? *Cancer Epidemiol Biomarkers Prev*. 2000;9:139–145.
131. Raderer M, Wrba F, Kornek G, et al. Association between Helicobacter pylori infection and pancreatic cancer. *Oncology*. 1998;55:16–19.
132. Stolzenberg-Solomon RZ, Blaser MJ, Limburg PJ, et al. Helicobacter pylori seropositivity as a risk factor for pancreatic cancer. *J Natl Cancer Inst*. 2001;93:937–941.

COMMENTARY

Miquel Porta, MD, PhD

Chapter 7 provides a comprehensive, accurate, and suggestive overview of the epidemiology of exocrine pancreatic cancer (EPC), including the presently limited knowledge on the causes of this lethal neoplasm. It is important for clinicians, public health practitioners, and other health professionals to keep in mind that knowledge on the causes of pancreatic cancer is essential for its primary prevention and for effective measures to reduce its incidence.[1] Although epidemiologic studies are really contributing to further our understanding of the causation of the disease, Chapter 7 by Li and Jiao is an invitation to think about both the difficulties faced by etiologic studies and how new avenues for knowledge and intervention could be opened. One clear way to do so is to integrate valid biological, clinical, and epidemiologic information better from unbiasedly selected groups of subjects with pancreatic cancer.[2,3] By developing briefly some of the clues offered in Chapter 7, much of what follows will try to show how such aim could be pursued.

Overcoming Biases Caused by Diagnostic Inaccuracies, Misclassification of Disease, and Patient Selection

One first path for progress stems from more critical uses of vital statistics on the incidence and mortality of pancreatic cancer. In such data, Li and Jiao appropriately find clues to suggest that environmental factors may be involved in the etiology of pancreatic cancer (because, for instance, mortality rates among US blacks are higher than those among African blacks). However, vital statistics may be biased because of differences across sociodemographic groups and over time in access to healthcare and, more specifically, because of differences in the accuracy of the diagnosis of pancreatic cancer. In fact, for new knowledge to accrue, it is important to overcome diagnostic inaccuracies—important for epidemiologic studies conducted *ad hoc* and for analyses of vital statistics, as well as for clinicopathologic and experimental studies.

Substantial differences have been reported in risk estimates for etiologic agents such as smoking among groups of patients whose diagnoses had different degrees of diagnostic certainty (e.g., patients with and without cytohistologic confirmation of pancreatic cancer). One example is a reanalysis done by Silverman et al.[4] of a study that they had previously conducted. The reanalysis by diagnostic certainty provided evidence that the risk of pancreatic cancer for "ever smokers" was 1.8 (95% confidence limits, 1.4 and 2.4) among cases microscopically confirmed and considered likely to have pancreatic cancer on clinical grounds; the risk estimate is close to what is generally considered true (smoking approximately doubles the risk of pancreatic cancer). Interestingly, the risk was only 1.3 (0.6–2.8) for "ever smokers" considered likely to have pancreatic cancer on clinical grounds but who lacked microscopic confirmation. Furthermore, the risk was 1.0 (0.4–2.4) for "ever smokers" who lacked both microscopic confirmation and clinical evidence in support of the diagnosis. This is a good example of how misclassification of disease may dilute etiologic estimates: If all three types of cases were lumped together, the true risk would spuriously appear closer to the null value of 1 than to the value of 1.8.

These differences in risk for smoking across strata of diagnostic certainty are remarkably in line with the results of the second example, a reanalysis conducted by Garabrant et al. for exposure to DDT (the pesticide dichlorodiphenyltrichloroethane) and related compounds. When they first looked at all subjects who supposedly had pancreatic cancer, the risk associated with past exposure to DDT compounds was 3.3 ($P = 0.02$).[5] However, a different picture emerged when the authors stratified by diagnostic certainty: Among cytologically confirmed cases, the risk was seen to be 21.0 ($P = 0.00052$). Among cytologically, surgically, or clinically confirmed cases, the risk was 8.5 ($P = 0.00106$); and, among cases diagnosed by death certificate only, the risk for DDT was null (odds ratio, 0.8; $P = 0.53$).[6,7]

Both examples tell us that studies ought to pay closer attention to the methods actually used in every geographic area and clinical setting to achieve a diagnosis of EPC. They also show that simple classifications of "diagnostic basis" or diagnostic certainty may suffice to make relevant findings come to light.

Clearly, hence, diagnostic inaccuracies may bias studies and jeopardize the acquisition of knowledge. Let us take one step forward by looking at another real epidemiologic study, whose authors wrote the following: "Case-control studies based exclusively on histologically confirmed cases may preferentially select cases with lower exposure to alcohol. Alcoholics may be more likely to be nonhistologically confirmed than nonalcoholics resulting from less access to medical care or cancer-related symptoms that are misdiagnosed as alcohol related. Because we included all likely cases, regardless of histological confirmation, our study was less prone to this type of selection bias."[8] Figures 7.1, A and B illustrate this reasoning, which seems to contradict conventional wisdom.

How comfortable should we feel excluding from studies patients without cytohistologic confirmation or those above a certain age?[9,10] Patients without confirmation may represent up to one fourth of the total number of EPC cases in the Sur-

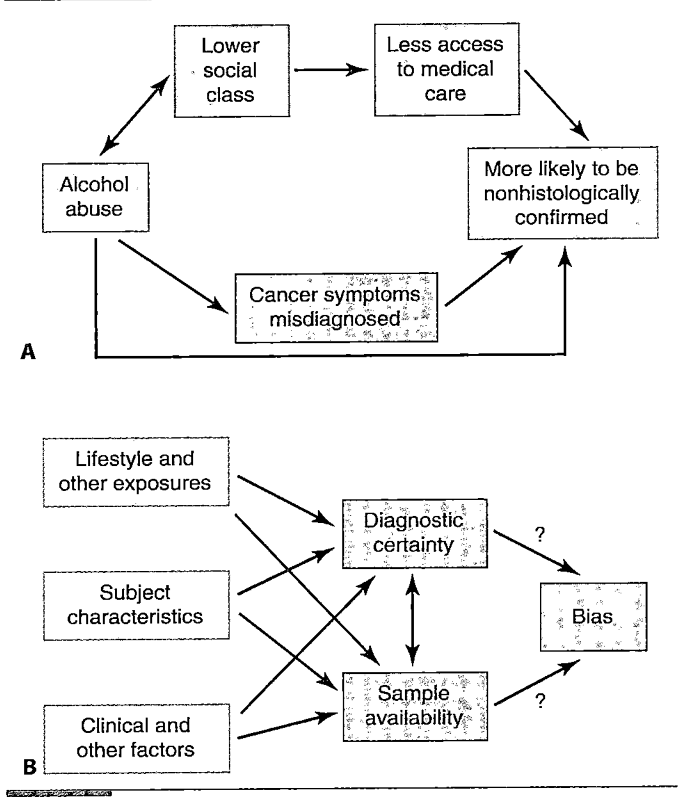

Figure 7.1
Diagnostic certainty and the availability of biological samples may be influenced by sociodemographic, clinical, lifestyle, and environmental factors. **(A)** Two paths through which alcohol exposure may influence the characteristics of patients included in the study. **(B)** A variety of factors may bias the study when they influence misclassification of disease or the availability of tumor tissue for pathologic analyses.

veillance, Epidemiology and End Results (SEER) program; in other US areas and demographic groups, the figure may be 60% or higher.[10] Of course, the proportion of cases without cytohistologic confirmation is even greater in some areas of other countries. Few clinicians would be surprised by these figures. In the United States, where the median age at diagnosis of EPC is close to 70 years, a significant proportion of cases are diagnosed after the age of 80 years (e.g., approximately 28% of white females).[10] In Europe, approximately 30% of male cases and 40% of female cases are 75 years or older at diagnosis. Furthermore, cytohistologic confirmation decreases markedly with age;[4,10-12] actually, in the United States and elsewhere, it also varies by gender, race, and geographic area.[10]

Differences in "confirmation" rates may vary over time; as used in routinely collected statistics, "microscopic confirmation" is sometimes a rather wide category. The cytologic and imaging techniques actually performed in countries also change with time and patients' age, and so do the staging procedures.[9-12] The specific origin of microscopic samples (pancreas, adjacent organs, lymph nodes) must also be judged. Hence, great caution is needed when assessing figures on the incidence, mortality, or distribution of stage at diagnosis. In the SEER program, 19% of EPC cases are unstaged, and 50% have distant dissemination at diagnosis.[10] A pathologic analysis of tissue obtained from an area other than the pancreas, particularly if based on cytology, may carry a significant degree of diagnostic uncertainty with respect to the tumor's primary site. This is why some classifications of diagnostic certainty pay particular attention to the origin of the sample.[9,10]

Restricting subject eligibility to patients less than 80 years with cytohistologic confirmation is reasonable but is not necessarily the best option. Such choice may provide internally valid estimates of risk, but at the expense of the external validity of the study (i.e., limiting the degree of generalizability of the results). Furthermore, it may not fully control the problem of misclassification of disease: Studies in Utah[13] and Spain[9] found significant room for misclassification among cases with cytohistologic confirmation. Therefore, a basis exists for the now common epidemiologic practice of including patients without cytohistologic confirmation but with a strong clinical evidence of EPC, provided that subsequently we assess whether heterogeneity exists in risk estimates across strata of diagnostic certainty[9] (as shown by the previous examples on smoking and DDT[4,7]). A true dilemma for all sorts of studies is "restriction a priory" (restricting the study only to patients with cytohistological confirmation) or "stratification a posteriori" (inclusion of patients with and without pathologic confirmation and stratification of risks by diagnostic certainty)? The latter option may be preferable when cytohistologic confirmation is not as highly practiced as one would wish in the study area (e.g., when it is available for, say, only 70% or less of eligible cases).[9]

The crucial point is that in EPC misclassification of disease status may have a great impact on etiologic and prognostic estimates.[9] This bias can also affect studies of the genetic, pathologic and clinical features of EPC subgroups.[2,3,14] However, information and selection biases can be more profound than anywhere else in studies that try to relate several types of information, such as those seeking associations among genetic alterations (e.g., in the *KRAS2*, *TP53*, and other genes), aspects of the patients' medical history, the molecular pathology of tumors, and environmental exposures.[2,3,15,16]

To avoid selection bias is equally important when planning the collection of biological samples, including tumor tissue. This is not easy, as completeness of the "biological study base" is frequently hampered by ethical, clinical, and logistic factors.[3,17] When the percentage of patients potentially eligible for inclusion who are finally analyzed in a study is low, doubts should arise about the validity of findings.

Valid information on tumor stage is also essential in any clinicomolecular epidemiologic study of clinically aggressive diseases such as pancreatic cancer. It is even more important when studying environmental exposures such as organochlorine compounds (OCs) because lipid mobilization (which might spuriously increase serum organochlorine concentrations) is more likely with increasing cancer dissemination.[15] Often it will also be of interest to have data on treatments given before blood sampling (because some treatments might alter levels of the environmental agents), changes in body mass index or weight loss, and clinical signs and symptoms before blood collection.[15]

Selection and information biases may blur our vision of causal agents. These problems ought to encourage a search for better methods to identify promptly eligible patients. Sometimes, the low percentage of cases analyzed may partly be due to the exclusion of large sections of patients with EPC; for instance, in some studies, two thirds of the patients without surgical tumor material were excluded.[2] One option may then be to retrieve cytohistologic samples from fine-needle aspiration and endoscopic or laparoscopic procedures, which most patients undergo[4,9] and which allow efficient analyses of many genetic alterations. The evolution of diagnostic technologies and clinical algorithms is a constant challenge to researchers trying to minimize selection biases. Readers of research reports deserve a fair description of the process followed to select cases.[2,3,14,18-21]

With these difficulties in mind, let us now turn to a few comments on some promising findings that—overcoming barriers—have been achieved through the molecular epidemiology approach.

The Possible Role of Gene–Environment Interactions in the Etiopathogenesis of EPC

Organochlorine Compounds (OCs)

Achieving a proper understanding of how genes and the environment interact to cause EPC and other human diseases is important both for primary prevention and to deepen our knowledge on the carcinogenic process.[22,23] Long viewed as a promising approach,[24] molecular epidemiology has for some time been contributing to both prevention and basic biological knowledge.[2,25-27] Li and Jiao are hence right in underscoring the relevance of advances in the field of molecular epidemiology for the primary prevention of this lethal disease. In my view, they are also correct in saying that both genetic and environmental factors may play significant roles in the etiology of pancreatic cancer.

Li and Jiao accurately review the epidemiologic evidence—presently, scant—on possible links between environmental exposures and *KRAS2* mutations. Over 15 years after their high prevalence at diagnosis was first reported, point mutations in the *KRAS2* gene remain the most consistent somatic genetic alteration in EPC.[28] Even more important, *KRAS2* mutations are one of the most common genetic alterations in human cancers and probably the most frequent somatic oncogene mutation. It is hence noteworthy that little evidence is available for or against the hypothesis that the occurrence and persistence of *KRAS2* mutations may be related to clinical, lifestyle, and environmental factors. Prominent among the latter are OCs.[19,20,29-30]

Li and Jiao comment that diabetes and pancreatic cancer might be "consequences of a common exposure" and that "obesity and diabetes may share some common mechanisms in contributing to cancer development." They also review studies on occupational or environmental exposure to OCs and pancreatic cancer. It is certainly possible that some OCs might increase the risk of diabetes.[31-38] Concentrations of these and other lipophilic compounds consistently increase with increasing body mass index. There are currently no more than three studies that directly measured blood concentrations of OCs in EPC, and varying degrees of risk were observed,[16,19,29] as noted in the previous chapter. Further studies should help refute or strengthen the hypothesis that OCs have an underlying, indirect etiologic role in EPC and diabetes, perhaps with obesity as a mediating process in subsets of the general population. Other lines of evidence also support the appropriateness of research along these lines. First, as noted by Li and Jiao, dietary studies in EPC have not established a single type of food source as a risk factor, but low concentrations of OCs are found in many fatty foods.[39] Dietary fats are the main source of OCs for humans. Therefore, OCs have been proposed as the agents underlying some food–EPC associations.[40] Second, OCs consistently increase with increasing age, and so does the risk of EPC. Third, the US black population's higher incidence and mortality from diabetes mellitus and pancreatic cancer are also consistent with the higher levels of many OCs among African Americans.[41] Finally, to name just one additional line of reasoning, experimental evidence has provided several mechanistic scenarios, genetic and epigenetic, to explain a possible association between OCs and EPC.[19,23]

Caffeine and Other Coffee Compounds

The epidemiologic evidence indicates that no overall association exists between the risk of EPC and regular coffee drinking at the doses widely used in most countries; nonetheless, studies have not excluded the possibility that the risk of EPC might be slightly increased among people who drink large amounts of coffee.[21,42-44] The issue is probably of little consequence in clinical and public health terms but could

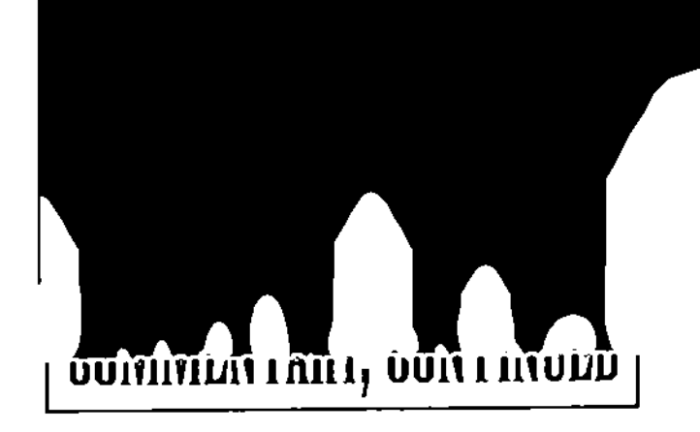

be of relevance for mechanistic research on pancreatic carcinogenesis, and it may hold a number of clues about endogenous and exogenous factors with which coffee can interact as a contributory cause of EPC.[23]

In this respect, it is worth noting that Slebos et al.[16] observed that EPC cases with a *KRAS2*–mutated tumor were almost three times more likely to be in the upper category of total coffee consumption than cases without a mutation (odds ratio, 2.78; $P = 0.11$). In fact, the study probably suffered from several biases, some of which would tend to underestimate the association between coffee and K-*ras*;[2] if so the mentioned OR of 2.78 might be even closer to the figure of 3.65 that we observed.[21,43] Odds ratios for the association between coffee drinking and K-*ras* mutations were above 6 and 19 in some subgroups.[43]

There are certainly good reasons to study the role of interactions between coffee and other lifestyle, environmental, and genetic factors in the pathogenesis of EPC.[21,42,43] First, conceptually, coffee could play a modulating role in a subgroup of patients with pancreatic cancer, an effect that would be diluted in the entire population of subjects with the disease. Second, the potential increased risk at higher levels of consumption is also compatible with several types of interaction. Third, new studies continue to report increased risks of developing EPC at moderate levels of coffee consumption. This suggests that such consumption may have an effect only among population groups with specific environmental or genetic characteristics. Fourth, the vast heterogeneity in results from different studies—that span from significant protection against to significant risk for pancreatic cancer at universally popular levels of coffee consumption—is another reason to suspect that causal estimates result from different interactions among different "component causes." Fifth, there is ample proof that many constituents of coffee—notably, but not solely, caffeine—exert strong effects on a wide variety of physiologic, cellular, and molecular systems. Such biologic evidence is in sharp contrast with the paucity of epidemiologic studies treating coffee as an effect modifier.[42] Of course, some of the reported associations, including coffee and K-*ras* activation, might totally or partly reflect the indirect action of factors with which coffee drinking is associated in a biologically irrelevant fashion.[21,42,43]

With respect to smoking and tobacco constituents, in EPC, the association between smoking and *KRAS2* mutations has not been established,[14,21,43] in spite of the fact that smoking is the best firmly established risk factor for the disease.

In closing, there is great promise in studying the role in the etiopathogenesis of pancreatic cancer of interactions among genetic processes and coffee, tobacco, alcohol, and other lifestyle and environmental exposures. Although a direct causal effect of such exposures is often unlikely, indirect causal effects are biologically plausible.[15,23,42,43] As pointed out by Trichopoulos et al.,[44] interactions must be viewed as part of the broader causal process, rather than as simply modifying the role of a cause in a subgroup of the population. Of course, great caution will always be warranted with initial findings on new gene–environment interactions; and, of course, such studies will continue to require close partnerships among a large variety of basic, clinical and public health specialties.

References

1. Hart AR. Pancreatic cancer: any prospects for prevention? *Postgrad Med J.* 1999;75:521–526.
2. Porta M, Malats N, Vioque J, et al. Incomplete overlapping of biological, clinical and environmental information in molecular epidemiologic studies: a variety of causes and a cascade of consequences. *J Epidemiol Community Health.* 2002;56:734–738.
3. Porta M, Malats N, Corominas JM, et al. Generalizing molecular results arising from incomplete biological samples: expected bias and unexpected findings. *Ann Epidemiol.* 2002;12:7–14.
4. Silverman DT, Schiffman M, Devesa S. Diagnostic certainty in pancreatic cancer. *J Clin Epidemiol.* 1996;49:601–602.
5. Garabrant DH, Held J, Langholz B, Peters JM, Mack TM. DDT and related compounds and risk of pancreatic cancer. *J Natl Cancer Inst.* 1992;84:764–771.
6. Malats N, Real FX, Porta M. DDT and pancreatic cancer. *J Natl Cancer Inst.* 1993;85:328.
7. Garabrant DH, Held J, Homa D. DDT and pancreatic cancer. *J Natl Cancer Inst.* 1993;85:328–329.
8. Silverman DT, Brown LM, Hoover RN, et al. Alcohol and pancreatic cancer in blacks and whites in the United States. *Cancer Res.* 1995;55:4899–4905.
9. Porta M, Malats N, Piñol JL, Rifà J, Andreu M, Real FX. Diagnostic certainty and potential for misclassification in exocrine pancreatic cancer. *J Clin Epidemiol.* 1994;47:1069–1079.
10. Porta M, Malats N, Piñol JL, Real FX, Rifà J. Relevance of misclassification of disease status in epidemiologic studies of exocrine pancreatic cancer. *J Clin Epidemiol.* 1996;49:602–603.
11. Alanen KA, Joensuu H. Long-term survival after pancreatic adenocarcinoma: often a misdiagnosis? *Br J Cancer.* 1993;68:1004–1005.
12. Nieman JL, Holmes FF. Accuracy of diagnosis of pancreatic cancer decreases with increasing age. *J Am Geriatr Soc.* 1989;37:97–100.
13. Lyon JL, Robison LM, Moser R Jr. Uncertainty in the diagnosis of histologically confirmed pancreatic cancer cases. *Int J Epidemiol.* 1989;18:305–308.
14. Malats N, Porta M, Corominas JM, et al. Ki-ras mutations in exocrine pancreatic cancer: association with clinico-pathological characteristics, and with tobacco and alcohol consumption. *Int J Cancer.* 1997;70:661–667.
15. Porta M. Role of organochlorine compounds in the etiology of pancreatic cancer: a proposal to develop methodological standards. *Epidemiology.* 2001;12:272–276.
16. Slebos RJC, Hoppin JA, Tolbert PE, et al. K-ras and p53 in pancreatic cancer: association with medical history, histopathology, and environmental exposures in a population-based study. *Cancer Epidemiol Biomark Prev.* 2000;9:1223–1232.
17. Slattery ML, Edwards SL, Palmer L, et al. Use of archival tissue in epidemiologic studies: collection procedures and assessment of potential sources of bias. *Mutat Res.* 2000;432:7–14.
18. Porta M, Costafreda S, Malats N, et al. Validity of the hospital discharge diagnosis in epidemiologic studies of biliopancreatic pathology. *Eur J Epidemiol.* 2000;16:533–541.

19. Porta M, Malats N, Jariod M, et al. Serum concentrations of organochlorine compounds and K-ras mutations in exocrine pancreatic cancer. *Lancet.* 1999;354:2125–2129.
20. Porta M, Jariod M, Malats N, et al. Prevalence of K-ras mutations at diagnosis and serum levels of DDT, DDE, PCBs and other organochlorine compounds in exocrine pancreatic cancer. In: Gress TM, ed. *Molecular Pathogenesis of Pancreatic Cancer.* Amsterdam: IOS Press; 2000:37–44.
21. Porta M, Malats N, Guarner L, et al. Association between coffee drinking and K-ras mutations in exocrine pancreatic cancer. *J Epidemiol Community Health.* 1999;53:702–709.
22. Vineis P, Malats N, Porta M, et al. Human cancer, carcinogenic exposures and mutational spectra. *Mutat Res.* 1999;436:185–194.
23. Porta M, Ayude D, Alguacil J, Jariod M. Exploring environmental causes of altered ras effects: fragmentation plus integration? *Mol Carcinog.* 2003;36:45–52.
24. Garner C. Epidemiology: molecular potential. *Nature.* 1992;360: 207–208.
25. Hunter DJ. The future of molecular epidemiology. *Int J Epidemiol.* 1999;28:S1012–S1014.
26. Vineis P, Porta M. Causal thinking, biomarkers and mechanisms of carcinogenesis. *J Clin Epidemiol.* 1996;49:951–956.
27. Mucci LA, Wedren S, Tamimi RM, et al. The role of gene–environment interaction in the etiology of human cancer: examples from cancers of the large bowel, lung and breast. *J Intern Med.* 2001; 249:477–493.
28. Gress TM, ed. *Molecular Pathogenesis of Pancreatic Cancer.* Amsterdam: IOS Press; 2000.
29. Hoppin JA, Tolbert PE, Holly EA, et al. Pancreatic cancer and serum organochlorine levels. *Cancer Epidemiol Biomark Prev.* 2000;9: 199–205.
30. Alguacil J, Porta M, Malats N, et al. Occupational exposure to organic solvents and K-ras mutations in exocrine pancreatic cancer. *Carcinogenesis.* 2002;23:101–106.
31. Morgan DP, Lin LI, Saikaly HH. Morbidity and mortality in workers occupationally exposed to pesticides. *Arch Environ Contam Toxicol.* 1980;9:349–382.
32. Takayama S, Sieber SM, Dalgard DW, et al. Effects of long-term oral administration of DDT on nonhuman primates. *J Cancer Res Clin Oncol.* 1989;125:219–225.
33. Henriksen GL, Ketchum NS, Michalek JE, et al. Serum dioxin and diabetes mellitus in veterans of Operation Ranch Hand. *Epidemiology.* 1997;8:252–258.
34. Axelson O, Persson B, Wingren G. Dioxin and diabetes mellitus. *Epidemiology.* 1998;9:358–359.
35. Longnecker MP, Michalek JE. Serum dioxin level in relation to diabetes mellitus among Air Force veterans with background levels of exposure. *Epidemiology.* 2000;11:44–48.
36. Remillard RB, Bunce NJ. Linking dioxins to diabetes: epidemiology and biologic plausibility. *Environ Health Perspect.* 2002;110:853–858.
37. Longnecker MP, Daniels JL. Environmental contaminants as etiologic factors for diabetes. *Environ Health Perspect.* 2001;109(Suppl 6):871–876.
38. Kraine MR, Tisch RM. The role of environmental factors in insulin-dependent diabetes mellitus: an unresolved issue. *Environ Health Perspect.* 1999;107(Suppl 5):777–781.
39. Schafer KS, Kegley SE. Persistent toxic chemicals in the food supply. *J Epidemiol Community Health.* 2002;56:813–817.
40. Stolzenberg-Solomon RZ, Pietinen P, Taylor PR, Virtamo J, Albanes D. Prospective study of diet and pancreatic cancer in male smokers. *Am J Epidemiol.* 2002;155:783–792.
41. Department of Health and Human Services, Centers for Disease Control and Prevention, National Center for Environmental Health. *Second National Report on Human Exposure to Environmental Chemicals.* NECH Pub. No. 03-002 / 02-0716. Atlanta: Centers for Disease Control and Prevention; 2003. http://www.cdc.gov/exposurereport.
42. Porta M, Vioque J, Ayude D, Alguacil A, Jariod M, Ruiz L, Murillo JA. Coffee drinking: the rationale for treating it as a potential effect modifier of carcinogenic exposures. *Eur J Epidemiol.* 2003;18:289–298.
43. Porta M, Malats N, Alguacil J, et al. Coffee, pancreatic cancer, and K-*ras* mutations: updating the research agenda. *J Epidemiol Community Health.* 2000;54:656–659.
44. Kuper HE, Mucci LA, Trichopoulos D. Coffee, pancreas cancer and the question of causation. *J Epidemiol Community Health.* 2000; 54:650–651.

CHAPTER 8

Hereditary Pancreatitis and Its Link to Pancreatic Cancer

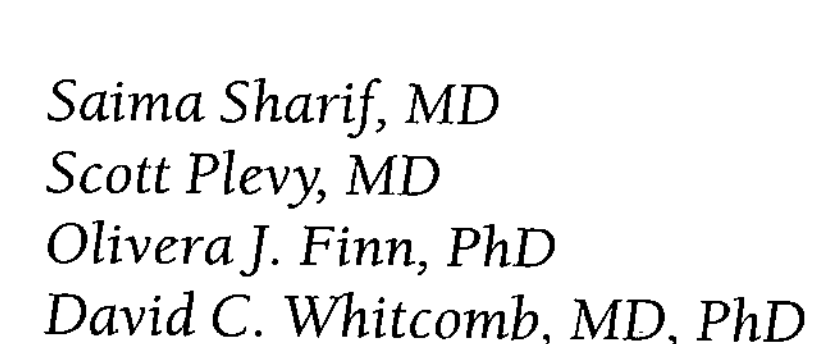

Saima Sharif, MD
Scott Plevy, MD
Olivera J. Finn, PhD
David C. Whitcomb, MD, PhD

Among the many risk factors for developing pancreatic cancer, few come close to the ~ 50-fold increased risk associated with hereditary pancreatitis. Investigation of these families reveals several striking features. First, most of the pancreatic cancers in patients with hereditary pancreatitis appear to be typical ductal adenocarcinomas of the pancreas. Second, these cancers arise about 20–30 years after chronic pancreatitis develops in the patients. Third, the most common gene associated with hereditary pancreatitis is the trypsinogen gene (*PRSS1*), a gene that is neither a typical oncogene nor a tumor suppressor gene, but instead codes for a digestive enzyme. Fourth, known risk factors, such as smoking, clearly modify the risk of pancreatic cancer in these families. Together, patients with hereditary pancreatitis represent a cohort of patients with a very high risk of pancreatic adenocarcinoma. Members of hereditary pancreatitis families serve as a useful model by which pancreatic cancer oncogenesis, early detection, and early diagnosis of pancreatic cancer (especially in patients with underlying pancreatic disease) can be studied and could be used to determine the utility of early intervention in prevention and treatment strategies.

Hereditary Pancreatitis as a Model

In many cases, the study of rare or unusual diseases provides key insights into common diseases. This has certainly been true for the study of hereditary pancreatitis as a model for understanding acute and chronic pancreatitis, as well as the relationship between inflammation and pancreatic cancer.[1-5] In this chapter, the biology of hereditary pancreatitis is briefly reviewed as a foundation for the discussion of inflammation in pancreatic disease. The importance of current observations is also discussed, as strategies for early detection, diagnosis, treatment, and prevention are developed.

Biology of Hereditary Pancreatitis

Hereditary pancreatitis is a rare syndrome of recurrent acute pancreatitis that follows an autosomal dominant inheritance pattern. The typical case is a patient who experiences recurrent episodes of abdominal pain from acute pancreatitis at the age of 10 years, who has chronic pancreatitis by the age of 20 (Fig. 8.1), and who dies of pancreatic cancer at the age of 65. The early age of onset and the distinct phenotypic features of typical acute and chronic pancreatitis

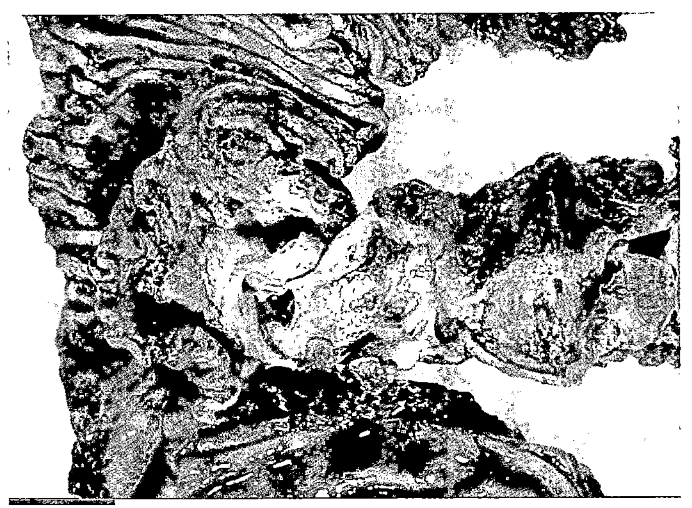

Figure 8.1
Gross photograph hereditary pancreatitis. Note the dramatic loss of pancreatic parenchyma. (Courtesy of Dr. Frederic B. Askin.)

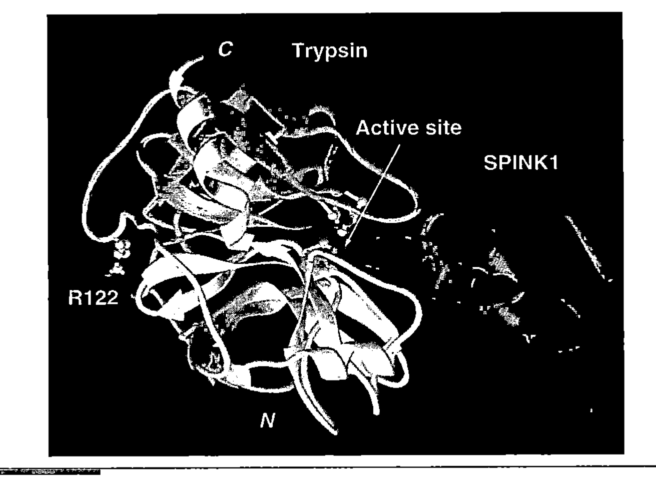

Figure 8.2
Model of trypsin and *SPINK1*. Trypsin is represented in blue and yellow with color transition at R122 to demonstrate the two globular domains of the active enzyme. The active site (*arrow*) is specifically inhibited when *SPINK1* (also known as pancreatic secretory trypsin inhibitor, PSTI), represented in red, binds to the active site and is neither released nor hydrolyzed. The R122 is a target for another trypsin (in the absence of calcium), which could potentially hydrolyze the bond, leading to division of the enzyme and autolysis. This self-destruct mechanism is important inside the acinar cells (where calcium levels are low) to protect the pancreas from autodigestion. Mutation of R122 to H122 in hereditary pancreatitis eliminates this autolysis site and renders these subjects susceptible to recurrent acute pancreatitis. Permission of the American Physiological Society.

allowed the disease gene to be mapped and cloned. The gene responsible for hereditary pancreatitis, in most cases, is the cationic trypsinogen gene, which codes for a digestive enzyme that is synthesized as a proenzyme (i.e., zymogen) within the pancreas and is delivered to the duodenum via the pancreatic duct, where it is activated into trypsin. The most common mutation is the cationic trypsinogen (*PRSS1*) R122H mutation,[5] which appears to be a gain-of-function mutation that disrupts the emergency self-destruction (autolysis) site in the trypsinogen protein, such that prematurely activated trypsinogen cannot be eliminated (Fig. 8.2). The persistence of active trypsin inside the pancreas is pathogenetic because active trypsin in turn prematurely activates the other zymogens inside the pancreas, leading to pancreatic autodigestion and pancreatitis. The discovery that trypsin is the central mediator of acute pancreatitis and that chronic pancreatitis develops in patients with recurrent acute pancreatitis proved to be key to unlocking the mystery of the etiology of these pancreatic disorders. Furthermore, it established hereditary pancreatitis as one of the most important models of human pancreatic disease.

The discovery of mutant trypsinogen as the hereditary pancreatitis disease gene provides tremendous new insights into acute and chronic pancreatitis but does not explain why these patients are at such high risk for pancreatic cancer. The pancreatic cancer risk, although very high, is realized only 30–40 years after the onset of pancreatitis.[6-8] Thus, important and progressive pathological processes must be ongoing before pancreatic cancer is detected. Understanding and identifying key steps in this process may provide opportunities for prevention or early detection, allowing intervention when treatment is most effective.

Hereditary Pancreatitis Increases the Risk of Pancreatic Cancer

A link between hereditary pancreatitis and pancreatic cancer has been suspected for some time. For example, two of the 22 patients with hereditary pancreatitis followed by Miller et al.[9] died of pancreatic cancer, Malik et al.[10] reported that one of his nine patients with hereditary pancreatitis developed pancreatic cancer and Kattwinkel et al.[11] reported that eight of 54 family members in three large kindreds with hereditary pancreatitis died of suspected pancreatic cancer. Similar high incidences of pancreatic cancer in hereditary pancreatitis families have been reported by others (Table 8.1).

In 1997 Lowenfels et al.[7] reported the results of an international study designed to formally define the relationship between hereditary pancreatitis and pancreatic cancer. Patients with hereditary pancreatitis were followed up for 8550 person years, and eight cases of pan-

Table 8.1 Incidence of Pancreatic Cancer in HP Kindreds

Author	Year	Patients, *N*	Cancers, *N*	Reference
Kindreds with definite and suspected cases				
Logan et al.[12]	1968	9	3	(12)
Davidson et al.[13]	1968	11	2	(13)
Kattwinkel et al.[11]	1973	81	2[a]	(11)
"(literature reviewed)"		150	11	(11)
Appel[14]	1974	7	0	(14)
Riccardi et al.[15]	1975	8	1	(15)
Malik et al.[10]	1977	9	1	(10)
Girard et al.[16]	1981	8	2	(16)
Lewis and Gazet[17]	1993	6	2	(17)
Case series/case control				
Miller et al.[9]	1992	22	2	(9)
Konzen et al.[18]	1993	42	0 (pediatric)	(18)
Lowenfels et al.[18]	1997	246	8	(7)
Keim et al.[19]	2001	101	3	(19)
Lowenfels et al.[8]	2001	497	19	(8)
Howes et al.[20]	2004	418	26	(20)

[a]Reported as intraabdominal cancers.

Abbreviation: HP, hereditary pancreatitis.

creatic cancer were observed against a background expected number of 0.15, resulting in a standardized incidence ratio of 53 (95% confidence interval [CI], 23–105). The estimated accumulated risk of pancreatic cancer by the age of 70 in these families is about 40%[7] (Fig. 8.3). These studies have been confirmed and extended.[1,6,21] A striking gene-environment interaction was noted that was related to tobacco smoking (Fig. 8.4). The age- and sex-adjusted odds ratio was doubled by tobacco smoking (odds ratio, 2.1; 95% CI, 0.7–6.1), and the median age of diagnosis of pancreatic cancer was 20 years earlier in smokers[8] (Fig. 8.4). Thus, hereditary pancreatitis clearly predisposes to pancreatic cancer, and smoking tobacco adds to this predisposition.

Several different types of cancer can develop in the pancreas. Patients with hereditary pancreatitis develop infiltrating ductal adenocarcinomas, with a presentation and clinical course typical of sporadic pancreatic ductal adenocarcinomas. Thus, the hereditary pancreatitis kindreds can serve as an important human cohort for studying the development of pancreatic adenocarcinoma.

Given this background information, several important questions arise. First, is the risk associated with the mutation that causes hereditary pancreatitis or with the long-standing inflammation that accompanies hereditary pancreatitis? Second, does inflammation alone predispose to pancreatic cancer? Third, is the risk of cancer in affected family members uniform? Fourth, are there methods for early detection, diagnosis, and effective interventions? Unfortunately, these are mostly research

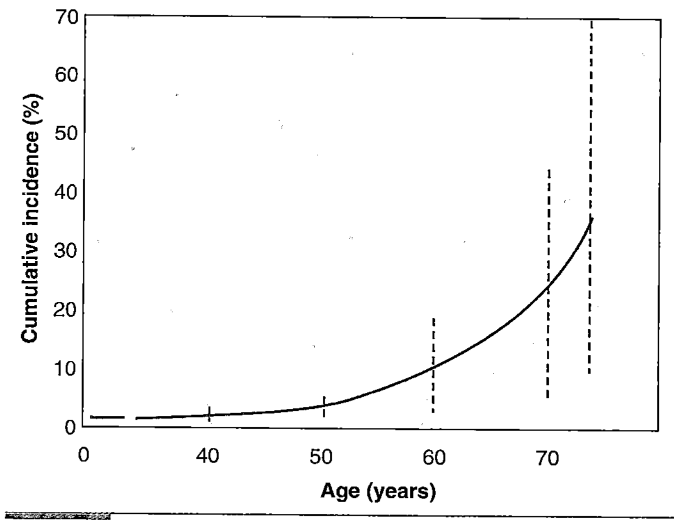

Figure 8.3
Cumulative incidence (%) of pancreatic cancer in subjects with hereditary pancreatitis. Vertical dotted lines are the 95% confidence intervals reported by Lowenfels et al.[7]

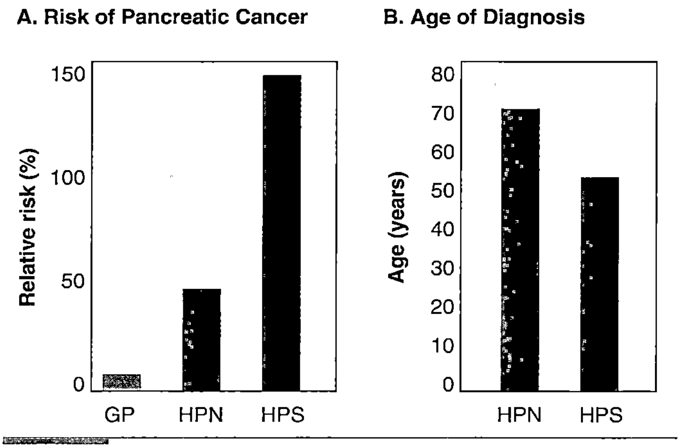

Figure 8.4
Smoking and cancer. **(A)** Estimated risk of pancreatic cancer in the general public (GP), subjects with hereditary pancreatitis who never smoked (HPN), and subjects who ever smoked (HPS). **(B)** Average age of diagnosis of pancreatic cancer in subjects with hereditary pancreatitis based on smoking status (From Lowenfels et al.[8]).

questions because the answers are only partially known. We review some of that information in the following sections.

1. Is the risk of pancreatic cancer in patients with hereditary pancreatitis associated with trypsinogen mutations or with long-standing inflammation?

The hereditary pancreatitis gene, in most cases, is mutant cationic trypsinogen.[5] This important discovery focused attention on the possible role of trypsin in the initiation of acute pancreatitis, and an understanding of the biology of trypsinogen, in turn, helped in an understanding of the biology of acute and chronic pancreatitis. This topic has been reviewed in detail elsewhere.[4,22,23] It now appears that acute pancreatitis starts with unregulated trypsinogen activation, and susceptibility to acute pancreatitis is directly related to environmental and genetic factors that enhance or diminish the activation of trypsinogen or the elimination of active trypsin inside the pancreas. The association between mutant trypsin and chronic pancreatitis is secondary. Recurrent acute pancreatitis (associated with trypsin activation) initiates an inflammatory process that eventually leads to chronic pancreatitis.[23,24] Factors that determine whether or not a patient with recurrent acute pancreatitis develops chronic pancreatitis include environmental and genetic risk factors that, among other things, modulate the immune system (unpublished observations). Because trypsinogen is not a typical oncogene or tumor suppressor gene, and because pancreatic cancer in patients with hereditary pancreatitis seems to follow the onset of chronic pancreatitis by >20 years, it appears that pancreatic cancer in these kindreds is tertiary to acute pancreatitis, with chronic pancreatitis as an important intermediate step. If this is true, then (1) mutations in pancreatitis susceptibility genes (e.g., trypsinogen, cystic fibrosis transmembrane conductance regulator [*CFTR*]) should *not* be associated with the development of sporadic pancreatic cancer in the absence of pancreatitis, and (2) there should be evidence of pancreatic cancer in patients with chronic pancreatitis from other etiologies.

At least two studies investigated common pancreatitis-associated mutations in the cationic trypsinogen gene (*PRSS1*) or *CFTR* gene in patients with pancreatic cancer but not the clinical syndrome of familial pancreatitis. Hengstler et al.[25] analyzed genomic DNA for R122H mutations in the trypsinogen gene in pancreatic cancer samples from 34 patients and corresponding normal tissue from 28 of these individuals. No *PRSS1* gene mutations were found. These data suggest that underlying trypsinogen gene mutations are uncommon in sporadic pancreatic cancers, and that trypsinogen R122H mutations are unlikely to be an important step in carcinogenesis. Malats et al.[26] investigated the possibility that common *CFTR* gene mutations were a risk factor for sporadic pancreatic cancers. However, the incidence of deltaF508 mutation and the 5T allele variant was similar in patients with pancreatic cancer and in control subjects. Although these two studies have limitations in size and scope, they suggest that pancreatitis-associated genes are in themselves not directly important in sporadic carcinogenesis. The increased risk of pancreatic cancer is likely due to a different mechanism.

The association between chronic pancreatitis and pancreatic cancer has been confirmed in numerous epidemiologic studies. During the 1970s and 1980s, small case-control studies noted an increased, but nonsignificant, number of pancreatic cancers in patients with chronic pancreatitis[27,28] (Table 8.2). Between 1990 and 1993, additional studies documented a small but significant increased risk of pancreatic cancer in patients with chronic pancreatitis.[29-31] In 1993, Lowenfels et al.[32] published a landmark paper reporting the results of the International Pancreatitis Study Group's multicenter historical cohort study of 2015 subjects with chronic pancreatitis. These subjects were recruited from clinical centers in six countries. A total of 56 pancreatic cancers were identified in these patients during a mean follow-up of 7.4 ± 6.2 years. The expected number of cases of cancer calculated from country-specific incidence data and adjusted for age and sex was 0.150. For subjects with a minimum of 5 years of follow-up, the standardized incidence ratio was 14.4. The

Table 8.2 Risk of Pancreatic Cancer in Subjects with Chronic Pancreatitis

Author	Year	Cancers/Subjects		RR	Comments
		Cases	Controls	(95% CI)	
Wynder et al.[35]	1973	4/142	0/307	ND	In 3/4 of cases, pancreatitis was diagnosed concurrent with PC.
Mohr et al.[36]	1975	1–2/146		ND	No control population.
Lin and Kessler[37]	1981	7/109	3/109	2.3 (0.5–11.7)	Pancreatitis >1 year before PC.
Gold et al.[27]	1985	2%	1%	NS	(Table 10: 201 cases)
Mack et al.[28]	1986	5/490	1/490	5.0 (0.7–116.5)	Risk higher in patients directly interviewed at 2/124 vs 0/124 (Table 5).
Farrow and Davis[29]	1990	5/148	0/188	Infinity	Pancreatitis >3 years before PC.
Jain et al.[30]	1991	11/249	5/505	8.0 (2.3–28.3)	No time window.
Bueno de Mesquita et al.[38]	1992	1/176	4/487	0.86 (0.1–7.9)	Population-based case-control from the Netherlands. No time window.
Kalapothaki et al.[31]	1993	4/181	1/188×2	8.2 (ND)	Two control series. No time window.
Lowenfels et al.[32]	1993	56/2015	2.13/2015 (exp)	16.5 (11.1–23.7)	SIR, pancreatitis >2 years before PC
Ekbom et al.[39]	1994	46/7956	21/7956 (exp)	2.2 SIR (1.6–2.9)	Swedish cancer registry, SIR 3.8 confidence interval 1.4–8.2 for discharge diagnosis of chronic pancreatitis.
Fernandez et al.[34]	1995	24/338	18/1390	5.1 (1.8–14.1)	Pancreatitis >5 years before PC
Bansal and Sonnenberg[40]	1995	93/2639	99/7774	2.9 (2.2–3.9)	Case-control from veterans administration database: data for chronic pancreatitis (Table 1).
Madeira et al.[41]	1998	3/379	0.12/279 (exp)	SMR 13.7 (ND)	Abstract. $P < 0.001$.

Modified from Fernandez et al.[34]

Abbreviations: ND, not done; NS, not significant; PC, pancreatic cancer; RR, relative risk; SIR, standardized incidence ratio; SMR, standardized mortality ratio; exp, expected; CI, confidence interval; VA, veterans administration.

cumulative risk of pancreatic cancer in subjects with chronic pancreatitis for 10 and 20 years was 1.8% and 4.0%, respectively. Furthermore, the risk of pancreatic cancer was independent of the underlying cause of chronic pancreatitis. Thus, the risk of pancreatic cancer in patients with chronic pancreatitis appeared to far exceed any other known risk factor, including cigarette smoking (relative risk from eight studies varied from 1.2 to 3.1[33]). To summarize, nearly all studies have demonstrated a significant risk of pancreatic cancer in patients with chronic pancreatitis (Table 8.2).

The incidence of pancreatic cancer is also high in other syndromes associated with chronic pancreatitis, such as cystic fibrosis and tropical pancreatitis.[3] In 1993, Sheldon et al.[42] reported on two cases of pancreatic cancer (0.008 expected) and one case of adenocarcinoma of the terminal ileum (<0.001 expected) among 412 subjects with cystic fibrosis. The increased incidence of digestive tract cancers, but not cancer in general, was then confirmed by Neglia et al.[43] among 28,511 cystic fibrosis patients in the United States and Canada (risk ratio, 6.5) and Europe (risk ratio, 6.4). Although only two pancreatic cancers were identified, pancreatic cancers developing during the third decade of life is exceedingly rare, resulting in an odds ratio of 31.5 compared with control subjects.[43] A combined analysis of all the information available suggests a relative risk of approximately 5–10 compared to relevant control populations.

Tropical pancreatitis is a form of idiopathic chronic pancreatitis seen in tropical Asia and Africa, characterized by abdominal pain, intraductal pancreatic calculi, and diabetes mellitus in young nonalcoholic individuals.[44] We identified pancreatitis-causing mutations[45,46] in the serine protease inhibitor Kazal type 1 (*SPINK1*) gene (also known as pancreatic secretory trypsin inhibitor; *PSTI*) in a significant subset of patients with tropical pancreatitis in Bangladesh.[47] This study suggested that a major underlying predisposing factor is genetic. Although the incidence of pancreatic cancer in India is about 10% of the incidence in the United States,[48] the incidence of pancreatic cancer in adult patients with tropical pancreatitis is striking. For example, in 1992, Augustine and Ramesh[49] reported on 22 pancreatic cancers among 266 patients with tropical pancreatitis over an 8-year period (8.3%). In this cohort, the risk was highest after age 40 years, and patients with tropical pancreatitis often had features of intraductal dysplasia (pancreatic intraepithelial neoplasia) as well as invasive cancer in resected pancreatic specimens. In 1994, Chari et al.[50] reported that over a 4.5-year period, 24 of 185 patients with tropical pancreatitis died, and six (25%) died of pancreatic cancer. The average age of onset was 45 ± 7 years, and the relative risk, compared with those without tropical pancreatitis, was 100.

Taken together, it appears that pancreatitis-associated gene mutations do not cause pancreatic cancer in the absence of the clinical syndrome of chronic pancreatitis. Second, all forms of chronic pancreatitis appear to markedly increase the risk of pancreatic cancer. Therefore, the increased risk of pancreatic cancer in patients with hereditary pancreatitis appears to be due to longstanding inflammation. Furthermore, patients with earlier age of onset of chronic pancreatitis (e.g., hereditary pancreatitis, cystic fibrosis, and tropical pancreatitis) have a higher incidence of pancreatic cancer than patients with adult-onset chronic pancreatitis (e.g., alcoholic chronic pancreatitis). This may be partly due to the longer duration of inflammation before the patients die of other diseases of old age.

2. Why does pancreatic inflammation predispose to pancreatic cancer?

Development of pancreatic cancer in any individual requires a progressive series of genetic events typically occurring within pancreatic duct cells.[51,52] In pancreatic cancer, there are many mutations that are commonly identified and others that appear to occur less commonly. If chronic pancreatic inflammation is associated with pancreatic cancer, then what are the common mutations and do they also occur in other cancers that arise in chronically inflamed tissues?

Cancer-associated mutated genes are broadly categorized as oncogenes, those that normally function to promote cell growth, and tumor suppressor genes that normally suppress cell growth and division. Mutations in the oncogene *KRAS2* and in the tumor suppressor genes *TP53*, *p16/CDKN2A*, and *DPC4/MADH4* have been demonstrated in most pancreatic cancers.[51] As the number of mutations accumulates in the cells, progressing toward adenocarcinoma, the morphology acquires characteristics of a more aggressive neoplasm. However, the exact sequence of mutation development, if necessary, and the complete repertoire of critical mutations have yet to be discovered.[51-56]

Specific genes that are known to be mutated in infiltrating ductal pancreatic adenocarcinoma can be divided into four groups on the basis of the frequency with which they occur. The *KRAS2* codon 12 and the *p16/CDKN2A* gene alterations are found in more than 90% of invasive pancreatic cancers.[57-60] These mutations appear to occur early because they are often detected in preinvasive lesions and may be found in patients with chronic pancreatitis.[61-64] The frequency of *KRAS2* mutation is approximately 90% in all infiltrating pancreatic adenocarcinomas and nearly 100% in ductal adenocarcinomas with a typical morphology.[58,59,65] The *p16/CDKN2A* gene product is also frequently altered or lost through homozygous deletions, intragenic mutations, and epigenetic alterations, including methylation that alters gene expression.[66] The fact that the *p16/CDKN2A* and *KRAS2* mutations occur early and that they are in the overwhelming majority of carcinomas suggests that these mutations are necessary but not sufficient for pancreatic cancer development.

A second group of genes in which mutations that occur in approximately half of pancreatic cancers include the *TP53* (50%–75%) and *DPC4/MADH4* (55%).[67,68] The third group includes less common germline mutations, such as those in the *BRCA2* gene. Mutations in the *BRCA2* gene occur in 7%–10% of pancreatic carcinomas.[69] A fourth group, which includes a group of genes that are mutated in 5% or less of pancreatic tumors, includes the *LKB1/STK11* and *MKK4* genes, the transforming growth factor-β receptors I or II genes, and the retinoblastoma (*RB1*) genes.[68,70-73] The information on the frequency and the timing of these less common mutations in individual cancers is being defined. Organization and classification of these data will lead to better understanding of the various forms of pancreatic cancer and how specific risk factors interact. Furthermore, as the pathway from normal ductal epithelium to invasive pancreatic cancer becomes clear, we can begin to investigate why the process is accelerated in patients with chronic pancreatitis. The approximate frequency of mutations in several of the major pancreatic cancer-associated genes is given in Table 8.3.

Table 8.3 Frequency of Mutations in Several of the Major Pancreatic Cancer-Associated Genes

	Gene Mutation*,†			
Type of Cancer	***KRAS2***	***TP53***	***p16***	***Cyclin D1***
Pancreas	~95% (61,95)	~40% (96-98)	~80% (76,99)	~95% (100)
Colon	~60% (101)	~60% (102)	~20% (101)	~60% (103)
Esophagus	~60% (104)	~60% (105)	~95% (106)	~40% (107)
Liver	~60% (108)	~60% (109)	~80% (110)	~20% (110)
Gallbladder	~60% (111)	~80% (112)	~80% (113)	~60% (114)

*Gene mutations shared by tumors of the gastrointestinal tract known to develop in the setting of chronic inflammation.
†Number in parentheses represents a relevant reference.

The progression from normal pancreas to pancreatic adenocarcinoma is associated with accumulation of mutations that are reflected in progressive morphologic changes in pancreatic cells. The current model for pancreatic ductal adenocarcinoma proposes a progression from normal cuboidal to low columnar epithelium through a series of lesions termed *pancreatic intraepithelial neoplasia* (PanIN) to invasive carcinoma.[52,54,74-76] Normal epithelium develops into PanIN-1A, which is a flat lesion composed of tall columnar cells with regular basally located nuclei and abundant supranuclear mucin, that is, mucinous cell hypertrophy. It progresses to PanIN-1B, which is characterized by cells similar to PanIN-1A, with a papillary, micropapillary, or basally pseudostratified architecture. The next stage, PanIN-2, is a flat or papillary epithelial lesion with mild-to-moderate nuclear atypia, that is, some nuclear stratification, crowding, enlargement, hyperchromatism, and occasional mitotic figures. PanIN-3 is severe atypia, that is, papillary, micropapillary, or cribriform architecture with budding and/or bridging, loss of nuclear polarity, pleomorphism, prominent nucleoli, frequent mitoses, and luminal necrosis.[52,74] PanIN-3 is thought to be at the highest risk for developing invasive carcinoma. The genetic alterations that occur in PanINs have been defined and include telomere shortening and mutations of *KRAS2* and $p21^{WAF1/CIP1}$ early in the development of PanIN, followed by Id-1/Id-2, *TP53*, cyclin D1, and *p16/CDKN2A*, with *DPC4/MADH4* and *BRCA2* abnormalities occurring late in the progression of PanIN. Continuing research into the preinvasive lesions with the use of an organized approach will provide the framework for understanding, diagnosing, and preventing pancreatic cancer.

We can now address the question of whether chronic pancreatic inflammation per se causes cancer. The focus of much of the earlier research in chronic pancreatitis and pancreatic cancer has been on the appearance of *KRAS2* gene mutations. Activating mutations of the *KRAS2* oncogene occur in more than 90% of pancreatic carcinomas. These mutations are generally not seen in normal pancreatic tissue and were thought to be specific for pancreatic neoplasia.[58,59,65] However, numerous reports suggest that *KRAS2* gene mutations are also common in chronic pancreatitis.[62-64,77,78] Indeed, the *KRAS2* gene mutations in patients with chronic pancreatitis may be localized to areas of the duct with PanINs,[79] suggesting focal progression toward carcinogenesis. Hingorani et al.[80] recently reported fascinating results from a mouse model with PanINs, confirming that both the level of *ras* expression and the cellular context determine biologic outcome. These mice have an identifiable serum proteomic signature, suggesting a means of detecting the presence of preinvasive lesions in patients.[80]

Intraductal dysplasia (PanIN) also appears to be increased in tropical pancreatitis. Augustine and Ramesh[49] observed dysplasia in two of five resected specimens in patients with tropical pancreatitis and cancer, whereas no dysplasia was seen in sporadic pancreatic cancers. Thus, focal areas of dysplasia, possibly harboring *KRAS2* mutations, frequently arise within the context of chronic pancreatitis. Together, these data suggest that the pathway to sporadic pancreatic cancer is similar to the pathway in patients with long-standing pancreatic inflammation and suggest that chronic pancreatitis is fertile ground for oncogenesis.

The mechanisms linking chronic inflammation with cancer remain the topic of intense investigation. An analogous area that may provide insight into the role of inflammation in the development of cancer is the development of colon cancer in patients with chronic colitis. Colonic mucosa is accessible through colonoscopy and biopsy, and the entire colon can be studied after colectomy. Hofseth et al.[81] highlighted the role of nitric oxide in the induction of cellular stress and the activation of a p53 response pathway during chronic inflammation in noncancerous colon tissues from patients with ulcerative colitis.[81] This process leads to apoptosis, which is a cellular defense against DNA damage. Macrophage migration inhibition factor, which is a potent pro-inflammatory cytokine and an essential component of an inflammatory response, can inhibit this p53-mediated apoptosis.[82,83] Levels of migration inhibition factor are increased in ulcerative colitis when compared with normal colon samples.[84,85] Eventually *TP53* gene mutations occur within inflammatory lesions of the ulcerative colitis colon.[86] Continued genomic damage from nitric oxide and other free radicals generated from activated macrophages and the stressed colonic epithelium could drive clonal selection and expansion of these *TP53* mutant cells that are resistant to free radical–induced growth arrest and apoptosis. Increased levels of migration inhibition factor are also described in hepatocellular cancers.[87] The process leading to cancer may also be accelerated by continual release of growth factors that are part of the repair process and by selection of clones with growth advantages (e.g., cells with mutations that increase the ability to repopulate injured areas).

Several other chronic inflammatory states are strongly associated with eventual cancer formation.[88,89] In addition to colon cancer in patients with ulcerative colitis,[90] esophageal cancer is linked to chronic esophagitis, and gastric cancer develops after chronic gastritis with *Helicobacter pylori* infection,[91,92] and hepatocellular cancer develops after chronic hepatitis B or hepatitis C virus infection.[93] In addition, gallbladder cancer is associated with a long-standing chronic cholecystitis from gallstones.[94] The association between hereditary chronic pancreatitis and pancreatic cancer therefore appears to be similar to observed associations of inflammation and cancer in other organs. The gene mutations found in pancreatic cancer are shared by other neoplasms that are known to have a strong association with chronic inflammation (see Table 8.3).

3. Is the risk of cancer uniform in hereditary pancreatitis-affected family members?

The high risk of pancreatic cancer in patients with hereditary, and likely other, forms of long-standing chronic pancreatitis implies an accelerated accumulation of cancer-causing mutations. However, some kindreds appear to have more cancer than others.[1] This suggests that risk factors other than inflammation are important in oncogenesis. Both the co-inheritance of oncogenic germline mutations and environmental factors must be carefully considered, especially because they represent risk-reducing preventative targets. Most of the work in this area focused on sporadic pancreatic cancers. In these studies, the probability that common occupational exposures significantly increase the risk of pancreatic cancer appears minimal. For example, a recent population-based, case-control study based on death certificates from 63,097 persons dying of pancreatic cancer and 252,386 controls from 24 US states, failed to identify industrial or occupational exposure as a major contributor to the etiology of pancreatic cancer.[115] Likewise, a population-based, case-control study of pancreatic cancer diagnosed in Atlanta, GA; Detroit, MI; and 10 New Jersey counties identified only mild risk or protection from dietary factors.[116] Thus, with the exception of cigarette smoking, common environmental factors appear to play a minor role in the development of pancreatic cancer. This should not be surprising because the pancreas is protected from exposure to most environmental factors, and neither filters nor concentrates xenobiotics and toxins, like the urinary tract, nor does it metabolize, solubilize, or eliminate these compounds, like the liver. However, the pancreas does express the important enzymes that metabolize tobacco smoke xenobiotics, including UDP glucuronosyltransferase 1A7 (UGT1A7).[117] Thus, inability of the pancreas to metabolize xenobiotics in tobacco smoke may contribute to this environmental risk and could contribute to the development of pancreatic cancer.

Cigarette smoking increases the risk of pancreatic cancer about twofold.[21,33] Recent evidence suggests that cigarette smoking and a positive family history of pancreatic cancer are synergistic. For example, Schenk et al.[118] examined the relative risk in smokers and in families with a positive family history of pancreatic cancer and found that each of these factors approximately doubled the risk of pancreatic cancer. The increased relative risk was 2.49 (95% CI, 1.32–4.49) for a positive family history and 2.04 (95% CI, 2.18–31.07) for individuals who had ever smoked. The relative risk of pancreatic cancer from smoking was dramatically increased to 8.23 in relatives of proband diagnosed with pancreatic cancer before the age of 60 years. A similar synergism between hereditary pancreatitis, pancreatic cancer, and smoking has also been reported.[7,8,21] As noted earlier, cigarette smoking doubles the risk of cancer among these very high-risk patients with hereditary pancreatitis and reduces the age of onset by about 20 years.[8] Therefore, smoking is an example of an environmental factor that alters the risk of pancreatic cancer in subjects with hereditary pancreatitis.

Co-inheritance of high-risk genetic factors with the cationic trypsinogen mutations or other chronic pancre-

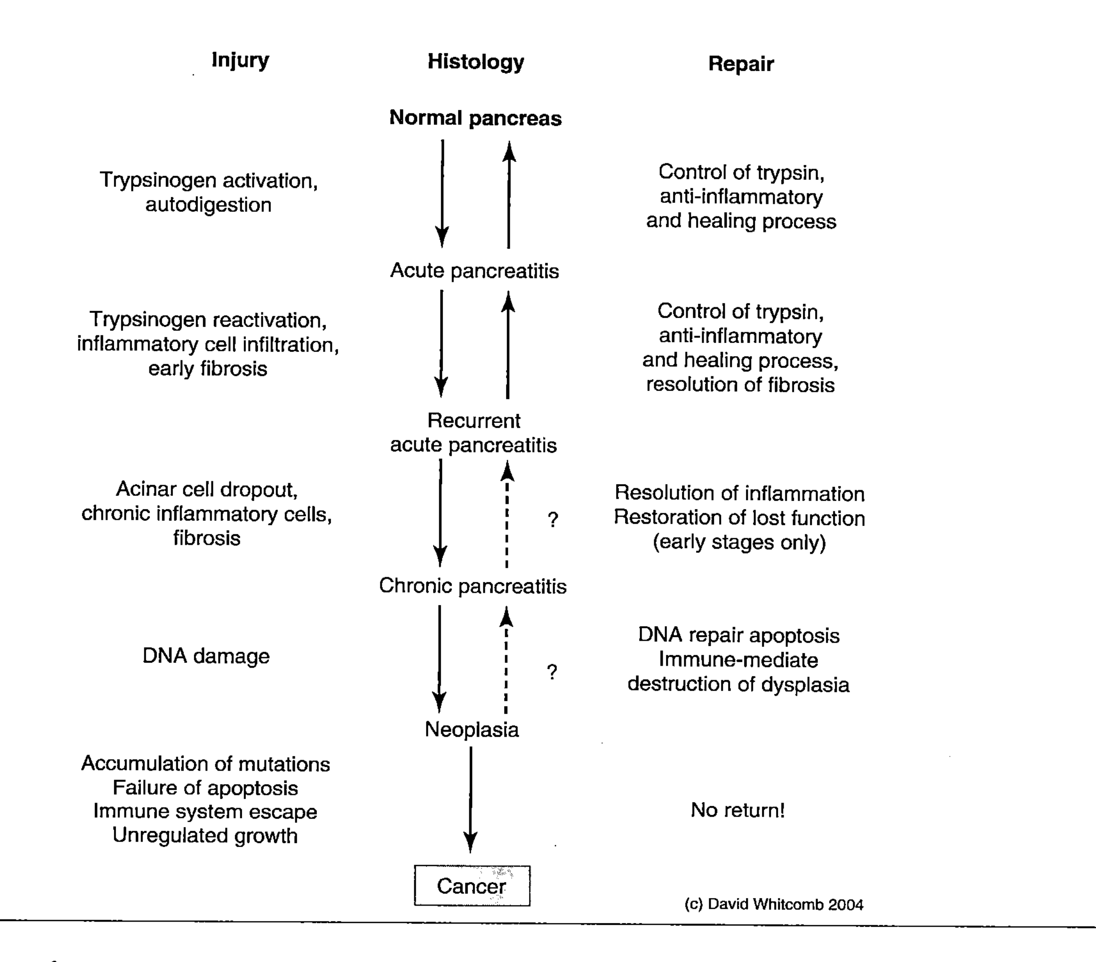

Figure 8.5
Injury and repair in the pathway from normal pancreas to pancreatic cancer. Chronic pancreatitis develops in subjects with hereditary pancreatitis because unregulated trypsin production leads to recurrent pancreatitis, chronic inflammation, and scarring. Pancreatic cancer develops in the context of chronic pancreatitis only after failure of the DNA repair mechanism, failure of apoptosis, and escape of dysplastic cells from the immune system. (Diagram courtesy of Dr. Whitcomb.) Permission of the American Physiological Society.

atitis susceptibility genes also alters the general risk of pancreatic cancer in patients with hereditary pancreatitis. To date, however, little investigation has occurred in this area. It is unlikely that the major familial cancer syndromes will be associated with most cases of pancreatic cancer in the hereditary pancreatitis kindreds. Rather, genomic mutations in various DNA repair pathways would likely lead to accelerated accumulation of mutations in some family members. The rate of mutation accumulation within clones of abnormal pancreatic cells would therefore determine in whom and when pancreatic cancer would develop. The process is illustrated in Fig. 8.5, which recognizes that multiple injuries and failed protective mechanisms can all contribute to the stepwise progression of normal pancreas to pancreatic adenocarcinoma. The effect of chronic pancreatic inflammation and smoking in hereditary pancreatitis in our lifetime risk model of pancreatic cancer development is presented in Fig. 8.6. Together, these data and conceptual models suggest that the risk of pancreatic cancer in patients with hereditary pancreatitis is not uniform and raises the possibility that the risk of pancreatic cancer can be modified.

4. Are there methods for early detection, diagnosis, and effective interventions?

Many patients with chronic pancreatitis, and especially chronic hereditary pancreatitis, are concerned about the high risk of pancreatic cancer. These concerns are shared by health care providers and raise questions about screening and early detection of preinvasive lesions or early cancers, as well as recommendations for effective therapy. However, the pancreas is difficult to evaluate by current imaging modalities, especially in the context of

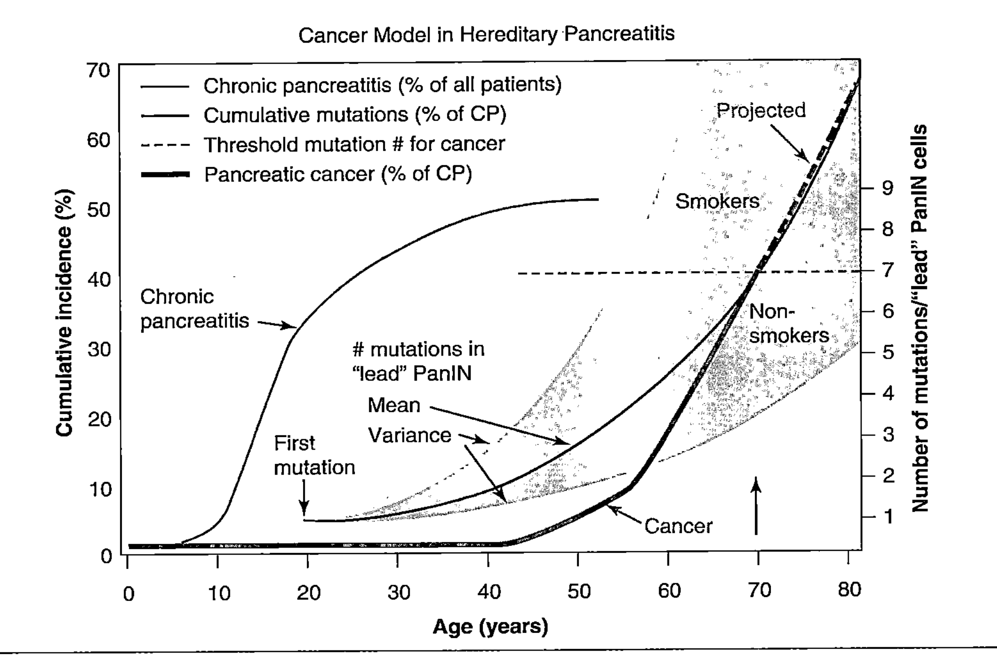

Figure 8.6
Pancreatic cancer model in hereditary pancreatitis. The model is based on current data from three sources that suggest that the cumulative incidence of pancreatic cancer in patients with hereditary pancreatitis and chronic pancreatitis begins rising between the ages of 40 and 50 years, with a rapid increase after age 60, reaching 40% by age 70 years (*red line*). Because chronic pancreatitis usually develops between ages 10 and 25 years (*thin brown line*), we modeled the first mutation in the eventual PanIN/cancer cell to occur at age 20. We also assumed that the rate of new mutation occurrence increases as mutations accumulate in the "lead" PanIN cells (*purple lines*). The rate of mutation accumulation is likely to be variable because of a variety of factors. This is illustrated by the area between the thin purple lines, with factors that increase the rate of mutation accumulation in orange (e.g., smoking) and factors that decrease mutation accumulation in light purple. Finally, the accumulation of key mutations (a total of seven was used only for illustrative purposes, y-axis, right side) is required for transformation of the lead PanIN lesion to cancer. Two observations were included in this model. First, the early PanIN lesions in this model develop between the ages of 30 and 50 years. Second, the rate of pancreatic cancer appearance is most rapid between the ages of 60 and 70 years. Because the pancreatic cancer in hereditary pancreatitis develops within the context of chronic pancreatitis, it is very difficult to detect early cancers in these patients. Thus, determining the optimal timing of intervention for screening and intervention remains challenging.

chronic pancreatitis, and it is the preinvasive lesion, rather than established, invasive cancers, that physicians prefer to identify. Furthermore, the only current therapy is pancreatectomy, which is associated with significant early and late mortality and morbidity.

In an effort to provide some guidelines for physicians caring for patients with hereditary pancreatitis, a consensus conference was sponsored by the International Association of Pancreatologists during the Third International Symposium on Inherited Diseases of the Pancreas[119] held in Milan, Italy on March 5–7, 2001. The consensus document has been published[120] and is available free of charge at several World Wide Web sites (e.g., www.pancreas.org or www.pancreatology.org). At the time of the consensus conference, it was the unanimous opinion of the participants that screening should be offered to patients with hereditary pancreatitis who were ≥ 40 years of age. Optimally, screening should be performed at medical centers expert in the care of patients with hereditary pancreatitis with state-of-the-art imaging technology.[120] In addition, screening should be considered yearly and within the context of multicenter protocols assessing the efficacy of endoscopic ultrasound or multiphasic helical computed tomography or magnetic resonance imaging/magnetic resonance cholangiopancreatography in conjunction with standardized collection and storage of blood/serum and pancreatic juice for future analysis.[120] The experts recognize the limitations of endoscopic ultrasound for the identification of suspicious lesions in the setting of chronic pancreatitis, and therefore, no recommendation of the modality of screening was reached.[120] Several investigators also argued for the use of endoscopic retrograde cholangiopancreatography because it facilitates detection and sampling of ductal pancreatic dysplasia/malignancy while allowing optimal collection of pancreatic juice.[120] However, other investigators believed that the same objectives could be accomplished with lower morbidity and mortality through endoscopic ultrasound with needle biopsy of suspicious lesions and aspiration of duodenal contents after secretin stimulation. Thus, the need for screening and counseling is recognized, but the mode and timing remain matters for future research.

Risk-factor determination for pancreatic cancer provides opportunities for prevention, delay, or early identification of pancreatic cancer. Inherited genetic factors cannot be altered, but identification of patients at high risk for pancreatic cancer affords the opportunity to eliminate or reduce other risks. For example, patients in families with a history of hereditary pancreatitis, pancreatic cancer, Peutz-Jeghers syndrome, familial atypical multiple mole melanoma, hereditary nonpolyposis colorectal cancer, *BRACA2* gene mutations, and other syndromes associated with pancreatic cancer should neither smoke cigarettes nor drink alcohol (which is associated with chronic pancreatitis).

Dietary factors play a small but perhaps significant role in altering risk for pancreatic cancer. However, attention to these factors may reduce the overall risk of pancreatic cancer in individual patients. The results of epidemiologic studies investigating different populations often conflict—obesity and excessive caloric intake increase risk, whereas consumption of fruits and vegetables reduces risk.[116,121,122] Thus, additional advice for patients at high risk for pancreatic cancer could include the reduction of caloric intake and the addition of more fruits and vegetables to their diets. Future risk reduction and preventative strategies will likely include chemoprevention[123] or vaccination.[124] Development of cancer vaccines for high-risk individuals is especially intriguing, but the vaccination process must overcome immune suppression exerted by the tumor, by previous therapy, or by the effects of advanced age of the patient, and these must elicit effective long-term memory without the potential of causing autoimmunity.[125] However, research in these areas is still very new, and no recommendations can yet be given.

Acknowledgments

This chapter is a modification and update of a previously published chapter.[1] This work was supported by a grant from the NIH DK54709 (D.C.W.) and the Lustgarten Foundation (D.C.W.).

References

1. Whitcomb DC, Applebaum S, Martin SP. Hereditary pancreatitis and pancreatic carcinoma. *Ann NY Acad Sci.* 1999;880:201–209.
2. Whitcomb DC. Chronic pancreatitis and pancreatic cancer. *Am J Physiol.* Gastointest Liver Physiol. 2004; 287:G315–G319.
3. Whitcomb DC, Pogue-Geile K. Pancreatitis as a risk for pancreatic cancer. *Gastroenterol Clin North Am.* 2002;31:663–678.
4. Whitcomb DC. Value of genetic testing in management of pancreatitis. *Gut* 2004.
5. Whitcomb DC, Gorry MC, Preston RA, et al. Hereditary pancreatitis is caused by a mutation in the cationic trypsinogen gene. *Nat Genet.* 1996;14:141–145.
6. Howes N, Wong T, Greenhalf W, et al. Pancreatic cancer risk in hereditary pancreatitis in Europe. *Digestion.* 2000;61:300.
7. Lowenfels A, Maisonneuve P, DiMagno E, et al. Hereditary pancreatitis and the risk of pancreatic cancer. *J Natl Cancer Inst.* 1997;89:442–446.
8. Lowenfels AB, Maisonneuve P, Whitcomb DC, Lerch MM, DiMagno EP. Cigarette smoking as a risk factor for pancreatic cancer in patients with hereditary pancreatitis. *JAMA.* 2001;286:169–170.
9. Miller AR, Nagorney DM, Sarr MG. The surgical spectrum of hereditary pancreatitis in adults. *Ann Surg.* 1992;215:39–43.
10. Malik SA, Van KH, Knight WJ. Inherited defect in hereditary pancreatitis. *Am J Dig Dis.* 1977;22:999–1004.
11. Kattwinkel J, Lapey A, Di SAP, Edwards WA. Hereditary pancreatitis: three new kindreds and a critical review of the literature. *Pediatrics.* 1973;51:55–69.
12. Logan AJ, Schlicke CP, Manning GB. Familial pancreatitis. *Am J Surg.* 1968;115:112–117.
13. Davidson P, Costanza D, Swieconek JA, Harris JB. Hereditary pancreatitis: a kindred without gross aminoaciduria. *Ann Intern Med.* 1968;68:88–96.
14. Appel MF. Hereditary pancreatitis: review and presentation of an additional kindred. *Arch Surg.* 1974;108:63–65.
15. Riccardi VM, Shih VE, Holmes LB, Nardi GL. Hereditary pancreatitis: nonspecificity of aminoaciduria and diagnosis of occult disease. *Arch Intern Med.* 1975;135: 822–825.
16. Girard RM, Dube S, Archambault AP. Hereditary pancreatitis: report of an affected Canadian kindred and review of the disease [review]. *Can Med Assoc J.* 1981;125:576–580.
17. Lewis MP, Gazet JC. Hereditary calcific pancreatitis in an English family. *Br J Surg.* 1993;80(4):487–488.
18. Konzen KM, Perrault J, Moir C, Zinsmeister AR. Long-term follow-up of young patients with chronic hereditary or idiopathic pancreatitis. *Mayo Clin Proc.* 1993;68: 449–453.
19. Keim V, Bauer N, Teich N, Simon P, Lerch MM, Mossner J. Clinical characterization of patients with hereditary pancreatitis and mutations in the cationic trypsinogen gene. *Am J Med.* 2001;111:622–626.
20. Howes N, Lerch MM, Greenhalf W, et al. Clinical and genetic characteristics of hereditary pancreatitis in Europe. *Clin Gastroenterol Hepatol.* 2004;2:252–261.
21. Lowenfels AB, Maisonneuve P, Whitcomb DC. Risk factors for cancer in hereditary pancreatitis: International Hereditary Pancreatitis Study Group. *Med Clin North Am.* 2000;84:565–573.
22. Whitcomb DC. Genetic predispositions to acute and chronic pancreatitis. *Med Clin North Am.* 2000;84:531–547.
23. Whitcomb DC. Hereditary pancreatitis: new insights into acute and chronic pancreatitis. *Gut.* 1999;45:317–322.

24. Schneider A, Whitcomb DC. Hereditary pancreatitis: a model for inflammatory diseases of the pancreas. *Best Pract Res Clin Gastroenterol*. 2002;16:347–363.
25. Hengstler JG, Bauer A, Wolf HK, et al. Mutation analysis of the cationic trypsinogen gene in patients with pancreatic cancer. *Anticancer Res*. 2000;20:2967–2974.
26. Malats N, Casals T, Porta M, Guarner L, Estivill X, Real FX. Cystic fibrosis transmembrane regulator (CFTR) DeltaF508 mutation and 5T allele in patients with chronic pancreatitis and exocrine pancreatic cancer. PANKRAS II Study Group. *Gut*. 2001;48:70–74.
27. Gold EB, Gordis L, Diener MD, et al. Diet and other risk factors for cancer of the pancreas. *Cancer*. 1985;55:460–467.
28. Mack TM, Yu MC, Hanisch R, Henderson BE. Pancreas cancer and smoking, beverage consumption and past medical history. *J Natl Cancer Inst*. 1986;76:49–60.
29. Farrow DC, Davis S. Risk of pancreatic cancer in relation to medical history and use of tobacco, alcohol and coffee. *Int J Cancer*. 1990;45:816–820.
30. Jain M, Howe GR, St Louis P, Miller AB. Coffee and alcohol as determinants of risk of pancreatic cancer: a case-control study from Toronto. *Int J Cancer*. 1991;47:384–389.
31. Kalapothaki V, Tzonou A, Hsieh CC, Toupadaki N, Trichopoulos D. Tobacco, ethanol, coffee, pancreatitis, diabetes mellitus, and cholelithiasis as risk factors for pancreatic carcinoma. *Cancer Causes Control*. 1993;4: 1433–1437.
32. Lowenfels AB, Maisonneuve P, Cavallini G, et al. Pancreatitis and the risk of pancreatic cancer: International Pancreatitis Study Group. *N Engl J Med*. 1993;328:1433–1437.
33. Gold EB. Epidemiology of and risk factors for pancreatic cancer [review]. *Surg Clin North Am*. 1995;75:819–843.
34. Fernandez E, La Vecchia C, Porta M, Negri E, D'Avanzo B, Boyle P. Pancreatitis and the risk of pancreatic cancer. *Pancreas*. 1995;11:185–189.
35. Wynder EL, Mabuchi K, Maruchi N, Fortner J. A case-control study of cancer of the pancreas. *Cancer*. 1973;31:641–648.
36. Mohr P, Ammann R, Largiader F, Knoblauch M, Schmid M, Akovbiantz A. Pancreatic carcinoma in chronic pancreatitis. *Schweiz Med Wochenschr*. 1975;105:590–592.
37. Lin RS, Kessler II. A multifactorial model for pancreatic cancer in man: epidemiologic evidence. *JAMA*. 1981; 245:147–152.
38. Bueno de Mesquita HB, Maisonneuve P, Moerman CJ, Walker AM. Aspects of medical history and exocrine carcinoma of the pancreas: a population-based case-control study in The Netherlands. *Int J Cancer*. 1992;52:17–23.
39. Ekbom A, McLaughlin JK, Karlsson BM, et al. Pancreatitis and pancreatic cancer: a population-based study. *J Natl Cancer Inst*. 1994;86:625–627.
40. Bansal P, Sonnenberg A. Pancreatitis is a risk factor for pancreatic cancer. *Gastroenterology*. 1995;109:247–251.
41. Madeira I, Pessione F, Malka D, Hammel P, Ruszniewski P, Bernades P. The risk of pancreatic adenocarcinoma in patients with chronic pancreatitis: myth or reality? *Gastroenterology*. 1998;114:A481.
42. Sheldon CD, Hodson ME, Carpenter LM, Swerdlow AJ. A cohort study of cystic fibrosis and malignancy. *Br J Cancer*. 1993;68:1025–1028.
43. Neglia JP, FitzSimmons SC, Maisonneuve P, et al. The risk of cancer among patients with cystic fibrosis: Cystic Fibrosis and Cancer Study Group. *N Engl J Med*. 1995;332:494–499.
44. Mohan V, Premalatha G, Pitchumoni CS. Tropical chronic pancreatitis: an update. *J Clin Gastroenterol*. 2003;36: 337–346.
45. Pfützer RH, Barmada MM, Brunskil APJ, et al. SPINK1/PSTI polymorphisms act as disease modifiers in familial and idiopathic chronic pancreatitis. *Gastroenterology*. 2000;119: 615–623.
46. Witt H, Luck W, Hennies HC, et al. Mutations in the gene encoding the serine protease inhibitor, Kazal type 1 are associated with chronic pancreatitis. *Nat Genet*. 2000;25: 213–216.
47. Rossi L, Pfützer RL, Parvin S, et al. SPINK1/PSTI mutations are associated with tropical pancreatitis in Bangladesh: a preliminary report. *Pancreatology*. 2001;1:242–245.
48. Dhir V, Mohandas KM. Epidemiology of digestive tract cancers in India IV: gall bladder and pancreas. *Ind J Gastroenterol*. 1999;18:24–28.
49. Augustine P, Ramesh H. Is tropical pancreatitis premalignant? *Am J Gastroenterol*. 1992;87:1005–1008.
50. Chari ST, Mohan V, Pitchumoni CS, Viswanathan M, Madanagopalan N, Lowenfels AB. Risk of pancreatic carcinoma in tropical calcifying pancreatitis: an epidemiologic study. *Pancreas*. 1994;9:62–66.
51. Yamano M, Fujii H, Takagaki T, Kadowaki N, Watanabe H, Shirai T. Genetic progression and divergence in pancreatic carcinoma. *Am J Pathol*. 2000;156:2123–2133.
52. Hruban RH, Wilentz RE, Kern SE. Genetic progression in the pancreatic ducts. *Am J Pathol*. 2000;156:1821–1825.
53. Kern S, Hruban R, Hollingsworth MA, et al. A white paper: the product of a pancreas cancer think tank. *Cancer Res*. 2001;61:4923–4932.
54. Wilentz RE, Iacobuzio-Donahue CA, Argani P, et al. Loss of expression of DPC4 in pancreatic intraepithelial neoplasia: evidence that DPC4 inactivation occurs late in neoplastic progression. *Cancer Res*. 2000;60:2002–2006.
55. Wong T, Howes N, Threadgold J, et al. Molecular diagnosis of early pancreatic ductal adenocarcinoma in high-risk patients. *Pancreatology*. 2001;1:480–503.
56. Shi X, Friess H, Kleef J, Ozawa F, Büchler MW. Pancreatic cancer: factors regulating tumor development, maintenance and metastasis. *Pancreatology*. 2001;1:511–518.
57. Caldas C, Hahn SA, Da Costa L, et al. Frequent somatic mutations and homozygous deletion of the p16 (MTS1) gene in pancreatic adenocarcinoma. *Nat Genet*. 1994;8: 27–32.
58. Tada M, Omata M, Ohto M. Clinical application of ras gene mutation for diagnosis of pancreatic adenocarcinoma. *Gastroenterology*. 1991;100:233–238.
59. Smit VTHB, Boot AJ, Smits AMM, Fleuren GJ, Cornelisse CJ, Bos JL. K-ras codon 12 mutations occur very frequently in pancreatic adenocarcinoma. *Nucleic Acids Res*. 1988;16:7773–7782.
60. Gerdes B, Ramaswamy A, Kersting M, et al. p16(INK4a) alterations in chronic pancreatitis: indicator for high-risk lesions for pancreatic cancer. *Surgery*. 2001;129:490–497.

61. Moskaluk CA, Hruban RH, Kern SE. p16 and K-ras mutations in the intraductal precursors of human pancreatic adenocarcinoma. *Cancer Res.* 1997;57:2140.
62. Yanagisawa A, Ohtake K, Ohashi K, et al. Frequent c-Ki-ras oncogene activation in mucous cell hyperplasias of pancreas suffering from chonic inflammation. *Cancer Res.* 1993;53:953–956.
63. Caldas C, Hahn SA, Hruban RH, Redston MS, Yeo CJ, Kern SE. Detection of K- ras mutations in the stool of patients with pancreatic adenocarcinoma and pancreatic ductal hyperplasia. *Cancer Res.* 1994;54:3568–3573.
64. Seki K, Suda T, Aoyagi Y, et al. Diagnosis of pancreatic adenocarcinoma by detection of human telomerase reverse transcriptase messenger RNA in pancreatic juice with sample qualification. *Clin Cancer Res.* 2001;7:1976–1981.
65. Almoguera C, Shibata D, Forrester K, Martin J, Arnheim N, Perucho M. Most human carcinomas of the exocrine pancreas contain mutant c-K-ras genes. *Cell.* 1988;53:549–554.
66. Schutte M, Hruban RH, Geradts J, et al. Abrogation of the Rb/p16 tumor-suppressive pathway in virtually all pancreatic carcinomas. *Cancer Res.* 1997;57:3126–3130.
67. Rozenblum E, Schutte M, Goggins M, et al. Tumor suppressive pathways in pancreatic carcinoma. *Cancer Res.* 1997;57:1731–1734.
68. Kern SE. Molecular genetic alteration in ductal pancreatic adenocarcinomas. In: Whitcomb DC, Cohn JA, Ulrich II CD, eds. *Inherited Diseases of the Pancreas.* Philadelphia: WB Saunders; 2000:691–696.
69. Goggins M, Schutte M, Lu J, et al. Germline BRCA2 gene mutations in patients with apparently sporadic pancreatic carcinomas. *Cancer Res.* 1996;56:5360–5364.
70. Su GH, Hruban RH, Bansal RK, et al. Germline and somatic mutations of the STK11/LKB1 Peutz-Jeghers gene in pancreatic and biliary cancers. *Am J Pathol.* 1999;154: 1835–1840.
71. Teng DH, Perry WL, Hogan JK, et al. Human mitogen-activated protein kinase 4 as a candidate tumor suppressor. *Cancer Res.* 1997;57:4177–4182.
72. Goggins M, Shekher M, Turnacioglu K, Yeo CJ, Hruban RH, Kern SE. Genetic alterations of the transforming growth factor beta receptor genes in pancreatic and biliary adenocarcinomas. *Cancer Res.* 1998;58:5329–5332.
73. Huang L, Lang D, Geradts J, et al. Molecular and immunochemical analyses of RB1 and cyclin D1 in human ductal pancreatic carcinomas and cell lines. *Mol Carcinog.* 1996;15:85–95.
74. Hruban RH, Adsay NV, Albores-Saavedra J, et al. Pancreatic intraepithelial neoplasia: a new nomenclature and classification system for pancreatic duct lesions. *Am J Surg Pathol.* 2001;25:579–586.
75. Hruban RH, Wilentz RE, Goggins M, Offerhaus GJ, Yeo CJ, Kern SE. Pathology of incipient pancreatic cancer. *Ann Oncol.* 1999;4:9–11.
76. Wilentz RE, Geradts J, Maynard R, et al. Inactivation of the p16 (INK4A) tumor-suppressor gene in pancreatic duct lesions: loss of intranuclear expression. *Cancer Res.* 1998;58:4740–4744.
77. Furuya N, Kawa S, Akamatsu T, Furihata K. Long-term follow-up of patients with chronic pancreatitis and K-ras gene mutation detected in pancreatic juice. *Gastroenterology.* 1997;113:595–598.
78. van Laethem JL. Ki-ras oncogene mutations in chronic pancreatitis: which discriminating ability for malignant potential? *Ann NY Acad Sci.* 1999;880:210–218.
79. Rivera JA, Fernandez-del Castillo C, Rall CJN, et al. Analysis of K-ras oncogene mutations in chronic pancreatitis with ductal hyperplasia. *Surgery.* 1997;121:42–49.
80. Hingorani SR, Petricoin EF, Maitra A, et al. Preinvasive and invasive ductal pancreatic cancer and its early detection in the mouse. *Cancer Cell.* 2003;4:437–450.
81. Hofseth LJ, Saito S, Hussain SP, et al. Nitric oxide-induced cellular stress and p53 activation in chronic inflammation. *Proc Natl Acad Sci USA.* 2003;100:143–148.
82. Mitchell RA, Liao H, Chesney J, et al. Macrophage migration inhibitory factor (MIF) sustains macrophage proinflammatory function by inhibiting p53: regulatory role in the innate immune response. *Proc Natl Acad Sci USA.* 2002;99:345–350.
83. Hudson JD, Shoaibi MA, Maestro R, Carnero A, Hannon GJ, Beach DH. A proinflammatory cytokine inhibits p53 tumor suppressor activity. *J Exp Med.* 1999;190:1375–1382.
84. Murakami H, Akbar SM, Matsui H, Onji M. Macrophage migration inhibitory factor in the sera and at the colonic mucosa in patients with ulcerative colitis: clinical implications and pathogenic significance. *Eur J Clin Invest.* 2001;31:337–343.
85. Shkolnik T, Livni E, Reshef R, Lachter J, Eidelman S. Comparison of two lymphokines (macrophage migration inhibition, leukocyte adherence inhibition factors) and carcinoembryonic antigen, in colorectal cancer and colonic premalignant lesions. *Am J Gastroenterol.* 1987;82:1275–1278.
86. Hussain SP, Amstad P, Raja K, et al. Increased p53 mutation load in noncancerous colon tissue from ulcerative colitis: a cancer-prone chronic inflammatory disease. *Cancer Res.* 2000;60:3333–3337.
87. Ren Y, Tsui HT, Poon RT, et al. Macrophage migration inhibitory factor: roles in regulating tumor cell migration and expression of angiogenic factors in hepatocellular carcinoma. *Int J Cancer.* 2003;107:22–29.
88. Balkwill F, Mantovani A. Inflammation and cancer: back to Virchow? *Lancet.* 2001;357:539–545.
89. Farrow B, Evers BM. Inflammation and the development of pancreatic cancer. *Surg Oncol.* 2002;10:153–169.
90. Ransohoff DF. Colon cancer in ulcerative colitis. *Gastroenterology.* 1988;94:1089–1091.
91. Eslick GD, Lim LL, Byles JE, Xia HH, Talley NJ. Association of *Helicobacter pylori* infection with gastric carcinoma: a meta-analysis. *Am J Gastroenterol.* 1999;94: 2373–2379.
92. Blaser MJ, Perez-Perez GI, Kleanthous H, et al. Infection with *Helicobacter pylori* strains possessing cagA is associated with an increased risk of developing adenocarcinoma of the stomach. *Cancer Res.* 1995;55:2111–2115.
93. Tagger A, Donato F, Ribero ML, et al. Case-control study on hepatitis C virus (HCV) as a risk factor for hepatocellular carcinoma: the role of HCV genotypes and the synergism with hepatitis B virus and alcohol. Brescia HCC Study. *Int J Cancer.* 1999;81:695–699.

94. Misra S, Chaturvedi A, Misra NC, Sharma ID. Carcinoma of the gallbladder. *Lancet Oncol.* 2003;4:167–176.
95. Hruban RH, van Mansfeld AD, Offerhaus GJ, et al. K-ras oncogene activation in adenocarcinoma of the human pancreas: a study of 82 carcinomas using a combination of mutant-enriched polymerase chain reaction analysis and allele-specific oligonucleotide hybridization. *Am J Pathol.* 1993;143:545–554.
96. DiGiuseppe JA, Hruban RH, Goodman SN, et al. Overexpression of p53 protein in adenocarcinoma of the pancreas. *Am J Clin Pathol.* 1994;101:684–688.
97. Apple SK, Hecht JR, Lewin DN, Jahromi SA, Grody WW, Nieberg RK. Immunohistochemical evaluation of K-ras, p53, and HER-2/neu expression in hyperplastic, dysplastic, and carcinomatous lesions of the pancreas: evidence for multistep carcinogenesis. *Hum Pathol.* 1999;30:123–129.
98. Heinmoller E, Dietmaier W, Zirngibl H, et al. Molecular analysis of microdissected tumors and preneoplastic intraductal lesions in pancreatic carcinoma. *Am J Pathol.* 2000;157:83–92.
99. Terhune PG, Phifer DM, Tosteson TD, Longnecker DS. K-ras mutation in focal proliferative lesions of human pancreas. *Cancer Epidemiol Biomarkers Prev.* 1998;7: 515–521.
100. Poch B, Gansauge F, Schwarz A, et al. Epidermal growth factor induces cyclin D1 in human pancreatic carcinoma: evidence for a cyclin D1-dependent cell cycle progression. *Pancreas.* 2001;23:280–287.
101. Guan RJ, Fu Y, Holt PR, Pardee AB. Association of K-ras mutations with p16 methylation in human colon cancer. *Gastroenterology.* 1999;116:1063–1071.
102. Samowitz WS, Holden JA, Curtin K, et al. Inverse relationship between microsatellite instability and K-ras and p53 gene alterations in colon cancer. *Am J Pathol.* 2001;158:1517–1524.
103. Sutter T, Doi S, Carnevale KA, Arber N, Weinstein IB. Expression of cyclins D1 and E in human colon adenocarcinomas. *J Med.* 1997;28:285–309.
104. Lord RV, O'Grady R, Sheehan C, Field AF, Ward RL. K-ras codon 12 mutations in Barrett's oesophagus and adenocarcinomas of the oesophagus and oesophagogastric junction. *J Gastroenterol Hepatol.* 2000;15:730–736.
105. Kobayashi S, Koide Y, Endo M, Isono K, Ochiai T. The p53 gene mutation is of prognostic value in esophageal squamous cell carcinoma patients in unified stages of curability. *Am J Surg.* 1999;177:497–502.
106. Bian YS, Osterheld MC, Fontolliet C, Bosman FT, Benhattar J. p16 inactivation by methylation of the CDKN2A promoter occurs early during neoplastic progression in Barrett's esophagus. *Gastroenterology.* 2002;122:1113–1121.
107. Jiang W, Zhang YJ, Kahn SM, et al. Altered expression of the cyclin D1 and retinoblastoma genes in human esophageal cancer. *Proc Natl Acad Sci USA.* 1993;90:9026–9030.
108. Weihrauch M, Benick M, Lehner G, et al. High prevalence of K-ras-2 mutations in hepatocellular carcinomas in workers exposed to vinyl chloride. *Int Arch Occup Environ Health.* 2001;74:405–410.
109. Tannapfel A, Busse C, Weinans L, et al. INK4a-ARF alterations and p53 mutations in hepatocellular carcinomas. *Oncogene.* 2001;20:7104–7109.
110. Azechi H, Nishida N, Fukuda Y, et al. Disruption of the p16/cyclin D1/retinoblastoma protein pathway in the majority of human hepatocellular carcinomas. *Oncology.* 2001;60:346–354.
111. Kim SW, Her KH, Jang JY, Kim WH, Kim YT, Park YH. K-ras oncogene mutation in cancer and precancerous lesions of the gallbladder. *J Surg Oncol.* 2000;75:246–251.
112. Wistuba II, Gazdar AF, Roa I, Albores-Saavedra J. p53 protein overexpression in gallbladder carcinoma and its precursor lesions: an immunohistochemical study. *Hum Pathol.* 1996;27:360–365.
113. Shi YZ, Hui AM, Li X, Takayama T, Makuuchi M. Overexpression of retinoblastoma protein predicts decreased survival and correlates with loss of p16INK4 protein in gallbladder carcinomas. *Clin Cancer Res.* 2000;6:4096–4100.
114. Hui AM, Li X, Shi YZ, Takayama T, Torzilli G, Makuuchi M. Cyclin D1 overexpression is a critical event in gallbladder carcinogenesis and independently predicts decreased survival for patients with gallbladder carcinoma. *Clin Cancer Res.* 2000;6:4272–4277.
115. Kernan GJ, Ji BT, Dosemeci M, Silverman DT, Balbus J, Zahm SH. Occupational risk factors for pancreatic cancer: a case-control study based on death certificates from 24 US states. *Am J Ind Med.* 1999;36:260–270.
116. Silverman DT, Swanson CA, Gridley G, et al. Dietary and nutritional factors and pancreatic cancer: a case-control study based on direct interviews. *J Natl Cancer Inst.* 1998;90:1710–1719.
117. Ockenga J, Vogel A, Teich N, Keim V, Manns MP, Strassburg CP. UDP glucuronosyltransferase (UGT1A7) gene polymorphisms increase the risk of chronic pancreatitis and pancreatic cancer. *Gastroenterology.* 2003;124:1802–1808.
118. Schenk M, Schwartz AG, O'Neal E, et al. Familial risk of pancreatic cancer. *J Natl Cancer Inst.* 2001;93:640–644.
119. Whitcomb DC, Ulrich DC, Learch MM, et al. Conference Report: Third International Symposium on Inherited Diseases of the Pancreas. *Pancreatology.* 2001;1:423–431.
120. Ulrich II CD. Pancreatic cancer in hereditary pancreatitis: consensus guidelines for prevention, screening, and treatment. *Pancreatology.* 2001;1:416–422.
121. Stolzenberg-Solomon RZ, Albanes D, Nieto FJ, et al. Pancreatic cancer risk and nutrition-related methyl-group availability indicators in male smokers. *J Natl Cancer Inst.* 1999;91:535.
122. Ghadirian P, Baillargeon J, Simard A, Perret C. Food habits and pancreatic cancer: a case-control study of the Francophone community in Montreal, Canada. *Cancer Epidemiol Biomarkers Prev.* 1995;4:895–899.
123. Hruban RH, Canto MI, Yeo CJ. Prevention of pancreatic cancer and strategies for management of familial pancreatic cancer. *Dig Dis.* 2001;19:76–84.
124. Finn OJ. Pancreatic tumor antigens: diagnostic markers and targets for immunotherapy. *Important Adv Oncol.* 1992;61–77.
125. Finn OJ. Cancer vaccines: between the idea and the reality. *Nat Rev Immunol.* 2003;3:630–641.

CHAPTER 9

Familial Pancreatic Cancer

Ralph H. Hruban, MD
Kieran Brune, BS
Alison Klein, PhD
Gloria M. Petersen, PhD

For years, anecdotal case reports have suggested that pancreatic cancer aggregates in some families, but the basis of this aggregation has only begun to become clear in the past decade. The most famous example of the aggregation of pancreatic cancer in a family is that of former President Jimmy Carter.[1] At least two of his siblings and one of his parents died of pancreatic cancer. The aggregation of a cancer in a family could be due to chance, it could be due to shared environmental exposures, it could have a genetic basis, or it could have a complex multifactorial basis. A growing body of evidence now makes it clear that some of the aggregation of pancreatic cancer in families has a genetic basis. As the genes responsible for this aggregation are discovered, they will provide a rational basis for genetic counseling, they will help identify those who would benefit most from screening for early cancer, and they will provide insight into the fundamental biology of pancreatic cancer.

Case Reports and Registries

The aggregation of pancreatic cancer in families has been reported in numerous well-documented case reports, including kindreds in which multiple siblings were affected and kindreds in which members of multiple generations died of the disease.[2-4] Several large familial pancreatic cancer registries have been established on the basis of these reports.[2] One of the largest of these registries is the National Familial Pancreas Tumor Registry (NFPTR) at Johns Hopkins.* As noted in Table 9.1, 1261 kindreds have enrolled in the NFPTR as of February 1, 2004. These include 501 kindreds in which at least a pair of first-degree relatives has been diagnosed with pancreatic cancer (referred to here as "familial pancreatic cancer kindreds"), and 760 kindreds in which at least one family member has been diagnosed with pancreatic cancer, but there is not a pair of affected first-degree relatives (referred here to as "sporadic pancreatic cancer kindreds"). Remarkably, the NFPTR includes a kindred in which seven family members were diagnosed with pancreatic cancer. Similar registries at the Mayo Clinic and at Creighton University have identified additional kindreds in which multiple family members are affected. Although these registries form an invaluable resource for the study of the genetic basis of pancreatic cancer, they cannot, by themselves, be

*The National Familial Pancreas Tumor Registry, Ross 632, Department of Pathology, The Johns Hopkins Medical Institution, Baltimore, MD 21205. Phone 410-955-3502.

Table 9.1 Kindreds Enrolled in the National Familial Pancreas Tumor Registry as of February 1, 2004

Characteristic	Number
Nonfamilial kindreds	760
Familial kindreds	501
Total	1261
Number of Pancreatic Cancers in Familial Kindreds	**Number of Kindreds**
7 pancreatic cancers	1
6 pancreatic cancers	5
5 pancreatic cancers	11
4 pancreatic cancers	38
3 pancreatic cancers	117
2 pancreatic cancers	329
Number of Incident Pancreatic Cancers	24

used to calculate the proportion of pancreatic cancer that has a familial basis. This is because most registries include clinician-referred and self-referred kindreds, introducing potential selection biases. Case-control and cohort studies of patients with pancreatic cancer and their families provide alternative research strategies to address familial aggregation.

Case-Control Studies

As summarized in Table 9.2, case-control studies from North America and Europe have demonstrated that a family history of pancreatic cancer is associated with a significantly increased risk of developing pancreatic cancer.[5-9] For example, in a case-control study from Italy, Fernandez et al.[6] found a 2.8-fold increased risk of pancreatic cancer in individuals who had a relative with pancreatic cancer. This increased risk remained even after investigators controlled for other risk factors, including smoking, diet, and chronic pancreatitis.[6] More recently, Silverman et al.[10] conducted a population-based, case-control study of pancreatic cancer in the United States. The study included 484 cases and 2099 control subjects. Pancreatic cancer was significantly associated with having a first-degree relative with pancreatic cancer (odds ratio = 3.2), colon cancer (odds ratio = 1.7), or ovarian cancer (odds ratio = 5.3).[10] In this study, personal history of diabetes mellitus or cholecystectomy were also found to be risk factors for pancreatic cancer.

Although the study populations and methodologies have varied, almost all case-control studies have found that a family history of pancreatic cancer is a significant risk factor for the disease (Table 9.2), adding strength to the hypothesis that there is an important inherited component that can contribute to the development of pancreatic cancer.

Cohort Studies

Prospective studies of large cohorts of subjects can overcome the problem of selection bias and can offer a unique opportunity to quantify the risk of pancreatic cancer. Klein et al.[11] recently completed a prospective study of more than 5000 individuals from 838 kindreds enrolled in the NFPTR. The study included more than 14,000 person-years of follow-up, and the number of incident pancreatic cancers that developed was compared with the number of those expected, based on the Surveillance, Epidemi-

Table 9.2 Case-Control Studies of Pancreatic Cancer Risk

First Author	Location of Study	Increased Risk Associated with a Family History of Pancreatic Cancer	Number of Study Participants	Reference
Falk	Louisiana, USA	OR = 5.3	363 cases, 1234 controls	[5]
Fernandez	Northern Italy	OR = 3	362 cases, 1408 controls	[6]
Ghadirian	Montreal, Canada	OR = 13	179 cases, 179 controls	[7]
Ghadirian	Montreal, Canada	OR = 5	174 cases, 136 controls	[8]
Schenk	Detroit, MI, USA	OR = 2.5, increased to 8.23 in smokers	247 cases, 420 controls	[9]
Silverman	3 areas in USA	OR = 3.2	484 cases, 2099 controls	[10]

Abbreviation: OR, Odds ratio.

ology, and End Results database. Remarkably, 24 incident pancreatic cancers were reported in NFPTR study participants.[11] The observed:expected ratio was significantly elevated in familial pancreatic cancer kindreds (observed:expected ratio = 9.0; 95% confidence interval, 4.5–16.1), but it was not elevated in sporadic pancreatic cancer kindreds (observed:expected ratio = 4.6, 95% confidence interval, 0.5–16.4). The risk of pancreatic cancer in the familial pancreatic cancer kindreds increased with the number of affected first-degree relatives of the study participant. The risk of pancreatic cancer was increased 32-fold in study participants with three first-degree relatives with pancreatic cancer, 6.4-fold in participants with two first-degree relatives, and 4.6-fold in participants with one first-degree relative with pancreatic cancer.[11] Risk was not increased among 369 spouses and other genetically unrelated relatives.[11] These data provide significant support to the case-control studies, and, importantly, they help quantify risk, an essential first step in identifying individuals who would most benefit from screening for early pancreatic cancer (see Chapter 17). For example, in this study, it was estimated that the incidence of pancreatic cancer in individuals who are members of a familial pancreatic cancer kindred and have three first-degree relatives with pancreatic cancer is 288 per 100,000 person-years (Fig. 9.1).[11]

In another large study, Coughlin et al.[12] followed up 483,109 men and 619,199 women who formed the American Cancer Society's Cancer Prevention Study II cohort. After 14 years of follow-up, 3751 study participants had been diagnosed with pancreatic cancer.[12] Cigarette smoking was associated with a 2.1-fold increased risk of pancreatic cancer, and family history of pancreatic cancer was associated with a 1.5-fold increased risk.[12] The familial risk persisted even after the analysis was adjusted for history of gallstones, body mass index, smoking history, alcohol consumption, history of diabetes, and several dietary factors.[12]

More recently, Hemminki and Li[13] reported a study based on the Swedish Family-Cancer database. This database includes more than 10.2 million people, 21,000 of whom have been diagnosed with pancreatic cancer.[13] Hemminki and Li[13] found that the offspring of patients with pancreatic cancer had a 1.73-fold increased risk of developing pancreatic cancer. Of interest, offspring of patients with lung, rectal, or endometrial cancer also had an increased risk of pancreatic cancer.[13]

Studies of large cohorts of twins have been conducted and support a genetic basis for the aggregation of pancreatic cancer. A study of 44,788 twins from Sweden, Denmark, and Finland found that the concordance of pancreatic cancer between monozygotic co-twins was greater than the concordance between dizygotic co-twins, but the finding was not as strong as it was for cancers of other organ sites.[14]

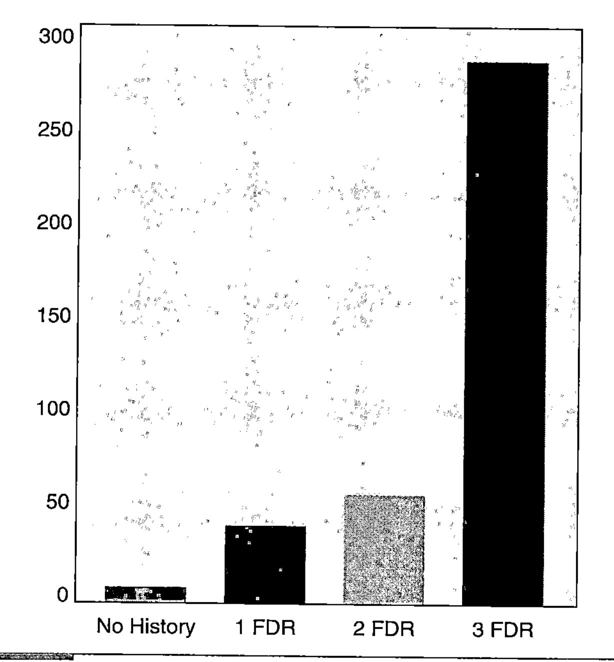

Figure 9.1
Expected annual incidence of pancreatic cancer per 100,000 for individuals without a family history of pancreatic cancer (no history) and individuals in a familial pancreatic cancer kindred (at least a pair of first-degree relatives with pancreatic cancer in the kindred). FDR, Number of first-degree relatives with pancreatic cancer.

Segregation Analysis

Although these case-control and cohort studies all point to a strong familial aggregation of pancreatic cancer, they have not defined the cause or causes of this aggregation. For example, an observed aggregation of a cancer in a family could be caused by a shared environmental exposure, it could have a genetic basis, or it could be due to a combination of environmental and genetic factors. Environmental factors have been known to increase the risk of pancreatic cancer. For example, in the prospective study conducted by Klein et al.,[11] cigarette smoking was shown to elevate risk to relatives in both the familial pancreatic cancer kindreds and the sporadic pancreatic cancer kindreds. Whether and how genetic susceptibility might interact with cigarette smoking is now being investigated.

Klein et al.[15] conducted a complex segregation analysis using families in which at least one family member

Table 9.3 Risk of Pancreatic Cancer in Selected Genetic Risk Categories

Risk Category	Relative Risk	Risk of PC by Age 50 Years	Risk of PC by Age 70 Years
No history of pancreatic cancer	1	0.05%	0.5%
Carrier of a germline *BRCA2* mutation	3.5–10×	0.5%	5%
Personal history of familial atypical multiple mole melanoma syndrome, or carrier of a germline *p16* mutation	20–34×	1%–2%	10%–17%
Three or more first-degree relatives with pancreatic cancer	32×	1.6%	16%
Personal history of familial pancreatitis	50–80×	2.5%–4%	25%–40%
Personal history of Peutz-Jeghers syndrome	75–132×	3.6%	36% (age 60 years)
Carrier of HNPCC-related germline mutation	?	?	<5%

Abbreviations: HNPCC, Hereditary nonpolyposis colorectal cancer; PC, Pancreatic cancer.

had been diagnosed with pancreatic cancer. Segregation analysis is a statistical methodology aimed at determining whether a major gene could cause the observed familial aggregation of a trait. Segregation analysis can also help determine the best explanatory model for how this gene is inherited (i.e., whether a gene that predisposes to pancreatic cancer is inherited in an autosomal dominant or autosomal recessive manner) and also estimate the frequency of the gene. Two hundred eighty-seven families were studied, and nongenetic transmission models were strongly rejected.[15] The most parsimonious explanatory model included the autosomal-dominant inheritance of a rare allele.[15] Klein et al.[15] further estimated that between 0.4% and 0.7% of the population has a higher risk of developing pancreatic cancer because of this putative gene.

Thus, case reports, case-control studies, and cohort studies all demonstrate the aggregation of pancreatic cancer in families, and segregation analyses suggest that this aggregation has a genetic basis. The next challenge is to find the genes!

To date, at least five genetic syndromes that significantly increase the risk of pancreatic cancer have been described (Table 9.3). These include familial breast cancer (caused by inherited mutations in the *BRCA2* gene), familial atypical multiple mole melanoma (caused by germline mutations in the *p16* gene), the Peutz-Jeghers syndrome (caused by inherited mutations in the *STK11* gene), familial pancreatitis (caused by germline mutations in the *PRSS1* gene), and hereditary nonpolyposis colorectal cancer syndrome ([HNPCC] usually caused by mutations in *hMLH1* or *hMSH2*). The following sections discuss each of these syndromes in greater detail.

Familial Breast Cancer

The discovery of the second breast cancer gene, *BRCA2*, was greatly facilitated by the finding of a small homozygous deletion on chromosome 13q in a pancreatic cancer.[16] Ever since this remarkable discovery, the *BRCA2* gene and pancreatic cancer have been reported to be associated.[17] Pancreatic cancers were noted in the early descriptions of *BRCA2* kindreds, and germline (inherited) *BRCA2* gene mutations have been shown to account for approximately 17% of highly familial pancreatic cancers.[18-20] Murphy et al.[21] analyzed 29 pancreatic cancer patients from familial pancreatic cancer kindreds in which at least three family members had been diagnosed with pancreatic cancer for germline *BRCA2* mutations. They found deleterious *BRCA2* gene mutations in five of these 29 patients (17%). Three of the five had the 6174delT mutation. This mutation is particularly common in individuals of Ashkenazi Jewish heritage.[22,23] Similarly, Hahn et al.[24] found germline *BRCA2* gene mutations in three of 26 (12%) European families in which at least two first-degree relatives had histologically confirmed pancreatic ductal adenocarcinoma.

A remarkable aspect of the families in these two studies is that most of the patients with a germline *BRCA2* gene mutation did not have families that look like typical hereditary breast cancer families. In fact, many had no history of breast cancer in their families at all. The incomplete penetrance of germline *BRCA2* gene mutations (i.e., the fact that all carriers of germline *BRCA2* mutations do not all develop cancer) suggests that a germline *BRCA2* gene mutation cannot be excluded just because

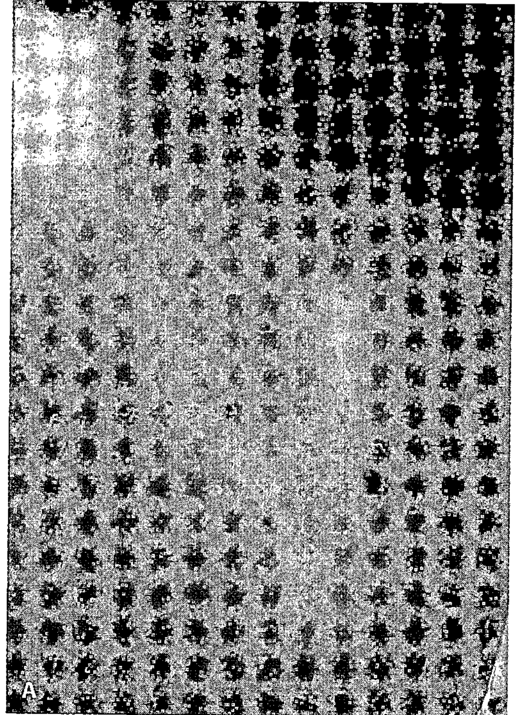

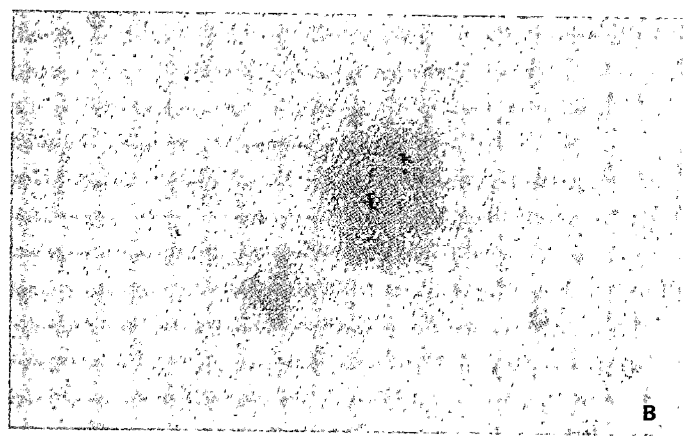

Figure 9.2
Familial atypical multiple mole melanoma (FAMMM) is characterized by numerous nevi (**A**) and atypical nevi (**B**). (Kindly provided by Dr. G.J.A. Offerhaus of the Academic Medical Center, Amsterdam, The Netherlands, and reprinted from Cameron JL, ed. *Pancreatic Cancer* 2001, BC Decker Inc, Hamilton, Ontario, Canada with permission of the American Cancer Society).

a person does not have a family history of breast cancer. Indeed, Goggins et al.[25] studied a large series of patients with apparently sporadic pancreatic cancer and found that 7% had a germline *BRCA2* gene mutation. Just as was true in the study by Murphy et al.,[21] breast cancer was not reported in many of these families with a germline *BRCA2* gene mutation.

Numerous studies have estimated the increased risk of pancreatic cancer in carriers of germline *BRCA2* gene mutations, and most estimates place the risk at between 3.5- and 10-fold greater than the general population.[22,26] This translates into a 5% risk of developing pancreatic cancer by the age of 70 years (see Table 9.3).

The protein product of the *BRCA2* gene has been shown to interact with protein products of several of the Fanconi anemia genes and to function in the repair of double-strand DNA breaks (see Chapter 3). van der Heijden et al.[27] hypothesized that if one member of a pathway is targeted for inactivation in a cancer, then the other members of the same pathway might also be targeted. They examined a series of pancreatic cancers for mutations in the Fanconi anemia genes *FANCC* and *FANCG*. In addition to somatic inactivation of the *FANCC* and *FANCG* genes, van der Heijden et al.[27] reported a probable germline mutation in the *FANCG* gene in a pancreatic cancer cell line. The finding that Fanconi anemia genes play an important role in some pancreatic cancers not only adds to our understanding of familial pancreatic cancer but it may also have therapeutic relevance (see Chapter 3).[27] Cancer cells with biallelic inactivation of one of the Fanconi anemia genes may be more sensitive to chemotherapeutic agents, such as mitomycin, that induce double-stranded DNA breaks.[27A]

Follow-up studies by Rogers et al.[28] examining the *FANCC* and *FANCG* genes in 38 patients with familial pancreatic cancer have not identified any additional deleterious germline mutations. Further studies are clearly needed to evaluate the other Fanconi anemia genes and to determine the full impact of germline Fanconi anemia gene mutations on the familial aggregation of pancreatic cancer.

Familial Atypical Multiple Mole Melanoma

The familial atypical multiple mole melanoma syndrome is an autosomal dominant disorder characterized by the familial occurrence of multiple melanocytic nevi, atypical nevi (Fig. 9.2), and an increased risk of both melanoma and pancreatic cancer.[17,29-37] Familial atypical multiple mole melanoma can be caused by germline mutations in the *p16/CDKN2A* gene on chromosome 9p.[38] For example, Vasen et al.[39] studied 19 kindreds with a germline *p16*-Leiden mutation.[39] Melanoma was the most common malignancy in these families, followed by pancreatic cancer. The mean age at diagnosis of the 15 patients with pancreatic cancer in these kindreds was 58 years (range, 38–77 years). Vasen et al.[39] further estimated that the risk that mutation carriers will develop pancreatic cancer by the age of 75 is 17%. The estimated magnitude of the increased risk varies from study to study. In a cohort of familial melanoma kindreds, Parker et al.[40] estimated that germline *p16/CDKN2A* gene mutation carriers have an 8.9- to 12.6-fold increased risk of developing pancreatic cancer, Borg et al.[31] estimated the risk to be 38-fold, and Goldstein et al.[41] estimated that the risk was between the two at 13- to 22-fold. In contrast to the incomplete penetrance of the *BRCA2* gene, most patients with pancreatic cancer with a germline *p16/CDKN2A* gene mutation have a family history of melanoma.

The demonstration that germline *p16/CDKN2A* gene mutations can cause pancreatic cancer has helped advance our understanding of the fundamental nature of pancreatic cancer. For example, the genes targeted for inactivation in the familial form of a cancer are also often targeted for inactivation in the sporadic form of the cancer. This is true for *p16/CDKN2A* gene mutations. As discussed in Chapter 3, the *p16/CDKN2A* gene is somatically inactivated in approximately 95% of sporadic pancreatic cancers. In 40%, this is by homozygous deletion of the gene, in 40% by an intragenic mutation coupled with loss of the second allele, and in 15% by hypermethylation of the *p16/CDKN2A* gene promoter.[42]

The demonstration that germline *p16/CDKN2A* gene mutations can cause pancreatic cancer also has a significant impact on screening.[43] Carriers of germline *p16/CDKN2A* gene mutations can be screened for dysplastic nevi and early melanomas, and lives can be saved. When a sensitive and specific screening test for early pancreatic cancer is developed, carriers of germline *p16/CDKN2A* gene mutations will be among the first to benefit from screening for early pancreatic cancer.[44]

Peutz-Jeghers Syndrome

The Peutz-Jeghers syndrome is an autosomal-dominant syndrome characterized by the familial occurrence of hamartomatous polyps of the gastrointestinal tract and mucocutaneous pigmentation (Fig. 9.3).[45,46] The polyps involve the stomach and the small and large intestines and have a characteristic morphologic appearance, with smooth muscle bundles intimately admixed with epithelial cells. Some polyps can grow large enough to cause intestinal obstruction, abdominal pain, or gastrointestinal bleeding. The mucocutaneous pigmentation typically involves the lips, buccal mucosa, eyelids, digits, and rarely, even the intestinal mucosa (see Fig. 9.3). The gene responsible for Peutz-Jeghers syndrome, *STK11* (also known as *LKB1*), has been discovered.[47,48] The *STK11/LKB1* gene on chromosome 19p13.3 encodes for a serine threonine kinase.

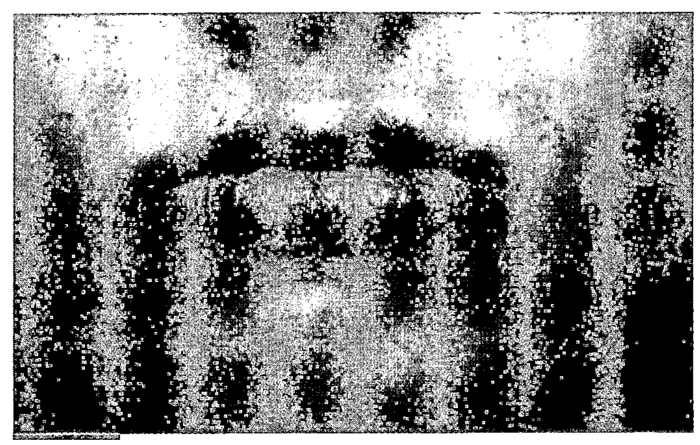

Figure 9.3
Peutz-Jeghers syndrome with numerous melanocytic macules on the lips. (Kindly provided by Dr. G.J.A. Offerhaus of the Academic Medical Center, Amsterdam, The Netherlands, and reprinted from Cameron JL, ed. *Pancreatic Cancer* 2001, BC Decker Inc, Hamilton, Ontario, Canada with permission of the American Cancer Society).

One of the patients originally described by Jeghers died of pancreatic cancer, and patients with the Peutz-Jeghers syndrome have been shown to have a markedly increased risk of developing pancreatic cancer.[45,46,49] For example, Giardiello et al.[50] conducted a meta-analysis of 210 patients with the Peutz-Jeghers syndrome reported in six papers and found that patients with the Peutz-Jeghers syndrome had a 132-fold increased risk of developing pancreatic cancer. The cumulative risk of pancreatic cancer in this group was 36% by the age of 64 years.[50]

Su et al.[51] studied a pancreatic cancer from a patient with the Peutz-Jeghers syndrome at the genetic level and demonstrated a germline *STK11/LKB1* gene mutation coupled with loss of the wild-type allele in the cancer. The demonstration of biallelic inactivation of the gene helps establish *STK11/LKB1* as a tumor-suppressor gene and helps establish a causal relationship between germline mutations in the *STK11/LKB1* gene and the development of pancreatic cancer.

The risk of pancreatic cancer in patients with the Peutz-Jeghers syndrome is so high that Dr. Canto at Johns Hopkins includes patients with the Peutz-Jeghers syndrome in her endoscopic ultrasound research screening study for the early detection of pancreatic cancer.[44] Remarkably, Canto et al.[44] found an asymptomatic intraductal papillary mucinous neoplasm (IPMN, see Chapter 51) in one of the patients with the Peutz-Jeghers syndrome. This IPMN was resected at a noninvasive stage, potentially saving the patient's life. The study by Canto et al.[44] not only highlights the potential value of screening for early pancreatic cancer, but it also suggests a possible association between the Peutz-Jeghers syndrome and IPMNs. Indeed, Sato et al.[52] have demonstrated loss of heterozygosity at 19p13.3 (the locus of the *STK11/LKB1* gene) in seven of 22 (32%) IPMNs.[52]

Familial Pancreatitis

Familial pancreatitis is discussed in detail in Chapter 8. Briefly, familial pancreatitis is characterized by the familial occurrence of pancreatitis with an early age of onset.[53] Germline mutations in the *PRSS1* gene cause an autosomal dominant form of the disease, whereas germline mutations in *SPINK1* lead to an autosomal recessive pattern of inheritance. Lowenfels et al.[54] have estimated that 40% of patients with familial pancreatitis will develop pancreatic cancer by the age of 70 years. This risk is even higher in smokers with familial pancreatitis.[54] Some patients with familial pancreatitis choose prophylactic pancreatectomy because their pancreas is essentially nonfunctional.

Matsubayashi et al.[55] studied a series of patients with sporadic and familial pancreatic cancer for germline polymorphisms in two other genes linked to pancreatitis, the *SPINK1* and *CFTR* genes.[55] The prevalence of the N34S polymorphism of *SPINK1* and the two most common polymorphisms of the *CFTR* gene, the Δ508 mutation and the 5T polymorphism, in patients with pancreatic cancer was similar to that in control subjects, suggesting that polymorphisms of *SPINK1* and *CFTR* genes do not predispose to the development of pancreatic cancer.[55]

Hereditary Nonpolyposis Colorectal Cancer

HNPCC is the most common hereditary disorder predisposing to colorectal carcinoma. In addition to colorectal carcinoma, patients with HNPCC have an increased risk of developing other cancers, including endometrial cancer, gastric carcinoma, ovarian carcinoma, transitional cell carcinoma of the ureter/renal pelvis, and hepatobiliary cancer. Pancreatic cancer has also been reported in some kindreds with HNPCC, and pancreatic cancers with microsatellite instability, the genetic hallmark of HNPCC, often have a distinct histologic appearance called a "medullary" histology.[56-58]

As noted in Chapter 3, the HNPCC syndrome is caused by germline mutations in one of the mismatch repair genes (including *hMSH2* and *hMLH1*). This suggests a scenario for identifying pancreatic cancers with microsatellite instability and patients who may have HNPCC.[57] Surgically resected pancreatic cancers with the medullary phenotype can be immunolabeled for the *hMSH2* and *hMLH1* gene products.[57] Patients with a cancer that shows a loss of expression of one of these two gene products can then be offered genetic counseling and possibly genetic testing for germline mutations in *hMSH2* or *hMLH1*.

As is true for most of the other genetic syndromes that predispose to pancreatic cancer, the recognition that a patient has HNPCC has a significant impact on other family members and will help guide the screening for pancreatic and extrapancreatic malignancies.

Other Genetic Syndromes

Several other syndromes deserve mention, even though their association with pancreatic cancer might not be strong or a genetic basis for their development has not been established.

A large kindred with multiple pancreatic cancers (called "family X") has been described by Brentnall and colleagues.[59] In addition to pancreatic cancer, many of the members of this family develop a distinctive fibrocystic atrophy of the pancreas with endocrine cell hyperplasia.[60] Recent linkage analysis has suggested that the gene responsible for the aggregation of pancreatic cancer in this family may be located on chromosome 4q22-24.[61]

Sina-Frey et al.[62] reported on three families with basal cell carcinoma and pancreatic cancer.[62] This association is of interest because germline mutations in the *PTCH* gene cause Gorlin syndrome (nevoid basal cell carcinoma syndrome), and Berman et al.[63] have reported *PTCH* activation in a series of pancreatic cancers. Although it is tempting to hypothesize that some germline *PTCH* gene mutations predispose to the development of pancreatic cancer, there is no solid evidence to do so at this time.

Both Giardiello et al.[64] and Spigelman et al.[65] have suggested a weak association between familial adenomatous polyposis and pancreatic cancer. Familial adenomatous polyposis is caused by germline mutations in the *APC* gene on chromosome 5q21,[66] and germline mutations greatly increase the risk of developing colorectal and small-intestinal adenomas. Some of the duodenal adenomas progress to invasive cancer, and these invasive duodenal cancers can mimic pancreatic cancer, possibly explaining some of the apparent association between familial adenomatous polyposis and pancreatic cancer.

Despite recent advances, the genetic basis for most cases of familial pancreatic cancer has not been discovered. In total, the aforementioned syndromes account for only 20% of the familial aggregation of pancreatic cancer. Although the familial pancreatic cancer gene remains elusive, several strides have been made that, taken together, may form the basis for its discovery. The two major hurdles to the discovery of the familial pancreatic cancer gene are a lack of families suitable for linkage and a lack of relatively pure cancer cell lines derived from patients with familial pancreatic cancer. G. Petersen recently established a multicenter consortium to identify kindreds that would be suitable for linkage analysis. This consortium, called "PACGENE," includes familial cancer registries at the Mayo Clinic; Johns Hopkins University; Creighton University; the University of Toronto; the Dana-Farber Cancer Institute; the Karmanos Cancer Institute; and M.D. Anderson Cancer Center. It is hoped that significant numbers of families suitable for linkage analyses will be obtained through this collaborative effort.

C. Iacobuzio-Donahue has started a second unique program to overcome the shortage of cancer cell lines derived from patients with familial pancreatic cancer. Called the "Gastrointestinal Cancer Rapid Medical Donation Program," this effort facilitates the rapid autopsy of patients with pancreatic cancer. Already, numerous pancreatic cancer xenografts and cell lines have been established through this program, and it is hoped that the inclusion of patients with familial pancreatic cancer will lead to the creation of renewable cell lines for genetic study.

Genes not Associated with Familial Pancreatic Cancer

Numerous genetic loci have been studied as possible candidates for the familial pancreatic cancer gene, but these were found not to be associated with familial pancreatic cancer. For example, germline mutations have not been found in the *DPC4/SMAD4*, *MAP2K4*, and *ACVR1β* genes in patients with familial pancreatic cancer.[21,67]

Screening for Early Cancer

Screening the general population for pancreatic cancer is not practical for the reasons discussed in Chapter 17. As the genetic basis for the aggregation of pancreatic cancer is defined, the genes discovered will help define populations of patients with an increased risk of developing pancreatic cancer and therefore will help guide screening for early pancreatic neoplasia.

Similarly, germline mutations in most cancer-associated genes do not just increase the risk of one cancer type. With few exceptions, multiple organs are at risk, and screening is available for these extrapancreatic malignancies. For example, individuals who carry germline *p16* mutations are at risk for both melanoma and pancreatic cancer. Recognition of this syndrome can therefore lead to the detection of early, curable melanomas.

Complex Multifactorial Traits

Although much of this chapter has focused on the notion that mutations in single genes cause the familial clustering of pancreatic cancer, the reality is certainly much more complex. It is likely that in some families, multiple genes contribute together to increase risk, and in others that environmental exposures, such as cigarette smoking, interact with genetic predisposition to greatly increase risk. The challenge is now to identify other yet-undiscovered genes, some of modest effect, and to define their relationship with environmental risk factors and the development of pancreatic cancer. In this regard, other research strategies, such as molecular epidemiologic studies that compare pancreatic cancer cases with control subjects, will be needed. These studies could examine, for example, candidate genes that encode for enzymes that are involved in metabolic activation of benzo[a]pyrene and other polycyclic aromatic hydrocarbons found in cigarette smoke and in some dietary sources. Such genes include cytochrome P450 1A1, glutathione *S*-transferase M1, and *N*-acetyl transferase 2. Polymorphisms in these genes have been analyzed in small studies to determine their associations with pancreatic cancer.[68-70] Although these studies have not reported substantial associations, most have lacked adequate power or lacked access to comprehensive collections of DNA specimens for genotyping. Further studies are planned or are ongoing to address these problems and will be positioned to examine both genetic and environmental factors in pancreatic cancer risk.

The ultimate goal of genetic and epidemiologic studies of familial pancreatic cancer is to identify the combination of genetic and environmental risk factors that lead to the aggregation of pancreatic cancer in families and to delineate susceptibility genes. When these are defined, patient lives can be saved because cancer risk will be better defined. High-risk individuals can be offered behavior modification, chemopreventive options, early detection of pancreatic cancer, and early detection of extrapancreatic cancers. In addition, patients with pancreatic cancer may eventually be offered therapies specifically targeting the genetic alterations that gave rise to their cancer.

References

1. Brinkley D. *The Unfinished Presidency: Jimmy Carter's Journey Beyond the White House*. New York: Penguin Group; 1998.
2. Lynch HT, Fitzsimmons ML, Smyrk TC, et al. Familial pancreatic cancer: clinicopathologic study of 18 nuclear families. *Am J Gastroenterol*. 1990;85:54–60.
3. Ehrenthal D, Haeger L, Griffin T, Compton C. Familial pancreatic adenocarcinoma in three generations: a case report and a review of the literature. *Cancer*. 1987;59:1661–1664.
4. MacDermott RP, Kramer P. Adenocarcinoma of the pancreas in four siblings. *Gastroenterology*. 1973;65:137–139.
5. Falk RT, Pickle LW, Fontham ET, et al. Life-style risk factors for pancreatic cancer in Louisana: a case-control study. *Am J Epidemiol*. 1988;128:324–336.
6. Fernandez E, La Vecchia C, D'Avanzo B, et al. Family history and the risk of liver, gallbladder, and pancreatic cancer. *Cancer Epidemiol Biomarkers Prev*. 1994;3:209–212.
7. Ghadirian P, Boyle P, Simard A, et al. Reported family aggregation of pancreatic cancer within a population-based case-control study in the francophone community in Montreal, Canada. *Int J Pancreatol*. 1991;10:183–196.
8. Ghadirian P, Liu G, Gallinger S, et al. A. Risk of pancreatic cancer among individuals with a family history of cancer of the pancreas. *Int J Cancer*. 2002;20;97:807–110.
9. Schenk M, Schwartz AG, O'Neal E, et al. Familial risk of pancreatic cancer. *J Natl Cancer Inst*. 2001;93:640–644.
10. Silverman DT, Schiffman M, Everhart J, et al. Diabetes mellitus, other medical conditions and familial history of cancer as risk factors for pancreatic cancer. *Br J Cancer*. 1999;80:1830–1837.
11. Klein AP, Brune K, Petersen GM, et al. Prospective risk of pancreatic cancer in familial pancreatic cancer kindreds. *Cancer Res*. 2004;64:2634-812.
12. Coughlin SS, Calle EE, Patel AV, Thun MJ. Predictors of pancreatic cancer mortality among a large cohort of United States adults. *Cancer Causes Control*. 2000;11:915–923.
13. Hemminki K, Li X. Familial and second primary pancreatic cancers: a nationwide epidemiologic study from Sweden. *Int J Cancer*. 2003;103:525–530.
14. Lichtenstein P, Holm NV, Verkasalo PK, et al. Environmental and heritable factors in the causation of cancer: analyses of cohorts of twins from Sweden, Denmark, and Finland. *N Engl J Med*. 2000;343:78–85.
15. Klein AP, Beaty TH, Bailey-Wilson JE, et al. Evidence for a major gene influencing risk of pancreatic cancer. *Genet Epidemiol*. 2002;23:133–149.
16. Schutte M, da Costa LT, Hahn SA, et al. Identification by representational difference analysis of a homozygous deletion in pancreatic carcinoma that lies within the *BRCA2* region. *Proc Natl Acad Sci USA*. 1995;92:5950–5954.
17. Lal G, Liu G, Schmocker B, et al. Inherited predisposition to pancreatic adenocarcinoma: role of family history and germ-line *P16*, *BRCA1*, and *BRCA2* mutations. *Cancer Res*. 2000;60:409–416.
18. Berman DB, Costalas J, Schultz DC, et al. A common mutation in *BRCA2* that predisposes to a variety of cancers is found in both Jewish Ashkenazi and non-Jewish individuals. *Cancer Res*. 1996;56:3409–3414.
19. Thorlacius S, Olafsdottir G, Tryggvadottir L, et al. A single *BRCA2* mutation in male and female breast cancer families from Iceland with varied cancer phenotypes. *Nat Genet*. 1996;13:117–119.
20. White K, Held KR, Weber BHF. A *BRCA2* germ-line mutation in familial pancreatic carcinoma. *Int J Cancer*. 2001; 91:742–744.
21. Murphy KM, Brune KA, Griffin CA, et al. Evaluation of candidate genes *MAP2K4*, *MADH4*, *ACVR1B*, and *BRCA2* in familial pancreatic cancer: deleterious BRCA2 mutations in 17%. *Cancer Res*. 2002;62:3789–3793.
22. Ozcelik H, Schmocker B, DiNicola N, et al. Germline *BRCA2* 6174delT mutations in Ashkenazi Jewish pancreatic cancer patients. *Nat Genet*. 1997;16:17–18.
23. Roa BB, Boyd AA, Volcik K, Richards CS. Ashkenazi Jewish population frequencies for common mutations in *BRCA1* and *BRCA2*. *Nat Genet*. 1996;14:185–187.
24. Hahn SA, Greenhalf B, Ellis I, et al. *BRCA2* germline mutations in familial pancreatic carcinoma. *J Natl Cancer Inst*. 2003;95:214–221.
25. Goggins M, Schutte M, Lu J, Moskaluk CA, et al. Germline *BRCA2* gene mutations in patients with apparently sporadic pancreatic carcinomas. *Cancer Res*. 1996;56:5360–5364.
26. Cancer risks in *BRCA2* mutation carriers. The Breast Cancer Linkage Consortium. *J Natl Cancer Inst*. 1999;91:1310–1316.
27. van der Heijden M, Yeo CJ, Hruban RH, Kern SE. Fanconi anemia gene mutations in young-onset pancreatic cancer. *Cancer Res*. 2003;63:2585–2588.

27A. van der Heijden MS, Brody JR, Gallmeier E, et al. Functional defects in the fanconi anemia pathway in pancreatic cancer cells. *Am J Pathol*. 2004;165:651–7.

28. Rogers CD, van der Heijden MS, Brune K, et al. The genetics of *FANCC* and *FANCG* in familial pancreatic cancer. *Cancer Biol Ther*. 2004;3:167-169.
29. Bartsch DK, Sina-Frey M, Lang S, et al. *CDKN2A* germline mutations in familial pancreatic cancer. *Ann Surg*. 2002;236:730–737.
30. Bergman W, Watson P, de Jong J, et al. Systemic cancer and the *FAMMM* syndrome. *Br J Cancer*. 1990;61:932–936.
31. Borg A, Sandberg T, Nilsson K, et al. High frequency of multiple melanomas and breast and pancreas carcinomas in *CDKN2A* mutation-positive melanoma families. *J Natl Cancer Inst*. 2000;92:1260–1266.
32. Ciotti P, Strigini P, Bianchi-Scarra G. Familial melanoma and pancreatic cancer. Ligurian Skin Tumor Study Group [letter; comment]. *N Engl J Med*. 1996;334:469–470.
33. Kefford RF, Newton Bishop JA, Bergman W, Tucker MA. Counseling and DNA testing for individuals perceived to be genetically predisposed to melanoma: a consensus statement of the Melanoma Genetics Consortium. *J Clin Oncol*. 1999;17:3245–32451.
34. Lynch HT, Fusaro RM. Pancreatic cancer and the familial atypical multiple mole melanoma (FAMMM) syndrome. *Pancreas*. 1991;6:127–131.
35. Lynch HT, Brand RE, Hogg D, et al. Phenotypic variation in eight extended *CDKN2A* germline mutation familial atypical multiple mole melanoma-pancreatic carcinoma-prone families: the familial atypical mole melanoma-pancreatic carcinoma syndrome. *Cancer*. 2002;94:84–96.

36. Parker JF, Florell SR, Alexander A, et al. Pancreatic carcinoma surveillance in patients with familial melanoma. *Arch Dermatol.* 2003;139:1019–1025.
37. Rulyak SJ, Brentnall TA, Lynch HT, Austin MA. Characterization of the neoplastic phenotype in the familial atypical multiple-mole melanoma-pancreatic carcinoma syndrome. *Cancer.* 2003;98:798–804.
38. Mantelli M, Barile M, Ciotti P, et al. High prevalence of the G101W germline mutation in the *CDKN2A* (p16(Ink4a)) gene in 62 Italian malignant melanoma families. *Am J Med Genet.* 2002;107:214–221.
39. Vasen HF, Gruis NA, Frants RR, et al. Risk of developing pancreatic cancer in families with familial atypical multiple mole melanoma associated with a specific 19 deletion of p16 (p16-Leiden). *Int J Cancer.* 2000;87:809–811.
40. Gruis NA, Sandkuijl LA, van der Velden PA, et al. *CDKN2* explains part of the clinical phenotype in Dutch familial atypical multiple-mole melanoma (FAMM) syndrome families. *Melanoma Res.* 1995;5:169-77
41. Goldstein AM, Fraser MC, Struewing JP, et al. Increased risk of pancreatic cancer in melanoma-prone kindreds with *p16INK4* mutations. *N Engl J Med.* 1995;333:970–974.
42. Schutte M, Hruban RH, Geradts J, et al. Abrogation of the Rb/*p16* tumor-suppressive pathway in virtually all pancreatic carcinomas. *Cancer Res.* 1997;57:3126–3130.
43. Lynch HT, Brand RE, Lynch JF, et al. Genetic counseling and testing for germline p16 mutations in two pancreatic cancer-prone families. *Gastroenterology.* 2000;119:1756–1760.
44. Canto MI, Goggins M, Yeo CJ, et al. Screening for pancreatic neoplasia in high-risk individuals: an EUS-based approach. *Clin Gastroenterol Hepatol.* 2004;2:606-21
45. Giardiello FM, Welsh SB, Hamilton SR, et al. Increased risk of cancer in the Peutz-Jeghers syndrome. *N Engl J Med.* 1987;316:1511–1514.
46. Jeghers H, McKusick V, Victor AMD, Katz KH. Generalized intestinal polyposis and melanin spots of the oral mucosa, lips and digits. *N Engl J Med.* 1949;241:992–1005.
47. Hemminki A, Markie D, Tomlinson I, et al. A serine/threonine kinase gene defective in Peutz-Jeghers syndrome. *Nature.* 1998;391:184–187.
48. Jenne DE, Reimann H, Nezu J, et al. Peutz-Jeghers syndrome is caused by mutations in a novel serine/threonine kinase. *Nat Genet.* 1998;18:38–43.
49. Bowlby LS. Pancreatic adenocarcinoma in an adolescent male with Peutz-Jeghers syndrome. *Hum Pathol.* 1986;17:97–99.
50. Giardiello FM, Brensinger JD, Tersmette AC, et al. Very high risk of cancer in familial Peutz-Jeghers syndrome. *Gastroenterology.* 2000;119:1447–1453.
51. Su GH, Hruban RH, Bova GS, et al. Germline and somatic mutations of the *STK11/LKB1* Peutz-Jeghers gene in pancreatic and biliary cancers. *Am J Pathol.* 1999;154:1835–1840.
52. Sato N, Rosty C, Jansen M, et al. *STK11/LKB1* Peutz-Jeghers gene inactivation in intraductal papillary-mucinous neoplasms of the pancreas. *Am J Pathol.* 2001;159:2017–2022.
53. Finch MD, Howes N, Ellis I, et al. Hereditary pancreatitis and familial pancreatic cancer. *Digestion.* 1997;58:564–569.
54. Lowenfels AB, Maisonneuve EP, Dimagno YE, et al. Hereditary pancreatitis and the risk of pancreatic cancer. *J Natl Cancer Inst.* 1997;89:442–446.
55. Matsubayashi H, Fukushima N, Sato N, et al. Polymorphisms of *SPINK1 N34S* and *CFTR* in patients with sporadic and familial pancreatic cancer. *Cancer Biol Ther.* 2003;2:652–655.
56. Lynch HT, Voorhees GJ, Lanspa SJ, et al. Pancreatic carcinoma and hereditary nonpolyposis colorectal cancer: a family study. *Br J Cancer.* 1985;52:271–273.
57. Wilentz RE, Goggins M, Redston M, et al. Genetic, immunohistochemical, and clinical features of medullary carcinomas of the pancreas: a newly described and characterized entity. *Am J Pathol.* 2000;156:1641–1651.
58. Goggins M, Offerhaus GJA, Hilgers W, et al. Pancreatic adenocarcinomas with DNA replication errors (RER+) are associated with wild-type K-*ras* and characteristic histopathology: poor differentiation, a syncytial growth pattern, and pushing borders suggest RER+. *Am J Pathol.* 1998;152:1501–1507.
59. Brentnall TA, Bronner MP, Byrd DR, et al. Early diagnosis and treatment of pancreatic dysplasia in patients with a family history of pancreatic cancer. *Ann Intern Med.* 1999;131:247–255.
60. Meckler KA, Brentnall TA, Haggitt RC, et al. Familial fibrocystic pancreatic atrophy with endocrine cell hyperplasia and pancreatic carcinoma. *Am J Surg Pathol.* 2001;25:1047–1053.
61. Eberle MA, Pfutzer R, Pogue-Geile KL, et al. A new susceptibility locus for autosomal dominant pancreatic cancer maps to chromosome 4q32-34. *Am J Hum Genet.* 2002;70:1044-8.
62. Sina-Frey M, Bartsch DK, Grundei T, et al. Pancreatic cancer and basal-cell carcinoma. *Lancet.* 2003;361:180.
63. Berman DM, Karhadkar SS, Maitra A, et al. Widespread requirement for Hedgehog ligand stimulation in growth of digestive tract tumours. *Nature.* 2003;425:846–851.
64. Giardiello FM, Offerhaus GJA, Lee DH, et al. Increased risk of thyroid and pancreatic carcinoma in familial adenomatous polyposis. *Gut.* 1993;34:1394–1396.
65. Spigelman AD, Farmer KC, James M, et al. Tumours of the liver, bile ducts, pancreas and duodenum in a single patient with familial adenomatous polyposis. *Br J Surg.* 1991;78:979–980.
66. Kinzler KW, Nilbert MC, Su LK, et al. Identification of FAP locus genes from chromosome 5q21. *Science.* 1991;253:661–669.
67. Moskaluk CA, Hruban RH, Schutte M, et al. Genomic sequencing of *DPC4* in the analysis of familial pancreatic carcinoma. *Diagn Mol Pathol.* 1997;6:85–90.
68. Bartsch H, Malaveille C, Lowenfels AB, et al. Genetic polymorphism of *N*-acetyltransferases, glutathione *S*-transferase M1 and NAD(P)H:quinone oxidoreductase in relation to malignant and benign pancreatic disease risk. The International Pancreatic Disease Study Group. *Eur J Cancer Prev.* 1998;7:215–223.
69. Liu G, Ghadirian P, Vesprini D, et al. Polymorphisms in *GSTM1, GSTT1* and *CYP1A1* and risk of pancreatic adenocarcinoma. *Br J Cancer.* 2000;82:1646–1649.
70. Duell EJ, Holly EA, Bracci PM, et al. A population-based, case-control study of polymorphisms in carcinogen-metabolizing genes, smoking, and pancreatic adenocarcinoma risk. *J Natl Cancer Inst.* 2002;94:297–306.

CHAPTER 10

Prevention

Marsha L. Frazier, PhD

Pancreatic cancer is the fourth leading cause of cancer deaths in the United States, with pancreatic adenocarcinoma being the most frequent form observed.[1] By the time of diagnosis, it has usually metastasized. Prognosis is grim, with a median survival time of 12 months, and a 5-year survival rate of 4%.[1] Men have a 50% higher incidence rate of pancreatic cancer than women, and the incidence of this disease is approximately 50% higher among blacks than whites.[2]

A first step in preventing pancreatic cancer requires an understanding of the risk factors for the disease. Identifying high-risk patients is important for increased surveillance but also for identifying patients who would be targeted for prevention trials. A small proportion of pancreatic cancers are a result of major genetic factors predisposing to familial cancer syndromes. The majority of pancreatic cancer cases are considered sporadic; however, it is generally thought that environmental and minor genetic factors play an important role. The identification of environmental and genetic risk factors as well as gene–environment interactions will be important for assessing susceptibility to pancreatic cancer and in developing strategies for prevention of pancreatic cancer. There are currently no biomarkers that are useful in early detection, and no other practical screening tools exist. Clearly, an improved understanding of the risk factors for pancreatic cancer will be important in its prevention. An overview of some of the risk factors for pancreatic cancer is shown in Table 10.1.

Genetic Factors and Pancreatic Cancer

A small proportion of pancreatic cancers arise as a result of germline mutations in genes causing familial predisposition to cancer. These genetic disorders are discussed in greater detail in Chapter 9. Among these mutated genes is

Table 10.1 Risk Factors for Pancreatic Cancer

Familial predisposition	Increased risk
Pancreatitis	Increased risk
Smoking	Increased risk
NSAIDs use	Conflicting results
Alcohol consumption	Increased risk in African Americans
Diabetes	Increased risk with increased duration of diabetes
Obesity	Increased risk
Organochlorines	Increased risk

the *p16* gene, which causes the familial atypical multiple mole melanoma syndrome, where patients are predisposed to melanoma and pancreatic cancer.[3] *LKB1* is mutated in Peutz-Jeghers syndrome, where family members are predisposed to a variety of cancers, including pancreatic cancer. Carriers of genetic alterations in *BRCA2* have an increased risk for cancers of the pancreas and breast.[4-6] In hereditary nonpolyposis colorectal cancer, which is caused by germline mutations in mismatch repair genes such as *MSH2* and *MLH1*, family members are predisposed to a variety of cancer types, including pancreatic cancer, although colorectal cancer is the most frequently seen cancer.[7]

Because pancreatic cancer in the population at large is not a frequent event, prevention trials for pancreatic cancer would likely target high-risk patients carrying germline mutations in genes causing a familial predisposition to cancer. A second group to be targeted might be patients with a hereditary form of pancreatitis. Patients with chronic pancreatitis are at an increased risk for pancreatic cancer.[8] In certain hereditary forms of pancreatitis, the risk for development of pancreatic cancer is as high as 40% in some families.[9] Genes that cause hereditary pancreatitis include the cationic trypsinogen (*PRSS1*) gene, the pancreatic secretory trypsin inhibitor (*SPINK1*) gene, and the cystic fibrosis transmembrane conductance regulator (*CFTR*) gene.[10] The link between hereditary pancreatitis and pancreatic cancer is discussed in Chapter 8.

The role of genetic and environmental factors for other forms of pancreatitis remains unknown. Although alcohol is a risk factor for pancreatitis, not all heavy drinkers develop alcoholic pancreatitis. Therefore, it is believed that genetic factors and/or other environmental factors are also involved.

Minor genetic factors such as biologically significant polymorphisms are believed to play a role in the risk for development of both alcoholic pancreatitis and pancreatic cancer. Unlike some of the other cancers, only a small handful of minor genetic factors has been reported in relationship to pancreatic cancer. Examples of minor genetic factors include polymorphisms in genes such as *GSTM1*, *UGT1A7*, and *XRCC1*; these are discussed further in this chapter. A compilation of patient information on these minor genetic factors, in combination with environmental factors, will eventually be useful in assessing the susceptibility to development of pancreatic cancer, as well as the response to preventive strategies such as chemoprevention.

Smoking

Although risk factors for sporadic pancreatic cancer have not been well characterized, cigarette smoking is known to be a major risk factor.[11-19] Tobacco exposure accounts for approximately one quarter to one third of pancreatic cancers, and long-term smoking (more than 20 years) doubles the risk.[19-21]

Studies by Fuchs et al.[21] used data from two large prospective cohort studies to quantify the affect of cigarette smoking on pancreatic cancer risk. One of the ongoing cohort studies is the Nurses' Health Study.[22] The second ongoing cohort study is the Health Professionals Follow-up Study.[23] The Nurses' Health Study began in 1976 when 121,700 American female registered nurses, aged 30–55 years, completed a mailed questionnaire on known or suspected risk factors for cancer and coronary heart disease. The Health Professionals Follow-up study began in 1986 when 51,529 American male dentists, optometrists, osteopaths, pharmacists, podiatrists, and veterinarians (aged 40–75 years) completed a mailed questionnaire on known or suspected risk factors of cancer and coronary heart disease. Both cohorts are updated biennially with follow-up questionnaires to update information about potential risk factors such as smoking status and to identify newly diagnosed cases of cancer and other diseases. Among smokers who had consumed cigarettes within the past 15 years, a positive association between cigarette smoking and risk of cancer was seen with both studies. The multivariate relative risk (RR) of pancreatic cancer for current smokers was found to be 2.5 (95% confidence interval [CI], 1.7–3.6). There was also a trend in increasing risk with increasing pack-years of smoking ($P = 0.004$). Former smokers had a 48% reduction in pancreatic cancer risk within 2 years of quitting. A significant linear trend between pack-years of smoking and pancreatic cancer risk was seen only among current smokers. When cigarette consumption was restricted to less than 15 years in the past, the RR of pancreatic cancer increased monotonically with increasing pack-years ($P = 0.01$). For consumption of 15 or more years in the past, no association was observed between pack-years and pancreatic cancer risk. The proportion of pancreatic cancer attributable to cigarette smoking was calculated to be roughly 25%.

In a case-control study of pancreatic cancers diagnosed in Atlanta, GA, Detroit, MI, and 10 New Jersey counties from August 1986 through April 1989, cigarette smokers were found to have a 70% increased risk of pancreatic cancer compared with nonsmokers. Direct interviews were conducted with 526 incident cases and 2,153 population control subjects.[24] Current smokers had an odds ratio (OR) of 2.0 (95% CI, 1.5–2.6) compared with control subjects. For those who quit smoking more than 2 years before the interview, the OR fell to 1.4 (95% CI, 1.1–1.9). Both men and women displayed increased risk with increasing duration smoked; however, women displayed a higher RR than men among those who smoked for 20–39 years and 40 years or more. In this study, cigarette smoking was estimated to account for 26% (95% CI, 12–48%) of pancreatic cancer in men and 29% (95% CI, 18–42%) in women.

Only a very small fraction of smokers develop pancreatic cancer, suggesting that other environmental factors and/or genetic factors interact with smoking to influence risk. Polymorphisms in the *GSTT1*, *XRCC1*, and *UGT1A7* have been shown to interact with smoking to increase the risk for pancreatic cancer as discussed later here.

The entire gene is deleted for the *GSTM1* polymorphism (the null allele). Therefore, patients who are homozygous for the polymorphism do not express the gene at all. Approximately 17%–18% of the population is homozygous for the null allele among whites. An interaction was observed between the *GSTT1* null genotype and cigarette smoking in whites, which was more prominent among women than men.[25] When compared with never smokers with the *GSTT1* present genotype, the age-adjusted ORs of pancreatic cancer for heavy smokers with the *GSTT1* null genotype were 5.0 (95% CI, 1.8–14.5) for women and 3.2 (95% CI, 1.3–8.1) for men. For heavy smokers with the *GSTT1*-present genotype, they were 2.0 (95% CI, 1.0–4.0) for women and 2.1 (95% CI, 1.1–3.9) for men.

A polymorphism in the x-ray repair cross-complimenting group 1 (*XRCC1*) gene has been reported to influence pancreatic cancer risk.[26] *XRCC1* is a base excision repair protein that plays a central role in the repair of DNA strand breaks and base damage from a variety of endogenous and exogenous oxidants, including tobacco smoke. A G-to-A polymorphism occurring at codon 399 results in an amino acid change from an arginine to a glutamine. This polymorphism occurs within a poly (ADP-ribose) polymerase-binding region and within the central breast cancer susceptibility gene 1 products COOH terminus domain-binding site of *XRCC1*.[27,28] In a population-based, case-control study of 309 cases of pancreatic adenocarcinoma and 964 control subjects in the San Francisco Bay area, the *XRCC1* genotype alone was not found to be associated with pancreatic cancer risk among whites, African Americans, or Asians. However, evidence was obtained for an interaction between *XRCC1* 399 Gln and smoking that was stronger among women than men.[26] Compared with never or passive smokers with the Arg/Arg genotype, the age- and race-adjusted ORs for heavy smoking (≥41 pack years) with the Gln/Gln or Arg/Gln genotypes were 7.0 (95% CI, 2.41–21) and 3.1 (95% CI, 0.03–6.2) for women and 2.4 (95% CI, 1.1–5.0) and 1.3 (95% CI, 0.20–2.8) for men, respectively. In addition, they studied the *GSTT1* null polymorphism and the *GSTM1* null polymorphism. Their findings suggested an interaction between *XRCC1* (Gln/Gln or Arg/Gln) and *GSTT1/GSTM1/*-null/null to increase risk for pancreatic cancer among women but not among men.[26]

Aspirin and Other Nonsteroidal Anti-Inflammatory Drugs

The use of aspirin and nonsteroidal anti-inflammatory drugs (NSAIDs) has been found to be associated with a reduced risk of colorectal cancer and adenomas. Epidemiologic studies on the influence of aspirin and other NSAIDs on pancreatic cancer have produced conflicting results. The association between the self-reported use of aspirin and other NSAIDs and the incidence of pancreatic cancer was examined from 1992 through 1999, in a prospective study on 28,283 postmenopausal women who lived in Iowa.[29] Eighty incident cases of pancreatic cancer were identified during 7 years of follow-up. The multivariate-adjusted RR of pancreatic cancer associated with any use of aspirin versus no use was 0.57 (95% CI, 0.36–0.90). A trend was observed of decreasing risk for pancreatic cancer incidence with increasing frequency of aspirin use per week ($P_{trend} = 0.005$). Nonaspirin NSAID use was not associated with the incidence of pancreatic cancer. These data suggest that aspirin may be chemopreventive for pancreatic cancer.

In contrast, as a part of the prospective Nurses' Health Study, the relationship between aspirin use and the development of pancreatic cancer was examined.[30] The design of the Nurses' Health Study was described previously here. The findings suggested that regular aspirin use was associated with a significantly increased pancreatic cancer risk among women.

One hundred sixty-one cases of pancreatic cancer were documented during the 18 years of follow-up of 88,378 women who were initially cancer free. Aspirin use was assessed in 1980 and was updated biannually thereafter. The multivariate RR of pancreatic cancer associated with current regular aspirin (two or more per week) was not associated with pancreatic cancer risk when compared with those taking less than two tablets per week. However, increasing the duration of regular use was associated with a significant increased risk. Women who reported 20 or more years of regular aspirin use experienced a RR of 1.58. Among women who reported aspirin use on at least two of three consecutive biannual questionnaires, the RR of pancreatic cancer was 1.11 for women who used one to three standard tablets per week, 1.29 for four to six tablets per week, 1.41 for 6 to 13 tablets per week, and 1.86 for 14 or more tablets per week when compared with consistent nonusers ($P_{trend} = 0.02$).

The opposite findings of the two studies were surprising. The studies of Anderson et al.[29] and Schernhammer et al.[30] both involved large numbers of participants. In the study of Anderson et al.,[29] 80 of 28,283 people developed pancreatic cancer, whereas 161 of 88,378 nurses developed pancreatic cancer in the Nurses' Health Study.[30] However, the study of Anderson et al.[29] focused on postmenopausal women, whereas the Nurses' Health Study captured data from women ranging in ages from 30 to 55 years during 1980. Therefore, at the start of the Nurses' Health Study, there were likely fewer postmenopausal women. Whether there might be a hormonal influence in the affects of aspirin use on cancer risk is not known, but this might possibly help to explain the different results of the two studies. It is also possible that some factor associated with aspirin use is associated with risk for pancreatic cancer, and this unknown is only significant in one of the studies. Factors associated with aspirin use in nurses might not be the same as those associated with aspirin use in midwestern women. An example of this type of confounding situation is seen when the frequency of alcohol use and smoking increases in tandem. People tend to smoke while drinking alcohol. These types of variables can be corrected for in the analysis if the confounder is known.

In a hospital-based, case-control study, 194 patients with pancreatic cancer were compared with 582 age- and sex-matched patients with nonneoplastic conditions to examine the association between aspirin use and the risk of pancreatic cancer.[31] Patients using at least one tablet per week for at least 6 months were classified as regular aspirin users. Unconditional logistic regression was used to compute crude and adjusted ORs with 95% CIs. Pancreatic cancer risk in aspirin users was not changed relative to nonusers, and no significant change in risk was found in relationship to greater frequency of prolonged duration of use in the total sample or in either gender. These data suggest that regular aspirin use may not be associated with a lower risk of pancreatic cancer.

There are a number of possible explanations for the differences in the findings of Menezes et al.[31] and the study of Anderson et al.[29] For example, it could be due to differences in the study populations or a different study design. Another possibility is that the amount and duration of aspirin use (at least one tablet per week for 6 months) that were used to define aspirin use may not have been enough to detect an influence of aspirin on pancreatic cancer risk.

As pointed out by Anderson et al.,[29] their findings are reasonable in view of laboratory findings. Studies on human cell lines suggest that NSAIDs may protect against pancreatic cancer. Further studies need to be conducted to explain the differences in conclusions among the different studies regarding the influence of aspirin on risk for pancreatic cancer. Because of the large focus on the use of NSAIDs in the prevention of other types of cancer, it will be important to understand whether aspirin use increases or decreases the risk for pancreatic cancer.[32]

Alcohol Consumption

There has been a lack of evidence to support a role for alcohol consumption in pancreatic cancer risk.[33] In the Atlanta–Detroit–New Jersey population-based, case-control study described previously here,[24] no evidence was found for an association of ever drinking alcohol for white or African American men. For white women, a 40% reduced risk was observed, whereas for African-American women, there was a 50% increased risk, but this was not significant. Trends in risk with increasing alcohol intake were significant for African-American men and women but not for whites. The increased risk for men was restricted to heavy drinkers, with those who drank 57 drinks per week having an OR of 2.2 (95% CI, 0.9–5.6) as compared with never drinkers. In contrast, for African-American women, there was an increase in risk with increasing levels of alcohol consumption. Those drinking 8 to less than 21 drinks per week had an OR of 1.8 (95% CI, 0.8–4.0) compared with never drinkers, and those who drank 21 drinks or more per week had an OR of 2.5 (95% CI, 1.02–5.9). Although evidence for a role of alcohol consumption has been weak, it is important to consider its possible role in the context of genetic background of the different ethnic groups.

Diabetes Mellitus

Diabetes mellitus has been shown to be associated with an increased risk for pancreatic cancer in a number of studies. In the population-based, case-control study by Silverman,[24] described previously here, pancreatic cancer cases with diabetes mellitus demonstrated a significant positive trend in risk with increasing years before diagnosis of pancreatic cancer ($P = 0.016$). For those with an onset of diabetes within 1 year of diagnosis of cancer, the risk was slightly elevated (OR, 1.3; 95% CI, 0.4–4.0). The risk was significantly increased for those with onset of diabetes within 5 to 9 years (OR, 1.7; 95% CI, 1.01–2.9) and 10 or more years before their cancer diagnosis (OR, 1.5; 95% CI, 1.01–2.2).

Everhart and Wright[34] reported that a history of diabetes mellitus preceding the diagnosis of pancreatic cancer by more than 1 year is associated with a twofold increased risk for pancreatic cancer, based on a meta-analysis of 20 case-control and cohort studies.

The explanation for the association between diabetes and pancreatic cancer is not clear. It is possible that the diabetes enhances the development of pancreatic cancer. However, it is also possible in some cases that diabetes is a consequence of the pathogenesis of pancreatic cancer.

Body Mass Index

Positive associations between the body mass index (BMI) and obesity in pancreatic cancer have been reported in at least four case-control studies[35-38] and two cohort studies.[39,40]

In a study of the Canadian National Enhanced Cancer Surveillance System, Hanley et al.[37] compared 312 patients with histologically confirmed pancreatic cancer with 2,919 control subjects in a population-based, case-control study in 7 of the 10 Canadian provinces. Men in the highest quartile of BMI (≥28.3 kg per m^2) 2 years before interview were at an increased risk of pancreatic cancer with an adjusted OR of 1.9 (95% CI, 1.08–1.35). In addition, men who reported a decrease in weight of at least 2.9% from their lifetime maximum were at reduced risk compared with those reporting a 2.9% or less loss. BMI values 2 years before interview were not associated with pancreatic cancer risk among women, although those reporting a 12.5% or more decrease in weight from their lifetime maximum had substantially lower risk compared with those in the baseline quartile (OR, 0.53; 95% CI, 0.29–0.99).

In the population-based study of 436 patients and 2,003 general-population control subjects from Atlanta GA, Detroit, MI, and New Jersey, Silverman et al.[38] report that obesity was observed to be associated with pancreatic cancer risk. For men and women combined, there was an increasing OR with each quartile for BMI (P = 0.003), and patients in the highest quartile had a 60% increase in risk of pancreatic cancer (95% CI, 1.1–2.1). Although the magnitude of risk associated with obesity was identical in African Americans and whites, a higher percentage of African Americans (38% in women, 27% in men) were obese than whites (16% in women, 22% in men). This finding may help to account for the higher risk for pancreatic cancer among African Americans as compared with whites. A significant trend was also observed for increasing risk of pancreatic cancer and increasing caloric intake. Patients in the highest quartile experienced a 70% higher risk than those in the lowest quartile (P = 0.001). Cases with the highest quartile of both BMI and caloric intake had a statistically significant 180% higher risk as compared with the lowest quartile (95% CI, 1.5–5.2).

In contrast to the previous findings, a study by Lee et al.[41] on 32,687 people who were either Harvard or University of Pennsylvania alumni did not detect a significant relationship between BMI with the risk of pancreatic cancer mortality in age- and sex-adjusted models. These participants provided information on body weight at baseline during, in 1962 or 1966, and with follow-up data collected two or three times up until 1993. The mean age at baseline was 47.1 years, and 93% of these were male. By 1995, 212 persons had died from pancreatic cancer.

Nutrition and Diet in Pancreatic Cancer

In the population-based, case-control study of Silverman et al.[38] described previously here, both men and women displayed a significant trend in risk with increasing consumption of cruciferous vegetables (P = 0.004 for men and 0.002 for women). ORs for men and women consuming more than four servings of cruciferous vegetables per week (the highest quartile of consumption) had a 50%–60% decrease in risk compared with subjects consuming less than 1.5 servings per week (the lowest quartile).

Studies on meat consumption can be complicated because the method of preparation can influence the risk for pancreatic cancer. Consumption of grilled or barbecued red meat has been shown to increase risk for pancreatic cancer in a case-control study.[42] When analyzed using quintiles, the risk increased with increasing intake. The OR for the fifth quintile relative to the reference group was 2.2 (95% CI, 1.4–3.4).

Other methods of cooking were also examined, including frying and broiling and degree of doneness (rare, medium, well done, and very well done), using photographs. None of these were significant; however, for fried red meat consumption, the risks associated with increasing intake were elevated but not statistically significant.

The explanation for these findings is thought to be due to the fact that unlike broiling, baking, or stewing, the process of grilling or barbecuing or frying meat produces high levels of carcinogens such as heterocyclic amines and polycyclic aromatic hydrocarbons.

Other studies have shown associations between meat intake and pancreatic cancer (e.g., pork and beef,[13,14] beef, chicken, and pork,[15] red meat and salted/smoked meat,[43] and daily meat consumption). The findings of Anderson et al.[29] suggest that the methods of preparation are also important in the assessment of meat consumption. Because methods of preparation vary among different countries, regions, and ethnic groups, the assessment of associations with meat and pancreatic cancer is difficult. A study on male smokers suggests that fat consumption is positively associated with pancreatic cancer, whereas carbohydrate intake is inversely associated with the disease.[44]

UGT1A7 Polymorphism in Pancreatic Cancer Risk

Human uridine 5′-diphosphate glucuronosyltransferases (UGTs) are a supergene family of proteins that play a major biologic role in cellular defense and detoxification.[45] They are able to glucuronidate dietary by-products, as well as many therapeutic drugs, and carcinogens such as heterocyclic and polycyclic hydrocarbons and heterocyclic amines and are therefore thought to protect the cell from damage caused by oxidative stress.[46-49] One member of this family of genes, *UGT1A7*, is expressed exclusively in the oropharynx,[50] esophagus,[51] stomach,[52] and pancreas,[53] but it is absent from the liver.[54]

UGT1A7 has five single nucleotide polymorphisms of the human *UGT1A7* gene (*UGT1A7*1*, *UGT1A7*2*, *UGT1A7*3*, *UGT1A7*4*, and *UGT1A7*5*). *UGT1A7*3* has three amino acid changes in it compared with the wild-type allele: *N129K*, *R131K*, and *W208R* and has functional significance, as it leads to a significant decrease in catalytic activity of the encoded protein.[55] Ockenga et al.[53] found *UGT1A7*3* to be associated with chronic pancreatitis. The allelic frequency was found to be 0.21 among 235 normal control subjects and 0.31 among 146 chronic pancreatitis patients (OR, 1.76; 95% CI, 1.26–2.46; $P = 0.0009$). A highly significant association of the *UGT1A7*3* allele was also seen among the 54 patients with pancreatic adenocarcinoma (OR, 1.98; 95% CI, 1.24–3.14, $P = 0.003$).

Because *UGT1A7*3* allele has also been associated with hepatocellular carcinoma,[56] oral cancer,[50] colorectal cancer,[57] in addition to pancreatic adenocarcinoma, *UGT1A7*3* may represent a general risk factor for predisposition to gastrointestinal cancer. Among the patients with pancreatic cancer, 44% were smokers. All 10 patients who developed pancreatic cancer under the age of 55 years were smokers and exhibited a highly significant association with *UGT1A7*3* (OR, 4.7; 95% CI, 1.9–11.8; $P = 0.0009$).

Among the patients with pancreatitis, there were three subgroups: those with alcoholic chronic pancreatitis, those with nonalcoholic pancreatitis carrying the *N34S* mutation of the pancreatic secretory trypsin inhibitor, and those with nonalcoholic pancreatitis without the *N34S* mutation. The *N34S* was chosen because *N34S* has been accepted as a defined genetic background marker for chronic pancreatitis. This group may therefore represent a homogenous group of patients in which toxic or metabolic reasons are less likely to play a significant role for the development of chronic pancreatitis. The significant association was evident in only the alcoholic group. The lack of association of the *UGT1A7*3* polymorphism with the two nonalcoholic pancreatitis subgroups supports a role of *UGT1A7*3* in modulating xenobiotic-induced pancreatic disease.

Exposure to Organochlorines and Cadmium

Exposures to organochlorines such as DDT (dichlorodiphenyltrichloroethane), DDD (dichlorodiphenyldichloroethane), and related PCB (polychlorinated biphenyls)compounds may increase the risk for pancreatic cancer. These compounds are found in some pesticides, and increased pancreatic cancer risk caused by pesticide exposure has been suggested in a variety of different studies.[58] DDT and PCBs were removed from the United States market in 1972 and Canada in 1989. The use of PCBs was banned in 1977 in the United States, and in Canada, as of 1977, PCBs were allowed only in existing closed electrical and hydraulic systems.[59] However, DDT and PCB are very stable, with half-lives of 10 years for DDT metabolites or derivatives and 30 years or more for some PCBs[60] and, therefore, have continued to persist in the food chain. DDT is still used in other parts of the world and, in particular, is used for control of malaria.[61]

In a population-based, case-control study in southeastern Michigan, pancreatic cancer cases were 10 times more likely to report having used ethylan, a DDT derivative, as a result of pesticide use than control subjects.[59] In a nested case-control study in a DDT manufacturing plant, workers whose average length of exposure to DDT was 47 months showed a sevenfold increased risk for pancreatic cancer.[61] The increased risk was also observed for the DDT derivatives ethylan and DDD.

Considering the substantial stability of DDT- and PCB-related compounds, there is reason for concern, as the consequences of the entry of organochlorines into the food chain are not clear.

Studies on serum lipid levels of organochlorines have supported the view that exposure to organochlorines results in increased risk for pancreatic cancer. In a study of

108 pancreatic cancer patients and 82 control subjects from the United States (San Francisco Bay Area in California), pancreatic cancer cases were found to have elevated serum levels of PCBs as compared with control subjects.[58] A less pronounced association of DDE (a metabolite of DDT) was observed in these patients. These findings were thought not to be due to direct exposure of the cases to DDT, but rather, the more likely explanation was that it was due to DDE exposure from food intake, where DDT in pesticides would have been metabolized to DDE.

Cadmium may also be responsible for an increased risk for pancreatic cancer. It is a heavy metal that is a known human carcinogen and acts by inhibiting mismatch repair.[62] Exposure to cadmium occurs in the environment and in occupational settings and is found in such things as nickel-cadmium batteries, pigments, chemical stabilizers, metal coatings, and alloys.[63] Cadmium exposure has been linked to cancers of the lung, prostate, and kidney.[64] It is known to accumulate in the pancreas and has therefore been hypothesized to increase the risk for pancreatic cancer.[65] A meta-analysis of cohorts with high exposure to cadmium is consistent with this hypothesis.[65]

Conclusion

Because pancreatic cancer is not very prevalent in the population at large, conducting chemoprevention trials for pancreatic cancer in the general population is impractical and cost prohibitive because of the large number of people that would be required for the study. Studies conducted with celecoxib as a chemopreventative agent for colorectal cancer were conducted on high-risk patients carrying germline mutations in the *APC* gene, which predisposes to familial adenomatous polyposis (FAP).[66] The studies showed a significant reduction in adenomas, and celecoxib is now Food and Drug Administration approved for treatment of FAP. A similar approach could be used to study people at high risk for developing pancreatic cancer.

As mentioned previously here, the influence of NSAIDs on risk for pancreatic cancer is controversial. Well-defined studies on patients at high risk for development of pancreatic cancer will be important for defining the role of NSAIDs in prevention of pancreatic cancer.

Metformin is another candidate agent that prevented the development of malignant lesions in Syrian golden hamsters that we fed a high-fat diet.[67] This agent has been shown to be effective in increasing glucose use, uptake, and oxidation as well as gluconeogenesis. Fifty percent of the animals that were fed the high-fat diet without metformin developed malignant lesions, whereas none were detected in the animals fed the high-fat diet and metiformin.

Other candidates for chemoprevention include somatostatin analogues, selective estrogen receptor modulators, and antiandrogenic agents.[68]

Initial clinical prevention trials for pancreatic cancer will likely focus on high-risk patients, such as those with germline mutations predisposing to familial pancreatic cancer. As both environmental and low penetrance genetic risk factors become better characterized, a panel of risk markers and factors might be assembled to allow identification of additional high-risk groups for prevention trials. For example, smokers with the *GSTT1* null genotype, the *XRCC1* 399 Gln genotype, and the *UGT1A7**3 genotype might serve as another at-risk group of patients for prevention trials.

References

1. Jemal, Tiwari RC, Murray T, et al. Cancer Statistics 2004. *CA Cancer J Clin.* 2004:52:23–47.
2. Ries LAG, Kosary CL, Hankey BF, et al (eds). *SEER Cancer Statistics Review, 1973–1996.* Bethesda, MD: National Cancer Institute; 1999.
3. Goldstein AM, Fraser MC, Struewing JP, et al. Increased risk of pancreatic cancer in melanoma-prone kindreds with *p16*INK4 mutations. *N Engl J Med.* 1995;333:970–974.
4. Thorlacius S, Olafsdottir G, Tryggvadottir L, et al. A single *BRCA2* mutation in male and female breast cancer families from zIceland with varied cancer phenotypes. *Nat Genet.* 1996;13:117–119.
5. Phelan CM, Lancaster J, Tonin P, et al. Mutation analysis of the *BRCA2* gene in 49 site-specific breast cancer families. *Nat Genet.* 1996;13:120–122.
6. Couch FJ, Farid LM, DeShano ML, et al. *BRCA2* germline mutations in male breast cancer cases and beast cancer families. *Nat Genet.* 1996;13:123–125.
7. Lynch HT, Voorhees GJ, Lanspa S, et al. Pancreatic carcinoma and hereditary nonpolyposis colorectal cancer: a family study. *Br J Cancer.* 1985;52:271–273.
8. Lowenfels AB, Maisonneuve P, Cavallini G, et al. Pancreatitis and the risk of pancreatic cancer. *N Engl J Med.* 1993; 328:1433–1437.
9. Hansel DE, Kern SE, Hruban RH. Molecular pathogenesis of pancreatic cancer. *Annu Rev Genomics Hum Genet.* 2003;4: 237–256.
10. Hanck C, Schneider A, Whitcomb DC. Genetic polymorphisms in alcoholic pancreatitis. *Best Practice Res Clin Gaastroenterol.* 2003;17:613–623.
11. Gold EB, Gordis L, Diener MD, et al. Diet and other risk factors for cancer of the pancreas. *Cancer.* 1985;55:460–467.
12. Mack TM, Yu MC, Hanisch R, Henderson BE. Pancreas cancer and smoking, beverage consumption, and past medical history. *J Natl Cancer Inst.* 1986;76:49–60.
13. Falk RT, Pickle LW, Fontham ET, et al. Life-style risk for pancreatic cancer in Louisiana: a case-control study. *Am J Epidemiol.* 1988;128:324–326.

14. Olsen GW, Mandel JS, Gibson RW, et al. A case-control study of pancreatic cancer and cigarettes, alcohol, coffee and diet. *Am J Public Health*. 1989;79:1016–1019.
15. Farrow DC, Davis S. Risk of pancreatic cancer in relation to medical history and the use of tobacco, alcohol and coffee. *Int J Cancer.* 1990;45:816–820.
16. Bueno de Mesquite HB, Maisonneuve P, Moerman CT, et al. Life-time history of smoking and exocrine carcinoma of the pancreas: a population-based case-control study in the Netherlands. *Int J Cancer.* 1991;49:816–822.
17. Zaponski WA, Boyle P, Przewozniak K, et al. Cigarette smoking, alcohol, tea and coffee consumption and pancreas cancer risk: a case-control study from Opole, Poland. *Int J Caner.* 1993;67:601–607.
18. Ghadirian P, Simard A, Baillargeon J. Tobacco, alcohol, and coffee and cancer of the pancreas: a population-based, case-control study in Quebec, Canada. *Cancer.* 1991;67:2664–2670.
19. Howe GR, Jain M, Burch JD, Miller AB. Cigarette smoking and cancer of the pancreas: evidence from a population-based case-control study in Toronto, Canada. *Int J Cancer.* 1991;47:323–328.
20. Silverman DT, Dunn JA, Hoover RN, et al. Cigarette smoking and pancreas cancer: a case-control study based on direct interviews. *J Natl Cancer Inst.* 1994;86:1510–1516.
21. Fuchs CS, Colditz GA, Stampfer MJ, et al. A prospective study of cigarette smoking and the risk of pancreatic cancer. *Arch Intern Med.* 1996;156:2255–2260.
22. Willett W, Green A, Stampfer M, et al. Relative and absolute excess risks of coronary heart disease among women who smoke cigarettes. *N Engl J Med.* 1987;317:1303–1309.
23. Rimm E, Giovannucci E, Willett W, et al. Prospective study of alcohol consumption and risk of coronary disease in men. *Lancet.* 1991;338:464–468.
24. Silverman D. Risk factors for pancreatic cancer: a case-control study based on direct interviews. *Teratog Carcinog Mutagen.* 2001;21:7–25.
25. Duell EJ, Holly EA, Bracci PM, et al. A population-based, case-control study of polymorphisms in carcinogen-metabolizing genes, smoking, and pancreatic adenocarcinoma risk. *J Natl Cancer Inst.* 2002;94:297–306.
26. Duell EJ, Holly EA, Bracci PM, et al. A population-based study of the *Arg399Gln* polymorphism in x-ray repair cross-complementing group 1 (*XRCC1*) and risk of pancreatic adenocarcinoma. *Cancer Res.* 2002;62:4630–4636.
27. Masson M, Niedergant C, Schreiber V, et al. *XRCC1* is specifically associated with poly (ADP-ribose) polymerase and negatively regulates its activity following DNA damage. *Mol Cell Biol.* 1998;18:3563–3571.
28. Callebaut I, Mornon J-P. From *BRCA1* to *RAP1:* a wide-spread *BRCT* module closely associated with DNA repair. *FEBS Lett.* 1997;400:25–30.
29. Anderson KE, Johnson TW, Lazovich D, Folsom AR. Association between nonsteroidal anti-inflammatory drug use and the incidence of pancreatic cancer. *J Natl Cancer Inst.* 2002;94:1168–1171.
30. Schernhammer E, Kang J-H, Chan AT, et al. A prospective study of aspirin use and risk of pancreatic cancer in women. *J Natl Cancer Inst.* 2004;96:22–28.
31. Menezes RJ, Huber KR, Mahoney MC, Moysich KB. Regular use of aspirin and pancreatic cancer risk. *BMC Public Health.* 2002;2:18–23.
32. Baron JA. What now for aspirin and cancer prevention? *J Natl Cancer Inst.* 2004;96:4–5.
33. Ye W, Lagergren J, Weiderpass E, Nyren O, Adami H, Ekbom A. Alcohol abuse and the risk of pancreatic cancer. *Gut.* 2002;51:236–239.
34. Everhart J, Wright D. Diabetes mellitus as a risk factor for pancreatic cancer: a meta-analysis. *JAMA.* 1995;273:1605–1609.
35. Freidman G, van den Eeden SK. Risk factors for pancreatic cancer: an exploratory study. *Int J Epidemiol.* 1993;22:30–37.
36. Ji BT, Hatch MC, Chow WH, et al. Anthropometric and reproductive factors and risk of pancreatic cancer. *Int J Cancer.* 1996;66:432–437.
37. Hanley AJG, Johnson KC, Villeneuve PJ, et al. Physical activity, anthropometric and risk of pancreatic cancer: results from the Canadian enhanced cancer surveillance system. *Int J Cancer.* 2001;94:140–147.
38. Silverman DR, Swanson CA, Gridley G, et al. Dietary and nutritional factors and pancreatic cancer: a case-control study based on direct interviews. *J Natl Cancer Inst.* 1998;90:1710–1719.
39. Moller H, Mellemgaard A, Kingvig K, Olsen JH. Obesity and cancer risk: a Danish record linkage study. *Eur J Cancer.* 1994;30A:344–350.
40. Gapstur SM, Gann PH, Lowe W, et al. Abnormal glucose metabolism and pancreatic cancer mortality. *JAMA.* 2000;283:2552–2558.
41. Lee IM, Sesso HD, Oguma Y, Paffenbarger RS. Physical activity, body weight, and pancreatic cancer mortality. *Br J Cancer.* 2003;88:679–683.
42. Anderson KE, Sinha R, Kulldorff M, et al. Meat intake and cooking techniques: associations with pancreatic cancer. *Mutat Res.* 2002;506–507:225–231.
43. Zheng W, McLaughlin JK, Gridley F, et al. A cohort study of smoking, alcohol consumption and dietary factors of pancreatic cancer (United States). *Cancer Causes Control.* 1993;4:477–482.
44. Stolzenberg-Solomon RZ, Pietinen P, Taylor PR, et al. Prospective study on diet and pancreatic cancer in male smokers. *Am J Epidemiol.* 2002;155:783–792.
45. Tukey RH, Strassburg CP. Human UDP-glucuronosyltransferases: metabolism, expression, and disease. *Annu Rev Pharmacol Toxicol.* 2000;40:581–616.
46. Strassburg CP, Strassburg A, Kneip S, et al. Developmental aspects of human hepatic drug glucuronidation in young children and adults. *Gut.* 2002:50:259–265.
47. Strassburg CP, Barut A, Obermayer-Straub P, et al. Identification of cyclosporine A and tacrolimus glucuronidation in human liver and the extrahepatic gastrointestinal tract by a differentially expressed UDP-glucuronosyltransferase: *UGT2B7. J Hepatol.* 2001:34:865–872.
48. Tukey RH, Strassburg CP. Genetic multiplicity of the human UDP-glucuronosyltransferase and regulation in the gastrointestinal tract. *Mol Pharmacol.* 2001;59:405–414.

49. Nowell SA, Massengill JS, Williams S, et al. Glucuronidation of 2-hydroxyamino-1-methyl-6-phenylimidazo[4,5-b]pyridine by human microsomal UDP-glucuronosyltransferases: identification of specific *UGT1A* family isoforms involved. *Carcinogenesis.* 1999;20:1107–1114.
50. Zheng Z, Park JY, Guillemette C, et al. Tobacco carcinogen-detoxifying enzyme UGT1A7 and its association with orolaryngeal cancer risk. *J Natl Cancer Inst.* 2001;93:1411–1418.
51. Strassburg CP, Strassburg A, Nguyen N, et al. Regulation and function of family 1 and family 2 UDP-glucuronosyltransferase genes (UGT1A, UGT2B) in human oesophagus. *Biochem J.* 1999;338:489–498.
52. Strassburg CP, Nguyen N, Manns MP, Tukey RH. Polymorphic expression of the UDP-glucuronosyltransferase *UGT1A* gene locus in human gastric epithelium. *Mol Parmacol.* 1998;54:647–654.
53. Ockenga J, Vogel A, Teich N, et al. UDP glucuronosyltransferase *(UGT1A7)* gene polymorphisms increase the risk of chronic pancreatitis and pancreatic cancer. *Gastroenterology.* 2003;124:1802–1808.
54. Strassburg CP, Nguyen N, Manns MP, Tukey RH. UDP-glucuronosyltransferase activity in human liver and colon. *Gastroenterology.* 1999;116:149–160.
55. Guillemette C, Ritter JK, Auyeung DJ, et al. Structural heterogeneity at the UDP-glucuronosyltransferase 1 locus: functional consequences of three novel missense mutations in the human *UGT1A7* gene. *Pharmacogenetics.* 2000; 10:629–644.
56. Vogel A, Kneip S, Barut S, et al. Genetic link of hepatocellular carcinoma with polymorphisms of the UDP-glucuronosyltransferase *UGT1A7* gene. *Gastroenterology.* 2001;121:1136–1144.
57. Strassburg CP, Vogel A, Kneip S, et al. Polymorphisms of the UDP-glucuronosyltransferase *(UGT)1A7* gene in colorectal cancer. *Gut.* 2002;50:851–856.
58. Hoppin JA, Tolbert PE, Holly EA, et al. Pancreatic cancer and serum organochlorine levels. *Cancer Epidemiol Biomark Prev.* 2000;9:199–205.
59. Fryzek JP, Garabrant DH, Harlow SD, et al. A case control study of self-reported exposures to pesticides and pancreas cancer in southeastern Michigan. *Int J Cancer.* 1997;72:62–67.
60. Porta M, Malats N, Jariod M, et al. Serum concentrations of organochlorine compounds and *K-ras* mutations in exocrine pancreatic cancer. *Lancet.* 1999;354:2125–2129.
61. Garabrant DH, Held J, Langholz B, Peters JM, Mack TM. DDT and related compounds and risk of pancreatic cancer. *J Natl Cancer Inst.* 1992;84:764–771.
62. Jin YH, Clark AB, Slebos RJ, et al. Cadmium is a mutagen that acts by inhibiting mismatch repair. *Nature Genet.* 2003; 34:326–329.
63. McMurray CT, Tainer JA. Cancer, cadmium and genome integrity. *Nature Genet.* 2003;34:239–241.
64. Waalkes MP. Cadmium carcinogenesis. *Mutat Res.* 2003; 533:107–120.
65. Schwartz GG, Reis IM. Is cadmium a cause of human pancreatic cancer? *Cancer Epidemiol Biomarkers Prev.* 2000;9: 139–145.
66. Steinbach G, Lynch PM, Phillips RKS, et al. *N Engl J Med.* 2000;342:1946–1952.
67. Schneider MB, Matsuzaki H, Haorah J, et al. Prevention of pancreatic cancer induction in hamsters by metformin. *Gastroenterology.* 2001;120:1263–1270.
68. Wolf RA. Chemoprevention for pancreatic cancer. *Int J Gastrointestinal Cancer.* 2003;33:27–42.

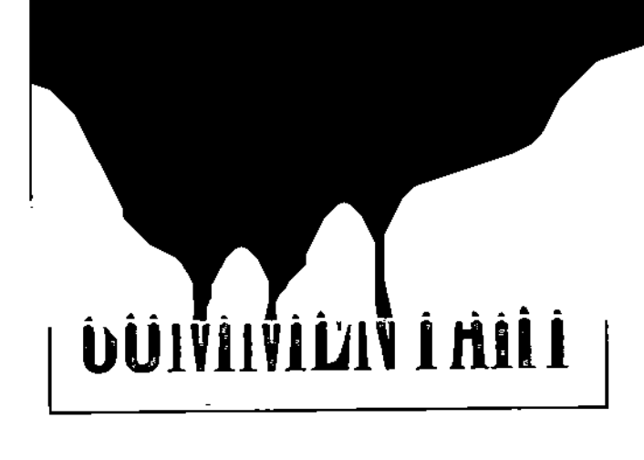

Diane M. Simeone, MD

Chapter 10 (on prevention of pancreatic cancer), which is nicely written by Dr. Frazier, provides a thorough review of what are the currently known risks factors for pancreatic cancer, as well as data regarding the use of chemoprevention agents in the treatment of pancreatic cancer. As can be surmised from the chapter, there remains a large gap in our knowledge regarding risks factors for pancreatic cancer, as the majority of patients have sporadic disease without a readily identifiable causative factor. Although we have identified a number of single genetic mutations that put individuals at high risk, such individuals account for less than 10% of all patients with pancreatic cancer. As Dr. Frazier pointed out, it is likely that environmental and minor genetic factors play an important role in the pathogenesis of this disease. However, the prevalence of pancreatic cancer in the population at large makes mass screening and chemoprevention trials cost prohibitive because of the large number of people that would be required for study. Based on these issues, it is imperative that we identify high-risk populations for further study.

Identification of the genetic and environmental factors that contribute to the development of pancreatic cancer is going to be essential for a decrease in the incidence of this disease. How can we approach such a daunting problem? Recent advances in the scientific arena suggest that the tools to tackle this problem may soon be at hand. The sequencing of the human genome and increasing information about the genome's function provide a robust foundation for the investigation of diseases such as pancreatic cancer.[1] In addition, results from the International HapMap Project[2] will provide powerful information to researchers regarding variations in human gene expression that may account for human disease. This information, in combination with innovations in cost-effective, high-throughput screening, will increase our ability to identify genetic factors important in the development of pancreatic cancer in large population samples.

A key component of these analyses will be the availability of large-scale cohort genetic studies—databases of individuals with detailed health histories along with repositories of matching DNA samples. Several large-scale cohort studies are already underway in a number of countries, including Iceland (deCODE), the United Kingdom (UK Biobank), Canada (CARTaGENE), Germany, and Japan.[3] A recent report by Frances Collins makes a strong case for the establishment of a United States prospective cohort study for the study of genes and environment.[1] Along with genetic analyses, advanced analytical methods for measuring environmental factors and nongenetic factors that contribute to disease have evolved. The development of these advanced methods will likely provide insight into the complex interplay between environmental and genetic factors in pancreatic cancer development. The goal will be to identify individuals at risk before disease has developed and to provide an opportunity for environmental modification (i.e., cessation of smoking), early preventative therapy, and targeted screening.

Another effective approach to define the numerous genes that have small but cumulative effects in disease is to first map them in mice and subsequently to study the role of their homologues in humans. This approach takes advantage of the fact that inbred strains of mice differ widely in susceptibility to different types of tumors and provides the parental strains for the crosses that are needed to map tumor-susceptibility genes through segregation analysis. Such an approach has been successful in identifying more than 100 cancer susceptibility loci in the mouse.[4] Together, these approaches may provide important insight into pathways of tumor development and may lead to more effective cancer prevention strategies.

Our broadening knowledge of the molecular aspects of pancreatic cancer has opened new avenues and targets for prevention trials. Alterations in several signal transduction pathways, including the epidermal growth factor, notch, and hedgehog signaling pathways, have been found to be critical in the early phases of pancreatic cancer development.[5] Efforts to develop small inhibitory molecules to target these pathways and validate their potential utility in in vivo mouse models may serve as an effective approach to develop new chemoprevention strategies.

The link between diet and cancer is well established, and new genomic technologies have made possible the investigation of nutritional modification of the carcinogenesis pathway with nutrients, micronutrients, and phytochemicals.[6] Current studies on the effects of nutrients on DNA damage and repair mechanisms, DNA methylation, responses to oxidant stress, and effects of target receptors and signaling pathways will likely provide new information on nutrient gene interactions and provide a framework for a contemporary paradigm for dietary intervention. With the identification of the PanIn (pancreatic intraephithelial neoplasia) lesions as preneoplastic lesions that develop into invasive pancreatic cancer,[7] we may be able to shift our target for chemoprevention to the intraepithelial stage of pancreatic tumorigenesis.

Over the last year, several mouse models that incorporate the genetic events and faithfully recapitulate the histologic and pathologic features of invasive pancreatic ductal adenocarcinoma have been developed (reviewed in Leach[8]). Hingorani and colleagues[9] reported that mice expressing Pdx-Cre–activated K-ras generated preneoplastic lesions (PanIn lesions) in the pancreas. Histologic review of these tumors could not distinguish them from human pancreatic adenocarcinoma;

however, they had a low incidence of metastatic disease. A subsequent report demonstrated an accelerated formation of PanIn lesions with rapid tumor progression and metastasis when PDx-Cre–activated K-ras mice were crossed with mice expressing a pancreas-specific Ink4a/ARF deficiency.[10] These models, along with others,[11,12] are likely to have a major impact on the development of strategies for early detection and chemoprevention. Although we do need to be cautious in interpreting data derived from mouse models to the human condition, they nevertheless do represent an important tool in gaining a deeper insight into the biology of pancreatic cancer.

Finally, new profiling technologies are being used to identify novel early detection biomarkers for pancreatic cancer. Microarrays can profile gene expression patterns containing tens of thousands of genes in a single experiment, thus permitting systematic analysis of DNA and RNA variations in biological samples from cancer and noncancer patients. In a similar way, proteomic analyses enable researchers to identify all of the proteins expressed in a cell or organ and detect changes in the protein expression pattern. These technologies are now being used by a number of laboratories and are also beginning to be applied clinically for use in early disease detection.

In summary, research efforts directed at identifying and quantifying risk factors as well as identifying individuals at high risk for pancreatic cancer development are critical to ultimately developing methods to prevent this disease. Recent advances in the understanding of the human genome, profiling technology, and development of mouse models of pancreatic cancer that accurately mimic human disease all provide a great deal of promise that significant strides in the field of prevention for this deadly disease will be made within the next decade.

References

1. Collins FS. The case for a US prospective cohort study of genes and environment. *Nature*. 2004;429:475–477.
2. The International HapMap Consortium. The International HapMap project. *Nature*. 2003;426:789–798.
3. Hagan H-E, Carlsted-Duke J. Building global networks for human disease: genes and populations. *Nat Med*. 2004;10:665–667.
4. Demant P. Cancer susceptibility in the mouse: genetics, biology and implications for human cancer. *Nat Rev Genet*. 2003;4:721–734.
5. Li D, Xie K, Wolff R, Abbruzzese JL. Pancreatic cancer. *Lancet*. 2004;363:1049–1057.
6. Go VL, Butrum RR, Wong DA. Diet, nutrition, and cancer prevention: the postgenomic era. *J Nutr*. 2003;133:3830S–3836S.
7. Hruban RH, Adsay NV, Albores-Saavedra J, et al. Pancreatic intraepithelial neoplasia: a new nomenclature and classification system for pancreatic duct lesions. *Am J Surg Pathol*. 2001;25:579–586.
8. Leach SD. Mouse models of pancreatic cancer: the fur is finally flying! *Cancer Cell*. 2004;5:7–11.
9. Hingorani SR, Petricoin EF, Maitra A, et al. Preinvasive and invasive ductal pancreatic cancer and its early detection in the mouse. *Cancer Cell*. 2003;4:437–450.
10. Aguirre AJ, Bardeesy N, Sinha M, et al. Activated Kras and Ink4a/Arf deficiency cooperate to produce metastatic pancreatic ductal adenocarcinoma. *Genes Dev*. 2003;17:3112–3126.
11. Lewis BC, Klimstra DS, Varmus HE. The c-myc and PyMT oncogenes induce different tumor types in a somatic mouse model for pancreatic cancer. *Genes Dev*. 2003;17:3127–3138.
12. Thayer SP, Di Magliano MP, Heiser PW, et al. Hedgehog is an early and late mediator of pancreatic cancer tumorigenesis. *Nature*. 2003;425:851–856.

CHAPTER 11

Pancreatic Cancer: Clinical Presentation

Vincent J. Picozzi, Jr., MD

Pancreatic cancer currently afflicts as many as 200,000 patients each year on a worldwide basis.[1] In the United States, pancreatic cancer is the ninth most common cancer, with an annual incidence of approximately 32,000 cases.[2] This equates to a lifetime risk for the development of pancreatic cancer in this country of approximately 1 in 130. Pancreatic cancer also has the poorest survival statistics of any major cancer in the United States, with a mortality/incidence ratio of 0.99.[3] Pancreatic cancer thus accounts for almost 5% of cancer deaths in the United States, making it the fourth leading cause of cancer mortality in the country. Surgery is generally regarded as being essential to curative therapy of pancreatic cancer, yet less than 15% of patients in the United States are considered surgical candidates at clinical presentation.[4] Unfortunately, pancreatic cancer represents a disease in our society that is both fairly common and highly lethal.

Despite its frequency and lethality, the diagnosis of pancreatic cancer can often prove difficult. Prevention and screening strategies for pancreatic cancer are still under evolution.[5] Presenting signs, symptoms, and laboratory values can be nonspecific, vague, absent, or normal. Nonetheless, a diagnostic delay in pancreatic cancer has been shown to relate directly to disease stage[6] and ultimately prognosis.[7] It is therefore imperative that the clinicians who are responsible for patients with pancreatic cancer both establish diagnosis and initiate therapy with optimum speed and accuracy. To do so requires a high "suspicion index" for the disease and a detailed understanding of its clinical presentation.

This chapter focuses on the clinical presentation of patients with pancreatic cancer. For greater understanding of other topics relevant to its diagnosis and initial evaluation (e.g., radiographic imaging and endoscopic evaluation), the reader is referred to other chapters of this book.

Epidemiology and Past Medical History

In reviewing the medical records of a patient with a potential diagnosis of pancreatic cancer, the astute clinician should bear several important epidemiologic facts in mind (Table 11.1). The first among these is the relationship of pancreatic cancer and patient age. Age is a very important risk factor for the development of pancreatic cancer.[2,5,8] Pancreatic cancer is rare among patients under 40 years of age, but 80% of patients present with this disease during the seventh and eighth decades of life. Demographic

Table 11.1 Epidemiology of Pancreatic Cancer for the Clinician

Risk Factor	Comment
Age	80% of patients diagnosed in seventh or eighth decade of life 1% of patients diagnosed under age 40
Diabetes mellitus	2× relative risk diabetic onset more than 3 years before diagnosis 3× relative risk diabetic onset less than 2 years before diagnosis Think particularly of pancreatic cancer diagnosis if new onset diabetes seen in a patient of "at-risk" age and with other clinical features of pancreas cancer (e.g., abdominal pain)
Abdominal surgery	2–5× the relative risk Both gastrectomy and cholecystectomy implicated
Pancreatitis	2–26× the relative risk The risk declines with time
Cigarette smoking	1.5× the relative risk if less than one-half a pack/day of cigarettes 10× the relative risk if more than two packs/day of cigarettes Risk declines (but not to baseline) over 10 years after smoking cessation
Family history	3× the relative risk with one first-degree relative with pancreatic cancer The risk increases as number of first-degree relatives increases

features of gender (more common in women than men) and race (slightly more common in African Americans and slightly less common in Asian Americans than whites) are usually not of practical assistance in diagnosis. Likewise, reports of pancreatic cancer as being more common among urban populations and in higher socioeconomic groups do not influence clinical decision making.[8]

With respect to a patient's past medical history, however, the presence of diabetes mellitus can be of major importance. Clinicians have long wondered whether diabetes was the cause or result of pancreatic cancer and about whatever concomitant pathophysiology existed. Analysis of this question has been made more difficult over time by varying definitions of diabetes and by poor characterization of the diabetic state in pancreatic cancer patients.

To attempt to address this, Gullo and colleagues[9] analyzed in detail the relationship between diabetes (using contemporary American Diabetes Association definitions) and pancreatic cancer. A comparison of 720 patients with pancreatic cancer and 720 control patients provided the following key observations: (1) Diabetes was present in 22.8% of patients with pancreatic cancer versus only 6.8% of control subjects (odds ratio, 3.0; 95% confidence interval, 2.2–4.2). (2) In the majority of patients with pancreatic cancer (56%), diabetes was diagnosed either concomitantly with the cancer (40%) or within 2 years before the diagnosis of cancer (16%). (3) The association between diabetes and pancreatic cancer, however, diminished with increasing time of diabetic onset to time of cancer diagnosis. When patients with diabetes of only 3 or more years were considered, the association became less significant (odds ratio, 1.4; 95% confidence interval, 1.0–2.1). The authors thus concluded that diabetes in patients with pancreas cancer is typically of recent onset and is presumably caused by the tumor. Diabetes itself was not considered a risk factor for pancreatic cancer.

Other authors, however, have found a stronger longitudinal association between diabetes and pancreatic cancer. Everhart and Wright[10] performed a meta-analysis of case control and cohort studies analyzing the relationship between diabetes mellitus and pancreatic cancer. A total of 20 studies that met two inclusion criteria (diagnosis of diabetes at least 1 year before pancreatic cancer diagnosis and/or death and the ability to calculate an appropriate relative risk estimate and variance) were included. The pooled results yield a relative risk of 2.1 (95% confidence interval, 1.6–2.8) for the association; patients with diabetes for more than 5 years resulted in a relative risk of 2.0 (95% confidence interval, 1.2–3.2). The authors concluded that pancreatic cancer occurs with increased frequency among persons with long-standing diabetes. In summary, both remote- and recent-onset diabetes are important risk factors for the development of pancreatic cancer, although the association seems particularly strong for the latter.

Permert et al.[11] have studied the pathophysiology of diabetes in pancreatic cancer in detail. High plasma levels of insulin and a state of pronounced insulin resistance characterize diabetes associated with pancreatic cancer. The insulin resistance seen in pancreatic cancer is associated with high levels of islet cell hormones in both fasting and hyperglycemic states, such as C-reactive peptide, islet amyloid polypeptide, glucagon, and somatostatin. Because not all islet cell hormones were found to be elevated, the elevations seen seemed to be due to a selective hypersecretion rather than a generalized hyperactivity of islet cells. This, in turn, might be due either to local influence of the tumor on islet cells or by secretion by islet cells in the tumor itself. A remote effect of the tumor that results in impaired glucose metabolism is also possible. Insulin sensitivity improves markedly after subtotal pancreatectomy, adding further weight to these hypotheses.

Two other conditions in a patient's past medical history are of particular importance in consideration of a potential diagnosis of pancreatic cancer. The first is a prior history of pancreatitis. Chronic pancreatitis is frequently associated with the development of pancreatic cancer. Relative risks as high as 26-fold have been found in some studies,[12] whereas other studies have found a more modest association.[13] Acute pancreatitis, particularly that which is unexplained by known etiologic factors, has been associated in up to 3% of cases with the development of pancreatic cancer.[14] The prevalence of pancreatitis with pancreatic cancer may also explain in part why cytologic diagnosis of this condition can be difficult.

The second important condition in the patient's past medical history is that of previous upper gastrointestinal surgery. Such patients typically have a 2-fold to 5-fold increased risk of pancreatic cancer. This risk typically manifests itself many years after surgery and is frequently seen in association with peptic ulcer disease.[15] Cholecystectomy has also been implicated as a potential risk.[16] Excessive gastrointestinal hormone secretion (gastrin, cholecystokinin) and decreased gastric digestion of carcinogens (nitrates) have been implicated as factors in the relationship.

The most important social/environmental factor associated with pancreatic cancer is tobacco smoking. Smoking can be implicated as a cause of pancreatic cancer in roughly 30% of cases. The relative risk of cigarette smoking depends on the number of cigarettes smoked, ranging from 1.5 in less than one-half pack per day smokers to 10 in people who smoke two or more packs of cigarettes per day. The risk does decrease with time (but does not reach baseline levels) when smoking ceases.[17] The risk of cigarette smoking is thought to relate to the release of nitrosamines as carcinogens.

Finally, a family history of pancreatic cancer is important in identifying risk. Up to 10% of patients diagnosed with pancreatic cancer will report the disease in a first-degree relative;[18] families with two or more first-degree relatives with pancreatic cancer have relative risks of 18-fold and higher.[19] A Canadian epidemiologic study assessed the lifetime risk of pancreatic cancer at approximately 1 in 25 for first-degree relatives of pancreatic cancer probands.[20] Pancreatic cancers have also been associated with a variety of other cancers, including ovarian and breast cancers and malignant melanoma.

Symptoms

At clinical presentation, pancreatic cancer is generally associated with the classic symptom triad of abdominal pain, weight loss, and jaundice. These symptoms are typically reported in clinical reviews of this subject to occur with very high (0%–90%) frequency.[21,22] Abdominal pain is often considered the most common of presenting symptoms of pancreatic cancer.[23] The pain is often insidious in onset and is gradually progressive over time, sometimes for many months. Although classically epigastric in location, the abdominal pain of pancreatic cancer may involve any of the abdominal quadrants.[24] It may also radiate to the sides or back. It is typically described as a gnawing or pressure sensation and may be described as worse in the supine position, with food, or at night. The progressive nature of this pain over time is often what first motivates a patient with pancreatic cancer to seek medical attention.

The pain associated with pancreatic cancer can have various causes. It may result from mechanical compression of proximate anatomic structures (e.g., the duodenum); this may explain why the pain of pancreatic cancer is sometimes positional in nature. Pain may also occur as a result of neural or neural sheath invasion.[24] Back pain represents a particular example of this pain mechanism, caused by splanchnic nerve and/or celiac invasion.[25] Postprandial pain exacerbation may arise from an increase in secretory ductal pressure caused by ductal compression or invasion.

Weight loss is often the symptom present for the greatest duration in pancreatic cancer patients.[26] Although common in all cancer patients, weight loss is particularly common in patients with this disorder. The weight loss associated with pancreatic cancer also is multifactorial. Decreased caloric intake, nausea and vomiting, and an increase in resting energy expenditure all play a role. However, pancreatic exocrine insufficiency caused by ductal obstruction is also often present, producing malabsorption. Fat malabsorption is typically more severe than protein malabsorption. The malabsorption associated with pancreatic cancer may be the most significant factor in the generation of weight loss in afflicted patients.

Jaundice is the final classic symptom of pancreatic cancer. Jaundice is most commonly seen because of direct compression of the distal common bile duct in the pancreatic head leading to extrahepatic biliary obstruction. Jaundice may also occur because of extensive liver metastases. The jaundice of pancreatic cancer is usually progressive in nature, unless biliary obstruction is anatomically corrected.

Table 11.2 Less Common Symptoms of Pancreatic Cancer
Anorexia
Back pain
Depression
Diarrhea or other change in bowel habits
Dyspepsia
Early satiety
Fever
Gastrointestinal bleeding
Intolerance to foods, wine, and tobacco
Malaise
Nausea/vomiting
New-onset diabetes mellitus
Pruritus
Pyrosis
Skin rash/changes
Sleep disorder
Thrombophlebitis

Although the cardinal symptoms of abdominal pain, weight loss, and jaundice are commonly thought of as nearly ubiquitous in pancreatic cancer patients, it is important to note that these symptoms often occur relatively late (or not at all) in the course of clinical evolution. A report from Nix et al.[27] from the Netherlands illustrates this point. Analyzing a series of 123 patients with carcinoma of the pancreatic head who underwent endoscopic retrograde cholangiopancreatography, Nix et al.[27] found the frequencies of abdominal pain, weight loss, and jaundice to be 71%, 80%, and 89%, respectively. However, their frequencies as initial symptoms were only 20%, 59%, and 4%, respectively.

The frequency of these cardinal symptoms (and other symptoms associated with pancreatic cancer) also vary based on patterns of care and type of practice. For example, the experience cited previously is in significant contrast to those from an Italian hospital[28] and from a university-affiliated regional oncology referral practice in the upper Midwestern United States.[29] In the former study, which consisted of 1,020 consecutive patients admitted because of a clinical suspicion of pancreatic cancer, the frequencies of the previously mentioned cardinal symptoms were all substantially less. In the latter study, performed retrospectively on 308 patients with a biopsy-proven diagnosis of pancreatic cancer that had already been established, abdominal pain and jaundice were much more common as initial symptoms (51% and 20%, respectively), weight loss much less so (7%).

Numerous other symptoms are seen in conjunction with pancreatic cancer (Table 11.2). Anorexia, back pain, diarrhea or other change in bowel habits, fever, malaise, sleep disorders, anorexia, pruritus, pyrosis, dyspepsia, dysgeusias (e.g., coffee), early satiety, nausea/vomiting, new-onset diabetes mellitus, unexplained acute pancreatitis, symptoms of gastrointestinal bleeding, skin rash or other skin changes, sleep disorders, thrombophlebitis, and depression are all symptoms mentioned at presentation in various clinical reviews. The plethora of symptoms associated with pancreatic cancer, many that are nonspecific in character, makes its detection based on clinical history even more difficult.

Physical Examination

The physical examination of patients with pancreatic cancer generally produces few useful clues. Significant physical findings beyond epigastric discomfort to deep palpation or jaundice (when present) usually represent manifestations of metastatic disease. The classic sign of a palpable gallbladder (Courvoisier's sign) is present in less than one third of patients.[21] Also uncommon are the presence of abdominal mass or periumbilical nodule (Sister Mary Joseph nodule), ascites, or other sites of adenopathy. Perhaps the most common physical finding is that of an enlarged liver, although this is nonspecific and is present in less than one half of patients.

Laboratory features of pancreatic cancer are also nonspecific at presentation. Anemia that is multifactorial in nature (chronic disease, blood loss, liver disease, and vitamin malabsorption) occurs in 25%–40% of patients. Routine laboratory tests are typically normal except for those associated with obstructive jaundice (e.g., alkaline phosphatase and conjugated bilirubin) or liver metastases (e.g., alkaline phosphatase, aspartate aminotransterase [AST]). Hypoalbuminemia is also occasionally detected, particularly in patients with more advanced disease.

Serologic tests may also be available to the clinician at clinical presentation. Among these, the most extensively studied in pancreatic cancer is a glycoprotein known as cancer antigen 19-9 (CA 19-9). Although detectable in 70–90% of patients with pancreatic carcinoma, it is also elevated in 10%–20% of patients with benign pancreatic diseases (e.g., chronic pancreatitis) and 25%–60% of patients with other malignancies. Thus, given the incidence of pancreatic cancer in the population, neither the specificity nor the predictive value of CA 19-9 is significant enough to be of primary use in establishing a diagnosis of pancreatic cancer.[30] Also, the CA 19-9 tends to rise in concert with both tumor volume[31] and disease stage,[32] further diminishing its value in the detection of early stage disease. Carcinoembryonic antigen can also be elevated in pancreatic cancer patients. However, its sensitivity in this disease is even less than that of CA 19-9 (30%–40%) and is likewise elevated in many other benign and malignant conditions. As a result, the measurement of carcinoembryonic antigen is even less useful than that of CA 19-9 in establishing a diagnosis in this setting.

Three unusual presentations of pancreatic cancer deserve particular mention. The first is that of thrombophlebitis. Thrombophlebitis associated with pancreatic cancer bears similarity with other hypercoagulability syndromes (migratory or recurrent, occurs in unusual sites, resistant to anticoagulants, especially Coumadin). The mechanism is thought to relate to extravascular activation of procoagulant cascades and/or alteration of fibrinolysis by tumor cells.[33] Mesenteric, splenic, or portal venous thromboses are of particular importance in the management of pancreatic cancer. Thrombophlebitis tends to occur in patients with more histologically differentiated cancers. This is a relatively rare (5%–15% of total presentations) presentation of pancreatic cancer; however, it is nonspecific, and tends to occur more often in advanced disease.[34,35]

The second unusual presentation of pancreatic cancer is that of depression. Depression, anxiety, and a premonition of impending doom have been reported.[36] Emotional and personality changes are known to occur as a prodrome of the disease or at the time of clinical presentation. The primary diagnosis is that of depression, apparently independent of pain levels.[37] Although the exact prevalence of depression in pancreatic cancer is difficult to ascertain, rates as high as 75% have been cited in comparison to a 20%–30% rate seen in other cancers.[38] Holland et al.[39] conducted a controlled study to compare the prevalence of depression in 107 patients with advanced pancreatic cancer with that of another gastrointestinal cancer (gastric cancer, 111 patients). The authors concluded from an analysis of both medical and psychosocial data that patients with pancreatic cancer had significantly greater psychologic distress (both depression and anxiety) than did patients with gastric cancer. Possible mechanisms advanced for an altered affective state include a tumor-mediated paraneoplastic syndrome and antibody interference of serotonin binding in the brain. Furthermore, like diabetes, there is evidence that these symptoms will abate if the cancer is excised.[40]

Finally, pancreatic cancer can be associated with a variety of cutaneous manifestations. Acquired ichthyosis ("fish-scale"–like drying of the skin) and other changes in hair and nail growth can be seen in association with pancreatic malabsorption. Palmar erythema can be a sign of liver metastases. Coagulopathy can produce signs of bleeding (e.g., purpura) or signs of cutaneous ischemia (e.g., splinter hemorrhages). Erythroderm and dermatomyositis have been reported as cutaneous manifestations of pancreatic cancer.[41] Pemphigoid, both cicatricial and bullous varieties, can also occur as a paraneoplastic phenomenon.[42] Finally, subcutaneous fat necrosis, sometimes associated with arthralgias and fevers, can be seen in acinar cell carcinomas of the pancreas as well as other benign pancreatic diseases.[43]

Other rare presentations of pancreatic cancer tend to be associated with either local tumor growth (e.g., pseudoachalasia, splenic rupture, and bile peritonitis) or hypercoagulability (e.g., cerebrovascular accident).

Diagnostic Challenges

Even with a detailed understanding of the clinical presentation of pancreatic cancer, a variety of diagnostic challenges present themselves to the managing clinician. These include the following:

Q. How is pancreatic cancer distinguished from other abdominal disorders?

A. Symptoms, signs, and basic laboratory manifestations of pancreatic cancer are frequently subtle or nonspecific. Patients may delay many months before seeking medical attention for their symptoms and/or have alternative explanations for symptoms. Twenty-five percent of patients with pancreatic cancer may have symptoms for 6 months or more before a diagnosis is established; 15% may have sought initial medical advice 6 months or more before diagnosis.[44,45] One review[46] cited a 57% incidence in pancreatic cancer patients of other medical problems (including benign pancreatic disorders, nonneoplastic abdominal disorders, and other forms of cancer) to explain their symptoms. The sage clinician must develop a strategy to assist in distinguishing pancreatic cancer from other conditions.

The following points may be useful in developing such a strategy (Table 11.3). First, a high degree of clinical awareness for the diagnosis is frequently necessary for success. Second, it is important to remember the key epidemiologic risks for pancreatic cancer, especially age at presentation, recent diabetic onset, heavy tobacco use, and positive family history in first-degree relatives. Third, multiple significant features of pancreatic cancer (e.g.,

Table 11.3 Differentiation of Pancreatic Cancer from Other Intraabdominal Disorders

1. High "index of suspicion"
2. Awareness of key epidemiologic risks (e.g., age, family history, intensive smoking)
3. Multiple key clinical features (abdominal pain, weight loss, jaundice, new-onset diabetes, unexplained pancreatitis) prompt immediate search for pancreatic cancer
4. Early high-resolution imaging (e.g., endoscopic ultrasound, high-resolution computed tomography) useful
5. Repetitive serologic and radiographic testing useful

abdominal pain, weight loss, jaundice, new-onset diabetes, unexplained pancreatitis) should trigger concern for this disorder. In particular, any form of abdominal pain (remembering its variability in pancreatic cancer) in conjunction with weight loss and/or jaundice should prompt a thorough search for pancreatic cancer. These are the symptoms most frequently associated with pancreatic cancer and occur much less commonly in other disorders (e.g., acute and chronic pancreatitis.) Fourth, any suspicion of the diagnosis should lead to early pancreatic imaging, particularly using techniques capable of detecting small-volume tumors (e.g., endoscopic ultrasound, endoscopic retrograde cholangiopancreatography, triphasic, and high-resolution helical computed tomography scanning). Finally, serial or repetitive evaluations may be necessary to establish a diagnosis of pancreatic cancer. This is particularly important for patients who have persistent, unexplained, or recurring symptoms. Repetitive laboratory (e.g., tumor markers)[47] and/or radiographic evaluations (e.g., computed tomography scanning) may be particularly helpful.

Q. How does one suspect/diagnose pancreatic cancer at the earliest possible time?

A. A second major concern for clinicians is the diagnosis of pancreatic cancer in the timeliest fashion possible. Two approaches have been used to sharpen the diagnostic acumen of clinicians in this regard. The first is to review retrospectively the clinical characteristics of patients with small-volume pancreatic cancer who underwent successful surgical resection. Multiple clinical series, mostly from Japan,[48-50] have been constructed with this objective in mind. Key findings from such series include the following: (1) Patients with small-volume pancreatic cancer tend to have similar symptoms to those with larger pancreatic cancers, but the frequency of symptoms such as abdominal pain and weight loss tend to be less. Up to 40% of such patients may be asymptomatic. Others have found a high incidence of jaundice among such patients.[51] (2) Such patients are often diagnosed via the evaluation of other diseases (e.g., diabetes mellitus and peptic ulcer disease). (3) Despite the presence of small-volume primary lesions, patients frequently have greater than stage I disease. For example, in the series by Furukawa et al., 58% of patients had nodal involvement, and 45% of patients had evidence of retroperitoneal invasion.

The second strategy used has been to examine patient histories retrospectively to investigate whether symptoms exist before abdominal pain and/or jaundice developed that could suggest the presence of pancreatic cancer and favor earlier diagnosis. Gullo et al.[52] in Italy used this approach. In their retrospective analysis, 305 patients with biopsy-proven pancreatic cancer were compared with an equal number of age-, gender-, and social class-matched control subjects. Approximately 35% of pancreatic cancer patients were found to have symptoms before the development of abdominal pain and/or jaundice; 14% did so more than 6 months before the development of these symptoms. Among such patients, the most important clinical features were anorexia and/or early satiety (22% of total), pruritus (7% of total), new-onset diabetes in the 2 years preceding diagnosis (6% of total), a change in oral taste/disgust (e.g., coffee, meat) (6% of total), and mood changes (3% of total). The first three of these features were statistically significant from the control group at the 0.001 level.

Information from these two approaches suggests once again that the classic symptoms of pancreatic cancer occur relatively late in the natural history of the disease. Early diagnosis depends on meticulous attention to subtle symptoms or more often the fortuitous mechanical result of a small-volume tumor (e.g., jaundice). However, even small-volume tumors may be associated with pathologic features that suggest metastatic spread.

Q. What information regarding pancreatic cancer disease stage and prognosis can be gained from the clinical presentation?

A. The clinical presentation of a patient with pancreatic cancer can also provide important information concerning cancer site, stage, and prognosis. As heads of pancreas lesions tend to present with earlier stage and are more often operable than those of the body and tail,[7] this information is also relevant to patient prognosis. Bakkevold et al.[6] specifically studied this question in a retrospective review of 472 biopsy-proven Norwegian patients with pancreatic and ampullary cancers accrued between 1984 and 1987. Important conclusions from this study included the following: (1) The presenting symptom of jaundice was more common in patients with pancreatic ampullary and head locations than in those of the body and tail ($p < 0.00001$). (2) Abdominal pain, however, was a more common presenting complaint of body and tail cancers than those of the ampulla and head ($P = 0.0001$). (3) Acute pancreatitis was the presenting complaint in 19% of patients with ampullary cancers. Approximately one third of all presentations (5 of 16) in this series attributed to acute pancreatitis were associated with ampullary cancers as opposed to pancreatic cancers (an approximate fivefold relative risk). (4) Jaundice was also statistically associated with earlier cancer stage when identified as the presenting symptom (stage I vs non-stage I) ($p < 0.0001$); conversely, abdominal pain and weight loss as presenting complaints were associated with more advanced stage ($P = 0.0001$ and $P = 0.004$, respectively). (5) The authors also found cancer stage to be related to diagnostic delay, defined as the time from symptom onset to first medical consultation (patient delay) plus the time from first medical consultation to diagnosis (physician delay). Stage I cancers had a mean diagnostic delay of 92 days versus a mean diagnostic delay of 118 days for stages II–IV ($P = 0.01$). The authors thus concluded that clinical presentation is useful in assessing cancer site, stage, and ultimately prognosis for pancreatic cancer patients.

Other authors have made observations relevant to this question. Kalser et al.[7] reviewed 393 patients with histologically proven pancreatic cancer accrued to Gastrointestinal Tumor Study Group trials between 1974 and 1978. As in the Bakkevold study, jaundice was more commonly associated with head of pancreas cancer and with resectable disease. Pain was more commonly associated with body and tail of pancreatic cancers and with unresectable disease, a finding confirmed by others.[53] Also, performance status (Eastern Cooperative Oncology Group 0 or 1) was statistically correlated with improved survival at the $P < 0.05$ level for all disease stages.

Symptoms are useful in predicting outcome even in advanced disease. Krech and Walsh[54] analyzed symptomatology in 39 patients with unresectable pancreatic cancer presenting to a palliative care service. Performance status once again was correlated with survival; performance status groups of 0, 1–2, and 3–4 had median survivorship of 7, 5, and 3 months, respectively. Among the most common symptoms seen were pain (82%), anorexia (64%), xerostomia (54%), and weight loss (51%), all symptoms of shortened survival time in previous hospice-based studies.[55] Another such symptom, dyspnea, was also found in 24% of patients and was similarly associated with shortened survival. Dyspnea was a particularly interesting symptom when it occurred; it did not seem to be associated with anemia, obstructive lung disease, pleural effusions or ascites, or venous thromboembolism. Finally, survival seemed to be inversely correlated with the number of the aforementioned symptoms present in a particular patient.

Table 11.4 Classification of Pancreatic Neoplasms for the Clinician

I. Ductal pancreatic cancer (65%)
II. Other periampullary cancers (25%)
1. Duodenal
2. Ampullary
3. Distal common bile duct
III. Other pancreatic exocrine cancers (5%)
1. Mucinous cystadenocarcinomas
2. Acinar-cell carcinomas
3. Undifferentiated cancers
4. Small-cell cancer
IV. Pancreatic neuroendocrine cancers (5%)
1. Islet cell cancers
2. Carcinoids
V. Other forms of cancer (<1%)
1. Lymphomas
2. Sarcomas

Q. How does one distinguish pancreatic cancer from other forms of cancer arising in the pancreas?

A. It is important to remember that not all cancers arising in or around the pancreas are ductal adenocarcinomas of ductal exocrine origin (Table 11.4). Approximately 70% of patients on whom pancreaticobiliary cancers are performed will have cancers arising from the exocrine pancreas itself; 90%–95% of these will be typical ductal adenocarcinomas.[51] Other forms of neoplasm seen in this site include: (1) other types of periampullary cancers (duodenal, ampullary, or distal common bile duct), (2) other forms of pancreatic cancer arising from the exocrine pancreas (mucinous cystadenocarcinomas, acinar cell cancers, undifferentiated cancers, small-cell cancer), (3) neuroendocrine tumors of the pancreas (islet cell cancers and carcinoid tumors), and (4) lymphomas and sarcomas. Although these tumors have overlapping clinical features with pancreatic cancers, specific clinical findings may suggest one diagnosis over the other.

Among periampullary cancers, duodenal cancers are most apt to present with symptoms of gastric outlet obstruction; they may also be associated with obstructive jaundice if the periampullary region is involved or with guaiac-positive stools. Ampullary cancers also tend to present with symptoms or signs of gastrointestinal bleeding as well as biliary obstruction; these symptoms can be intermittent because of spontaneous tumor necrosis and cell sloughing. Cancers of the distal common bile duct present with jaundice up to 90% of the time; other symptoms typically associated with pancreatic cancer are comparatively infrequent, occurring in only approximately one-third of the cases.[56] As different treatment strategies and prognoses may evolve for these conditions, it is important to distinguish among the various forms of periampullary cancer as best as possible, although this sometimes proves difficult in practice.

With respect to rarer forms of pancreatic exocrine cancer, mucinous cystadenocarcinomas tend to occur in younger patients (median age of approximately 50 years), preferentially involve the body and tail of the pancreas, and produce symptoms typical of this location (e.g., abdominal pain).[57] Kitagawa et al.[58] further characterized clinical presentation of mucinous cystadenocarcinomas in 28 patients. Patients frequently had a long symptom prodrome (a median of 15 months). Abdominal pain (83%), jaundice (43%), a history of pancreatitis (43%), liver function test elevation (57%), and CA 19.9 elevation (75%) were relatively frequent findings; weight loss (36%) was relatively uncommon. Acinar cell cancers tend to be relatively asymptomatic. They often present as an abdominal mass. As previously mentioned, acinar carcinomas can also present with subcutaneous fat necrosis (panniculitis) often in association with arthralgias, eosinophilia, and high levels of serum lipase secreted by the tumor.[59] Undifferentiated cancers of the pancreas can exist in large cell, spindle cell, or small-cell forms; they tend to be seen in males and have a predilection for hematogenous spread and a poor prognosis.

Nonexocrine pancreatic cancers include islet cell cancers, carcinoids, sarcomas, and lymphomas. Islet cell cancers (approximately 5%–10% as frequent as pancreatic exocrine cancers) typically present in the pancreatic body or tail and are slow growing. They of course can also present with their associated ectopic hormonal syndrome (e.g., gastrinomas, gastric acid hypersecretion causing peptic ulcer disease, and diarrhea). Carcinoids are rarely (<1% of cases) found in the pancreas. Although technically foregut in character (carcinoid syndrome rare, predilection for bone metastases), variability in clinical behavior can occur. Primary sarcomas and lymphomas of the pancreas are exceedingly rare.

Q. What is the relationship between pancreatic cancer and adenocarcinomas of unknown primary site?

A. The final aspect of the clinical presentation of pancreatic cancer worthy of mention is its relationship to adenocarcinoma of unknown primary site. Adenocarcinoma is the most frequent light microscopic diagnosis among patients with carcinoma of unknown primary site, accounting for approximately 60% of all such patients[60] or as many as 50,000 patients annually in the United States. Pancreatic carcinoma is disproportionately represented as a primary site among such patients. Although rarely detected antemortem, autopsy studies confirm the pancreas as the site of origin in 25%–40% of cases.[61] Such studies suggest an atypical metastatic pattern for pancreatic cancer in such cases, with atypical sites of hematogenous spread (lung, pleura, and bone) seemingly more common.[62] A detailed search for pancreatic cancer among cancers of unknown primary origin has not been demonstrated to be of benefit at this time. However, common chemotherapeutic approaches to adenocarcinomas of unknown primary origin[63] (e.g., paclitaxel, carboplatin, and etoposide) may differ significantly from those being used for advanced pancreatic cancer (e.g., gemcitabine with or without other drugs). Thus, consideration should be given to the possibility of occult pancreatic cancer among patients with intra-abdominal presentations of adenocarcinomas of unknown primary (especially in males and those with liver-predominant disease). If the patient elects chemotherapy, a regimen appropriate for advanced pancreatic cancer is a consideration.

Conclusion

In summary, the clinical presentation of pancreatic cancer frequently can be elusive, even to experienced clinicians. A high level of clinical suspicion, a practical understanding of clinical epidemiology, a keen awareness of vagaries of presentation, a rapid progression to appropriate diagnostic tests, and a diligence in serial observation are all important to the physician attempting to establish a diagnosis of pancreatic cancer. Diagnostic speed is essential for the maximization of clinical outcomes for this highly lethal disease. New strategies involving a variety of molecular, clinical, and radiographic techniques will likely be necessary to advance the timetable of pancreatic cancer diagnosis to a point where meaningful improvements in outcome can be achieved as a result.

References

1. Parkin DM, Pisani P, Ferlay J. Estimates of the worldwide incidence of eighteen major cancers in 1985. *Int J Cancer.* 1993;54:594–606.
2. Jemal A, Tiwani, RC, Murray T, et al. Cancer statistics 2004. *CA Cancer J Clin.* 2004;54:8–29.
3. Niederhuber JE, Brennan MF, Menck HR. The National Cancer Database report on pancreas cancer. *Cancer.* 1995;76:1671–1677.
4. Pisters WT, Picozzi VJ, Abrams RA. Therapy for localized pancreatic adenocarcinoma: one, two, or three modalities? *ASCO Educational Book.* 2003;39:397–418.
5. Konner J, O'Reilly E. Pancreatic cancer: epidemiology, genetics and approaches to screening. *Oncology.* 2002;16: 1615–1622.
6. Bakkevold KE, Arnesio B, Kamestad B. Carcinoma of the pancreas and papilla of Vater: presenting symptoms, signs and diagnosis related to stage and tumour site. *Scand J Gastroenterol.* 1992;27:317–325.
7. Kalser MH, Barkin J, MacIntyre JM. Pancreatic cancer: assessment of prognosis by clinical presentation. *Cancer.* 1985;56:397–402.
8. Ahlgren JD. Epidemiology and risk factors in pancreatic cancer. *Semin Oncol.* 1996;23:241–250.
9. Gullo L, Pezzilli R, Moriselli-Labate AM. Diabetes and the risk of pancreatic cancer. *N Engl J Med.* 1994;331:81–84.
10. Everhart J, Wright D. Diabetes mellitus as a risk factor for pancreatic cancer. *JAMA.* 1995;273:1605–1609.
11. Permert J, Larsson J, Fruin AB, et al. Islet hormone secretion in pancreatic cancer patients with diabetes. *Pancreas.* 1997;15:60–68.
12. Lowenfels AB, Maissonneuve P, Cavallini G, et al. Pancreatitis and the risk of pancreatic cancer. *N Engl J Med.* 1993;328:1433–1437.
13. Karlson BM, Ekbom A, Josefsson S, et al. The risk of pancreatic cancer following pancreatitis: an association due to confounding? *Gastroenterology.* 1997;113:587–592.
14. Lin A, Feller ER. Pancreatic carcinoma as a cause of unexplained pancreatitis: a report of ten cases. *Ann Intern Med.* 1990;113:116–117.
15. Offerhaus GJA, Tersmette AC, Tersmette KWF, et al. Gastric, pancreatic and colorectal carcinogenesis following remote peptic ulcer surgery. *Mod Pathol.* 1988;1:352–356.
16. Hyvarinen H, Partanen S. Association of cholecystectomy with abdominal cancers. *Hepatogastroenterology.* 1987;34: 280–284.
17. Silverman DT, Dunn JA, Hoover RN, et al. Cigarette smoking and pancreas cancer: a case-control study based on direct interviews. *J Nat Cancer Inst.* 1994;86:1510–1516.
18. Hruban RH, Petersen GM, Goggins M, et al. Familial pancreatic cancer. *Ann Oncol.* 1999;10(Suppl 4):69–73.
19. Lynch HT, Smyrk T, Kern SE, et al. Familial pancreatic cancer: a review. *Semin Oncol.* 1996;23:251–275.
20. Ghadirian P, Liu G, Gallinger S, et al. Risk of pancreatic cancer among individuals with a family history of cancer of the pancreas. *Int J Cancer.* 2002;97:807–810.
21. Howard JM, Jordan GL. Cancer of the pancreas. *Curr Prob Cancer.* 1977;2:2–52.
22. Warshaw AL, Fernandez-del Castillo C. Pancreatic carcinoma. *N Engl J Med.* 1992;326:455–465.
23. Modollel I, Guarner J, Malageda JR. Vagaries of clinical presentation of pancreatic and biliary tract cancer. *Ann Oncol.* 1999;10(Suppl 4):82–84.
24. Gambrill EE. Pancreatic and ampullary carcinoma: diagnosis and prognosis in relation to symptoms, physical findings and elapse of time as observed in 255 patients. *South Med J.* 1970;63:1119–1122.
25. Bockman DL, Buchler M, Beger HG. Interaction of pancreatic ductal carcinoma with nerves leads to nerve damage. *Gastroenterology.* 1994;107:219–230.
26. Malagelada JR. Pancreatic cancer: an overview of epidemiology, clinical presentation and diagnosis. *Mayo Clin Proc.* 1979;54:459–467.
27. Nix GAJ, Schmitz PJM, Wilson HP, et al. Carcinoma of the head of the pancreas. *Gastroenterology.* 1984;87:37–43.
28. Maringhini, A, Ciambra M, Raimondo M, et al. Clinical presentation and ultrasonography in the diagnosis of pancreatic cancer. *Pancreas.* 1993;8:146–150.
29. Ganti AP, Potti A, Koch M, et al. Predictive value of clinical features at initial presentation in pancreatic adenocarcinoma. *Med Oncol.* 2002;4:233–237.
30. Steinberg W. The clinical utility of the CA 19.9 tumor associated antigen. *Am J Gastroenterol.* 1990;85:350–355.
31. Sakahara H, Endo K, Nakajima K, et al. Serum CA 19.9 concentrations and computerized tomography findings in patients with pancreatic carcinoma. *Cancer.* 1986;57: 1324–1326.
32. Tian F, Appert HE, Myles J, et al. Prognostic value of serum CA 19.9 levels in pancreatic adenocarcinoma. *Ann Surg.* 1992;215:350–355.
33. Rickles FR, Edwards RL. Activation of blood coagulation in cancer: Trousseau syndrome revisited. *Blood.* 1983;62:14–31.
34. Pinzon R, Drewinko B, Trujillo JM, et al. Pancreatic carcinoma and Trousseau's syndrome: experience at a large cancer center. *J Clin Oncol.* 1986;4:509–514.
35. Cubilla A, Fitzgerald PJ. Pancreas cancer: I: ductal adenocarcinoma: a clinico-pathologic study of 380 patients. *Pathol Annu.* 1978;13:2241–2289.
36. Green AI, Auston CP. Pathophysiology of pancreatic cancer: a psychobiologic probe. *Psychosomatics.* 1993;34:208–212.
37. Joffe RT, Rubinow DR, Denicoff KD. Depression and carcinoma of the pancreas. *Gen Hosp Psychiatry.* 1986;8:241–245.
38. Fras I, Litin EM, Pearson JS. Comparison of psychiatric symptoms in patients with carcinoma of the pancreas with those in some other intra-abdominal neoplasms. *Am J Psychiatry.* 1967;123:1553–1562.
39. Holland JC, Korzun AH, Tross S, et al. Comparative psychological disturbance in patients with pancreatic and gastric cancer. *Am J Psychiatry.* 1986;143:982–986.
40. Shakin EJ, Holland JC. Depression and pancreatic cancer. *J Pain Symptom Manage.* 1988;3:194–198.
41. Hill CL, Zhang Y, Sigurgeirsson B, et al. Frequency of specific cancer types in dermatomyositis and polymyositis: a population-based study. *Lancet.* 2001;357:96–100.
42. Osterle LS, Branfoot AC, Staughton ACD. Cicatricial pemphigoid and carcinoma of the pancreas. *Clin Exp Dermatol.* 1192;17:67–68.

43. Dahl PR, Winkelman RK, Connolly SM. The vascular calcification-cutaneous necrosis syndrome. *J Am Acad Dermatol.* 1995;53:33–37.
44. Tarpila E, Borch K, Kullman E, et al. Pancreatic cancer. *Ann Chir Gynaecol.* 1986;75:146–150.
45. DiMagno EP. Pancreatic cancer: clinical presentation, pitfalls, and early clues. *Ann Oncol.* 1999;10(Suppl 40):140–142.
46. DiMagno EP, Malagelada JR, Taylor WP, et al. A prospective comparison of current diagnostic tests in pancreatic cancer. *N Engl J Med.* 1977;97:737–742.
47. Tanaka N, Okada S, Ueno H, et al. The usefulness of serial changes in serum CA 19-9 levels in the diagnosis of pancreatic cancer. *Pancreas.* 2000;20:378–381.
48. Tsuchiya R, Noda T, Harada N, et al. Collective review of small carcinomas of the pancreas. *Ann Surg.* 1986;203:77–81.
49. Manabe T, Miyashita T, Ohshio G, et al. Small carcinoma of the pancreas. *Cancer.* 1988;62:135–141.
50. Furukawa H, Okada S, Siacho H, et al. Clinicopathologic features of small pancreatic adenocarcinoma. *Cancer.* 1996;78:986–990.
51. Yeo CJ, Cameron JL. The Johns Hopkins experience. In: Traverso LW, ed. *Problems in General Surgery.* pp. 93–103, Vol. 14. Lippincot–Raven, Philadelphia, PA, 1997.
52. Gullo L, Tomassetti P, Migliori M, et al. Do early symptoms of pancreatic cancer exist that can allow an earlier diagnosis? *Pancreas.* 2001;22:210–213.
53. Ridder GJ, Klempnauer J. Back pain in patients with ductal pancreatic cancer: its impact on resectability and prognosis after resection. *Scand J Gastroenterol.* 1195;30:1216–1220.
54. Krech RL, Walsh D. Symptoms of pancreatic cancer. *J Pain Symptom Manage.* 1991;6:360–367.
55. Reuben DB, Mor V, Hiris J. Clinical symptoms and length of survival in patients with terminal cancer. *Arch Intern Med.* 1988;148:1586–1591.
56. Fong Y, Blumgart LH, Lin E, et al. Outcome of treatment for distal bile duct cancer. *Br J Surg.* 1996;83:1712–1715.
57. Hashimoto L, Walsh RW, Vogt D, et al. Malignant cystic neoplasms of the pancreas. *J Gastrointest Surg.* 1998;2:504–508.
58. Kitagawa Y, Unger T, Taylor S, et al. Mucus is a predictor of better prognosis and survival in patients with intraductal papillary mucinous tumor of the pancreas. *J Gastrointest Surg.* 2003;7:12–19.
59. van Klaveren RJ, de Mulder PMH, Boerbooms AMT, et al. Pancreatic carcinoma with polyarthritis, fat necrosis, and high serum lipase and trypsin activity. *Gut.* 1990;31: 953–955.
60. Hainsworth JD, Greco FA. Treatment of patients with cancer of an unknown primary site. *N Engl J Med.* 1993;329:257–263.
61. Nystrom JS, Weiner JM, Heffelfinger-Juttner J, et al. Metastatic and histologic presentations in unknown primary cancer. *Semin Oncol.* 1977;4:53–58.
62. Mayordomo J, Guerra JM, Guijarro C, et al. Neoplasms of unknown primary site: a clinicopathological study of autopsied patients. *Tumori.* 1993;79:321–324.
63. Hainswroth JD, Erland JB, Kalman LA, et al. Carcinoma of unknown primary site: treatment with 1-hour paclitaxel, carboplatin and extended-schedule etoposide. *J Clin Oncol.* 1998;16:3918–3919.

CHAPTER

12

Radiographic Imaging: CT/MRI/PET

Eric P. Tamm, MD
Evelyne M. Loyer, MD
Janio Szklaruk, MD
Haesun Choi, MD
Silvana C. Faria, MD
Chusilp Charnsangavej, MD

Noninvasive cross-sectional imaging (computed tomography [CT] and magnetic resonance imaging [MRI]), with confirmation by biopsy, serves as the primary means for establishing the diagnosis of pancreatic ductal adenocarcinoma and for staging this disease before surgery. The poor prognosis for this devastating disease demands high accuracy for both diagnosis and staging. At the time of diagnosis, approximately 60% of patients have liver metastases, peritoneal carcinomatosis, or locally advanced disease and are therefore not candidates for surgery, the only option for cure.[1] Of those who undergo surgery, only 18%–21% are alive 5 years after surgery.[1-4] For those who cannot undergo surgery, the median survival is 3–6 months. High accuracy in the interpretation of cross-sectional imaging is necessary to avoid needless surgery for those whose life expectancy is markedly short and to avoid excluding surgery in the small group for whom this treatment can offer cure.

Positron emission tomography (PET) imaging, in contrast to CT and MRI, is based on the imaging of glucose metabolism. The technique offers new opportunities for assessing response to chemotherapy and radiation therapy. The technique, which typically images the entire body during a given examination, offers the potential to detect unexpected sites of metastases. The very recent development of CT-PET offers the ability to use both physiologic and anatomic information by combining these two modalities.

Technique

CT

The primary goal of oncologic imaging, irrespective of modality, is to maximize contrast between tumor and surrounding normal structures. For cross-sectional techniques, additional goals are to maximize in-plane resolution and to minimize slice thickness to avoid volume averaging artifact; these latter goals are important for precisely delineating the relationship of tumor to adjacent structures, such as vessels and solid organs.

For CT, the contrast between pancreatic ductal adenocarcinoma and normal pancreatic parenchyma is enhanced by injecting contrast rapidly and by imaging during the appropriate temporal phase of contrast enhancement. The timing to peak pancreatic enhancement varies with the rate of injection and the total amount of iodinated contrast that has been injected.[5,6] The period of peak pancreatic enhancement has been shown to occur during what has been termed the *pancreatic parenchymal phase*, which occurs after the time of maximum arterial enhancement but before

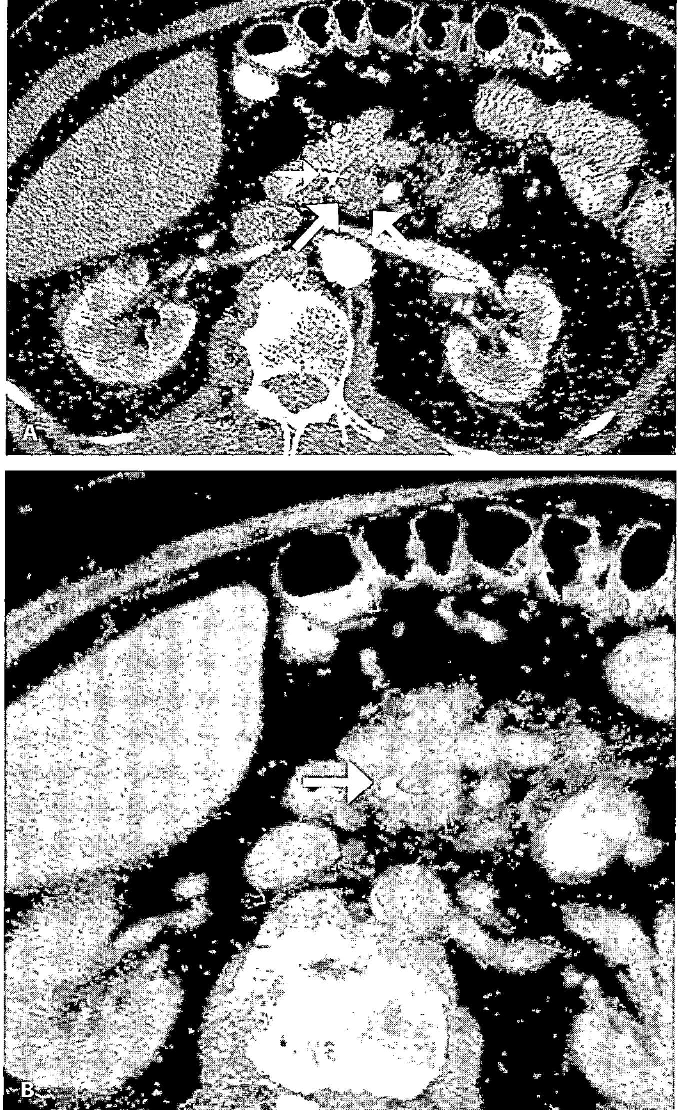

Figure 12.1
Patient with ductal adenocarcinoma. Axial contrast-enhanced images during (**A**) the pancreatic parenchymal phase and (**B**) the portal venous phase. Tumor is identified in the pancreatic head (*large white arrows in A*) on the pancreatic parenchymal phase. A stent (*small white arrow in B*) is present. On the portal venous phase, the tumor can no longer be identified.

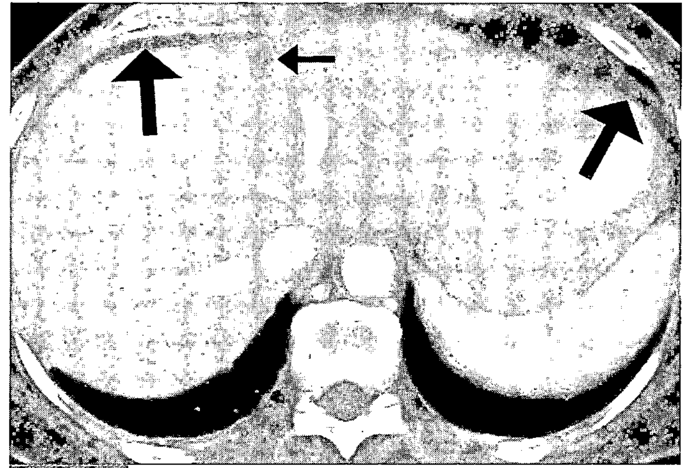

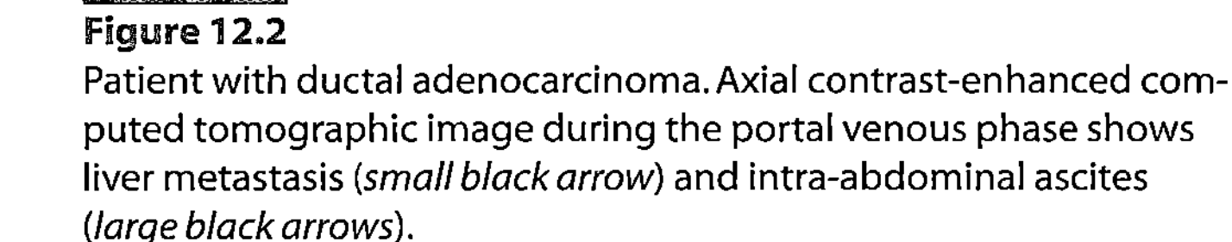

Figure 12.2
Patient with ductal adenocarcinoma. Axial contrast-enhanced computed tomographic image during the portal venous phase shows liver metastasis (*small black arrow*) and intra-abdominal ascites (*large black arrows*).

the period of peak portal venous enhancement. Using an injection rate of 4–5 mL/sec, for a volume of 140–150 mL of intravenous iodinated contrast, the peak pancreatic parenchymal phase occurs between 35 and 50 seconds after the start of contrast injection.[5,6] This phase has also been shown to maximize contrast between tumor and normal pancreatic parenchyma[7,8] (Fig. 12.1). Most of the literature that has been available has been based on single-detector-row helical CT. The recent development of multidetector-row CT has allowed for far more rapid imaging of the abdomen; this capability can be used to obtain images of unprecedented thinness of the abdomen within a single breath hold. Thinner sections would potentially decrease obscuration of tumor by volume averaging artifact, and the more rapid acquisition of images during each phase of imaging would allow for more uniform enhancement of all images within a given phase. A recent study by McNulty et al.[9] used multidetector-row, CT-confirmed peak parenchymal enhancement during the typical pancreatic parenchymal phase, although they did not show a significant difference in tumor conspicuity between the pancreatic and the portal venous phases of contrast enhancement. A study by Fletcher et al.[10] of 39 patients evaluated imaging of the pancreas during the arterial, pancreatic parenchymal, and hepatic phases of contrast enhancement. The timing of the onset of each phase varied with the injection rate used per patient. For the arterial phase, imaging started 20 seconds after the start of contrast injection when an injection rate of 5 mL/sec was used and started at 30 seconds after contrast injection when a rate of 3 mL/sec was used. Similarly, the pancreatic parenchymal and hepatic phases of imaging started at 40 and 60 seconds for an injection rate of 5 mL/sec and at 50 and 70 seconds, respectively, for an injection rate of 3 mL/sec. They found the sensitivity for detecting tumor to be 0.63, 0.97, and 0.93 for the arterial, pancreatic parenchymal, and hepatic phases, respectively. The sensitivity for detecting vascular invasion was 0.25, 0.58 and 0.83 for the arterial, pancreatic parenchymal, and hepatic phases.

In contrast, pancreatic ductal adenocarcinoma metastases to the liver are best visualized during the portal venous phase of contrast enhancement (Fig. 12.2). This phase

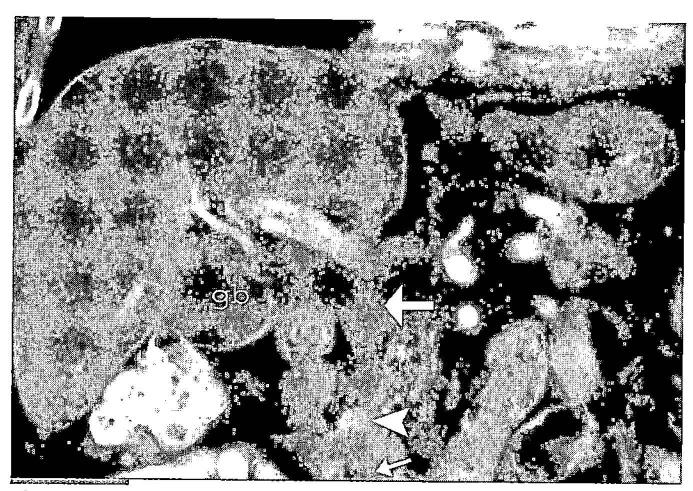

Figure 12.3
Patient with distal common bile duct cholangiocarcinoma identified during workup for presumed pancreatic cancer. Multiplanar reformation image created in the coronal plane shows common bile duct (*large white arrow*) dilatation. The distal cholangiocarcinoma obstructs the distal common bile duct (*white arrowhead*). Choledochocele, partially visualized, extended below the limits of coverage on this computed tomographic examination (*small white arrow*). gb = gallbladder.

of contrast enhancement typically occurs 60–70 seconds after the start of contrast injection. Other advantages of imaging during the portal venous phase include optimal opacification of the superior mesenteric vein, portal vein, and splenic vein and ability to evaluate the relationship of tumor to these venous structures. The use of a dual-phase imaging technique optimizes the ability to detect tumor and to provide information for staging.

Another means to improve tumor conspicuity is to obtain images as thin as possible to eliminate obscuration of tumor due to the effect of volume averaging, which occurs when both tumor and pancreatic tissue are within the same voxel because of the thickness of the image slice volume. For a single-detector helical CT unit, images are typically obtained at a 3- to 5-mm slice thickness with a pitch of 1.5–2[11-14]; because of the limitations of this type of CT scanner, typically only the pancreas can be imaged at this slice thickness. Such limitations are essentially eliminated when multidetector CT technology is used. At our institution, with the use of a four-detector-row multidetector CT scanner, images are obtained of the abdomen from the level of the diaphragm through to the horizontal portion of the duodenum during both the pancreatic parenchymal phase and the portal venous phase. These images are obtained at a slice thickness of 2.5 mm and are reconstructed to 1.25 mm. The 2.5-mm-thick images are used for diagnostic review, and the 1.25-mm-thick images are used for problem solving and for advanced postprocessing, that is, multiplanar reconstructions, curved planar reformations, and volume-rendered and maximum intensity projection reconstructions.

Postprocessing The development of multidetector CT, and therefore the ability to acquire very thin section images, has greatly improved the quality of postprocessed images. Thin-section images can be stacked, a viewing perspective chosen, and images rendered from any perspective with the use of a variety of algorithms, including ray sum (average intensity) for multiplanar or curved planar reformations, as well as maximum-intensity projection, minimum-intensity projection, and volume-rendered reconstructions.

Multiplanar images have the closest appearance to those of the axial source images. We typically reconstruct such images at 2.5-mm slice thickness and often obtain images in the coronal oblique plane that passes through both the portal venous confluence and the common bile duct to visualize structures in the hepatoduodenal ligament (Fig. 12.3). Multiplanar images can display soft tissue structures in relationship to tumor and adjacent vessels. A study by Itoh et al.[15] reported that multiplanar reformation images obliqued to encompass the length of the pancreatic duct improved visualization of the relationship of the tumor to the duct.

In contrast, curved planar reformations allow the user to create a complex curving section through the length of a structure, that is, the pancreatic duct[16] or the superior mesenteric artery. A single image can therefore show the entire length of a structure that would otherwise require multiple axial images for its entire length to be depicted. This technique can be used to create pictures that can summarize the relationship of tumor to vessels or other structures (Fig. 12.4); however, anatomic knowledge is required for accurate tracing of structures, and knowledge of the tumor is necessary to provide an accurate image. A recent comparison of axial images and curved planar reformations showed them to be equivalent for the detection of pancreatic tumors and for the determination of surgical resectability.[17]

Maximum-intensity projection images display the pixel with the highest density along a given ray, corresponding with the perspective chosen by the user, projected through the stack of axial source images. It is best used for high-density structures, such as contrast-enhanced vasculature, stents, and bones. The effects of tumor are visualized, rather than the hypodense tumor itself. It is most commonly used to depict vasculature and to show the narrowing and irregularity of contour of

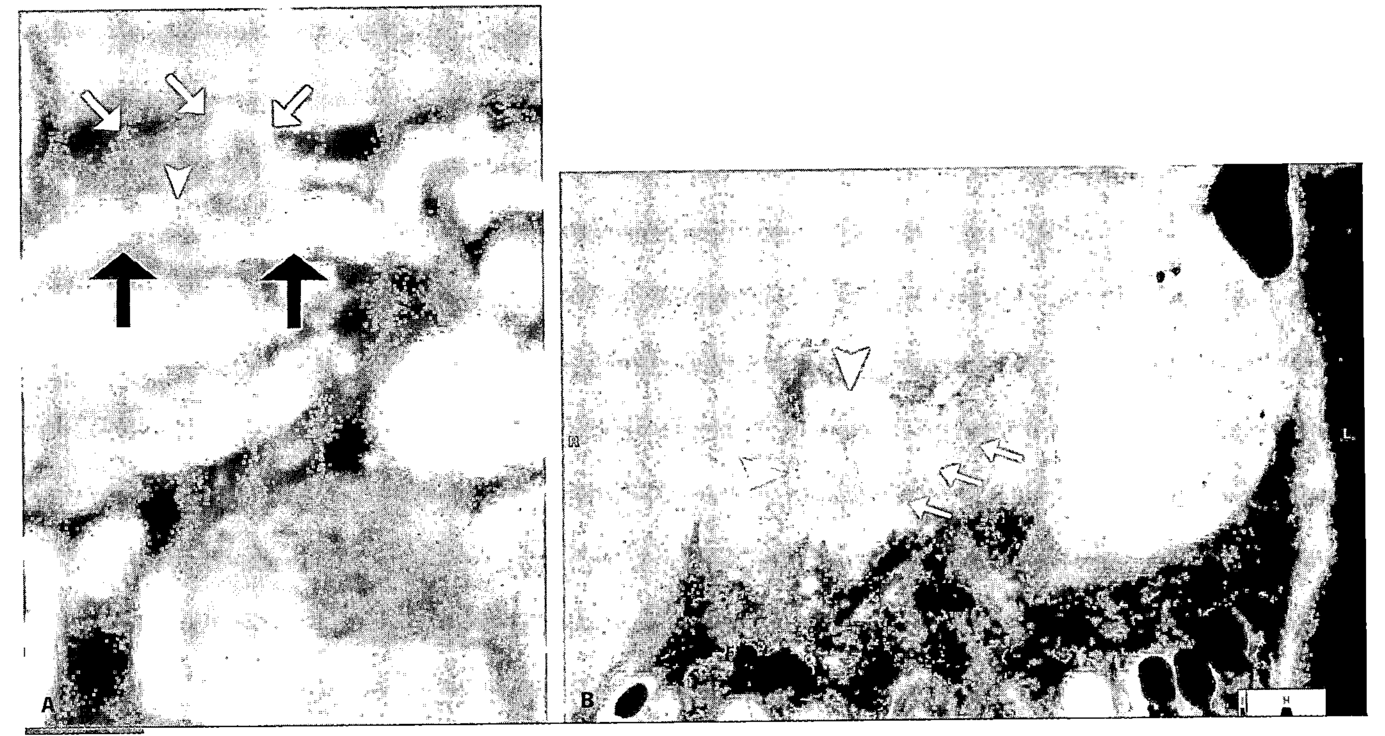

Figure 12.4
Postprocessed image in a patient with a history of pancreatic cancer. **(A)** Curved planar reformation of the common and proper hepatic arteries (*large black arrows*) shows tumor (*small white arrows*) engulfing these vessels. Tumor has caused narrowing of the junction of the common and proper hepatic arteries (*white arrowhead*). **(B)** Minimum-intensity projection image, 10 mm thick, created in a coronally oriented plane, shows the tumor in the pancreatic head (*white arrowheads*) obstructing the pancreatic duct (*short white arrows*).

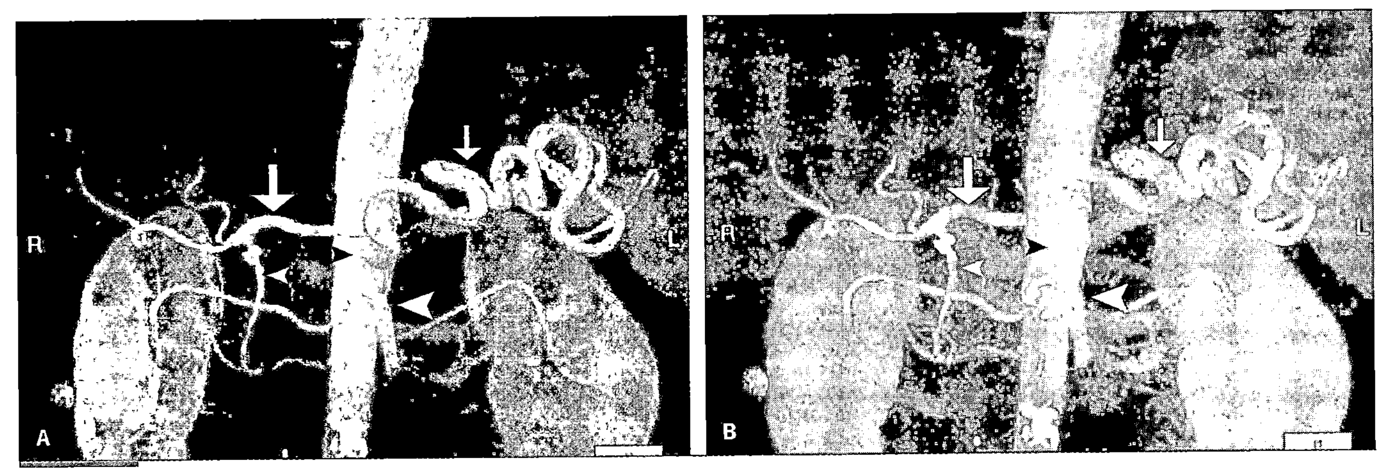

Figure 12.5
Volume-rendered image **(A)** and maximum intensity projection image **(B)** showing the celiac axis and superior mesenteric artery. The splenic artery (*small white arrow*) and the common hepatic artery (*large white arrow*) are identified arising from the celiac trunk (*small black arrowhead*). The superior mesenteric artery origin can be identified (*large white arrowhead*), as can the gastroduodenal artery (*small white arrowhead*). Note that the celiac artery origin is essentially indistinguishable from the aorta on the maximum intensity projection image.

vessels due to tumor involvement. A study of 89 patients in which maximum-intensity projection was used did not show improved accuracy in assessing vascular involvement by tumor when compared with axial-source images alone.[11] A more recent study in which readers could interact with a three-dimensional maximum-intensity projection model cross-referenced with corresponding axial images showed improved accuracy for venous invasion (92% vs 69% for helical CT alone) but no improvement in detection of arterial invasion.[18]

In contrast, the newer technique of volume rendering allows the user, through a combination of settings

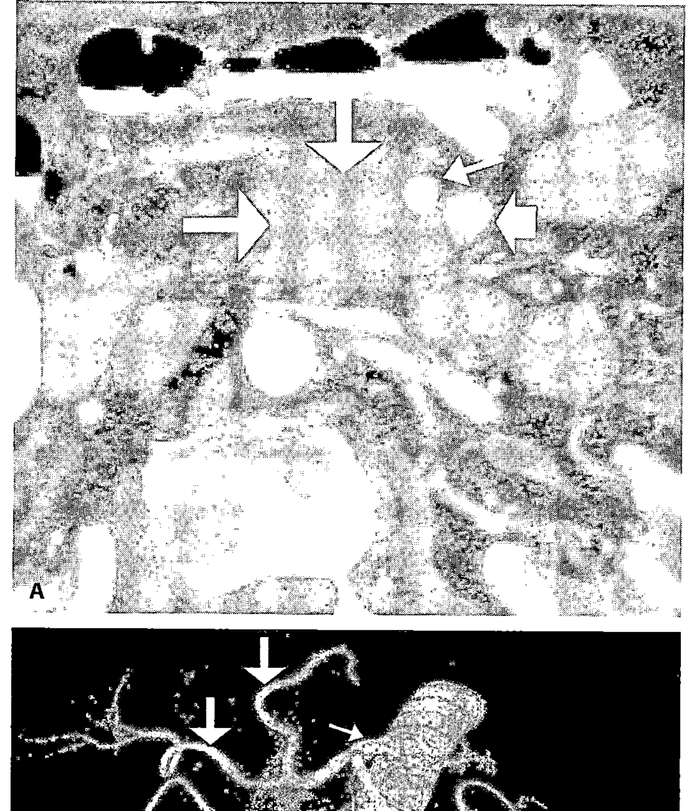

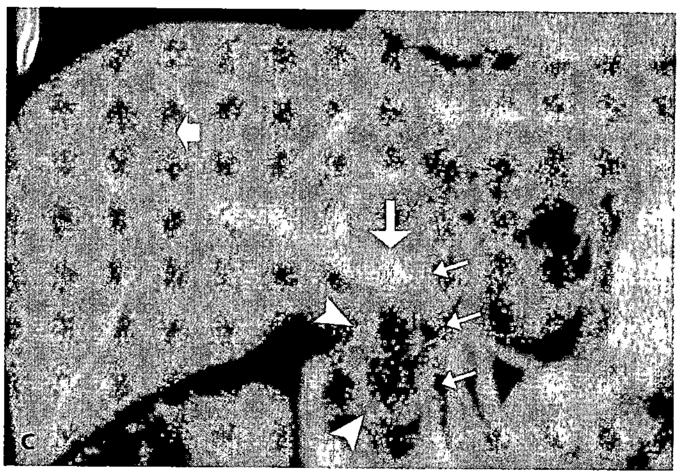

Figure 12.6
Patient with ductal adenocarcinoma. **(A)** Axial computed tomographic image showing pancreatic head tumor (*large white arrows*) involving the superior mesenteric artery (*small white arrow*) and a normal-variant left-sided superior mesenteric vein (*thick white arrow*). **(B)** Volume-rendered image, in an oblique coronal-axial orientation, optimized to show vasculature, shows a replaced right hepatic artery (*white arrowhead*) arising from the superior mesenteric artery (*thick white arrow*). The left hepatic arteries (*large white arrows*) are supplied by the celiac trunk (*small white arrow*). **(C)** Volume-rendered image, coronal plane, 20-mm-thick slab, optimized to show tumor, normal soft tissues, and vasculature, shows primary tumor in pancreatic head (*white arrowheads*) markedly narrowing the superior mesenteric vein (*small white arrows*). Main portal vein (*large white arrow*) can be seen above the level of the tumor. A metastatic focus to the liver (*thick white arrow*) is also identified.

for multiple variables, to assign a variety of opacities, colors, and brightness to different ranges of densities. The technique can be used to show tumor alone, vasculature alone, ductal anatomy alone, or any combination of any of the anatomic structures (Figs. 12.5 and 12.6). It is this ability to show vasculature and the soft tissue surrounding them that gives volume rendering an advantage over maximum-intensity projection.[19] Volume rendering has been used to depict the distal branches of the superior mesenteric artery in the evaluation of ischemic bowel disease[20] and has been used, in combination with an oral cholecystographic agent, to demonstrate the biliary tree.[21,22] Johnson et al.[23] even described the use of volume rendering techniques to successfully display the length of the intrahepatic and extrahepatic biliary tree without the use of a cholecystographic agent. Volume rendering has also been used to demonstrate pancreaticoduodenal arcades,[24] as well as tumor involvement of superior mesenteric and portal venous structures.[25]

Minimum-intensity projection images use the lowest density value along a given ray and are therefore the opposite of maximum-intensity projections. This technique is typically used to visualize the biliary and pancreatic ducts (Fig. 12.4) and can therefore provide images of utility similar to that of images obtained by cholangiography; the technique has been named CT cholangiopancreatography. A study by Raptopoulos et al.[26] showed that CT cholangiopancreatography image quality was similar to that of endoscopic retrograde cholangiopancreatography and that the determination of duct caliber on CT cholangiopancreatography correlated

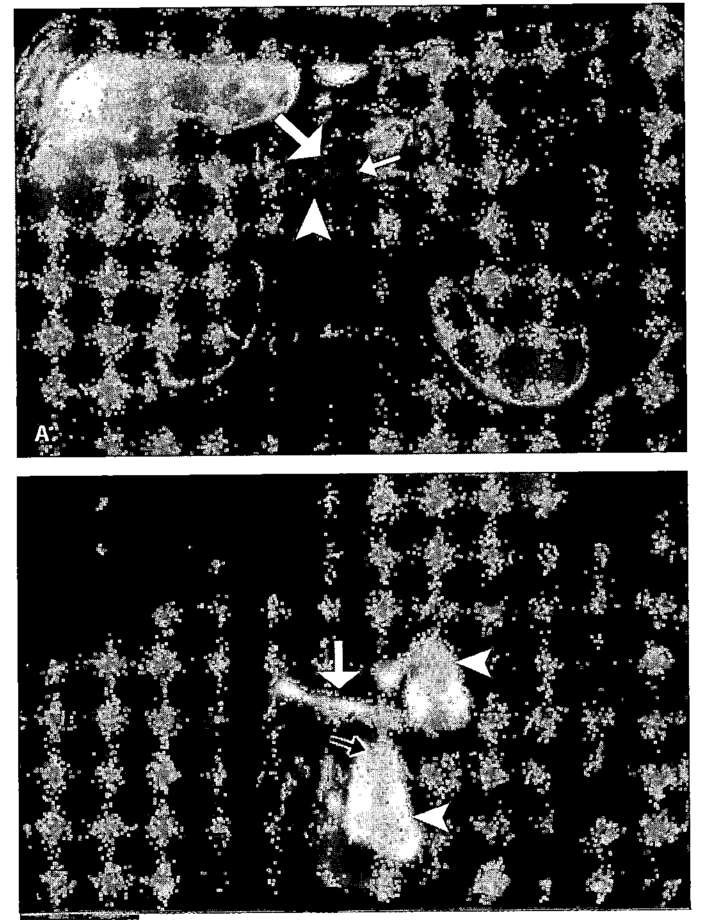

Figure 12.7
Patient with normal pancreas undergoing imaging to evaluate for liver metastases. **(A)** Dynamically enhanced magnetic resonance T1-weighted image, obtained with a three-dimensional (3-D) volumetric acquisition. Image shows the normal pancreatic head (*large white arrow*), normal caliber common bile duct (*white arrowhead*), and normal caliber pancreatic duct (*small white arrow*). **(B)** Coronal oblique reconstructed image from dynamically enhanced 3-D T1-weighted MRI sequence. The normal portal vein (*white arrow*), pancreas (*white arrowheads*), and pancreatic duct (*black arrow*) are visualized.

with results from endoscopic retrograde cholangiopancreatography.[26] Park et al.[27] found that when compared with percutaneous cholangiography, CT cholangiopancreatography could identify the level of obstruction and in most cases was able to diagnose the cause.[27]

MRI

Although multidetector CT offers higher image resolution (typically 512 × 512 pixels for CT vs 256 × 128–192 for MRI) and thinner sections, MRI offers inherently better soft tissue contrast before the administration of intravenous contrast. MRI can be performed in patients for whom the administration of iodinated contrast agents is contraindicated (allergy or renal insufficiency).

Imaging of the pancreas requires systems that have high signal-to-noise ratios; therefore, systems with high field strengths (1.5 T or higher) and, optimally, phased-array surface coils are recommended. A typical MRI protocol for imaging the pancreas may include, before the administration of intravenous gadolinium, breath-hold multiplanar spoiled gradient or respiratory-averaged T1-weighted images, with and/or without fat suppression, and fat-suppressed, breath-hold, fast-recovery, fast spin echo or respiratory-triggered or -averaged fast spin echo T2-weighted images. On the administration of intravenous gadolinium, images can be obtained dynamically with the use of either two- or three-dimensional gradient echo T1-weighted images (Figs. 12.7 and 12.8). The latter offers overlapping thin-section (4–6 mm) images through the liver and pancreas within a single breath-hold with fat suppression; images acquired in this fashion can also be used for advanced postprocessing, such as multiplanar reformations (Fig. 12.7). Dynamically obtained images have been shown to increase the conspicuity of tumor.[28-34]

Mangafodipir trisodium (MnDPDP), originally developed as a hepatocyte-specific contrast agent, has been found to also be taken up by normal pancreatic parenchyma; however, pancreatic parenchyma typically shows greater enhancement with gadolinium than with MnDPDP.[35] Images are typically obtained 15–20 minutes after the injection of contrast and can be obtained with either a breath-hold technique, to eliminate respiratory motion artifact, or a respiratory averaged technique, such as in spin echo T1-weighted images. The ability to use the latter technique is useful in patients who cannot suspend respiration, such as patients under sedation and children.

Magnetic resonance cholangiopancreatography allows for noninvasive imaging of the pancreatic and biliary ductal systems. This technique uses heavily T2-weighted fast spin echo sequences with or without fat suppression. These can be acquired during free breathing with the use of respiratory triggering.[36] Recent advances, such as half-Fourier T2-weighted fast spin echo techniques (HASTE, Siemens AG, Munich, Germany) and single-shot fast spin echo (General Electric, Milwaukee, WI), allow for thick-slab or multiple thin-slab images to be obtained within the time of a single breath-hold, although they can be acquired with the use of respiratory-triggered techniques.[37,38] More recent developments include the use of rapid high-performance,

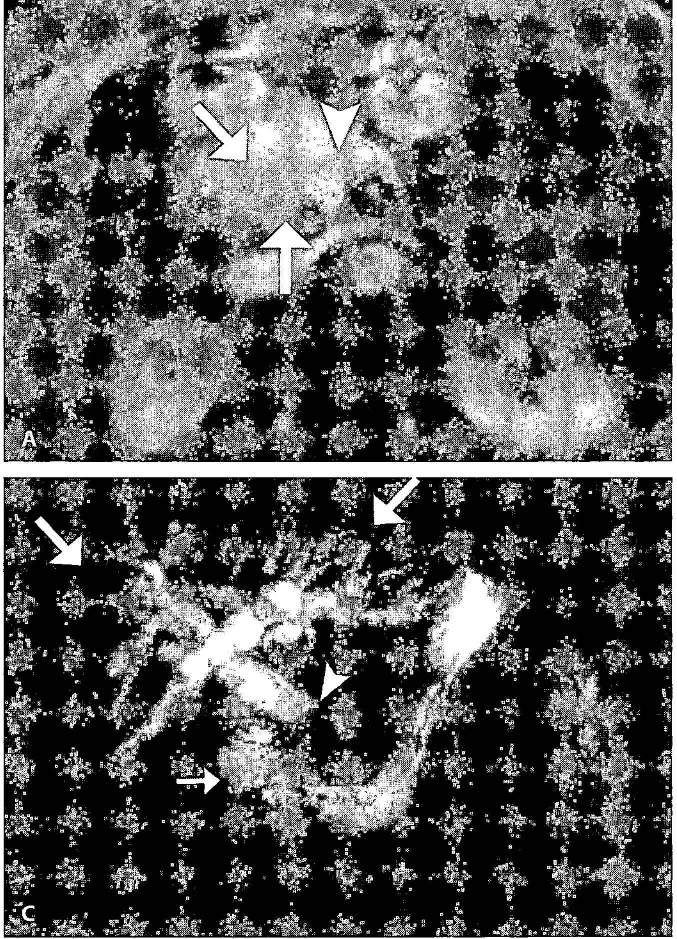
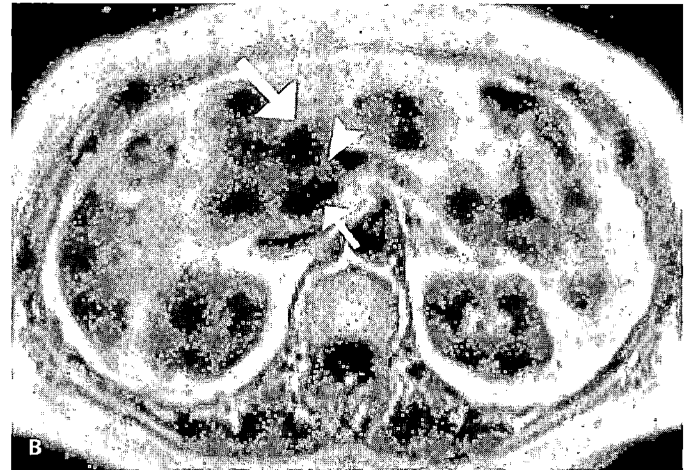
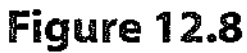

Figure 12.8
Patient with ductal adenocarcinoma involving the pancreatic head. **(A)** Dynamically enhanced fat-suppressed axial T1-weighted magnetic resonance image of patient with ductal adenocarcinoma. Tumor (*large white arrows*) involves the superior mesenteric vein (*white arrowhead*). **(B)** T1-weighted unenhanced axial image shows tumor (*large white arrow*) involving the pancreatic head, with obliteration of the fat plane (*small white arrowhead*) between the tumor and the superior mesenteric vein (*small white arrow*). **(C)** Thick-section (50-mm) magnetic resonance cholangiopancreatographic image of same patient. Abrupt termination of the distal common bile duct (*white arrowhead*) is secondary to pancreatic cancer (not visualized). There is moderately severe intrahepatic ductal dilatation (*large white arrows*). Fluid in the duodenum is also visualized (*small white arrow*).

gradient-based echo planar imaging. Wielopolski et al.[39] reported improved visualization of the common bile duct and hepatic ducts, but blurring and incomplete suppression of signal from background soft tissues limited visualization of the pancreatic duct.[39] Other techniques, such as three-dimensional fast recovery, fast spin echo are being developed, but their utility has yet to be reported. Thick slabs, measuring approximately 50 mm, can be obtained in multiple projections to provide an overview of biliary and pancreatic ductal anatomy (Fig. 12.8) and to conduct dynamic magnetic resonance cholangiopancreatography.[38] This approach reportedly can improve visualization of the pancreatic main duct and its side branches.[40-42] Multiple thin slabs, varying between 3 and 6 mm, provide a better means to visualize findings within the biliary and the pancreatic ductal systems, such as stones and polypoid growths. A combination of thick- and thin-slab imaging has been used in several studies assessing the efficacy of magnetic resonance cholangiopancreatography.[40,43]

PET

PET typically uses the intravenously administered ^{18}F-labeled agent fluorodeoxy-D-glucose (FDG). Imaging is usually obtained between 40 minutes and 3 hours after injection.[44,45] Patients should be screened for hyperglycemia before imaging to avoid false-negative results, and for pancreatitis to avoid false-positive results.[44] Imaging of the whole body is typically obtained with the use of a volumetric technique, and the data are typically reconstructed in the axial, coronal, and sagittal planes for review (Fig. 12.9). Standard uptake values are calculated for semiquantitative assessment of lesions. The recent development of CT-PET combines a multidetector CT unit with a PET unit; this improves the determination of the anatomic location of foci of increased metabolic activity.

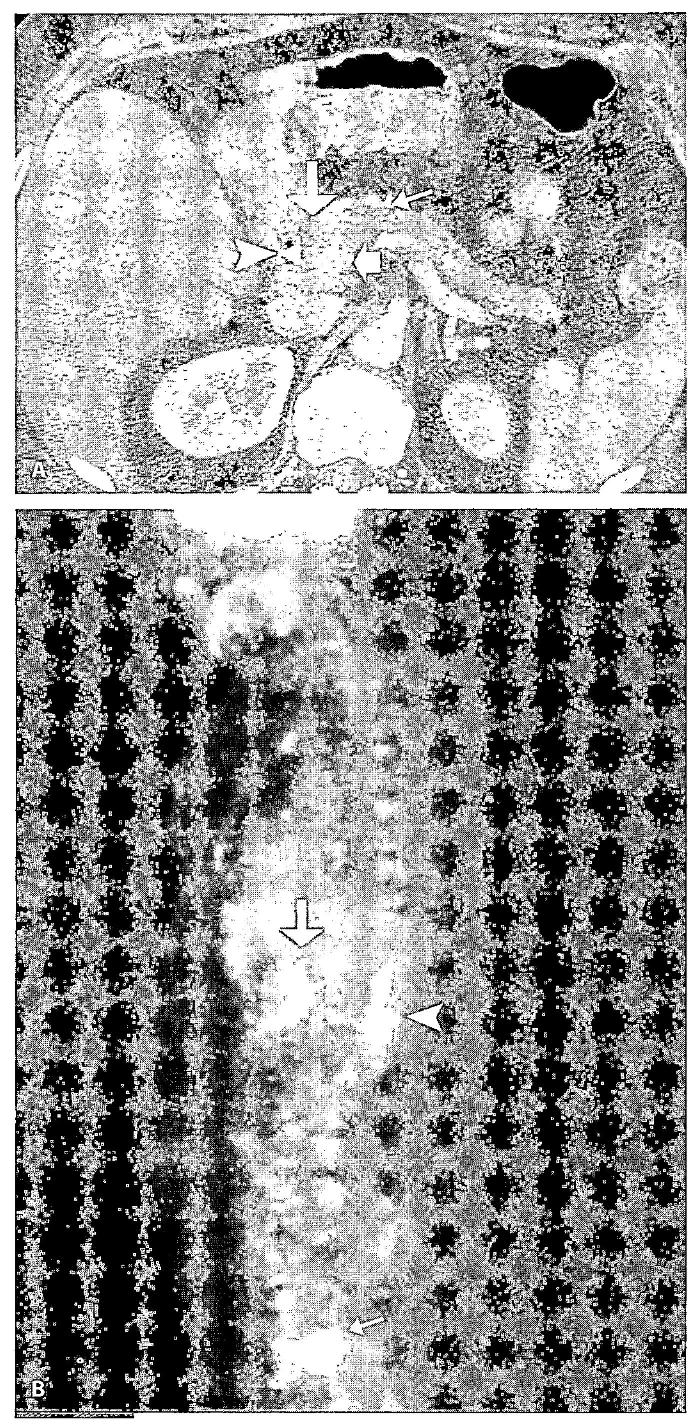

Figure 12.9
Patient with pancreatic ductal adenocarcinoma of the pancreatic head. **(A)** Axial contrast-enhanced computed tomographic image. Pancreatic head tumor (*large white arrow*) obstructs the dilated pancreatic duct (*small white arrow*) and markedly narrows the portal vein (*white arrowhead*). A biliary stent is present (*white arrowhead*). **(B)** Sagittal image from a positron emission tomographic scan shows pancreatic head tumor (*large white arrow*), kidneys (*white arrowhead*), and bladder (*small white arrow*).

Diagnosis

CT

Pancreatic ductal adenocarcinoma typically has a hypodense appearance on contrast-enhanced CT. Close attention to technique is vital; approximately 40% of tumors that are hypodense on the initial pancreatic parenchymal phase are isodense to the remainder of the pancreas on later phases of imaging (Fig. 12.1). A recent study of 53 patients reported that up to 11% of tumors can be isoattenuating to normal pancreas on both pancreatic parenchymal and portal venous phases.[46] For this reason, close attention must be paid to secondary signs when a mass is not readily detectable. Secondary signs include dilatation of the pancreatic duct and/or the common bile duct, interruption of the pancreatic duct, atrophy of the pancreas distal to the site of tumor, distortion of the pancreatic contour, narrowing of adjacent vascular structures (Fig. 12.10), soft tissue density infiltrating the fat surrounding vascular structures, and, in later stages of disease, adenopathy, peritoneal implants, and liver metastases. Unfortunately, small tumors and tumors located in the uncinate process may not produce significant secondary signs. Small tumors may not even distort the contour of the pancreas, and therefore, a subtle finding of hypodensity may be all that is present to indicate the possibility of tumor.

The literature on single-detector helical CT indicates a detection rate of approximately 78%–100% for tumors 2 cm or greater and 40%–100% for those less than 2 cm.[14,31,33,47,48] Overall, single-detector CT has an accuracy of between 86% and 91%, a specificity of 54%–100%, and a sensitivity of 76%–97% for the detection of pancreatic cancer.[11,13,14,30,33,48] Early published data regarding multidetector CT shows a detection rate of approximately 96%–97%.[9,10] Our unpublished data support this improvement in sensitivity.

Pitfalls in the diagnosis of pancreatic cancer include small tumors, uncinate process tumors, and diseases that can mimic ductal adenocarcinoma, including chronic pancreatitis, cholangiocarcinoma of the distal common bile duct, lymphoma, and disease metastatic to the pancreas. Biopsy is typically necessary to confirm the diagnosis of pancreatic ductal adenocarcinoma.

MRI

The findings for pancreatic ductal adenocarcinoma on MRI parallel those for CT. Pancreatic ductal adenocarcinoma typically shows relatively lower signal on precontrast and postcontrast, dynamically enhanced, T1-weighted images

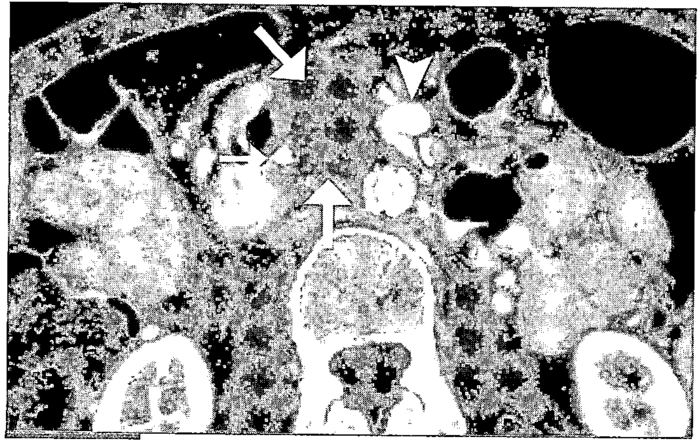

Figure 12.10
Pancreatic ductal adenocarcinoma involving the pancreatic head (*large white arrows*) distorts the superior mesenteric vein (*white arrowhead*) causing the "tear drop" sign. The point of contact between tumor and vein is concave in geometric configuration. Stent (*small white arrow*) is incidentally identified.

than normal pancreatic parenchyma (Figs. 12.7 and 12.8). On delayed phases of imaging, tumor can become indistinguishable from normal pancreatic parenchyma. Therefore, as with CT, optimum technique, particularly for dynamic imaging, is vital. Tumor is typically best visualized on immediate postgadolinium, dynamically obtained, breath-hold, T1-weighted images and pregadolinium fat-suppressed, T1-weighted images.[49-54] The detection rate for pancreatic carcinoma on MRI is reportedly between 80% and 95%.[13,30,33] In the study by Nishiharu et al.,[13] MRI had a specificity of 71%–78% and an accuracy of 79%–81%.[13] The differential diagnosis for the findings on MRI are the same as those for CT. Chronic pancreatitis is particularly problematic for both modalities because it can mimic all of the findings of ductal adenocarcinoma.

MnDPDP, which is taken up by normal pancreatic parenchyma but not by tumor, has been studied for its possible role in the detection of pancreatic ductal adenocarcinoma.[55] Imaging with this agent can be performed with or without breath-holding, a characteristic that increases the pool of patients that can be evaluated. Results have been mixed when MnDPDP has been compared with multiphase CT. Studies have shown the sensitivity of detecting malignancy to be 88%–100%.[56-58]

The magnetic resonance cholangiopancreatographic findings for ductal adenocarcinoma are essentially the same as those seen on endoscopic retrograde cholangiopancreatography. Tumors located in the pancreatic body and tail typically involve the pancreatic duct alone, whereas those involving the head, neck, or pancreas diffusely can involve both the common bile duct and the pancreatic duct (Fig. 12.8). Tumor may cause an abrupt "cut off" appearance of an involved duct, or an irregular stricture with a shelf-like appearance; unfortunately, a normal caliber pancreatic duct may be present in up to 20% of patients with pancreatic cancer.[59] Stricture typically associated with chronic pancreatitis usually has a smooth, tapered appearance, but its appearance can also overlap that seen with cancer; the presence of side-branch ectasia can increase the likelihood that a stricture is secondary to chronic pancreatitis.[40,59] Although malignant strictures are typically seen with pancreatic ductal adenocarcinoma, they may occur with other malignant processes, including metastases.

PET

As typically occurs with malignancies in other regions of the body, pancreatic ductal adenocarcinoma usually has the appearance of a focus of intense radiotracer uptake (Fig. 12.9). Unfortunately, tumors less than 1 cm in diameter, highly differentiated tumors, and tumors that are imaged in patients who are hyperglycemic ($>$130 mg/dL) at the time of imaging may not be detectable.[60-62] The intense metabolic activity of an acute episode of pancreatitis at the time of imaging can have the appearance of tumor.[60] Standardized uptake values have been used to quantitatively differentiate pancreatitis from tumor. However, there is considerable overlap in the standardized uptake values of pancreatic ductal adenocarcinoma and pancreatitis.[62-64] A variety of parameters, including measurements at delayed imaging and assessment of FDG kinetics, have been used with mixed results.[63,65] In a recent study by Kalady et al.[66] of the utility of PET in the diagnosis and management of periampullary tumors in a group of 54 patients, sensitivity was 88%, specificity was 86%, positive predictive value was 95%, and negative predictive value was 71%, whereas dual-phase CT had a sensitivity of 90%, a specificity of 62%, a positive predictive value of 88%, and a negative predictive value of 67%.[66] A review of the literature by Zimny and Schumpelick[67] indicated a median sensitivity of 92% and a specificity of 82% for PET for the detection of pancreatic cancer. Only very limited information is available on the recent development of CT-PET.

Staging

Vascular Involvement

Several criteria have been developed to predict vascular involvement by tumor on evaluation with CT. These criteria are able to predict resectability of tumor in 80%–85%

of cases and are based on the relationship of tumor to adjacent vessels.[68,69] Studies that have examined the relationship of the degree of circumferential involvement of a vessel by tumor have shown that tumor that encompassed more than half the circumference of a vessel was predictive of tumor involvement of that vessel, with a sensitivity of 46%–84% and a specificity of 97%.[11,69,70]

A study by Loyer et al.[68] examined instead the geometric configuration of tumor to adjacent vasculature. When either a fat plane or normal-appearing pancreatic tissue separated tumor from adjacent vessel, resectability of tumor was possible in 95% of cases. When tumor was inseparable from adjacent vasculature and the point of contact between tumor and vasculature formed a convexity against the vessel, it was not possible to reliably predict tumor involvement of vasculature. In contrast, when the point of contact formed a concavity against a vessel (partial encirclement), irresectability of arterial vasculature was identified in 47% of cases; in the case of venous structures, venous resection was necessary for tumor removal (Fig. 12.10). When tumor completely encircled or occluded a vessel, tumor could not be resected with a negative margin.

Phoa et al.[71] evaluated the effectiveness of combining criteria from various systems for detecting vascular involvement by tumor; they showed the most effective combination for predicting tumor involvement of vasculature to be tumor either circumferentially involving a vessel or having a concave relationship of more than 90 degrees of a vessel's surface. With this combination of findings, they showed a sensitivity of 60%, a specificity of 90%, and a positive predictive value of 90% for determining irresectability.

A study by Diehl et al.[11] that evaluated the overall assessment of irresectability showed a sensitivity of 91%, a specificity of 90%, a positive predictive value of 96%, a negative predictive value of 79%, and an accuracy of 91%. Similar negative predictive values have been obtained in other studies.[72,73]

MRI

As with CT, the relationship of tumor to adjacent vasculature has been analyzed with MRI to determine irresectability. Sironi et al.[74] defined tumor-vessel contiguity as present when tumor infiltrated the perivascular fat planes to within 5 mm of a vessel wall and encompassed <180 degrees of its circumference. Encasement was identified when tumor obliterated perivascular fat planes and involved 180 degrees or more of the circumference of a vessel wall (Fig. 12.8). The accuracy for identifying encasement was 91% on precontrast and 94% on postcontrast spin echo, T1-weighted images, with lower accuracies for corresponding breath-hold, gradient-recalled images (74% and 76%, respectively). However, gradient echo techniques for breath-hold T1-weighted imaging have improved since the time of this study. A recent comparison study of MRI, MRI with magnetic resonance angiography, and dual-phase CT showed comparable accuracies (87%, 90%, and 90%, respectively), specificities, and sensitivities between the three modalities,[75] an improvement over earlier studies that showed lower accuracies (58%–86%) for MRI for detection of vascular invasion.[13,30,76,77]

PET

PET, and the recent development of CT-PET, has a very limited role in detecting vascular involvement by tumor. This is because PET provides markedly limited anatomic information. Although it provides anatomic information that far more accurately localizes foci of increased metabolic activity than PET alone, CT-PET is currently performed without intravenous contrast and typically without oral or rectal contrast. Discrimination of tumor from vessel is therefore markedly limited when compared with contrast-enhanced CT or MRI. Therefore, complete staging is not possible with PET or CT-PET and typically requires a follow-up examination with either contrast-enhanced CT or MRI.

Metastases

Liver

A high percentage of patients with pancreatic ductal adenocarcinoma have advanced disease at presentation. The sensitivity for CT for the detection of liver metastases (Fig. 12.11) has been reported to be between 75%-87%.[11,77-79] A study directly comparing spiral CT with MRI showed an accuracy of 93.5% for MRI for detecting liver metastases, compared with 87% for CT.[77] Sensitivity for both modalities decreases with a decrease in the size of metastases. Early studies that evaluated for the detection of small metastases (<2 cm) to the surface of liver showed sensitivities as low as 26%–42% for both modalities; however, these studies included information from early, conventional, nonhelical CT.[80,81] To our knowledge, no data have been published comparing state-of-the-art multidetector-row CT with state-of-the-art MRI (with three-dimensional gradient echo–enhanced imaging).

Only limited information is available regarding detection by PET of pancreatic cancer metastatic to the liver (Fig. 12.12). An evaluation of 159 patients showed

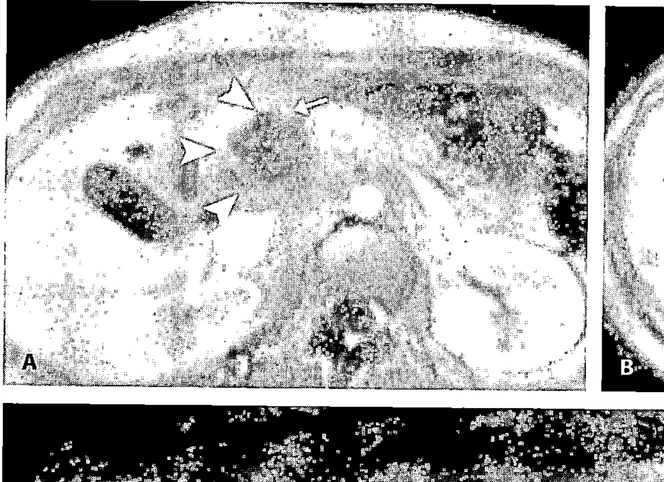

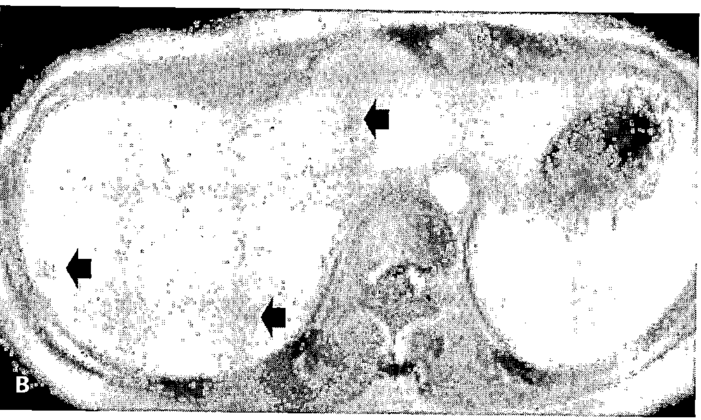

Figure 12.11
Patient with metastatic pancreatic ductal adenocarcinoma. **(A)** Axial dynamically enhanced T1-weighted image shows tumor in the pancreatic head (*white arrowheads*) involving the superior mesenteric vein (*small white arrow*). **(B)** Axial dynamically enhanced T1-weighted image of the liver during the portal venous phase shows three metastatic foci to the liver (*thick black arrows*). **(C)** Axial fat-suppressed T2-weighted image also shows metastatic foci within the liver but not as clearly as on the dynamically enhanced images (*thick white arrows*).

a sensitivity of 70% and a specificity of 95% for the detection of liver metastases.[82] As expected, sensitivity for liver metastases decreases with decrease in size of the lesions in question; a study of 168 patients showed a detection rate of only 43% for tumors less than or equal to 1 cm in diameter.[83] False-positive results can occur in patients with metabolically active benign disease, such as abscesses or severe cholestasis.[83] Pulmonary findings, such as pulmonary metastases, may be misrepresented as being within the liver.[83] False-positive results should be reduced with the advent of CT-PET because of the additional anatomic information provided by this modality; however, because the CT information is obtained during suspended respiration and the PET information is obtained during free respiration, misregistration of the PET and CT data can occur.

Nodal and Peritoneal Disease

CT and MRI have traditionally been limited in their detection of peritoneal disease (Fig. 12.13) and have had limited accuracy in the identification of nodal metastases because size is the primary criterion (>1 cm in short axis) for identifying nodal metastases.[11,84] The study by Diehl et al.[11] reported a sensitivity for detecting nodal metastases of 54% for single-detector CT,[11] whereas a study by Zeman et al.[85] showed an accuracy for determining the N (nodal) stage of 58% for single-detector CT.[85] A recent study showed an overall accuracy of 73% but a sensitivity of only 14% for single-detector CT when the criterion of short axis being >10 mm (as indicative of metastatic nodal disease) was used; other criteria (ovoid nodal shape, clustering of nodes, absence of a fatty hilum) were not found to be useful.[86] For this reason, laparoscopic surgery and use of laparoscopic ultrasound have been suggested as a means to improve the detection of small peritoneal and hepatic metastases. Studies have shown increased sensitivity over CT for detecting peritoneal metastases.[87-89] A study by Jimenez et al.[89] showed that of 125 patients identified as having resectable disease on CT between 1994 and 1998, nearly 25% had liver or peritoneal metastases. A subsequent review of the literature by Pisters et al.[90] noted that several studies on laparoscopic staging had included patients with M0 but

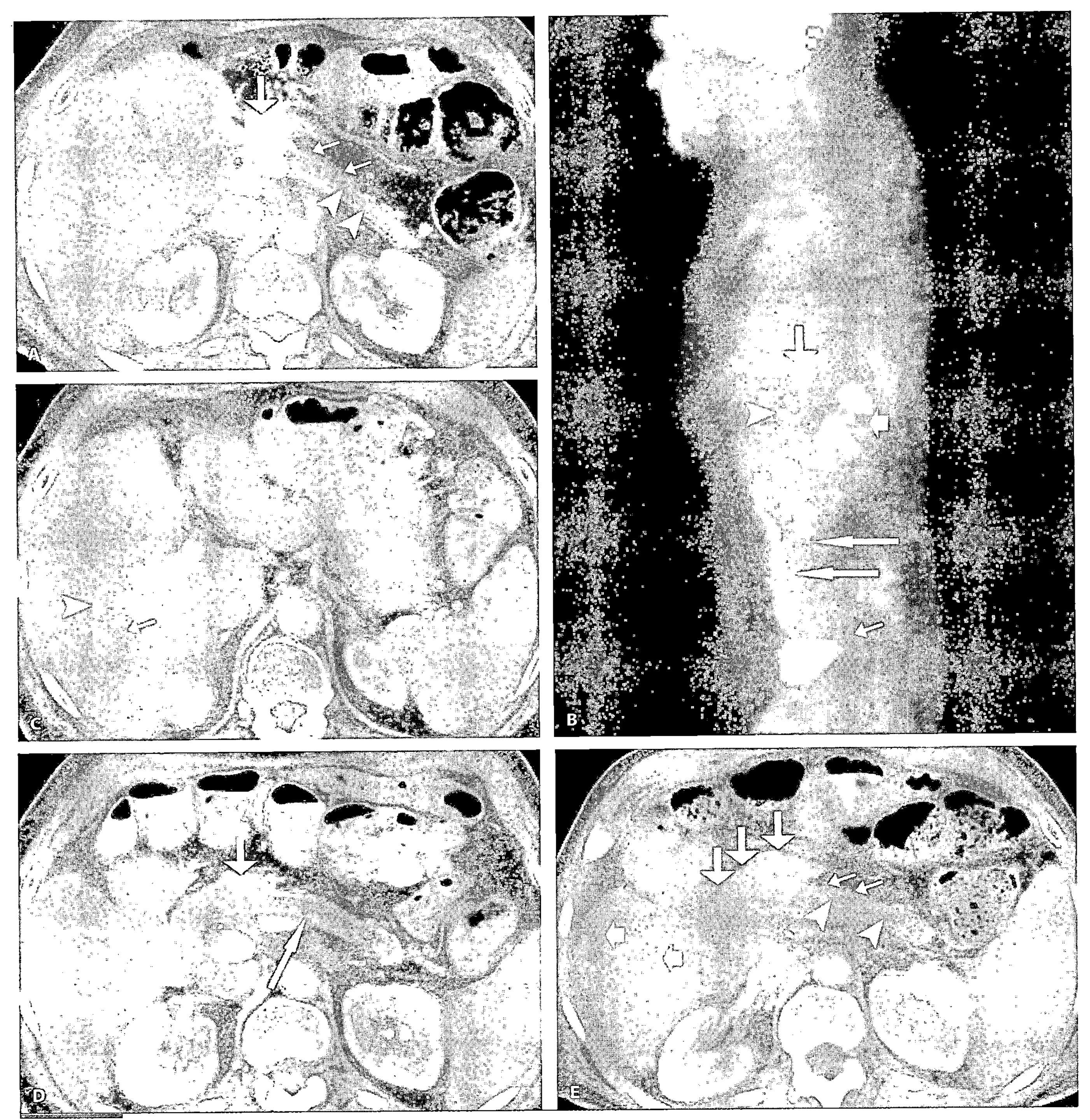

Figure 12.12
Patient who has undergone Whipple procedure for pancreatic ductal adenocarcinoma. **(A)** Axial baseline postoperative computed tomographic image shows pancreatic remnant (*small white arrows*) and dilated pancreatic duct (*white arrowheads*) anastomosed to loops of jejunum (*large white arrow*). **(B)** Sagittal positron emission tomographic image 2 years later shows abnormal increased metabolic activity within the liver (*large white arrow*) and near the pancreatic remnant (*white arrowhead*). Normal physiologic activity is identified within the kidneys (*thick white arrow*), bowel (*long white arrows*), and bladder (*small white arrow*). **(C)** and **(D)** Axial computed tomographic images confirm metastatic disease to the right lobe of liver (*white arrowhead*) with associated biliary dilatation (*small white arrow*) as well as increasing dilatation of the pancreatic duct (*long white arrow*) and possible increased prominence of soft tissue density at the pancreaticojejunostomy (*large white arrow*) at the level of the anastomosis between pancreatic remnant and jejunum. **(E)** Axial computed tomographic image from an examination 4 months after C and D shows progression of the mass at the pancreaticojejunostomy (*large white arrows*) and persistent dilatation of the pancreatic duct (*white arrowheads*) of the pancreatic remnant (*small white arrows*). Liver metastases (*thick white arrows*) and associated perfusion abnormalities have progressed in the interim as well.

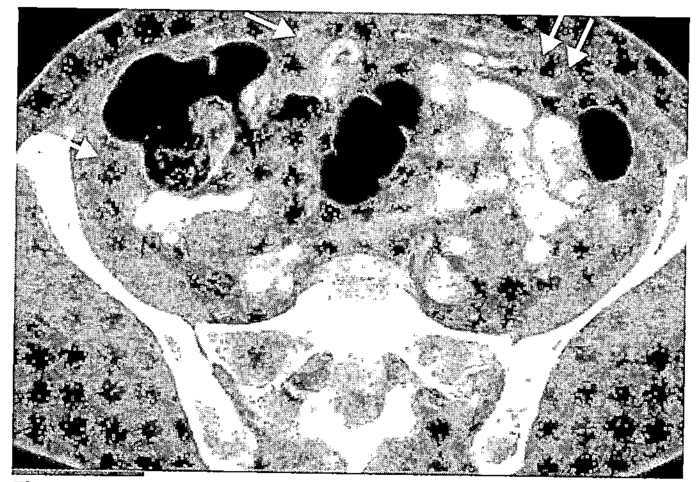

Figure 12.13
Axial image from contrast-enhanced computed tomography in patient with pancreatic cancer. Multiple peritoneal implants (*white arrows*) from widely metastatic pancreatic cancer are identified.

identifiable locally advanced disease or had used CT equipment or techniques of limited quality when compared with modern systems.[90] Pisters et al.[90] concluded that only 4%–13% of patients identified as having resectable disease on optimized CT examinations could potentially benefit from laparoscopic assessment. Another limitation of this invasive technique is that it cannot be used to monitor response to treatment.

In their study of 159 patients by PET, Diederichs et al.[82] showed a sensitivity of 49% and a specificity of 63% for lymph node staging and a detection rate of 25% for peritoneal metastases. They reported that PET missed poorly localized microscopic spread of tumor. These findings appear to be supported by the more recent study of periampullary tumors by Kalady et al.[66] who concluded that PET imaging "did not change clinical management in the vast majority of patients previously evaluated by CT." No published data are yet available on CT-PET, which would improve accuracy in localizing sites of increased FDG activity by combining the anatomic information of an unehanced CT examination with the physiologic information available with PET.

Treatment Response

At our institution, patients typically undergo chemotherapy and radiation therapy before surgery. Cross-sectional imaging, typically with CT, is used to monitor the response to therapy, as well as to evaluate for the possible progression of disease or interval development of metastases that could render a case inoperable. Patients in whom contrast-enhanced CT may be contraindicated are then evaluated by MRI. The role of PET or CT-PET has yet to be determined, but limited published data suggest that PET could be useful in the assessment of early response to therapy or in the early detection of distant metastases.[91]

Recurrence

The role of postoperative imaging is to detect complications, local recurrence, and development of distant metastases. In our institution, as in the case of monitoring treatment response, patients typically undergo imaging by CT or MRI. CT is the preferred modality at our institution, especially in patients who may be quite ill in the immediate postoperative period because of abscess, anastomotic leak, pancreatitis, or possibly intra-abdominal hemorrhage. This is because of the ability of CT to acquire images rapidly, freezing bowel, and often respiratory, motion, and because of the routine use of a water-soluble contrast agent to discriminate bowel from abscess or other extraluminal fluid collections.

The findings for tumor recurrence can be subtle (Fig. 12.12). Patients at our institution typically undergo a baseline postoperative examination to serve as a comparison for follow-up examinations to aid in the detection of small-volume recurrence. In our experience, thin-section imaging, 2.5–5 mm in thickness, can improve detection of recurrent disease in the surgical bed and can be used to provide guidance for fine-needle aspiration. PET or CT-PET may be of assistance in discriminating postoperative changes from local recurrence on the basis of metabolic activity; however, the low volume of tumor in early recurrence may not show sufficient uptake of FDG to be readily detectable. Early data suggest that PET may have utility in detecting early recurrence.[91] Further investigation into the utility of PET and CT-PET is necessary.

Conclusion

CT, MRI, and PET each have an important role in the diagnosis and staging of pancreatic cancer, the assessment of treatment response, the detection of treatment complications, and the detection of tumor recurrence. Each of these techniques continue to rapidly evolve.

References

1. Douglass HJ, Kim S, Meropol N. Neoplasms of the exocrine pancreas. In: Holland J, Frei EI, Bast RJ, eds. *Cancer Medicine*. 4th ed. Baltimore: Williams & Wilkins; 1997:1989–2018.
2. Evans DB, Abbruzzese JL, Rich T. Cancer of the pancreas. In: Devita VJ, Hellman S, Rosenberg S, eds. *Cancer Principles and Practice of Oncology*. 5th ed. Philadelphia: Lippincott-Raven; 1997:1054–1087.
3. Lowenfels A, Maisonneuve P, Boyle P. Epidemiology of pancreatic cancer. In: Howard J, Idezuki Y, Ihse I, Prinz R, eds. *Surgical Disease of the Pancreas*. 3rd ed. Baltimore: Williams & Wilkins; 1998:433–437.

4. Trede M, Schwall G, Saeger H-D. Survival after pancreatoduodenectomy. *Ann Surg*. 1990;211:447–458.
5. Tublin ME, Tessler FN, Cheng SL, Peters TL, McGovern PC. Effect of injection rate of contrast medium on pancreatic and hepatic helical CT. *Radiology*. 1999;210:97–101.
6. Kim T, Murakami T, Takahashi S, et al. Pancreatic CT imaging: effects of different injection rates and doses of contrast material. *Radiology*. 1999;212:219–225.
7. Lu D, Vedantham S, Krasny RM, et al. Two-phase helical CT for pancreatic tumors: pancreatic versus hepatic phase enhancement for tumor, pancreas and vascular structures. *Radiology*. 1996;199:697–701.
8. Boland GW, O'Malley ME, Saez M, Fernandez-del-Castillo C, Warshaw AL, Mueller PR. Pancreatic-phase versus portal vein-phase helical CT of the pancreas: optimal temporal window for evaluation of pancreatic adenocarcinoma. *AJR Am J Roentgenol*. 1999;172:605–608.
9. McNulty NJ, Francis IR, Platt JF, Cohan RH, Korobkin M, Gebremariam A. Multi-detector row helical CT of the pancreas: effect of contrast-enhanced multiphasic imaging on enhancement of the pancreas, peripancreatic vasculature, and pancreatic adenocarcinoma. *Radiology*. 2001;220:97–102.
10. Fletcher JG, Wiersema MJ, Farrell MA, et al. Pancreatic malignancy: value of arterial, pancreatic, and hepatic phase imaging with multi-detector row CT. *Radiology*. 2003;229:81–90.
11. Diehl SJ, Lehmann KJ, Sadick M, Lachmann R, Georgi M. Pancreatic cancer: value of dual-phase helical CT in assessing resectability. *Radiology*. 1998;206:373–378.
12. Ichikawa T, Haradome H, Hachiya J, Nitatori T, Araki T. Perfusion-weighted MR imaging in the upper abdomen: preliminary clinical experience in 61 patients. *AJR Am J Roentgenol*. 1997;169:1061–1066.
13. Nishiharu T, Yamashita Y, Abe Y, et al. Local extension of pancreatic carcinoma: assessment with thin-section helical CT versus with breath-hold fast MR imaging: ROC analysis. *Radiology*. 1999;212:445–452.
14. Tabuchi T, Itoh K, Ohshio G, et al. Tumor staging of pancreatic adenocarcinoma using early- and late-phase helical CT. *AJR Am J Roentgenol*. 1999;173:375–380.
15. Itoh S, Ikeda M, Ota T, Satake H, Takai K, Ishigaki T. Assessment of the pancreatic and intrapancreatic bile ducts using 0.5-mm collimation and multiplanar reformatted images in multislice CT. *Eur Radiol*. 2003;13:277–285.
16. Takeshita K, Furui S, Yamauchi T, et al. [Minimum intensity projection image and curved reformation image of the main pancreatic duct obtained by helical CT in patients with main pancreatic duct dilation]. *Nippon Igaku Hoshasen Gakkai Zasshi*. 1999;59:146–148.
17. Prokesch RW, Chow LC, Beaulieu CF, et al. Local staging of pancreatic carcinoma with multi-detector row CT: use of curved planar reformations initial experience. *Radiology*. 2002;225:759–765.
18. Lepanto L, Arzoumanian Y, Gianfelice D, et al. Helical CT with CT angiography in assessing periampullary neoplasms: identification of vascular invasion. *Radiology*. 2002;222:347–352.
19. Fishman EK, Horton KM, Urban BA. Multidetector CT angiography in the evaluation of pancreatic carcinoma: preliminary observations. *J Comput Assist Tomogr*. 2000;24:849–853.
20. Fishman EK. From the RSNA refresher courses: CT angiography: clinical applications in the abdomen. *Radiographics*. 2001;21:S3–S16.
21. Stabile Ianora AA, Scardapane A, Midiri M, Rotondo A, Angelelli G. [Pre- and postoperative study of the bile ducts with spiral computerized tomography]. *Radiol Med (Torino)*. 2000;100:152–159.
22. Caoili EM, Paulson EK, Heyneman LE, et al. Helical CT cholangiography with three-dimensional volume rendering using an oral biliary contrast agent: feasibility of a novel technique. *AJR Am J Roentgenol*. 2000;174:487–492.
23. Johnson PT, Heath DG, Hofmann LV, Horton KM, Fishman EK. Multidetector-row computed tomography with three-dimensional volume rendering of pancreatic cancer: a complete preoperative staging tool using computed tomography angiography and volume-rendered cholangiopancreatography. *J Comput Assist Tomogr*. 2003;27:347–353.
24. Hong KC, Freeny PC. Pancreaticoduodenal arcades and dorsal pancreatic artery: comparison of CT angiography with three-dimensional volume rendering, maximum intensity projection, and shaded-surface display. *AJR Am J Roentgenol*. 1999;172:925–931.
25. Graf O, Boland GW, Kaufman JA, Warshaw AL, Fernandez del Castillo C, Mueller PR. Anatomic variants of mesenteric veins: depiction with helical CT venography. *AJR Am J Roentgenol*. 1997;168:1209–1213.
26. Raptopoulos V, Prassopoulos P, Chuttani R, McNicholas MM, McKee JD, Kressel HY. Multiplanar CT pancreatography and distal cholangiography with minimum intensity projections. *Radiology*. 1998;207:317–324.
27. Park SJ, Han JK, Kim TK, Choi BI. Three-dimensional spiral CT cholangiography with minimum intensity projection in patients with suspected obstructive biliary disease: comparison with percutaneous transhepatic cholangiography. *Abdom Imaging*. 2001;26:281–286.
28. Murakami T, Tsuda K, Nakamura H, et al. 3DFT-flash MR imaging of pancreatic cancer with gadopentetate dimeglumine. *Acta Radiol*. 1996;37:190–194.
29. Irie H, Honda H, Kaneko K, Kuroiwa T, Yoshimitsu K, Masuda K. Comparison of helical CT and MR imaging in detecting and staging small pancreatic adenocarcinoma. *Abdom Imaging*. 1997;22:429–433.
30. Ichikawa T, Haradome H, Hachiya J, et al. Pancreatic ductal adenocarcinoma: preoperative assessment with helical CT versus dynamic MR imaging. *Radiology*. 1997;202:655–662.
31. Tervahartiala P, Kivisaari L, Lamminen A, Maschek A, Wohling H, Standertskjold-Nordenstam CG. Dynamic fast-gradient echo MR imaging of pancreatic tumours. *Eur J Radiol*. 1997;25:74–80.
32. Murakami K, Nawano S, Moriyama N, Onuma Y. Usefulness of magnetic resonance imaging with dynamic contrast enhancement and fat suppression in detecting a pancreatic tumor. *Jpn J Clin Oncol*. 1998;28:107–111.
33. Sheridan MB, Ward J, Guthrie JA, et al. Dynamic contrast-enhanced MR imaging and dual-phase helical CT in the preoperative assessment of suspected pancreatic cancer: a

comparative study with receiver operating characteristic analysis. *AJR Am J Roentgenol.* 1999;173:583–590.
34. Spencer JA, Ward J, Guthrie JA, Guillou PJ, Robinson PJ. Assessment of resectability of pancreatic cancer with dynamic contrast-enhanced MR imaging: technique, surgical correlation and patient outcome. *Eur Radiol.* 1998;8:23–29.
35. Kettritz U, Warshauer DM, Brown ED, Schlund JF, Eisenberg LB, Semelka RC. Enhancement of the normal pancreas: comparison of manganese-DPDP and gadolinium chelate. *Eur Radiol.* 1996;6:14–18.
36. Papanikolaou N, Karantanas AH, Heracleous E, Costa JC, Gourtsoyiannis N. Magnetic resonance cholangiopancreatography: comparison between respiratory-triggered turbo spin echo and breath hold single-shot turbo spin echo sequences. *Magn Reson Imaging.* 1999;17:1255–1260.
37. Fulcher AS, Turner MA. Magnetic resonance pancreatography (MRP). *Crit Rev Diagn Imaging.* 1999;40:285–322.
38. Takehara Y. Fast MR imaging for evaluating the pancreaticobiliary system. *Eur J Radiol.* 1999;29:211–232.
39. Wielopolski PA, Gaa J, Wielopolski DR, Oudkerk M. Breath-hold MR cholangiopancreatography with three-dimensional, segmented, echo-planar imaging and volume rendering. *Radiology.* 1999;210:247–252.
40. Fulcher AS, Turner MA. MR pancreatography: a useful tool for evaluating pancreatic disorders. *Radiographics.* 1999;19:5–24; discussion 41–44; quiz 148–149.
41. Irie H, Honda H, Tajima T, et al. Optimal MR cholangiopancreatographic sequence and its clinical application. *Radiology.* 1998;206:379–387.
42. Yamashita Y, Abe Y, Tang Y, Urata J, Sumi S, Takahashi M. In vitro and clinical studies of image acquisition in breath-hold MR cholangiopancreatography: single-shot projection technique versus multislice technique. *AJR Am J Roentgenol.* 1997;168:1449–1454.
43. Masui T, Takehara Y, Ichijo K, et al. Evaluation of the pancreas: a comparison of single thick-slice MR cholangiopancreatography with multiple thin-slice volume reconstruction MR cholangiopancreatography. *AJR Am J Roentgenol.* 1999;173:1519–1526.
44. Diederichs CG, Shreve PD. Pancreatic cancer. In: Wieler HJ, Coleman RE, eds. *PET in Clinical Oncology.* Darmstadt: Steinkopff Verlag; 2000:211–224.
45. Steinert HC, Kubik-Huch R, Kacl G. Tumors of the abdomen and pelvis. In: von Schulthess GK, ed. *Clinical Positron Emission Tomography: Correlation with Morphological Cross-Sectional Imaging.* Philadelphia: Lippincott Williams & Wilkins; 2000:195–206.
46. Prokesch RW, Chow LC, Beaulieu CF, Bammer R, Jeffrey RB Jr. Isoattenuating pancreatic adenocarcinoma at multidetector row CT: secondary signs. *Radiology.* 2002;224:764–768.
47. Choi BI, Chung MJ, Han JK, Han MC, Yoon YB. Detection of pancreatic adenocarcinoma: relative value of arterial and late phases of spiral CT. *Abdom Imaging.* 1997;22:199–203.
48. Legmann P, Vignaux O, Dousset B, et al. Pancreatic tumors: comparison of dual-phase helical CT and endoscopic sonography. *AJR Am J Roentgenol.* 1998;170:1315–1322.
49. Gabata T, Matsui O, Kadoya M. Small pancreatic adenocarcinomas: efficacies of MR imaging with fat suppression and gadolinium enhancement. *Radiology.* 1994;193:683–688.
50. Semelka R, Kelekis N, Molina P. Pancreatic masses with inconclusive findings on spiral CT: is there a role for MRI? *J Magn Reson Imag.* 1996;6:585–588.
51. Bret PM, Reinhold C, Taourel P, et al. Evaluation with MR pancreatography. *Radiology.* 1996;199:521–527.
52. Buetow PC, Parrino TV, Buck JL, et al. Pathologic-imaging correlation among size, necrosis and cysts, calcification, malignant behavior and functional status. *AJR Am J Roentgenol.* 1995;165:1175–1179.
53. Semelka RC, Cummings M, Shoenut JP, et al. MRI of the pancreas—state of the art. *Radiology.* 1993;188:593–602.
54. Semelka RC, Simm FC, Recht M, et al. MRI of the pancreas at high field strength: a comparison of six sequences. *J Comput Asssist Tomogr.* 1991;15:966–971.
55. Gehl HB, Urhahn R, Bohndorf K, et al. Mn-DPDP in MR imaging of pancreatic adenocarcinoma: initial clinical experience. *Radiology.* 1993;186:795–798.
56. Romijn MG, Stoker J, van Eijck CH, van Muiswinkel JM, Torres CG, Lameris JS. MRI with mangafodipir trisodium in the detection and staging of pancreatic cancer. *J Magn Reson Imaging.* 2000;12:261–268.
57. Schima W, Fugger R, Schober E, et al. Diagnosis and staging of pancreatic cancer: comparison of mangafodipir trisodium-enhanced MR imaging and contrast-enhanced helical hydro-CT. *AJR Am J Roentgenol.* 2002;179:717–724.
58. Rieber A, Tomczak R, Nussle K, Klaus H, Brambs HJ. MRI with mangafodipir trisodium in the detection of pancreatic tumours: comparison with helical CT. *Br J Radiol.* 2000;73:1165–1169.
59. Vitellas KM, Keogan MT, Spritzer CE, Nelson RC. MR cholangiopancreatography of bile and pancreatic duct abnormalities with emphasis on the single-shot fast spin-echo technique. *Radiographics.* 2000;20:939–957; quiz 1107–1108, 1112.
60. Diederichs CG, Staib L, Glatting G, et al. Differentiation of malignant and benign pancreatic disease [abstract]. *J Nucl Med.* 1997;38:257P.
61. Diederichs CG, Staib L, Glatting G, Beger HG, Reske SN. FDG PET: elevated plasma glucose reduces both uptake and detection rate of pancreatic malignancies. *J Nucl Med.* 1998;39:1030–1033.
62. Zimny M, Bares R, Fass J, et al. Fluorine-18 fluorodeoxyglucose positron emission tomography in the differential diagnosis of pancreatic carcinoma: a report of 106 cases. *Eur J Nucl Med.* 1997;24:678–682.
63. Nitzsche EU, Hoegerle S, Mix M, et al. Non-invasive differentiation of pancreatic lesions: is analysis of FDG kinetics superior to semiquantitative uptake value analysis? *Eur J Nucl Med.* 2002;29:237–242.
64. Zimny M, Buell U. 18FDG-positron emission tomography in pancreatic cancer. *Ann Oncol.* 1999;10[suppl 49]:S28–S32.
65. Nakamoto Y, Higashi T, Sakahara H, et al. Delayed (18)F-fluoro-2-deoxy-D-glucose positron emission tomography scan for differentiation between malignant and benign lesions in the pancreas. *Cancer.* 2000;89:2547–2554.

66. Kalady MF, Clary BM, Clark LA, et al. Clinical utility of positron emission tomography in the diagnosis and management of periampullary neoplasms. *Ann Surg Oncol.* 2002;9:799–806.
67. Zimny M, Schumpelick V. [Fluorodeoxyglucose positron emission tomography (FDG-PET) in the differential diagnosis of pancreatic lesions]. *Chirurgie.* 2001;72:989–994.
68. Loyer EM, David CL, Dubrow RA, Evans DB, Charnsangavej C. Vascular involvement in pancreatic adenocarcinoma: reassessment by thin-section CT. *Abdom Imaging.* 1996;21:202–206.
69. Lu DS, Reber HA, Krasny RM, Kadell BM, Sayre J. Local staging of pancreatic cancer: criteria for unresectability of major vessels as revealed by pancreatic-phase, thin-section helical CT. *AJR Am J Roentgenol.* 1997;168:1439–1443.
70. O'Malley ME, Boland GW, Wood BJ, Fernandez-del Castillo C, Warshaw AL, Mueller PR. Adenocarcinoma of the head of the pancreas: determination of surgical unresectability with thin-section pancreatic-phase helical CT. *AJR Am J Roentgenol.* 1999;173:1513–1518.
71. Phoa SS, Reeders JW, Stoker J, Rauws EA, Gouma DJ, Lameris JS. CT criteria for venous invasion in patients with pancreatic head carcinoma. *Br J Radiol.* 2000;73:1159–1164.
72. Valls C, Andia E, Sanchez A, et al. Dual-phase helical CT of pancreatic adenocarcinoma: assessment of resectability before surgery. *AJR Am J Roentgenol.* 2002;178:821–826.
73. McCarthy MJ, Evans J, Sagar G, Neoptolemos JP. Prediction of resectability of pancreatic malignancy by computed tomography. *Br J Surg.* 1998;85:320–325.
74. Sironi S, De Cobelli F, Zerbi A, et al. Pancreatic adenocarcinoma: assessment of vascular invasion with high-field MR imaging and a phased-array coil. *AJR Am J Roentgenol.* 1996;167:997–1001.
75. Arslan A, Buanes T, Geitung JT. Pancreatic carcinoma: MR, MR angiography and dynamic helical CT in the evaluation of vascular invasion. *Eur J Radiol.* 2001;38:151–159.
76. Hochwald S, Rofsky N, Dobryansky M. Magnetic resonance imaging with magnetic resonance cholangiopancreatography accurately predicts resectability of pancreatic carcinoma. *J Gastrointest Surg.* 1999;3:506–511.
77. Trede M, Rumstadt B, Wendl K, et al. Ultrafast magnetic resonance imaging improves the staging of pancreatic tumors. *Ann Surg.* 1997;226:393–405; discussion 405–407.
78. Richter GM, Simon C, Hoffmann V, et al. [Hydrospiral CT of the pancreas in thin section technique]. *Radiologe.* 1996;36:397–405.
79. Calculli L, Casadei R, Diacono D, et al. [Role of spiral computerized tomography in the staging of pancreatic carcinoma]. *Radiol Med (Torino).* 1998;95:344–348.
80. Megibow A, Zhou X, Rotterdam H, et al. Pancreatic adenocarcinoma: CT versus MR imaging in the evaluation of resectability: Report of the Radiology Diagnostic Oncology Group. *Radiology.* 1995;195:327–332.
81. Freeny P, Marks W, Ryan JA. Pancreatic ductal adenocarcinoma: diagnosis and staging with dynamic CT. *Radiology.* 1988;166:125–133.
82. Diederichs CG, Staib L, Vogel J, et al. Values and limitations of 18F-fluorodeoxyglucose-positron-emission tomography with preoperative evaluation of patients with pancreatic masses. *Pancreas.* 2000;20:109–116.
83. Frohlich A, Diederichs CG, Staib L, Vogel J, Beger HG, Reske SN. Detection of liver metastases from pancreatic cancer using FDG PET. *J Nucl Med.* 1999;40:250–255.
84. Murakami K, Nawano S, Moriyama N, et al. [Staging of pancreatic ductal adenocarcinoma using dynamic MR imaging]. *Nippon Igaku Hoshasen Gakkai Zasshi.* 1997;57:596–601.
85. Zeman RK, Cooper C, Zeiberg AS, et al. TNM staging of pancreatic carcinoma using helical CT. *AJR Am J Roentgenol.* 1997;169:459–464.
86. Roche CJ, Hughes ML, Garvey CJ, et al. CT and pathologic assessment of prospective nodal staging in patients with ductal adenocarcinoma of the head of the pancreas. *AJR Am J Roentgenol.* 2003;180:475–480.
87. van Delden OM, de Wit LT, Nieveen van Dijkum EJ, Reeders JW, Gouma DJ. Laparoscopic ultrasonography for abdominal tumor staging. *Eur Radiol.* 1998;8:1405–1408.
88. Jimenez RE, Warshaw AL, Fernandez-Del Castillo C. Laparoscopy and peritoneal cytology in the staging of pancreatic cancer. *J Hepatobiliary Pancreat Surg.* 2000;7:15–20.
89. Jimenez RE, Warshaw AL, Rattner DW, Willett CG, McGrath D, Fernandez-del Castillo C. Impact of laparoscopic staging in the treatment of pancreatic cancer. *Arch Surg.* 2000;135:409–414; discussion 414–415.
90. Pisters PW, Lee JE, Vauthey JN, Charnsangavej C, Evans DB. Laparoscopy in the staging of pancreatic cancer. *Br J Surg.* 2001;88:325–337.
91. Rose DM, Delbeke D, Beauchamp RD, et al. 18Fluorodeoxyglucose-positron emission tomography in the management of patients with suspected pancreatic cancer. *Ann Surg.* 1999;229:729–737; discussion 737–738.

CHAPTER

13

Endoscopic Staging: EUS, ERCP

Richard A. Erickson, MD

The advances in cross-sectional imaging made in the last decade by spiral computed tomography (CT) and magnetic resonance imaging (MRI) have been impressive. These technologies have rightly become the cornerstones of abdominal imaging, especially in patients with suspected pancreatic cancer. However, endoscopic procedures, such as endoscopic retrograde cholangiopancreatography (ERCP) and endoscopic ultrasound (EUS), continue to play an important and sometimes central role in many of these patients (Table 13.1). In fact, before the advent of high-resolution CT and MRI, ERCP was the primary diagnostic procedure in the evaluation of pancreatic neoplasms.[1,2] Now, the primary utility of ERCP is therapeutic in patients with pancreatic cancer and obstructive jaundice or to help diagnose lesions that are difficult to diagnose, such as intraductal papillary mucinous tumors (IPMT) of the pancreas. On the other hand, where high-quality EUS is readily available, it is often a very useful procedure because it simultaneously provides primary diagnosis, biopsy, and important staging information for patients with pancreatic cancer.[3] Assessing the most appropriate roles for CT, MRI, EUS, and ERCP in the diagnosis, staging, and treatment of pancreatic cancer is difficult. The technologies for each procedure are changing so quickly that comparative studies are rapidly out of date relative to state-of-the-art techniques. In addition, few institutions have the same level of expertise in each procedure to make truly comparative studies. Finally, they are in practice quite different procedures performed by radiologists versus gastroenterologists, such that only parts of the capabilities of each procedure are truly comparable in studies. Thus, deciding which algorithms to use in the management of the pancreatic cancer patient often depends more on local expertise, interest, and equipment than on published comparative data.

Endoscopic Ultrasound

Technologic Issues

EUS was developed by placing small, high-frequency ultrasound transducers on the tips of fiberoptic and subsequently video endoscopes.[4] A variety of transducer designs have been used, but the two main varieties are a 360-degree rotating radial array and nonmoving, convex linear, and radial array transducers. By placing the transducer within the gut lumen, EUS overcomes the two major technologic problems for pancreatic imaging by transcutaneous ultrasound: obscuring overlying gas-filled bowel and the necessity to use low-frequency and therefore low-resolution ultrasound to penetrate to the depth of the pancreas. With

Table 13.1 Summary of EUS and ERCP Utilities for Pancreatic Cancer

	EUS	ERCP
Primary diagnosis	Nearly 100%	>90% with ductal neoplasms
Tissue diagnosis	80%–93%	~ 50%
Staging	About 80% accurate at T staging Only 60%–80% accurate at nodal staging Occasional M-staging information from finding occult liver metastases, remote nodal disease, or malignant ascites	Does not generally add new staging information
Therapeutic applications	Celiac neurolysis EUS-guided tumor injection	Placement of biliary stents Pancreatic stents for relief of pain from pancreatic obstruction
Special advantages	Biopsy of pancreatic head lesions includes potential resection tract Assessment of venous involvement around portal, SMV, and splenic venous confluence Detection and biopsy of occult metastatic disease Screening in familial pancreatic cancer	Diagnosis of IPMT Intraductal ultrasonography, peroral pancreatography, and biopsy
Special disadvantages	Technically difficult Poor at assessing tumor involvement of SMA and at detecting deep mesenteric adenopathy	Technically difficult High morbidity

Abbreviations: ERCP, endoscopic retrograde cholangiopancreatography; EUS, endoscopic ultrasound; IPMT, intraductal papillary mucinous tumor; SMV, superior mesenteric vein; SMA, superior mesenteric artery.

the use of ultrasonic imaging through the stomach and duodenum, the whole of the pancreas can be brought to within a few centimeters of a 5- to 20-MHz ultrasound transducer, providing resolutions in the few tenths of millimeter range. Like transcutaneous ultrasound, EUS is a "live" procedure that offers the advantage of being an interactive examination of the pancreas and surrounding tissues, where subtle abnormalities can be imaged by the endoscopist from different perspectives and at different frequencies and ultimately cytologically sampled, if necessary. In addition, as clinicians, endosonographers usually have the advantage of bringing much more clinical information to the procedure than the typical radiologist has in performing an abdominal CT or MRI. Furthermore, EUS now allows combining of the biopsy (EUS-guided fine-needle aspiration [FNA]) and therapeutic capabilities of EUS (e.g., tumor injection therapy or celiac neurolysis) with the initial diagnostic procedure. Finally, when EUS is combined with its sister endoscopic procedure, therapeutic ERCP, it results in a powerfully efficient combination of diagnostic, staging, and therapeutic techniques that are very difficult to match with any other set of procedures.

The first echoendoscopes were developed in the early 1980s.[5,6] Commercial radial echoendoscopes became available in the mid- to late 1980s, offering a 360-degree view of the gastrointestinal tract wall and surrounding structures, with imaging depths of about 12 cm from the endoscope tip. By the early 1990s, echoendoscopes with curved-linear array ultrasonic transducers were produced.[7] These so-called linear echoendoscopes have the ultrasound transducer imaging in the plane of the biopsy channel of the echoendoscope. This modification resulted in a significant advance in the utility of EUS because needles could be precisely directed in "real time" into lesions, resulting in EUS-guided FNA (EUS-FNA).[8-13] Curved-linear array instruments also have color flow and Doppler capabilities, which often permit better assessment of vascular anatomy during procedures. EUS-FNA techniques have advanced from a few tentative case reports and series in the early 1990s[14-16] to its current role of providing the primary means of tissue diagnosis of pancreatic neoplasms in many institutions.[8,13] Like transcutaneous ultrasound, CT, and MRI, EUS imaging has advanced with improvements in the computing power.

EUS is obviously, by its very nature, more invasive than CT or MRI. It is performed, as are most endoscopic procedures, with the use of conscious sedation with a benzodiazepine (e.g., midazolam) and a narcotic (e.g., meperi-

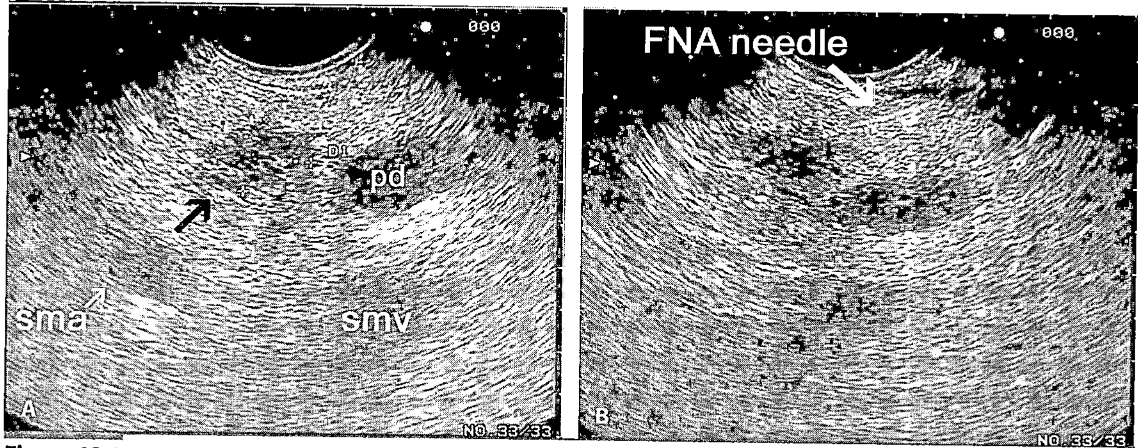

Figure 13.1
(A) Linear EUS image of a small 12- × 9-mm pancreatic head adenocarcinoma (*arrow*) presenting with mild biliary obstruction (T1N0M0) and not visible to multidetector, dual-phase, spiral computed tomography. **(B)** EUS-FNA of lesion showed moderately differentiated adenocarcinoma. All radial images were produced using the Olympus UM20 or UM130 echoendoscope at 7.5 MHz, and all linear images were produced using the Pentax FG-36UX echoendoscope at 7.5 MHz. EUS, endoscopic ultrasound; FNA, fine-needle aspiration; pd, pancreatic duct; sma, superior mesenteric artery; smv, superior mesenteric vein.

dine or fentanyl). There has also been considerable recent interest in using propofol for endoscopic sedation in long procedures, such as EUS and ERCP.[17] The major morbidity of EUS is similar (0.05%) to that of diagnostic endoscopy.[4] A possible exception to this is gut perforation, which may be higher than standard endoscopy because of the more rigid tips of echoendoscopes.[9,10,18] This is especially true when endosonographers try to force an echoendoscope around a duodenum stenosed by a pancreatic neoplasm.[19] However, despite the increased perforation risk, EUS is much less morbid than its counterpart endoscopic procedure, ERCP, which has a 5%–10% risk of major morbidity, primarily pancreatitis. In the United States, the charges for diagnostic EUS are generally at the level of a therapeutic colonoscopy and are similar to those of a therapeutic ERCP for EUS-FNA. EUS also has a long learning curve,[20] especially in the area of pancreatic cancer diagnosis, EUS-FNA, and staging.[21]

Diagnosis of Pancreatic Neoplasms

The utility of EUS in visualizing pancreatic neoplasms was apparent soon after its clinical introduction in the mid-1980s in Japan[22] and Germany.[23] Since then, many series have demonstrated the superiority of EUS over CT and MRI in the diagnosis of pancreatic disorders and especially neoplasms.[8-13,24-26] Even for lesions less than 3 cm, EUS diagnosis rates have been consistently in the range of 95%–100%. Another powerful aspect of EUS is that its specificity for ruling out pancreatic neoplasia is nearly 100%, as long as the patient does not have underlying chronic pancreatitis.[27] Although ERCP is not generally used anymore as a diagnostic technique for pancreatic neoplasms, EUS is also superior to ERCP in the diagnosis of small pancreatic neoplasms,[3] although they have similar sensitivities in detecting pancreatic head lesions.[28]

With the advent of multidetector, high-speed spiral CT, the advantage of EUS over CT in the diagnosis of pancreatic cancer is narrowing (see Chapter 12). Series comparing state-of-the-art helical CT with high-quality EUS are still few.[27] Spiral CT has overall detection rates of greater than 90%; however, EUS still seems to be superior at detecting small (<2 to 3 cm) pancreatic carcinomas[29] (Fig. 13.1, A and B).

Numerous problems confound series comparing EUS and CT. Rarely do institutions have similar levels of expertise in both procedures. In addition, in almost all series, the endosonographers are not blinded to the results of prior imaging or clinical information, whereas radiologists rarely have access to the EUS information because it is usually performed after CT.[30] Clinical assessment has an accuracy similar to that of imaging procedures in patients with suspected pancreatic cancer.[31] Patient groups may also not be the same when studies of the two procedures are compared. In endosonographic series, patients presenting with metastatic liver disease (about one third of patients) or large, unresectable tumors are generally not included, because there is little indication for EUS in these patients. However, these patients are often included in series assessing the diagnostic accuracy of CT.[32,33] This inclusion can increase the overall diagnostic sensitivity of CT in pancreatic cancer detection by 5%–15% compared with series focused only on those patients undergoing both EUS and CT.[34]

There are few comparative data for EUS versus MRI in pancreatic cancer.[18] Because series comparing CT with MRI for the detection of pancreatic masses (see Chapter 12) show CT to have a slight advantage over MRI, it would be reasonable to presume that EUS is superior to MRI at least for small masses. MRI has the additional advantage of being able to show ductal anatomy using magnetic resonance cholangiopancreatography.

When patients have underlying chronic pancreatitis, all diagnostic modalities (CT, MRI, EUS, ERCP, and positron emission tomography) are poor at detecting a superimposed pancreatic malignancy. EUS rarely misses pancreatic neoplasm when the pancreas is normal; however, this is not the case when chronic pancreatitis is present.[14,24,25,35-37] When faced with this kind of patient, one has to use multiple diagnostic modalities, such as FNA,[38] tumor markers,[39] close clinical follow-up, and occasionally empiric resection[40] to find underlying pancreatic cancers in chronic pancreatitis. Molecular diagnostic techniques on FNA specimens may hold some promise in this area.[41,42]

Despite the superior diagnostic capabilities of EUS, the frequency of its use in patients with suspected pancreatic neoplasms in the United States is still disappointingly low.[8-13] This is a multifactorial problem. Initially, this problem was primarily caused by a lack of expert endosonographers at many institutions. However, in the past few years, high-quality EUS has become available at most major institutions caring for significant volumes of patients with cancer. Education of primary care practitioners, oncologists, radiologists, and surgeons about the capabilities of EUS and its appropriate role in patients with suspected pancreatic cancer is a priority.

EUS-Guided Fine-Needle Aspiration

Technique The first EUS-FNA of a pancreatic cancer was reported in 1994,[16] and there have been numerous series since then.[8,25,35,37,43-54] EUS-FNA techniques have been described extensively elsewhere[37,48,51,55,56] and involve passing an 18- to 25- (usually 22-) gauge stainless steel, echogenic aspiration needle through the biopsy port of an echoendoscope under real-time guidance into an endosonographically visualized pancreatic mass, lymph node, liver metastasis, or fluid collection (Fig. 13.2, B, C, E, and G). The needle is moved back and forth through the lesion with varying degrees of suction applied to it, and the sample is deposited on a cytology slide or slides for immediate staining and cytopathologic examination.

Yield EUS-FNA can provide a cytologic diagnosis in 80%–93% or more of pancreatic malignancies,[8,25,35,37,43-56] even in patients with previously negative attempts at tissue diagnosis.[57] As with FNA techniques in other organs,[58] the diagnostic yield of EUS-FNA depends on the technique used,[56] especially the training of the endosonographer[60] and the active involvement of a cytopathologist.[60] Having a cytopathologist available in the room or close enough to give immediate feedback on the adequacy and preliminary cytologic diagnosis of an aspirate is a common clinical practice in endosonography centers in the United States.[19,35,37,43,44,47-50,60] Cytopathologic feedback during the EUS-FNA probably increases the yield of a definitive cytologic diagnosis by about 10%.[37,46,50,60] As long as the lesion is visible, similar definitive cytologic yields are possible with transcutaneous ultrasound or CT-guided FNA of pancreatic masses, especially if a cytopathologist participates in the procedure. However, because EUS still seems superior for small lesions, the net overall yield of a definitive cytologic diagnosis is higher with EUS-FNA than with CT-guided techniques. An additional advantage of EUS-FNA is that because it is a real-time procedure, when an abnormality is found in the pancreas, one can proceed directly on to FNA at that time rather than scheduling a separate procedure, as with CT. This may just be a matter of patient inconvenience in an ambulatory setting, but it may add additional days of hospitalization for inpatients. False-positive EUS-FNA cytologic results of pancreatic samples do occur rarely, mainly because of interpretation errors.[61]

It takes an average of three to four passes to provide a definitive cytologic diagnosis of a pancreatic malignancy.[37,46,57,59,62] However, malignant lymph nodes and liver metastases generally require only one or two EUS-FNA passes for a definitive diagnosis.[37] There are no clinical or endosonographic features that predict when a patient's lesion may take more FNA passes to make a diagnosis. The major determinant of FNA pass number is the differentiation of the tumor,[37,63] with some masses taking up to 10 or more passes or more to make a definitive diagnosis in well-differentiated tumors.[64] If a cytopathologist is not immediately available, generally five to six passes into the lesion are recommended, but this approach may still result in a nondiagnostic specimen 15%–20% of the time.[37,55] Larger needles and "Tru-Cut" designs have been used obtain actual tissue biopsies[65-67];

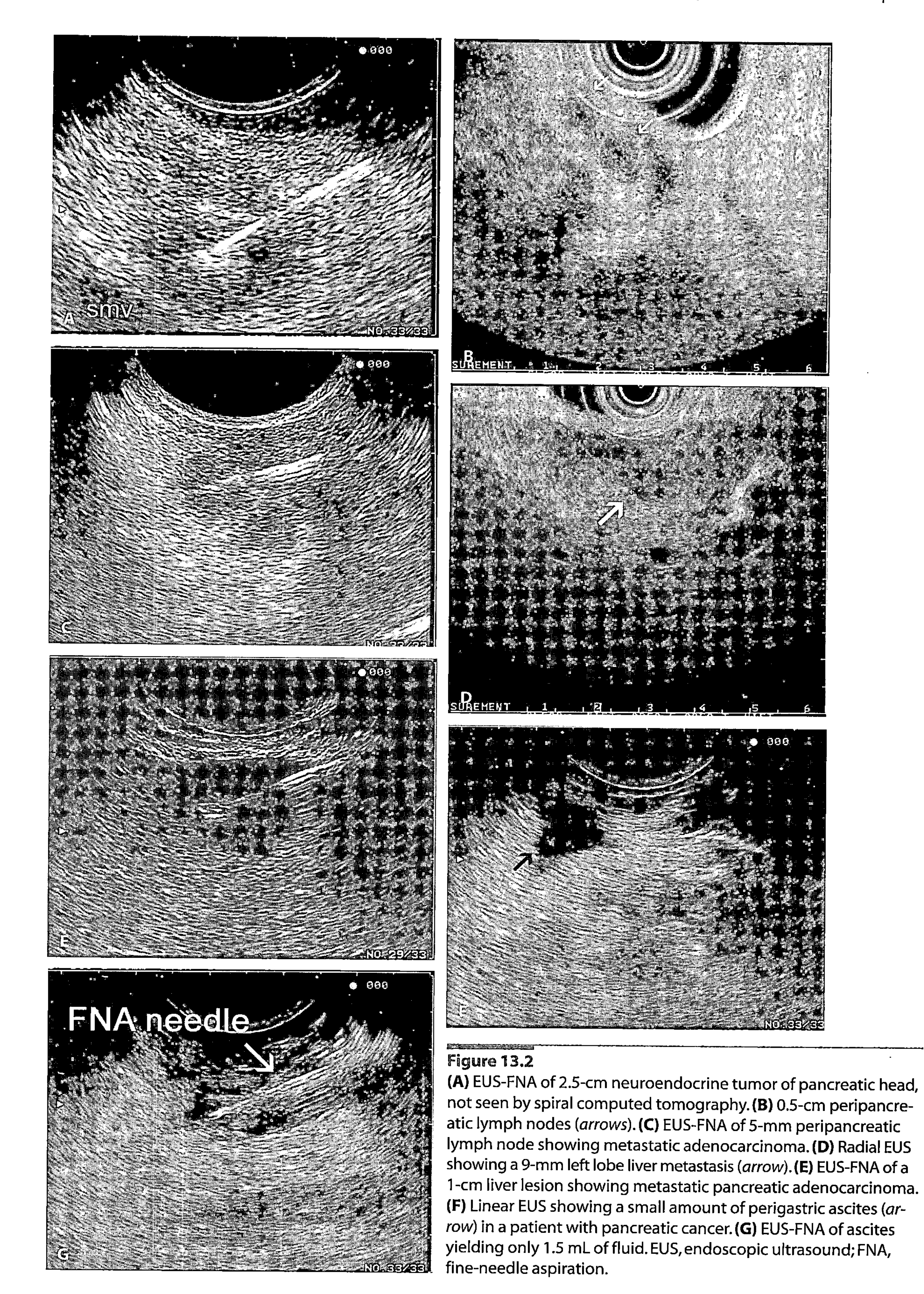

Figure 13.2

(A) EUS-FNA of 2.5-cm neuroendocrine tumor of pancreatic head, not seen by spiral computed tomography. **(B)** 0.5-cm peripancreatic lymph nodes (*arrows*). **(C)** EUS-FNA of 5-mm peripancreatic lymph node showing metastatic adenocarcinoma. **(D)** Radial EUS showing a 9-mm left lobe liver metastasis (*arrow*). **(E)** EUS-FNA of a 1-cm liver lesion showing metastatic pancreatic adenocarcinoma. **(F)** Linear EUS showing a small amount of perigastric ascites (*arrow*) in a patient with pancreatic cancer. **(G)** EUS-FNA of ascites yielding only 1.5 mL of fluid. EUS, endoscopic ultrasound; FNA, fine-needle aspiration.

however, these larger needles have failed to significantly improve diagnostic accuracy,[67,68] except perhaps in the case of unusual histology.[56] Using cell surface markers also makes it possible to make a cytologic characterization of pancreatic lymphomas, as long as enough cells are obtained.[69,70] EUS-FNA of cystic tumors of the pancreas present special challenges because cytology is often nondiagnostic and must be supplemented by chemical analysis of fluid for tumor markers, such as carcinoembryonic antigen or CA19-9 and amylase.[71-75]

Whether a cytologic diagnosis is necessary in all patients with a pancreatic mass visualized by EUS, CT, MRI, or ERCP is a topic of significant debate,[8-13,76] with some physicians[77,78] believing that attempts at obtaining a tissue diagnosis in potentially resectable pancreatic masses do not change management and therefore are of little use. Other physicians[34,79] believe there are numerous rationales for attempting to make a preoperative tissue diagnosis in all of these patients.

Complications The overall complication rate of EUS-FNA is approximately 0.5%–3%,[8,19,25,35,37,43-57,62] similar to that reported with CT or ultrasound-guided FNA or biopsy.[80-82] The major complications reported with EUS-FNA are pancreatitis[83] and bleeding,[55,84] with rare deaths having been reported from cholangitis associated with biopsy of a liver metastasis in a patient with poorly drained biliary obstruction from a pancreatic cancer[85] and uncontrolled bleeding from a pseudoaneurysm.[47] Bile peritonitis[86] and acute portal vein thrombosis[87] have also been reported with pancreatic EUS-FNA. As of yet, there have been no published cases of peritoneal seeding with EUS-FNA; however, seeding has been reported with CT-guided biopsy or ultrasound-guided biopsy.[88] In addition, a recent study reported peritoneal recurrence significantly higher in patients having had CT or ultrasound-guided pancreatic biopsy than with EUS-FNA.[89] Clinically significant bacteremia following EUS-FNA is rare[90]; however, EUS-FNA of cystic lesions may have a higher risk complication due to the risk of infecting the cyst with luminal bacteria.[91] Because of this, intravenous antibiotics with oral antibiotics are routinely used for a few days for EUS-FNA of pancreatic cystic lesions.[8-13,71,73,75] In addition, we use transluminal povidone-iodine solution to minimize bacterial contamination during EUS-FNA of cystic pancreatic lesions.[92]

Pancreatic Cancer Staging

Overview The primary impact of endosonography on the management of pancreatic cancer is in detection and cytologic diagnosis. Early in its introduction, there was considerable excitement about the use of EUS as an accurate staging tool in these patients.[8-13,21,93-95] However, more recent studies[30,96] have tempered the initial enthusiasm for EUS as a staging procedure. In addition, the progressive technologic advances in cross-sectional imaging have largely overshadowed many of the perceived advantages of EUS staging. Despite this, EUS does provide some potentially unique staging information in patients with pancreatic cancer, primarily in the detection of occult metastatic disease and in the evaluation of splanchnic venous-involvement by tumors near the portal vein/superior mesenteric vein/splenic vein confluence.

Numerous staging systems exist for pancreatic cancer, but the most frequently used in the United States is the recently modified,[97] sixth edition of the American Joint Committee on Cancer tumor, node, metastasis (TNM)–based staging system. To address the evolution of surgical approaches to pancreatic cancer,[98-100] the most recent modification of this staging system has made involvement of the splanchnic venous system less relevant to advanced staging. How this modification will affect the accuracy and utility of EUS in overall staging is unclear.

T staging The accuracy of EUS for T staging of pancreatic cancer is generally reported to be about 80%–85% at all stages,[21,59,93-95,101-103] although other studies report an accuracy of only 70%.[104] This is similar to the accuracy of CT and MRI; however, the degree of accuracy is dependent on the experience of the endosonographer[21] and the fact that clinical data are accessible to the endosonographer at the time of the procedure.[30,96] Because the small (<2-cm) T1 lesions are difficult to image by other cross-sectional techniques, EUS by default would be expected to have an advantage in T staging of these lesions. Patients presenting with jaundice generally have bile duct compression by encasement or direct invasion. The region of the ampulla and the pancreatic portion of the common bile duct are very easily seen by EUS, although distinguishing between encasement (T1 or T2) and invasion of the bile duct (T3) can be difficult. However, this distinction is largely irrelevant to management. Duodenal wall invasion also is a T3 criteria, and this is usually easily visualized both endoscopically and endosonographically at EUS.

Many major oncologic centers no longer consider splanchnic venous involvement as an absolute contraindication to resection,[99,100,105] because patients with this condition appear to have the same postoperative survival rates as those who undergo successful resections without venous involvement. To reflect this trend, the new American Joint Committee on Cancer staging criteria changed splanchnic venous involvement from a T4-stage lesion to a T3-stage lesion.[98] However, many surgeons still consider significant splanchnic involvement to be a relative or absolute contraindication to an attempt at curative resection.[102,106,107] Thus, depending on the institution and the available surgical expertise, accurate information regarding splanchnic involvement with a tumor may still significantly affect management, although it may not affect staging.

The interface between the portal and superior mesenteric vein and a pancreatic head tumor is usually well visualized by both radial and linear endosonography (Fig. 13.3A through F). The overall accuracy of various endosonographic criteria for invasion has been assessed in detail[108] and include an irregular venous wall (87%) (Fig. 13.3D), loss of acoustic interface (78%) (Figs. 13.3C and 13.4A), proximity of mass to the portal vein (73%), and absolute tumor size (39%). Using these criteria, EUS was more accurate (78%) than angiography (60%) at assessing portal vein involvement.[108] Another recent large study reported an overall accuracy of 93% for vascular invasion[21] but also noted a considerably poorer accuracy from endosonographers who had staged less than 100 tumors. The presence of collateral formation, as evidenced by the presence of peripancreatic head or periportal venous collaterals (Figs. 13.3D, 13.3E), invariably indicates extensive portal vein involvement with tumors. The presence of gastric varices can indicate portal or splenic vein obstruction by tumors. As discussed in Chapter 12, dual-phase spiral CT and gadolinium-contrasted MRI show similar or better accuracies than EUS at assessing major venous invasion.[108,109]

Some anatomic regions relevant to T staging are difficult to assess by EUS. The distal superior mesenteric vein and especially the superior mesenteric artery are often too far from the duodenal lumen to visualize adequately by EUS (Fig. 13.3F). Because major arterial (superior mesenteric, hepatic, or celiac) invasion is a T4-stage criteria, the ability to consistently assess these vessels is a significant advantage of CT or MRI over EUS. EUS also has trouble assessing colonic invasion because most of this organ is out of range of the echoendoscope or visualization is limited because ultrasound cannot penetrate the air in the colonic lumen. Peritumor edema or pancreatitis can result in overstaging by EUS[21]; however, this problem is not unique to ultrasound. The T-staging criteria have not been validated for nonadenocarcinomas. Thus, my own practice is to be very conservative in diagnosing portal vein invasion with neuroendocrine tumors (Fig. 13.4A).

In summary, T staging of pancreatic cancer by EUS is correct about 80%–85% of the time, an accuracy similar to that of CT and MRI. It has unique staging advantages in small tumors and lesions of the pancreatic head but has the disadvantage of being highly operator dependent and being unable to enable visualization of deep areas of mesenteric root and pancreatico-colonic interface. EUS provides T-stage information that is often complimentary to CT, MRI, and angiography, but it cannot usually replace these procedures.

N staging EUS can detect very small (<0.5-cm) lymph nodes in the regions around the celiac axis, porta hepatis, and pancreatic head, neck, body, and tail. However, nodes at the root of the small bowel mesentery and subduodenal periaortic regions are often poorly seen. Visualizing a lymph node by EUS does not make it malignant. For example, benign nodes around the porta hepatis are a common finding, especially in the setting of previous inflammatory processes, such as cholecystitis or pancreatitis. Endosonographic criteria for malignant adenopathy have been established[110,111] and include lymph node size greater than 1 cm, echolucency, homogeneity, round shape, and sharp edges. However, even if all of these criteria are present, they have an overall accuracy of only about 80%–90%. Use of computerized analysis of nodal appearance has not improved this accuracy.[112]

Although it is uniformly superior to CT or MRI, there have been multiple series showing the N stage accuracy of EUS in pancreatic cancer to be disappointingly low, at 65%–70%.[21,93-95] This poor result is due to the lack of specificity of endosonographic criteria for malignant adenopathy,[111-113] undetectable micrometastatic nodal disease, and the inability to visualize some anatomic regions where metastatic nodes are found such as the small-bowel mesenteric root. The addition of EUS-FNA has greatly enhanced the specificity of N staging by EUS for pancreatic and other cancers,[94,111] even in nodes as small as 5 mm (Figs. 13.2B, C).

Pancreatic surgeons debate the relevance of cytologically documented nodal disease.[105] Some argue that cytologically documented nodal metastases is a contraindication to resection because of the poor survivals in such patients.[113,114] However, others argue that although survivals are poor in patients with nodal metastases, they are still better after resection than with no resection at all.[115,116] All agree that nodal disease remote to the primary tumor, such as the mediastinum,[117] should mitigate against resection. Thus, the significance of EUS-FNA documentation of nodal spread depends on the institutional approach to such patients. If malignant adenopathy is considered a contraindication to resection, EUS and EUS-FNA can result in significant cost savings when they are used for

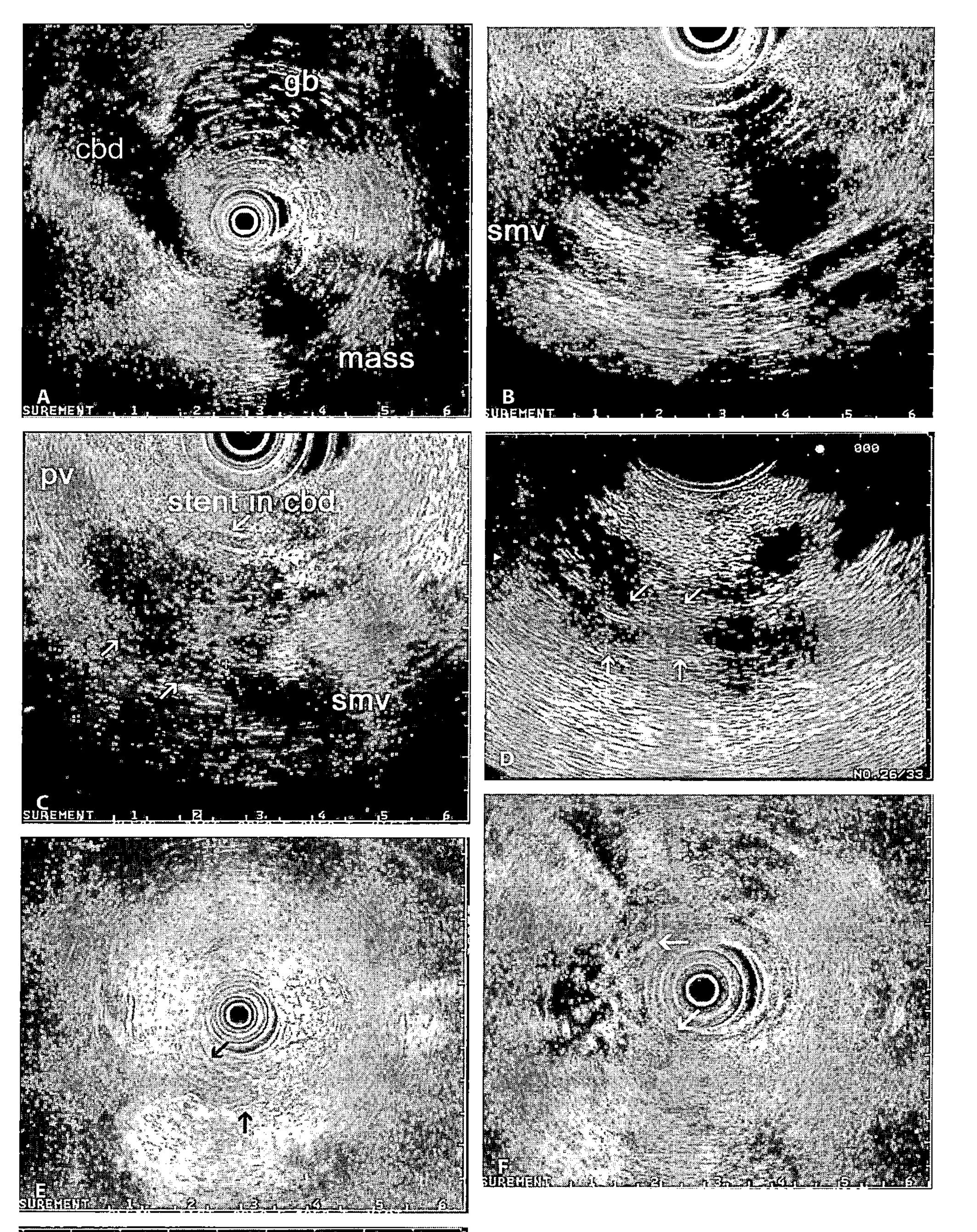

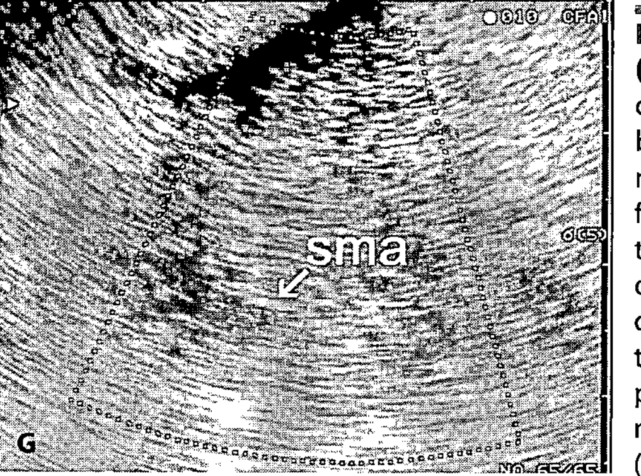

Figure 13.3
(A) Radial EUS image of a 3-cm pancreatic head adenocarcinoma obstructing the common bile duct (cbd) resulting in a massively distended and sludge-filled gallbladder (gb). **(B)** Radial image of a 4-cm adenocarcinoma, well clear of the superior mesenteric vein (smv). **(C)** Radial EUS showing a significant region of loss of interface and vein irregularity (*arrows*) between the portal vein (pv) and superior mesenteric vein (smv) and the tumor. **(D)** Linear EUS showing encasement and irregularity of superior mesenteric vein (*arrows*) by a pancreatic head adenocarcinoma. **(E)** Radial EUS showing periportal collaterals (*arrows*) around common bile duct in a patient with portal vein obstruction by pancreatic adenocarcinoma. **(F)** Radial EUS of perisplenic collaterals in a patient with splenic vein obstruction by pancreatic adenocarcinoma. **(G)** Linear EUS showing encasement of the superior mesenteric artery (sma), a T4 finding. EUS, endoscopic ultrasound.

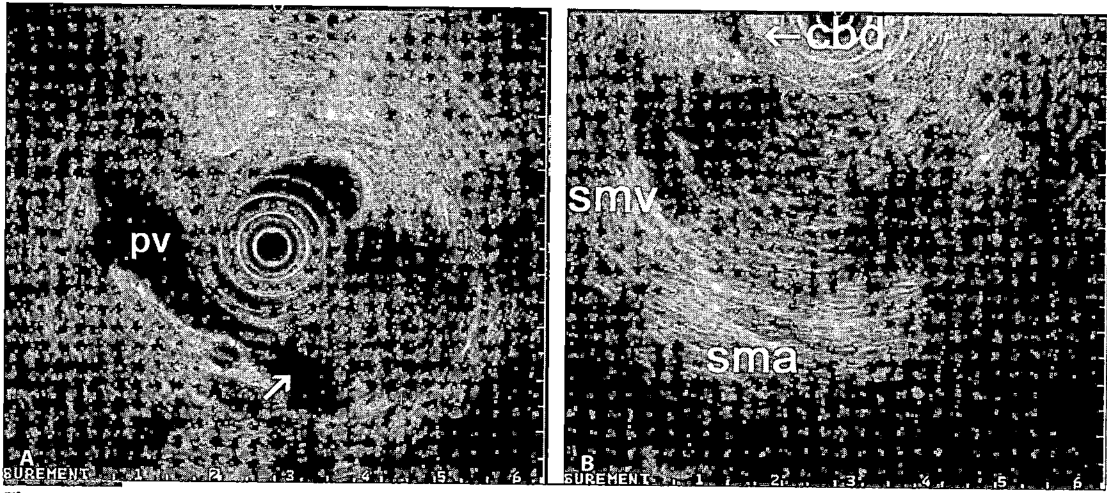

Figure 13.4
(A) Radial EUS image of a pancreatic neuroendocrine tumor showing a large segment of loss of acoustic interface with the portal vein (pv). However, at operation, the portal vein was free of adherent tumor. **(B)** Radial EUS of a B-cell lymphoma of the pancreatic head diagnosed by EUS-FNA and cell surface marker analysis. EUS, endoscopic ultrasound; FNA, fine-needle aspiration; cbd, common bile duct; sma, superior mesenteric artery; smv, superior mesenteric vein.

pancreatic cancer assessment.[50] In our own series of EUS-FNA for pancreatic cancer, approximately 8% of patients who underwent diagnostic and staging EUS were found to have nodal spread by EUS-FNA.[37] The relevance of EUS and EUS-FNA nodal staging may be significantly increased by the advent of molecular diagnosis of occult malignancy within nodes that are cytologically negative by EUS-FNA.[118,119] In addition, as effective neoadjuvant regimens are developed for locally advanced disease, EUS-FNA demonstration of nodal metastases may have greater clinical significance.

M staging EUS is limited in its ability to assess metastatic disease to only those regions that are accessible to EUS-FNA. About 80% of the liver is visible to EUS, with the far right lobe and the high dome of the liver usually being inaccessible to endosonographic imaging. However, only 4–6 cm of the left lobe and periduodenal right lobe are amenable to EUS-FNA. Liver metastases as small as 5 mm can be seen by EUS and sampled by EUS-FNA[37,45,85,94,120] (Figs. 13.2D, E). If cytologically positive, these findings would obviate any attempt at curative resection and thus dramatically change the approach to treating that patient. Likewise, small amounts of peritoneal fluid can be easily aspirated by EUS-FNA[121,122] (Figs. 13.2F, G) and if found to contain malignant cells represent metastatic, inoperable disease. However, only about 10% of peritoneal aspirates has a positive cytologic result.[122] Because ultrasound does not penetrate into air, the lungs cannot be examined for metastatic disease. However, small, right pleural effusions are easily seen and tapped by EUS-FNA.[121] Again, in our series,[37] we found occult metastatic disease in about 7% of our patients, primarily small liver metastases.

Conclusion EUS is probably inferior to CT and MRI in overall T-staging accuracy because of its inability to visualize the superior mesenteric artery. EUS may still have an advantage over these procedures in detecting occult malignant adenopathy. It can be considered only a supplementary procedure for M staging. If it will obviate operative intervention, cytologically documenting occult remote nodal disease or metastatic disease can dramatically and cost-effectively[48,123,124] affect the treatment of the patient with pancreatic cancer. If EUS is used purely as a staging procedure, its findings have to be considered complimentary, not superior, to those from CT and MRI. However, if EUS is being used primarily for its diagnostic, biopsy, and/or therapeutic capabilities, then the staging information obtained is an added bonus of the procedure.

Therapeutic EUS in Pancreatic Cancer

EUS also has therapeutic applications in pancreatic cancer. Celiac neurolysis can be performed through the posterior gastric wall under direct endosonographic guidance with the use of bupivacaine and absolute alcohol injected on either side of the celiac artery.[125,126] This is a relatively simple approach to the procedure compared with radiologic transabdominal or anesthesiologic transthoracic

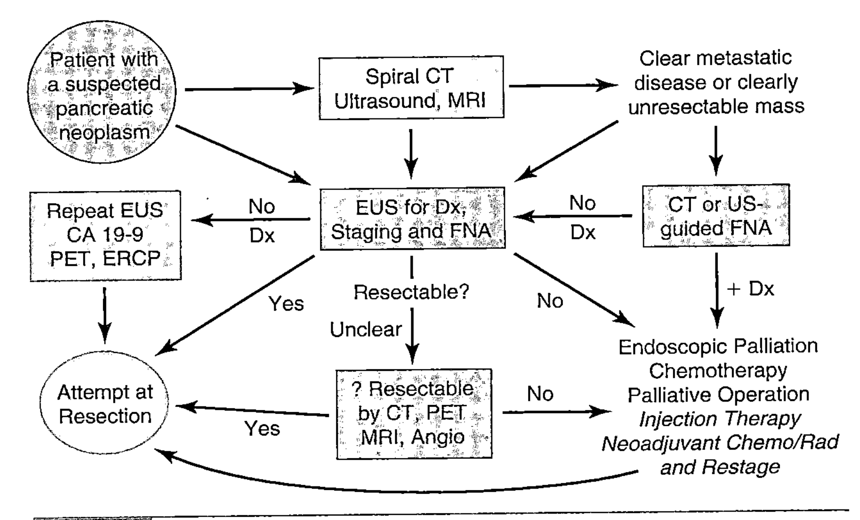

Figure 13.5
Algorithm used for incorporating EUS and EUS-FNA into the management of the patient with suspected pancreatic cancer at Scott & White Clinic and Hospital. EUS, endoscopic ultrasound; FNA, fine-needle aspiration.

approaches to celiac neurolysis. EUS celiac neurolysis takes about 10 minutes and can be performed under the same sedation after a diagnostic EUS or EUS-FNA. EUS-guided fine-needle injection is now also being used experimentally for tumor injection therapy using activated lymphocytes[127] and viral gene vectors.[128]

Screening for Pancreatic Cancer in High-Risk Patients

Five percent to 10% of all pancreatic cancer appears to be familial.[129] In rare kindreds, the risk of developing pancreatic cancer is very high.[130] How to screen for presumed precursors[131] of neoplastic transformation, pancreatic intraepithelial neoplasia, and IPMTs in these families is unclear. Imaging, cytologic, and molecular techniques are being used,[130,132] with EUS and EUS-FNA usually being the cornerstone of this kind of surveillance. Decision analysis studies have suggested that this type of survey can be cost-effective when compared with other accepted forms of cancer screening.[133]

The Role of EUS in Pancreatic Cancer

Where high-quality EUS and EUS-FNA is readily available, EUS can play a central and early role in the evaluation of the patient with suspected pancreatic cancer.[3,8-13,27,103,134-136] Its superiority as a diagnostic tool and its very high specificity make it an ideal definitive test for patients suspected to have any pancreatic abnormality by CT, transcutaneous ultrasound, or clinical evaluation. Because cytologic diagnosis and staging information can also be obtained at the same time, EUS with EUS-FNA usually provides most, if not all, of the data needed to provide definitive stage-specific therapy. State-of-the-art staging CT or MRI can be used before or after EUS to compliment the EUS staging information provided, especially in equivocal operative cases, and to rule out occult liver metastases. In the rare situation in which CT, EUS, and EUS-FNA have failed to provide a definitive diagnosis, other modalities, such as CA 19-9,[137] ERCP, repeat EUS a month or two later, positron emission tomography, or laparoscopy, can be used, depending on the clinical situation. Our own approach to incorporating EUS and EUS-FNA into the management of pancreatic cancer is summarized in Fig. 13.5. Using EUS as an imaging procedure of last resort minimizes the clinical impact and cost-effectiveness of this powerful procedure by placing it at the end of the evaluation instead of near the beginning.

Endoscopic Retrograde Cholangiopancreatography

Technologic Considerations and Complications

Endoscopic retrograde cholangiopancreatography is a technically demanding procedure[90] that was first introduced in the late 1960s.[138] The first therapeutic sphincterotomies were reported in 1974 from Japan and Germany.[139,140] In the hands of a skilled endoscopist, ERCP should have success rates in excess of 90% for visualizing the duct or ducts of interest. ERCP has the highest complication rates of any endoscopic procedure, with 5%–10% of patients having a major complication after diagnostic or therapeutic ERCP.[141] More than half of these complications are related to ERCP-induced pancreatitis, and most of the rest are complications specific to endoscopic sphincterotomy, such as perforation, cholangitis, and bleeding. The risk of cholangitis in patients with obstructive jaundice can be minimized by placing a biliary stent and using prophylactic antibiotics when performing ERCP in patients with this condition.[141,142] Many trials of various ways of preventing ERCP-induced pancreatitis have been

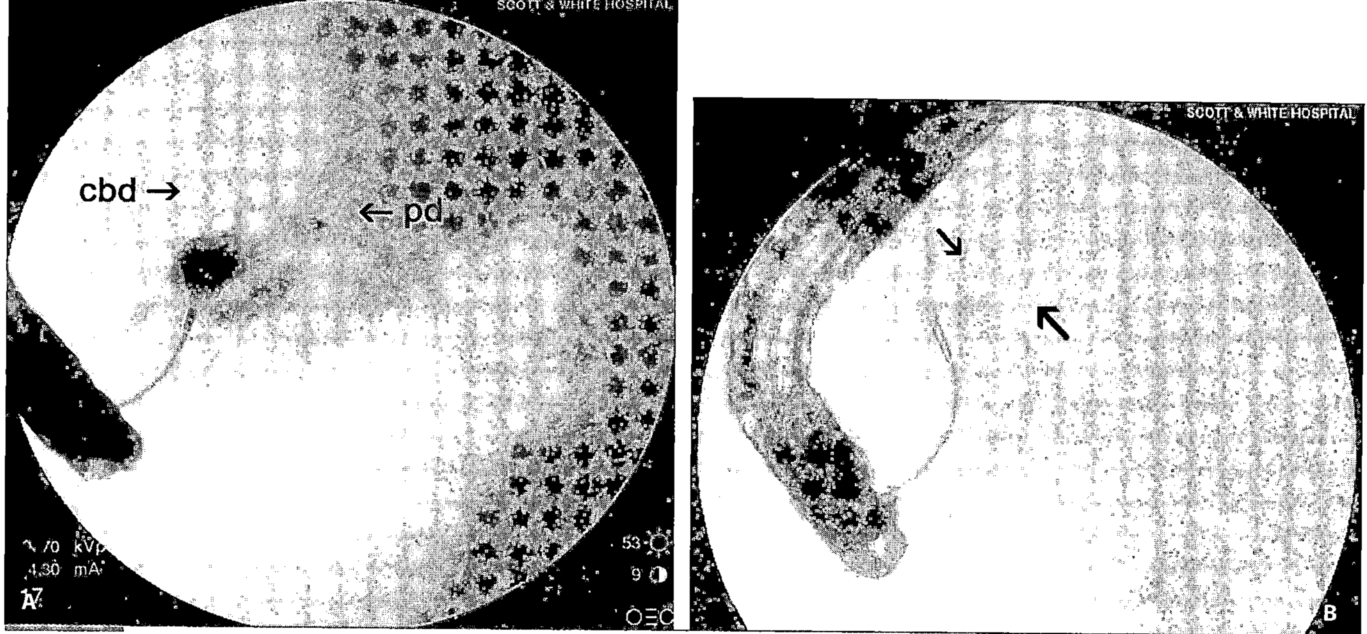

Figure 13.6
(A) Demonstrates a classic endoscopic retrograde cholangiopancreatography (ERCP) "double-duct cut-off" sign (*arrows*) of pancreatic head cancer. **(B)** Pancreatogram showing an irregularly strictured pancreatic duct in a patient with a small (<2 cm) pancreatic cancer (*arrows*). Both of these findings also occur in chronic pancreatitis.

studied[143]; however, to date, no intervention has been consistently effective, except perhaps placement of a temporary pancreatic duct stent after complicated cannulations or in high-risk patients.[144]

Diagnosis of Pancreatic Neoplasms

Morphologic changes in the bile and/or pancreatic duct occur in 90%–100% of patients with pancreatic adenocarcinoma (Figs. 13.6A, B),[145-148] even in small pancreatic carcinomas.[149,150] However, these ductal changes are nonspecific, especially in chronic pancreatitis, leading to an overall accuracy ranging from 60% to 80% for diagnosing pancreatic cancer by ERCP alone. Even classic ductographic appearances, such as the "double-duct cutoff" sign (Fig. 13.6A), are not specific for pancreatic carcinoma and can occur in chronic pancreatitis.[151-153] A normal pancreatogram does not exclude the possibility of an underlying pancreatic carcinoma, because this can occur in about 7% of patients.[154] Half of these normal pancreatograms may have missed the cancer because Santorini's duct was not visualized. Additionally, nonadenocarcinomas of the pancreas do not generally arise from ductal tissue, and therefore, patients may have normal pancreatograms until the tumors get large enough to compress or invade the duct.

Tissue Diagnosis of Pancreatic Neoplasms

There has been considerable interest in using ERCP to provide a tissue diagnosis in pancreatic cancer.[146,147,155-162] However, success rates are extremely variable, running from 20% to 80%, with most series having yields of diagnostic specimens in the range of 40%–50% for pancreatic carcinomas. Many techniques have been developed to try to improve obtaining diagnostic cytologic or biopsy specimens at the time of ERCP.[161,162] These include transpapillary biopsy,[163-167] new brush devices,[168,169] transductal FNA,[113,166,170] dilation of strictures before brush cytology,[171,172,173] cytology from removed stents[174] or the addition of flow cytometry,[175] or K-*ras* or other molecular markers analysis of pancreatic juice.[176-180] However, none of these has brought the rate of definitive tissue diagnosis of pancreatic cancer by ERCP to anywhere near that provided by EUS-FNA.

A problem common to many ERCP cytologic series is that they somewhat artificially increase the reported cytologic yield with ERCP by counting a "suspected" or a "suspicious" diagnosis as being positive for cancer. This makes it difficult to compare to EUS, CT, or ultrasound series where a suspicious cytologic diagnosis is not generally reported as a positive result. A suspicious pancreatic cytologic result usually does mean that an underlying pancreaticobiliary malignancy is present,[181,182] and this may be enough information to proceed to surgery. However, a suspicious cytologic result is usually not sufficient to allow the delivery of nonsurgical therapy, such as chemotherapy, radiation therapy, or palliative therapy, such as placing a permanent metallic biliary or enteral stent.

The complication rate for CT, ultrasound, or EUS-FNA of pancreatic masses is reasonably low at about 1%–2%; however, the complication rate for ERCP cytologic brushing is as high as 11% for the biliary tree and 21% for pancreatic strictures.[161,162,183] If ERCP is being performed for another indication (e.g., stent placement for obstructive jaundice) and no tissue diagnosis is yet available, attempting transductal brush cytology or biopsy is worthwhile. However, performing ERCP just for tissue diagnosis in suspected pancreatic malignancy can no longer be justified when ultrasound, CT, and especially EUS-FNA have much higher yields of a definitive diagnosis and with much lower morbidities. At our institution, we routinely perform EUS-FNA before ERCP in patients with malignant obstruction from pancreatic cancer[184] to eliminate the need for attempting a cytologic diagnosis by ERCP when a stent is being placed.

Staging of Pancreatic Neoplasms

ERCP generally has little utility as a staging procedure. Patients presenting with obstructive jaundice and having a biliary stricture by ERCP may have a T1, T2, or T3 lesion, depending on the size of the primary tumor and whether biliary compression or invasion is present. The only other staging information provided by ERCP is some rough information on tumor size. Pancreatic or biliary duct stricture length does correlate with tumor size as measured by other imaging modalities.[185,186] Because tumor size does affect prognosis and tumor stage,[187] stricture length at ERCP does have some relevance. Yet this information is at best supplementary to the much more accurate size information provided by ultrasound, CT, MRI, or EUS. A normal pancreatogram in a patient with pancreatic cancer does not imply a better prognosis or a smaller tumor,[154] because the tumor may be arising from an unseen duct of Santorini or a secondary ductule. One area where ERCP still plays a role is in diagnosing IPMTs of the pancreas. ERCP techniques can be used for ductal imaging, direct pancreatoscopy, transductal biopsy, or intraductal ultrasound.[167,188-189]

Therapeutic ERCP for Pancreatic Neoplasms

Although early in its history, ERCP was used as a powerful diagnostic tool in pancreatic cancer, its primary role now in pancreatic cancer is for the palliation of obstructive jaundice,[190,191] using endoscopically placed plastic or expandable metallic stents (see Chapter 31). There has also been some limited interest in stenting the obstructed pancreatic duct for pain relief in selected patients with pancreatic cancer.[192-195] However, this invasive technique may require repeated ERCPs to maintain stent patency, and the pain relief provided appears to be more temporary than that reported with the better-studied approach of celiac neurolysis.

The Role of ERCP in Pancreatic Cancer and Interface with EUS

Even with the high sensitivity of ERCP for detecting ductal abnormalities in pancreatic cancer, because of its higher cost, its invasiveness, and especially its morbidity, it has little role as a primary diagnostic modality in pancreatic neoplasia, except when it is being used as a therapeutic modality. Since the introduction of spiral CT, MRI, and EUS, the role for purely diagnostic ERCP in pancreatic cancer should be limited to the occasional patient in whom pancreatic cancer is still suspected despite a nondiagnostic EUS/EUS-FNA, CT, and/or MRI or for the diagnosis of the rare patient with suspected IPMT.

ERCP has traditionally been considered the procedure of choice in patients with obstructive jaundice from a presumed pancreatic malignancy.[190-191] However, if EUS is going to be performed, it is probably preferable to perform EUS/EUS-FNA first.[184] EUS can accurately diagnose almost all the causes of obstructive jaundice, including pancreaticobiliary malignancies[196-199] and choledocholithiasis,[200-202] with the same or better accuracy than ERCP. Additionally, EUS-FNA provides a tissue diagnosis of underlying pancreaticobiliary malignancy with a much higher success rate (80%–93%) than ERCP (30%–60%). Unlike ERCP, EUS provides significant staging information if a pancreaticobiliary malignancy is found, and the diagnostic, cytologic, and staging information provided by EUS and EUS-FNA does not carry the significant risk of pancreatitis or cholangitis associated with ERCP. Further EUS/EUS-FNA does not mandate placing a biliary stent[141,142,184] or using prophylactic antibiotics,[203,204] except in the case of EUS-FNA of liver metastases in a patient with an undrained biliary tree.[85] Anecdotally, stents can make T staging by EUS more difficult by casting acoustic shadows in the pancreatic head. Finally, ERCP can always be performed after EUS (and CT) if it is needed as a therapeutic procedure. Because there is little evidence that preoperative endoscopic biliary decompression is advantageous in malignant obstruction,[205] if the patient is going to go on directly to surgery for a resectable pancreatic cancer, ERCP with stent may not even be needed if EUS/EUS-FNA has been performed for diagnosis, cytology, and staging.[184]

The diagnostic capabilities and lower morbidity of EUS/EUS-FNA have led our institution[184] and others[206,207] to propose that the ideal endoscopic approach to obstructive jaundice of unknown origin is the combination of EUS/EUS-FNA followed directly by ERCP if necessary for therapy. This may be especially true for patients with possible malignant obstructive jaundice because pancreatic cancer is the most common cause of malignant biliary obstruction, and EUS/EUS-FNA has already been shown to be highly cost-effective in the management of pancreatic carcinoma.[50] In our own study,[184] using EUS/EUS-FNA before ERCP in obstructive jaundice saved $1000–$2500 in medical costs per patient. These costs savings were even higher in patients with pancreatic cancer.

Conclusion

EUS with EUS-FNA can cost-effectively play an early central role in the diagnosis, cytologic assessment, staging, and treatment of patients with pancreatic cancer. ERCP should now be used primarily as a palliative therapeutic procedure in patients with unresectable pancreatic cancer and obstructive jaundice. Ideally, EUS/EUS-FNA is best performed before therapeutic ERCP because this would optimize the utility of both procedures and would minimize patient morbidity. Where these powerful endoscopic procedures fit into the algorithm of the evaluation and treatment of patients with suspected pancreatic cancer varies significantly between institutions. This variation results from differences in the availability of these procedures, institutional biases, local expertise, equipment, and the institutional approach to the medical and surgical management of patients with pancreatic cancer.

References

1. Niederau C, Grendell JH. Diagnosis of pancreatic carcinoma. Imaging techniques and tumor markers. *Pancreas*. 1992;7:66–86.
2. Alvarez C, Livingston EH, Ashley SW, et al. Cost-benefit analysis of the work-up for pancreatic cancer. *Am J Surg*. 1993;165:53–58.
3. Baron PL, Kay C, Hoffman B. Pancreatic imaging. *Surg Oncol Clin North Am*. 1999;8:35–58.
4. Dancygier H, Lightdale CJ, Stevens PD. Endoscopic ultrasonography of the upper gastrointestinal tract and colon. In: Dancygier H, Lightdale CJ, eds. *Endosonography in Gastroenterology: Principles, Techniques, Findings*. Stuttgart: Thieme; 1999:13–22.
5. Strohm WD, Philip J, Hagenmuller F, et al. Ultrasonic tomography by means of an ultrasonic fiberendoscope. *Endoscopy*. 1980;12:241–244.
6. DiMagno EP, Buxton JL, Regan PT, et al. Ultrasonic endoscope. *Lancet*. 1980;1:629–631.
7. Vilmann P, Khattar S, Hancke S. Endoscopic ultrasound examination of the upper gastrointestinal tract using a curved array transducer: a preliminary report. *Surg Endosc*. 1991;5:79–82.
8. Chang KJ. Endoscopic ultrasound-guided fine needle aspiration in the diagnosis and staging of pancreatic tumors. *Gastrointest Endosc Clin North Am*. 1995;5:723–734.
9. Hawes RH. Endoscopic ultrasound. *Gastrointest Endosc Clin North Am*. 2000;10;161–174.
10. Antillon MR, Chang KJ. Endoscopic and endosonography guided fine-needle aspiration. *Gastrointest Endosc Clin North Am*. 2000;10:619–636.
11. Bhutani MS. Endoscopic ultrasonography. *Endoscopy*. 2000;32:853–862.
12. Kochman ML. EUS in pancreatic cancer. *Gastrointest Endosc*. 2002;56:S6–S12.
13. Hunt GC, Faigel DO. Assessment of EUS for diagnosing, staging, and determining resectability of pancreatic cancer: a review. *Gastrointest Endosc*. 2002;55:232–237.
14. Vilman P, Jacobsen GK, Henriksen FW, et al. Endoscopic ultrasonography with guided fine needle aspiration biopsy in pancreatic disease. *Gastrointest Endosc*. 1992;38:172–173.
15. Wiersema MJ, Kochman ML, Chak A, et al. Real-time endoscopic ultrasound-guided fine-needle aspiration of a mediastinal lymph node. *Gastrointest Endosc*. 1993;39:429–431.
16. Chang KJ, Albers CG, Erickson RA, et al. Endoscopic ultrasound guided fine needle aspiration of pancreatic carcinoma. *Am J Gastroenterol*. 1994;89:263–266.
17. Vargo JJ, Zuccaro G, Dumot JA, et al. Gastroenterologist-administered propofol versus meperidine and midazolam for advanced upper endoscopy: a prospective, randomized trial. *Gastroenterology*. 2002;123:8–16.
18. Das A, Sivak MV, Chak A. Cervical esophageal perforation during EUS: a national survey. *Gastrointest Endosc*. 2001;53:599–602.
19. Raut CP, Grau AM, Staerkel GA, et al. Diagnostic accuracy of endoscopic ultrasound-guided fine-needle aspiration in patients with presumed pancreatic cancer. *J Gastrointest Surg*. 2003;7:118–126.
20. Van Dam J, Brady PG, Freeman M, et al. Guidelines for training in endoscopic ultrasound: guidelines for clinical application. From the ASGE. American Society for Gastrointestinal Endoscopy. *Gastrointest Endosc*. 1999;49:829–833.
21. Gress FG, Hawes RH, Savides TJ, et al. Role of EUS in the preoperative staging of pancreatic cancer: a large single-center experience. *Gastrointest Endosc*. 1999;50:786–791.
22. Yasuda K, Mukai H, Fujimoto S, et al. The diagnosis of pancreatic cancer by endoscopic ultrasonography. *Gastrointest Endosc*. 1988;34:1–8.
23. Rösch T, Lorenz R, Braig C, et al. Endoscopic ultrasound in pancreatic tumor diagnosis. *Gastrointest Endosc*. 1991;37:347–352.

24. Muller MF, Meyenberger C, Bertschinger P, Schaer R, Marincek B. Pancreatic tumors: evaluation with endoscopic US, CT and MR imaging. *Radiology*. 1994;190:745–751.
25. Bhutani MS. Endoscopic ultrasonography in pancreatic disease. *Semin Gastroint Dis*. 1998;9:51–60.
26. Yasuda K, Mukai H, Nakajima M. Endoscopic ultrasonography diagnosis of pancreatic cancer. *Gastrointest Endosc Clin North Am*. 1995;5:699–712.
27. Wiersema MJ. Identifying contraindications to resection in patients with pancreatic carcinoma: the role of endoscopic ultrasound. *Can J Gastroenterol*. 2002;16:109–114.
28. Glasbrenner B, Schwarz M, Pauls S, et al. Prospective comparison of endoscopic ultrasound and endoscopic retrograde cholangiopancreatography in the preoperative assessment of masses in the pancreatic head. *Dig Surg*. 2000;17:468–474.
29. Legmann P, Vignaux O, Dousset B, et al. Pancreatic tumors: comparison of dual-phase helical CT and endoscopic sonography. *Am J Radiol*. 1998;170:1315–1332.
30. Meining A, Dittler HJ, Wolf A, et al. You get what you expect? A critical appraisal of imaging methodology in endosonographic cancer staging. *Gut*. 2002;50:599–603.
31. Rosch T, Schusdziarra V, Born P, et al. Modern imaging methods versus clinical assessment in the evaluation of hospital in-patients with suspected pancreatic disease. *Am J Gastroenterol*. 2000;95:2261–2270.
32. Van Hoe L, Baert AL. Pancreatic carcinoma: applications for helical computed tomography. *Endoscopy*. 1997;29:539–560.
33. Qian X, Hecht JL. Pancreatic fine needle aspiration: a comparison of computed tomographic and endoscopic ultrasonographic guidance. *Acta Cytol*. 2003;47:723–726.
34. Erickson RA. Endoscopic diagnosis and staging: endoscopic ultrasound, endoscopic retrograde cholangiopancreatography. In: Evans DB, Pisters PWT, Abbruzzese JL, eds. *Pancreatic Cancer*. New York: Springer; 2002:97–114.
35. Bhutani MS, Hawes RH, Baron PL, et al. Endoscopic ultrasound guided fine needle aspiration of malignant pancreatic lesions. *Endoscopy*. 1997;29:854–858.
36. Barthet M, Portal I, Boujaoude J, et al. Endoscopic ultrasonographic diagnosis of pancreatic cancer complicating chronic pancreatitis. *Endoscopy*. 1996;28:487–491.
37. Erickson RA, Sayage-Rabie L, Beisner RS. Factors impacting endoscopic ultrasound-guided fine needle aspiration passes for pancreatic malignancies. *Gastrointest Endosc*. 2000;51:184–190.
38. Marchevsky AM, Nelson V, Martin SE, et al. Telecytology of fine-needle aspiration biopsies of the pancreas: a study of well-differentiated adenocarcinoma and chronic pancreatitis with atypical epithelial repair changes. *Diagn Cytopathol*. 2003;28:147–152.
39. Hayakawa T, Naruse S, Kitagawa M, et al. A prospective multicenter trial evaluating diagnostic validity of multivariate analysis and individual serum marker in differential diagnosis of pancreatic cancer from benign pancreatic diseases. *Int J Pancreatol*. 1999;25:23–29.
40. Abraham SC, Wilentz RE, Yeo CJ, et al. Pancreaticoduodenectomy (Whipple resections) in patients without malignancy: are they all "chronic pancreatitis"? *Am J Surg Pathol*. 2003;27:110–120.
41. Tada M, Komatsu Y, Kawabe T, et al. Quantitative analysis of K-*ras* gene mutation in pancreatic tissue obtained by endoscopic ultrasonography-guided fine needle aspiration: clinical utility for diagnosis of pancreatic tumor. *Am J Gastroenterol*. 2002;97:2263–2270.
42. Buchler P, Conejo-Garcia JR, Lehmann G, et al. Real-time quantitative PCR of telomerase mRNA is useful for the differentiation of benign and malignant pancreatic disorders. *Pancreas*. 2001;22:331–340.
43. Chang KJ, Katz KD, Durbin TE, et al. Endoscopic ultrasound guided fine needle aspiration. *Gastrointest Endosc*. 1994;40:694–699.
44. Wiersema MJ, Kouchman ML, Cramer HM, et al. Endosonography-guided real-time fine-needle aspiration biopsy. *Gastrointest Endosc*. 1994;40:700–707.
45. Giovannini M, Seitz JF, Monges F, et al. Fine-needle aspiration cytology guided by endoscopic ultrasonography: results in 141 patients. *Endoscopy*. 1995;27:171–177.
46. Wiersema MJ, Vilmann P, Giovannini M, et al. Endosonography-guided fine-needle aspiration biopsy: diagnostic accuracy and complication assessment. *Gastroenterology*. 1997;112:1087–1095.
47. Gress FG, Hawes RH, Savides TJ, et al. Endoscopic ultrasound-guided fine-needle aspiration biopsy using linear array and radial scanning endosonography. *Gastrointest Endosc*. 1997;45:243–250.
48. Erickson RA, Sayage-Rabie L, Avots-Avotins A. Clinical utility of endoscopic ultrasound-guided fine needle aspiration. *Acta Cytol*. 1997;41:1647–1653.
49. Faigel DO, Ginsberg GG, Bentz JS, et al. Endoscopic ultrasound guided real time fine needle aspiration biopsy of the pancreas in cancer patients with pancreatic lesions. *J Clin Oncol*. 1997;15:1439–1443.
50. Chang KJ, Nguyen P, Erickson RA, et al. The clinical utility of endoscopic ultrasound-guided fine-needle aspiration in the diagnosis and staging of pancreatic carcinoma. *Gastrointest Endosc*. 1997;45:387–393.
51. David O, Green L, Reddy V, et al. Pancreatic masses: a multi-institutional study of 364 fine-needle aspiration biopsies with histopathologic correlation. *Diagn Cytopathol*. 1998;19:423–427.
52. Afify AM, al-Khafaji BM, Kim B, et al. Endoscopic ultrasound-guided fine needle aspiration of the pancreas: diagnostic utility and accuracy. *Acta Cytol*. 2003;47: 341–348.
53. Harewood GC, Wiersema MJ. Endosonography-guided fine needle aspiration biopsy in the evaluation of pancreatic masses. *Am J Gastroenterol*. 2002;97:1386–1391.
54. Ylagan LR, Edmundowicz S, Kasal K, et al. Endoscopic ultrasound guided fine-needle aspiration cytology of pancreatic carcinoma: a 3-year experience and review of the literature. *Cancer*. 2002;96:362–369.
55. Erickson RA. EUS-guided FNA. *Gastrointest Endosc*. 2004:60;267–279.
56. Binmoeller KF, Rathod VD. Difficult pancreatic mass FNA: tips for success. *Gastrointest Endosc*. 2002;56:S86–S91.

57. Gress F, Gottlieb K, Sherman S, Lehman G. Endoscopic ultrasonography-guided fine-needle aspiration biopsy of suspected pancreatic cancer. *Ann Intern Med.* 2001;134:459–464.
58. Frable WJ. Needle aspiration biopsy: past, present, and future. *Hum Pathol.* 1989;20:504–517.
59. Harewood GC, Wiersema LM, Halling AC, et al. Influence of EUS training and pathology interpretation on accuracy of EUS-guided fine needle aspiration of pancreatic masses. *Gastrointest Endosc.* 2002;55:669–673.
60. Klapman JB, Logrono R, Dye CE, et al. Clinical impact of on-site cytopathology interpretation on endoscopic ultrasound-guided fine needle aspiration. *Am J Gastroenterol.* 2003;98:1289–1294.
61. Schwartz DA, Unni KK, Levy MJ, et al. The rate of false-positive results with EUS-guided fine-needle aspiration. *Gastrointest Endosc.* 2002;56:868–872.
62. O'Toole D, Palazzo L, Arotcarena R, et al. Assessment of complications of EUS-guided fine-needle aspiration. *Gastrointest Endosc.* 2001;53:470–474.
63. Molino D, Perrotti P, Antropoli C, et al. Analysis of factors influencing the diagnostic failure of intraoperative fine needle aspiration cytology in pancreatic cancer. *Chir Ital.* 2002;54:289–294.
64. Lin F, Staerkel G. Cytologic criteria for well differentiated adenocarcinoma of the pancreas in fine-needle aspiration biopsy specimens. *Cancer.* 2003;99:44–50.
65. Harada N, Kouzu T, Arima M, et al. Endoscopic ultrasound-guided histologic needle biopsy: preliminary results using a newly developed endoscopic ultrasound transducer. *Gastrointest Endosc.* 1996;44:327–330.
66. Matsui M, Goto H, Niwa Y, et al. Preliminary results of fine needle aspiration biopsy histology in upper gastrointestinal submucosal tumors. *Endoscopy.* 1998;30: 750–755.
67. Binmoeller KF, Thul R, Rathod V, et al. Endoscopic ultrasound-guided 18-gauge, fine needle aspiration biopsy of the pancreas using a 2.8 mm channel convex array echoendoscope. *Gastrointest Endosc.* 1998;47:121–127.
68. Solmi L, Muratori R, Bacchini P, Primerano A, Gandolfi L. Comparison between echo-guided fine needle aspiration cytology and microhistology in diagnosing pancreatic masses. *Surg Endosc.* 1992;6:222–224.
69. Henrique RM, Sousa ME, Godinho MI, et al. Immunophenotyping by flow cytometry of fine needle aspirates in the diagnosis of lymphoproliferative disorders: a retrospective study. *J Clin Lab Anal.* 1999;13:224–228.
70. Bouvet M, Staerkel GA, Spitz FR, et al. Primary pancreatic lymphoma. *Surgery.* 1998;123:382–390.
71. Bounds BC, Brugge WR. EUS diagnosis of cystic lesions of the pancreas. *Int J Gastrointest Cancer.* 2001;30:27–31.
72. Brandwein SL, Farrell JJ, Centeno BA, et al. Detection and tumor staging of malignancy in cystic, intraductal, and solid tumors of the pancreas by EUS. *Gastrointest Endosc.* 2001;53:722–727.
73. Hernandez LV, Mishra G, Forsmark C, et al. Role of endoscopic ultrasound (EUS) and EUS-guided fine needle aspiration in the diagnosis and treatment of cystic lesions of the pancreas. *Pancreas.* 2002;25:222–228.
74. Bounds BC. Diagnosis and fine needle aspiration of intraductal papillary mucinous tumor by endoscopic ultrasound. *Gastrointest Endosc Clin North Am.* 2002:12;735–745.
75. Frossard JL, Amouyal P, Amouyal G, et al. Performance of endosonography-guided fine needle aspiration and biopsy in the diagnosis of pancreatic cystic lesions. *Am J Gastroenterol.* 2003;98:1516–1524.
76. Brugge WR. Fine needle aspiration of pancreatic masses: the clinical impact. *Am J Gastroenterol.* 2002;97:2701–2702.
77. Warshaw AL, Fernandez-del Castillo C. Pancreatic carcinoma. *N Engl J Med.* 1992;326:455–465.
78. Nakamura R, Machado R, Amikura K, et al. Role of fine needle aspiration cytology and endoscopic biopsy in the preoperative assessment of pancreatic and peripancreatic malignancies. *Int J Pancreatol.* 1994;16:17–21.
79. Evans DB, Staley CA, Lee JE, et al. Adenocarcinoma of the pancreas: recent controversies, current management, and future therapies. *Gastrointest Cancer.* 1996;1:149–161.
80. Smith EH. Complications of percutaneous abdominal fine-needle biopsy. *Radiology.* 1991;178:253–258.
81. Fornari F, Buscarini L. Ultrasonically-guided fine-needle biopsy of gastrointestinal organs: indications, results and complications. *Dig Dis.* 1992;10:121–133.
82. Brandt KR, Charboneau JW, Stephens DH, et al. CT and US guided biopsy of the pancreas. *Radiology.* 1993;187:99–104.
83. Gress F, Michael H, Gelrud D, et al. EUS-guided fine-needle aspiration of the pancreas: evaluation of pancreatitis as a complication. *Gastrointest Endosc.* 2002;56:864–867.
84. Affi A, Vazquez-Sequeiros E, Norton ID, et al. Acute extraluminal hemorrhage associated with EUS-guided fine needle aspiration: frequency and clinical significance. *Gastrointest Endosc.* 2001;53:221–225.
85. ten Berge J, Hoffman BJ, Hawes RH, et al. EUS-guided fine needle aspiration of the liver: indications, yield, and safety based on an international survey of 167 cases. *Gastrointest Endosc.* 2002;55:859–862.
86. Chen HY, Lee CH, Hsieh CH. Bile peritonitis after EUS-guided fine-needle aspiration. *Gastrointest Endosc.* 2002;56:594–596.
87. Matsumoto K, Yamao K, Ohashi K, et al. Acute portal vein thrombosis after EUS-guided FNA of pancreatic cancer: case report. *Gastrointest Endosc.* 2003;57:269–271.
88. Lundstedt C, Stridbeck H, Andersson R, et al. Tumor seeding occurring after fine-needle biopsy of abdominal malignancies. *Acta Radiol.* 1991;32:518–520.
89. Micames CG, Jowell P, White R, et al. Lower frequency of peritoneal carcinomatosis in patients with pancreatic cancer diagnosed by EUS-guided FNA vs. percutaneous FNA. *Gastrointest Endosc.* 2003;58:690–695.
90. Levy MJ, Norton ID, Wiersema MJ, et al. Prospective risk assessment of bacteremia and other infectious complications in patients undergoing EUS-guided FNA. *Gastrointest Endosc.* 2003;57:672–678.
91. Catalano MF, Hoffman B, Bhutani M, et al. American Endosonography Club. Endoscopic ultrasound (EUS) guided fine needle aspiration (FNA) of gastrointestinal (GI) tract lesions: multicenter assessment of accuracy, complication rate and technical competence [abstract]. *Gastrointest Endosc.* 1997;45:AB26.

92. Sing JT, Erickson RA, Fader R. An in-vitro analysis of microbial transmission during endoscopic ultrasound guided fine-needle aspiration and the utility of sterilization agents [abstract]. *Am J Gastroenterol.* 2003;98:S284.
93. Rösch T. Staging of pancreatic cancer. Analysis of literature results. *Gastrointest Endosc Clin North Am.* 1995;5: 735–739.
94. Chang KJ. Endoscopic ultrasound guided fine needle aspiration in the diagnosis and staging of pancreatic tumors. *Gastrointest Endosc Clin North Am.* 1995;5:723–734.
95. Tio TL, Sie LH, Kallimanis G, et al. Staging of ampullary and pancreatic carcinoma: comparison between endosonography and surgery. *Gastrointest Endosc.* 1996;44:706–713.
96. Rosch T, Dittler HJ, Strobel K, et al. Endoscopic ultrasound criteria for vascular invasion in the staging of cancer of the head of the pancreas: a blind reevaluation of videotapes. *Gastrointest Endosc.* 2000;52:469–477.
97. Exocrine pancreas. In: Greene FL, Page DL, Fleming ID, et al., eds. *AJCC Cancer Staging Handbook.* New York: Springer-Verlag; 2002:179–188.
98. Harrison LE, Brennan MF. Portal vein resection for pancreatic adenocarcinoma. *Surg Oncol Clin North Am.* 1998;7:165-181.
99. Harrison LE, Klimstra DS, Brennan MF. Isolated portal vein involvement in pancreatic adenocarcinoma: a contraindication for resection? *Ann Surg.* 1996;224:342–347.
100. Leach SD, Lee JE, Charnsangavej C, et al. Survival following pancreaticoduodenectomy with resection of the superior mesenteric portal vein confluence for adenocarcinoma of the pancreatic head. *Br J Surg.* 1998;85: 611–717.
101. Protiva P, Sahai AV, Agarwal B. Endoscopic ultrasonography in the diagnosis and staging of pancreatic neoplasms. *Int J Gastrointest Cancer.* 2001;30:33–45.
102. Mertz HR, Sechopoulos P, Delbeke D, et al. EUS, PET, and CT scanning for evaluation of pancreatic adenocarcinoma. *Gastrointest Endosc.* 2000;52:367–371.
103. Levy MJ, Wiersema MJ. Endoscopic ultrasound in the diagnosis and staging of pancreatic cancer. *Oncology.* 2002;16:29–38.
104. Ahmad NA, Lewis JD, Ginsberg GG, et al. EUS in preoperative staging of pancreatic cancer. *Gastrointest Endosc.* 2000;52:463–468.
105. Sasson AR, Hoffman JP, Ross EA, et al. En bloc resection for locally advanced cancer of the pancreas: is it worthwhile? *J Gastrointest Surg.* 2002;6:147–157.
106. Roder JD, Stein HJ, Siewert JR. Carcinoma of the periampullary region: who benefits from portal vein resection? *Am J Surg.* 1996;171:170–174.
107. Launois B, Franci J, Bardaxoglou E, et al. Total pancreatectomy for ductal adenocarcinoma of the pancreas with special reference to resection of the portal vein and multicentric cancer. *World J Surg.* 1993;17:122–126.
108. Brugge WR, Lee MJ, Kelsey PB, et al. The use of EUS to diagnose malignant portal venous system invasion by pancreatic cancer. *Gastrointest Endosc.* 1996;43:561–567.
109. Bluemke DA, Fishman EK. CT and MR evaluation of pancreatic cancer. *Surg Oncol Clin North Am.* 1998;7:103–124.
110. Catalano MF, Sivak MV Jr, Rice T, et al. Endosonographic features predictive of lymph node metastasis. *Gastrointest Endosc.* 1994;40:442–446.
111. Bhutani MS, Hawes RH, Hoffman BJ. A comparison of the accuracy of echo features during endoscopic ultrasound (EUS) and EUS guided fine needle aspiration for diagnosis of malignant lymph node invasion. *Gastrointest Endosc.* 1997;45:474–479.
112. Loren DE, Seghal CM, Ginsberg GG, et al. Computer-assisted analysis of lymph nodes detected by EUS in patients with esophageal carcinoma. *Gastrointest Endosc.* 2002;56:742–746.
113. Nitecki SS, Sarr MG, Colby TV, et al. Long term survival after resection for ductal adenocarcinoma of the pancreas: is it really improving? *Ann Surg.* 1995;221:59–66.
114. Johnstone PA, Sindelar WF. Lymph node involvement and pancreatic resection: correlation with prognosis and local disease control in a clinical trial. *Pancreas.* 1993;8:535–539.
115. Delcore R, Rodriguez FJ, Forster J, et al. Significance of lymph node metastases in patients with pancreatic cancer undergoing curative resection. *Am J Surg.* 1996;172:463–468.
116. Huguier M, Baumel H, Manderscheid JC. Cancer of the exocrine pancreas: a plea for resection. *Hepatogastroenterology.* 1996;43:721–729.
117. Hahn M, Faigel DO. Frequency of mediastinal lymph node metastases in patients undergoing EUS evaluation of pancreaticobiliary masses. *Gastrointest Endosc.* 2001;54: 331–335.
118. Wallace MB, Block M, Hoffman BJ, et al. Detection of telomerase expression in mediastinal lymph nodes of patients with lung cancer. *Am J Respir Crit Care Med.* 2003:167;1670–1675.
119. Mitas M, Cole DJ, Hoover L, et al. Real-time reverse transcription-PCR detects KS1/4 mRNA in mediastinal lymph nodes from patients with non-small cell lung cancer. *Clin Chem.* 2003:49;312–315.
120. Nguyen P, Feng JC, Chang KJ. Endoscopic ultrasound (EUS) and EUS-guided fine-needle aspiration (FNA) of liver lesions. *Gastrointest Endosc.* 1999;50:357–361.
121. Chang KJ, Albers CG, Nguyen P. Endoscopic ultrasound guided fine needle aspiration of pleural and ascitic fluid. *Am J Gastroenterol.* 1995;90:148–150.
122. Nguyen PT, Chang KJ. EUS in the detection of ascites and EUS-guided paracentesis. *Gastrointest Endosc.* 2001;54:336–339.
123. Powis ME, Chang KJ. Endoscopic ultrasound in the clinical staging and management of pancreatic cancer: its impact on cost of treatment. *Cancer Control.* 2000;7:413–420.
124. Mortensen MB, Pless T, Durup J, et al. Clinical impact of endoscopic ultrasound-guided fine needle aspiration biopsy in patients with upper gastrointestinal tract malignancies: a prospective study. *Endoscopy.* 2001:33;478–483.
125. Harada N, Wiersema MJ, Wiersema LM. Endosonography guided celiac plexus neurolysis. *Gastrointest Endosc Clin North Am.* 1997;7:237–245.
126. Gunaratnam NT, Sarma AV, Norton ID, et al. A prospective study of EUS-guided celiac plexus neurolysis for pancreatic cancer pain. *Gastrointest Endosc.* 2001;54:316–324.

127. Chang KJ, Nguyen PT, Thompson JA, et al. Phase I clinical trial of allogeneic mixed lymphocyte culture (cytoimplant) delivered by endoscopic ultrasound-guided fine-needle injection in patients with advanced pancreatic carcinoma. *Cancer*. 2000;88:1325–1335.
128. Hecht JR, Bedford R, Abbruzzese JL, et al. A phase I/II trial of intratumoral endoscopic ultrasound injection of ONYX-015 with intravenous gemcitabine in unresectable pancreatic carcinoma. *Clin Cancer Res*. 2003;9:555–561.
129. Rulyak SJ, Lowenfels AB, Maisonneuve P, et al. Risk factors for the development of pancreatic cancer in familial pancreatic cancer kindreds. *Gastroenterology*. 2003;124:1292–1299.
130. Rulyak SJ, Brentnall TA. Inherited pancreatic cancer: surveillance and treatment strategies for affected families. *Pancreatology*. 2001;1:477–485.
131. Biankin AV, Kench JG, Dijkman FP, et al. Molecular pathogenesis of precursor lesions of pancreatic ductal adenocarcinoma. *Pathology*. 2003;35:14–24.
132. Kimmey MB, Bronner MP, Byrd DR, Brentnall TA. Screening and surveillance for hereditary pancreatic cancer. *Gastrointest Endosc*. 2002;56:S82–S86.
133. Rulyak SJ, Kimmey MB, Veenstra DL, et al. Cost-effectiveness of pancreatic cancer screening in familial pancreatic cancer kindreds. *Gastrointest Endosc*. 2003;57:23–29.
134. Soetikno RM, Chang KJ. Endoscopic ultrasound guided diagnosis and therapy in pancreatic disease. *Gastrointest Endosc Clin North Am*. 1998;8:237–247.
135. Stevens PD, Lightdale CJ. The role of endosonography in the diagnosis and management of pancreatic cancer. *Surg Oncol Clin North Am*. 1998;7:125–133.
136. Barkin JS, Goldstein JA. Diagnostic approach to pancreatic cancer. *Gastroenterol Clin North Am*. 1999;28:709–722.
137. Ritts RE, Pitt HA. CA 19 9 in pancreatic cancer. *Surg Oncol Clin North Am*. 1998;7:93–101.
138. McCune WS, Shorb PE, Moscowitz H. Endoscopic cannulation of the ampulla of Vater: a preliminary report. *Ann Surg*. 1968;167:752.
139. Kawai K, Akasaka Y, Murakami K, et al. Endoscopic sphincterotomy of the ampulla of Vater. *Gastrointest Endosc*. 1974;20:148–151.
140. Classen M, Demling L. Endoscopic sphincterotomy of the papilla of Vater and extraction of stones from the choledochal duct (author's transl.). *Dtsch Med Wochenschr*. 1974;496–497.
141. Aliperti G. Complications related to diagnostic and therapeutic ERCP. *Gastrointest Endosc Clin North Am*. 1996;6:379–407.
142. Baillie J. Complications of ERCP. In: Jacobson IM, ed. *ERCP and Its Applications*. Philadelphia: Lippincott-Raven; 1998:37–54.
143. Baillie J. Predicting and preventing post-ERCP pancreatitis. *Curr Gastroenterol Rep*. 2002;4:112–119.
144. Fazel A, Quadri A, Catalano MF, et al. Does a pancreatic duct stent prevent post-ERCP pancreatitis? A prospective randomized study. *Gastrointest Endosc*. 2003;57:291–294.
145. Hatfield AR, Smithies A, Wilkins R, et al. Assessment of endoscopic retrograde cholangiopancreatography (ERCP) and pure pancreatic juice cytology in patients with pancreatic disease. *Gut*. 1976;17:14–21.
146. Harada H, Sasaki T, Yamamoto N, et al. Assessment of endoscopic aspiration cytology and endoscopic retrograde cholangipancreatography (ERCP) in patients with cancer of the pancreas. Part I. *Gastroenterol Jpn*. 1977;12:52–58.
147. Gilinsky NH, Bornman PC, Girdwood AH, et al. Diagnostic yield of endoscopic retrograde cholangiopancreatography in carcinoma of the pancreas. *Br J Surg*. 1986;73:539–543.
148. Nix GA, Van Overbeeke IC, Wilson JH, et al. ERCP diagnosis of tumors in the region of the head of the pancreas: analysis of criteria and computer-aided diagnosis. *Dig Dis Sci*. 1988;33:577–586.
149. Bakkevold KE, Arnesjo B, Kambestad B. Carcinoma of the pancreas and papilla of Vater: assessment of resectability and factors influencing resectability in stage I carcinomas. A prospective multicentre trial in 472 patients. *Eur J Surg Oncol*. 1992;18:494–507.
150. Ishikawa O, Ohigashi H, Imaoka S, et al. Minute carcinoma of the pancreas measuring 1 cm or less in diameter: collective review of Japanese case reports. *Hepatogastroenterology*. 1999;46:8–15.
151. Ralls PW, Halls J, Renner I, et al. Endoscopic retrograde cholangiopancreatography (ERCP) in pancreatic disease: a reassessment of the specificity of ductal abnormalities indifferentiating benign from malignant disease. *Radiology*. 1980;134:347–352.
152. Plumley TF, Rohrmann CA, Freeny PC, et al. Double duct sign: reassessed significance in ERCP. *AJR Am J Roentgenol*. 1982;138:31–35.
153. Low VH. Retrograde cholangiography of malignant biliary strictures: spectrum of appearances and pitfalls. *Abdom Imaging*. 1997;22:421–425.
154. Hewitt PM, Beningfield SJ, Bornman PC, et al. Pancreatic carcinoma: diagnostic and prognostic implications of a normal pancreatogram. *Surg Endosc*. 1998;12:867–869.
155. Osnes M, Serck-Hanssen A, Kristensen O, et al. Endoscopic retrograde brush cytology in patients with primary and secondary malignancies of the pancreas. *Gut*. 1979;20:279–284.
156. Roberts-Thomson IC, Hobbs JB. Cytodiagnosis of pancreatic and biliary cancer by endoscopic duct aspiration. *Med J Aust*. 1979;1:370–372.
157. Klapdor R, Soehendra N, Kloppel G, et al. Diagnosis of pancreatic carcinoma by means of endoscopic retrograde pancreatography and pancreatic cytology. *Hepatogastroenterology*. 1980;27:227–230.
158. Goodale RL, Gajl-Peczalska K, Dressel T, et al. Cytologic studies for the diagnosis of pancreatic cancer. *Cancer*. 1981;47[6 suppl]:1652–1655.
159. Kameya S, Kuno N, Kasugai T. The diagnosis of pancreatic cancer by pancreatic juice cytology. *Acta Cytol*. 1981;25:354–360.
160. Hunt DR, Blumgart LH. Preoperative differentiation between carcinoma of the pancreas and chronic pancreatitis: the contribution of cytology. *Endoscopy*. 1982;14:171–173.
161. de Bellis M, Sherman S, Fogel EL, et al. Tissue sampling at ERCP in suspected malignant biliary strictures (Part 1). *Gastrointest Endosc*. 2002;56:552–561.

162. de Bellis M, Sherman S, Fogel EL, et al. Tissue sampling at ERCP in suspected malignant biliary strictures (Part 2). *Gastrointest Endosc.* 2002;56:720–730.
163. Aabakken L, Karesen R, Serck-Hanssen A, et al. Transpapillary biopsies and brush cytology from the common bile duct. *Endoscopy.* 1986;18:49–51.
164. Kubota Y, Takaoka M, Tani K, et al. Endoscopic transpapillary biopsy for diagnosis of patients with pancreaticobiliary ductal strictures. *Am J Gastroenterol.* 1993;88:1700–1704.
165. Schoefl R, Haefner M, Wrba F, et al. Forceps biopsy and brush cytology during endoscopic retrograde cholangiopancreatography for the diagnosis of biliary stenoses. *Scand J Gastroenterol.* 1997;32:363–368.
166. Jailwala J, Fogel EL, Sherman S, et al. Triple-tissue sampling at ERCP in malignant biliary obstruction. *Gastrointest Endosc.* 2000;51:383–390.
167. Hurwitz LK, Daniels A, Barkin JS, et al. Preoperative diagnosis of intraductal papillary mucinous tumors of the pancreas by endoscopic pancreatic biopsy. *Gastrointest Endosc.* 2001;53:510–513.
168. Venu RP, Geenen JE, Kini M, et al. Endoscopic retrograde brush cytology. A new technique. *Gastroenterology.* 1990;99:1475–1479.
169. Parasher VK, Huibregtse K. Endoscopic retrograde wire-guided cytology of malignant biliary strictures using a novel scraping brush. *Gastrointest Endosc.* 1998;48:288–290.
170. Farrell RJ, Jain AK, Brandwein SL, et al. The combination of stricture dilation, endoscopic needle aspiration, and biliary brushings significantly improves diagnostic yield from malignant bile duct strictures. *Gastrointest Endosc.* 2001;54:587–594.
171. Mohandas KM, Swaroop VS, Gullar SU, et al. Diagnosis of malignant obstructive jaundice by bile cytology: results improved by dilating the bile duct strictures. *Gastrointest Endosc.* 1994;40:150–154.
172. de Bellis M, Fogel EL, Sherman S, et al. Influence of stricture dilation and repeat brushing on the cancer detection rate of brush cytology in the evaluation of malignant biliary obstruction. *Gastrointest Endosc.* 2003;58:176–182.
173. Farrell RJ, Jain AK, Brandwein SL, et al. The combination of stricture dilation, endoscopic needle aspiration, and biliary brushings significantly improves diagnostic yield from malignant bile duct strictures. *Gastrointest Endosc.* 2001;54:587–594.
174. Devereaux BM, Fogel EL, Bucksot L, et al. Clinical utility of stent cytology for the diagnosis of pancreaticobiliary neoplasms. *Am J Gastroenterol.* 2003;98:1028–1031.
175. Ryan ME, Baldauf MC. Comparison of flow cytometry for DNA content and brush cytology for detection of malignancy in pancreaticobiliary strictures. *Gastrointest Endosc.* 1994;40:133–139.
176. Trumper LH, Burger B, von Bonin F, et al. Diagnosis of pancreatic adenocarcinoma by polymerase chain reaction from pancreatic secretions. *Br J Cancer.* 1994;70:278–284.
177. Lee JG, Leung JW, Cotton PB, et al. Diagnostic utility of K-*ras* mutational analysis on bile obtained by endoscopic retrograde cholangiopancreatography. *Gastrointest Endosc.* 1995;42:317–320.
178. McGuire DE, Venu RP, Brown RD, et al. Brush cytology for pancreatic carcinoma: an analysis of factors influencing results. *Gastrointest Endosc.* 1996;44:300–304.
179. Van Laethem JL, Bourgeois V, Parma J, et al. Relative contribution of K-*ras* gene analysis and brush cytology during ERCP for the diagnosis of biliary and pancreatic diseases. *Gastrointest Endosc.* 1998;47:479–485.
180. Pugliese V, Pujic N, Saccomanno S, et al. Pancreatic intraductal sampling during ERCP in patients with chronic pancreatitis and pancreatic cancer: cytologic studies and k-ras-2 codon 12 molecular analysis in 47 cases. *Gastrointest Endosc.* 2001;54:595–599.
181. Enayati PG, Traverso LW, Galagan K, et al. The meaning of equivocal pancreatic cytology in patients thought to have pancreatic cancer. *Am J Surg.* 1996;171:525–528.
182. Lee JG, Leung JW, Baillie J, et al. Benign, dysplastic, or malignant–making sense of endoscopic bile duct brush cytology: results in 149 consecutive patients. *Am J Gastroenterol.* 1995;90:722–726.
183. Vandervoort J, Soetikno RM, Montes H, et al. Accuracy and complication rate of brush cytology from bile duct versus pancreatic duct. *Gastrointest Endosc.* 1999;49:322–327.
184. Erickson RA, Garza AA. EUS with EUS-guided fine needle aspiration as the first endoscopic test for the evaluation of obstructive jaundice. *Gastrointest Endosc.* 2001;53:475–484.
185. Nix GA, Schmitz PI, Wilson JH, et al. Carcinoma of the head of the pancreas: therapeutic implications of endoscopic retrograde cholangiopancreatography findings. *Gastroenterology.* 1984;87:37–43.
186. Shah SA, Movson J, Ransil BJ, et al. Pancreatic duct stricture length at ERCP predicts tumor size and pathological stage of pancreatic cancer. *Am J Gastroenterol.* 1997;92:964–967.
187. Tsuchiya R, Oribe T, Noda T. Size of the tumor and other factors influencing prognosis of carcinoma of the head of the pancreas. *Am J Gastroenterol.* 1985;80:459–462.
188. Mansfield JC, Griffin SM, Wadehra V, et al. A prospective evaluation of cytology from biliary strictures. *Gut.* 1997;40:671–677.
189. Hara T, Yamaguchi T, Ishihara T, et al. Diagnosis and patient management of intraductal papillary-mucinous tumor of the pancreas by using peroral pancreatoscopy and intraductal ultrasonography. *Gastroenterology.* 2002;122:34–43.
190. Kozarek RA. Endoscopy in the management of malignant obstructive jaundice. *Gastrointest Endosc Clin North Am.* 1996;6:153–176.
191. Rossi RL, Traverso LW, Pimentel F. Malignant obstructive jaundice: evaluation and management. *Surg Clin North Am.* 1996;76:63–70.
192. Costamagna G, Gabbrielli A, Mutignani M, et al.Treatment of "obstructive" pain by endoscopic drainage in patients with pancreatic head carcinoma. *Gastrointest Endosc.* 1993;39:774–777.
193. Ashby K, Lo SK. The role of pancreatic stenting in obstructive ductal disorders other than pancreas divisum. *Gastrointest Endosc.* 1995;42:306–311.

194. Costamagna G, Alevras P, Palladino F, et al. Endoscopic pancreatic stenting in pancreatic cancer. *Can J Gastroenterol.*1999;13:481–487.
195. Tham TC, Lichtenstein DR, Vandervoort J, et al. Pancreatic duct stents for "obstructive type" pain in pancreatic malignancy. *Am J Gastroenterol.* 2000;95:956–960.
196. Amouyal P, Palazzo L, Amouyal G, et al. Endosonography: promising method for diagnosis of extrahepatic cholestasis. *Lancet.* 1989;2:1195–1198.
197. Snady H, Cooperman A, Siegel J. Endoscopic ultrasonography compared with computed tomography with ERCP in patients with obstructive jaundice or small peri pancreatic mass. *Gastrointest Endosc.* 1992;38:27–34.
198. Dancygier H, Nattermann C. The role of endoscopic ultrasonography in biliary tract disease: obstructive jaundice. *Stadtische Kliniken Endosc.* 1994;26:800–802.
199. Caletti G, Fusaroli P, Bocus P. Endoscopic ultrasonography. *Digestion.* 1998;59:509–529.
200. Palazzo L, Girollet PP, Salmeron M, et al. Value of endoscopic ultrasonography in the diagnosis of common bile duct stones: comparison with surgical exploration and ERCP. *Gastrointest Endosc.* 1995;42:225–231.
201. Norton SA, Alderson D. Prospective comparison of endoscopic ultrasonography and endoscopic retrograde cholangiopancreatography in the detection of bile duct stones. *Br J Surg.* 1997;84:1366–1369.
202. Canto MI, Chak A, Stellato T, et al. Endoscopic ultrasonography versus cholangiography for the diagnosis of choledocholithiasis. *Gastrointest Endosc.* 1998;47:439–448.
203. Motte S, Deviere J, Dumonceau JM, et al. Risk factors for septicemia following endoscopic biliary stenting. *Gastroenterology.* 1991;101:1374–1381.
204. Niederau C, Pohlmann U, Lubke H, Thomas L. Prophylactic antibiotic treatment in therapeutic or complicated diagnostic ERCP: results of a randomized controlled clinical study. *Gastrointest Endosc.* 1994;40:533–537.
205. Saleh MM, Norregaard P, Jorgensen HL, et al. Preoperative endoscopic stent placement before pancreaticoduodenectomy: a meta-analysis of the effect on morbidity and mortality. *Gastrointest Endosc.* 2002;56:529–534.
206. Stevens PD, Lightdale CJ. Endoscopic ultrasound for pancreatic and biliary disease. Impact on the role of diagnostic ERCP. In: Jacobson IM, ed. *ERCP and Its Applications.* Philadelphia: Lippincott-Raven; 1998:55–64.
207. Dancygier H, Lightdale CJ. *Endosonography in gastroenterology.* New York: Thieme; 1999;148–153.

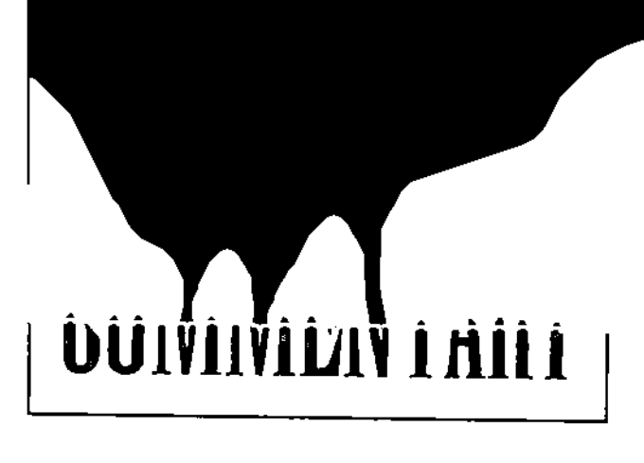

Kenneth J. Chang, MD

In this chapter, Dr. Erickson presents a thorough and comprehensive overview of endoscopic ultrasound (EUS) and endoscopic retrograde cholangiopancreatography (ERCP) in the diagnosis, staging, and treatment of pancreatic cancer. It was elegantly pointed out that the primary impact of endosonography on the management of pancreatic cancer is currently in detection and cytologic diagnosis. Currently existing modalities still cannot rival EUS/fine-needle aspiration (FNA) in its unique diagnostic capabilities. Staging of pancreatic cancer, however, is no longer considered to be championed by EUS/FNA. Most recent studies suggest that the EUS T- and N-staging accuracy is considerably lower than the initial studies. How can one explain a decrease in staging accuracy when the technology and training have dramatically improved? Does the recent literature truly confirm that computed tomography (CT) and magnetic resonance imaging (MRI) are superior to EUS in staging pancreatic cancer? This is worth examining further.

The initial studies on the staging accuracy of EUS for pancreatic cancer were very encouraging. These results showed that EUS had a T-stage accuracy of 85%–94% and an N-stage accuracy of 72%–80%.[1-3] During this time, EUS T and N-stage accuracy was superior to conventional imaging with either transabdominal ultrasound (US) or CT. Thus, in the early 1990s, it was stated that "EUS is the single best modality for the pre-operative local staging of pancreatic cancer." However, over the last 5 years, this notion has been challenged. The T-stage accuracy for EUS in the recent literature (1999 to present) ranges from 69%–85%.[4-6] Taking the combined accuracy of these studies, the mean accuracy for EUS T-stage accuracy is 77%, with a 95% confidence interval between 70% and 83% (Table 1). The N-stage accuracy ranged from 54%–72%. The calculated combined nodal accuracy was 69%, with a 95% confidence interval between 56% and 71% (Table 2). Thus, there is an obvious discrepancy between the earlier and more recent articles with regard to staging accuracy of EUS (Table 3).

Several possible explanations for these discrepancies exist. The earlier studies had relatively small numbers of patients enrolled, and almost all of these patients went to surgery. However, the recent studies had larger numbers of patients, with less than 50% of the EUS patients going on to surgery. Those patients who were determined to be "unresectable" by EUS did not go to surgery and obviously could not be included in the accuracy calculation. In addition, patients in the recent studies would most likely have had better imaging for metastatic disease, namely helical CT (HCT). These patients would also not be included in the surgical correlation group, whereas in the early 1990s, these metastases may have been missed by non-helical CT. It would be reasonable to assume that pa-

Table 1 EUS T-Stage Accuracy

Author	# of Patients Staged by EUS	# of Surgical Patients	Staging Accuracy	% Accuracy
Buscail et al.[4]	73	26	19/26	73%
Gress et al.[5]	151	75	64/75	85%
Ahmad et al.[6]	—	89	55/79	69%
Total		190	138/180	77% (95% CI = 70%–83%)

Table 2 N-Stage Accuracy

Author	# of Patients Staged by EUS	# of Surgical Patients	Staging Accuracy	% Accuracy
Buscail et al.[4]	73	26	18/26	69%
Gress et al.[5]	151	71	51/71	72%
Ahmad et al.[6]	—	89	35/67	54%
Total		186	104/164	63% (95% CI = 56%–71%)

Table 3 Comparison of Early and Recent Studies on EUS Staging Accuracy

Author	Year	n	# of Surgical Patients	T Stage (%)
Grimm et al.[1]	1990	—	26	85
Tio et al.[2]	1990	43	36	92
Rosch et al.[3]	1992	46	40	94
Buscail et al.[4]	1999	73	26	73
Gress et al.[5]	1999	151	75	85
Ahmad et al.[6]	2000	—	89	69

Table 4 T- and N-Stage Accuracy from Ahmad et al.[7]

	Surgical Stage		
EUS Stage	T4 (N = 41)	T3 (N = 38)	Tx (N = 10)
T4 (41)	25 (61%)	9 (22%)	7 (17%)
T3 (46)	15 (33%)	28 (61%)	3 (6%)
Tx (2)	1 (50%)	1 (50%)	—
	N1 (N = 43)	N0 (N = 24)	Nx (N = 22)
N1 (42)	20 (48%)	9 (21%)	13 (31%)
N0 (45)	21 (47%)	15 (33%)	9 (20%)
Nx (2)	2 (100%)	—	—

tients who were deemed "unresectable" by EUS were more "clear-cut" cases where the endosonographer had a high level of certainty that these patients were truly unresectable. If these patients were added to the surgical correlation group, it may reduce the bias of the staging accuracy results.

However, there is still a major concern regarding the apparent "overstaging" by EUS in the more recent articles. Specifically, the article by Ahmad et al.[7] showed a 23% overstaging by EUS where patients were called T4 (unresectable) by EUS, only to go to surgery and ultimately be found to have T3 (resectable) lesions. A summary of the T- and N-stage data from this study is shown on Table 4.

A more detailed analysis of these overstaged patients shows that all nine patients were staged as T4 based on vascular invasion. It is important to look carefully at the staging criteria used to determine vascular invasion. Five of nine patients were assessed to have vascular invasion based on "loss of interface" only. Seven of the nine tumors were large (>3 cm). Four of nine had chronic pancreatitis changes on pathology. It is important, then, to review the studies that have been used to establish the vascular invasion criteria for EUS. These studies are summarized in Table 5.

The relatively small number of patients and the lack of concordance in these studies stand out. Certainly, there is a trade-off between sensitivity and specificity. However, the most appropriate criterion to adopt clinically is one with the highest specificity, even if it means accepting a lower sensitivity. Based on these studies, the EUS criteria of irregular vein wall, tumor in the vessel lumen, or formation of collaterals should be the only ones used because they have the highest specificity. The loss of hyperechoic interface, based on these studies and confirmed by Ahmad et al.[7] should be considered "marginal" criteria for predicting vascular invasion. Further studies are certainly necessary to refine our current vascular staging by EUS.

EUS Versus HCT

More important than the explanation for seemingly decreased staging accuracy for EUS, is the question concerning what are the recent comparison studies between EUS versus CT and MRI for staging pancreatic cancer? A recent review of studies comparing EUS with HCT for pancreatic cancer by Hunt and Faigel[8] is summarized in Table 6. This review shows that the pooled data among the four recent studies show superiority of EUS to HCT in detection of pancreatic tumor (97% vs 73%), in accuracy for resectability (91% vs 83%), and sensitivity for vascular invasion (91% vs 64%). Although the gap is certainly closing, EUS is still the most accurate modality for tumor detection, with a relatively high accuracy for local staging. In addition, as a single modality, EUS, especially when combined with EUS-guided FNA, has been shown to be cost-efficient.[9]

MRI Versus HCT and EUS

Four clinical studies have recently been published comparing the utility of MRI to HCT in the vascular staging of pancreatic cancer. Nishiharu et al.[10] reported on 57 patients, 31 of whom were confirmed at surgery to have pancreatic cancer. All patients underwent both HCT and MRI (turbo spin-echo and fast low-angle shot) studies. Pancreatic enhancement by HCT and MRI was comparable, but depiction of vessels was superior with HCT. Detection of tumor was comparable. However, HCT was significantly superior to MRI in showing invasion into the peripancreatic tissue, portal vein, and/or adjacent arteries ($P < 0.01$). The authors concluded that HCT is more sensitive than MRI for detection of peripancreatic and vascular invasion in patients with pancreatic cancer. Sheridan et al.,[11] however, in a series of 33 patients, concluded that MRI was superior to HCT in pre-

Table 5 Summary of Studies Determining EUS Criteria for Vascular Invasion

Author	# of Patients	Criteria	Sensitivity (%)	Specificity (%)	Accuracy (%)
Yasuda et al.[20]	37	Rough edged vessel with compression	79	87	81
Rosch et al.[3]	40	Close contact, abnormal contour, loss of interface	91	96	94
Snady et al.[21]	33	Venous collateral	19	100	55
		Tumor in lumen	38	100	66
		Loss of hyperechoic interface	33	100	63
Brugge[22]	28	Irregular vein wall	40	100	85
		Loss of hyperechoic interface	50	85	77
		Proximity of mass	87	55	73
		Size of mass	80	23	33

Table 6 Summary of Studies Comparing EUS to HCT in Pancreatic Cancer

	Detection		Accuracy for Resectability		Sensitivity for Vascular Invasion	
Series	EUS	CT	EUS	CT	EUS	CT
Legmann et al.[23]	27/27	25/27	20/22	19/22	6/7	7/7
Midwinter et al.[24]	33/34	26/34	25/30	23/30	13/16	9/16
Tierney et al.[25]			30/31	25/31	16/16	10/16
Mertz et al.[26]	29/31	16/31	16/16	13/16	6/6	3/6
Total	97%	73%	91%	83%	91%	64%
P value*	<0.001		0.02		<0.001	

* Fisher exact test.

dicting resectability (87% vs 76%; $P = 0.02$). The two most recent studies concluded that there was no significant difference between the two modalities: that HCT and MRI had similar accuracies for staging vascular invasion. Romijn et al.[12] compared HCT with MRI (with and without mangafodipir trisodium infusion). Vascular staging accuracy was 81%, 75%, and 81% for HCT, MRI alone, and MRI with mangafodipir trisodium infusion, and overall staging accuracies were 57%, 54%, and 54%, respectively. Arslan et al.[13] reported that among 31 patients with pancreatic cancer who had surgical staging, MRI, MRI angiography, and HCT had vascular staging accuracies of 87%, 90% and 90%, respectively. Thus, the 4 studies comparing HCT with MRI are inconclusive as to which modality is superior for staging pancreatic cancer. There was one study by Ahmad et al.[6] that compared MRI with EUS among 63 patients with adenocarcinoma of the pancreas. They concluded that neither MRI nor EUS alone were highly sensitive (73% vs 61%) or predictive (positive predictive value (PPV) = 77% vs 69%) of resectability. However, when both tests agreed on resectability, nearly all patients (89%) were found to be resectable at surgery.

M-Staging by EUS

It has long been thought that EUS cannot be used for metastatic staging of pancreatic cancer. Recent studies have shown that EUS combined with FNA may be quite effective at assessing the majority of the liver, detecting and taking tissue samples of suspected metastatic lesions within both the left and right hepatic lobes.[14] In addition, EUS/FNA can also sample scant amounts of ascitic fluid to assess for peritoneal metastasis.[15] Newer generation echoendoscopes will be able to penetrate further into the liver and potentially assess the entire liver for possible metastasis. If this occurs, EUS may become even more effective in the diagnosis and staging of these patients. Furthermore, therapeutic interventions with EUS-guided celiac nerve block and/or simultaneous ERCP with stent placement for palliation of jaundice could be performed during the same endoscopy session.

Therapeutic EUS

Erickson includes a brief paragraph on therapeutic applications of EUS. This needs to be underscored as a promising new "delivery system" for anti-tumor agents. Patients with significant abdominal pain who have unresectable pancreatic cancer may be candidates for EUS-guided celiac plexus neurolysis (CPN). Wiersema and Wiersema[16] described this novel technique and the impact on pancreatic cancer patients' pain management. After visualizing the celiac trunk by the linear array echoendoscope and using a 22-gauge needle, an injection of bupivacaine (0.25%) followed by ethyl alcohol (98%) can then be performed on either side of the vessel. Up to 88% of patients had persistent improvement in their pain score. Only minor complications were seen and consisted of transient diarrhea in four patients.[16] This anterior transgastric approach for performing CPN is considered theoretically safer when compared with the traditional CT-guided posterior method. This is because of the rare reported cases of paraplegia that occurred with the posterior approach due to its proximity to the spinal column.

We have examined the feasibility and safety of direct injection of allogenic mixed lymphocyte culture (cytoimplant) in pancreatic adenocarcinoma under EUS guidance.[17] In a phase I clinical trial, eight patients with unresectable pancreatic adenocarcinoma underwent EUS-guided fine-needle injection (FNI) of cytoimplants. Four patients were stage II, three stage III, and one stage IV. The escalating doses of cytoimplants 3-, 6-, or 9-billion cells were implanted using a novel EUS-guided FNI technique. The median survival was 13.2 months with two partial responders and one minor response. Major complications, including bone marrow toxicity, hemorrhagic, infectious, renal, or cardiopulmonary toxicity, were absent. Low-grade fever was encountered in seven of the eight patients and was symptomatically treated with acetaminophen. Our study showed that local immunotherapy is feasible and safe. The technique of EUS-guided FNI was recently also used to deliver anti-tumor viral therapy.[19] ONYX-015 (dl1520) is an E1B 55-kD gene-deleted replication-selective adenovirus that preferentially replicates in and kills malignant cells. Twenty-one patients with locally advanced adenocarcinoma of the pancreas or with metastatic disease, but minimal or absent liver metastases, underwent eight sessions of ONYX-015 delivered by EUS injection into the primary pancreatic tumor over 8 weeks. The final four treatments were given in combination with gemcitabine (intravenously, 1000 mg/m^2). After combination therapy, 2 patients had partial regressions of the injected tumor, 2 had minor responses, 6 had stable disease, and 11 had progressive disease. No clinical pancreatitis occurred despite mild, transient elevations in lipase in a minority of patients. Two patients had sepsis before the institution of prophylactic oral antibiotics. Two patients had duodenal perforations from the rigid endoscope tip. No perforations occurred after the protocol was changed to transgastric injections only.

The most recent EUS-guided anti-tumor therapy involves a novel gene therapy.[19] TNFerade is a replication-deficient adenovector containing the human tumor necrosis factor-α (TNF-α) gene, regulated by a radiation-inducible promoter Egr-1. The study design consisted of a 5-week treatment of weekly intratumoral injections of TNFerade ($4 \times 10^{9-11}$ particle units in 2 mL). EUS-guided FNI was compared to percutaneous approaches (PTAs) (CT or US). TNFerade was combined with continuous intravenous 5-FU (200 mg/m^2/day $\times$ 5 days/week) and radiation (50.4 Gy). TNFerade was delivered with a single–needle pass at a single site in the tumor for PTAs, whereas up to four injections were given by EUS. The clinical endpoints included safety and tumor response on spiral CT by a core lab. Of 37 patients, 17 had EUS and 20 had PTA (similar TNFerade doses). Baseline tumor stage, nodal staging, tumor size, and CA 19-9 levels were similar in the EUS and PTA groups. One dose-limiting toxicity (grade 3 hypotension) was noted in a PTA patient; all other adverse events potentially related to TNFerade were grades 1–2. Procedure-related adverse events were all grades 1–2 and were similar between the two groups, except for injection site pain: 35% PTA versus 0% EUS ($P = 0.01$). Tumor responses and disease control were similar. Four patients underwent resection; one, an EUS patient, had a complete pathologic response. These initial studies have established that EUS-guided FNI is an effective delivery system for anti-tumor agents.

Thus, despite improvement in other imaging modalities, EUS/FNA still plays an important role for both the diagnosis and staging of pancreatic cancer. Recent reports of the role for EUS in M–staging as well as simultaneous biopsy and therapeutic interventions will further expand the importance of this modality in the management of patients with pancreatic cancer.

References

1. Grimm H, Maydeo A, Soehendra N. Endoluminal ultrasound for the diagnosis and staging of pancreatic cancer. *Baillieres Clin Gastroenterol.* 1990;4:869–888.
2. Tio TL, Tytgat GN, Cikot RJ, Houthoff HJ, Sars PR. Ampullopancreatic carcinoma: preoperative TNM classification with endosonography. *Radiology*. 1990;175:455–461.
3. Rosch T, Braig C, Gain T, et al. Staging of pancreatic and ampullary carcinoma by endoscopic ultrasonography: comparison with conventional sonography, computed tomography, and angiography. *Gastroenterology*. 1992;102:188–199.

4. Buscail L, Pages P, Berthelemy P, Fourtanier G, Frexinos J, Escourrou J. Role of EUS in the management of pancreatic and ampullary carcinoma: a prospective study assessing resectability and prognosis. *Gastrointest Endosc.* 1999;50:34–40.
5. Gress FG, Hawes RH, Savides TJ, et al. Role of EUS in the preoperative staging of pancreatic cancer: a large single-center experience. *Gastrointest Endosc.* 1999;50:786–791.
6. Ahmad NA, Lewis JD, Siegelman ES, Rosato EF, Ginsberg GG, Kochman ML. Role of endoscopic ultrasound and magnetic resonance imaging in the preoperative staging of pancreatic adenocarcinoma. *Am J Gastroenterol.* 2000;95:1926–1931.
7. Ahmad NA, Lewis JD, Ginsberg GG, Rosato EF, Morris JB, Kochman ML. EUS in preoperative staging of pancreatic cancer. *Gastrointest Endosc.* 2000;52:463–468.
8. Hunt GC, Faigel DO. Assessment of EUS for diagnosing, staging, and determining resectability of pancreatic cancer: a review. *Gastrointest Endosc.* 2002;55:232–237.
9. Harewood GC, Wiersema MJ. A cost analysis of endoscopic ultrasound in the evaluation of pancreatic head adenocarcinoma. *Am J Gastroenterol.* 2001;96:2651–2656.
10. Nishiharu T, Yamashita Y, Abe Y, et al. Local extension of pancreatic carcinoma: assessment with thin-section helical CT versus with breath-hold fast MR imaging–ROC analysis. *Radiology.* 1999;212:445–452.
11. Sheridan MB, Ward J, Guthrie JA, et al. Dynamic contrast-enhanced MR imaging and dual-phase helical CT in the preoperative assessment of suspected pancreatic cancer: a comparative study with receiver operating characteristic analysis. *AJR Am J Roentgenol.* 1999;173:583–590.
12. Romijn MG, Stoker J, van Eijck CH, van Muiswinkel JM, Torres CG, Lameris JS. MRI with mangafodipir trisodium in the detection and staging of pancreatic cancer. *J Magn Reson Imaging.* 2000;12:261–268.
13. Arslan A, Buanes T, Geitung JT. Pancreatic carcinoma: MR, MR angiography and dynamic helical CT in the evaluation of vascular invasion. *Eur J Radiol.* 2001;38:151–159.
14. Nguyen P, Feng JC, Chang KJ. Endoscopic ultrasound (EUS) and EUS-guided fine-needle aspiration (FNA) of liver lesions. *Gastrointest Endosc.* 1999;50:357–361.
15. Nguyen P, Chang KJ. Endoscopic ultrasound (EUS) in the detection of ascites and EUS-guided paracentesis. *Gastrointest Endosc.* 2001;54:336–339.
16. Wiersema M, Wiersema L. Endosonography guided celiac plexus neurolysis (EUS CPN) in patients with pain due to intra-abdominal malignancy (IAM) [abstract]. *Gastrointest Endosc.* 1996;43:A565.
17. Chang KJ, Nguyen PT, Thompson JA, et al. Phase I clinical trial of allogeneic mixed lymphocyte culture (cytoimplant) delivered by endoscopic ultrasound-guided fine-needle injection in patients with advanced pancreatic carcinoma. *Cancer.* 2000;88:1325–1335.
18. Hecht JR, Bedford R, Abbruzzese JL, et al. A phase I/II trial of intratumoral endoscopic ultrasound injection of ONYX-015 with intravenous gemcitabine in unresectable pancreatic carcinoma. *Clin Cancer Res.* 2003;9:555–561.
19. Chang KC, Senzer N, Chung T, et al. A novel gene transfer therapy against pancreatic cancer (TNFerade) delivered by endoscopic ultrasound (EUS) and percutaneous guided fine needle injection (FNI) [abstract]. *Gastrointest Endosc.* (in press).
20. Yasuda K, Mukai H, Fujimoto S, Nakajima M, Kawai K. The diagnosis of pancreatic cancer by endoscopic ultrasonography. *Gastrointest Endosc.* 1988;34:1–8.
21. Snady H, Bruckner H, Siegel J, Cooperman A, Neff R, Kiefer L. Endoscopic ultrasonographic criteria of vascular invasion by potentially resectable pancreatic tumors. *Gastrointest Endosc.* 1994; 40:326–333.
22. Brugge WR. Pancreatic cancer staging: endoscopic ultrasonography criteria for vascular invasion. *Gastrointest Endosc Clin N Am.* 1995; 5:741–753.
23. Legmann P, Vignaux O, Dousset B, et al. Pancreatic tumors: comparison of dual-phase helical CT and endoscopic sonography. *AJR Am J Roentgenol.* 1998;170:1315–1322.
24. Midwinter MJ, Beveridge CJ, Wilsdon JB, Bennett MK, Baudouin CJ, Charnley RM. Correlation between spiral computed tomography, endoscopic ultrasonography and findings at operation in pancreatic and ampullary tumours. *Br J Surg.* 1999;86:189–193.
25. Tierney WM, Francis IR, Eckhauser F, Elta G, Nostrant TT, Scheiman JM. The accuracy of EUS and helical CT in the assessment of vascular invasion by peripapillary malignancy. *Gastrointest Endosc.* 2001;53:182–188.
26. Mertz HR, Sechopoulos P, Delbeke D, Leach SD. EUS, PET, and CT scanning for evaluation of pancreatic adenocarcinoma. *Gastrointest Endosc.* 2000;52:367–371.

14

Laparoscopic Staging

Olga N. Tucker, MD
Kevin C. Conlon, MD, MBA

Accurate staging of disease is of paramount importance in planning treatment approaches to upper gastrointestinal cancer. Staging procedures should accurately define the extent of disease, direct appropriate therapy, and avoid unnecessary interventional techniques in a cost-efficient and safe manner. This chapter focuses on the role of laparoscopy in the management of patients with pancreatic cancer. Despite the concerns of Bernard Bernheim,[1] of Johns Hopkins University in 1911 that "a structure lying as deeply as the pancreas could not be inspected," laparoscopic staging has become an important tool in the assessment of patients with pancreatic cancer.

Historical Perspective

Laparoscopic staging examination for abdominal malignancies has evolved over the past century. George Kelling,[2] a German physicist, introduced the concept of laparoscopy with his description of "endoscopy of an unopened abdominal cavity" in dogs with the use of a Nitze cystoscope. A Russian gynecologist, Dimitri Von Ott,[3] performed the first human procedure in 1901. Cystoscopic examination of the abdominal cavity was described in 1910 by Jacobaeus.[4] During that same year, Bernheim,[1] of John Hopkins University, conducted experimental work in the Hunterian library using a proctoscope of 0.5-inch bore with blunting of the distal end by a metal collar to perform inspection of the abdominal cavity. In 1911, Bernheim[1] staged a patient of W.S. Halstead with presumed pancreatic cancer before laparotomy. In his seminal paper *Organoscopy. Cystoscopy of the Abdominal Cavity* he stated that "In cases of ordinary exploratory operations for carcinoma, before having recourse to the usual large incision, the cystoscope is introduced through a very small and relatively unimportant incision, possibly made with cocaine, which may reveal general metastases or a secondary nodule in the liver, thus rendering further procedures unnecessary and saving the patient a rather prolonged convalescence."[1]

The term *laparoscopy* was first coined in 1911 by Jacobaeus,[5,6] who published a series of 97 laparoscopic cases performed between 1910 and 1912 at Stockholm's Community Hospital. Kelling[7] continued to develop the procedure in experimental work with dogs. Further work in the 1930s led to the concept of creating a pneumoperitoneum with carbon dioxide or oxygen[8] and the design of the spring-loaded Veress needle.[9] However, the technique was not widely adopted.[10] The introduction of the fiber optic bundle, improved instrumentation, and advances in video endoscopy led to improved visualization; however, the procedure was not embraced until the advent of laparoscopic cholecystectomy.[11,12] Worldwide acceptance of the technique of laparoscopic cholecystectomy led to an explosion of interest in minimally invasive techniques.[13,14]

Indications for Laparoscopy in Pancreatic Cancer

The National Cancer Institute Surveillance, Epidemiology, and End Results Program estimated 30,700 new cases of pancreatic cancer in 2003 in the United States.[15] The most common malignant tumor is ductal adenocarcinoma, accounting for 90% of cases. It remains one of the most lethal malignancies. Its mortality rate is in excess of 95% of its incidence rate, and it has the lowest 5-year survival rate of any cancer.[16] Unfortunately, most patients present at a late stage when locally advanced or metastatic disease precludes curative therapy. At the time of diagnosis, only 15%–20% of patients have disease confined to the pancreas, 20%–30% have locally advanced disease, and >50% have distant spread. The median survival in unresectable disease is 4.1 months, and the overall 5-year survival is 2%–3%.[17,18] Surgical resection remains the only therapy to result in long-term survival, albeit in a small percentage of patients.[19-21] In patients with advanced local or metastatic disease, the role of surgery is more controversial. Many authors have argued that nonoperative palliative procedures can be performed, eliminating the need for laparotomy.

Several reported studies have demonstrated the value of laparoscopy in the staging of intraabdominal malignancies. Staging laparoscopy is used as a technique to decrease the number of unnecessary open exploratory laparotomies. Avoidance of unnecessary open operations should in theory lead to decreased perioperative morbidity and mortality, shorter hospital stay, reduced time to appropriate therapy, improved quality of life, and reduced hospital costs.

The role of laparoscopy in the management of pancreatic cancer has evolved over many years. Proponents of laparoscopic staging have argued that because of the poor prognosis in patients with unresectable disease, avoidance of a laparotomy is beneficial, with the reduced hospital stay and the reduced time to administration of chemotherapy or chemoradiation.[22] In many centers, laparoscopic staging has been made an integral component of the preoperative workup of patients with radiologic resectable disease. From 1983 to 1992, before the introduction of laparoscopic staging at Memorial Sloan-Kettering, 1135 patients with potentially resectable pancreatic cancer were explored, and only 35% underwent resection. Laparoscopy was attempted in 243 patients with radiologically resectable disease from 1993 to 1996. One hundred eighty-five patients underwent exploratory surgery, and 74% underwent resection.[23] Laparoscopy can be performed for definitive diagnosis and biopsy in patients with suspected liver or peritoneal metastases that are inaccessible or too small to undergo biopsy with the use of interventional radiologic techniques. Laparoscopic ultrasound can aid in obtaining sufficient tissue for diagnosis when metastatic lesions are located deep in the liver parenchyma. Despite advances in radiologic techniques for preoperative imaging, patients thought to have resectable pancreatic cancer have unsuspected metastases in 20%–35% of cases.[22,24-26]

In addition to the determination of resectability, laparoscopic staging may play a role in the accurate stratification of patients with unresectable pancreatic cancer before treatment is initiated for locally advanced or metastatic disease. Staging laparoscopy can be used in patients undergoing neoadjuvant treatment regimens before planned resection to assess tumor response and the presence or absence of metastatic disease. The technique could also play a role in the accurate assessment of response in patients with advanced disease who are undergoing novel chemotherapeutic approaches as part of experimental protocols. Clinical and radiographic responses may result in the need for restaging and resection.

Technique of Laparoscopic Staging

The technique of laparoscopic staging should mimic the operative assessment performed at laparotomy. We favor an extended laparoscopic technique in the staging of pancreatic cancer (Table 14.1).[27] A multiport technique under general anesthesia in the operating room is

Table 14.1 Laparoscopic Assessment

Examination of the peritoneal cavity
Insertion of laparoscopic trocars
Instillation of 200 mL of normal saline and aspiration of specimen for cytology
Assessment of primary tumor
Examination of the liver
Examination of regional lymph nodes
Identification of the ligament of Treitz, inspection of the mesocolon, duodenum, and jejunum
Laparoscopic ultrasound

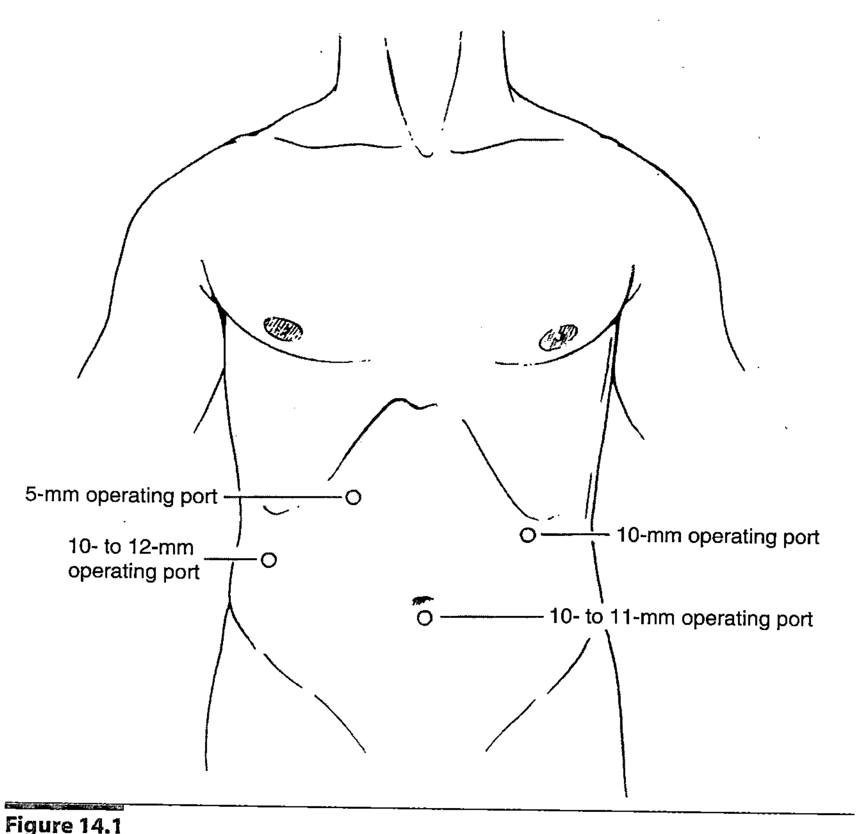

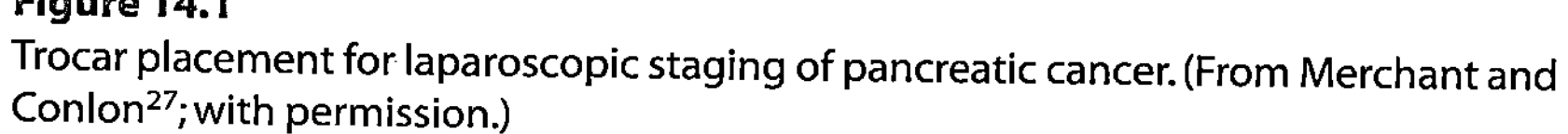

Figure 14.1
Trocar placement for laparoscopic staging of pancreatic cancer. (From Merchant and Conlon[27]; with permission.)

recommended; this approach allows for a thorough examination of the peritoneal cavity.

The patient is placed supine on the operating table. Access to the peritoneal cavity is achieved by an open Hasson technique through a subumbilical incision. The initial 1- to 2-cm incision is extended down to the fascia, which is incised in a vertical manner with the peritoneum under direct vision. A blunt port is inserted through the umbilical incision and attached to a high-flow insufflator at a set flow rate of 10-15L /min. A 5- to 10-mm 30-degree angled telescope is used. Secondary 5- to 10-mm trocars are placed in the right (10-mm and 5-mm) and left (5-mm) upper quadrants along the line of a bilateral subcostal incision (Fig. 14.1).

A four-quadrant systematic examination of the peritoneal cavity is performed for obvious peritoneal extension of disease. Peritoneal washings for cytologic examination are taken from the right and left upper quadrants after instillation of 200 mL into the peritoneal cavity before manipulation of the primary or metastatic tumor. The primary tumor is assessed. Local extent, size, and fixation are noted. Extension to contiguous organs, such as the colon, duodenum, spleen, and stomach, are identified. The patient is placed in a 20-degree reverse Trendelenburg position with 10 degrees of left lateral tilt. The anterior and posterior surfaces of the left lateral segment of the liver are examined, followed by examination of the anterior and inferior surface of the right lobe. Palpation of the liver is achieved with the use of a 10-mm instrument (Fig. 14.2).

Improved visualization of diaphragmatic and posterior surfaces may be achieved by placing the camera in the right upper quadrant port. The hilum of the liver, hepatoduodenal ligament, and foramen of Winslow are examined (Fig. 14.3). Periportal nodes undergo biopsy, if required. The patient is then positioned in a 10-degree Trendelenburg position without lateral tilt, and the omentum is retracted toward the left upper quadrant. The transverse colon is elevated to examine the transverse mesocolon and the ligament of Treitz. The mesocolon is carefully inspected, with particular attention being paid to the middle colic vein, which is usually visible. Any nodes around the middle colic vein are noted. The patient is then returned to a supine position, the left lobe of the liver is elevated, and the gastrohepatic omentum is incised to gain entrance into the lesser sac (Fig. 14.4). This exposes the caudate lobe of the liver, inferior vena cava, and celiac axis. Even in obese patients,

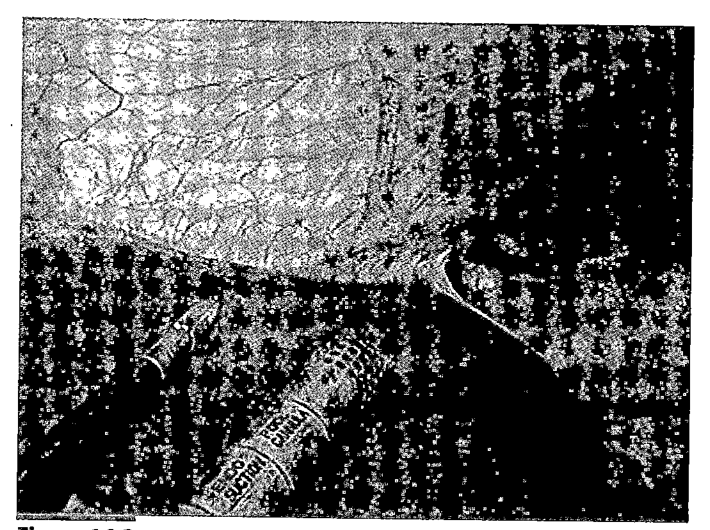

Figure 14.2
Two-instrument technique for palpation of liver surface for detection of liver metastases.

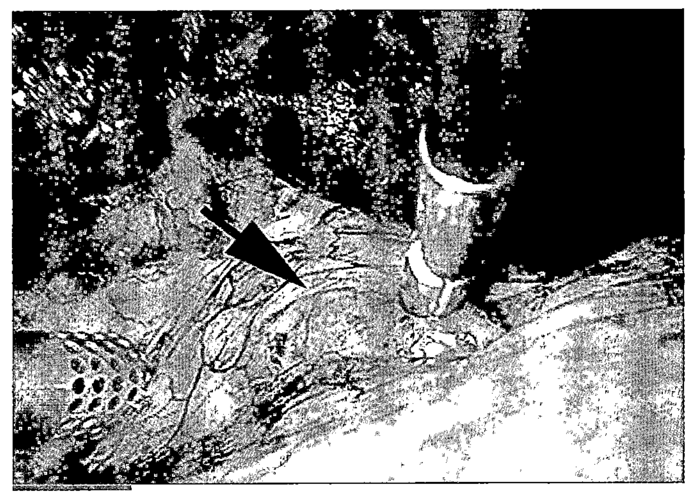

Figure 14.3
Two-instrument technique for palpation of enlarged hepatoduodenal lymph nodes complemented by assessment with intraoperative ultrasound. The arrow points to metastatic hepatoduodenal lymphadenopathy.

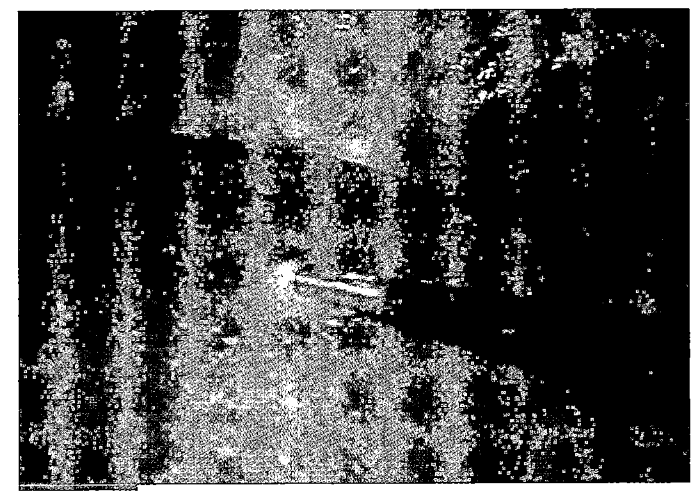

Figure 14.5
Biopsy of liver metastases.

the part of the lesser omentum overlying the caudate lobe is transparent, rendering safe access to the lesser sac.

The lesser sac is entered with the camera in the right upper quadrant port for evaluation of the primary tumor. The anterior aspect of the pancreas, hepatic artery, and left gastric artery are visualized. The course of the hepatic artery is visualized to the porta. Celiac, portal, perigastric, and hepatogastric nodes can be sampled if they are suspicious in appearance. During the examination, biopsy of suspicious peritoneal or hepatic lesions can readily be performed with cup forceps (Fig. 14.5).

Laparoscopic ultrasound (LUS) is then performed with a 7.5-MHz flexible probe to systematically evaluate the liver and pancreas. Full examination of the liver, portal pedicles, and hepatic veins is possible through the 10-mm right upper quadrant port. Laparoscopic ultrasound evaluates

1. The liver for small intraparenchymal lesions
2. The primary tumor's relationship to surrounding vasculature, in particular invasion into portal vein, superior mesenteric vein, or superior mesenteric artery (Fig. 14.6)
3. Peripancreatic extension of tumor

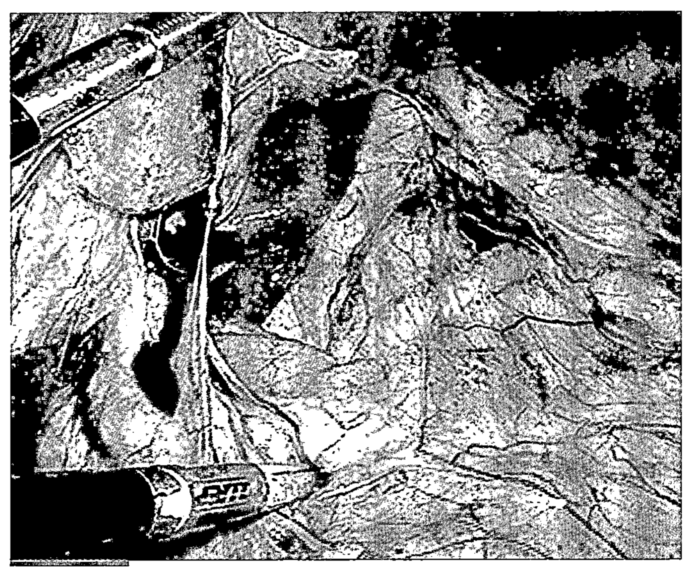

Figure 14.4
Division of the gastrohepatic (lesser) omentum.

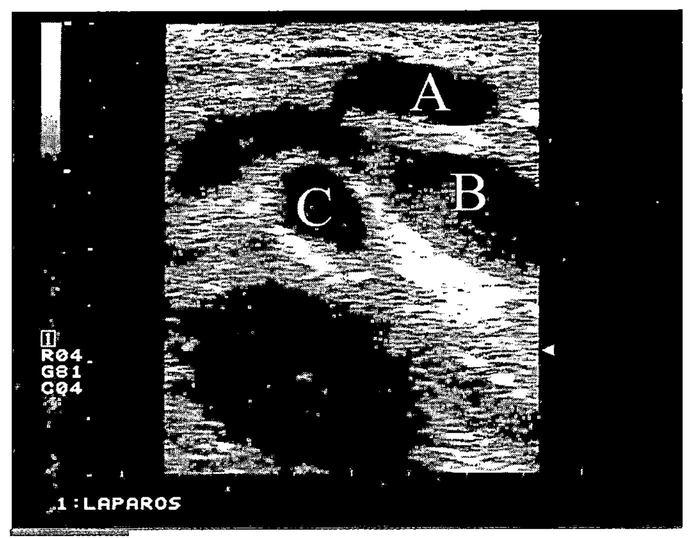

Figure 14.6
A transverse view at laparoscopic ultrasound demonstrating dilated pancreatic duct (A), portal vein (B), and common hepatic artery (C).

Table 14.2 Criteria for Unresectability at Staging Laparoscopy

1. Histologically confirmed hepatic, serosal, peritoneal, or omental metastases
2. Extrapancreatic extension of tumor
3. Histologically confirmed celiac or high portal node involvement by tumor
4. Invasion or encasement of the celiac axis, hepatic artery, or superior mesenteric artery[a]

[a]Cases of portal or superior mesenteric vein encasement are considered potentially resectable and undergo exploratory laparotomy.

Abnormal findings are photographed, and the laparoscopic ultrasound findings are recorded. Frozen section examination is performed on all biopsy samples taken during the procedure.

Patients are considered to have unresectable disease (Table 14.2) in the presence of

1. Histologically confirmed hepatic, serosal, peritoneal, or omental metastases
2. Extrapancreatic extension of tumor, such as mesocolic involvement
3. Celiac or high portal node involvement by tumor confirmed by frozen section
4. Invasion or encasement of the celiac axis, hepatic artery, or superior mesenteric artery

Cases of portal or superior mesenteric vein encroachment by tumor are considered potentially resectable and undergo exploratory laparotomy. This procedure can be performed in 25–40 minutes in experienced hands.

Perioperative Staging Techniques

Accurate preoperative staging is essential. Helical computed tomography (CT) scan is the diagnostic and staging investigation of choice for patients with pancreatic cancer. It has an accuracy rate of about 95%–97% for the detection of carcinomas and of virtually 100% for staging unresectable carcinomas.[28] However, its ability to predict tumor resectability ranges from 57% to 88% in reported series.[22,28,29] For metastatic disease, the resolution of helical CT is limited to lesions larger than 2–3 mm. This results in nondetection of small-volume surface liver and peritoneal metastases. The identification of these lesions before consideration of open exploration is the major advantage of staging laparoscopy (Figs. 14.7, 14.8).

The yield of positive laparoscopic results that avoid unnecessary laparotomy is highly dependent on the quality of the preoperative radiologic studies. The yield of laparoscopy cannot be assessed from studies that have not included state-of-the-art CT.[29] Earlier reports of Memorial Sloan-Kettering Cancer Centers experience with laparoscopic staging of peripancreatic malignancy reported an improvement in resectability from 50% on the basis of CT alone, to 92% when staging laparoscopy was performed. Compared with previous reports, improvements in technology and better patient selection have reduced the benefit of laparoscopy. However, laparoscopy continues to upstage 15%–20% of patients with perioperative radiologic evidence of resectable disease.[22,30-33]

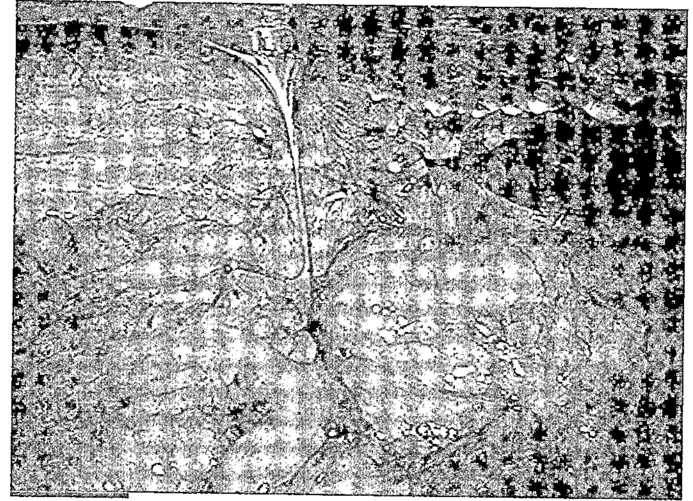

Figure 14.7
Peritoneal carcinomatosis.

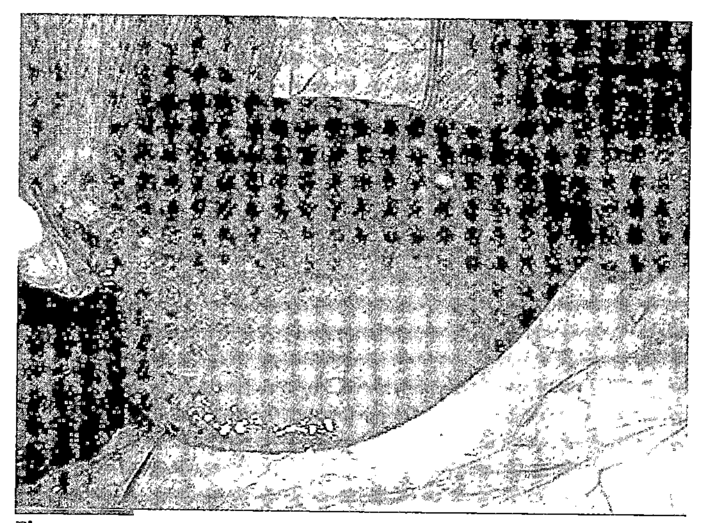

Figure 14.8
Laparoscopic examination reveals multiple small liver metastases not detected on preoperative imaging studies.

To study the accuracy of preoperative staging techniques for assessing resectability of peripancreatic malignancies, Warshaw et al.[34] compared the results of contrast-enhanced dynamic CT, MRI, angiography, and laparoscopy. In 88 patients considered to have resectable disease, preoperative CT was 92% accurate in determining unresectability, but it predicted resectability in only 45% of cases. CT failed to identify liver metastases of 1- to 3-mm diameter in 23 patients. MRI findings were similar to those of CT and conferred no benefit. Angiography predicted unresectability in 95%, but it predicted resectability in only 54% of cases. The overall accuracy of predicting unresectability by laparoscopy was 98%.

CT correctly predicted unresectability in 100% of patients but predicted resectability in only 67% in a prospective analysis of 213 patients with pancreatic cancer by Freeny et al.[35] The missed cases included tumor invasion into the root of the mesocolon and small-bowel mesentery, posterior extension of tumor, and metastatic portal adenopathy. Eight years later, the same group reported an accuracy rate of 95%–97% for detecting carcinomas, 100% for predicting unresectability, and 80%–85% for predicting resectability by helical CT.[28] Yoshida et al.[36] retrospectively analyzed 45 patients with radiologically resectable pancreatic head cancer on the basis of preoperative helical CT to clarify the role of staging laparoscopy. Laparoscopy identified four patients (9%) with localized unresectable disease and 12 (27%) with metastatic disease.

Fernandez-del Castillo[33] of Massachusetts General Hospital performed laparoscopy in 114 patients with pancreatic cancer with no evidence of metastatic disease on a preoperative CT. Unsuspected intraabdominal metastases were detected in 24% of the patients. None of these patients underwent further surgery. Angiography demonstrated unresectable vascular involvement in a further 42 patients. Forty patients underwent exploratory surgery, and 30 of those underwent resection. Staging laparoscopy missed peritoneal disease in two patients, resulting in a false-negative rate of 7%. The addition of cytology of peritoneal lavage upstaged a further 17% (16/92) of patients. In contrast, Fuhrman et al.[37] reported a predictive value of 88% for CT in determining resectability. However, this study included patients with all periampullary malignancies, of which some nonpancreatic tumors may be associated with a lower incidence of peritoneal metastases.

Selective laparoscopy has been recommended in patients thought to have a high risk of occult M1 disease.[29] Critics of routine laparoscopy argue that the value of laparoscopy has been overestimated because it fails to account for patients who require open procedures for palliation of unresectable disease. In addition, false-negative rates of 3%–9% are reported for laparoscopic detection of CT-occult intraperitoneal M1 disease.[22,24,30] Pisters et al.[29] reported a high radiographic resectabiltiy rate of 80% with the use of high-quality CT alone. The authors proposed that the maximum positive yield of routine staging laparoscopy in patients with potentially resectable disease on high-quality CT would be 20%, assuming a false-negative result of zero. Based on other published series, they determined that laparoscopy may prevent unnecessary laparotomy in only 4%–13% of patients judged to have resectable disease by high-quality CT. Importantly, this group does not perform routine staging laparoscopy but rather advocates selective laparoscopy at the time of planned laparotomy for tumor resection in patients with localized disease on CT and in patients at high risk for occult M1 disease.[38] In a study by the same group published in 1997, CT-occult M1 disease was found in 15% of the patients whose disease was considered resectable by high-quality CT.[39] Thus, a laparotomy could have been avoided in these 18 patients (15%) if laparoscopy had been used routinely.

Obertop and Gouma[40] tested two possible strategies for the diagnosis and staging of patients with suspected biliopancreatic cancer in a decision analysis. The strategies included (1) a "surgical strategy" of ultrasonography and CT followed by open exploration in radiologically resectable disease and (2) a "nonsurgical" strategy of endoscopic retrograde cholangiopancreatography and biliary stenting, laparoscopy, laparoscopic ultrasonography followed by laparotomy in resectable disease. The "nonsurgical" strategy using laparoscopy and laparoscopic ultrasonography was suggested to have a higher utility than the "surgical strategy" of CT followed by laparotomy only in a situation in which laparoscopy is predicted to yield a high level of unresectable disease.

A paper by Nieveen van Dijkum at el.[41] compared laparoscopic staging in patients with periampullary tumors versus standard radiologic staging with helical CT scan. Laparoscopic staging identified biopsy-proven unresectable disease in only 13% of 297 patients, with a detection rate of 35%. Based on these findings, the authors proposed that laparoscopic staging should not be performed routinely in patients with peripancreatic malignancy. However, in this study, overall resectability rates at laparotomy were low, at 74%. Also, at laparoscopy, the procedure was unsuccessful in 11 patients, and complications occurred in a further 11 patients, including a small-bowel and a gastric perforation. Peritoneal washings for cytologic examination for M1 disease were not performed. There was a very high rate of negative histology for suspected metastatic disease. Only 31 of 89 suspected liver metastases and 12 of 44 suspected peritoneal metastases were biopsy proved. LUS was unsuccessful in six patients (2.1%). Suspected tumor ingrowth around the superior mesenteric vein in 15% and portal vein in 8.4% seen at LUS was unconfirmed by biopsy. Only 10 of 27 suspected liver metastases seen at LUS were confirmed by biopsy, and none of eight suspect lymph nodes were confirmed. Also, the length of hospital stay after staging laparoscopy was prolonged, at 2–26 days (average, 4.3 days). The authors were also biased toward surgical palliation as the preferred form of treatment in patients with an unresectable tumor. Only 27 patients were randomly assigned to surgical palliation or endoscopic palliation. Five of the 27 patients were not treated according to the protocol, yet all five were included in the final analysis. The average survival and hospital-free survival was higher for patients who underwent surgical palliation. However, the numbers are very small, and therefore, the conclusions have to be interpreted with caution.

Some authors believe that preoperative angiography plays a role in staging.[34,42] High false-positive rates have been reported.[42] Others believe that angiography adds little additional staging information to dynamic CT. Squillaci et al.[43] prospectively compared the ability of spiral CT angiography (CTA) and digital subtraction angiography (DSA) to detect vascular involvement in 50 patients with pancreatic carcinoma.[43] Complete concordance was obtained in 20 patients without vascular involvement. Of 30 patients with vascular involvement, there was complete concordance between CTA and DSA in 22 and discordance in eight patients. CTA was superior in two cases with periadventitial infiltration and in five patients with splenoportal confluence thrombosis. DSA was superior in one case with infiltration of the superior mesenteric vein. After surgical evaluation, sensitivity of CTA and DSA was 97% and 77%, respectively, and the negative predictive values were 95% and 74%. However, given the accuracy of contrast-enhanced thin-cut CT, we do not routinely recommend angiography as part of the preoperative staging in patients with pancreatic cancer.

Contrast-enhanced dynamic thin-cut CT of the pancreas is the radiologic investigation of choice in all patients presenting with suspected pancreatic cancer in our practice. Those considered to have resectable disease by radiologic criteria undergo laparoscopic staging before open exploration. An extended-staging laparoscopy is advocated that involves examination of the peritoneal cavity, liver, lesser sac, porta hepatis, duodenum, transverse mesocolon, and celiac and portal vessels to mimic the assessment performed at open exploration. Extended laparoscopy was performed at Memorial-Sloan Kettering between 1993 and 1998 in 577 patients with radiologically resectable peripancreatic tumors before planned curative resection.[44] Of these patients, 366 were considered to have resectable disease after laparoscopic staging and subsequently underwent open exploration, with 92% (338 patients) being resected. In the remaining patients, vascular invasion precluded resection in only three patients, emphasizing the utility of CT to determine vascular encasement. Minor complications were seen in <1% of patients. This compares with results from 1983–1992 in the decade before the introduction of laparoscopic staging, when 1135 patients at Memorial Sloan-Kettering Cancer Center with potentially resectable disease underwent exploratory surgery but only 35% underwent resection.

It has been suggested that recent advances in CT technology may improve the diagnostic accuracy of preoperative radiologic staging. Reports claim that the introduction of multidetector helical CT has created a new dimension of temporal and spatial resolution in pancreatic imaging, with clear differentiation of pancreatic perfusion phases and better delineation of small structures, resulting in improvements in its diagnostic value.[45-49] Volume rendering, a postprocessing computer algorithm, can create three-dimensional images from intravenous contrast-enhanced abdominal CT datasets.[47] Catalano et al.[50] examined the role of multislice CT in 46 patients with a suspected pancreatic tumor. The sensitivity, specificity, and accuracy of the multislice CT were 97%, 80%, and 96%, respectively. The procedure correctly predicted unresectability with a sensitivity of 96%, a specificity of 86%, and an accuracy of 93%. In another report, the use of multislice CT with a biphasic technique and creation of three-dimensional volume-rendered images in 27 patients yielded a correct diagnosis in 20 cases (sensitivity, 95%; specificity, 100%). Positive predictive values for resectability and unresectability were 80% and 93.3%, respectively. Despite these data, contemporary studies continue to show an approximate 15%–20% yield for laparoscopic staging.

Staging laparoscopy can aid in the stratification of patients for appropriate treatment regimens in the presence of unresectable disease. Patients with locally advanced pancreatic cancer are frequently considered as candidates for chemoradiotherapy. Radiotherapy is not routinely administered in patients with metastatic disease. At Memorial Sloan-Kettering, a prospective study was performed involving 100 patients with locally advanced pancreatic cancer who underwent laparoscopic staging from 1994 to 2000 (Shoup, Conlon 2004). All patients were considered candidates for palliative chemoradiotherapy. All patients underwent high-quality thin-cut helical CT scans or MRI. Metastatic disease was detected in 37% of patients. None of the patients with metastatic disease were offered radiotherapy.

Laparoscopic Ultrasonography

LUS was initially developed for the assessment of hepatic disease. It has been used extensively in benign biliary tract disease and in staging of upper gastrointestinal malignancies.[51,52] Several studies have demonstrated that LUS improves diagnostic accuracy of staging laparoscopy alone, providing additional information in 14%–25% of patients.[32,53-55] LUS allows the assessment of liver metastases, regional nodal disease, and local vascular involvement.

In 1993, Murugiah et al.[56] reported their experience using a rigid 7.5-MHz linear array probe in 12 patients with suspected resectable pancreatic head cancer. Laparoscopy identified advanced disease in four patients. Laparoscopic ultrasonography detected advanced disease in an additional two patients and predicted resectable disease in six patients (50%). Only 27% of patients who underwent laparotomy had unresectable disease due to lymph node metastases. Further work from this group using LUS in 40 patients with pancreatic cancer demonstrated factors confirming unresectable tumor in 59%, provided staging information in addition to that of laparoscopy alone in 53%, and altered management in 25%.[30] Staging laparoscopy with laparoscopic ultrasonography was more specific and accurate in predicting tumor resectability than laparoscopy alone (88% and 89%, respectively, vs 50% and 65%, respectively).

Some groups use LUS to improve the sensitivity of laparoscopic staging in predicting resectability of pancreatic and periampullary tumors. Several groups have reported an improvement in resection rates in patients with carcinoma of the head of the pancreas with the use of this approach.[32] Callery et al.[32] analyzed the effect of routine implementation of laparoscopy with LUS. Staging laparoscopy with LUS was performed in 50 consecutive patients who had radiologically resectable hepatic, pancreatic or biliary malignancies. Laparoscopy with laparoscopic ultrasonography predicted resectable tumors in 28 patients. At laparotomy, 26 of 28 cases were actually resectable, resulting in a false-negative rate of 4%. Staging laparoscopy with laparoscopic ultrasonography indicated unresectability in 22 patients. Staging laparoscopy alone demonstrated previously unrecognized occult metastases in 11 patients. In 11 other patients, LUS established unresectability from vascular invasion, lymph node metastases, or intraparenchymal hepatic tumor.

Minnard et al.[54] reported the benefit of LUS over laparoscopy alone in evaluating the primary tumor and the presence of vascular involvement. LUS findings resulted in a change in surgical treatment in 14% of patients in whom standard laparoscopic examination was equivocal. A further study by Schachter et al.[57] demonstrated a change in surgical intervention in 36% of patients, and unnecessary laparotomy was avoided in 31%. Merchant and Conlon[27] concluded that the addition of laparoscopic ultrasound during laparoscopic staging enhances the ability of laparoscopy to determine resectability and approaches the accuracy of open exploration without significantly increasing morbidity or mortality.

Peritoneal Cytologic Examination

The use of peritoneal cytology enhances the sensitivity of staging laparoscopy.[58] Recurrence in the peritoneum occurs in up to 50% of patients after a potentially curative pancreaticoduodenectomy. Laparoscopy combined with peritoneal cytology is reported to upstage an additional 8% of patients with positive cytology and advanced unresectable pancreatic cancer.[59,60] Leach et al.[61] studied a consecutive series of patients between 1991 and 1993 with suspected or biopsy-proven radiologically resectable adenocarcinoma of the pancreatic head. Peritoneal washings were obtained at the time of staging laparoscopy and/or at subsequent laparotomy. Seven percent had positive peritoneal cytologic findings, and all had metastatic disease at a median of 4.8 months.

Merchant et al.[59] examined 228 patients with radiographically resectable pancreatic adenocarcinoma who underwent laparoscopic staging. Peritoneal washings were taken from both upper quadrants at the beginning of laparoscopy. Positive peritoneal cytology (PPC) was identified in 15% of patients. Twenty percent of patients who had undergone a preoperative fine-needle aspiration had PPC, and 13% of those who had not undergone a previous fine-needle aspiration had PPC. Seventy-six percent of patients with PPC had stage IV disease, and only 24% had no metastases. Overall survival was significantly higher in patients who had negative peritoneal cytology. PPC had a positive predictive value of 94.1%, a specificity of 98.1%, and a sensitivity of 25.6% for determining unresectability of pancreatic adenocarcinoma.

Laparoscopic Palliation

Controversy exists regarding the treatment of patients with unresectable disease. Critics of staging laparoscopy believe that inoperable disease secondary to local extension and vascular encasement can be determined only by laparotomy. "Truly accurate assessment of local resectability is possible only by the means of the traditional surgical approach of open exploration."[62]

Palliative measures to minimize symptoms and maximize quality of life are vitally important in this group of patients. Intervention is most commonly required for symptoms associated with biliary obstruction, gastric outlet obstruction, and/or relief of pain. The decision to perform nonoperative versus surgical palliative procedures for unresectable pancreatic cancer is influenced by the patient's symptoms, overall health status, projected length of survival, and expected procedure-related morbidity and mortality.

Critics of staging laparoscopic have argued that the procedure is of minimal benefit because patients with unresectable disease would require a subsequent bypass procedure for biliary or gastric outlet obstruction. Historically, prophylactic bypasses have been supported by reports of the development of obstructive jaundice in as many as 70% of patients and gastric outlet obstruction in up to 25% of patients with unresectable pancreatic adenocarcinoma.[63-65] More recent reports suggest that gastric outlet and biliary obstruction occur much less frequently. Data from Memorial Sloan-Kettering reported a 10% rate of gastric outlet obstruction in patients with unresectable disease.[66] Surgical bypass is not without risk. In that same study, de Rooij at al.[66] retrospectively examined 117 patients with pancreatic cancer who underwent exploratory laparotomy as a single procedure between October 1983 and November 1989. Twenty-four patients underwent gastric bypass; 38, biliary bypass; and 118, both gastric and biliary bypass. The postoperative in-hospital mortality rate was 4.4%, and the overall morbidity was 29.7%. Survival was decreased in patients who underwent a therapeutic gastric bypass (median survival, 136 days) or a combination of two therapeutic bypasses (median survival, 93 days).

The Johns Hopkins Medical Institute group does not routinely use staging laparoscopy, and they recommend full open surgical exploration by an experienced surgeon to assess true unresectability. They contend that by performing a laparotomy, the tumor can be accurately staged, resected, or bypassed. They advocate surgical palliation at initial laparotomy to relieve jaundice, pain, and potential gastric outlet obstruction. However, in a study by Sohn et al.,[67] 33% of the patients who underwent surgical exploration did not undergo resection, and of these, 69% had liver or peritoneal metastases. These lesions would have been detected at laparoscopy, and most could have been managed nonoperatively by biliary stenting. Of the 256 patients, 51% underwent double bypass (hepaticojejunostomy and gastrojejunostomy), 11% underwent hepaticojejunostomy alone, 19% underwent gastrojejunostomy alone, and 19% did not undergo bypass. Celiac block was performed in 75% of patients. Palliative bypass carried a mortality of 3%, a morbidity of 22%, and a 10.3-day postoperative length of stay. In a further study from the Johns Hopkins Medical Institute, 709 patients with radiologically resectable periampullary malignancies underwent exploratory laparotomy with the purpose of performing a pancreaticoduodenectomy.[68] On the basis of preoperative symptoms, preoperative radiologic investigations, and intraoperative findings, a gastrojejunostomy was performed in 107 patients. Other palliative procedures, including cholecystectomy, hepaticojejunostomy, and chemical splanchnicectomy, were performed at the discretion of the attending surgeon. The remaining 87 patients were thought to lack a significant risk for duodenal obstruction and were randomly assigned during surgery to receive either a retrocolic gastrojejunostomy or no gastrojejunostomy. Late gastric outlet obstruction requiring intervention developed in eight of 43 patients (18.6%) who did not receive a gastrojejunostomy at a median of 2 months from initial exploration. However, obstructive jaundice was present in only 70% of this group. This finding implies that patient selection may have been biased toward those with uncinate process tumors located distal to the ampulla, which would be associated with a high risk of late duodenal obstruction as the tumor enlarges.

van Heek at al.[69] published data from a prospective randomized multicenter trial to evaluate the effect of a prophylactic gastrojejunostomy on the development of gastric outlet obstruction and quality of life in patients with unresectable periampullary cancer found at exploratory laparotomy. Between December 1998 and March 2002, patients with a periampullary malignancy found to be unresectable during laparotomy were randomly assigned to receive a double bypass (hepaticojejunostomy and gastroenterostomy) or a single bypass (hepaticojejunostomy). Primary endpoints were development of clinical gastric outlet obstruction and surgical intervention for gastric outlet obstruction. Of 65 patients, 36 underwent a double bypass and 29 a single bypass. All patients underwent hepaticojejunostomy, cholecystectomy, and chemical splanchnicectomy with 50% alcohol. During follow-up, clinical symptoms of gastric outlet obstruction developed in two patients (5.5%) who had undergone a double bypass and 12 patients (41.4%) who had undergone a single bypass. One patient (2.8%) in the double-bypass group and six patients (20.7%) required reoperation during follow-up. Again, in this study, obstructive jaundice was reported in only 78% of patients, and only 78% had pancreatic head carcinomas. A biliary bypass procedure was performed in all patients, although only 78% of patients in the double-bypass group and 79% in the single-bypass group had jaundice. The indication for biliary bypass in the absence of jaundice must be questioned, particularly with the reported morbidity of 11% in the double-bypass group and 8% in the single-bypass group. Although differences were not statistically different, there was a trend for higher morbidity, longer median postoperative length of stay, and reduced median survival in the double-bypass group. Because the study was terminated early to perform an interim analysis without achieving the planned sample size of 140, the statistical power of the analysis should be interpreted with caution. Moreover, the rate of late gastric outlet obstruction in the single-bypass group is very high compared with other recently reported series.[66,70]

The most convincing argument against prophylactic palliative surgical bypass is that it may be unnecessary. Espat et al.[70] analyzed the outcome of 155 patients with laparoscopically staged, unresectable, histologically proven pancreatic cancer who did not undergo open enteric or biliary bypass at the time of initial laparoscopic staging. Only 3% of the patients required a subsequent surgical bypass. The mean postoperative length of stay was 2 days, compared with the 10.3-day length of stay after open surgery at Johns Hopkins Hospital. As a result, we propose that surgical biliary bypass be performed in patients with obstructive jaundice who do not respond to endoscopic stent placement, and open gastroenterostomy should be reserved for those who experience documented gastric outlet obstruction.

It has been suggested that laparoscopy could be used to stratify patients with locally advanced unresectable disease who would be expected to have a longer survival from those with metastatic disease in whom survival is very limited. This approach could assist in the evaluation of indications for surgical palliation and to determine the optimal palliative technique.

Various nonsurgical procedures are available to manage symptomatic unresectable pancreatic cancer. Several randomized trials have demonstrated that placement of endoscopic biliary endoprosthesis is equally as effective as surgical biliary bypass in the relief of obstructive jaundice.[71-73] Malignant gastric outlet obstruction can also be alleviated by placement of self-expanding metal stents. Adler et al.,[74] of the Mayo Clinic, analyzed data from 36 patients with malignant gastric outlet obstruction. Only 25% required reintervention for recurrent symptoms. Sixteen of the 36 patients (44%) had concomitant or subsequent development of biliary obstruction, of which 15 were successfully treated with endoscopic decompression.

Laparoscopic palliative bypass procedures are feasible and safe. Reported procedures performed laparoscopically include cholecystojejunostomy, choledochojejunostomy, choledochoduodenostomy, hepatojejunostomy, and gastroenterostomy.[75] Cholecystojejunostomy is the most popular laparoscopic biliary bypass procedure. Accurate patient selection is vital. A low insertion of the cystic duct into the common bile duct or tumor impingement within 1 cm of the duct are predictors of early technical failure. The anastomosis can be performed with either a stapled or a hand-sewn technique. Laparoscopic gastroenterostomy can be performed without difficulty. Rothlin et al. compared the outcome of 14 patients who underwent laparoscopic gastroenterostomy and hepaticojejunostomy with that of 14 matched patients who underwent palliative open procedures. Postoperative morbidity was 7%, versus 43% for laparoscopic and open palliation, respectively ($P < 0.05$). There were no mortalities in the laparoscopic group, compared with 29% in the group who had open bypass surgery ($P < 0.05$). The average postoperative stay was 9 days in the laparoscopic group and 21 days in the open group ($P < 0.06$). Operating time was shorter and analgesic requirements were reduced in the laparoscopic group.

Pain can be managed effectively by celiac plexus block under CT guidance. Surgery for pain relief is limited to thoracoscopic splanchnicectomy or an intraoperative celiac plexus block, which appears to be an important part of palliative surgery.[76,77] Lillemoe et al.[78] performed a prospective, randomized, double-blind study comparing intraoperative chemical splanchnicectomy with 50% alcohol versus a placebo injection of saline in patients with unresectable pancreatic cancer. Alcohol significantly reduced pain scores in patients without significant preoperative pain and delayed or prevented the subsequent onset of pain. In patients with significant preoperative pain, alcohol significantly reduced existing pain. Interestingly, patients with preexisting pain who received alcohol showed a significant improvement in survival when compared with control patients. Neurolytic celiac plexus block is feasible at laparoscopy.[79]

Laparoscopic Resection

Laparoscopic resection of the pancreas was initially described in the early 1990s.[80-82] Laparoscopic distal or subtotal pancreatectomy with or without preservation of the splenic vessels and spleen for neuroendocrine and cystic tumors of low-grade malignancy and for some patients with chronic pancreatitis, and laparoscopic enucleation of neuroendocrine tumors has been reported to be feasible and safe.[83-86] Using a lateral approach the splenic vessels can be isolated from the pancreatic tail.[87] Transection of the gland is achieved by use of a linear stapler. In experienced hands, the laparoscopic approach reduces postoperative hospital stay and expedites recovery. However, median operating times of 3.7–5 hours have been reported, and total morbidity rates of 20%–40% with the development of a pancreatic fistula in 0%–33% of patients.[88-90] This compares with pancreatic fistula rates of 12.5% after open pancreaticoduodenectomy.[91]

Jossart and Gagner[92] reported on their experience with 10 attempted laparoscopic pancreatic resections, of which eight were for malignant disease (pancreatic cancer, $N = 4$; ampullary, $N = 3$; and cholangiocarcinoma, $N = 1$).[92] The open conversion rate was 40%. In comparing the cases completed laparoscopically with those converted to open laparotomy, median operating time was 8.5 vs 4.6 hours, respectively, and the average hospital stay was 22.3 vs 20.1 days, respectively. Complications were reported in three of the patients in the laparoscopic resection group. Currently, routine laparoscopic resection of pancreatic malignancies is not recommended, because it does not appear to confer an advantage over the open procedure.[93] The procedure should be performed only in a specialized center as part of an institutional trial. Other approaches, including a hand-assisted laparoscopic approach, have been described, which may expand the role of laparoscopic resection in the future.[94,95]

Cost-Effectiveness of Laparoscopic Staging

Critics of staging laparoscopy argue that the procedure results in increased total operative expenditure for patients who have undergone resection and argue that a more selective approach should be undertaken to ensure cost-effectiveness. Andren-Sandberg et al.[96] suggested selective use of laparoscopy in patients with radiologically resectable tumors. They suggested that the selective use of laparoscopy could reduce hospital costs in 30% to 50% of patients with pancreatic cancer.

In a study from Memorial Sloan-Kettering, patients undergoing laparoscopic staging alone for unresectable disease had a significantly reduced median hospital stay of 2 days, compared with 7 days in those undergoing open exploration, 9.5 days in those undergoing biliary bypass, and 12 days in those undergoing gastric and biliary bypass.[22] Furthermore, in the same institution, a prospective study was conducted to determine the effect of laparoscopic staging on hospital charges in patients with pancreatic adenocarcinoma.[97] Patients were divided into three groups: (1) open procedure, (2) laparoscopy and open procedure, and (3) laparoscopy only. There was no increase in hospital charges with the addition of laparoscopic staging to an open procedure. Overall hospital charges were 25% lower in the laparoscopy-only group. Considerable savings were achieved in patients found to have unresectable disease at laparoscopy because an open procedure was avoided.

Morbidity of Laparoscopic Staging

Morbidity following laparoscopy remains low, and major complications are uncommon. Minor complications, including urinary retention, wound infection, and port-site incisional hernia, are also uncommon.

Concerns exist regarding the use of laparoscopy in staging malignant disease because of the risk of port-site metastases. Etiologic mechanisms thought to be the cause of port-site recurrences include indirect contamination caused by pneumoperitoneum, aerosolization, or intraperitoneal spread, and direct contamination by physical trocar seeding.[98] Experimental animal studies using the transplantable VX-2 rabbit carcinoma model have demonstrated a higher frequency of recurrence at laparoscopic working ports than in the open wound ($P < 0.02$) or laparoscopic video-port groups ($P < 0.007$).[99] No significant difference existed in recurrence between the open incision and the laparoscopic video-port ($P > 0.5$). In this model, trocar recurrence is due to direct contamination between viable tumor cells and surgical instruments.

Barrat et al.[98] suggested that peritoneal spread and tumor manipulation are important factors in the occurrence of port-site metastases. However, recent reports suggest that port-site recurrences occur infrequently. Shoup et al.[100] prospectively compared the occurrence of port-site metastases from 1650 laparoscopic procedures for upper gastrointestinal malignancies in 1548 patients with wound recurrence after 1040 open procedures. Port-site implantation for all laparoscopies occurred in 13 (0.79%) of 1650 procedures, with a median time to recurrence of 8.2 months. After laparotomy, open-incision-site recurrence occurred in nine (0.86%) of 1040 procedures. Five (0.60%) of 830 port-site recurrences and seven (0.84%) of 830 open-incision-site recurrences occurred in patients who had undergone resection. At the time of diagnosis of recurrence, all patients with port-site and five of seven with open-site implantation also had distant or local disease or a combination of the two. These data agree with data from Pearlstone et al.[101] at M.D. Anderson Cancer Center, who noted recurrence at port sites in only 0.8% of patients who underwent staging laparoscopy for malignant disease. Three of the patients who experienced a port-site recurrence had advanced disease at the time of diagnosis. None of the patients with pancreatic cancer in the series experienced a port site recurrence.

Port-site implantation after staging laparoscopy for upper gastrointestinal malignancy is uncommon and does not appear to significantly differ in pathophysiology or incidence from open-incision-site recurrence. It also tends to occur in patients found to have progression of stage of disease at other sites.

The Role of Laparoscopy in Other Pancreatic Lesions

Reported studies have concentrated on the role of staging laparoscopy in pancreatic adenocarcinoma. However, the technique may also be beneficial in investigating other pancreatic lesions. Metastatic disease has been found at exploratory laparotomy in >50% of patients with nonfunctioning islet cell tumors of the pancreas.[102-104] Hochwald et al.[105] demonstrated a high incidence of occult metastases at laparoscopy in patients with nonfunctioning islet cell tumors. CT followed by laparoscopy was significantly more sensitive than CT alone in predicting resectability (93% vs 50%; $P = 0.03$) with similar specificity (both 100%). A high false-negative rate was obtained for CT because of its failure to detect small-volume metastatic disease. Predicted tumor resectability was 95% for CT followed by laparoscopy, compared with 74% for CT alone. The value of resecting an asymptomatic metastatic nonfunctioning islet cell tumor is controversial. However, in the case of detection of metastases at laparoscopy in patients with functional tumors, patients can be stratified to numerous treatment options, including hormonal therapy, tumor embolization, chemotherapy, and surgery. Brooks et al.[106] examined the role of laparoscopy in patients with radiologically resectable periampullary nonpancreatic adenocarcinoma. Laparoscopy increased the resectability rate from 83% to 92% based on CT alone. The added yield of laparoscopy for predicting resectability was 5%–9% in duodenal and ampullary tumors and 12% for distal bile duct tumors. Selective laparoscopy was recommended in patients with distal bile duct tumors to assess resectability and avoid unnecessary surgery, and in patients with very large duodenal or ampullary tumors where metastatic spread is more likely.

Conclusion

Laparoscopic staging of pancreatic malignancy in conjunction with laparoscopic ultrasound and peritoneal fluid cytology accurately predicts tumor resectabilty. In patients with laparoscopically diagnosed unresectable disease, significant morbidity and mortality are minimized by the avoidance of unnecessary laparotomy. The role of laparoscopy has expanded to include palliative procedures in malignant disease and pancreatic resections for benign or low-grade tumors. With future technologic advances, the role of laparoscopy in the management of pancreatic cancer will undergo further refinement.

References

1. Bernheim BM. Organoscopy. *Ann Surg*. 1911;53:764–767.
2. Kelling G. Ueber oesophagoskopie, gastroskopie und kolioskopie. *Munch Med Wochenschr*. 1902;49:21–24.
3. Von Ott DO. Ventoroscopic illumination of the abdominal cavity in pregnancy. *Zh Akrestierstova I Zhenskikh Boloznei*. 1901; 7.
4. Jacobaeus HC. *Munch Med Wochenschr*. 1910;40.
5. Jacobaeus HC. Kurze Ubersicht uber meine Erfahrungen mit der Laparoskopie. *Munch Med Wochenschr*. 1911;58: 2017–2019.
6. Jacobaeus HC. Uber laparo- und tharaoskopie. *Beitr Klin Tuberk*. 1912;25:185.
7. Kelling G. Zur Celioskopie. *Arch Klin Chir*. 1923;126: 226–229.
8. Fervers C. Die laparoskopie mit dem Zytoskope. *Med Klin*. 1933;29:1042–1045.
9. Verres J. Neus instrument zur Ausfuhrung Von Brust oder Bauchpunktionen. *Dtsch Med Wochenschr*. 1938;41: 1480–1481.
10. Lau WY, Leow CK, Li AK. History of endoscopic and laparoscopic surgery. *World J Surg*. 1997;21:444–453.
11. Litynski GS. Erich Muhe and the rejection of laparoscopic cholecystectomy (1985): a surgeon ahead of his time. *Journal of the Society of Laparoenscopic Surgeons*. 1998;2:341–346.
12. Litynski GS. Profiles in laparoscopy. Mouret, Dubois, and Perissat: the laparoscopic breakthrough in Europe (1987-1988). *Journal of the Society of Laparoenscopic Surgeons*. 1999;3:163–167.
13. Fuchs KH. Minimally invasive surgery. *Endoscopy*. 2002;34:154–159.
14. Litynski GS. Endoscopic surgery: the history, the pioneers. *World J Surg*. 1999;23:745–753.
15. Gloeckler Ries LA, Reichman ME, Lewis DR, Hankey BF, Edwards BK. Cancer survival and incidence from the Surveillance, Epidemiology, and End Results (SEER) Program. *Oncologist*. 2003;8:541–552.
16. Ahlgren JD. Epidemiology and risk factors in pancreatic cancer. *Semin Oncol*. 1996;23:241–250.
17. Brennan MF. Cancer of the pancreas. In: DeVita VHSaRSe, ed. *Principles and Practice of Oncology*. 5th ed. Philadelphia: J.B. Lippincott; 1993:849–882.

18. Carter DC. Cancer of the pancreas. *Gut*. 1990;31:494–496.
19. Conlon KC, Klimstra DS, Brennan MF. Long-term survival after curative resection for pancreatic ductal adenocarcinoma: clinicopathologic analysis of 5-year survivors. *Ann Surg*. 1996;223:273–279.
20. Cameron JL, et al. Factors influencing survival after pancreaticoduodenectomy for pancreatic cancer. *Am J Surg*. 1991;161:120–124.
21. Sohn TA, et al. Resected adenocarcinoma of the pancreas-616 patients: results, outcomes, and prognostic indicators. *J Gastrointest Surg*. 2000;4:567–579.
22. Conlon KC, et al. The value of minimal access surgery in the staging of patients with potentially resectable peripancreatic malignancy. *Ann Surg* 1996;223:134–140.
23. Conlon KC, Minnard EA. The value of laparoscopic staging in upper gastrointestinal malignancy. *Oncologist*. 1997;2:10–17.
24. Jimenez RE, et al. Impact of laparoscopic staging in the treatment of pancreatic cancer. *Arch Surg*. 2000;135:409–414.
25. Reddy KR, et al. Experience with staging laparoscopy in pancreatic malignancy. *Gastrointest Endosc*. 1999;49:498–503.
26. Catheline JM, Turner R, Rizk N, Barrat C, Champault G. The use of diagnostic laparoscopy supported by laparoscopic ultrasonography in the assessment of pancreatic cancer. *Surg Endosc*. 1999;13:239–245.
27. Merchant NB, Conlon KC. Laparoscopic evaluation in pancreatic cancer. *Semin Surg Oncol*. 1998;15:155–165.
28. Freeny PC. Pancreatic carcinoma: imaging update 2001. *Dig Dis*. 2001;19:37–46.
29. Pisters PW, Lee JE, Vauthey JN, Charnsangavej C, Evans DB. Laparoscopy in the staging of pancreatic cancer. *Br J Surg*. 2001;88:325–337.
30. John TG, Greig JD, Carter DC, Garden OJ. Carcinoma of the pancreatic head and periampullary region: tumor staging with laparoscopy and laparoscopic ultrasonography. *Ann Surg*. 1995;221:156–164.
31. Bemelman WA, et al. Diagnostic laparoscopy combined with laparoscopic ultrasonography in staging of cancer of the pancreatic head region. *Br J Surg*. 1995;82:820–824.
32. Callery MP, Strasberg SM, Doherty GM, Soper NJ, Norton JA. Staging laparoscopy with laparoscopic ultrasonography: optimizing resectability in hepatobiliary and pancreatic malignancy. *J Am Coll Surg*. 1997;185:33–39.
33. Fernandez-del Castillo C, Rattner DW, Warshaw AL. Further experience with laparoscopy and peritoneal cytology in the staging of pancreatic cancer. *Br J Surg*. 1995;82:1127–1129.
34. Warshaw AL, Gu ZY, Wittenberg J, Waltman AC. Preoperative staging and assessment of resectability of pancreatic cancer. *Arch Surg*. 1990;125:230–233.
35. Freeny PC, Traverso LW, Ryan JA. Diagnosis and staging of pancreatic adenocarcinoma with dynamic computed tomography. *Am J Surg*. 1993;165:600–606.
36. Yoshida T, et al. Staging with helical computed tomography and laparoscopy in pancreatic head cancer. *Hepatogastroenterology*. 2002;49:1428–1431.
37. Fuhrman GM, et al. Thin-section contrast-enhanced computed tomography accurately predicts the resectability of malignant pancreatic neoplasms. *Am J Surg*. 1994;167:104–111.
38. Abdalla EK, et al. Subaquatic laparoscopy for staging of intraabdominal malignancy. *J Am Coll Surg*. 2003;196:155–158.
39. Spitz FR, et al. Preoperative and postoperative chemoradiation strategies in patients treated with pancreaticoduodenectomy for adenocarcinoma of the pancreas. *J Clin Oncol*. 1997;15:928–937.
40. Obertop H, Gouma DJ. Essentials in biliopancreatic staging: a decision analysis. *Ann Oncol*. 1999;10[suppl 4]:150–152.
41. Nieveen van Dijkum EJ, et al. Laparoscopic staging and subsequent palliation in patients with peripancreatic carcinoma. *Ann Surg*. 2003;237:66–73.
42. Dooley WC, et al. Is preoperative angiography useful in patients with periampullary tumors? *Ann Surg*. 1990;211:649–654.
43. Squillaci E, et al. Vascular involvement in pancreatic neoplasm: a comparison between spiral CT and DSA. *Dig Dis Sci*. 2003;48:449–458.
44. Conlon KC, Brennan MF. Laparoscopy for staging abdominal malignancies. *Adv Surg*. 2000;34:331–350.
45. Prokesch RW, Schima W, Chow LC, Jeffrey RB. Multidetector CT of pancreatic adenocarcinoma: diagnostic advances and therapeutic relevance. *Eur Radiol*. 2003;13:2147–2154.
46. Itoh S, et al. Assessment of the pancreatic and intrapancreatic bile ducts using 0.5-mm collimation and multiplanar reformatted images in multislice CT. *Eur Radiol*. 2003;13:277–285.
47. Johnson PT, Heath DG, Hofmann LV, Horton KM, Fishman EK. Multidetector-row computed tomography with three-dimensional volume rendering of pancreatic cancer: a complete preoperative staging tool using computed tomography angiography and volume-rendered cholangiopancreatography. *J Comput Assist Tomogr*. 2003;27:347–353.
48. Merkle EM, Boll DT, Fenchel S. Helical computed tomography of the pancreas: potential impact of higher concentrated contrast agents and multidetector technology. *J Comput Assist Tomogr*. 2003;27[suppl 1]:S17–S22.
49. Nino-Murcia M, Tamm EP, Charnsangavej C, Jeffrey RB Jr. Multidetector-row helical CT and advanced postprocessing techniques for the evaluation of pancreatic neoplasms. *Abdom Imaging*. 2003;28:366–377.
50. Catalano C, et al. Pancreatic carcinoma: the role of high-resolution multislice spiral CT in the diagnosis and assessment of resectability. *Eur Radiol*. 2003;13:149–156.
51. Cuesta MA, Meijer S, Borgstein PJ, Sibinga ML, Sikkenk AC. Laparoscopic ultrasonography for hepatobiliary and pancreatic malignancy. *Br J Surg*. 1993;80:1571–1574.
52. Ascher SM, Evans SR, Zeman RK. Laparoscopic cholecystectomy: intraoperative ultrasound of the extrahepatic biliary tree and the natural history of postoperative transabdominal ultrasound findings. *Semin Ultrasound CT MR*. 1993;14:331–337.
53. John TG, et al. Laparoscopy with laparoscopic ultrasonography in the TNM staging of pancreatic carcinoma. *World J Surg*. 1999;23:870–881.

54. Minnard EA, et al. Laparoscopic ultrasound enhances standard laparoscopy in the staging of pancreatic cancer. *Ann Surg.* 1998;228:182–187.
55. Pietrabissa A, et al. Laparoscopy and laparoscopic ultrasonography for staging pancreatic cancer: critical appraisal. *World J Surg.* 1999;23:998–1002.
56. Murugiah M, Paterson-Brown S, Windsor JA, Miles WF, Garden OJ. Early experience of laparoscopic ultrasonography in the management of pancreatic carcinoma. *Surg Endosc.* 1993;7:177–181.
57. Schachter PP, et al. The impact of laparoscopy and laparoscopic ultrasonography on the management of pancreatic cancer. *Arch Surg.* 2000;135:1303–1307.
58. Jimenez RE, Warshaw AL, Fernandez-del Castillo C. Laparoscopy and peritoneal cytology in the staging of pancreatic cancer. *J Hepatobiliary Pancreat Surg.* 2000;7:15–20.
59. Merchant NB, Conlon KC, Saigo P, Dougherty E, Brennan MF. Positive peritoneal cytology predicts unresectability of pancreatic adenocarcinoma. *J Am Coll Surg.* 1999;188:421–426.
60. Fernandez-del Castillo CL, Warshaw AL. Pancreatic cancer: laparoscopic staging and peritoneal cytology. *Surg Oncol Clin North Am.* 1998;7:135–142.
61. Leach SD, et al. Significance of peritoneal cytology in patients with potentially resectable adenocarcinoma of the pancreatic head. *Surgery.* 1995;118:472–478.
62. Rumstadt B, Schwab M, Schuster K, Hagmuller E, Trede M. The role of laparoscopy in the preoperative staging of pancreatic carcinoma. *J Gastrointest Surg.* 1997;1:245–250.
63. Singh SM, Longmire WP Jr, Reber HA. Surgical palliation for pancreatic cancer: the UCLA experience. *Ann Surg.* 1990;212:132-139.
64. Warshaw AL, Swanson RS. Pancreatic cancer in 1988: possibilities and probabilities. *Ann Surg.* 1988;208:541–553.
65. Sarr MG, Cameron JL. Surgical palliation of unresectable carcinoma of the pancreas. *World J Surg.* 1984;8:906–918.
66. de Rooij PD, Rogatko A, Brennan MF. Evaluation of palliative surgical procedures in unresectable pancreatic cancer. *Br J Surg.* 1991;78:1053–1058.
67. Sohn TA, et al. Surgical palliation of unresectable periampullary adenocarcinoma in the 1990s. *J Am Coll Surg.* 1999;188:658–666.
68. Lillemoe KD, et al. Is prophylactic gastrojejunostomy indicated for unresectable periampullary cancer? A prospective randomized trial. *Ann Surg.* 1999;230:322–328.
69. van Heek NT, et al. The need for a prophylactic gastrojejunostomy for unresectable periampullary cancer: a prospective randomized multicenter trial with special focus on assessment of quality of life. *Ann Surg.* 2003;238:894–902.
70. Espat NJ, Brennan MF, Conlon KC. Patients with laparoscopically staged unresectable pancreatic adenocarcinoma do not require subsequent surgical biliary or gastric bypass. *J Am Coll Surg.* 1999;188:649–655.
71. Andersen JR, Sorensen SM, Kruse A, Rokkjaer M, Matzen P. Randomised trial of endoscopic endoprosthesis versus operative bypass in malignant obstructive jaundice. *Gut.* 1989;30:1132–1135.
72. Smith AC, Dowsett JF, Russell RC, Hatfield AR, Cotton PB. Randomised trial of endoscopic stenting versus surgical bypass in malignant low bileduct obstruction. *Lancet.* 1994;344:1655–1660.
73. Shepherd HA, et al. Endoscopic biliary endoprosthesis in the palliation of malignant obstruction of the distal common bile duct: a randomized trial. *Br J Surg.* 1988;75:1166–1168.
74. Adler DG, Baron TH. Endoscopic palliation of malignant gastric outlet obstruction using self-expanding metal stents: experience in 36 patients. *Am J Gastroenterol.* 2002;97: 72–78.
75. Tinoco R, El Kadre L, Tinoco A. Laparoscopic choledochoduodenostomy. *J Laparoendosc Adv Surg Tech A.* 1999;9:123–126.
76. Russell RC. Palliation of pain and jaundice: an overview. *Ann Oncol.* 1999;10[suppl 4]:S165–S169.
77. Sakorafas GH, Tsiotou AG, Sarr MG. Intraoperative celiac plexus block in the surgical palliation for unresectable pancreatic cancer. *Eur J Surg Oncol.* 1999;25:427–431.
78. Lillemoe KD, et al. Chemical splanchnicectomy in patients with unresectable pancreatic cancer: a prospective randomized trial. *Ann Surg.* 1993;217:447–455.
79. Underwood RA, Wu JS, Quasebarth MA, Brunt LM. Development of a laparoscopic approach to neurolytic celiac plexus block in a porcine model. *Surg Endosc.* 2000;14: 839–843.
80. Cuschieri A. Laparoscopic surgery of the pancreas. *J R Coll Surg Edinb.* 1994;39:178–184.
81. Gagner M, Pomp A, Herrera MF. Early experience with laparoscopic resections of islet cell tumors. *Surgery.* 1996;120:1051–1054.
82. Salky BA, Edye M. Laparoscopic pancreatectomy. *Surg Clin North Am.* 1996;76:539–545.
83. Tagaya N, et al. Laparoscopic resection of the pancreas and review of the literature. *Surg Endosc.* 2003;17:201–206.
84. Ammori BJ. Pancreatic surgery in the laparoscopic era. *JOP.* 2003;4:187–192.
85. Mori T, Abe N, Sugiyama M, Atomi Y. Laparoscopic hepatobiliary and pancreatic surgery: an overview. *J Hepatobiliary Pancreat Surg.* 2002;9:710–722.
86. Sussman LA, Christie R, Whittle DE. Laparoscopic excision of distal pancreas including insulinoma. *Aust NZ J Surg.* 1996;66:414–416.
87. Barlehner E, Anders S, Schwetling R. Laparoscopic resection of the left pancreas: technique and indication. *Dig Surg.* 2002;19:507–510.
88. Patterson EJ, et al. Laparoscopic pancreatic resection: single-institution experience of 19 patients. *J Am Coll Surg.* 2001;193:281–287.
89. Cuschieri SA, Jakimowicz JJ. Laparoscopic pancreatic resections. *Semin Laparosc Surg.* 1998;5:168–179.
90. Gagner M, Pomp A. Laparoscopic pancreatic resection: is it worthwhile? *J Gastrointest Surg.* 1997;1:20–26.
91. Conlon KC, et al. Prospective randomized clinical trial of the value of intraperitoneal drainage after pancreatic resection. *Ann Surg.* 2001;234:487–493.

92. Jossart GH, Gagner M. Pancreaticoduodenal resection. *J Hepatobiliary Pancreat Surg*. 2000;7:21–27.
93. Ceulemans R, Henri M, Leroy J, Marescaux J. Laparoscopic surgery for cancer: are we ready? *Acta Gastroenterol Belg*. 2003;66:227–230.
94. Posner MC, Alverdy J. Hand-assisted laparoscopic surgery for cancer. *Cancer J*. 2002;8:144–153.
95. Gagner M, Gentileschi P. Hand-assisted laparoscopic pancreatic resection. *Semin Laparosc Surg*. 2001;8:114–125.
96. Andren-Sandberg A, Lindberg CG, Lundstedt C, Ihse I. Computed tomography and laparoscopy in the assessment of the patient with pancreatic cancer. *J Am Coll Surg*. 1998;186:35–40.
97. Conlon KC, Dougherty E, Brennan MF. *Proceedings of the 50th Annual Cancer Symposium Society of Surgical Oncology*. 1997;25.
98. Barrat C, Champault G, Catheline JM. Is laparoscopic evaluation of digestive cancers legitimate? A prospective study of 109 cases. *Ann Chir*. 1998;52:602–606.
99. Wilkinson NW, Shapiro AJ, Harvey SB, Stack RS, Cornum RL. Port-site recurrence reproduced in the VX-2 rabbit carcinoma model: an in vivo model comparing laparoscopic port sites and open incisions. *JSLS*. 2001;5:221–226.
100. Shoup M, et al. Port site metastasis after diagnostic laparoscopy for upper gastrointestinal tract malignancies: an uncommon entity. *Ann Surg Oncol*. 2002;9:632–636.
101. Pearlstone DB, Feig BW, Mansfield PF. Port site recurrences after laparoscopy for malignant disease. *Semin Surg Oncol*. 1999;16:307–312.
102. Thompson GB, van Heerden JA, Grant CS, Carney JA, Ilstrup DM. Islet cell carcinomas of the pancreas: a twenty-year experience. *Surgery*. 1988;104:1011–1017.
103. Solorzano CC, et al. Nonfunctioning islet cell carcinoma of the pancreas: survival results in a contemporary series of 163 patients. *Surgery*. 2001;130:1078–1085.
104. Evans DB, et al. Nonfunctioning islet cell carcinoma of the pancreas. *Surgery*. 1993;114:1175–1181.
105. Hochwald SN, Weiser MR, Colleoni R, Brennan MF, Conlon KC. Laparoscopy predicts metastatic disease and spares laparotomy in selected patients with pancreatic nonfunctioning islet cell tumors. *Ann Surg Oncol*. 2001;8:249–253.
106. Brooks AD, Mallis MJ, Brennan MF, Conlon KC. The value of laparoscopy in the management of ampullary, duodenal, and distal bile duct tumors. *J Gastrointest Surg*. 2002;6:139–145.

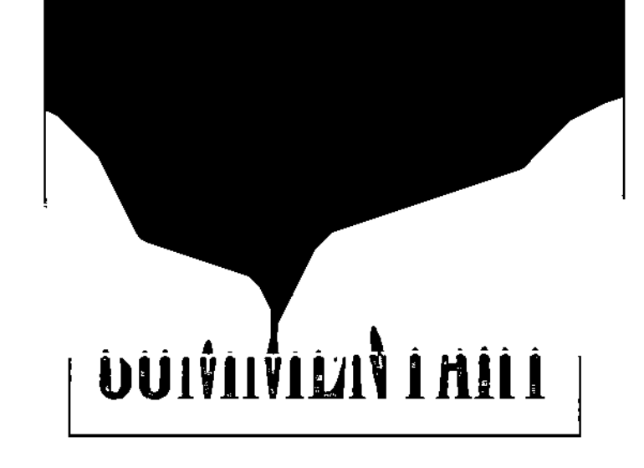

Charles M. Vollmer, Jr., MD
Mark P. Callery, MD

Accurate staging in patients with pancreatic cancer is essential for proper treatment. We must be able to differentiate as many patients as possible that should undergo laparotomy from those who should not. Futile unnecessary laparotomy should be avoided whenever and however possible so that we can maintain quality and comfort in the final stages of a patient's life. This applies in all malignancies, especially pancreatic cancer. This is not to say surgical palliation of unresectable disease is not valuable. It is in many cases, but not all. Today we have minimally invasive options for disease staging and palliation that cannot be overlooked. Many are detailed in Chapter 14 on laparoscopic staging.

Short of surgery, we have traditionally depended on radiologic staging. We still can but must accept that a major hurdle remains. Despite high accuracy in predicting unresectable disease, today's spectacular imaging technology still falls short in predicting resectable disease. A complementary staging method to overcome this shortfall is necessary, and it should ideally be one that accurately upstages a patient's pancreatic cancer with the least physical insult. Over the last 15 years, this has been the central hypothesis driving the acceptance of staging laparoscopy. However, not all agree, and two intellectual camps seem to have emerged: Those who conceptually embrace laparoscopy believe that palliation is best achieved nonoperatively, and others, taking the opposite approach, believe that all forms of disease presentation are palliated best using open surgical techniques. As with any good debate, neither camp has all the right answers.

Kevin Conlon, now writing with Olga Tucker, was appropriately selected to provide the definitive word on laparoscopic staging of pancreatic cancer. The authors have rendered a thorough, evidence-based chapter that is beautifully written and supported by vivid illustrations and today's most important citations. Professor Conlon became an authority on this subject during years of experience, innovation, and clinical research while at Memorial Sloan-Kettering Cancer Center. Collectively, he has provided the largest defined series in the world literature on the subject. His insight and detailed cost-comparison analyses have also helped us to evaluate critically the economic benefits of laparoscopic staging.

The authors' historic perspective suggests that promising concepts often cannot be manifest until technology is able to catch up. Although considered a modern technique, laparoscopic staging for pancreatic cancer was initially proposed over a century ago, but really did not resurface until approximately 70 years later. In regards to technique, they outline and illustrate a systematic, reproducible, and thorough approach akin to an open laparotomy. When properly performed, this is not a cursory "spin-through" of the abdomen. Rather, key areas of tumor spread are examined, including inside the lesser sac, along the falciform ligament, and under the transverse mesocolon. In skilled hands, this is regularly performed in less than 1 hour and burns no bridges for subsequent resection. In addition, Conlon emphasizes both the staging and diagnostic impact of laparoscopy—especially for those patients considering investigational approaches such as neoadjuvant chemoradiation therapy.

We too have strived to clarify the benefits of staging laparoscopy for hepatobiliary and pancreatic malignancies.[1-3] Early work from Washington University in St. Louis, MO, demonstrated that laparoscopy alone could obviate laparotomy in 22% of patients. Furthermore, the routine addition of laparoscopic ultrasound (LUS) could prevent even more patients from undergoing an unnecessary open exploration, all within a low false-negative rate of 4%. Tucker and Conlon reaffirm these findings, citing the numerous studies over the last decade that show that up to a third of those patients felt to be resectable by state-of-the-art imaging will consistently have advanced local/regional disease revealed by laparoscopic staging.

Like Professor Conlon, who beautifully describes his technique, we remain strong proponents of LUS in staging. LUS is valuable at identifying intrahepatic metastatic lesions, the degree of tumor involvement on the portal vein (as well as at the PV/SMV [portal vein / superior mesenteric vein] confluence), involvement of structures of the porta hepatis superior to the pancreas, major arterial involvement (celiac, hepatic, and SMA [superior mesenteric artery]), and pathologically involved lymph nodes beyond the boundaries of dissection. It also provides advanced visualization for controlled biopsies if they are warranted. In contrast, LUS is limited in its ability to delineate tumor involvement on the left side of the PV or distally along the SMV proper. We do not use LUS for every staging procedure, however, because the technologic prowess of today's computed tomography–angiography probably makes it redundant and unnecessary in certain cases.

We are not as convinced as the authors that the addition of cytologic analysis of peritoneal fluid is valuable. We remain skeptical of excluding a patient for resection based on positive cytology alone. Just as in the case of the cytologic evaluation of bile duct cytology washings, the precision of diagnosis is variable. A broad endorsement of cytologic analysis could be considered if equivalent accuracy existed in all centers, but it does not. The utility of peritoneal washing may be refined with ongoing progress in molecular and genetic marker analysis.

There has been an evolution, as delineated in the literature, from generalized laparoscopy for all upper gastrointestinal malignancies to selective application. We proposed in our 2002 manuscript in the *Annals of Surgery* that patients with distinct subsets of peripancreatic tumors derive benefit from laparoscopic staging, whereas others do not.[3] Specifically, staging laparoscopy, when combined with LUS, improved resectability rates dramatically for cancers of the pancreatic head (including intrapancreatic cholangiocarcinoma), as well as gallbladder cancer. No additional value was demonstrated for ampullary and duodenal malignancies. Furthermore, all distal pancreatic adenocarcinomas should be staged laparoscopically given the 40%–50% chance of local/regional spread from these tumors. These findings attest to the different biologic virulence of the various "periampullary" tumors. Simply put, laparoscopic staging is sometimes entirely unnecessary, as in focal periampullary lesions. These results in pancreatic tumor staging are mirrored by similar data collected by the Memorial group, led by William Jarnigan, that show high rates of unresectability for gallbladder cancer and cholangiocarcinoma—tumors of the same tissue origin that behave in a similarly aggressive clinical manner.[4]

Conlon aptly quotes morbidity and mortality rates for open palliative approaches that rival those for a Whipple's resection. We believe that the majority of patients can be adequately palliated in a minimally invasive manner, whether by endoscopic or laparoscopic means or a combination thereof. We feel that staging laparoscopy dovetails nicely with this philosophy, and it is therefore our default mode. However, like the majority of specialists in this field, we strive to remain flexible when it comes to options for palliation of jaundice, duodenal obstruction, and chronic pain. We depend entirely on constant multidisciplinary consultation to be certain that all of our palliative services are available, reliable, and in agreement. In those patients who obviously would benefit from open surgical palliation, laparoscopy is not warranted.

Finally, just as the rise of technology allowed laparoscopy to flourish, so too may it lead to its obsolescence. The recent advances in sensitivity of multichannel computed tomography–angiography as well as functional (i.e., physiologic) imaging such as PET (positron emission tomography) scanning may obviate the value of laparoscopy in the future. Just as laparoscopy and mutidetector CT rendered angiography obsolete for the preoperative assessment of patients with pancreatic cancer, so might it be surpassed as well? Going forward, we should welcome opportunities to validate new staging modalities and to confirm prospectively their clinical utility.

References

1. Callery MP, Strasberg SM, Doherty GM, et al. Staging laparoscopy with laparoscopic ultrasonography: optimizing resectability in hepatobiliary and pancreatic malignancy. *J Am Coll Surg.* 1997;185: 33–39.
2. Potter MW, Shah SA, McEnaney P, Chari RS, Callery MP. A critical appraisal of laparoscopic staging in hepatobiliary and pancreatic malignancy. *Surg Oncol.* 2000;9:103–110.
3. Vollmer CM, Drebin JA, Middleton WD, et al. Utility of staging laparoscopy in subsets of peripancreatic and biliary malignancies. *Ann Surg.* 2002;235:1–7.
4. Jarnigan WR, Bodniewicz J, Dougherty E, Conlon K, Blumgart LH, Fong Y. A prospective analysis of staging laparoscopy in patients with primary and secondary hepatobiliary malignancies. *J Gastrointest Surg.* 2000;4:34–43.

CHAPTER 15

Fine-Needle Aspiration Biopsy of the Pancreas: Indications and Interpretations

Gregg A. Staerkel, MD

Fine-needle aspiration (FNA) is fast becoming the preferred method for evaluating a lesion of the pancreas suspected of being neoplastic.[1] The selection of FNA as a diagnostic tool has occurred because of radiologic advances.[2] In addition, the utility of FNA has improved sensitivity and specificity for tumor detection while decreasing complications that occurred in traditionally performed biopsy procedures.[3,4]

Before FNA, cutting needle or wedge biopsy and endoscopic exfoliative cytology were widely used. For the pancreas, cutting needle and wedge biopsies yield complications that include hemorrhage, fistula formation, pancreatitis, and death in 5%–20% of cases.[3-5] Furthermore, obtaining representative tissue for histologic examination can be problematic in up to half of cases sampled.[3,5,6] In addition, histologic tissues obtained for frozen-section evaluation can yield a false-positive rate of 3%.[3] Although endoscopic exfoliative cytology is a relatively safe method for tissue acquisition, sensitivity rates are low, approximately 50%.[7] Reaching the level of a stricture for sampling can be difficult because of the small size of pancreatic ducts.[7]

The use of FNA, in conjunction with computed tomography and ultrasonography, has maintained the reliability of diagnosing pancreatic carcinoma with specificity rates near 100%, while increasing sensitivity to 80%-90%.[3] Percutaneous computed tomographic guided–FNA is technically easier to use than percutaneous ultrasound because it is unaffected by gas within the bowels and excessive adipose tissue[4,8] However, the lack of real-time imaging increases procedure time.[8] The arrival of endoscopic ultrasonography eliminates the aforementioned problem with percutaneous ultrasound. It also allows for the evaluation of the primary pancreatic lesion and, if malignant, simultaneous staging of the disease.[4,8] In addition, smaller lesions can be detected and/or can undergo biopsy in less time with real-time imaging.[2] With any technique that is used, overall accuracy increases with aspirator experience and with the availability of a cytopathologist for immediate specimen adequacy assessment.[1] Major complications for FNA are reported at less than a tenth of 1%.[4] The relative noninvasive detection of malignancy by FNA causes little or no change in the performance status of the patient for subsequent surgery or chemoradiation.

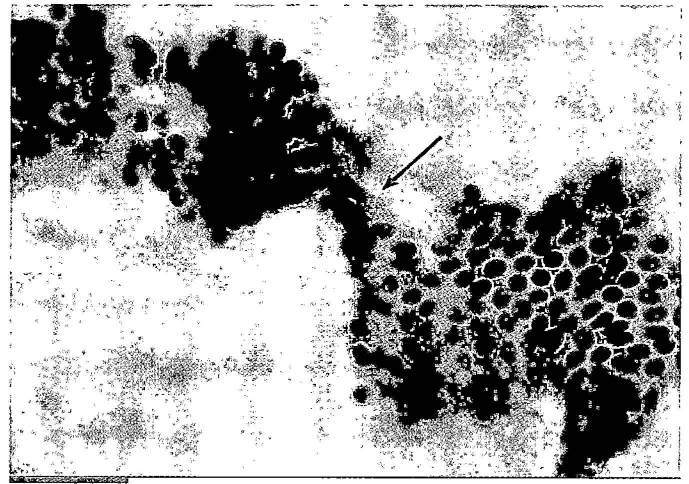

Figure 15.1
Ductal epithelium in glandular (columnar cells) "honeycomb" sheets. Where epithelium is twisted, columnar cells show profile consistent with a "picket fence" arrangement (*arrow*). Cells are uniform with nuclei appearing round/oval and evenly distributed within fragment (Papanicolaou, ×250).

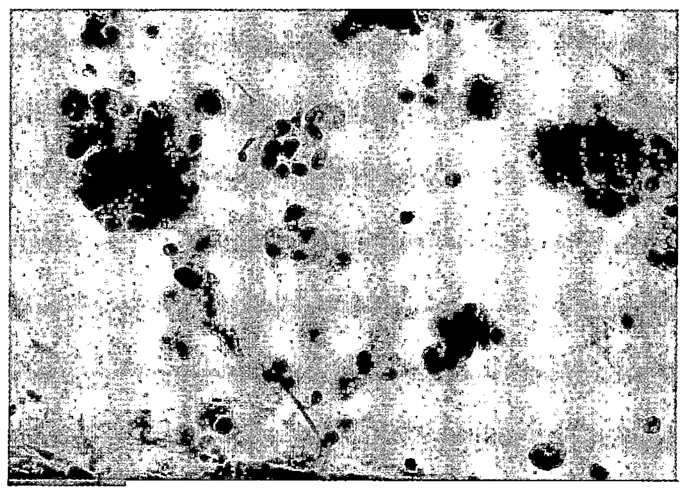

Figure 15.2
Acinar epithelial cells arranged in raspberry-like clusters with occasional dispersed single cells (Papanicolaou, ×250).

Interpretation of Pancreatic Fine-Needle Aspirations

Normal Anatomy

The pancreas is composed of exocrine tissue (acini and excretory ducts) and endocrine tissue (islets of Langerhans). In aspiration preparations only, the exocrine tissue is readily identified. Endocrine tissue is not recognized because of its sparse distribution and its similarity to acinar cells.[3,7] Special stains for cytoplasmic neurosecretory granules are required for identification.[3]

Surgically excised tissue, when processed for interpretation, provides cross-sections of cells that maintain their spacial relationship within surrounding connective tissue. In contrast, cytologic preparations consist of these same cells but are detached from surrounding connective tissue. As a result, architectural information is lost. Cells are fragmented into groups that consist of whole cells rather than cross-sectioned cells. FNA obtains a disproportionate amount of epithelial tissue to connective tissue. Although some architectural features are lost, the increased cellularity and complete cell profiles provide advantage to the interpreting pathologist.

Ductal cells typically appear as monolayer sheets of uniform columnar cells ("honeycomb" pattern) with round to oval, smooth nuclei with fine chromatin and indistinct nucleoli. When viewed sideways, these columnar cells display a "picket fence" appearance.[9] (Fig. 15.1). Acinar cells are typically displayed in small, cohesive, raspberry-like groups with indistinct cell borders. Nuclei are eccentrically placed, small, and round to oval with evenly distributed chromatin. Cytoplasm is moderate in quantity and is granular, a reflection of the presence of zymogen granules, that is, digestive enzymes[9] (Fig. 15.2). Caution must be exercised when aspiration smears are prepared because aggressive smearing can result in disruption of normal acinar cell groups into single cells, thereby creating a cytomorphologic appearance that can be mistaken for a pancreatic endocrine tumor.

Reactive/Inflammatory Cell Changes

The distinction between reactive ductal epithelial cell changes and well-differentiated adenocarcinoma can be problematic when nuclear atypia is minimal and cellularity is limited.[10] Each diagnosis is based on the same constellation of cytologic features, which become more extreme when the diagnosis shifts from pancreatitis to well-differentiated adenocarcinoma to poorly differentiated adenocarcinoma. Consequently, to guard against a misdiagnosis, it is wise to adjust one's threshold upward, demanding more cytologic evidence of malignancy before rendering a diagnosis of adenocarcinoma, when clinical and radiologic input favor an inflammatory process (e.g., young patient, history of excessive alcohol intake or abdominal trauma, hereditary pancreatitis, autoimmune sialoadenitis or primary sclerosing cholangitis, no discrete pancreatic mass, diffuse gland involvement, prior stent placement, and/or no worsening of clinical/radiologic findings over a prolonged period of time).[11-13] Cy-

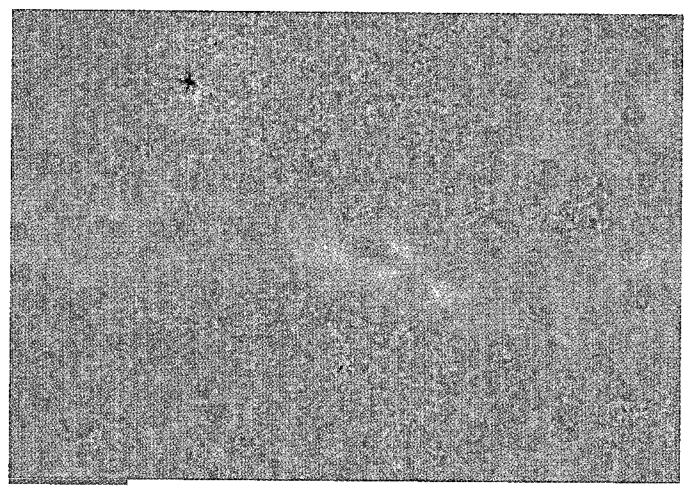

Figure 15.3
Pancreatitis. Cells display cytologic atypia with a mild increase in nuclear size and crowding; however, complete features of malignancy are absent (Papanicolaou, ×300).

tologic preparations of pancreatitis are typically sparse in cellularity, frequently displaying both benign and atypical epithelial cell fragments admixed with variable amounts of acute and chronic inflammation. The atypical epithelial cell fragments are cohesive and two-dimensional, with relatively orderly spaced nuclei. Nuclei are mildly enlarged, at times showing a prominent nucleolus. Infrequent mitotic figures can be seen, as well as necrotic debris. Although the nuclear to cytoplasmic ratio of most cells is unaltered, a small degree of nuclear pleomorphism and nuclear membrane irregularity can be identified.[10,14,15] Although most of these findings are on a continuum with features of well-differentiated adenocarcinoma, the changes in pancreatitis fall short of a diagnosis of adenocarcinoma when they are assessed as a group (Fig. 15.3). The diagnosis of pancreatitis is also more likely when the cellular atypia is only focal.

Mass Lesions of the Pancreas

Nonneoplastic Cysts

Pseudocyst The pseudocyst, the most common cyst of the pancreas, yields turbid dark brown fluid on aspiration.[16] The fluid most commonly results from inflammation, trauma, or prior surgery that produce a spillage of digestive enzymes.[16] The pseudocyst is not a true cyst because it does not have an epithelial lining. Aspirates contain no epithelium, displaying mostly variable amounts of acute and chronic inflammatory cells, histiocytes, granular (necrotic) debris, and fibroblasts.[16-19] To provide further confirmation of this cytologic diagnosis, the serous/turbid fluid obtained may be sent for biochemical analysis. The findings of high amylase and lipase levels, normal carcinoembryonic antigen levels, and viscosity less than serum separate the pseudocyst from other cystic neoplasms.[10,20-22]

Congenital cyst/retention cyst In contrast to the pseudocyst, congenital and retention cysts are true cysts, lined by glandular epithelium of ductal cell origin.[3,16] In the patient with a congenital cyst, multiple unilocular cysts occur both in the pancreas and in other organs of the body, such as the liver and kidneys.[3] Retention cysts are the result of cystic dilatation from focal duct obstruction.[3] They are unilocular and small.[11] Epithelial lining cells, derived via aspiration from these two types of cysts, are sparse or nonexistent and show columnar-to-cuboidal cell morphology. Few inflammatory cells and histiocytes can be seen in obtained fluid that may grossly appear clear, turbid, serous, or mucoid.[3,16] Aspirates from these cysts can incorrectly suggest pseudocyst if there is a failure to sample the cyst wall epithelium, particularly in larger lesions in which the epithelial lining is atrophic. Also, aspirates from cysts lined by epithelium that has undergone mucinous metaplasia show features similar to those of mucinous neoplasms. Consequently, cytologic findings require correlation with available clinical/radiologic data to help ensure diagnostic accuracy. Findings such as small tumor size, peripheral location, cysts involving other organs of the body, uniloculation, and complete collapse of the cyst after aspiration are features favoring a nonneoplastic cyst.

Lymphoepithelial cyst The lymphoepithelial cyst, another true cyst, is large, often greater than 5 cm, and occurs in middle-aged or older men.[23] They are detected as a result of the patient's complaint of abdominal pain or incidentally on abdominal scans for unrelated disease.[23] Although these lesions are composed of mature keratinizing squamous epithelium surrounded by lymphoid tissue, it is the squamous epithelial tissues that accumulate within this lesion, dominating the lymphoid component.[23,24] Consequently, aspiration needles quickly penetrate the lymphoid layer and therefore acquire almost exclusively the squamous (keratinous) debris found in the center of these lesions. Slide preparations show benign nucleated and anucleated squamous cells in a background of necrotic debris[23,24] (Fig. 15.4). Small, mature lymphocytes can at times be seen, although they are frequently overlooked because peripheral blood, a normal

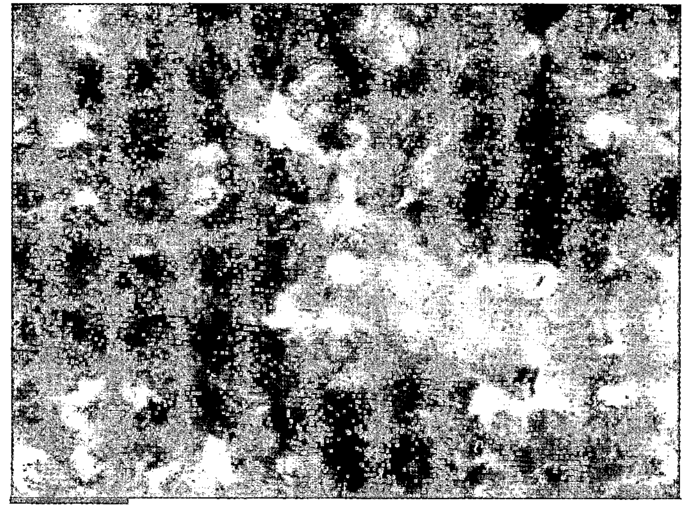

Figure 15.4
Lymphoepithelial cyst. Anucleated squamous cells are embedded within necrotic keratinous debris (Papanicolaou, ×200).

component of all aspirations, also contains lymphocytes. Cholesterol crystals, from the breakdown of cell membranes, have also been reported.[23]

Neoplastic Cysts

Serous cystadenoma Serous cystadenoma, also referred to as microcystic adenoma or glycogen-rich cystadenoma, commonly affects elderly women.[3] These patients typically do not experience bile duct obstruction with resulting jaundice, even when lesions are found in the head of the pancreas.[3] When these lesions are clinically discovered, they are often large and composed of numerous small cysts, giving this tumor the gross appearance of a sponge.[3,11] The classic radiologic appearance is that of a central scar with the presence of post–contrast media enhancement, indicating the vascular nature of the neoplasm.[25] These findings, when present, suggest serous cystadenoma rather than a mucinous cystic neoplasm. As the individual cysts enlarge, the lining epithelium progresses from low columnar to cuboidal to flattened. Consequently, aspirates are frequently hypocellular, with the few epithelial cells present arranged in monolayer sheets composed of cells with small, round nuclei showing evenly dispersed chromatin, nonprominent nucleoli, and no crowding. The modest cytoplasm of these cells is clear because of significant accumulation of glycogen[16,26,28] (Fig. 15.5A). When cells are more columnar and have clear cytoplasm, an erroneous diagnosis of a mucinous neoplasm can be made. In addition, this incorrect diagnosis is facilitated when conventional cytology stains, that is, the Papanicolaou and Diff-Quik stains, suggest the presence of mucinous fluid by displaying a light blue-green or magenta matrix, respectively, in the background of prepared slides when they are examined microscopically. Consequently, it is prudent for the pathologist to perform two ancillary stains, using periodic acid–Schiff with and without the addition of diastase. A positive result without diastase that is eliminated with the addition of diastase indicates the presence of glycogen and not mucin (Fig. 15.5B), thereby suggesting the diagnosis of serous cystadenoma.[26,28]

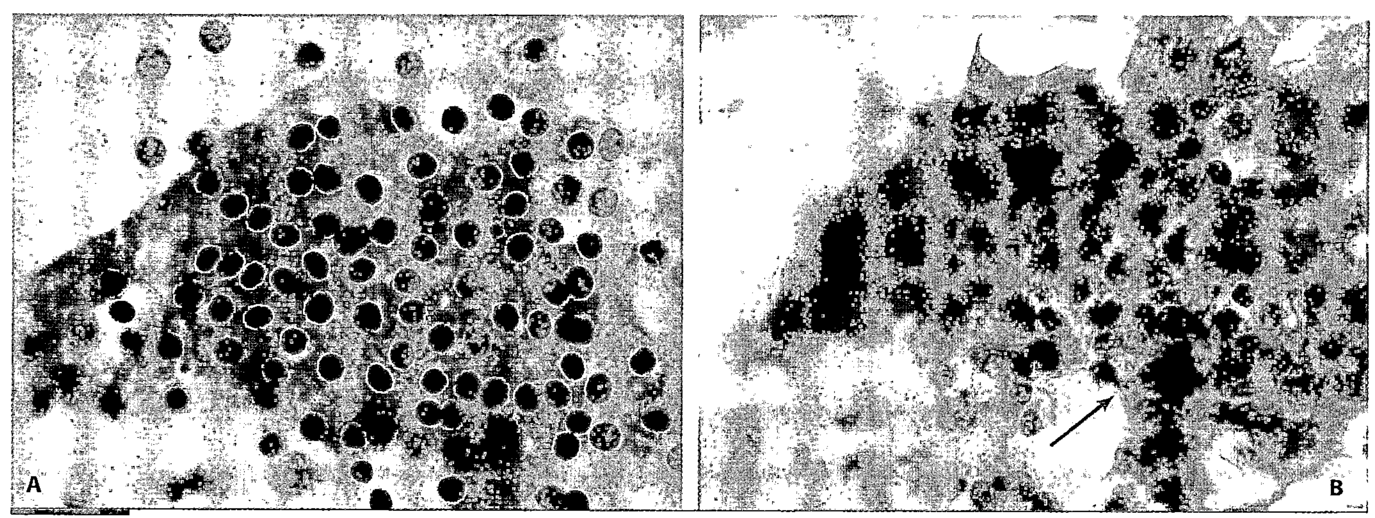

Figure 15.5
(A) Serous cystadenoma. Monolayer sheet of cuboidal cells with defined cytoplasmic borders and focal zones of perinuclear clearing (Papanicolaou, ×300). **(B)** Serous cystadenoma. Cells demonstrating focal, reddish, cytoplasmic periodic acid-Schiff (PAS) positive granules (*arrow*). Reaction was eliminated with addition of diastase; findings consistent with glycogen (PAS, ×300).

Mucinous cystic neoplasm Typically, a mucinous cystic neoplasm is quite large when discovered.[3,11] It most commonly affects middle-aged women and involves the body or tail of the pancreas.[3,11] These lesions can be uniloculated or multiloculated.[3] Aspirates from these neoplasms show two-dimensional epithelial cell groups composed of columnar epithelium with mucinous cell changes, identified by clear cytoplasm or a slight purple-magenta coloration of the cytoplasm that has a tissue-paper textured look (i.e., goblet cell–like appearance). Background mucin should be abundant[19,27,28] (Fig. 15.6A). When this mucin is viscous, it is easy to recognize cytologically. However, if the mucin is thin, the aspirate bears similarity to serous cystadenoma. Ancillary stains for the detection of mucin can be helpful. The most commonly employed stains are the mucicarmine stain and the periodic acid–Schiff stain with and without diastase.[29] Unlike the cells in a serous cystadenoma, the cells from a mucinous cystic neoplasm remain positive with the addition of diastase. When lesions that occur in the body and tail of the pancreas are aspirated, the use of endoscopic ultrasound–guided FNA requires that the aspirating needle be passed through the stomach.[9,27] Therefore, great care must be taken to stylet the aspirating needle when knowingly penetrating the stomach. In addition, the aspirator should not inadvertently repenetrate the stomach when the needle is moved back and forth while aspirating, particularly for lesions close to the stomach. Superficial gastric epithelium is composed of mucin-secreting columnar cells, and if acquired accidentally, these nonneoplastic cells can lead to a misdiagnosis of mucinous neoplasm. Consequently, before a diagnosis of a mucinous neoplasm is made, it is important to radiologically establish the presence of a cystic lesion within the pancreatic body or tail. In addition, in this setting, the identification of significant mucinous cell changes and excellular mucin on repeated aspirations is more indicative of a mucinous neoplasm rather than mere stomach contamination. As described in Chapter 54, the differential diagnosis of the pathological interpretation of mucinous cystic neoplasm includes mucinous cyst adenoma and mucinous cystadenocarcinoma. Recognition of the cytologic features delineated in the section on "pancreatic (ductal) adenocarcinoma" points to the diagnosis of mucinous cystadenocarcinoma[25,28] (Fig. 15.6B). However, making the diagnosis of mucinous cystadenoma on a cytologic preparation is another matter.[30] A potential cystadenoma must be thoroughly sampled to evaluate for a focal malignant component.[30,31] This can be accomplished only on excision of the entire mass. Hence, for aspirates of a mucinous nature that lack overt malignant cell features, a definitive subclassification cannot be made.

Intraductal papillary mucinous neoplasm The cytologic presentation of intraductal papillary mucinous neoplasm shares criteria with the lesions outlined in the section on mucinous cystic neoplasm. The intraductal papillary mucinous neoplasm is characterized by an area of ectatic pancreatic duct that is lined by mucinous papillary epithelium. Both benign and malignant neoplasms

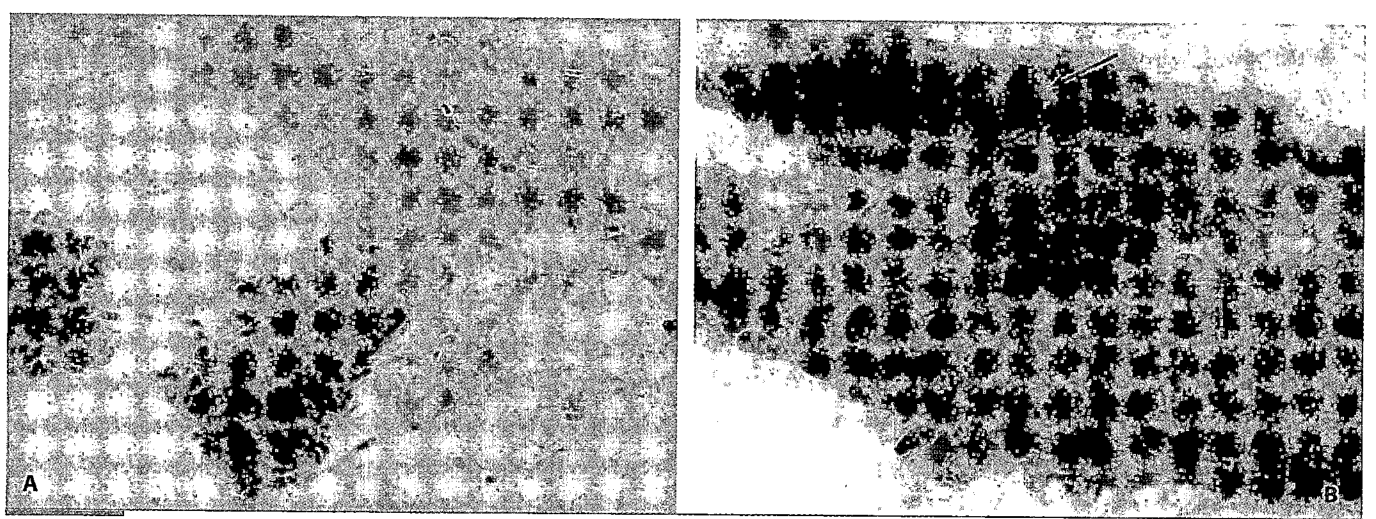

Figure 15.6
(A) Mucinous cystic neoplasm. Ductal epithelial cell groups embedded in a gelatinous-appearing polychromatic (blue-green to magenta) matrix, consistent with mucin (Papanicolaou, ×100). **(B)** Mucinous cystic neoplasm. Fragment of ductal epithelium raising some concern for malignancy by demonstrating a degree of nuclear crowding and nuclear volume ratio differences that are 4:1 or greater (*arrow*) (Papanicolaou, ×300).

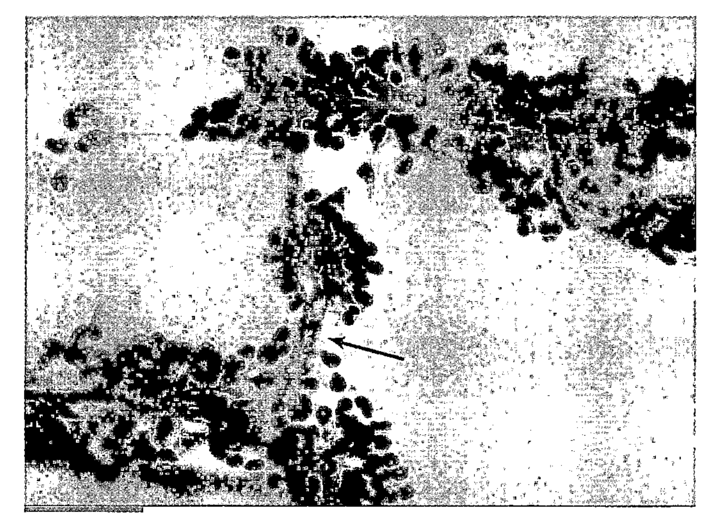

Figure 15.7
Solid-pseudopapillary neoplasm. Neoplastic cells radiate out from a central fibrovascular core, recognized by the perpendicularly placed spindled endothelial cells (*arrow*) (Papanicolaou, ×200).

are seen in this category, as reflected by the criteria stated in the section on pancreatic (ductal) adenocarcinoma.[4,8,16] It has been reported that intraductal papillary mucinous neoplasm differs from mucinous cystic neoplasm in that the former displays a greater abundance of mucin and cellularity that includes complex papillary formations.[32] However, these differences are difficult to appreciate in the isolated case. Most significantly, intraductal papillary mucinous neoplasms are differentiated from mucinous cystic neoplasms by virtue of their communication with the pancreatic duct.[4,8,16] At times, the endoscopist performing the FNA procedure can suggest the intraductal nature of these tumors by identifying mucin exuding from the ampulla, the terminal point of drainage for the pancreatic duct.[33] This finding, along with the identification of duct ectasia on radiologic imaging and the appropriate cytologic features of mucinous cell changes and excellular mucin, allows one to favor this diagnosis.[33]

Solid Neoplasms

Solid-pseudopapillary tumor Solid-pseudopapillary tumors characteristically arise within the tail of the pancreas in adolescent girls and young women.[3,11] The neoplasm grows as a solid mass of cells; however, in areas where cells are furthest from the tumor's delicate capillary blood supply, the cells become dishesive. As a result, papillary, albeit pseudopapillary, structures are seen.[11] Cytologic smears are cellular, showing slender papillary-like fonds that are composed of a delicate endothelial-lined capillary and attached epithelial cells. The noncohesive cells present as single cells in the background[34,35] (Fig. 15.7). Epithelial cells are bland in appearance and can resemble the cells seen in a pancreatic endocrine tumor. Nuclei are small and round, possess fine chromatin and inconspicuous nucleoli, and are eccentrically placed within modest amounts of cytoplasm.[34,35] Globules of myxoid stroma, with and without surrounding neoplastic cells, have been reported.[16,34]

Pancreatic (ductal) adenocarcinoma Pancreatic (ductal) adenocarcinoma (not otherwise specified) accounts for at least 90% of all pancreatic malignancies.[3] A predominance of these neoplasms arise in the head region, and as a result, even small lesions often give rise to obstructive jaundice.[3] The diagnosis of ductal adenocarcinoma is made when ductal epithelium displays cytologic atypia consisting of nuclear enlargement with anisonucleosis (defined as nuclear volume variation of 4:1 or greater in cells seen within the same cell group), nuclear crowding leading to squeezed or angulated nuclei, nuclear overlap (three dimensionality), irregular nuclear contours, irregular distribution of nuclei within an epithelial fragment, chromatin clumping, and nuclear hyperchromasia[10,14,36] (Fig. 15.8). Additional features, such as the presence of single cells, necrosis, and mitotic figures, are helpful when seen in abundance.[10,14,36] Nuclear atypia can be subtle and focal, especially in well-differentiated lesions. Consequently, the better differentiated the carcinoma, the more cytologic tissue the pathologist will require to render a definitive diagnosis of malignancy.

Pancreatic endocrine neoplasm (islet cell tumor) Pancreatic endocrine neoplasms can occur at any point along the length of the pancreas. The greatest number of islets are found in the body and tail; therefore, the largest percentage of islet cell neoplasms arise in these areas.[3] In rare cases, they can present as a largely cystic mass.[17,19] Aspirates are typically cellular, consisting of a relatively even mixture of single cells and small, cohesive cell groups. Individual cells are round to cuboidal with dense, homogeneous, well-defined cytoplasm. Nuclei are small; are round to oval; contain fine, evenly dispersed chromatin and an inconspicuous nucleolus; and are eccentrically placed within the cytoplasm[37-40] (Fig. 15.9A). Acinar-like formations and thin, delicate vessels can be seen.[38] Endocrine neoplasms are typically hormonally functional as a result of the presence of neurosecretory granules.[8] These diagnostic granules can be identified via electron mi-

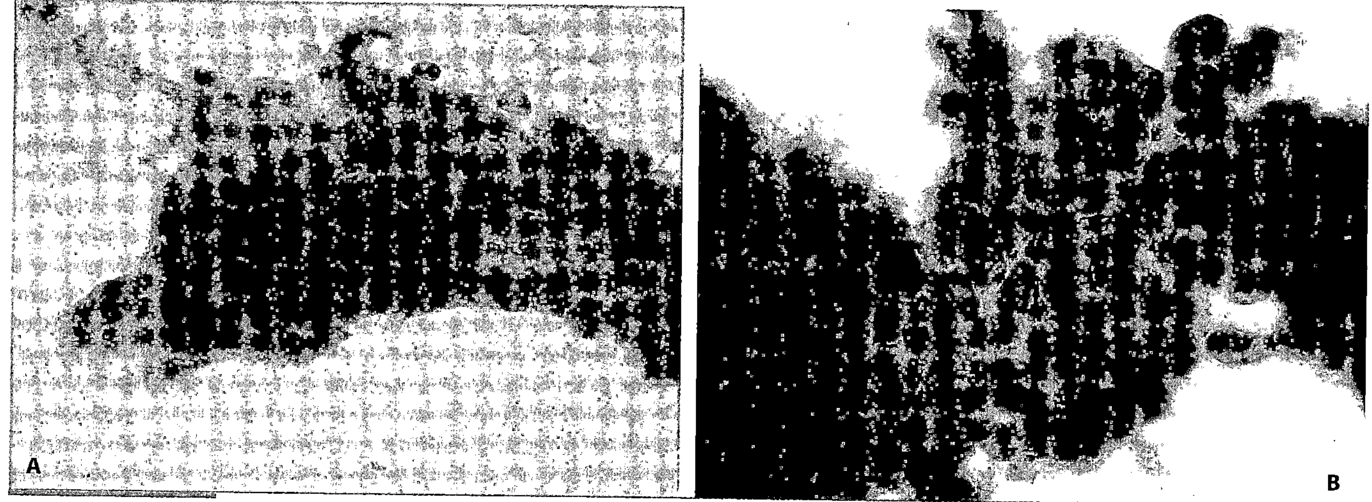

Figure 15.8, A and B
Ductal adenocarcinoma. Epithelial cell groups demonstrate malignant cell features consisting of nuclear enlargement, anisonucleosis, nuclear crowding and irregularity, chromatin clumping, nuclear hyperchromasia, and the irregular distribution of nuclei (Papanicolaou, ×300 and ×400).

croscopy, presenting as small (0.14- to 0.4-μm), electron-dense, membrane-bound structures with or without a clear zone beneath the membrane[37,41] (Fig. 15.9B). Immunolabeling for neuroendocrine differentiation, such as chromogranin and synaptophysin, also confirms the presence of neurosecretory granules.[8,39,40] The demonstration of neurosecretory granules differentiates pancreatic endocrine neoplasm from acinar cell carcinoma and solid pseudopapillary tumor.

Acinar cell carcinoma Although exocrine (acinar) tissues dominate the substance of the pancreas, acinar cell carcinomas are relatively rare.[11] The acinar cell carcinoma aspiration is similar to that of an islet cell tumor in that cells are displayed singly and in small cell groups; nuclei are relatively small, are round to oval, and can be arranged in loosely cohesive acinar structures.[40,42,43] Conversely, the acinar cell carcinoma smear differs in that the cytoplasm within cell groups is granular in appearance

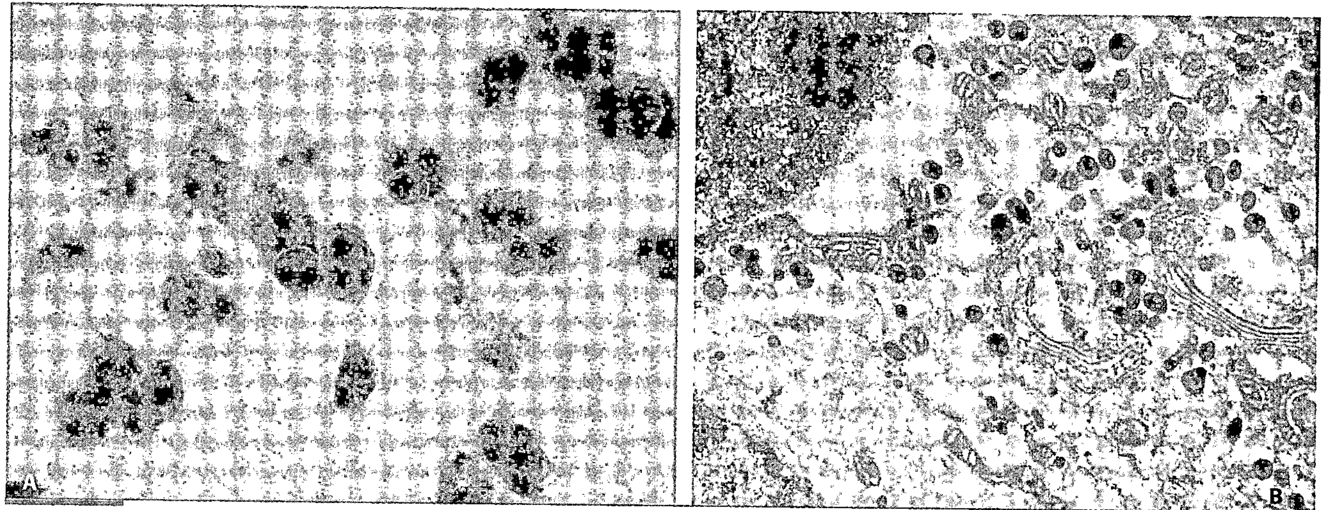

Figure 15.9
(A) Pancreatic endocrine tumor. Single cells display small, round nuclei with inconspicuous nucleoli and fine, evenly distributed chromatin. Nuclei are eccentrically placed within homogeneous, well-defined cytoplasm (Papanicolaou, ×800). **(B)** Pancreatic endocrine tumor. Electron micrograph (EM) showing small, electron-dense, neurosecretory granules (EM, ×28,000).

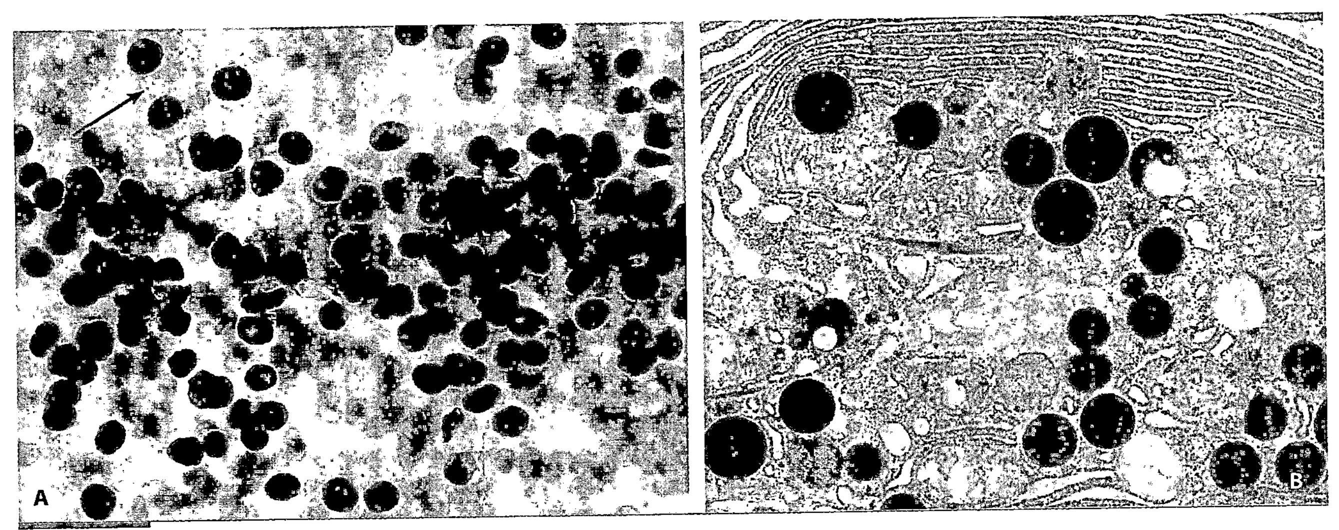

Figure 15.10
(A) Acinar cell carcinoma. Loosely cohesive cells display poorly formed acinar-like structures. Cell cytoplasm is granular in appearance (*arrow*) (Diff-Quik, ×600). **(B)** Acinar cell carcinoma. Electron micrograph (EM) demonstrating abundant linear endoplasmic reticulum and large, round, electron-dense, zymogen granules (EM, ×12,000).

due to the presence of zymogen (enzyme) granules[40,42,44] (Fig. 15.10A). Via electron microscopy, these tumors show abundant rough endoplasmic reticulum and the diagnostic feature of zymogen granules.[41,43,44] These structures present as large (up to 2 μm), electron-dense, membrane-bound vesicles with no clear zone beneath their membrane[41] (Fig. 15.10B). Immunolabeling for trypsin, chymotrypsin, and lipase support the diagnosis of acinar cell carcinoma.[11,40,42,45]

Other Malignant Neoplasms

Other malignant neoplasms have been reported in the general pathology literature, but because of their rarity and the relative recent use of FNA, their presence in the cytology literature has been given little coverage and is mentioned here only for completeness. Pancreatoblastoma, a malignant neoplasm with acinar differentiation and squamoid nests, is seen in the head of the pancreas, usually as a very large mass in young children.[11] Histologically, polygonal cells are found in nests partitioned by fibrous connective tissue bands. Cells vary from undifferentiated to a tubuloglandular and/or squamoid morphology.[11] Thus far, in the rare reported aspirations of this tumor, a cell morphology similar in appearance to islet cell tumor and acinar cell carcinoma has been reported.[46] This similarity was also seen at the ultrastructural level by neoplastic cells showing bidirectional differentiation, with both neurosecretory and zymogen granules being identified.[46] Pleomorphic giant cell carcinoma, adenosquamous carcinoma, and signet ring cell carcinoma are rare variants of pancreatic (ductal) carcinoma that prominently display the cytomorphology denoted in the name of the neoplasm. Consequently, in addition to showing malignant nuclear features, as outlined in the section on pancreatic (ductal) carcinoma, the pleomorphic giant cell carcinoma shows poorly cohesive, irregularly shaped, bizarre giant cells, with some cells showing multinucleation.[11,47,48] In addition to features of adenocarcinoma, the adenosquamous carcinoma has a coexistent malignant component showing squamous differentiation.[49,50] Presumably, this squamous cell component is a malignant metaplasia of the adenocarcinoma.[41] Signet ring cell carcinoma shows noncohesive single cells that display prominent cytoplasmic mucin that displaces the nucleus to the far periphery of the cell and frequently deforms the nucleus into a crescent shape.[11] Although this malignancy has been reported in histologic tissues, no aspiration cases have yet been reported in the cytology literature. Undifferentiated small cell carcinoma is a high grade carcinoma with neuroendocrine differentiation that is morphologically similar to small cell carcinoma occurring in the lung.[45] Lastly, metastatic tumors and lymphomas can involve the pancreas and should be placed in the differential diagnosis when the cytomorphology is not consistent with typical pancreatic lesions or when the patient has a known history of prior malignancy.[51-53]

References

1. Hajdu SI. The value and limitations of aspiration cytology in the diagnosis of primary tumors: a symposium. *Acta Cytol.* 1989;33:741–790.
2. Chang KJ, Nguyen P, Erickson RA, et al. The clinical utility of endoscopic ultrasound-guided fine needle aspiration in the diagnosis and staging of pancreatic carcinoma. *Gastrointest Endosc.* 1997;45:387–393.
3. DeMay RM. Pancreas. In: DeMay RM, ed. *The Art and Science of Cytopathology: Aspiration Cytology*. Chicago: ASCP Press; 1996:1054–1082.
4. Deshpande V. Pancreas. In: Gray W, McKee GT, eds. *Diagnostic Cytopathology*. 2nd ed. Edinburgh: Churchill Livingstone; 2003:427–446.
5. Lightwood R, Reber HA, Way LW. The risk and accuracy of pancreatic biopsy. *Am J Surg.* 1976;132:189–194.
6. Bowden M. The fallibility of pancreatic biopsy. *Ann Surg.* 1954;139:403–408.
7. Layfield LJ, Wax TD, Lee JF, et al. Accuracy and morphologic aspects of pancreatic and biliary duct brushings. *Acta Cytol.* 1995;39:11–18.
8. Weinstein LJ. Pancreas. In: Cibas ES, Ducatman BS, eds. *Cytology: Diagnostic Principles and Clinical Correlates*. 2nd ed. New York: Saunders; 2003:367–382.
9. Pitman MB. Normal pancreas. In: Centeno BA, Pitman MB, eds. *Fine Needle Aspiration Biopsy of the Pancreas*. Boston: Butterworth-Heinemann; 1999:17–30.
10. Robins DB, Katz RL, Evans DB, et al. Fine needle aspiration of the pancreas: in quest of accuracy. *Acta Cytol.* 1995;39:1–10.
11. Solcia EN, Capella C, Kloppel G. Tumors of the pancreas. *In Atlas of Tumor Pathology*. 3rd series. Washington DC: Armed Forces Institute of Pathology; 1997:fascicle 20.
12. Furukawa N, Muranaka T, Yasumori K, et al. Autoimmune pancreatitis: radiologic findings in three histologically proven cases. *J Comput Assist Tomogr.* 1998;22:880–883.
13. Van Dyke JA, Stanley RJ, Berland LL. Pancreatic imaging. *Ann Intern Med.* 1985;102:212–217.
14. Cohen MB, Egerter DP, Holly EA, et al. Pancreatic adenocarcinoma: regression analysis to identify improved cytologic criteria. *Diagn Cytopathol.* 1991;7:341–345.
15. Pitman MB. Pancreatitis. In: Centeno BA, Pitman MB, eds. *Fine Needle Aspiration Biopsy of the Pancreas*. Boston: Butterworth-Heinemann; 1999:31–51.
16. Centeno BA. Cystic lesion. In: Centeno BA, Pitman MB, eds. *Fine Needle Aspiration Biopsy of the Pancreas*. Boston: Butterworth-Heinemann; 1999:53–108.
17. Centeno BA, Warshaw AL, Mayo-Smith W, et al. Cytologic diagnosis of pancreatic cystic lesions: a prospective study of 28 percutaneous aspirates. *Acta Cytol.* 1997;41:972–980.
18. Young NA, Villani MA, Khoury P, Naryshkin S. Differential diagnosis of cystic neoplasms of the pancreas by fine-needle aspiration. *Arch Pathol Lab Med.* 1991;115:571–577.
19. Centeno BA, Lewandrowski KB, Warshaw AL, et al. Cyst fluid cytologic analysis in the differential diagnosis of pancreatic cystic lesions. *Am J Clin Pathol.* 1994;101:483–487.
20. Pinto MM, Avila NA, Criscuolo EM. Fine needle aspiration of the pancreas: a five-year experience. *Acta Cytol.* 1988;32:39–42.
21. Hammel P, Levy P, Voitot H, et al. Preoperative cyst fluid analysis is useful for the differential diagnosis of cystic lesions of the pancreas. *Gastroenterology.* 1995;108:1230–1235.
22. Lewandrowski KB, Southern JF, Pins MR, et al. Cyst fluid analysis in the differential diagnosis of pancreatic cysts: a comparison of pseudocysts, serous cystadenomas, mucinous cystic neoplasms, and mucinous cystadenocarcinoma. *Ann Surg.* 1993;217:41–47.
23. Liu J, Shin HJ, Rubenchik I, et al. Cytologic features of lymphoepithelial cyst of the pancreas: two preoperatively diagnosed cases based on fine-needle aspiration. *Diagn Cytopathol.* 1999;21:346–350.
24. Mandavilli SR, Prot J, Ali SZ. Lymphoepithelial cyst (LEC) of the pancreas: cytomorphology and differential diagnosis on fine-needle aspiration (FNA). *Diagn Cytopathol.* 1999;20:371–374.
25. Vellet D, Leiman G, Mair S, et al. Fine needle aspiration cytology of mucinous cystadenocarcinoma of the pancreas. *Acta Cytol.* 1988;32:43–48.
26. Hittmair A, Pernthaler H, Totsch M, et al. Preoperative fine needle aspiration cytology of a microcystic adenoma of the pancreas. *Acta Cytol.* 1991;35:546–548.
27. Jones EC, Suen KC, Grant DR, et al. Fine-needle aspiration cytology of neoplastic cysts of the pancreas. *Diagn Cytopathol.* 1987;3:238–243.
28. Laucirica R, Schwartz MR, Ramzy I. Fine needle aspiration of pancreatic cystic epithelial neoplasms. *Acta Cytol.* 1992;36:881–886.
29. Wilentz RE, Albores-Saavedra J, Hruban RH. Mucinous cystic neoplasms of the pancreas. *Semin Diagn Pathol.* 2000;17:31–42.
30. Dodd LG, Farrell TA, Layfield LJ. Mucinous cystic tumor of the pancreas: an analysis of FNA characteristics with an emphasis on the spectrum of malignancy associated features. *Diagn Cytopathol.* 1995;12:113–119.
31. Hyde GL, Davis JB Jr., McMillin RD, McMillin M. Mucinous cystic neoplasm of the pancreas with latent malignancy. *Am Surg.* 1984;50:225–229.
32. Shabaik A. Endoscopic ultrasound-guided fine needle aspiration cytology of intraductal papillary mucinous tumor of the pancreas. *Acta Cytol.* 2003;47:657–662.
33. Yamaguchi K, Tanaka M. Mucin-hypersecreting tumor of the pancreas with mucin extrusion through an enlarged papilla. *Am J Gastroenterol.* 1991;86:835–839.
34. Bondeson L, Bondeson AG, Genell S, et al. Aspiration cytology of a rare solid and papillary epithelial neoplasm of the pancreas. *Acta Cytol.* 1984;28:605–609.
35. Pelosi G, Iannucci A, Zamboni G, et al. Solid and cystic papillary neoplasm of the pancreas: a clinico-cytopathologic and immunocytochemical study of five new cases diagnosed by fine-needle aspiration cytology and a review of the literature. *Diagn Cytopathol.* 1995;13:233–246.
36. Lin F, Staerkel G. Cytologic criteria for well differentiated adenocarcinoma of the pancreas in fine-needle aspiration biopsy specimens. *Cancer (Cancer Cytopathol).* 2003;99:44–50.
37. Al-Kaisi N, Weaver MG, Abdul-Karim FW, et al. Fine needle aspiration cytology of neuroendocrine tumors of the pancreas: a cytologic, immunocytochemical and electron microscopic study. *Acta Cytol.* 1992;36:655–660.

38. Sneige N, Ordonez NG, Veanattukalathil S, et al. Fine needle aspiration cytology in pancreatic endocrine tumors. *Diagn Cytopathol*. 1987;3:35–40.
39. Collins BT, Cramer HM. Fine-needle aspiration cytology of islet cell tumors. *Diagn Cytopathol*. 1996;15:37–45.
40. Labate AM, Klimstra DS, Zakowski MF. Comparative cytologic features of pancreatic acinar cell carcinoma and islet cell tumor. *Diagn Cytopathol*. 1997;16:112–116.
41. Walker PD. Pancreas. In: Karcioğlu ZA, Someren A, eds. *Practical Surgical Pathology*. Lexington, MA: The Collamore Press; 1985:309–338.
42. Samuel LH, Frierson HF. Fine needle aspiration cytology of acinar cell carcinoma of the pancreas: a report of two cases. *Acta Cytol*. 1996;40:585–591.
43. Villanueva RR, Nguyen-Ho P, Nguyen GK: Needle aspiration cytology of acinar-cell carcinoma of the pancreas: report of a case with diagnostic pitfalls and unusual ultrastructural findings. *Cytopathology*. 1994;10:362–364.
44. Ishihara A, Sanda T, Takanari H, et al. Elastage-1-secreting acinar cell carcinoma of the pancreas: a cytologic, electron microscopic and histochemical study. *Acta Cytol*. 1989;33:157–163.
45. Centeno BA, Pitman MB. Neoplasms of the exocrine and endocrine pancreas. In: Centeno BA, Pitman MB, eds. *Fine Needle Aspiration of the Pancreas*. Boston: Butterworth-Heinemann; 1999:109–160.
46. Silverman JF, Holbrook CT, Pories WJ, et al. Fine needle aspiration cytology of pancreatoblastoma with immunocytochemical and ultrastructural studies. *Acta Cytol*. 1990;34:632–640.
47. Pinto MM, Monteiro NL, Tizol DM. Fine needle aspiration of pleomorphic giant-cell carcinoma of the pancreas: case report with ultrastructural observations. *Acta Cytol*. 1986;30:430–434.
48. Silverman JF, Finley JL, Bern L, et al. Significance of giant cells in fine-needle aspiration biopsies of benign and malignant lesions of the pancreas. *Diagn Cytopathol*. 1989;5:388–391.
49. Smit W, Mathy JP, Donaldson E. Pancreatic cytology and adenosquamous carcinoma of the pancreas. *Pathology*. 1993;25:420–422.
50. Wilczynski SP, Valente PT, Atkinson BF. Cytodiagnosis of adenosquamous carcinoma of the pancreas: use of intraoperative fine needle aspiration. *Acta Cytol*. 1984;28:733–736.
51. Carson HJ, Green LK, Castelli MJ, et al. Utilization of fine-needle aspiration biopsy in the diagnosis of metastatic tumors to the pancreas. *Diagn Cytopathol*. 1995;12:8–13.
52. Benning TL, Silverman JF, Berns LA, et al. Fine needle aspiration of metastatic and hematologic malignancies clinically mimicking pancreatic carcinoma. *Acta Cytol*. 1992;36:471–476.
53. David O, Green L, Reddy V, et al. Pancreatic masses: a multi-institutional study of 364 fine-needle aspiration biopsies with histopathologic correlation. *Diagn Cytopathol*. 1998;19:423–427.

CHAPTER

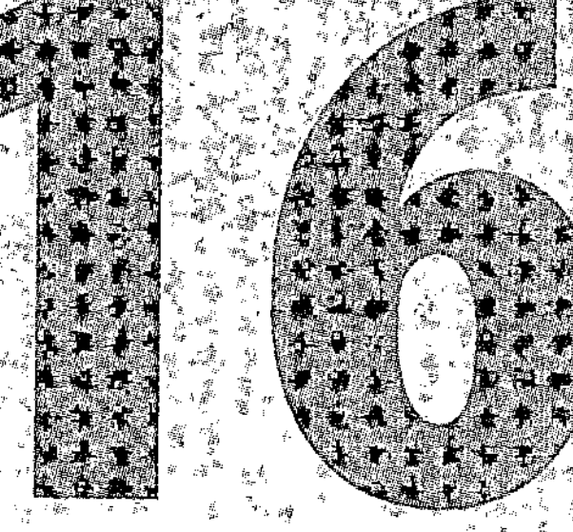

Serologic Diagnosis of Pancreatic Cancer

Matthew H. Katz, MD
Abdool R. Moosa, MD
Michael Bouvet, MD

For patients with ductal adenocarcinoma of the pancreas, long-term survival is dependent upon complete surgical tumor resection by pancreaticoduodenectomy or total pancreatectomy, which currently provides these patients with their only chance for cure.[1] Over the past 3 decades, advances in the surgical treatment and perioperative care of patients with pancreatic cancer have resulted in a sharp decline in the perioperative morbidity and mortality associated with these complex surgical operations.[2,3] Nonetheless, the ability of surgeons to perform these procedures safely and thereby to achieve prolonged survival in selected patients[4-6] is complicated by the fact that only 10%–15% of patients with pancreatic cancer are found to have localized, resectable disease at the time of diagnosis.[7] Because most individuals diagnosed with pancreatic cancer are therefore ineligible for attempted curative resection, the overall outlook for these patients remains grim. Each year, approximately 30,000 individuals will die of this disease in the United States alone, ranking pancreatic cancer among the top five causes of adult cancer deaths nationwide.[8,9]

These statistics suggest that the overall outcome for patients with pancreatic cancer may be impacted most significantly by improvements in diagnostic accuracy, especially in the early stages of the disease when surgical resection is most feasible. Data from numerous studies identifying advanced tumor size, stage, and the presence of nodal and distant metastases among the most important predictors of patient outcome[5,10,11] support this hypothesis. Similarly, subset analyses of patients undergoing resection for pancreatic cancer demonstrating that 5-year survival rates up to 40%–50% may be achieved in selected patients with small[12] and node-negative[3] disease emphasize the need for improved diagnostic ability at an earlier stage, when more effective surgical resection is permitted.

Unfortunately, the diagnosis of pancreatic cancer, particularly in its early stages, remains a considerable challenge. The deep anatomic location of the pancreas in the retroperitoneum is largely responsible for a paucity of symptoms in the early stages of the disease and makes its early detection by routine physical exam difficult. Typically, an aggressive search for a pancreatic mass is initiated only after the development of abdominal pain, unexplained weight loss, or obstructive jaundice, all of which are symptoms that may occur relatively late in its natural history and are not specific to pancreatic malignancy.[13] Furthermore, pancreatic adenocarcinoma appears to be particularly aggressive, rapidly leading to extensive locoregional or distant dissemination before detection. For these reasons, up to 60% of patients with pancreatic cancer are found to have liver metastases or peritoneal carcinomatosis at the time of diagnosis.[14] A short window of opportunity therefore exists after the onset of symptoms within which a pancreatic tumor can be identified at a resectable stage.

Further difficulty is due to limitations associated with current technology and the imaging modalities routinely used to detect pancreatic malignancy. Transabdominal ultrasound, traditionally one of the first diagnostic tests used in the evaluation of jaundice, has relatively poor sensitivity and specificity in the diagnosis of pancreatic cancer.[15] Likewise, the clinical efficacy of computed tomography (CT) is somewhat limited in the identification of small primary tumors, liver metastases, peritoneal deposits, and occult vascular invasion.[14,16,17] Advances in CT technology and the introduction of new diagnostic modalities, such as endoscopic ultrasound[18] and magnetic resonance imaging promise to increase our ability to detect smaller tumors. Nevertheless, all of these techniques are associated with considerable expense, particularly when used in combination. Moreover, the use of such imaging modalities may be operator or interpreter dependent, may require the use of intravenous contrast agents, and may be invasive to the patient.

The recent increased interest in and use of serologic markers of pancreatic malignancy is thus clearly based on an urgent need for improvement in the diagnosis of pancreatic cancer. Over the past 2 decades, advancements in technology and the development and isolation of monoclonal antibodies using hybridoma techniques have led to the identification of a number of potentially promising serological markers that could theoretically be used to diagnose, to determine the prognosis of, and to monitor the therapeutic course of patients with this disease. Unfortunately, only one of these markers—CA 19-9—has gained widespread clinical acceptance, and it has so far proven largely unsuccessful at enhancing the ability to detect early pancreatic malignancy. Nevertheless, CA 19-9, as well as several other serum markers, may be employed successfully as a valuable part of the evaluation and management of patients with pancreatic cancer. Moreover, the promise of an objective, easy-to-perform serologic assay that is inexpensive, accurate, and reproducible continues to drive active investigation in this area. In this chapter, we review the serologic markers associated with pancreatic cancer, with a special emphasis on the widely used monoclonal antibody CA 19-9.

Overview of Serologic Markers of Pancreatic Cancer

Definition and Classification

Serum tumor markers may be defined as those substances that are selectively released by tumor cells into the blood stream and are readily detected in the serum for the clinical monitoring of various malignancies.[19] A more general definition would include any measurable biologic material, the concentration of which is abnormally elevated in the serum in association with malignant disease.[20] Two broad groups of tumor markers have historically been defined. Specifically expressed by a single malignant cell population, tumor-specific antigens related to pancreatic cancer have yet to be identified. These markers are uncommon in oncology but have been discovered in association with several B-cell lymphomas and virus-induced malignancies.[21] Because they are tumor specific, such markers are found only in the serum of patients harboring an associated cancer. In contrast, low concentrations of tumor-associated antigens may exist in unaffected populations and nonmalignant tissues; serum concentrations above a normal reference range connote a positive marker. A wide range of tumor-associated markers for pancreatic cancer has been reported and has been classified using a variety of schemes based on their natural properties or biological activities.[19-23] In general, the serum markers associated with pancreatic cancer may be grouped into five broad categories (Table 16.1).

Some of the oldest and best studied tumor markers of pancreatic cancer are the oncofetal antigens, normal fetal proteins such as carcinoembryonic antigen (CEA),[24] or pancreatic oncofetal antigen (POA),[25] which are absent or present in reduced quantities in the normal adult but which may be released into the serum in states of cellular dedifferentiation and malignancy. Complex glycoconjugates and blood group related-antigens are large glycoprotein or glycolipid macromolecules such as CA 19-9,[26] CA 50,[27] and CA 242,[27] which can be identified and measured in the serum through the binding of specifically developed antibodies. Many of these antigens have epitopes consisting of sialylated carbohydrate structures, and they are often associated with blood group antigens. Mutations of oncogenes and tumor suppressor genes such as *K-ras*[28] and *p53*,[29] which are frequently associated with pancreatic malignancy, have been measured in the serum and have been recently reported as possible markers of pancreatic malignancy. The overexpression of certain enzymes such as elastase[30] and tumor-associated trypsin inhibitor[31] has been studied, as these could be potential serum markers for pancreatic cancer. Finally, elevations

Table 16.1 Serologic Tumor-Associated Markers of Pancreatic Cancer

Marker	Reference
Oncofetal proteins	
CEA	Gold and Freedman[24]
POA	Banwo et al.[25]
Complex glycoconjugates	
CA 19-9	Koprowski et al.[26]
CA 50	Lindholm et al.[27]
CA 242	Lindholm et al.[27]
CAM 17.1	Parker et al.[119]
DUPAN-2	Metzgar et al.[131]
Span-1	Chung et al.[132]
TPA	Bjorklund and Bjorklund[124]
TPS	Bjorklund[126]
Oncogenes and suppressor genes	
K-ras	Mulcahy et al.[28]
p53	Laurent-Puig et al.[29]
Enzymes/Isoenzymes	
Elastase I	Banga[30]
TATI	Stenman et al.[31]
Hormones and other peptides	
TIMP-1	Zhou et al.[32]
PTHrP	Bouvet et al.[34]

Classification system adapted from Moossa et al.[20] and Suresh.[21]
Abbreviations: TPS, tissue polypeptide-specific antigen; TATI, tumor-associated trypsin inhibitor; TIMP-1, tissue inhibitor of metalloproteinase type 1; PTHrP, parathyroid hormone-related protein.

in the serum level of certain hormones and peptides such as tissue inhibitor of metalloproteinase type 1[32] and parathyroid hormone related protein[33-36] have also been described in patients with exocrine pancreatic malignancy.

The Ideal Serologic Marker and Its Potential Clinical Applications

The ideal serologic tumor marker of pancreatic cancer would be inexpensive, reproducible, and easily measured. Its detection in serum would reflect the presence of minimal tumor burden, and its concentration would accurately reflect tumor load.[19] Such a marker could be effectively employed for any of five clinically valuable applications: screening, diagnosis, assessment of prognosis, monitoring of therapy, and detection of recurrent disease[37] (Table 16.2). Unfortunately, despite the large number of new serologic markers that have been identified over the past 2 decades, none has proven to be ideal, and therefore, the ability of these markers to serve each of these purposes is highly variable. Furthermore, it is unlikely that one of the most potentially beneficial uses of these markers—as a screening test of early pancreatic malignancy in the asymptomatic population—will ever be realized.[38,39] This is because the prevalence of pancreatic cancer in the asymptomatic population is so low that the specificity of a screening test would need to be 100% in order to reduce the number of false-positive test results in the general population to a reasonable level[40] and thereby achieve a useful positive predictive value. Podolsky[22] noted that with an estimated prevalence of pancreatic cancer in the general population over 50 years of 0.05%, even a test with 95% specificity and sensitivity would yield 100 false-positive results for every true-positive result when used to test this general population. Attempts to improve the case-finding potential of serum markers by using them to screen asymptomatic subpopulations at high risk of pancreatic cancer have been complicated by a difficulty in identifying a meaningful, well-defined subgroup at high risk for this disease.[41]

Table 16.2 Potential Clinical Applications for Serologic Markers of Pancreatic Cancer

Population screening*
Diagnosis
Assessment of prognosis
Therapeutic monitoring
Detection of recurrence

* Not shown to be of value in pancreatic cancer.

Although unsuitable for screening asymptomatic individuals in the general population, serum tumor markers have shown considerable promise in other clinical settings, particularly in the evaluation and management of patients for whom a high suspicion of pancreatic malignancy exists or in whom the presence of malignancy is known. In these groups, a substantial disease prevalence allows several markers with high specificity and sufficient predictive value to be clinically useful.[41] Of particular value in these groups of patients is the ability of a tumor marker to assist in the differential diagnosis of obstructive jaundice and abdominal pain, a diagnostic dilemma that is not always straightforward. Serum markers have also been shown to be beneficial in assessing prognosis, monitoring the course of therapy, and detecting recurrences in patients with known disease. In each of these settings, the utility of serologic markers is maximized by their incorporation into a comprehensive diagnostic and therapeutic strategy. Combined with conventional imaging techniques,[42] the results of other serologic marker tests,[43,44] and clinical data,[45] serum markers may contribute valuable information with which decisions can be made regarding the care of patients with pancreatic cancer.

Table 16.3 Reference Values and Performance Characteristics of Selected Serologic Markers of Pancreatic Cancer

Marker	Suggested Reference	Sensitivity (%)	Specificity
CEA	5 ng/ml	30–80	58–95
CA 19-9	37 U/ml	68–90	70–98
CA 50	17 U/ml	71–96	48–71
CA 242	20 U/ml	68–81	65–95
CAM 17.1	37–39 U/ml	67–86	76–91
p53	Presence	18–28	90–96
K-ras	Presence	70–81	92–100

Reference Values and Performance Characteristics of Serologic Markers

Because the tumor-associated markers of pancreatic cancer can be present in the serum of normal patients or those with other benign or malignant diseases, the reference cut-off of a marker is of paramount importance in determining whether a test result should be interpreted as "positive" or "negative" (Table 16.3). These reference values are established empirically through the use of prospective and retrospective studies and have been determined so as to maximize their sensitivity and specificity in the samples reported. It is therefore important to realize that these cut-offs are not absolute; indeed, a marker may be associated with several reference values that may be used for different applications[46] and that may be associated with different sensitivities and specificities relevant to the intended clinical use of the marker.[47] Moreover, the reference cut-off of a serum marker may be adjusted, but doing so will change the performance characteristics of the test. Specifically, increasing the reference cut-off for a positive test will invariably decrease sensitivity and increase specificity.[48] Cut-offs may thus be manipulated in order to accentuate either the sensitivity or specificity according to the relative importance of each in a specific clinical scenario.[19]

As a final comment, it should be noted that the studies used to evaluate serum markers for pancreatic cancer, as for all malignancies, have historically used different cut-off levels and have identified sensitivity and specificity in various patient populations,[49] making evaluation and comparison of such studies and their associated markers difficult.[41] A receiver operating characteristic curve analysis[50] may be used as a standardized approach to the assessment of serum tumor markers.[51] Using this statistical method, the sensitivity of a serum marker is measured and plotted at various specificity levels, thus describing a curve that describes the discriminative power of a marker test independently of cut-off levels. Such curves facilitate meaningful evaluation and comparison of potential markers and are therefore routinely used in the tumor marker literature.

Selected Serologic Markers of Pancreatic Cancer

CA 19-9

CA 19-9 is presently the most clinically useful serologic marker for pancreatic cancer and has become the "gold standard" to which newly discovered markers are compared. First described in 1979,[26] the CA 19-9 antigen was originally defined by a monoclonal antibody produced by hybridomas obtained from a mouse inoculated with the human colon cancer cell line SW 1116. The epitope of this antibody was subsequently identified as a sialylated lacto-N-fucopentaose II[52] related to the Lewis^a blood group antigen. In tissue samples, CA 19-9 has been found to be associated with normal tissues of the pancreas, stomach, and biliary tract, bronchial, and salivary glands[53,54] and pancreatic secretions.[55] In serum, the antigen is associated with circulating mucins[56] and is detectable at basal levels in normal patients using a radioimmunometric assay.[57]

Although originally reported as a potential marker for colorectal cancer,[58] Ritts et al.[59] subsequently demonstrated that elevation of CA 19-9 was frequently associated with tumors of the upper gastrointestinal tract, particularly with those of the pancreas. In this study, serum samples from over 1,600 patients from the National Cancer Institute/Mayo Clinic Serum Bank were analyzed for the presence of CA 19-9. Only 18% of patients with colon cancer were found to have CA 19-9 levels above 40 U/ml; in contrast, 67% of patients with adenocarcinomas of the upper gastrointestinal tract had levels above this value, including 70% of those patients with pancreatic cancer,

Table 16.4 Sensitivity of CA 19-9 in the Diagnosis of Gastrointestinal Malignancies

	Pancreas		Esophagus		Stomach		Biliary		Colon/Rectum		Liver	
	n	%	n	%	n	%	n	%	n	%	n	%
Del Villano et al.[57]	80	79			24	50			189	41		
Ritts et al.[59]	43	70	8	13	21	62	12	67	95	18		
Jalanko et al.[60]	25	76			50	42	11	73		18	22	
Andriulli et al.[61]	76	79	5	20	21	33	15	36	67	45	14	71
Safi et al.[64]	145	87	47	21	122	39	31	84	309	29	16	44
Ritts et al.[42]	84	74	26	15	62	18	30	77	245	17	5	20
Nazli et al.[63]	40	90			15	53	10	60			10	70
Carpelan-Holmstrom et al.[62]	30	80			16	44	22	86	28	36	19	47

67% of those with hepatobiliary cancer, and 62% of those with gastric cancer. The highest mean CA 19-9 levels in the series were found in patients with pancreatic cancer.

Caveats to the use of CA 19-9 Further experience with the serum marker acknowledged the presence of elevated levels of CA 19-9 in patients with a variety of gastrointestinal malignancies (Table 16.4).[42,57,60-64] The greatest potential for CA 19-9, however, lies in the evaluation of patients with pancreatic cancer. Over the past 2 decades, an extensive world experience with CA 19-9 has demonstrated it to have a sensitivity of up to 90% and a specificity of up to 98% in the diagnosis of this malignancy (Table 16.5).[42,57,60-71] Nonetheless, several caveats to its use have been identified. First, patients genotypically Lewis^{a-b-} are unable to synthesize CA 19-9

Table 16.5 Performance Characteristics of CA 19-9 in the Diagnosis of Pancreatic Cancer

	Sensitivity (Cut-off)				Specificity (Cut-off)				
	PC n	37–40	100–120	1000	Controls	n	37–40	100–120	1000
Del Villano et al.[57]	80	79%			B + EPM	557	83%		
					B only	323	98%		
Jalanko et al.[60]	25	76%	68%	64%	B + EPM	221	80%	87%	94%
					B only	145	92%	98%	100%
Sakahara et al.[65]	55	80%	73%	37%	B	22	91%	100%	100%
Steinberg et al.[66]	37	89%	84%	24%	B	147	86%	95%	99%
Piantino et al.[67]	99	83%	60%		B	151	92%	100%	
Haglund et al.[68]	91	78%	73%		B	111	78%	94%	100%
Malesci et al.[69]	63	90%	64%		B	49	90%	98%	
Safi et al.[64]	145	87%	73%		B + EPM	1772	80%	93%	
					B only	1081	86%	98%	
Pleskow et al.[70]	54	76%	63%	39%	B + EPM	207	77%	90%	99%
					B only	161	78%	93%	100%
Malesci et al.[71]	54	83%	61%		B + EPM	56	68%	89%	
Ritts et al.[42]	84	77%	61%		B + EPM	1570	88%	95%	
					B only	915	93%	99%	
Nazli et al.[63]	40	90%	73%	23%	B + EPM	60	70%	90%	100%
					B only	25	84%	100%	100%

Sensitivity and specificity are related to the selected reference cut-off value. Specificity also depends on the control group selected for comparison.
Abbreviations: PC, pancreatic cancer; B, benign disease; EPM, extrapancreatic malignancy.

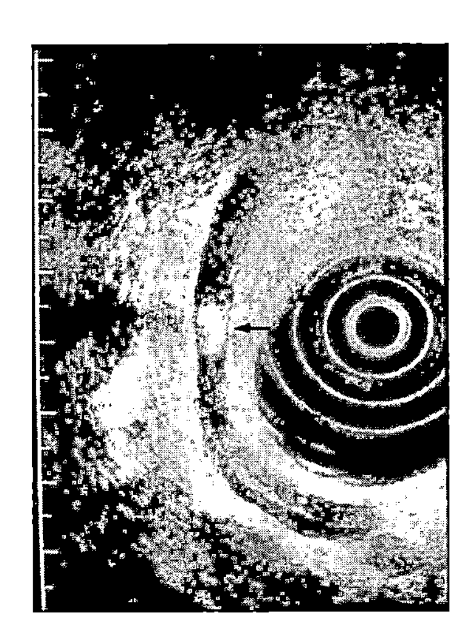

Figure 16.1
Endoscopic ultrasound findings of choledocholithiasis *(arrow)* in a 63-year-old patient with abdominal pain and jaundice and a serum CA 19-9 level of more than 1000 U/ml. The patient underwent endoscopic retrograde pancreatography with sphincterotomy and stone extraction, followed by laparoscopic cholecystectomy. Her CA 19-9 level fell within normal limits within 1 month.

because of a deficiency in a fucosyltransferase specified by the *Le* gene, which is involved in its synthesis.[72,73] Serum levels of those patients with pancreatic cancer among the 5%–15% of the general population with the Lewis^{a-b-} genotype will therefore be falsely low even in the presence of a large, disseminated pancreatic tumor.[74,75] For this reason, the maximum sensitivity of this marker falls short of 100%.[23] A second caveat to the use of this marker is that, in addition to being elevated in patients with other gastrointestinal malignancies, CA 19-9 elevations may also be found in patients with benign disease, particularly when associated with obstructive jaundice or cirrhosis.[42,60,66,68,76-81] Several studies have noted falsely positive CA 19-9 elevations in patients with benign biliary obstruction, and a correlation between serum bilirubin and CA 19-9 levels has frequently been demonstrated in such cases,[77,78] although others have found no such correlation.[68] Furthermore, it has been demonstrated that CA 19-9 levels fall, in many cases to normal levels, after appropriate biliary decompression (Fig. 16.1).[76-81] These data are consistent with the belief that a progressive impairment in hepatic metabolism of the antigen in the face of cholestasis is responsible for an elevation in serum CA 19-9.

Several studies have demonstrated that these potentially confounding effects of cholestasis may reduce the discriminative power of the serum CA 19-9 test. In an evaluation of 164 patients with elevated CA 19-9 levels, Mann et al.[77] found that a single elevated serum CA 19-9 level was unreliable in discriminating between benign and malignant pancreatic disease in the face of obstructive jaundice. Likewise, Haglund et al.[68] were unable to distinguish benign from malignant sources of CA 19-9 and hyperbilirubinemia using a reference cut-off of 37 or 100 U/ml. Noting that malignant causes of obstruction were typically associated with significantly higher CA 19-9 levels than benign causes, however, both Haglund et al.[68] and Benamouzig et al.[79] were able to discriminate satisfactorily between these etiologies in jaundiced patients by employing a higher reference cut-off value (200–500 U/ml). Other methods of increasing the accuracy of CA 19-9 in jaundiced patients have also been suggested, including the use by Schlieman et al.[80] of an "adjusted CA 19-9" calculated by dividing the serum CA 19-9 level by the total bilirubin level in patients with a bilirubin greater than 2.0 mg/dl. The data from these studies suggest that, although the serum CA 19-9 level may still be valuable in patients with hyperbilirubinemia, the results of this marker test must be evaluated carefully in the jaundiced patient.

As a final qualification to its use, CA 19-9 appears to hold little promise as a screening tool for the early diagnosis of pancreatic malignancy, as previously suggested. A prospective study by Frebourg et al.[82] of 866 individuals admitted to an internal medicine unit for a variety of benign diseases clearly demonstrated this limitation. Among this cohort, 117 individuals were found to have an elevated CA 19-9 level on admission and therefore underwent an appropriate investigation for cancer with a CT scan and other diagnostic tests. After 2 years of observation, 115 of these patients were determined to have had falsely positive elevations of CA 19-9. Over the course of the study, only two patients developed malignancies—one pancreatic and one pulmonary. Based on these findings, the authors concluded that CA 19-9 was an ineffective tool for the early detection of pancreatic cancer in the general population. A similar conclusion was drawn by Satake et al.,[83] who identified only four cases of pancreatic cancer—only one of which was resectable—using a mass screening protocol employing diagnostic serum CA

19-9, serum elastase, and abdominal ultrasound in over 10,000 asymptomatic patients.

Diagnosis and preoperative characterization of pancreatic malignancy Despite these shortcomings, a wealth of investigations performed both in the United States and Europe has conclusively demonstrated that the serum marker CA 19-9 can be a valuable tool in the diagnosis, assessment, and follow-up of patients with pancreatic cancer. With regard to diagnosis, this serum marker is most useful in the evaluation of patients with signs and symptoms suspicious for the disease. Piantino et al.[67] analyzed patients with pancreatic cancer and compared them with patients with chronic pancreatitis, a typical and often difficult differential diagnosis.[84] In this series, a CA 19-9 reference value of 37 U/ml was associated with an 83% specificity, 96% sensitivity, and 95% positive predictive value when comparing these two populations. Similarly, in a study comparing 63 patients with pancreatic cancer with 49 patients with chronic pancreatitis, Malesci et al.[71] used a CA 19-9 reference cut-off of 40 U/ml to achieve a 90% sensitivity and specificity in diagnosing pancreatic cancer and distinguishing it from chronic pancreatitis among all patients. It is important to keep in mind, however, that use of the low recommended cut-off value of approximately 37 U/ml sacrifices specificity for sensitivity. As could be expected, the use of a higher reference cut-off value would be associated with a further increase in specificity. A finding of a serum CA 19-9 value over 1000 U/ml in the face of a clinical presentation suspicious for pancreatic cancer is therefore virtually diagnostic for malignancy (Table 16.5).[46,48,70]

The most impressive performance by CA 19-9 can be achieved when the marker is combined with traditional imaging modalities. By itself, the diagnostic accuracy of CA 19-9 is nearly comparable to that of CT scan alone;[65] a combination of these two studies has been identified by Ritts et al.[42] as a cost-effective and diagnostically accurate workup for pancreatic cancer. In his prospective study of 356 patients undergoing laparotomy and found to have pancreaticobiliary disease, the predictive value of a positive preoperative CT or transabdominal ultrasound study of a nonjaundiced patient with suspected pancreatic malignancy was enhanced from 71% and 62%, respectively, to 100% in both cases by the addition of a CA 19-9 level greater than 100. CA 19-9 was especially helpful in patients with equivocal imaging findings, in whom the positive predictive value was likewise increased to 100%. Similar findings have been reported by Malesci et al.[69] who concluded from their data that the best use for the CA 19-9 test was to confirm the results of ultrasound and CT scan in patients with a strong clinical suspicion of pancreatic carcinoma. In a separate study analyzing the cost-effectiveness of the inclusion of a serum CA 19-9 test in the workup of patients presenting with symptoms suspicious for pancreatic cancer, Richter et al.[85] found that its use did not enhance diagnostic accuracy relative to a more traditional diagnostic strategy employing ultrasound followed by CT scan and acquisition of a tissue diagnosis. Nonetheless, use of the serum CA 19-9 test did diminish the use of other potentially invasive diagnostic modalities and therefore led to a significant reduction in both complication rates and healthcare costs.

These findings demonstrate significant potential benefit to including the CA 19-9 test in the diagnostic workup of patients presenting with signs and symptoms suspicious for pancreatic cancer. Unfortunately, however, the efficacy of this marker as a diagnostic tool appears to be limited in the presence of early disease. Malesci et al.[71] were unable to discriminate adequately between patients with small (T1 or T2) disease and chronic pancreatitis because the majority of these patients had only modestly elevated serum antigen levels.[71] A similar dilemma was faced by Fabris et al.,[86] who found CA 19-9 ineffective at discriminating between pancreatic cancer and chronic pancreatitis in the early stages of disease and who therefore concluded that early diagnosis of pancreatic cancer was not significantly improved by the use of this serum marker.

Several studies have confirmed that small pancreatic tumors are frequently associated with normal or only slightly elevated levels of CA 19-9 but that levels increase in both frequency and extent with disease progression. Sakahara et al.[65] found CA 19-9 levels greater than 37 U/ml in only 13% of tumors less than 3 cm in size, although elevated levels have been reported in as many 73% of patients with small tumors.[87] In contrast, elevated CA 19-9 values are routinely found in patients with advanced disease, the highest serum levels typically being reported in association with metastatic, stage IV cancers.[64,88] An inverse correlation could therefore be expected between the serum CA 19-9 level and tumor resectability in patients with pancreatic cancer. In an analysis of prior studies,[55,66,71,78,89-91] Steinberg[48] found that CA 19-9 was elevated in only 67% of patients with resectable pancreatic cancer, but in 87% of patients with unresectable disease. Moreover, this analysis also identified 249 patients with both pancreatic cancer and CA 19-9 values greater than 1000 U/ml and found 96% of these patients to have unresectable disease.

Based on these findings, several authors have subsequently attempted to define a reference cut-off to determine resectability.[92-94] Most recently, Schlieman et al.[80]

examined 89 patients who underwent surgical exploration for presumably resectable pancreatic adenocarcinoma based on preoperative imaging. Preoperatively, serum CA 19-9 was drawn from all patients and adjusted for hyperbilirubinemia as previously described. Thirty-three patients were found to have an adjusted CA 19-9 value greater than 150 U/ml, of whom 29 (88%) were found on exploration to harbor unresectable tumors and of whom 16 (49%) were found to have metastatic disease that was missed on preoperative imaging. The authors therefore concluded that an adjusted CA 19-9 value greater than 150 U/ml can be used as a marker of unresectability in patients otherwise presumed to be resectable on the basis of traditional imaging and encouraged the use of additional diagnostic modalities such as laparoscopy in this group of patients to prevent potentially unnecessary laparotomy.

Assessment of prognosis The apparent correlation between CA 19-9 serum concentration and tumor load has led many authors to investigate the potential of this marker to assess prognosis and therefore to assist in patient management and therapeutic decision making. Among patients with resectable tumors, median survival after surgical resection was demonstrated by both Safi et al.[94] and Lundin et al.[95] to be significantly longer in those patients with low preoperative CA 19-9 values, although the reference cut-offs (400 and 210 U/ml) used in their analyses differed. In both series, an elevated CA 19-9 level was associated with postoperative survival of 13 months or less despite attempted curative resection. In contrast, median survival of patients with lower CA 19-9 levels was upwards of 18 months. In Lundin's series, a similar discrepancy in survival was found in patients with unresectable disease that underwent palliation. Interestingly, the overall survival rate of patients with a high preoperative CA 19-9 who underwent attempted curative resection was similar to that of patients with unresectable disease treated palliatively.

CA 19-9 can also be determined preoperatively to assess the prognosis of patients undergoing non-operative therapies. In an analysis of patients with advanced, inoperable pancreatic cancer treated with split-course radiotherapy and combination chemotherapy, Gattani et al.[96] found that patients with a CA 19-9 level greater than 2000 U/ml before therapy had a significantly shorter survival (8 months) than those with a lower level (13 months). Moreover, this study identified CA 19-9 as a superior indicator of prognosis after therapy than either tumor size or performance status. These studies clearly indicate that in addition to assessing resectability in patients with pancreatic cancer, preoperative CA 19-9 levels can be used before either surgical or nonsurgical therapy to effectively assess post-therapeutic survival and overall prognosis.

Assessment of therapeutic efficacy, monitoring, and detection of recurrence The serum CA 19-9 level is also of value in the evaluation of patients with pancreatic malignancy when measured after therapeutic intervention has been completed. Surgical resection, but not palliative bypass procedures, is typically accompanied by a reduction in preoperatively determined CA 19-9 values within 2 weeks. Furthermore, a persistent elevation of the serum CA 19-9 after surgery for resectable disease is indicative of residual tumor mass. Postoperative CA 19-9 levels can therefore be used to predict patients' responses to therapy, as demonstrated by Tian et al.[97] In 7 of 11 patients in whom preoperatively pathologic CA 19-9 values returned to normal after radical tumor resection, median postoperative survival was greater than 21 months. In contrast, survival was only 8 months in patients in whom CA 19-9 levels remained elevated. These findings are similar to those of Safi et al.[94] and others. CA 19-9 can also be used as an index of response to chemotherapy, as demonstrated in the neoadjuvant setting by Willett et al.[98]

In addition, CA 19-9 can be used to monitor patients' post-therapeutic course as a marker of tumor recurrence. Tian et al.[97] described 11 Lewis-positive patients who survived radical tumor resection, 6 of whom later developed local or distant tumor recurrence. Each of these recurrences was predicted between 2 and 9 months before by a secondary elevation of CA 19-9 after an initial postoperative decline. Beretta et al.[99] similarly demonstrated that a secondary rise in CA 19-9 is indicative of recurrence and showed that CA 19-9 could detect recurrence earlier than ultrasound. Therefore, although reports exist to the contrary,[88] measurement of serum CA 19-9 preoperatively, postoperatively, and then periodically thereafter would appear to be a sensible diagnostic strategy.

In summary, the use of CA 19-9 does not enhance our ability to diagnose pancreatic cancer at an earlier stage. This marker does, however, have important roles in the diagnosis, management, and follow-up of patients with this disease.

CA 50 and CA 242

The CA 50 and CA 242 antigens are similar in many respects both to CA 19-9 and to each other and, therefore, are considered together. Both antigens are defined by monoclonal antibodies, C-50 and C-242, respectively, which were originally raised in mice against the inoculated human colon cancer cell line COLO 205.[27] The C-50 antibody binds to the same Lewis^a epitope as the CA 19-9 antibody but also recognizes the related sialyllacto-N-tetraose, which lacks a fucose component.[100,101] The CA 242 epitope is also a sialylated carbohydrate structure related to those of both CA 19-9 and CA 50.[102] In serum, these three related antigens are collocated on the same macromolecular mucin complex.[103] In accordance with their structural similarity, a high correlation has been found between the serum levels of these serum markers[43,104,105] in states of disease. For this reason, there appears to be little utility to using two or more of these markers in concert for patient evaluation.

Neither CA 50 nor CA 242 is tumor specific for pancreatic cancer; indeed, both have been found in association with a variety of other malignancies as well as benign disorders.[105,106] Nonetheless, both have respectable performance characteristics. With regard to pancreatic cancer, the sensitivity and specificity of CA 50 have been reported as high as 69%–96% and 71%–98%, respectively, using a variety of patient populations and reference cut-off values.[105,107-111] Using a reference value of 20 U/ml, Palsson et al.[45] found the best features of the marker to be its sensitivity and negative predictive value (both 96%) in a prospective study of 512 patients presenting with signs and symptoms suspicious for pancreatic cancer. He also demonstrated, however, that the initial clinical suspicion based on history and physical was about equal in this regard and was even better than CA 50 in terms of specificity and positive prediction. Although at the suggested reference cut-off of 17 U/ml the specificity of CA 50 is less than satisfactory, two studies[50,112] have demonstrated that it can be significantly improved by using a higher reference cut-off value.

The advantage of CA 242 over CA 50 appears to be its specificity. In an in-depth analysis of the receiver operating characteristic curves of both CA 242 and CA 50, Pasanen et al.[50] found that CA 242 was significantly more sensitive than CA 50 at specificity levels greater than 90% and only slightly less sensitive at low specificity levels. Haglund et al.[104] used a similar analysis and found CA 242 to be more sensitive than CA 50 at all specificity levels.

Unfortunately, as with CA 19-9, the ability to detect pancreatic cancer in its early stages does not appear to have been enhanced by the development of either of these markers. The levels of both markers in the serum are correlated to tumor load; values are elevated in the presence of positive lymph nodes, distant metastases, and in general, a higher stage of disease,[113,114] whereas lower levels or even normal values are often found in patients with early disease. Haglund et al.[104] found that only 60% of patients with resectable disease had an elevated CA 242, in contrast to 67% of patients with CA 19-9. Only 50% of patients with resectable disease were identified by Kuusela et al.[109] to have an elevated serum CA 50 level. However, because of the association of tumor marker and tumor burden, the markers have been shown to play a role in the assessment of prognosis[95,115] and as a marker of a disease recurrence.[116]

Finally, it should be noted that although CA 242 levels appear to be less affected by benign cholestasis than CA 50,[105,107,110,112] biliary obstruction does appear to have an incompletely defined effect on the serum levels of both markers. In a study of 70 cholestatic patients, 35 with pancreatic cancer and 35 with benign biliopancreatic diseases, Palsson et al.[112] identified a significant correlation between total bilirubin and both CA 50 and CA 242 in cholestatic patients, in findings similar to those of Pasanen et al.[117,118] Moreover, their data demonstrated that in patients with benign, but not malignant disease, relief of cholestasis and normalization of bilirubin was followed by an acute drop in both serum tumor marker levels. Nonetheless, serum levels of both markers were appreciably higher in patients with pancreatic cancer. These data suggest that both CA 50 and CA 242 are affected by cholestasis to some degree, but a significantly elevated CA 50 or CA 242 level in a symptomatic patient is nonetheless highly indicative of pancreatic malignancy.

Despite the incremental increase in specificity associated with CA 242, advantages sufficient to warrant displacement of CA 19-9 as the routine serologic marker of pancreatic cancer by either CA 242 or CA 50 have not yet been identified.

CAM 17-1

The recently described CAM-1/WGA assay[119] uses the monoclonal antimucin antibody CAM 17-1, which, like CA 19-9, was developed by the inoculation of mice with a human colorectal cancer cell line (Coll 2-23) and has as its epitope a sialylated blood group antigen.[120] In a study of patients with benign and malignant pancreatic diseases, Gansauge et al.[121] reported that the marker is associated with a higher specificity and comparable sensitivity to CA 19-9. In a subsequent prospective study[122] of 250 patients with suspected pancreatic cancer, the marker was found to have even higher performance characteristics, particularly in patients without jaundice, in whom a sensitivity and specificity of 89% and 94%, respectively, were reported. This analysis also demonstrated that the diagnostic accuracy of CAM 17-1 exceeded that of conventional imaging modalities, and when used in conjunction with abdominal ultrasound, the marker identified 100% of resectable pancreatic tumors. Although clinical experience with this marker has to this point been limited, CAM 17-1 thus appears to be a promising marker in the evaluation of patients with pancreatic cancer.

Other Complex Glycoconjugates and Blood Group-Associated Markers

Other potential serological markers in this category have been described but have not been put to routine clinical use. Tissue polypeptide antigen (TPA)[123,124] is released in the process of cell division and thus is considered an index of cell proliferation. Tissue polypeptide-specific antigen[125,126] is an epitope of the TPA molecule detectable with a monoclonal antibody. Although it has been suggested that these markers could be used in combination with other markers,[127] neither has been found to be clinically useful in practice.[128,129]

Like CA 19-9 and others, both the DUPAN-2[130,131] and Span-1[132] antigens are present in the serum on mucins and are recognized by monoclonal antibodies. DUPAN-2 has been shown to be a precursor of CA 19-9[133] but, unlike that marker, may be found in patients with a Lewis-negative genotype.[134,135] The marker has been reported to have a performance profile somewhat less favorable than that of CA 19-9, and it also shares that marker's susceptibility to the effects of cholestasis.[136-138] Span-1 is likewise affected by jaundice[139] and appears to possess similar performance characteristics to CA 19-9. Significantly, both Span-1 and CA 19-9 were found to have a sensitivity of 73% in the identification of small pancreatic cancers less than 4 cm in size,[87] significantly greater to that of DUPAN-2. Nevertheless, neither DUPAN-2 nor Span-1 has yet been definitively demonstrated to be more useful than CA 19-9,[136,137,140] and therefore, neither has been put to routine clinical use.

Oncofetal Antigens

Until the advent of hybridoma technology, the development of monoclonal antibody assays, and the widespread clinical acceptance of CA 19-9, CEA was the only serologic marker in routine use in the evaluation of patients with pancreatic cancer. First described in 1965,[24] the marker still remains applicable in the evaluation of patients with colorectal malignancy. Although CEA is still frequently ordered in many centers, however, neither the sensitivity nor specificity of this marker justify its continued use in the care of patients with pancreatic cancer.[141,142] Likewise, another of the early serum tumor markers found to be elevated in certain patients with pancreatic cancer, alpha-fetoprotein currently plays no role in the evaluation of patients with this disease,[143] although it remains relevant in the evaluation of patients with hepatocellular carcinoma.

Derived from the immunization of rabbits with human fetal pancreas, POA, appeared to hold promise in the diagnosis of pancreatic cancer when it was first reported in 1974[25] and subsequently evaluated in patients.[144,145] Nonetheless, like that of CEA, the clinical utility of POA has subsequently been shown to be inferior than that of the newer markers based on monoclonal antibodies.[44] Other oncofetal antigens, such as the feto-acinar pancreatic protein[146] have likewise not proven useful.

K-ras Oncogene

The well-described *K-ras* oncogene is associated with point mutations at codon 12 in over 90% of pancreatic cancers,[147] and such mutations occur early in the evolution of pancreatic neoplasia.[148,149] For these reasons, interest has accumulated in the use of mutated *K-ras* as a potential tissue tumor marker for pancreatic cancer in cytological specimens.[150] The finding of high levels of circulating DNA in the plasma of patients with pancreatic cancer[151] subsequently directed attention to the possibility of using mutated *K-ras* as a serum marker. Using polymerase chain reaction analysis of sera taken from 21 individuals with advanced pancreatic cancer, Mulcahy et al.[28] found an 81% sensitivity for this marker. Moreover, four of these cases were found to have *K-ras* mutations in their sera from 5–14 months before a definitive diagnosis of pancreatic cancer. In contrast, zero of five healthy subjects and zero of three patients with chronic pancreatitis were found to harbor *K-ras* gene mutations. Dianxu et al.[152] recently reported similar findings and also demonstrated that the marker was elevated in two of two patients with stage I resectable disease in that series. In both this study and another by Theodor et al.,[153] the use of the serologic marker *K-ras* was complimentary to CA 19-9. These studies and others suggesting a role for *K-ras* detection in the assessment of prognosis and efficacy of treatment[154] have identified *K-ras* as a promising serum marker in the evaluation of patients with pancreatic cancer, even in its early stages.

p53 Tumor Suppressor Gene

Although frequently associated with pancreatic cancer, the tumor suppressor gene *p53* appears to have limited potential as a serologic marker of pancreatic cancer. Located on chromosome 17, the *p53* gene encodes a nuclear protein involved in the inhibition of cellular proliferation and induction of apoptosis. Mutations of the gene are found in a variety of human malignancies, including that of the pancreas, in which they have been associated with enhanced biological aggressiveness.[155] Encouraged by reports describing the detection of circulating *p53* autoantibodies in patients with other cancers, Raedle et al.[156] and Laurent-Puig et al.[29] measured antibodies to *p53* in patients with pancreatic cancer but found the test to be neither sensitive nor specific for pancreatic malignancy. Using a different approach, Suwa et al.[157] measured *p53* protein in the serum using enzyme-linked immunosorbent assay. Although the *p53* serum concentration did correlate with disease progression and dissemination in patients with pancreatic cancer, elevated levels were found in only 22% of patients with the disease and only 12% of patients with localized pancreatic cancer.

Conclusion

The past 2 decades have seen a virtual explosion in the number of serologic tests evaluated for use in the diagnosis and management of patients with pancreatic cancer. Unfortunately, none of these markers has yet proven ideal, and importantly, none has significantly advanced our ability to detect pancreatic malignancy at an earlier, treatable stage. Nevertheless, the use of serologic markers in the evaluation of patients with pancreatic cancer has merit. Particularly when used as one part of a comprehensive diagnostic and therapeutic strategy, the best established serologic marker CA 19-9 has been shown to be valuable in the differential diagnosis, assessment of prognosis, and follow-up of patients with pancreatic cancer. This and other serologic markers may therefore play a considerable role in patient management. Moreover, as a more complete understanding of the molecular genetics behind both pancreatic cancer and its precursor lesions evolves and as technological advancements and high-throughput techniques for marker identification improve, it is increasingly likely that an early marker for the disease will be found. Until such time, active investigation should continue in this area, and the established serum tumor marker, CA 19-9, should be put to its best possible clinical use.

References

1. Stojadinovic A, Brooks A, Hoos A, et al. An evidence-based approach to the surgical management of resectable pancreatic adenocarcinoma. *J Am Coll Surg.* 2003;196:954–964.
2. Shapiro TM. Adenocarcinoma of the pancreas: a statistical analysis of biliary bypass vs Whipple resection in good risk patients. *Ann Surg.* 1975;182:715–721.
3. Yeo CJ, Cameron JL, Lillemoe KD, et al. Pancreaticoduodenectomy for cancer of the head of the pancreas. 201 patients. *Ann Surg.* 1995;221:721–731; discussion 721–731.
4. Breslin TM, Hess KR, Harbison DB, et al. Neoadjuvant chemoradiotherapy for adenocarcinoma of the pancreas: treatment variables and survival duration. *Ann Surg Oncol.* 2001;8:123–132.
5. Bouvet M, Gamagami RA, Gilpin EA, et al. Factors influencing survival after resection for periampullary neoplasms. *Am J Surg.* 2000;180:13–17.
6. Yeo CJ, Cameron JL, Sohn TA, et al. Six hundred fifty consecutive pancreaticoduodenectomies in the 1990s: pathology, complications, and outcomes. *Ann Surg.* 1997;226:248–257; discussion 257–260.
7. Sener SF, Fremgen A, Menck HR, et al. Pancreatic cancer: a report of treatment and survival trends for 100,313 patients diagnosed from 1985–1995, using the National Cancer Database. *J Am Coll Surg.* 1999;189:1–7.
8. Jemal A, Murray T, Samuels A, et al. Cancer statistics, 2004. *CA Cancer J Clin.* 2003;53:5–26.
9. Bouvet M, Binmoeller KF, Moossa AR. The diagnosis of adenocarcinoma of the pancreas. In: Cameron JL, ed. *Atlas of Clinical Oncology: Pancreatic Cancer.* London: BC Decker; 2001:67–85.
10. Sohn TA, Yeo CJ, Cameron JL, et al. Resected adenocarcinoma of the pancreas—616 patients: results, outcomes, and prognostic indicators. *J Gastrointest Surg.* 2000;4:567–579.
11. Cameron JL, Crist DW, Sitzmann JV, et al. Factors influencing survival after pancreaticoduodenectomy for pancreatic cancer. *Am J Surg.* 1991;161:120–124; discussion 124–125.
12. Furukawa H, Okada S, Saisho H, et al. Clinicopathologic features of small pancreatic adenocarcinoma: a collective study. *Cancer.* 1996;78:986–990.
13. DiMagno EP, Malagelada JR, Taylor WF, et al. A prospective comparison of current diagnostic tests for pancreatic cancer. *N Engl J Med.* 1977;297:737–742.
14. Tamm E, Charnsangavej C. Pancreatic cancer: current concepts in imaging for diagnosis and staging. *Cancer J.* 2001;7:298–311.
15. Rosch T, Braig C, Gain T, et al. Staging of pancreatic and ampullary carcinoma by endoscopic ultrasonography: comparison with conventional sonography, computed tomography, and angiography. *Gastroenterology.* 1992;102:188–199.
16. Rumstadt B, Schwab M, Schuster K, et al. The role of laparoscopy in the preoperative staging of pancreatic carcinoma. *J Gastrointest Surg.* 1997;1:245–250.
17. Friess H, Kleeff J, Silva JC, et al. The role of diagnostic laparoscopy in pancreatic and periampullary malignancies. *J Am Coll Surg.* 1998;186:675–682.
18. Nakaizumi A, Uehara H, Iishi H, et al. Endoscopic ultrasonography in diagnosis and staging of pancreatic cancer. *Dig Dis Sci.* 1995;40:696–700.
19. Magdelenat H. Tumour markers in oncology: past, present and future. *J Immunol Methods.* 1992;150:133–143.
20. Moossa AR, Mackie CR, Gelder FB, et al. The value of tumor markers in the diagnosis and management of nonendocrine tumors of the pancreas. In: Moossa AR, ed. *Tumors of the Pancreas.* Baltimore: Williams & Wilkins; 1980:397–414.
21. Suresh MR. Classification of tumor markers. *Anticancer Res.* 1996;16:2273–2277.

22. Podolsky DK. Serologic markers in the diagnosis and management of pancreatic carcinoma. *World J Surg.* 1984;8: 822–830.
23. Plebani M, Basso D, Panozzo MP, et al. Tumor markers in the diagnosis, monitoring and therapy of pancreatic cancer: state of the art. *Int J Biol Markers.* 1995;10:189–199.
24. Gold P, Freedman S. Demonstration of tumor-specific antigens in human colonic carcinomata by immunological tolerance and absorption techniques. *J Exp Med.* 1965;121: 439–462.
25. Banwo O, Versey J, Hobbs JR. New oncofetal antigen for human pancreas. *Lancet.* 1974;1:643–645.
26. Koprowski H, Steplewski Z, Mitchell K, et al. Colorectal carcinoma antigens detected by hybridoma antibodies. *Somatic Cell Genet.* 1979;5:957–971.
27. Lindholm L, Holmgren J, Svennerholm L, et al. Monoclonal antibodies against gastrointestinal tumour-associated antigens isolated as monosialogangliosides. *Int Arch Allergy Appl Immunol.* 1983;71:178–181.
28. Mulcahy HE, Lyautey J, Lederrey C, et al. A prospective study of *K*-ras mutations in the plasma of pancreatic cancer patients. *Clin Cancer Res.* 1998;4:271–275.
29. Laurent-Puig P, Lubin R, Semhoun-Ducloux S, et al. Antibodies against *p53* protein in serum of patients with benign or malignant pancreatic and biliary diseases. *Gut.* 1995;36:455–458.
30. Banga I. Isolation and crystallisation of elastase from the pancreas of cattle. *Acta Physiol Acad Sci Hung.* 1958;3: 317–324.
31. Stenman UH, Huhtala ML, Koistinen R, et al. Immunochemical demonstration of an ovarian cancer-associated urinary peptide. *Int J Cancer.* 1982;30:53–57.
32. Zhou W, Sokoll LJ, Bruzek DJ, et al. Identifying markers for pancreatic cancer by gene expression analysis. *Cancer Epidemiol Biomarkers Prev.* 1998;7:109–112.
33. Rasnake MS, Glanton C, Ornstein D, et al. Hypercalcemia mediated by parathyroid hormone-related protein as an early manifestation of pancreatic adenocarcinoma metastasis: a case report. *Am J Clin Oncol.* 2001;24:416–417.
34. Bouvet M, Nardin SR, Burton DW, et al. Parathyroid hormone-related protein as a novel tumor marker in pancreatic adenocarcinoma. *Pancreas.* 2002;24:284–290.
35. Cavestro GM, Mantovani N, Coruzzi P, et al. Hypercalcemia due to ectopic secretion of parathyroid related protein from pancreatic carcinoma: a case report. *Acta Biomed Ateneo Parmense.* 2002;73:37–40.
36. Abraham P, Ralston SH, Hewison M, et al. Presentation of a PTHrP-secreting pancreatic neuroendocrine tumour, with hypercalcaemic crisis, pre-eclampsia, and renal failure. *Postgrad Med J.* 2002;78:752–753.
37. Lamerz R. Role of tumour markers, cytogenetics. *Ann Oncol.* 1999;10(Suppl 4):S145–S149.
38. Aziz DC. Clinical use of tumor markers based on outcome analysis. *Lab Med.* 1996;27:760–764.
39. Posner MR, Mayer RJ. The use of serologic tumor markers in gastrointestinal malignancies. *Hematol Oncol Clin North Am.* 1994;8:533–553.
40. Brand R. The diagnosis of pancreatic cancer. *Cancer J.* 2001;7:287–297.
41. Roulston JE. Novel tumour markers: a diagnostic role in pancreatic cancer? *Br J Cancer.* 1994;70:389–390.
42. Ritts RE Jr, Nagorney DM, Jacobsen DJ, et al. Comparison of preoperative serum CA19-9 levels with results of diagnostic imaging modalities in patients undergoing laparotomy for suspected pancreatic or gallbladder disease. *Pancreas.* 1994; 9:707–716.
43. Pasanen PA, Eskelinen M, Partanen K, et al. A prospective study of serum tumour markers carcinoembryonic antigen, carbohydrate antigens 50 and 242, tissue polypeptide antigen and tissue polypeptide specific antigen in the diagnosis of pancreatic cancer with special reference to multivariate diagnostic score. *Br J Cancer.* 1994;69:562–565.
44. Schmiegel WH, Eberl W, Kreiker C, et al. Multiparametric tumor marker (CA 19-9, CEA, AFP, POA) analyses of pancreatic juices and sera in pancreatic diseases. *Hepatogastroenterology.* 1985;32:141–145.
45. Palsson B, Masson P, Andren-Sandberg A. Tumour marker CA 50 levels compared to signs and symptoms in the diagnosis of pancreatic cancer. *Eur J Surg Oncol.* 1997;23: 151–156.
46. Ritts RE, Pitt HA. CA 19-9 in pancreatic cancer. *Surg Oncol Clin N Am.* 1998;7:93–101.
47. Aziz K. Tumour markers: current status and future applications. *Scand J Clin Lab Invest Suppl.* 1995;221:153–155.
48. Steinberg W. The clinical utility of the CA 19-9 tumor-associated antigen. *Am J Gastroenterol.* 1990;85:350–355.
49. Eskelinen M, Haglund U. Developments in serologic detection of human pancreatic adenocarcinoma. *Scand J Gastroenterol.* 1999;34:833–844.
50. Pasanen PA, Eskelinen M, Partanen K, et al. Receiver operating characteristic (ROC) curve analysis of the tumour markers CEA, CA 50 and CA 242 in pancreatic cancer: results from a prospective study. *Br J Cancer.* 1993;67:852–855.
51. Van der Schouw YT, Segers MFG, Smits L, et al. Towards a more standardized assessment of diagnostic tumour markers. *Int J Oncol.* 1993;3:979–985.
52. Magnani JL, Nilsson B, Brockhaus M, et al. A monoclonal antibody-defined antigen associated with gastrointestinal cancer is a ganglioside containing sialylated lacto-N-fucopentaose II. *J Biol Chem.* 1982;257:14365–14369.
53. Atkinson BF, Ernst CS, Herlyn M, et al. Gastrointestinal cancer-associated antigen in immunoperoxidase assay. *Cancer Res.* 1982;42:4820–4823.
54. Dietel M, Arps H, Klapdor R, et al. Antigen detection by the monoclonal antibodies CA 19-9 and CA 125 in normal and tumor tissue and patients' sera. *J Cancer Res Clin Oncol.* 1986;111:257–265.
55. Schmiegel WH, Kreiker C, Eberl W, et al. Monoclonal antibody defines CA 19-9 in pancreatic juices and sera. *Gut.* 1985;26:456–460.
56. Magnani JL, Steplewski Z, Koprowski H, et al. Identification of the gastrointestinal and pancreatic cancer-associated antigen detected by monoclonal antibody 19-9 in the sera of patients as a mucin. *Cancer Res.* 1983;43:5489–5492.

57. Del Villano BC, Brennan S, Brock P, et al. Radioimmunometric assay for a monoclonal antibody-defined tumor marker, CA 19-9. *Clin Chem.* 1983;29:549–552.
58. Koprowski H, Herlyn M, Steplewski Z, et al. Specific antigen in serum of patients with colon carcinoma. *Science.* 1981;212:53–55.
59. Ritts RE, Jr, Del Villano BC, Go VL, et al. Initial clinical evaluation of an immunoradiometric assay for CA 19-9 using the NCI serum bank. *Int J Cancer.* 1984;33:339–345.
60. Jalanko H, Kuusela P, Roberts P, et al. Comparison of a new tumour marker, CA 19-9, with alpha-fetoprotein and carcinoembryonic antigen in patients with upper gastrointestinal diseases. *J Clin Pathol.* 1984;37:218–222.
61. Andriulli A, Gindro T, Piantino P, et al. Prospective evaluation of the diagnostic efficacy of CA 19-9 assay as a marker for gastrointestinal cancers. *Digestion.* 1986;33:26–33.
62. Carpelan-Holmstrom M, Louhimo J, Stenman UH, et al. CEA, CA 19-9 and CA 72-4 improve the diagnostic accuracy in gastrointestinal cancers. *Anticancer Res.* 2002;22:2311–2316.
63. Nazli O, Bozdag AD, Tansug T, et al. The diagnostic importance of CEA and CA 19-9 for the early diagnosis of pancreatic carcinoma. *Hepatogastroenterology.* 2000;47: 1750–1752.
64. Safi F, Roscher R, Beger HG. Tumor markers in pancreatic cancer: sensitivity and specificity of CA 19-9. *Hepatogastroenterology.* 1989;36:419–423.
65. Sakahara H, Endo K, Nakajima K, et al. Serum CA 19-9 concentrations and computed tomography findings in patients with pancreatic carcinoma. *Cancer.* 1986;57:1324–1326.
66. Steinberg WM, Gelfand R, Anderson KK, et al. Comparison of the sensitivity and specificity of the CA19-9 and carcinoembryonic antigen assays in detecting cancer of the pancreas. *Gastroenterology.* 1986;90:343–349.
67. Piantino P, Andriulli A, Gindro T, et al. CA 19-9 assay in differential diagnosis of pancreatic carcinoma from inflammatory pancreatic diseases. *Am J Gastroenterol.* 1986;81:436–439.
68. Haglund C, Roberts PJ, Kuusela P, et al. Evaluation of CA 19-9 as a serum tumour marker in pancreatic cancer. *Br J Cancer.* 1986;53:197–202.
69. Malesci A, Montorsi M, Mariani A, et al. Clinical utility of the serum CA 19-9 test for diagnosing pancreatic carcinoma in symptomatic patients: a prospective study. *Pancreas.* 1992;7:497–502.
70. Pleskow DK, Berger HJ, Gyves J, et al. Evaluation of a serologic marker, CA19-9, in the diagnosis of pancreatic cancer. *Ann Intern Med.* 1989;110:704–709.
71. Malesci A, Tommasini MA, Bonato C, et al. Determination of CA 19-9 antigen in serum and pancreatic juice for differential diagnosis of pancreatic adenocarcinoma from chronic pancreatitis. *Gastroenterology.* 1987;92:60–67.
72. Koprowski H, Brockhaus M, Blaszczyk M, et al. Lewis blood-type may affect the incidence of gastrointestinal cancer. *Lancet.* 1982;1:1332–1333.
73. Takasaki H, Uchida E, Tempero MA, et al. Correlative study on expression of CA 19-9 and DU-PAN-2 in tumor tissue and in serum of pancreatic cancer patients. *Cancer Res.* 1988;48:1435–1438.
74. Tempero MA, Uchida E, Takasaki H, et al. Relationship of carbohydrate antigen 19-9 and Lewis antigens in pancreatic cancer. *Cancer Res.* 1987;47:5501–5503.
75. von Rosen A, Linder S, Harmenberg U, et al. Serum levels of CA 19-9 and CA 50 in relation to Lewis blood cell status in patients with malignant and benign pancreatic disease. *Pancreas.* 1993;8:160–165.
76. Albert MB, Steinberg WM, Henry JP. Elevated serum levels of tumor marker CA19-9 in acute cholangitis. *Dig Dis Sci.* 1988;33:1223–1225.
77. Mann DV, Edwards R, Ho S, et al. Elevated tumour marker CA19-9: clinical interpretation and influence of obstructive jaundice. *Eur J Surg Oncol.* 2000;26:474–479.
78. Del Favero G, Fabris C, Plebani M, et al. CA 19-9 and carcinoembryonic antigen in pancreatic cancer diagnosis. *Cancer.* 1986;57:1576–1579.
79. Benamouzig R, Buffet C, Fourre C, et al. Serum levels of carbohydrate antigenic determinant (CA 19.9) in obstructive jaundice. *Dig Dis Sci.* 1989;34:1640–1642.
80. Schlieman MG, Ho HS, Bold RJ. Utility of tumor markers in determining resectability of pancreatic cancer. *Arch Surg.* 2003;138:951–955; discussion 955–956.
81. Barone D, Onetto M, Conio M, et al. CA 19-9 assay in patients with extrahepatic cholestatic jaundice. *Int J Biol Markers.* 1988;3:95–100.
82. Frebourg T, Bercoff E, Manchon N, et al. The evaluation of CA 19-9 antigen level in the early detection of pancreatic cancer: a prospective study of 866 patients. *Cancer.* 1988;62:2287–2290.
83. Satake K, Takeuchi T, Homma T, et al. CA19-9 as a screening and diagnostic tool in symptomatic patients: the Japanese experience. *Pancreas.* 1994;9:703–706.
84. Kim T, Murakami T, Takamura M, et al. Pancreatic mass due to chronic pancreatitis: correlation of CT and MR imaging features with pathologic findings. *AJR Am J Roentgenol.* 2001;177:367–371.
85. Richter JM, Christensen MR, Rustgi AK, et al. The clinical utility of the CAL9-9 radioimmunoassay for the diagnosis of pancreatic cancer presenting as pain or weight loss: a cost-effectiveness analysis. *Arch Intern Med.* 1989;149:2292–2297.
86. Fabris C, Del Favero G, Basso D, et al. Serum markers and clinical data in diagnosing pancreatic cancer: a contrastive approach. *Am J Gastroenterol.* 1988;83:549–553.
87. Satake K, Chung YS, Umeyama K, et al. The possibility of diagnosing small pancreatic cancer (less than 4.0 cm) by measuring various serum tumor markers: a retrospective study. *Cancer.* 1991;68:149–152.
88. van den Bosch RP, van Eijck CH, Mulder PG, et al. Serum CA19-9 determination in the management of pancreatic cancer. *Hepatogastroenterology.* 1996;43:710–713.
89. Satake K, Kanazawa G, Kho I, et al. Evaluation of serum pancreatic enzymes, carbohydrate antigen 19-9, and carcinoembryonic antigen in various pancreatic diseases. *Am J Gastroenterol.* 1985;80:630–636.

90. Safi F, Beger HG, Bittner R, et al. CA 19-9 and pancreatic adenocarcinoma. *Cancer.* 1986;57:779–783.
91. Wang TH, Lin JT, Chen DS, et al. Noninvasive diagnosis of advanced pancreatic cancer by real-time ultrasonography, carcinoembryonic antigen, and carbohydrate antigen 19-9. *Pancreas.* 1986;1:219–223.
92. Forsmark CE, Lambiase L, Vogel SB. Diagnosis of pancreatic cancer and prediction of unresectability using the tumor-associated antigen CA19-9. *Pancreas.* 1994;9:731–734.
93. Yasue M, Sakamoto J, Teramukai S, et al. Prognostic values of preoperative and postoperative CEA and CA19.9 levels in pancreatic cancer. *Pancreas.* 1994;9:735–740.
94. Safi F, Schlosser W, Falkenreck S, et al. Prognostic value of CA 19-9 serum course in pancreatic cancer. *Hepatogastroenterology.* 1998;45:253–259.
95. Lundin J, Roberts PJ, Kuusela P, et al. Prognostic significance of serum CA 242 in pancreatic cancer: a comparison with CA 19-9. *Anticancer Res.* 1995;15:2181–2186.
96. Gattani AM, Mandeli J, Bruckner HW. Tumor markers in patients with pancreatic carcinoma. *Cancer.* 1996;78:57–62.
97. Tian F, Appert HE, Myles J, et al. Prognostic value of serum CA 19-9 levels in pancreatic adenocarcinoma. *Ann Surg.* 1992;215:350–355.
98. Willett CG, Daly WJ, Warshaw AL. CA 19-9 is an index of response to neoadjunctive chemoradiation therapy in pancreatic cancer. *Am J Surg.* 1996;172:350–352.
99. Beretta E, Malesci A, Zerbi A, et al. Serum CA 19-9 in the postsurgical follow-up of patients with pancreatic cancer. *Cancer.* 1987;60:2428–2431.
100. Mansson JE, Fredman P, Nilsson O, et al. Chemical structure of carcinoma ganglioside antigens defined by monoclonal antibody C-50 and some allied gangliosides of human pancreatic adenocarcinoma. *Biochim Biophys Acta.* 1985;834:110–117.
101. Nilsson O, Mansson JE, Lindholm L, et al. Sialosyllactotetraosylceramide, a novel ganglioside antigen detected in human carcinomas by a monoclonal antibody. *FEBS Lett.* 1985;182:398–402.
102. Johansson C, Nilsson O, Baeckstrom D, et al. Novel epitopes on the CA50-carrying antigen: chemical and immunochemical studies. *Tumour Biol.* 1991;12:159–170.
103. Johansson C, Nilsson O, Lindholm L. Comparison of serological expression of different epitopes on the CA50-carrying antigen CanAg. *Int J Cancer.* 1991;48:757–763.
104. Haglund C, Lundin J, Kuusela P, et al. CA 242, a new tumour marker for pancreatic cancer: a comparison with CA 19-9, CA 50 and CEA. *Br J Cancer.* 1994;70:487–492.
105. Kuusela P, Haglund C, Roberts PJ. Comparison of a new tumour marker CA 242 with CA 19-9, CA 50 and carcinoembryonic antigen (CEA) in digestive tract diseases. *Br J Cancer.* 1991;63:636–640.
106. Holmgren J, Lindholm L, Persson B, et al. Detection by monoclonal antibody of carbohydrate antigen CA 50 in serum of patients with carcinoma. *Br Med J.* 1984;288:1479–1482.
107. Haglund C, Kuusela P, Jalanko H, et al. Serum CA 50 as a tumor marker in pancreatic cancer: a comparison with CA 19-9. *Int J Cancer.* 1987;39:477–481.
108. Paganuzzi M, Onetto M, Marroni P, et al. CA 19-9 and CA 50 in benign and malignant pancreatic and biliary diseases. *Cancer.* 1988;61:2100–2108.
109. Kuusela P, Haglund C, Roberts PJ, et al. Comparison of CA-50, a new tumour marker, with carcinoembryonic antigen (CEA) and alpha-fetoprotein (AFP) in patients with gastrointestinal diseases. *Br J Cancer.* 1987;55: 673–676.
110. Nilsson O, Johansson C, Glimelius B, et al. Sensitivity and specificity of CA242 in gastro-intestinal cancer: a comparison with CEA, CA50 and CA 19-9. *Br J Cancer.* 1992;65: 215–221.
111. Haglund C, Roberts PJ, Jalanko H, et al. Tumour markers CA 19-9 and CA 50 in digestive tract malignancies. *Scand J Gastroenterol.* 1992;27:169–174.
112. Palsson B, Masson P, Andren-Sandberg A. The influence of cholestasis on CA 50 and CA 242 in pancreatic cancer and benign biliopancreatic diseases. *Scand J Gastroenterol.* 1993;28:981–987.
113. Rothlin MA, Joller H, Largiader F. CA 242 is a new tumor marker for pancreatic cancer. *Cancer.* 1993;71:701–707.
114. Palsson B, Andren-Sandberg A, Masson P. Plasma concentrations of CA-50 in relation to tumour burden in exocrine pancreatic cancer. *Eur J Cancer.* 1991;27:1279–1282.
115. Plebani M, Basso D, Navaglia F, et al. Is CA242 really a new tumour marker for pancreatic adenocarcinoma? *Oncology.* 1995;52:19–23.
116. Von Rosen A, Linder S, Harmenberg U, et al. Clinical relevance of tumour markers CA 19-9 and CA-50 in sera from patients with pancreatic duct carcinoma. *Surg Oncol.* 1992;1:109–113.
117. Pasanen PA, Eskelinen M, Partanen K, et al. Clinical value of serum tumour markers CEA, CA 50 and CA 242 in the distinction between malignant versus benign diseases causing jaundice and cholestasis: results from a prospective study. *Anticancer Res.* 1992;12:1687–1693.
118. Pasanen PA, Eskelinen M, Partanen K, et al. Multivariate analysis of six serum tumor markers (CEA, CA 50, CA 242, TPA, TPS, TATI) and conventional laboratory tests in the diagnosis of hepatopancreatobiliary malignancy. *Anticancer Res.* 1995;15:2731–2737.
119. Parker N, Makin CA, Ching CK, et al. A new enzyme-linked lectin/mucin antibody sandwich assay (CAM 17.1/WGA) assessed in combination with CA 19-9 and peanut lectin binding assay for the diagnosis of pancreatic cancer. *Cancer.* 1992;70:1062–1068.
120. Eccleston DW, Milton JD, Hoffman J, et al. Pancreatic tumour marker anti-mucin antibody CAM 17.1 reacts with a sialyl blood group antigen, probably I, which is expressed throughout the human gastrointestinal tract. *Digestion.* 1998;59:665–670.
121. Gansauge F, Gansauge S, Parker N, et al. CAM 17.1: a new diagnostic marker in pancreatic cancer. *Br J Cancer.* 1996; 74:1997–2002.
122. Yiannakou JY, Newland P, Calder F, et al. Prospective study of CAM 17.1/WGA mucin assay for serological diagnosis of pancreatic cancer. *Lancet.* 1997;349:389–392.
123. Ochi Y, Ura Y, Hamazu M, et al. Immunological study of tissue polypeptide antigen (TPA): demonstration of keratin-like sites and blood group antigen-like sites on TPA molecules. *Clin Chim Acta.* 1985;151:157–167.
124. Bjorklund B, Bjorklund V. Antigenity of pooled human malignant and normal tissues by cyto-immunological tech-

nique: presence of an insoluble, heatlabile tumor antigen. *Int Arch Allergy.* 1957;10:153–184.
125. Marino P, Buccheri G, Preatoni A, et al. Tissue polypeptide specific antigen (TPS) and objective response to treatment in solid tumors. *Int J Biol Markers.* 1992;7:65–67.
126. Bjorklund B. On the nature and clinical use of tissue polypeptide antigen (TPA). *Tumor Diagn.* 1980;1:9–20.
127. Pasanen PA, Eskelinen M, Partanen K, et al. Clinical evaluation of tissue polypeptide antigen (TPA) in the diagnosis of pancreatic carcinoma. *Anticancer Res.* 1993;13: 1883–1887.
128. Plebani M, Basso D, Del Favero G, et al. Clinical utility of TPS, TPA and CA 19-9 measurement in pancreatic cancer. *Oncology.* 1993;50:436–440.
129. Basso D, Fabris C, Panucci A, et al. Tissue polypeptide antigen, galactosyltransferase isoenzyme II and pancreatic oncofetal antigen serum determination: role in pancreatic cancer diagnosis. *Int J Pancreatol.* 1988;3(Suppl 1):S95–S100.
130. Lan MS, Finn OJ, Fernsten PD, et al. Isolation and properties of a human pancreatic adenocarcinoma-associated antigen, DU-PAN-2. *Cancer Res.* 1985;45:305–310.
131. Metzgar RS, Rodriguez N, Finn OJ, et al. Detection of a pancreatic cancer-associated antigen (DU-PAN-2 antigen) in serum and ascites of patients with adenocarcinoma. *Proc Natl Acad Sci USA.* 1984;81:5242–5246.
132. Chung YS, Ho JJ, Kim YS, et al. The detection of human pancreatic cancer-associated antigen in the serum of cancer patients. *Cancer.* 1987;60:1636–1643.
133. Kawa S, Tokoo M, Oguchi H, et al. Epitope analysis of SPan-1 and DUPAN-2 using synthesized glycoconjugates sialyllact-N-fucopentaose II and sialyllact-N-tetraose. *Pancreas.* 1994;9:692–697.
134. Kawa S, Oguchi H, Kobayashi T, et al. Elevated serum levels of Dupan-2 in pancreatic cancer patients negative for Lewis blood group phenotype. *Br J Cancer.* 1991;64: 899–902.
135. Tempero M, Takasaki H, Uchida E, et al. Co-expression of CA 19-9, DU-PAN-2, CA 125, and TAG-72 in pancreatic adenocarcinoma. *Am J Surg Pathol.* 1989;13(Suppl 1):S89–S95.
136. Ohshio G, Manabe T, Watanabe Y, et al. Comparative studies of DU-PAN-2, carcinoembryonic antigen, and CA19-9 in the serum and bile of patients with pancreatic and biliary tract diseases: evaluation of the influence of obstructive jaundice. *Am J Gastroenterol.* 1990;85:1370–1376.
137. Ferrara C, Basso D, Fabris C, et al. Comparison of two newly identified tumor markers (CAR-3 and DU-PAN-2) with CA 19-9 in patients with pancreatic cancer. *Tumori.* 1991;77:56–60.
138. Fabris C, Malesci A, Basso D, et al. Serum DU-PAN-2 in the differential diagnosis of pancreatic cancer: influence of jaundice and liver dysfunction. *Br J Cancer.* 1991;63:451–453.
139. Kiriyama S, Hayakawa T, Kondo T, et al. Usefulness of a new tumor marker, Span-1, for the diagnosis of pancreatic cancer. *Cancer.* 1990;65:1557–1561.
140. Takeda S, Nakao A, Ichihara T, et al. Serum concentration and immunohistochemical localization of SPan-1 antigen in pancreatic cancer: a comparison with CA19-9 antigen. *Hepatogastroenterology.* 1991;38:143–148.
141. Benini L, Cavallini G, Zordan D, et al. A clinical evaluation of monoclonal (CA19-9, CA50, CA12-5) and polyclonal (CEA, TPA) antibody-defined antigens for the diagnosis of pancreatic cancer. *Pancreas.* 1988;3:61–66.
142. Molina LM, Diez M, Cava MT, et al. Tumor markers in pancreatic cancer: a comparative clinical study between CEA, CA 19-9 and CA 50. *Int J Biol Markers.* 1990;5: 127–132.
143. Wood RA, Moossa AR. The prospective evaluation of tumour-associated antigens for the early diagnosis of pancreatic cancer. *Br J Surg.* 1977;64:718–720.
144. Gelder FB, Reese CJ, Moossa AR, et al. Purification, partial characterization, and clinical evaluation of a pancreatic oncofetal antigen. *Cancer Res.* 1978;38:313–324.
145. Gelder F, Reese C, Moossa AR, et al. Studies on an oncofetal antigen, POA. *Cancer.* 1978;42:1635–1645.
146. Fujii Y, Albers GH, Carre-Llopis A, et al. The diagnostic value of the foetoacinar pancreatic (FAP) protein in cancer of the pancreas: a comparative study with CA19/9. *Br J Cancer.* 1987;56:495–500.
147. Almoguera C, Shibata D, Forrester K, et al. Most human carcinomas of the exocrine pancreas contain mutant *c-K-ras* genes. *Cell.* 1988;53:549–554.
148. Lemoine NR, Jain S, Hughes CM, et al. *Ki*-ras oncogene activation in preinvasive pancreatic cancer. *Gastroenterology.* 1992;102:230–236.
149. Hruban RH, Iacobuzio-Donahue C, Wilentz RE, et al. Molecular pathology of pancreatic cancer. *Cancer J.* 2001;7: 251–258.
150. Shibata D, Almoguera C, Forrester K, et al. Detection of *c-K*-ras mutations in fine needle aspirates from human pancreatic adenocarcinomas. *Cancer Res.* 1990;50:1279–1283.
151. Shapiro B, Chakrabarty M, Cohn EM, et al. Determination of circulating DNA levels in patients with benign or malignant gastrointestinal disease. *Cancer.* 1983;51: 2116–2120.
152. Dianxu F, Shengdao Z, Tianquan H, et al. A prospective study of detection of pancreatic carcinoma by combined plasma *K*-ras mutations and serum CA19-9 analysis. *Pancreas.* 2002;25:336–341.
153. Theodor L, Melzer E, Sologov M, et al. Diagnostic value of *K*-ras mutations in serum of pancreatic cancer patients. *Ann N Y Acad Sci.* 2000;906:19–24.
154. Yamada T, Nakamori S, Ohzato H, et al. Detection of *K*-ras gene mutations in plasma DNA of patients with pancreatic adenocarcinoma: correlation with clinicopathological features. *Clin Cancer Res.* 1998;4:1527–1532.
155. Yokoyama M, Yamanaka Y, Friess H, et al. *p53* expression in human pancreatic cancer correlates with enhanced biological aggressiveness. *Anticancer Res.* 1994;14:2477–2483.
156. Raedle J, Oremek G, Welker M, et al. *p53* autoantibodies in patients with pancreatitis and pancreatic carcinoma. *Pancreas.* 1996;13:241–246.
157. Suwa H, Ohshio G, Okada N, et al. Clinical significance of serum *p53* antigen in patients with pancreatic carcinomas. *Gut.* 1997;40:647–653.

CHAPTER

17

The Molecular Diagnosis of Pancreatic Cancer

Michael G. Goggins, MD

Current Approaches for Diagnosing Pancreatic Cancer

Most pancreatic ductal adenocarcinomas (~ 85%) are diagnosed at a late, incurable stage. Since complete resection of small cancers may improve the outcome of this deadly disease, there is great interest in improving the early detection of pancreatic cancer.[1] Improving diagnostic tests for pancreatic cancer would help achieve two major goals. First, better diagnostic strategies would ensure that patients with symptoms suspicious of pancreatic cancer are diagnosed rapidly and their disease managed optimally. This goal can be achieved through improved diagnostic imaging and the discovery of more accurate molecular markers of pancreatic cancer. Depending on their diagnostic attributes, molecular markers could be used to detect pancreatic cancer in a variety of clinical situations using specimens such as serum, pancreatic juice, stool, fine-needle aspirates of pancreatic masses, or in brush cytology specimens of the pancreatic duct. Second, accurate diagnostic tests for pancreatic cancer are needed to detect early symptomless pancreatic neoplasms as part of clinical screening protocols for individuals at high risk of pancreatic cancer, such as those individuals with a strong family history of pancreatic cancer and carriers of genetic alterations known to predispose to the development of pancreatic cancer (see Chapters 8 and 9). The optimal approach for detecting these asymptomatic pancreatic neoplasms as well as diagnosing symptomatic patients is still under investigation.

Currently pancreatic cancer diagnosis relies heavily on imaging tests, including CT, MRI/MRCP, endoscopic ultrasonography (EUS) and endoscopic retrograde cholangiopancreaticography (ERCP) (see Chapters 12 and 13). The accuracy of CT, MRI, and EUS has improved over the last decade but these tests are still not sufficiently sensitive to diagnose small potentially curable cancers. This is particularly true of standard radiologic imaging tests that are used in the community. High-quality CT imaging is available in larger centers and such scanners can often detect small cancers.[2]

EUS can detect small pancreatic lesions [3,4] and in experienced hands, EUS may have a greater accuracy than dual-phase helical CT for diagnosing small pancreatic cancers in patients with pancreatic masses.[5] Furthermore, fine-needle aspirates (FNA) can be performed during EUS procedures and can help to establish a diagnosis of malignancy, although the diagnostic yield from cytology in this setting is modest. Importantly, even the best CT or

EUS investigation of the pancreas may not detect 1- to 2-cm-lesions of the pancreas. ERCP is less likely to detect small tumors than EUS, but like EUS, is useful for acquiring tissue (i.e., pancreatic juice, pancreatic fine-needle aspirates) for molecular diagnosis. ERCP complements EUS in interpreting abnormal findings by EUS imaging and it also can be used for palliative therapy. Unfortunately, all too often high-quality spiral CT or EUS imaging tests of the pancreas are performed late in the clinical evaluation of patients with pancreatic cancer. The recognition that delayed diagnosis of pancreatic cancer is common and probably contributes to the excess mortality of this disease has encouraged efforts to identify accurate markers of pancreatic cancer.

An accurate marker of pancreatic cancer could help the many patients with pancreatic cancer who present with nonspecific symptoms. As discussed in greater detail in Chapter 16, CA19-9, the only widely used tumor marker for patients with suspected pancreatic cancer, is valuable for following the therapeutic response of patients with pancreatic cancer that have an elevated serum CA19-9 level.[6] CA19-9 is, however, not considered a diagnostic marker. First, 10%–15% of the general population do not secrete CA19-9 because of their Lewis antigen status. In addition, CA19-9 levels may be within the normal range in patients with small and asymptomatic cancers. For example, only two thirds of patients presenting with a resectable pancreatic cancer at The Johns Hopkins Hospital had an elevated CA19-9 level.[7] Conversely, CA19-9 can be elevated in benign biliary or pancreatic conditions. Other investigational pancreatic markers have had similar problems with their diagnostic accuracy.

Diagnosing Precancerous Lesions of the Pancreas

The recognition that invasive pancreatic ductal adenocarcinomas arise from noninvasive intraductal precursors has highlighted the need for more accurate molecular markers that can not only accurately diagnose pancreatic cancer but can ultimately also identify these precancerous lesions. Preinvasive pancreatic lesions include microscopic pancreatic intraepithelial neoplasia (so-called PanIN), and macroscopic intraductal papillary mucinous neoplasms (IPMNs). IPMNs are being recognized more frequently and they are ideal lesions for early detection because they appear to go through a long non-invasive stage before they progress to invasive cancer. Although PanINs are also important precursor lesions, they usually are too small to give rise to symptoms. Molecular markers are needed to identify asymptomatic individuals that have PanIN or IPMN lesions with the highest likelihood of progressing to invasive cancer. Ideally, the same molecular tests that identify small pancreatic ductal adenocarcinomas not visible with conventional imaging tests would also identify advanced PanIN and IPMN lesions.[8] Useful markers would also be able to distinguish lesions with a significant risk of progressing from the more prevalent low-grade PanINs that have much lower malignant potential.

Screening High-Risk Individuals for Pancreatic Cancer

Individuals with a family history of pancreatic cancer and those who inherit a germline mutation in tumor-suppressor genes such as *BRCA2*, have been shown to have a significantly increased risk of developing pancreatic cancer, and they are already being screened for the presence of asymptomatic pancreatic cancer in several centers with an interest in pancreatic cancer diagnosis. Current approaches to screen such individuals have used a combination of approaches including EUS of the pancreas, multidetector CT with thin sections of the pancreas, and serum CA19-9 measurements. ERCP, EUS-FNA, and other investigations are often reserved for when abnormalities are found on EUS, because of the higher morbidity of these procedures. A number of precursor lesions have been found in an ongoing clinical trial at The Johns Hopkins University using this approach in at-risk relatives from familial pancreatic cancer kindreds, and in patients with the Peutz-Jeghers syndrome (who have a high lifetime risk of developing pancreatic adenocarcinoma). Thirty-seven asymptomatic individuals were screened by EUS and an invasive pancreatic cancer, an IPMN with in situ carcinoma and 2 mucinous cystic neoplasms were detected.[9] Two additional patients went to surgery for atypical cytological changes suggestive of cancer, but they did not have invasive cancer in the pancreaticoduodenectomy resection specimen. These data highlight the risks and benefits of screening high-risk groups by EUS. Some early curable lesions will be found, but there is a risk of false-positive tests. The experience of T. Brentnall and colleagues is also helpful. They reported their experience of screening high-risk families.[10] Of 14 patients from 3 families surveyed primarily by EUS, 7 were found to have EUS and ERCP abnormalities. Pathologic analysis of pancreatectomy resection specimens in these patients revealed pancreatic duct lesions (PanINs) and chronic pancreatitis. The most severe abnormalities were found in a large pedigree with early-onset pancreatic insufficiency and diabetes (called Family "X"). The clinical presentation of the affected members of this kindred is not typical of most patients who have a strong family history of pancreatic cancer.

These initial studies provide evidence for the value of screening of high-risk populations, but the risks and benefits of such screening need to be defined in larger studies. Most patients currently enrolled in screening are individuals with a strong family history of pancreatic cancer and not those with known germline mutations in tumor-suppressor genes. Since the individuals in these families that undergo screening are selected based on family history, many are, in fact, not gene carriers. The identification of the gene(s) responsible for the aggregation of pancreatic cancer in families will help identify those individuals who will benefit most from screening studies. This is important because the diagnostic value of a screening test is highly dependent on the prior probability of disease in the population under study. In symptomatic individuals, the prior probability of disease such as pancreatic cancer is usually quite high (such as 20%–90%), and diagnostic tests with excellent accuracy will help facilitate diagnosis. On the other hand, even in a high-risk screening population, although the risk of disease over an extended period may be moderately high, the risk of cancer at any one point in time is very low. For example, while the lifetime risk for an individual with an increased risk of pancreatic cancer may be 10% or more, this risk of cancer may be spread over a 30-year period. As a result at any one time, the prior probability of disease will be lower, and may be only ~1%. Applying diagnostic tests to individuals with a low prior probability of disease is problematic. Let us look at an example. In a scenario where a population of 1000 patients has a prior probability of pancreatic cancer of 1% that undergoes diagnostic evaluation with a test with a sensitivity and specificity of 90%, one would expect to identify 9 patients with cancer with a positive test, 1 patient with cancer that would be missed by the test, 100 patients whose test would be falsely positive for cancer, and 890 patients that did not have cancer at the time of the test whose test would be negative. These figures highlight the need for highly accurate diagnostic tests and for very careful evaluation of the diagnostic significance of emerging molecular tests when they are applied to a high-risk population. Given these limitations, a sound clinical strategy, particularly one that identifies the right population to screen, along with sensitive and specific markers is needed.

In addition to better identifying subjects at risk there remains uncertainty and caution about the best surgical approach for managing the lesions discovered in asymptomatic individuals. For example, even if the suspicious portion of the gland is removed, cancer can develop in the remnant pancreas. Removing the entire pancreas might seem reasonable, but total pancreatectomy is associated with significant morbidity (including brittle diabetes mellitus) and mortality.

In addition to imaging protocols, current screening protocols often include the banking of pancreatic juice in the hope that molecular assays applied to the tissues will be discovered that can sensitively and specifically identify early pancreatic neoplasia. Given the very high accuracy required of any molecular marker in the screening setting, newer molecular markers will have to first demonstrate diagnostic accuracy in patients with symptoms suggestive of pancreatic cancer.

Investigations to Identify Improved Diagnostic Markers of Pancreatic Cancer

When attempting to diagnose pancreatic cancer using molecular markers an important consideration is the clinical specimens being assayed. Clinical specimens that can be used for pancreatic cancer diagnosis include serum, pancreatic juice, stool, or fine-needle aspirates of pancreatic masses. Each tissue has its own advantages and disadvantages, and each requires different degrees of diagnostic accuracy.

Many patients would benefit from the availability of a serum marker such as a protein marker with superior diagnostic performance to CA19-9. Serum is easily obtainable with minimal morbidity and, once developed, most blood tests are readily performed at most centers. At the same time, the need to identify very small pancreatic lesions has also led to interest in identifying novel markers of pancreatic cancer that can be applied to other types of samples such as samples obtained directly from the pancreas. Highly specific molecular markers of pancreatic cancer would be valuable for evaluating patients with suspected pancreatic cancer in whom cytological or biopsy specimens are inconclusive for cancer.[11] Samples of pancreatic secretions ("pancreatic juice") are also attractive targets for screening because they have high concentrations of neoplastic DNA and proteins. Pancreatic juice is a potentially optimal specimen to use when diagnosing symptomatic patients as well as when screening high-risk individuals for pancreatic cancer, analogous to using sputum to aid in the diagnosis of lung cancer[12] or nipple aspirates for breast cancer.[13] As shown in Fig. 17.1, pancreatic juice samples can be analyzed for DNA

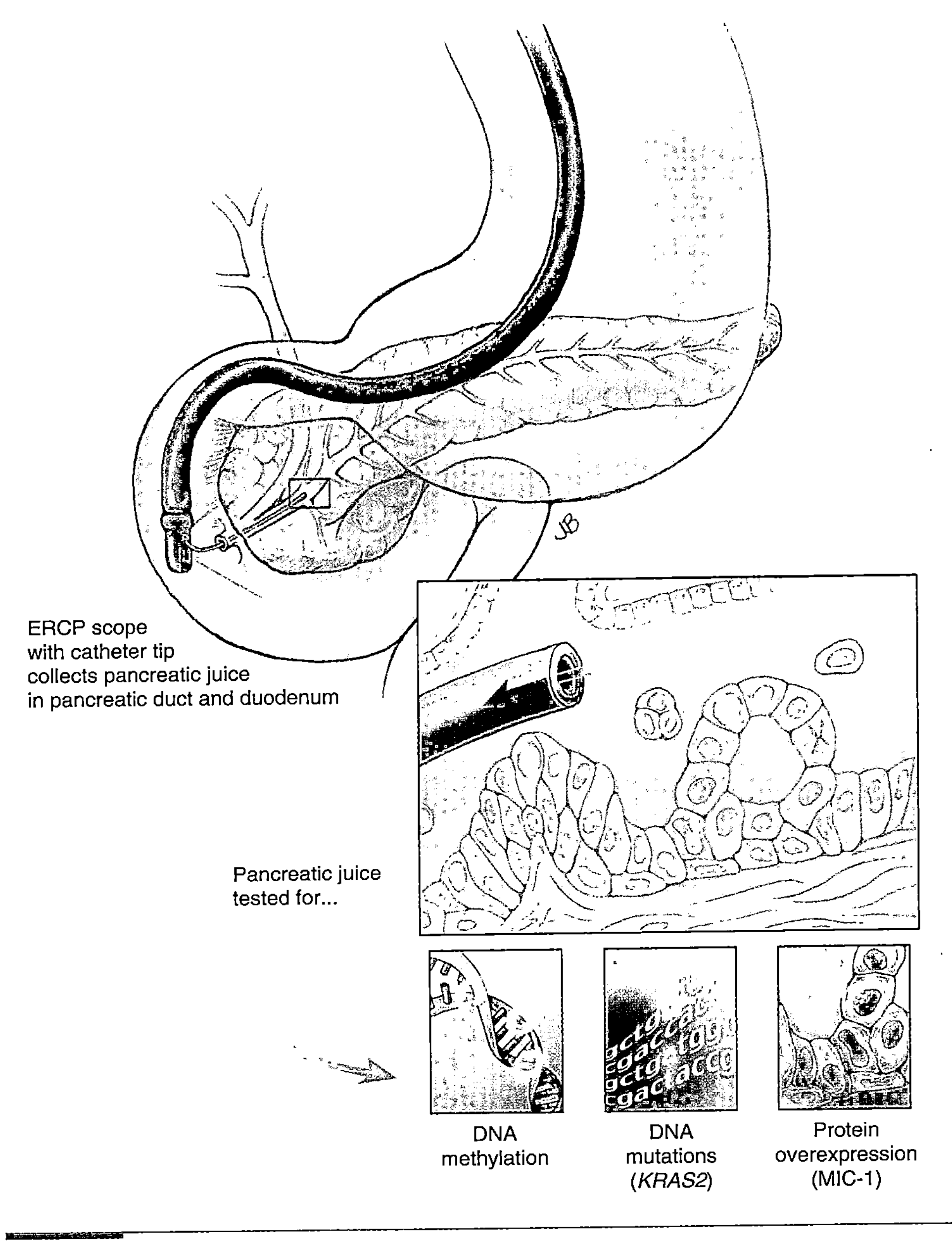

Figure 17.1
Direct sampling of pancreatic juice at the time of ERCP can yield material suitable for screening. This fluid is enriched in cells, DNA, RNA, and protein from the tumor. It can be evaluated for changes in DNA methylation, for DNA mutations, and for protein overexpression. "*Artwork by Jennifer Parsons Brumbaugh*".

methylation changes, for DNA mutations, and for protein overexpression. For example, mutant *KRAS2* genes are readily detected in pancreatic juice but these mutations are usually not detectable in plasma until relatively late in the course of the disease, more often in patients with inoperable cancers.[14-16] Pure pancreatic juice collection requires ERCP, but pancreatic juice can also be collected in the duodenum and assayed for the presence of cancer DNA during routine upper gastrointestinal endoscopy after secretin stimulation without the need for ERCP. Recombinant secretin has been available for several years for this purpose. Fluid collected from the duodenum following secretin stimulation will contain a mixture of pancreatic juice and duodenal juice contents, and will therefore require the use of assays that have greater sensitivity than is required for the analysis of pure pancreatic juice alone. In one study the analysis of *KRAS2* gene mutations in duodenal fluid obtained peri-operatively from patients with pancreatic cancer identified mutations in only 24% of the samples.[17] This low prevalence of mutant *KRAS2* genes may reflect the timing of collection as endoscopic collection of duodenal juice during secretin stimulation enables the collection of purer pancreatic juice. Stool is another sample type that could potentially be used for screening. Stool-based DNA assays have been used to detect neoplasia in the gastrointestinal tract, however, stool would obviously contain a very small amount of material from the pancreas. Stool-based assays would therefore need to be able to detect very rare mutant alleles in the presence of much larger quantities of normal DNA.

DNA Alterations as Markers of Pancreatic Cancer

Potential markers of pancreatic cancer can be divided into three categories of targets: DNA-based (both nuclear and mitochondrial), RNA-based, and protein-based targets. DNA-based assays aim to detect cancer-specific DNA alterations. The diagnostic potential of both DNA- and RNA-based markers has improved in recent years with technologic developments such as chip-based technology and quantitative polymerase chain reaction (qPCR).[18] Besides the improvements in technologies for assessing DNA alterations, the detection of DNA mutations has another theoretical advantage which is that mutations can be detected at very low concentrations even when a mutant allele is admixed with many hundreds, potentially even thousands, of wild-type alleles. In contrast, the best protein markers often have only moderate sensitivity and specificity for cancer. Despite such improvements and the tremendous accuracy of many DNA-based detection methods, few somatic mutations have been identified that have ideal diagnostic characteristics. An ideal genetic marker would be present in all pancreatic cancers and would be readily detectable. The easiest mutations to detect are those that are limited to a single codon or to a very specific portion of the gene targeted. When mutations are limited to a specific portion of a gene, very specific probes can be developed just for that portion of the genome. Examples of potential useful cancer markers include mutations in the *KRAS2* and *BRAF* genes.[19-23] The *BRAF* gene is frequently mutated in melanomas and in papillary thyroid carcinomas and the detection of mutant *BRAF* is a promising diagnostic strategy for these cancers.[20-22] *KRAS2* gene mutations occur in ~ 90% of pancreatic cancers and these mutations almost always target codon 12. Unfortunately *KRAS2* gene mutations are not specific for invasive pancreatic cancer; they occur in individuals with chronic pancreatitis, individuals who smoke, and in PanINs from patients without pancreatic cancer.[24-28] Not surprisingly, the detection of *KRAS2* gene mutations, whether in pancreatic juice or in stool, has not proven to be a specific test for pancreatic cancer diagnosis.[24-28]

TP53 gene mutations generally occur relatively late in cancer development and the detection of *TP53* gene mutations has been widely investigated as a potentially specific diagnostic marker in a variety of cancers. In pancreatic ductal adenocarcinoma, *TP53* gene mutations are found in ~ 70% of invasive cancers.[29] Although a few nucleotide hot spots of *TP53* gene mutation are known to exist, the mutations can be spread across the entire gene.[30] In one study, assaying for eight common *TP53* mutations in stool using a mismatch ligation assay, investigators identified 59% of stool samples from patients with colon cancer,[31] but other studies have found a much lower percentage of recurrent *TP53* mutations.[32] Several hot spots of *TP53* mutation arise because of specific environmental exposures such as smoking or aflatoxin exposure, and so the prevalence of hot spots of *TP53* gene mutation will vary with the population under study.[30] Any strategy of *TP53* gene mutation detection involving only the common nucleotide mutations will require inclusion of assays of mutations in other genes to improve diagnostic sensitivity.

Since specific nucleotide detection strategies for *TP53* gene mutations are not sufficiently sensitive for cancer detection, investigators have used other laboratory approaches that have the potential to identify the complete spectrum of *TP53* gene mutations. Assays with this capability are not as sensitive as strategies that detect single nucleotide mutations, but they can detect most mutations, and some of these assays are amenable to clinical use. These assays include chip technologies such as the Affymetrix platform,[31] single-strand conformational polymorphism (SSCP), temperature gradient gel electrophoresis (TGGE) and TGCE (temperature gradient capillary electrophoresis), and p53 immunohistochemistry. The latter assay detects p53 protein and this strategy is based on the property of mutant p53 proteins to heterodimerize and to resist degradation. P53 immunohistochemistry is the simplest but least accurate of the approaches for identifying *TP53* gene mutations. In addition, immunolabeling for p53 obviously requires tissue, usually in the form of a biopsy. Assays such as SSCP and TGCE can detect mutations that are present in at least 1%–10% of the total DNA and using SSCP.[33,34] Using these techniques investigators have reported the presence of

TP53 gene mutations, within exons 5–8, in pancreatic juice samples and in brush cytology specimens of 40%–50% of patients with pancreatic cancers—a figure close to the number of mutations one would expect to find in the primary pancreatic cancers from these patients.[35]

Chronic pancreatitis can be difficult to distinguish from pancreatic cancer using clinical, imaging, and biochemical parameters, and *TP53* gene mutation detection is particularly useful in this regard because it can help distinguish pancreatic lesions due to pancreatic cancer from those due to chronic pancreatitis. One study using TGGE demonstrated that pancreatic juice from patients with chronic pancreatitis rarely harbor *TP53* gene mutations.[36] Gene chip technology has the advantage that it can in a single assay identify a large percentage of possible *TP53* gene mutations in a given DNA sample as long as the mutation is present in the sample at sufficient concentration relative to normal DNA (>1% of DNA).[31] Such gene chips, which rely on exact hybridizations of DNA between the chip and PCR products from a clinical sample, are very effective in identifying missense mutations, but may miss the small deletions and insertions which represent ~10%–20% of all *TP53* gene mutations. In studies using Affymetrix *p53* gene chips investigators were able to identify ~ 80% of all *TP53* gene mutations in non–small-cell lung cancer tissues.[32,37]

Refinements of technology are likely to soon permit the facile detection of mutations in multiple genes in clinical specimens in a single assay. For example, gene chip technologies can now be used to array sufficient amounts of DNA that multiple genes can be probed on a single chip, which will enable investigators to search for mutations in genes that are infrequently targeted for mutation in human cancer. Since chip-based assays can detect mutations as long as mutant DNA is present in at least 1% of total DNA,[38] such assays could work well in pancreatic juice (but not in stool). Given the spectrum of known genes targeted for point mutations in pancreatic cancer, it is possible that a single chip assay could detect point mutations not only of *KRAS2* and *TP53*, but also of the *p16/INK4A* and *SMAD4/DPC4* genes. The *p16/INK4A* gene has point mutations in ~ 40% of pancreatic cancers (another 40% of pancreatic cancers harbor homozygous deletion of *p16*, but these deletions would not be detectable in clinical specimens). The *SMAD4/DPC4* gene harbors point mutations in ~15%–25% of pancreatic cancers (an additional 40% inactivate SMAD4 by homozygous deletion).[39] Thus, a gene chip platform that assayed for mutations in the *TP53*, *SMAD4/DPC4*, and *p16/INK4A* genes would be expected to have a far higher sensitivity and specificity than any single genetic assay alone.

The emergence of powerful DNA technologies has also facilitated investigations into the diagnostic utility of mitochondrial mutations. Mitochondrial mutations are commonly found in multiple cancer types.[40-43] One advantage of mitochondrial DNA as a marker is that in every cell there are many more copies of the mitochondrial genome than of nuclear DNA and in cancers, the amount of mitochondrial DNA is several-fold more abundant than it is in normal tissues.[43] In addition, a hot spot of mitochondrial mutations has been identified that is a frequent site of mutations.[44] One obstacle to assaying mitochondrial DNA for mutations is the biological variation in mitochondrial sequences present within each cell. Each cell has hundreds of mitochondria, each with their own DNA, and individual mitochondria can have DNA sequence variants. Such variation in the mitochondrial DNA within a cell is termed *"heteroplasmy."* Variant mitochondrial DNA sequences identified in cancers may reflect the clonal outgrowth of mitochondria with a particular DNA sequence (*"homoplasmy"*). This tendency to homoplasmy in cancers may not be due to selection, however they still may be useful for early detection.[42] Even if most such mitochondrial mutations found in cancer do not contribute to disease, they will reflect the presence of a dominant clone and these features make mitochondrial DNA mutations potentially useful markers of cancer. Mitochondrial DNA is ~16 kilobases in length and the mitochondrial genome has been evaluated in only a few cancers to date.[40,42-47] A "MitoChip" has recently been developed by Dr. A. Maitra, and initial studies suggest that mitochondrial mutations can be detected in pancreatic juice samples obtained from patients with pancreatic cancer.[41]

DNA Methylation

Abnormal DNA methylation occurs during the development of pancreatic cancer, and abnormally methylated DNA may prove to be a useful diagnostic marker of pancreatic cancer. DNA methylation abnormalities may be particularly suitable for use in early detection strategies for a number of reasons. Aberrant hypermethylation of tumor-suppressor genes is common during carcinogenesis (e.g., methylation of the *hMLH1*, *VHL*, *E-cadherin*, and *p16/INK4A* genes).[48] The aberrant methylation of normally unmethylated genes is associated with the silencing of tumor-suppressor genes and the silencing of many other genes with important biological functions.[49] In human cells, methylation of DNA is restricted to the cytosines at CG dinucleotides. CG dinucleotides (often referred to as CpGs) are often found in regions of DNA rich in CG dinucleotides known as CpG islands. CpG islands are commonly located in the 5′ regulatory regions of genes, and most CpG islands are normally unmethylated. Aberrant methylation changes at CpG islands are readily identifiable in clinical samples using the very sensitive methylation-specific PCR (MSP) technique.[50,51] To perform MSP, a chemical modification of the DNA is performed converting all unmethylated cytosines to uracils using bisulfite. Methylated cytosines do not convert. After this bisulfite conversion, unmethylated and methylated regions of DNA can be distinguished using PCR. MSP has been used successfully to identify methylated DNA in most biological fluids including blood, fine-needle aspirates, saliva, prostatic fluid, and sputum of patients with cancers.[52] In addition, quantification of the methylated DNA using real-time MSP may help to accurately distinguish cancers from nonneoplastic diseases. Several dozen genes have been identified as aberrantly methylated in pancreatic carcinomas, such as *SPARC*, *ppENK*, *p16/INK4A*, *TSLC1*, *p14* and others (see Table 17.1).[49,51,53-57] Initial studies have demonstrated that such aberrant methylation patterns can be detected in pancreatic juice samples from patients with pancreatic cancer.[11,51] These changes are not present in samples from patients without pancreatic cancer. Although these data are promising, there are several biological features of DNA methylation that need to be considered before it can be applied to clinical practice.

One potential obstacle towards using DNA methylation as a diagnostic tool in the pancreas is the problem of tissue-specific differences in normal methylation patterns. Several groups have highlighted partial methylation of the CpG islands of tumor-suppressor genes in normal tissues. In addition, for some genes the likelihood of finding methylation increases with patient age.[53,58-61] For example, some genes that appear to be specific markers of pancreatic cancer because they are not normally methylated in the pancreas but are aberrantly methylated in pancreatic cancers, are methylated in normal duodenum.[11] This suggests that pure pancreatic juice collected directly from the pancreatic duct will be needed to avoid duodenal contamination (see Fig. 17.1).[11] Another concern with PCR-based assays, such as MSP, is one that was observed with mutant *KRAS2* gene detection-methylation assays being "too sensitive"—the detection of a few methylated copies of DNA may identify lesions of low or even no malignant potential. For example, low-grade pancreatic intraepithelial neoplasias (PanINs) develop with increasing frequency in the pancreata of people as they age and some of these PanINs harbor methylation changes that are not found in normal pancreatic epithelium. Despite this theoretical concern, initial studies of pancreatic juice have not identified aberrant methylation changes in the pancreatic juice of patients without pancreatic cancer. Although some of these patients would be expected to harbor low-grade PanINs, small low-grade PanINs probably do not shed significant quantities of DNA and if they do, this DNA may be present at concentrations below the limit of detection of methylation-specific PCR. Ultimately, the diagnostic utility of using DNA hypermethylation as a diagnostic tool will be strengthened by the quantitative measurement of the level of methylated DNA. The diagnostic utility of quantitative MSP has recently been demonstrated for *GSTP* gene methylation in prostate cancer. Adding the *GSTP* gene methylation status of prostatic fine-needle biopsies provided additional diagnostic information over using PSA and FNA cytology alone.[62] Because MSP requires a bisulfite modification step that causes DNA degradation, MSP is not as sensitive as simple PCR, having a lower limit of detection of ~10–20 copies.[11] Modifications of the basic MSP assay have been developed to improve assay sensitivity including one method coined, interestingly enough, "Heavy Methyl."[63]

In addition to interest in aberrant hypermethylated genes as cancer markers, several genes have been identified that are methylated in normal tissues and become abnormally "hypomethylated" during cancer development. Such loss of DNA methylation is associated with induction of gene expression. The hypomethylation of several genes with oncogenic properties (such as *S100A4*

Table 17.1 Select Genes Aberrantly Hypermethylated in Pancreatic Cancer

Gene	
ppENK	FOXE1
SPARC	WNT7A
HLTF	CDH3
CCD2	hpp1
TSLC1	LHX1
p14	Reprimo
p73	CLDN5
p16	UCHL1
RARbeta	NPTX2
Ecad	St14
SOCS1	UCHL1
THBS	SRBC
hMLH1	TJP2
APC	PIG11

and others) has been described in pancreatic and other cancers.[64-67] While hypomethylation and overexpression of these genes may have important biological consequences, the detection of such aberrantly hypomethylated templates is also possible using the MSP assay. One study demonstrated that serum from patients with testicular neoplasms contained hypomethylated copies of the *XIST* gene which were not present in the serum of healthy individuals.[68]

RNA Alterations in Pancreatic Cancer and their Diagnostic Utility

The expression of hundred of genes is altered during pancreatic cancer development and knowledge of such alterations can help in the design of pancreatic cancer markers (see Chapter 36).[66,69-73] This information can be used to identify the protein products of these overexpressed genes, and these proteins can, in turn, be suitable targets for protein-based diagnostic tests. In addition, the direct assaying of pancreatic specimens for changes in specific RNA levels has the potential to assist in diagnosis. Such an approach is important because many of the proteins overexpressed in pancreatic and other cancers are not secreted proteins and therefore may not be present in serum. Quantification of mRNA levels in samples to be screened can be achieved using qRT-PCR or global gene expression profiling using chip-based assays. With the appropriate RNA marker, such assays could be applied to secretin stimulated pancreatic juice collected during endoscopy or to fine-needle aspirates of pancreatic masses. Although RNA-based assays must take into account the abundance of RNases in pancreatic tissues, RNA analysis of clinical pancreatic tissue specimens is achievable.[71]

The best studied RNA-based marker to date has been the human telomerase reverse transcriptase gene (*hTERT*). About 90% of cancers express the telomerase subunit *hTERT*, and ~ 90% of patients with pancreatic cancer have detectable telomerase activity in their pancreatic juice.[74] The detection of telomerase enzymatic activity or the *hTERT* subunit may be helpful in differentiating pancreatic cancer from benign pancreatic diseases; however telomerase is also expressed in inflammatory cells, suggesting that it may not be sufficiently specific for use as a cancer-screening marker.

Gene expression profiling has led to the identification of hundreds of genes overexpressed at the RNA level in primary pancreatic cancer tissues compared to normal pancreas (see Table 17.2 and Chapter 36).[66,69-73,75] Some of the differentially expressed genes in pancreatic cancers arise from expression changes in nonneoplastic stromal cells. For this reason, it is critical to determine the cell of origin of genes tentatively identified as overexpressed in pancreatic cancer. This can be accomplished using assays that can be correlated with cell morphology, such as immunohistochemistry or in situ hybridization.

The use of gene expression profiling coupled with confirmatory analysis of expression changes in the tissues has led to the identification of hundreds of genes that are overexpressed in pancreatic cancer cells relative to normal pancreas. Examples of such genes include *mesothelin, prostate stem cell antigen (PSCA), 14-3-3 sigma, S100P, S100A4, osteopontin, MMP-7, Muc4, kallikrein 10, fascin, keratin 17, and others*.[66,69,75,76,77] For example, mesothelin and PSCA are expressed in the majority of pancreatic cancers,[78] and immunolabeling for mesothelin and PSCA can be used to aid in the interpretation of diagnostically challenging pancreatic biopsies.[79] It is likely

Table 17.2 Select Genes Identified as Overexpressed in Pancreatic Adenocarcinomas

Gene	Source of overexpression
MIC-1	Cancer, Stroma
PSCA	cancer
Mesothelin	cancer
14-3-3 sigma	cancer
TFF2	cancer
osteopontin	stroma
HIP/PAP	acinar
s100a4	cancer
claudin 4	cancer
s100p	cancer
mmp7	cancer
fascin	cancer
timp1	cancer
c-myc	cancer
her-2	cancer
uPA	stroma
inhibin	cancer
IL-8	cancer
kallekrein 10	cancer
cyclin D1	cancer
Akt2	cancer
uPAR	cancer
biglycan	cancer
hsp47	stroma
keratin 17	cancer
keratin 19	cancer
igfbp3	cancer

that the expression patterns of other overexpressed genes in cytological specimens, identified using approaches such as immunohistochemistry, qRT-PCR, or gene chip profiling, could be used to distinguish fine-needle aspirates of pancreatic cancers from noncancerous aspirates. Mesothelin is also overexpressed in mesotheliomas and in ovarian cancers, cancers that also secrete a version of the protein that can be detected in serum. Unfortunately, only the nonsecreted isoform of mesothelin is expressed in pancreatic cancers (unpublished observation).

Overall, only a minority of the protein products of overexpressed genes are generally suitable for use in serologic diagnosis. In addition, while some genes may be abundantly expressed in pancreatic cancer cells relative to the normal pancreas, in other tissues the expression of such genes may be normal (such as for 14-3-3 sigma). Finally, many genes that are overexpressed in pancreatic cancer cells are also overexpressed in chronic pancreatitis tissues.[71,80] Therefore, a careful characterization of the genes whose overexpression is most sensitive and specific for cancer is needed when designing assays to detect the protein products of overexpressed genes. Thus, to translate an overexpressed protein into a serum-based marker of pancreatic cancer, a marker should be a secreted protein, it should be overexpressed in pancreatic cancers, it should not be expressed in nonneoplastic pancreas, and it should have a restricted pattern of expression in other organs and tissues.

One gene that fulfills these criteria is macrophage inhibitory cytokine (*MIC-1*). *MIC-1* is overexpressed in pancreatic cancer cells relative to normal pancreas, and the protein product of *MIC-1* is secreted. MIC-1 protein has been shown to be detectable in the serum by enzyme linked immunosorbent assay at levels more than 2 standard deviations above the normal range in ~ 80% of patients with resectable pancreatic cancer.[81] Serum levels of MIC-1 can be elevated in chronic pancreatitis and overall MIC-1 has a similar diagnostic usefulness to CA19-9.[81] Of interest, the combination of serum CA19-9 and MIC-1 measurements is a better predictor of pancreatic cancer than using CA19-9 alone.[81] Another potential marker identified through gene expression profiling is osteopontin. Osteopontin is expressed in peritumoral macrophages, and is usually elevated in the serum of patients with pancreatic cancer.[82]

Proteomics Profiling to Detect Markers of Pancreatic Cancer

Protein-based markers are the most widely used diagnostic markers. The overriding goal for investigators attempting to identify pancreatic cancer diagnostic markers is to identify a "PSA-test" for pancreatic cancer. While gene expression profiling has been a useful tool for identifying overexpressed proteins such as mesothelin, PSCA, MIC-1 and osteopontin, the direct analysis of unknown proteins in pancreatic cancer tissues is important because many novel cancer protein alterations are posttranscriptional alterations that would not be evident from RNA analysis. The large-scale analysis of unknown proteins in biological fluids or cells is called *"Proteomics."*

Several technologies have been employed to carry out proteomics studies. Studies commonly involve the characterization of the unknown proteins using mass spectrometry after separating proteins using techniques such as 2D gel electrophoresis, or liquid chromatography. One approach that has been applied to pancreatic and other cancer specimens is SELDI (surface enhanced laser desorption ionization) mass spectrometry. SELDI involves the analysis of protein profiles of samples applied to protein chips.[83] SELDI protein profiling will identify protein peaks of a certain mass:charge ratio. Further identification of protein peaks requires subsequent analysis and as a result most initial SELDI studies have focused on identifying protein peaks with diagnostic potential leaving the identification of these proteins to subsequent studies. SELDI profiling of pancreatic juice led to the demonstration that hepatocarcinoma-intestine-pancreas/pancreatitis-associated protein I (HIP/PAP) levels are elevated in pancreatic juice samples from patients with pancreatic cancer compared to patients with other pancreatic diseases.[83] Serum profiling using SELDI and other mass spectrometry approaches is being explored as a diagnostic tool in a variety of cancers and a recent study has demonstrated that serum from patients with pancreatic cancer have several protein peak alterations that can be used to accurately distinguish between serum from patients with pancreatic cancer and normal serum or serum from patients with periampullary diseases. These proteins added to the diagnostic yield of serum CA19-9 measurement in predicting the presence of pancreatic cancer.[7] Other investigations have profiled cell culture supernatants of pancreatic cancer cells in an attempt to identify secreted proteins. Using this approach a fragment of DMBT1 was identified in supernatants of five of 15 pancreatic cancer cell lines but not in other cancer cell supernatants or in pancreatic nonneoplastic cell line supernatants.[84] Further improvements in SELDI profiling technology may improve the discovery and diagnostic utility of SELDI profiling.

Mass spectrometry approaches have also been used to identify pancreatic cancer proteins in serum (matrix assisted laser desorption ionization [MALDI]),[85] and in pancreatic juice using liquid chromatography tandem mass spectrometry (LC-MS/MS).[86]

Beyond Molecular Diagnosis: Diagnosing Subtypes of Pancreatic Cancer Using Molecular Markers

The deadly nature of the majority of invasive pancreatic ductal adenocarcinomas has meant that identifying molecular markers that predict pancreatic cancer behavior has not been a research priority. This is in contrast to cancers of other organs where prognosticating the biological behavior of the cancer is either part of clinical practice or is under investigation. Examples of such markers include knowledge of estrogen receptor status in breast cancer and the use of global gene expression profiles to predict the behavior of lymphomas, leukemias, myeloma, breast cancer, and others. In these cancers such information can influence clinical decision making, while in pancreatic cancer such information has largely been of academic interest. Knowledge of markers that are truly predictive of tumor behavior can guide more effective research into treatment options. It is likely that use of molecular profiles for prognosticating tumor behavior will increase in the future.

Not surprisingly, given the deadly nature of pancreatic ductal adenocarcinoma, it has been difficult to identify markers that are predictive of prognosis independent of known clinical and pathologic factors that predict tumor behavior such as tumor size, stage, and differentiation.[87] One molecular marker that does appear to provide independent modest prognostic information is Smad4 expression status. In one study of patients with resectable pancreatic adenocarcinoma, those patients with cancers that did not express the tumor-suppressor gene product, Smad4 (also known as Dpc4), had a poorer prognosis by multivariate analysis than those patients whose tumors retained Smad4 expression.[88]

Another useful genetic classification of cancers is the stratification of cancers based on whether they demonstrate chromosomal or microsatellite instability.[89] A small percentage of pancreatic adenocarcinomas display microsatellite instability, and these microsatellite unstable cancers have a unique medullary morphology[90-91] and appear to have a better prognosis.[92]

One clinical situation where prognostication of pancreatic neoplasms is particularly important is in the predicting (and understanding) of the behavior of the less aggressive pancreatic neoplasms such as intraductal papillary mucinous neoplasms (IPMNs), and mucinous cystic neoplasms (MCNs) (see Chapter 51). These neoplasms have a much higher rate of cure after surgical resection.[93,94] The single most important determinant of IPMN and MCN prognosis is pathologic assessment of the presence or absence of invasion in the resection specimen. Thus, molecular profiles that predict the presence or absence of early invasion could help predict which patients could be observed over time with a view to avoiding surgery if symptoms permitted and if the neoplasm remained noninvasive. Recent studies suggest this may be possible as several proteins that are overexpressed in a subset of IPMNs predict invasiveness (claudin 4, CXCR4, S100A4, and mesothelin).[95] Thus, it may ultimately prove useful to assay pancreatic IPMNs preoperatively for the expression of these genes to help determine whether or not an IPMN has already invaded or not.[95]

Perhaps more important than simple prognostication of tumor behavior is the identification of targets of novel therapies. There is considerable hope that the future of pancreatic cancer diagnosis will include molecular profiling to identify therapeutic targets for novel therapies. Several novel chemotherapeutics that target specific signaling pathways are now available as anti-cancer agents including EGFR inhibitors[96] and rapamycin (an inhibitor of mTOR).[97] These novel therapies are under investigation in pancreatic and other cancers. For many of these agents, therapeutic response may depend on identifying which patients have the cancers with the appropriate genetic background for the drug to respond. One recent and hopeful example of this paradigm is the recent identification of genetic inactivation of the Fanconi anemia pathway in a small percentage of pancreatic adenocarcinomas (see Chapter 3).[98,99] The Fanconi anemia pathway includes at least nine genes (*FANCA*, *FANCC*, *FANCD1* [*BRCA2*], *FANCD2*, *FANCE*, *FANCF*, *FANCG*, *FANCL*) that respond to DNA damage.[100,101] Cells with inactivation of this pathway are hypersensitive to certain chemotherapeutics such as mitomycin C which may explain previous clinical evidence of occasional treatment responses to mitomycin C. These encouraging findings highlight the need to identify which pancreatic cancers harbor inactivation of the Fanconi anemia pathway.

In conclusion, recent years have seen an explosion of new information about molecular alterations of pancreatic cancer. This knowledge provides tremendous hope that there will soon be better diagnostic tests for pancreatic cancer and other pancreatic neoplasms, as well as a better ability to predict the biological behavior of these lesions, and to use molecular profiling information of individual cancers to predict which therapies are the ones that are most likely to be effective in destroying each individual pancreatic cancer.

References

1. Ariyama J, Suyama M, Ogawa K, et al. The detection and prognosis of small pancreatic carcinoma. *Int J Pancreatol.* 1990;7:37–47.
2. Fishman EK, Horton KM, Urban BA. Multidetector CT angiography in the evaluation of pancreatic carcinoma: preliminary observations. *J Comput Assist Tomogr.* 2000;24:849–853.
3. Bluemke DA, Cameron JL, Hruban RH, et al. Potentially resectable pancreatic adenocarcinoma: spiral CT assessment with surgical and pathologic correlation. *Radiology.* 1995;197:381–385.
4. Rosch T, Braig C, Gain T, et al. Staging of pancreatic and ampullary carcinoma by endoscopic ultrasonography: comparison with conventional sonography, computed tomography, and angiography. *Gastroenterology.* 1992;102:188–199.
5. Legmann P, Vignaux O, Dousset B, et al. Pancreatic tumors: comparison of dual-phase helical CT and endoscopic sonography. *AJR Am J Roentgenol.* 1998;170:1315–1322.
6. Abrams RA, Grochow LB, Chakravarthy A, et al. Intensified adjuvant therapy for pancreatic and periampullary adenocarcinoma: survival results and observations regarding patterns of failure, radiotherapy dose and CA19-9 levels. *Int J Radiat Oncol Biol Phys.* 1999;44:1039–1046.
7. Koopmann JZZ, White N, Rosenzweig J, et al. Serum diagnosis of pancreatic adenocarcinoma using surface-enhanced laser desorption and ionization mass spectrometry. *Clin Cancer Res.* 2004;10:860–868.
8. Hruban RH, Adsay NV, Albores-Saavedra J, et al. Pancreatic intraepithelial neoplasia: a new nomenclature and classification system for pancreatic duct lesions. *Am J Surg Pathol.* 2001;25:579–586.
9. Canto MI, Goggins M, Yeo CJ, et al. Screening for pancreatic neoplasia in high-risk individuals: a pilot study. *Clin Gastroenterol Hepatol.* 2004;2:606–621.
10. Brentnall TA, Bronner MP, Byrd DR, Haggitt RC, Kimmey MB. Early diagnosis and treatment of pancreatic dysplasia in patients with a family history of pancreatic cancer. *Ann Intern Med.* 1999;131:247–255.
11. Fukushima N, Walter KM, Uek T, et al. Diagnosing pancreatic cancer using methylation specific PCR analysis of pancreatic juice. *Cancer Biol Ther.* 2003;2:78–83.
12. Belinsky SA, Nikula KJ, Palmisano WA, et al. Aberrant methylation of p16(INK4a) is an early event in lung cancer and a potential biomarker for early diagnosis. *Proc Natl Acad Sci USA.* 1998;95:11891–11896.
13. Evron E, Dooley WC, Umbricht CB, et al. Detection of breast cancer cells in ductal lavage fluid by methylation-specific PCR. *Lancet.* 2001;357:1335–1336.
14. Castells A, Puig P, Mora J, et al. K-ras mutations in DNA extracted from the plasma of patients with pancreatic carcinoma: diagnostic utility and prognostic significance. *J Clin Oncol.* 1999;17:578–584.
15. Mulcahy HE, Lyautey J, Lederrey C, et al. A prospective study of K-ras mutations in the plasma of pancreatic cancer patients. *Clin Cancer Res.* 1998;4:271–275.
16. Yamada T, Nakamori S, Ohzato H, et al. Detection of K-ras gene mutations in plasma DNA of patients with pancreatic adenocarcinoma: correlation with clinicopathological features. *Clin Cancer Res.* 1998;4:1527–1532.
17. Wilentz RE, Chung CH, Sturm PD, et al. K-ras mutations in the duodenal fluid of patients with pancreatic carcinoma. *Cancer.* 1998;82:96–103.
18. Harden SV, Sanderson H, Goodman SN, et al. Quantitative GSTP1 methylation and the detection of prostate adenocarcinoma in sextant biopsies. *J Natl Cancer Inst.* 2003; 95:1634–1637.
19. Calhoun ES, Jones JB, Ashfaq R, et al. BRAF and FBXW7 (CDC4, FBW7, AGO, SEL10) mutations in distinct subsets of pancreatic cancer: potential therapeutic targets. *Am J Pathol.* 2003;163:1255–1260.
20. Cohen Y, Xing M, Mambo E, et al. BRAF mutation in papillary thyroid carcinoma. *J Natl Cancer Inst.* 2003;95:625–627.
21. Davies H, Bignell GR, Cox C, et al. Mutations of the BRAF gene in human cancer. *Nature.* 2002;417:949–954.
22. Kimura ET, Nikiforova MN, Zhu Z, et al. High prevalence of BRAF mutations in thyroid cancer: genetic evidence for constitutive activation of the RET/PTC-RAS-BRAF signaling pathway in papillary thyroid carcinoma. *Cancer Res.* 2003;63:1454–1457.
23. Wang L, Cunningham JM, Winters JL, et al. BRAF mutations in colon cancer are not likely attributable to defective DNA mismatch repair. *Cancer Res.* 2003;63:5209–5212.
24. Berger DH, Chang H, Wood M, et al. Mutational activation of K-ras in nonneoplastic exocrine pancreatic lesions in relation to cigarette smoking status. *Cancer.* 1999;85:326–332.
25. Caldas C, Hahn SA, Hruban RH, Redston MS, Yeo CJ, Kern SE. Detection of K-ras mutations in the stool of patients with pancreatic adenocarcinoma and pancreatic ductal hyperplasia. *Cancer Res.* 1994;54: 3568–3573.
26. Kalthoff H, Schmiegel W, Roeder C, et al. p53 and K-RAS alterations in pancreatic epithelial cell lesions. *Oncogene.* 1993;8:289–298.
27. Moskaluk CA, Hruban RH, Kern SE. p16 and K-ras mutations in the intraductal precursors of human pancreatic adenocarcinoma. *Cancer Res.* 1997;57:2140–2143.
28. Tada M, Omata M, Kawai S, et al. Detection of ras gene mutations in pancreatic juice and peripheral blood of patients with pancreatic adenocarcinoma. *Cancer Res.* 1993;53:2472–2474.
29. Redston MS, Caldas C, Seymour AB, et al. p53 mutations in pancreatic carcinoma and evidence of common involvement of homocopolymer tracts in DNA microdeletions. *Cancer Res.* 1994;54:3025–3033.
30. Hollstein M, Sidransky D, Vogelstein B, Harris CC. p53 mutations in human cancers. *Science.* 1991;253:49–53.
31. Dong SM, Traverso G, Johnson C, et al. Detecting colorectal cancer in stool with the use of multiple genetic targets. *J Natl Cancer Inst.* 2001;93:858–865.
32. Ahrendt SA, Hu Y, Buta M, et al. p53 mutations and survival in stage I non-small-cell lung cancer: results of a prospective study. *J Natl Cancer Inst.* 2003;95:961–970.
33. Yamaguchi Y, Watanabe H, Yrdiran S, et al. Detection of mutations of p53 tumor suppressor gene in pancreatic juice and its application to diagnosis of patients with pancreatic cancer: comparison with K-ras mutation. *Clin Cancer Res.* 1999;5:1147–1153.

34. Kaino M, Kondoh S, Okita S, et al. Detection of K-ras and p53 gene mutations in pancreatic juice for the diagnosis of intraductal papillary mucinous tumors. *Pancreas.* 1999;18:294–299.
35. Sturm PD, Hruban RH, Ramsoekh TB, et al. The potential diagnostic use of K-ras codon 12 and p53 alterations in brush cytology from the pancreatic head region. *J Pathol.* 1998;186:247–253.
36. Lohr M, Muller P, Mora J, et al. p53 and K-ras mutations in pancreatic juice samples from patients with chronic pancreatitis. *Gastrointest Endosc.* 2001;53:734–743.
37. Ahrendt SA, Halachmi S, Chow JT, et al. Rapid p53 sequence analysis in primary lung cancer using an oligonucleotide probe array. *Proc Natl Acad Sci USA.* 1999;96: 7382–7387.
38. Wikman FP, Lu ML, Thykjaer T, et al. Evaluation of the performance of a p53 sequencing microarray chip using 140 previously sequenced bladder tumor samples. *Clin Chem.* 2000;46:1555–1561.
39. Hahn SA, Schutte M, Hoque ATMS, et al. DPC4, a candidate tumor-suppressor gene at 18q21.1. *Science.* 1996;271: 350–353.
40. Polyak K, Li Y, Zhu H, et al. Somatic mutations of the mitochondrial genome in human colorectal tumours. *Nat Genet.* 1998;20:291–293.
41. Maitra A, Cohen Y, Gillespie SED, et al. The human mitochip: a high-throughput sequencing microarray for mitochondrial mutation detection. *Genome Res.* 2004;14: 814–819.
42. Jones JB, Song JJ, Hempen PM, Parmigiani G, Hruban RH, Kern SE. Detection of mitochondrial DNA mutations in pancreatic cancer offers a "mass"-ive advantage over detection of nuclear DNA mutations. *Cancer Res.* 1304; 61:1299–1304.
43. Fliss MS, Usadel H, Caballero OL, et al. Facile detection of mitochondrial DNA mutations in tumors and bodily fluids. *Science.* 2000;287:2017–2019.
44. Sanchez-Cespedes M, Parrella P, Nomoto S, et al. Identification of a mononucleotide repeat as a major target for mitochondrial DNA alterations in human tumors. *Cancer Res.* 2001;61:7015–7019.
45. Jeronimo C, Nomoto S, Caballero OL, et al. Mitochondrial mutations in early stage prostate cancer and bodily fluids. *Oncogene.* 2001;20:5195–5198.
46. Parrella P, Xiao Y, Fliss M, et al. Detection of mitochondrial DNA mutations in primary breast cancer and fine-needle aspirates. *Cancer Res.* 2001;61:7623–7626.
47. Nomoto S, Yamashita K, Koshikawa K, et al. Mitochondrial D-loop mutations as clonal markers in multicentric hepatocellular carcinoma and plasma. *Clin Cancer Res.* 2002;8:481–487.
48. Jones PA, Baylin SB. The fundamental role of epigenetic events in cancer. *Nat Rev Genet.* 2002;3:415–428.
49. Sato N, Fukushima N, Maehara N, et al. SPARC/osteonectin is a frequent target for aberrant methylation in pancreatic adenocarcinoma and a mediator of tumor–stromal interactions. *Oncogene.* 2003;22:5021–5030.
50. Herman JG, Graff JR, Myohanen S, Nelkin BD, Baylin SB. Methylation-specific PCR: a novel PCR assay for methylation status of CpG islands. *Proc Natl Acad Sci USA.* 1996;93:9821–9826.
51. Sato N, Fukushima N, Maitra A, et al. Discovery of novel targets for aberrant methylation in pancreatic carcinoma using high-throughput microarrays. *Cancer Res.* 2003; 63:3735–3742.
52. Esteller M, Corn PG, Baylin SB, Herman JG. A gene hypermethylation profile of human cancer. *Cancer Res.* 2001;61:3225–3229.
53. Matsubayashi H, Sato N, Fukushima N, et al. Methylation of cyclin D2 is observed frequently in pancreatic cancer but is also an age-related phenomenon in gastrointestinal tissues. *Clin Cancer Res.* 2003;9:1446–1452.
54. Sato N, U T., Fukushima N, et al. Aberrant methylation of CpG islands in intraductal papillary mucinous neoplasms of the pancreas increases with histological grade. *Gastroenterology.* 2002;123:1365–1372.
55. Ueki T, Toyota M, Sohn T, et al. Hypermethylation of multiple genes in pancreatic adenocarcinoma. *Cancer Res.* 2000;60:1835–1839.
56. Ueki T, Toyota M, Skinner H, et al. Identification and characterization of differentially methylated CpG islands in pancreatic carcinoma. *Cancer Res.* 2001;61:8540–8546.
57. Jansen M, Fukushima N, Rosty C, et al. Aberrant Methylation of the 5′ CpG island of TSLC1 is common in pancreatic ductal adenocarcinoma and is first manifest in high-grade PanlNs. *Cancer Biol Ther.* 2002;1:293–296.
58. Issa JP, Ahuja N, Toyota M, Bronner MP, Brentnall TA. Accelerated age-related CpG island methylation in ulcerative colitis. *Cancer Res.* 2001;61:3573–3577.
59. Issa JP, Ottaviano YL, Celano P, Hamilton SR, Davidson NE, Baylin SB. Methylation of the oestrogen receptor CpG island links ageing and neoplasia in human colon. *Nat Genet.* 1994;7:536–540.
60. Pao MM, Tsutsumi M, Liang G, Uzvolgyi E, Gonzales FA, Jones PA. The endothelin receptor B (EDNRB) promoter displays heterogeneous, site specific methylation patterns in normal and tumor cells. *Hum Mol Genet.* 2001;10: 903–910.
61. Nguyen C, Liang G, Nguyen TT, et al. Susceptibility of nonpromoter CpG islands to de novo methylation in normal and neoplastic cells. *J Natl Cancer Inst.* 2001;93: 1465–1472.
62. Harden SV, Sanderson H, Goodman SN, et al. Quantitative GSTP1 methylation and the detection of prostate adenocarcinoma in sextant biopsies. *J Natl Cancer Inst.* 2003;95:1634–1637.
63. Cottrell SE, Distler J, Goodman NS, et al. A real-time PCR assay for DNA-methylation using methylation-specific blockers. *Nucleic Acids Res.* 2004;32:e10.
64. Sato N, Maitra A, Fukushima N, et al. Frequent hypomethylation of multiple genes overexpressed in pan-

creatic ductal adenocarcinoma. *Cancer Res.* 2003;63: 4158–4166.

65. Rosty C, Ueki T, Argani P, et al. Overexpression of S100A4 in pancreatic ductal adenocarcinomas is associated with poor differentiation and DNA hypomethylation. *Am J Pathol.* 2002;160:45–50.
66. Iacobuzio-Donahue CA, Maitra A, Olsen M, et al. Exploration of global gene expression patterns in pancreatic adenocarcinoma using cDNA microarrays. *Am J Pathol.* 2003;162:1151–1162.
67. Jang SJ, Soria JC, Wang L, et al. Activation of melanoma antigen tumor antigens occurs early in lung carcinogenesis. *Cancer Res.* 2001;61:7959–7963.
68. Kawakami T, Okamoto K, Ogawa O, Okada Y. XIST unmethylated DNA fragments in male-derived plasma as a tumour marker for testicular cancer. *Lancet.* 2004;363:40–42.
69. Iacobuzio-Donahue CA, Maitra A, Shen-Ong GL, et al. Discovery of novel tumor markers of pancreatic cancer using global gene expression technology. *Am J Pathol.* 2002;160:1239–1249.
70. Ryu B, Jones J, Blades NJ, et al. Relationships and differentially expressed genes among pancreatic cancers examined by large-scale serial analysis of gene expression. *Cancer Res.* 2002;62:819–826.
71. Logsdon CD, Simeone DM, Binkley C, et al. Molecular profiling of pancreatic adenocarcinoma and chronic pancreatitis identifies multiple genes differentially regulated in pancreatic cancer. *Cancer Res.* 2003;63:2649–2657.
72. Crnogorac-Jurcevic T, Efthimiou E, Capelli P, et al. Gene expression profiles of pancreatic cancer and stromal desmoplasia. *Oncogene.* 2001;20:7437–7446.
73. Crnogorac-Jurcevic T, Efthimiou E, Nielsen T, et al. Expression profiling of microdissected pancreatic adenocarcinomas. *Oncogene.* 2002;21:4587–4594.
74. Iwao T, Hiyama E, Yokoyama T, et al. Telomerase activity for the preoperative diagnosis of pancreatic cancer. *J Natl Cancer Inst.* 1997;89:1621–1623.
75. Iacobuzio-Donahue CA, Ashfaq R, Maitra A, et al. Highly expressed genes in pancreatic ductal adenocarcinomas: a comprehensive characterization and comparison of the transcription profiles obtained from three major technologies. *Cancer Res.* 2003;63:8614–8622.
76. Argani P, Rosty C, Reiter RE, et al. Discovery of new markers of cancer through serial analysis of gene expression: prostate stem cell antigen is overexpressed in pancreatic adenocarcinoma. *Cancer Res.* 2001;61:4320–4324.
77. Maitra A, Iacobuzio-Donahue C, Rahman A, et al. Immunohistochemical validation of a novel epithelial and a novel stromal marker of pancreatic ductal adenocarcinoma identified by global expression microarrays: sea urchin fascin homolog and heat shock protein 47. *Am J Clin Pathol.* 2002;118:52–59.
78. Argani P, Iacobuzio-Donahue C, Ryu B, et al. Mesothelin is overexpressed in the vast majority of ductal adenocarcinomas of the pancreas: identification of a new pancreatic cancer marker by serial analysis of gene expression (SAGE). *Clin Cancer Res.* 2001;7:3862–3868.
79. McCarthy DM, Maitra A, Argani P, et al. Novel markers of pancreatic adenocarcinoma in fine-needle aspiration: mesothelin and prostate stem cell antigen labeling increases accuracy in cytologically borderline cases. *Appl Immunohistochem Mol Morphol.* 2003;11:238–243.
80. Friess H, Ding J, Kleeff J, et al. Identification of disease-specific genes in chronic pancreatitis using DNA array technology. *Ann Surg.* 2001;234:769–778; discussion 778–779.
81. Koopmann J , Buckhaults P, Brown DA, et al. Serum macrophage inhibitory cytokine 1 as a marker of pancreatic and other periampullary cancers. *Clin Cancer Res.* 2004;10:2386–2392.
82. Koopmann J, Fedarko N, Jain A, et al. Evaluation of osteopontin as biomarker for pancreatic adenocarcinoma. *Cancer Epidemiol Biomarkers Prev.* 2004;13:487–491.
83. Rosty C, Christa L, Kuzdzal S, Baldwin WM, et al. Identification of hepatocarcinoma-intestine-pancreas/pancreatitis-associated protein I as a biomarker for pancreatic ductal adenocarcinoma by protein biochip technology. *Cancer Res.* 2002;62:1868–1875.
84. Sasaki K, Sato K, Akiyama Y, Yanagihara K, Oka M, Yamaguchi K. Peptidomics-based approach reveals the secretion of the 29-residue COOH-terminal fragment of the putative tumor suppressor protein DMBT1 from pancreatic adenocarcinoma cell lines. *Cancer Res.* 2002;62: 4894–4898.
85. Valerio A, Basso D, Mazza S, et al. Serum protein profiles of patients with pancreatic cancer and chronic pancreatitis: searching for a diagnostic protein pattern. *Rapid Commun Mass Spectrom.* 2001;15:2420–2425.
86. Gronborg M, Bunkenborg J, Kristiansen TZ, Jensen ON, Yeo CJ, Hruban RH, Maitra A, Goggins MG, Pandey A. Comprehensive proteomic analysis of human pancreatic juice. *J Proteom Res.* 2004; 3:1042-1055.
87. Yeo CJ, Cameron JL. Prognostic factors in ductal pancreatic cancer. *Langenbecks Arch Surg.* 1998;383: 129–133.
88. Tascilar M, Skinner HG, Rosty C, et al. The SMAD4 protein and prognosis of pancreatic ductal adenocarcinoma. *Clin Cancer Res.* 2001;7:4115–4121.
89. Lengauer C, Kinzler KW, Vogelstein B. Genetic instability in colorectal cancers. *Nature.* 1997;386:623–627.
90. Goggins M, Offerhaus GJ, Hilgers W, et al. Pancreatic adenocarcinomas with DNA replication errors (RER+) are associated with wild-type K-ras and characteristic histopathology: poor differentiation, a syncytial growth pattern, and pushing borders suggest RER+. *Am J Pathol.* 1998;152:1501–1507.
91. Wilentz RE, Goggins M, Redston M, et al. Genetic, immunohistochemical, and clinical features of medullary carcinoma of the pancreas: a newly described and characterized entity. *Am J Pathol.* 2000;156:1641–1651.

92. Yamamoto H, Itoh F, Nakamura H, et al. Genetic and clinical features of human pancreatic ductal adenocarcinomas with widespread microsatellite instability. *Cancer Res.* 2001;61:3139–3144.
93. Sohn TA, Yeo CJ, Cameron JL, et al. Intraductal papillary mucinous neoplasms of the pancreas: an increasingly recognized clinicopathologic entity. *Ann Surg.* 2001;234: 313–321; discussion 321–322.
94. Tollefson MK, Libsch KD, Sarr MG, et al. Intraductal papillary mucinous neoplasm: did it exist prior to 1980? *Pancreas.* 2003;26:e55–e58.
95. Sato N, Fukushima N, Maitra A, et al. Gene expression profiling identifies genes associated with invasive intraductal papillary mucinous neoplasms of the pancreas. *Am J Pathol.* 2004;164:903–914.
96. Kris MG, Natale RB, Herbst RS, et al. Efficacy of gefitinib, an inhibitor of the epidermal growth factor receptor tyrosine kinase, in symptomatic patients with non-small cell lung cancer: a randomized trial. *JAMA.* 2003;290:2149–2158.
97. Mita MM, Mita A, Rowinsky EK. The molecular target of rapamycin (mTOR) as a therapeutic target against cancer. *Cancer Biol Ther.* 2003;2:S169–S177.
98. van der Heijden MS, Yeo CJ, Hruban RH, Kern SE. Fanconi anemia gene mutations in young-onset pancreatic cancer. *Cancer Res.* 2003;63:2585–2588.
99. Rogers CD, van der Heijden MS, Brune K, et al. The genetics of FANCC and FANCG in familial pancreatic cancer. *Cancer Biol Ther.* 2004;3:167–169.
100. D'Andrea AD. The Fanconi road to cancer. *Genes Dev.* 2003;17:1933–1936.
101. Meetei AR, de Winter JP, Medhurst AL, et al. A novel ubiquitin ligase is deficient in Fanconi anemia. *Nat Genet.* 2003;35:165–170.

CHAPTER

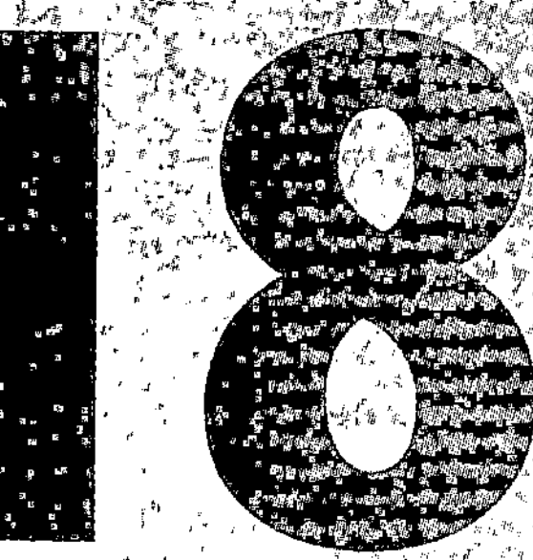

Pancreaticoduodenectomy

Tina W. F. Yen, MD
Eddie K. Abdalla, MD
Peter W. T. Pisters, MD
Douglas B. Evans, MD

The standard surgical treatment for localized, potentially resectable adenocarcinoma of the pancreatic head is pancreaticoduodenectomy, which involves the removal of the pancreatic head, duodenum, gallbladder, and bile duct, with or without the gastric antrum. In 1935, Whipple et al.[1] originally described this as a two-stage procedure consisting of biliary diversion and gastrojejunostomy during the first operation, followed by resection of the pancreatic head and duodenum after the patient recovered (approximately 3 weeks later).[1] By 1941, the world experience totaled 41 cases, with a perioperative mortality rate of 30%.[2] Because the original technique did not include reanastomosis of the pancreatic remnant to the small bowel, the high mortality rate was largely due to the development of a pancreatic fistula from the oversewn pancreatic remnant. In 1941, Whipple subsequently modified his operation to a one-stage procedure, with reconstruction including a pancreaticojejunostomy.[2] In 1946, Waugh and Claggett modified the one-stage procedure to its current form.[3]

Today, when performed at high-volume centers by experienced surgeons, the 30-day in-hospital mortality rate for pancreaticoduodenectomy is less than 2% (Table 18.1).[4-10] In contrast, recently reported mortality rates range from 7.8% to more than 10% from other university centers and Department of Veterans Affairs hospitals.[11-14] The most compelling data demonstrating that higher hospital volume and individual surgeon volume are associated with lower perioperative mortality and longer long-term survival after pancreatic resection come from Birkmeyer et al.[15-19] and are reviewed in detail by Drs. Lambert and Birkmeyer in Chapter 23.

Current treatment strategies for patients with localized pancreatic cancer are based on our understanding of the natural history and treatment failure patterns of this disease. Exocrine pancreatic cancer is characterized by infiltration of surrounding blood vessels and perineural tissues, spread to regional lymph nodes, and early vascular dissemination.[20] Patients who undergo surgical resection for localized, nonmetastatic adenocarcinoma of the pancreatic head have a long-term survival rate of approximately 20% and a median survival of 17–21 months (Table 18.2).[8,21-23] Because clinically occult metastases are present in most patients at the time of operation, disease recurrence (local or distant) after a potentially curative pancreaticoduodenectomy is common. Local recurrence occurs in up to 50% of patients, peritoneal recurrence in approximately 25%, and liver metastases in a minimum of 50%.[24-28] As pretreatment

Table 18.1 Recently Reported Perioperative Mortality Rates in Patients Who Underwent Pancreaticoduodenectomy*

Author	No. of Patients	Perioperative Mortality (%)
Balcom et al.[4]	489	1.0
Martignoni et al.[5]	257	2.3
Pisters et al.[6]	300	1.3
Sewnath et al.[7]	290	1.0
Sohn et al.[8]	564†	2.3†
Povoski et al.[9]	240	5.0
Yeo et al.[10]	650	1.4

* Includes patients who did and did not receive preoperative or postoperative chemotherapy, external-beam radiation therapy, or both.

† Includes 526 patients who underwent pancreaticoduodenectomy and 38 who underwent total pancreatectomy.

staging improves and multimodality treatment strategies enhance local control rates, liver metastases and other distant sites become the dominant form of tumor recurrence.[8,21,29,30] Therefore, current and future treatment strategies emphasize novel systemic therapies designed to treat micrometastases that are responsible for disease recurrence after a potentially curative pancreaticoduodenectomy.

Pretreatment Diagnostic Evaluation

Diagnosis and staging are covered in detail in Chapters 11–17; however, a few points deserve special comment. There is now general consensus that resectability should be assessed before laparotomy. The accurate preoperative assessment of resectability (local and distant disease) is the most critical aspect of the diagnostic evaluation in patients with pancreatic cancer. Indiscriminate use of laparotomy in all patients with presumed localized pancreatic cancer will result in low resectability rates. Patients found to have unresectable disease at the time of laparotomy have a perioperative morbidity rate of 20%–30%, a mean hospital stay of 1–2 weeks, and a median survival after surgery of approximately six months depending on disease extent and performance status.[31-33] Similarly, once the intraoperative decision has been made to proceed with pancreaticoduodenectomy, it is critically important to perform a complete resection. Patients who undergo an incomplete resection leaving grossly positive margins (R2 resection) have a survival duration of less than 1 year (Table 18.3),[8,22,28,34-37] which is no different than the survival duration seen in patients with locally advanced, unresectable disease who are treated with palliative chemotherapy and radiation.[38,39] Therefore, in contrast to the situation in selected patients with gastric or colorectal cancer, there are no data supporting palliative resection (i.e., R2) for adenocarcinoma of the pancreas.

We currently use multidetector (multislice) computed tomography (CT) to define accurately the relationship of the tumor to the celiac axis and the superior mesenteric vessels. We strongly encourage the use of objective CT criteria to define a potentially resectable carcinoma of the pancreatic head. Such criteria are mandatory for the conduct of clinical trials and are critically important for all surgeons to prevent margin-positive resections. The intraoperative finding of gross tumor encasing the superior mesenteric artery (SMA) after pancreatic transection is a preventable situation if high-

Table 18.2 Recently Reported Survival Durations in Patients with Localized Pancreatic Adenocarcinoma Who Underwent Surgical Resection of the Primary Tumor*

Author	No. of Patients	Follow-up (Months)	Median Survival (Months)	Estimated 4- or 5-Year Survival (%)
Breslin et al.[21]	132	14†	21	23
Sohn et al.[8]	612	13†	17	17
Nitecki et al.[22]	174	22‡	17.5	6.8
Geer and Brennan[23]	146	28†	18	24

* Includes patients who did and did not receive preoperative or postoperative chemotherapy, external-beam radiation therapy, or both.

† Median.

‡ Mean.

Table 18.3 Median Patient Survival Following Surgical Resection for Pancreatic Adenocarcinoma with Positive Resection Margin*

Author	No. of Patients	Margin Status	Median Survival (Months)
Neoptolemos et al.[34]	101	R1	11
Sohn et al.[8]	184	R1/2	12
Millikan et al.[35]	22	R1	8
Nishimura et al.[36]	70	R1/2	6
Sperti et al.[37]	19	R1/2	7
Nitecki et al.[22]	28	R2	9
Willett et al.[28]	37	R1/2	11

Abbreviations: R1, microscopically positive margin; R2, grossly positive margin.
* Many patients received postoperative 5-fluorouracil–based chemoradiation therapy.

quality imaging is performed before surgery. The CT findings defining a potentially resectable pancreatic cancer (American Joint Committee on Cancer [AJCC] Stages I or II; Fig. 18.1) are (1) the absence of extrapancreatic disease, (2) a patent superior mesenteric-portal vein (SMPV) confluence, assuming that it is technically possible to resect and reconstruct isolated involvement of the superior mesenteric vein (SMV) or SMPV confluence, and (3) no direct tumor extension to the celiac axis or SMA. A patient is deemed to have locally advanced, unresectable disease (AJCC Stage III) when there is clear evidence on CT images of tumor encasement of the celiac axis or SMA, defined as anything more than short-segment abutment of these vessels.

We prefer to use the term "borderline resectable" to describe a tumor that abuts the SMA or hepatic artery on one or two CT images. Surgery may be considered in such situations based on patient age and comorbidities, especially if performed as a multimodality treatment approach to include some form of neoadjuvant therapy. Short-segment occlusion of the SMV or SMPV confluence may also be classified as borderline resectable. Very rarely, a patient may have short-segment occlusion of the SMV or SMPV without arterial extension and have suitable venous anatomy for resection and reconstruction, as discussed in Chapter 22. However, occlusion of the SMPV confluence is a sign of unresectability in the majority of patients in whom this is found. Such venous occlusion is usually accompanied by arterial encasement caused by the close proximity of these vascular structures, and venous reconstruction is impossible in the absence of a patent SMV caudal to the site of obstruction, and a patent portal vein (PV) cephalad to the site of obstruction.

The accuracy of CT in predicting unresectability is well established; it is not necessary to perform a laparotomy to assess local tumor resectability.[40-42] In the absence of extrapancreatic disease, the main goal of preoperative imaging studies is to determine the relationship of the low-density tumor mass to the SMA and celiac axis, as this relationship cannot be accurately assessed at the time of laparotomy before gastric and pancreatic transection. The loss of the normal tissue plane

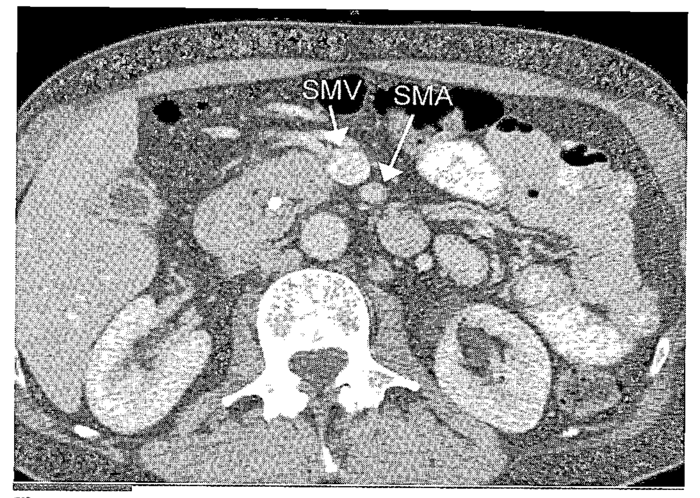

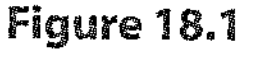

Figure 18.1
Multidetector CT scan demonstrating a resectable adenocarcinoma of the pancreatic head. The normal fat plane between the pancreatic tumor and both the SMA and the SMV is shown. Note the normal contour of the SMV at the level of the gastroepiploic vein.

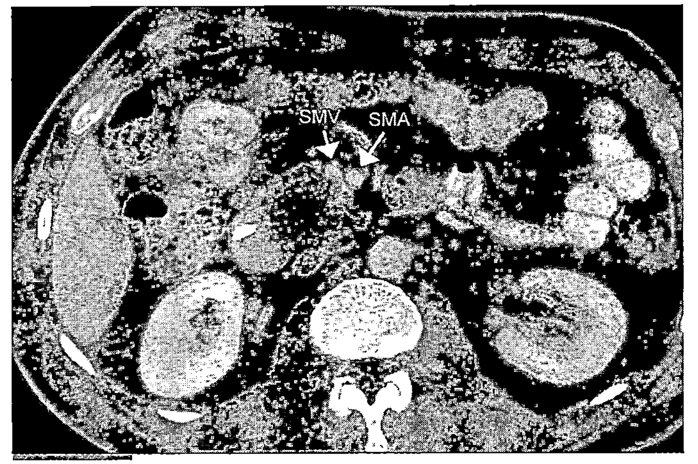

Figure 18.2
A multidetector CT scan demonstrating tumor extension to the posterior wall of the SMV. This patient will likely require venous resection and reconstruction at the time of pancreaticoduodenectomy. The tumor comes very close to the postereolateral wall of the SMA, which added further to the surgical complexity of this case.

between the tumor and the SMV (Fig. 18.2) should alert the surgeon preoperatively to the potential for direct tumor invasion of the vessel wall. If the tumor is inseparable from the lateral or posterolateral wall of the SMV or PV on preoperative CT scans, surgery should not be undertaken unless the surgeon has developed a technical strategy for the intraoperative management of this condition (see Chapter 22). When performing pancreaticoduodenectomy for malignant tumors of the pancreatic head or uncinate process, the finding of tumor adherence to the lateral or posterior walls of the SMV or SMPV confluence should not be unexpected.

Our current algorithm for the diagnosis and treatment of patients with presumed or biopsy-proven adenocarcinoma of the pancreatic head or periampullary region is illustrated in Fig. 18.3. We strongly encourage the use of protocol-based multimodality therapy and favor the delivery of chemotherapy and/or chemoradiation before surgery. This treatment strategy requires tissue confirmation of cancer and often biliary decompression. Pancreatic biopsy and endobiliary decompression are reviewed in detail in Chapters 13–15. Patients with extrahepatic biliary obstruction in the absence of a mass in the pancreas undergo diagnostic endoscopic ultrasonography (EUS), as well as diagnostic and therapeutic endoscopic retrograde cholangiopancreatography (ERCP). EUS may identify a CT-occult pancreatic mass in some patients, thereby allowing fine-needle aspiration (FNA) biopsy, followed by protocol-based neoadjuvant therapy if malignancy is confirmed.[43] Patients without a tissue diagnosis of malignancy who have clinical and radiologic findings suggestive of a pancreatic or periampullary neoplasm undergo pancreaticoduodenectomy; in general, we do not consider neoadjuvant therapy in the absence of a positive biopsy result. Such patients often have a neoplastic stricture of the intrapancreatic portion of the common bile duct on ERCP in the absence of a mass seen on CT or EUS. When possible, high-quality CT should always be performed before ERCP because ERCP-induced pancreatitis may interfere with accurate radiographic assessment of the local–regional extent of disease.

Diagnostic and therapeutic endoscopic biliary decompression is performed in most pancreatic cancer patients before definitive treatment planning. However, as discussed in Chapter 13, controversy does exist regarding the use of preoperative biliary drainage in patients with potentially resectable disease, given the potential for increased pancreaticoduodenectomy-associated morbidity and mortality.[9,44] However, the largest study examining the risk for postoperative morbidity and mortality showed an increase only in the risk of postoperative wound infection in patients who underwent preoperative biliary stent placement.[45] Furthermore, in a recently completed retrospective analysis of 300 consecutive patients who underwent pancreaticoduodenectomy, we demonstrated no increase in the risk of major postoperative complications or death associated with preoperative stent placement.[6] Others have confirmed this finding.[5] Moreover, even the subset of patients who undergo neoadjuvant chemoradiation with indwelling biliary stents do not have significant biliary stent-related complications if the duration of neoadjuvant therapy is two months or less.[46] As the duration of neoadjuvant therapy increases, metal stents will assume a greater role in the biliary management of these patients. Thus, endobiliary decompression as a part of an organized staging evaluation does not increase the risk associated with subsequent therapies, including chemoradiation and surgery. It is important to remember that the quality of the CT images will be better if CT is performed before the placement of an endobiliary stent.

Pancreaticoduodenectomy

Pancreaticoduodenectomy involves removal of the pancreatic head, duodenum, gallbladder, and bile duct, with or without removal of the gastric antrum. It represents the standard surgical procedure for neoplasms of the pancreatic head and periampullary region. Our recommended technique for pancreaticoduodenectomy uses a midline

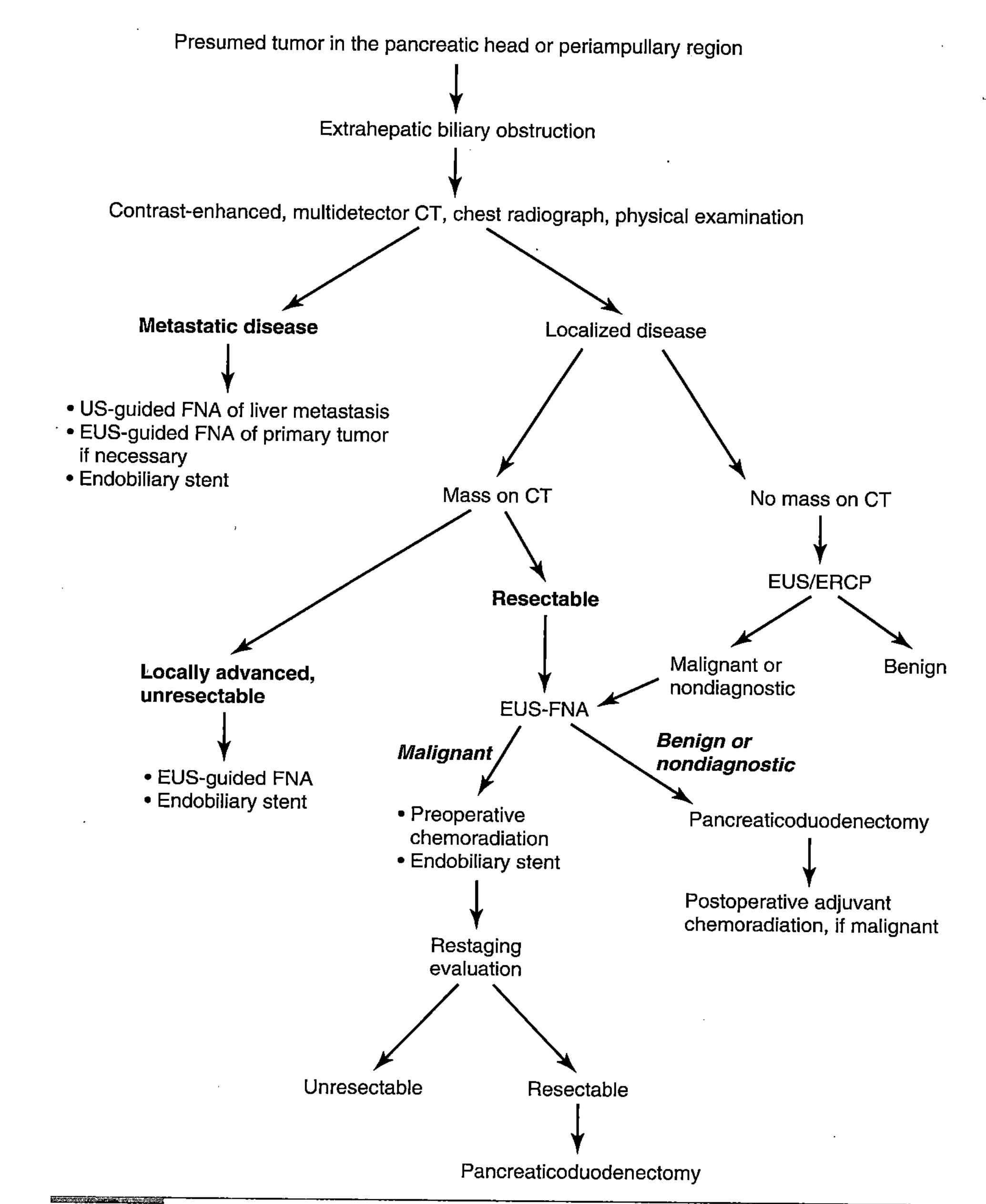

Figure 18.3
Management algorithm employed at the University of Texas M. D. Anderson Cancer Center for patients with suspected or biopsy-proven adenocarcinoma of the pancreatic head or periampullary region. Patients without a histologic or cytologic diagnosis of adenocarcinoma who have a low-attenuation, resectable mass in the pancreatic head on contrast-enhanced CT undergo EUS-guided FNA biopsy. The development of EUS-guided FNA has greatly simplified tissue acquisition in patients with localized, nonmetastatic pancreatic cancer. In the absence of a mass on CT, diagnostic EUS and ERCP are usually performed. When there is no obvious mass to biopsy or if pretreatment biopsies are nondiagnostic, patients who have clinical and radiologic findings suggestive of a pancreatic or periampullary neoplasm undergo pancreaticoduodenectomy.

or bilateral subcostal incision. When opening the abdomen, we carefully preserve the falciform ligament for later use as coverage of the gastroduodenal artery (GDA) stump. Exposure is achieved with a Thompson retractor (Thompson Surgical Instruments, Inc., Traverse City, MI) or other self-retaining retractor. The abdomen is first carefully explored to exclude extrapancreatic metastatic disease. The liver and peritoneal surfaces are examined, and intraoperative ultrasonography of the liver is used if preoperative CT findings are indeterminate but suggestive of hepatic metastasis. Suspected liver or peritoneal metastatic lesions are biopsied, and the material is submitted for frozen-section histologic analysis. We do not proceed with tumor resection when biopsy-proven liver or peritoneal metastases are found.

There is no indication for routine intraoperative pancreatic biopsy in patients who have resectable disease. One reason is that tumor cells can be disseminated in the peritoneum during surgical manipulation and intraoperative large-needle pancreatic biopsy.[47] In addition, intraoperative pancreatic biopsy has been associated with significant complications, such as pancreatitis, pancreatic fistula formation, and hemorrhage.[48] Nevertheless, because many surgeons perceive that preoperative EUS–FNA is unnecessary, patients who have presumed periampullary or pancreatic neoplasms are often brought to the operating room for a planned intraoperative diagnostic biopsy followed by extirpative surgery. If the frozen-section findings are negative, many surgeons do not proceed with pancreatic resection because they are concerned about unnecessarily performing an extensive operation for benign disease.[48,49] Unnecessary and preventable patient morbidity occurs when laparotomy and/or an open pancreatic biopsy are used as diagnostic studies. In addition, if a preoperative or intraoperative FNA result is benign or nondiagnostic, it may be a mistake to assume that the patient does not have cancer when the clinical presentation and imaging studies indicate otherwise.[43]

Whether to perform lymph node biopsy for frozen-section analysis remains controversial. Although positive lymph nodes are a prognostic factor (along with positive resection margins and increased tumor size) that predicts decreased survival,[8,21] microscopic metastases are found in regional lymph nodes on permanent-section pathologic evaluation in 60%-90% of patients who undergo pancreaticoduodenectomy. In a good-risk patient with localized, resectable pancreatic cancer, we do not currently view lymph node metastases as an absolute contraindication to pancreaticoduodenectomy when surgical resection of the pancreas is part of a combined-modality treatment approach.[50] Therefore, we do not generally perform random lymph node sampling for frozen-section analysis at the time of pancreaticoduodenectomy. However, each case should be considered individually. For example, when a patient is high risk because of medical comorbidities or oncologic concerns (such as a very high CA 19-9 level) and has suspicious adenopathy, a positive regional lymph node may be viewed as a contraindication to pancreaticoduodenectomy.

In contrast to historical teaching, we do not feel that local tumor resectability can be accurately assessed at the time of operation before gastric and pancreatic transection. Therefore, we do not begin the operation with a Kocher maneuver (Fig. 18.4). The relationship of the tumor to the right lateral wall of the SMA cannot be accurately assessed intraoperatively after a Kocher maneuver, particularly in the case of larger tumors, tumors with significant peritumoral fibrosis, and reoperation after a previous unsuccessful attempt at pancreaticoduodenectomy. Accurate preoperative CT imaging has replaced the Kocher maneuver for assessment of possible SMA involvement. Another maneuver traditionally performed to assess resectability involves dissection between the anterior surface of the SMPV confluence and the posterior surface of the pancreatic neck to exclude tumor involvement of the SMV or SMPV confluence (Fig. 18.5). Such tumor involvement precludes resection in the opinion of many surgeons. However, tumors of the pancreatic head or uncinate process are prone to invade the lateral or posterior wall of the SMPV confluence. The anterior wall of the

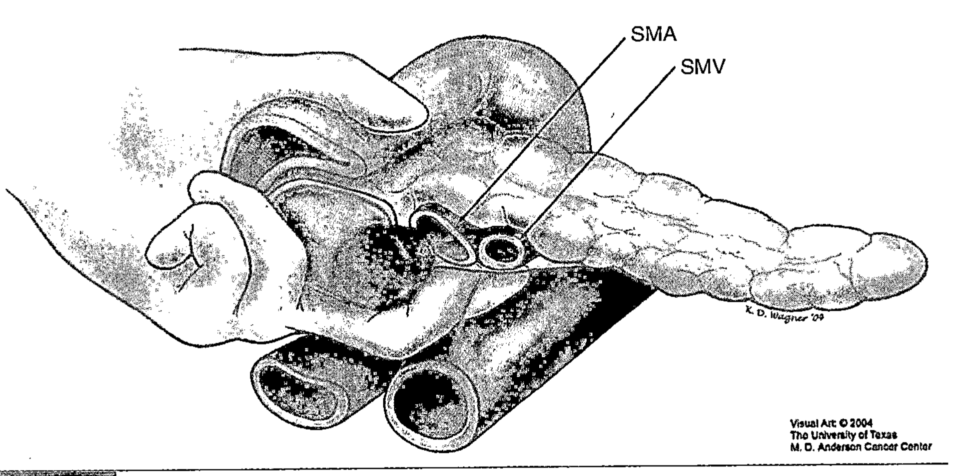

Figure 18.4
Intraoperative palpation to determine the relationship of the tumor to the mesenteric vessels at the time of the Kocher maneuver; a maneuver illustrated for historical interest. We do not perform this maneuver, as it is difficult or impossible to assess accurately the relationship of the tumor to the posterior pulsation of the SMA by palpation. Importantly, it may convey to the surgeon incorrect information, suggesting that the tumor is resectable or unresectable. Preoperative assessment of this critical tumor–vessel relationship is the goal of preoperative CT imaging, which is much more accurate than intraoperative palpation.

SMV or SMPV confluence is rarely involved in the absence of encasement of the celiac axis or SMA origin, as seen with locally advanced tumors of the pancreatic neck or body. The relationship of a pancreatic head tumor to the lateral and posterior walls of the SMPV confluence and the SMA can be directly assessed only after gastric and pancreatic transection, at which point the surgeon is already committed to resection. Again, preoperative imaging using high-quality, contrast-enhanced CT can alert the surgeon to the possible need for venous resection and reconstruction.[50,51]

The technique of pancreaticoduodenectomy currently used at our institution emphasizes the importance of removing all soft tissue to the right of the SMA.[50] The surgical resection is divided into the following steps:

1. Separation of the colon and its mesentery from the duodenum and pancreatic head and isolation of the infrapancreatic SMV (Fig. 18.6): The lesser sac is entered by separating the greater omentum from the transverse colon. The right colon and hepatic flexure are mobilized from their retroperitoneal attachments. The right colon mobilization is extended to include the visceral peritoneum of the small bowel up to the ligament of Treitz, as initially described by Cattell and Braasch.[52] When complete, this maneuver allows cephalad retraction of the right colon and small bowel, exposing the third and fourth portions of the duodenum. Such exposure facilitates the subsequent mobilization of the duodenum (Step 2) and dissection of the duodenum from the root of the mesentery (Step 5). The mesentery along the inferior border of the pancreas from a point medial to (to the patient's left of) the middle colic vessels is incised and carried out laterally and inferiorly to expose the junction of the middle colic vein and the SMV. The middle colic vein may enter directly into the anterior surface of the infrapancreatic SMV or arise as a common trunk with the gastroepiploic vein (gastrocolic trunk). If the middle colic vein and gastroepiploic vein share a common trunk, the common trunk can be divided; otherwise, the gastroepiploic vein is left intact and divided after pancreatic transection. The middle colic vein is usually divided proximal to its junction with the SMV. Division of the middle colic vein often allows greater exposure of the infrapancreatic SMV and prevents iatrogenic traction injury to the SMV during dissection of the middle colic vein–SMV junction, especially when dealing with large tumors or tumors extending inferiorly from the uncinate process. In fact, the base of the transverse mesocolon and the anterior leaf of the small bowel mesentery can be left attached to the tumor and resected en bloc with the pancreatic head. Such caudal or inferior tumor extension is not a contraindication to pancreaticoduodenectomy but does add complexity to the operation

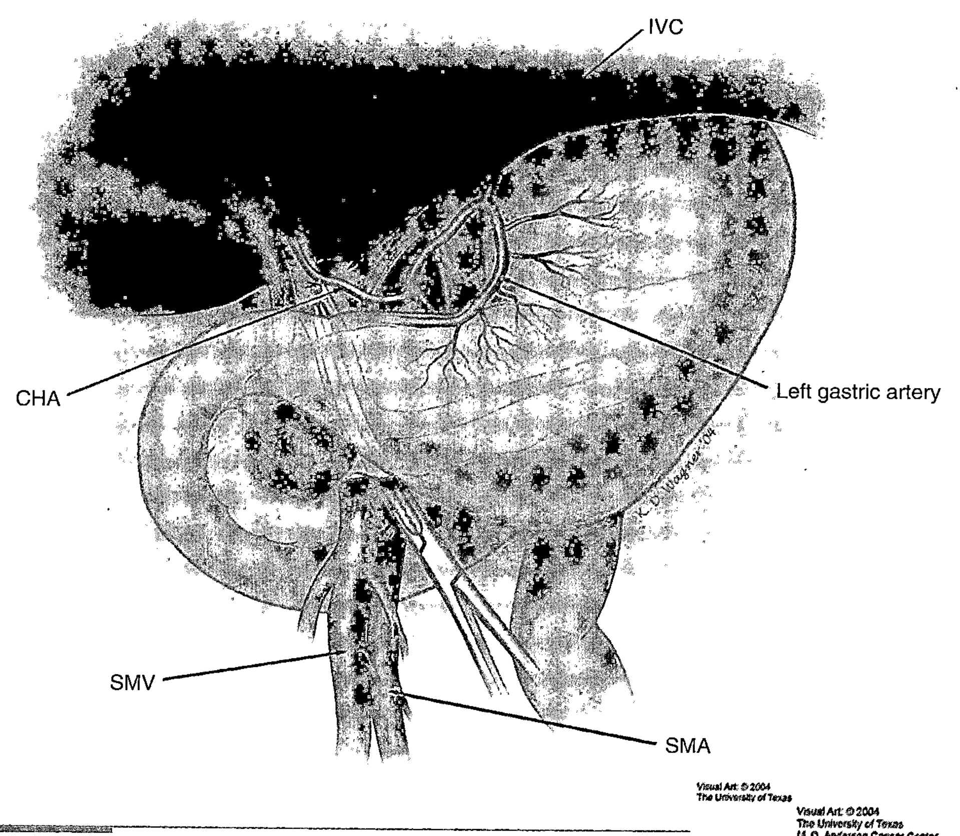

Figure 18.5
An illustration demonstrating a maneuver commonly performed early in pancreaticoduodenectomy to detect tumor invasion of the SMV or SMPV confluence. We do not perform this maneuver because a tumor-free plane often can be developed despite fixation of the tumor to the lateral wall of the SMV. This maneuver may incorrectly suggest that tumor adherence to the SMV does not exist and may result in unnecessary bleeding if the SMV or PV is injured. CHA = common hepatic artery; IVC = inferior vena cava.

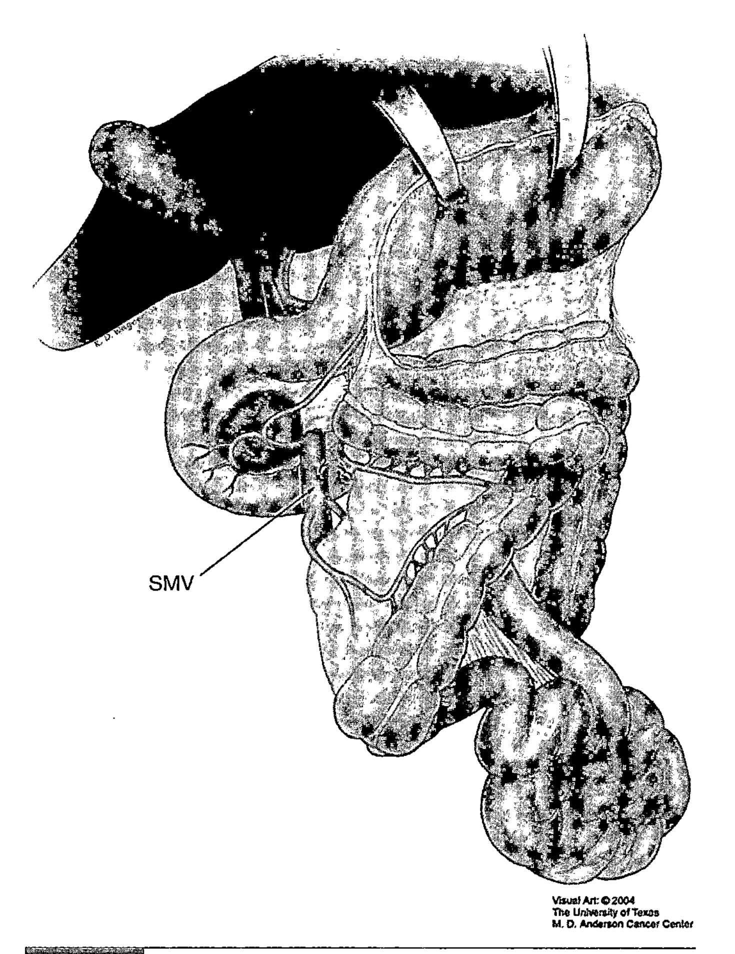

Figure 18.6
An illustration of Step 1. The lesser sac is entered, and the colon and the root of the small bowel mesentery are mobilized in the fashion of Cattell and Braasch.[52] This involves incision of the visceral peritoneum of the small bowel to the ligament of Treitz. This allows anterior reflection of the colon off of the duodenum and pancreatic head. The middle colic vein may be divided, and the SMV is exposed at the inferior border of the neck of the pancreas adjacent to the uncinate process.

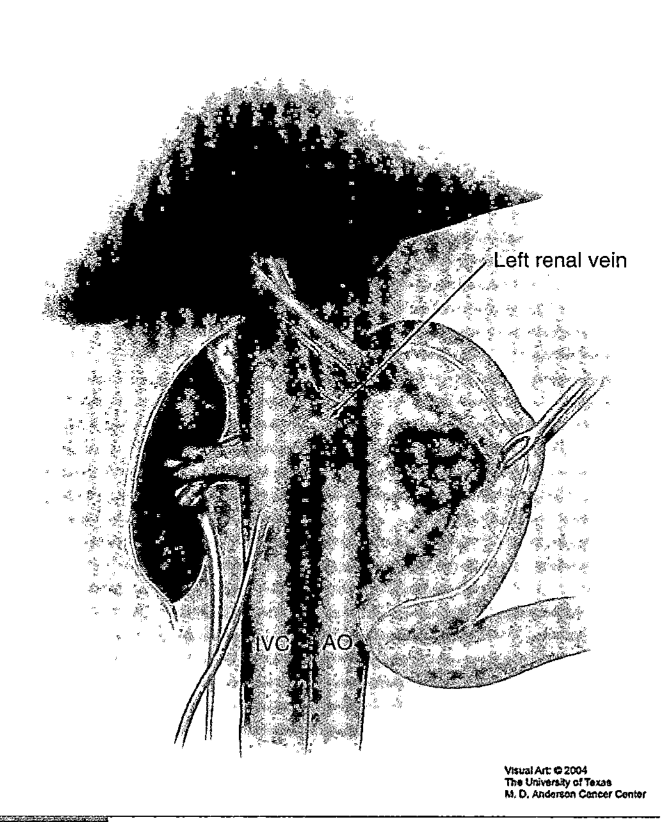

Figure 18.7
An illustration of Step 2. An extended Kocher maneuver has been performed. The right gonadal vein is usually preserved if possible, as it serves as a good landmark to help prevent inadvertent injury to the underlying ureter (which is usually posterior and slightly lateral to the gonadal vein). The Kocher maneuver is extended to the left lateral border of the aorta (AO). IVC = inferior vena cava.

during this step when the infrapancreatic SMV needs to be identified.

2. Extended Kocher maneuver: This maneuver is begun at the transverse portion (third portion) of the duodenum by identifying the inferior vena cava. All fibrofatty and lymphatic tissue medial to the right ureter and anterior to the inferior vena cava is elevated, along with the pancreatic head and duodenum (Fig. 18.7). The Kocher maneuver is continued to the left lateral edge of the aorta, with care to identify the left renal vein. The right gonadal vein is usually preserved as it courses anterior to the right ureter and serves as a good landmark to help prevent inadvertent injury to the ureter. A complete Kocher maneuver is necessary for the subsequent dissection of the pancreatic head from the SMA (Step 6). Particularly important is the division of the leaf of peritoneum that is posterior to the mesenteric vessels; incision of this portion of peritoneum is necessary before performing the SMA dissection.
3. Dissection of the porta hepatis: The portal dissection is initiated by removing the lymph node that lies directly anterior to the common hepatic artery (CHA) proximal to the right gastric artery and GDA. This facilitates exposure of the CHA proximal and distal to the GDA. The right gastric artery and GDA are then ligated and divided

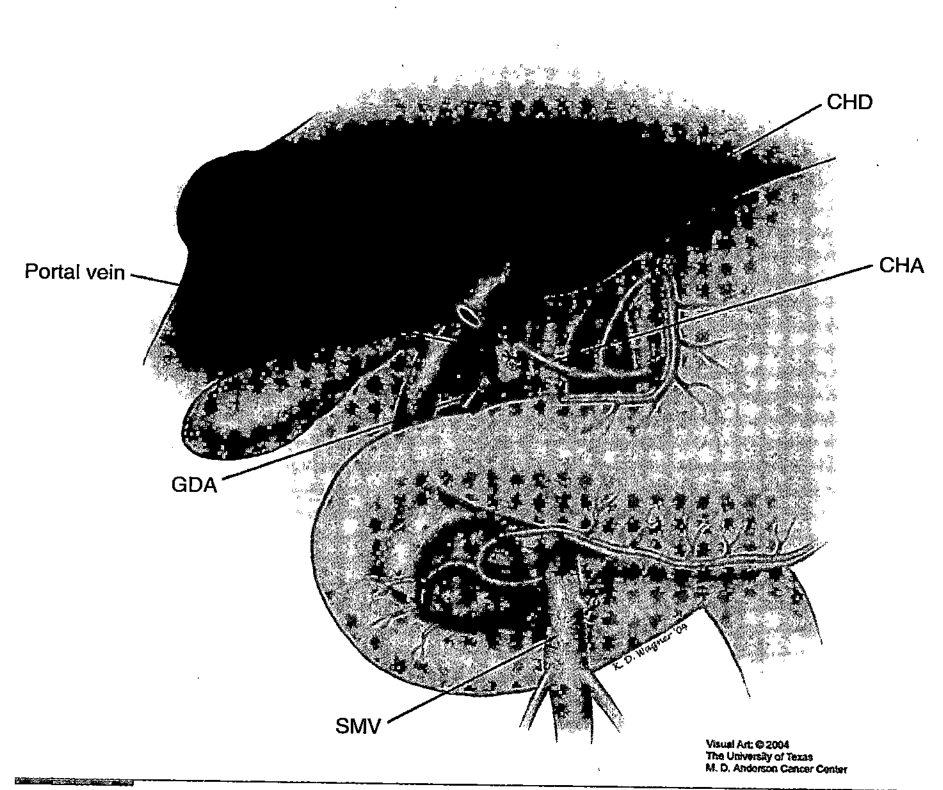

Figure 18.8
An illustration of Step 3. Dissection of the porta hepatis begins with identification of the CHA, followed by ligation and division of the right gastric artery (not shown) and the GDA. This allows the CHA-proper hepatic artery to be mobilized cephalad and medial. The anterior surface of the PV is then easily identified before division of the common hepatic duct (CHD). Careful palpation before division of the bile duct should alert one to the possibility of an accessory or replaced right hepatic artery traveling posterior to the bile duct. The CHD is divided at the level of the cystic duct. Step 3 and Step 6 are the most technically difficult parts of pancreaticoduodenectomy.

(Fig. 18.8). If the tumor extends to within a few millimeters of the GDA, one should obtain proximal and distal control of the hepatic artery and then divide the GDA flush at its origin. The resulting arteriotomy can be closed primarily with interrupted 6–0 Prolene sutures, often using a small vascular pledget, as the hepatic artery can be quite fragile. Dissection of the hepatic artery should be performed with gentle, sharp dissection, especially in patients who have received prior chemotherapy or chemoradiation and in those with extensive peritumoral inflammation from a previous laparotomy or stent-related pancreatitis. Blunt dissection at the GDA origin can result in intimal dissection of the hepatic artery. Division of the GDA allows mobilization of the hepatic artery and exposure of the anterior surface of the PV directly posterior to the inferior border of the CHA. The PV should always be exposed in this way before dividing the common hepatic duct. Cholecystectomy is then performed, and the common hepatic duct is transected at its junction with the cystic duct. Biliary fluid cultures are sent, and the indwelling biliary stent, when present, is removed. We place a gentle bulldog clamp on the transected bile duct to prevent bile spillage until the time of bile duct reconstruction. When this is not possible because of portal soft tissue fibrosis secondary to radiation treatment or prior surgery, Surgicel (Ethicon, Inc., Somerville, NJ) can be packed into the ostium of the common hepatic duct to prevent ongoing peritoneal contamination.

Review of the preoperative CT scan and careful palpation of the porta hepatis before division of the bile duct should alert one to the possibility of anomalous hepatic arterial circulation. A replaced or accessory right hepatic artery arising from the proximal SMA may course posterolateral to the PV. Rarely, the entire CHA may arise from the SMA (type IX hepatic arterial anatomy). Fatal hepatic necrosis can result if this is unrecognized and the vessel is sacrificed. If the foramen of Winslow was initially closed because of adhesions, it should have been re-established at the time of the Kocher maneuver (Step 2). Access to the foramen of Winslow is necessary to palpate the porta hepatis and appreciate anomalous hepatic arterial circulation. Rarely, the right hepatic artery arising from the proper hepatic artery courses posterior to the PV. In addition, a low-lying right hepatic artery (arising from the CHA) may be injured when the bile duct is divided in an inflamed porta hepatis.

The anterior wall of the PV is further exposed after division of the common hepatic duct and medial retraction of the CHA. The PV itself should be identified but not extensively mobilized until Step 6, at which time the stomach and pancreas have been divided. The superior pancreaticoduodenal vein is a constant venous tributary of the PV,

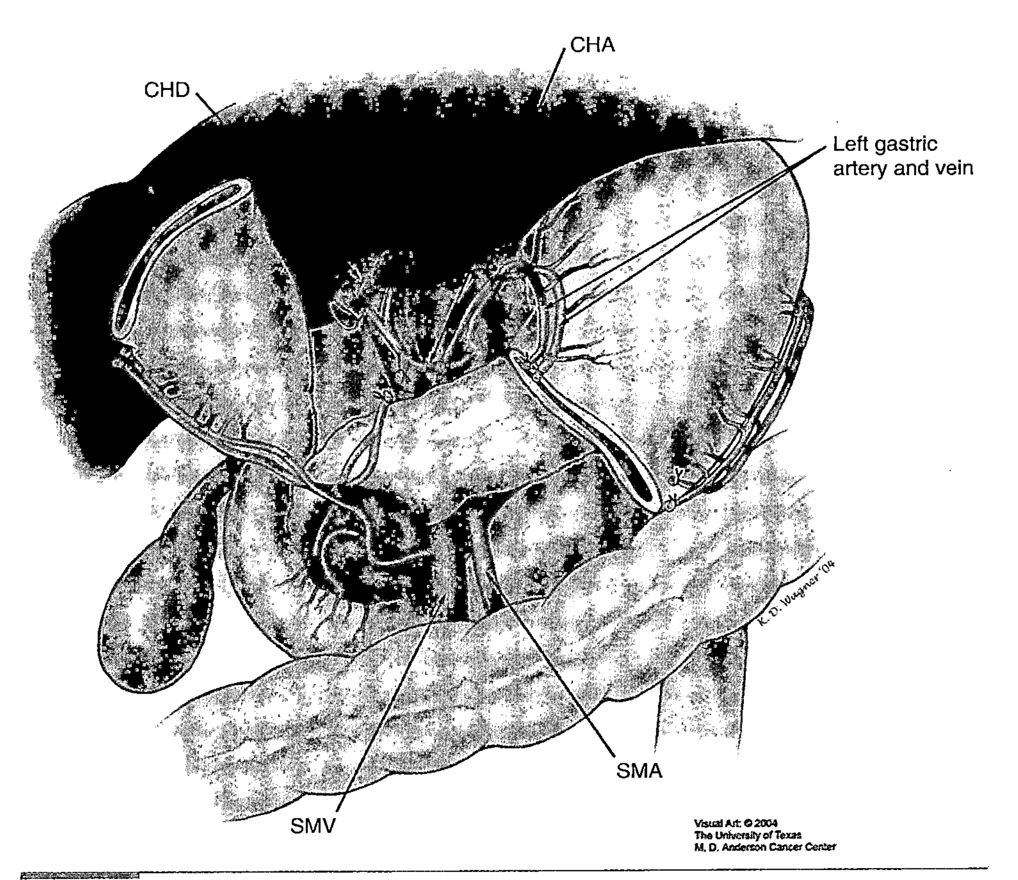

Figure 18.9
An illustration of Step 4. The antrum of the stomach is resected with the main specimen by dividing the stomach at the level of the third or fourth transverse vein on the lesser curvature. CHA = common hepatic artery; CHD = common hepatic duct.

which drains the cephalad aspect of the pancreatic head and is located at the superolateral aspect of the PV. Bleeding caused by traction injury to this venous tributary may be difficult to control at this time in the operation.

4. Transection of the gastric antrum (or the duodenum if pylorus preservation is planned): The terminal branches of the left gastric artery along the lesser curvature of the stomach are ligated and divided. The stomach is then transected with a linear gastrointestinal stapler (Ethicon, Inc.) at the level of the third or fourth transverse vein on the lesser curvature and at the confluence of the gastroepiploic veins on the greater curvature so as to perform a standard antrectomy (Fig. 18.9). The omentum is divided at the level of the greater curvature transection with the harmonic scalpel (Ethicon, Inc.). Pylorus preservation may be considered in patients with small periampullary neoplasms but should not be performed in patients with bulky pancreatic head tumors, duodenal tumors involving the first or second portions of the duodenum, or lesions associated with grossly positive pyloric or peripyloric lymph nodes. To ensure adequate blood supply to the duodenojejunostomy (if pylorus preservation is performed), the anastomosis is created 1.0–1.5 cm from the pylorus (please refer to Chapter 21 for a complete discussion of pylorus preservation).
5. Transection of the jejunum: The loose attachments of the ligament of Treitz are taken down with care to avoid injury to the inferior mesenteric vein. The jejunum is then transected with a linear gastrointestinal stapler approximately 10 cm distal to the ligament of Treitz, and its mesentery is sequentially ligated and divided (Fig. 18.10). We prefer to tie the mesenteric side (staying side) and use the harmonic scalpel on the serosal (bowel) side. This dis-

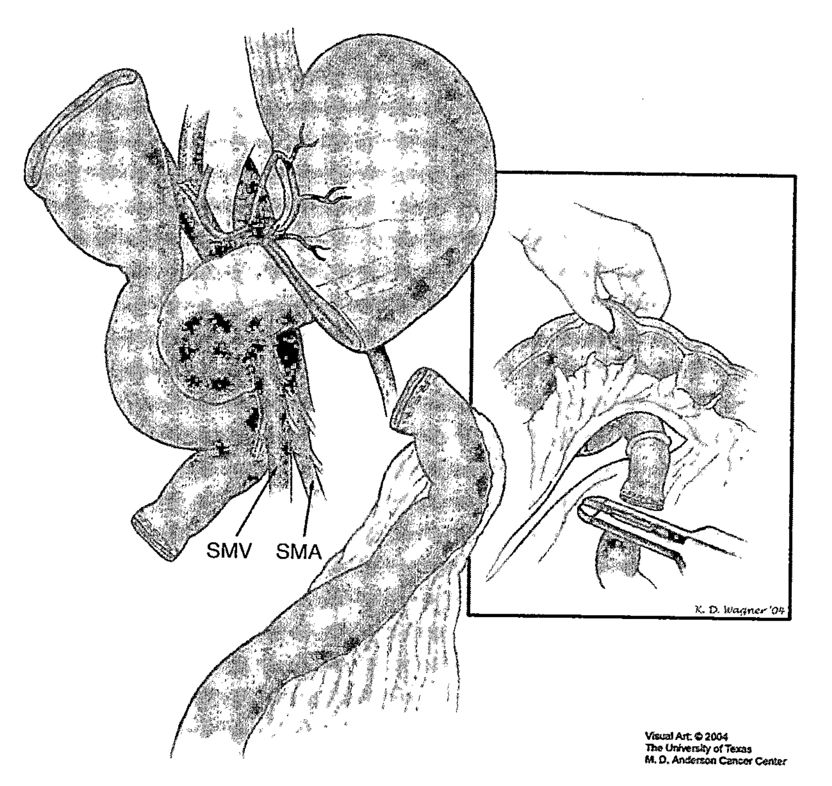

Figure 18.10
An illustration of Step 5. Transection of the jejunum is followed by ligation and division of its mesentery. The loose attachments of the ligament of Treitz are taken down, and the fourth and then third portions of the duodenum are mobilized by dividing their short mesenteric vessels. The duodenum and jejunum are then reflected underneath the mesenteric vessels in preparation for the final and most important step of pancreaticoduodenectomy.

section is continued proximally to involve the fourth and then third portions of the duodenum. The duodenal mesentery is similarly divided to the level of the aorta, allowing the devascularized segment of duodenum and jejunum to be reflected beneath the mesenteric vessels.

6. Transection of the pancreas and completion of the retroperitoneal dissection: The most oncologically important and difficult part of the operation involves the complete mobilization of the SMPV confluence and separation of the specimen from the right lateral border of the SMA. After traction sutures are placed on the superior and especially inferior borders of the pancreatic neck, the pancreas is transected with electrocautery in an anterior to posterior direction down to the anterior surface of the SMPV confluence. Bleeding from the cut surface of the pancreas should not be a problem if the small artery along the inferior border of the pancreas is ligated before pancreatic transection. If there is evidence of tumor adherence to the PV or SMV, the pancreas can be divided at a more distal location (along the left or medial border of the SMPV confluence) in preparation for segmental venous resection, as discussed in Chapter 22. The pancreas is separated from the SMV by reflecting the specimen laterally and separating it from the PV and SMV by the ligation and division of the small venous tributaries to the uncinate process and pancreatic head (Fig. 18.11). The uncinate process must be completely removed from the SMV and its first jejunal branch to ensure full mobilization of the SMPV confluence and subsequent identification of the SMA. Failure to mobilize fully the SMPV confluence risks injury to the SMA and usually results in a positive margin of resection caused by incomplete removal of the uncinate process and the mesenteric soft tissue adjacent to the SMA (Fig. 18.12). In more complicated situations, such as those usually requiring venous resection, the SMA can be identified medial to the SMV; however, the traditional approach for a standard pancreaticoduodenectomy is to expose the SMA posterolateral to the SMV by fully mobilizing the SMPV confluence.

Proper mobilization of the SMV involves identification of the first jejunal branch of the SMV. This branch originates from the right posterolateral aspect of the SMV (at the level of the

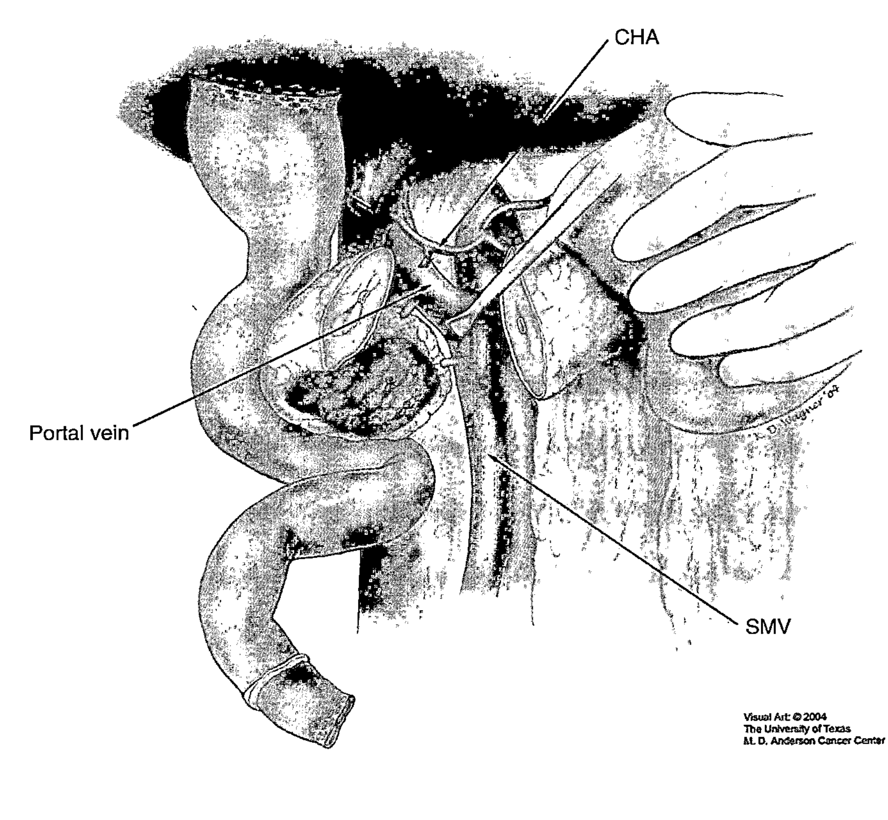

Figure 18.11
An illustration of Step 6. The pancreatic head and uncinate process are separated from the SMPV confluence. The pancreas has been transected at the level of the portal vein and reflected laterally, allowing identification of small venous tributaries to the portal vein and SMV. These tributaries are ligated and divided. CHA = common hepatic artery.

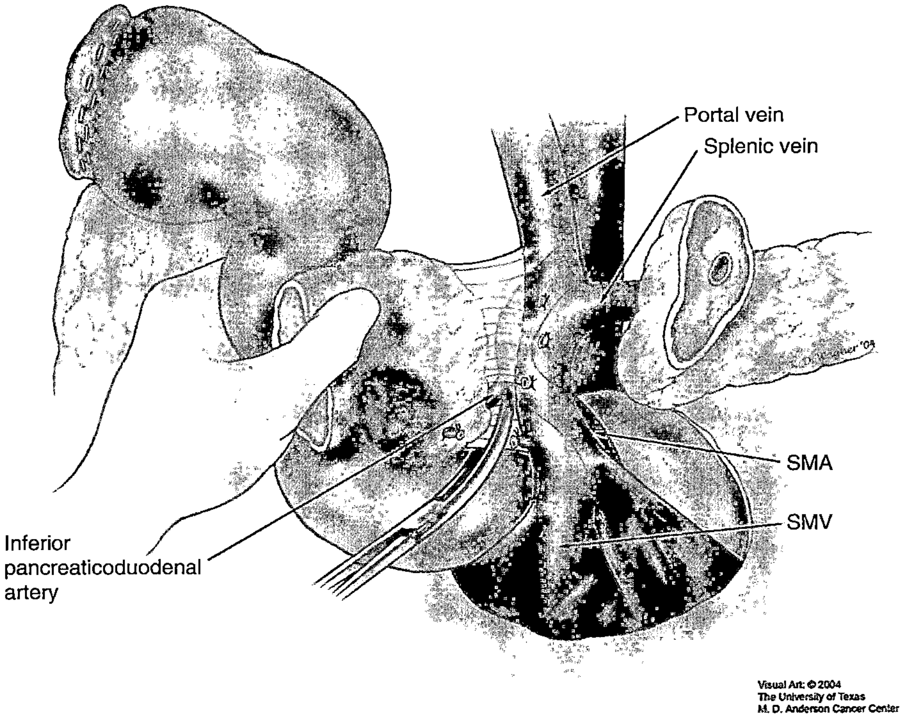

Figure 18.12
An illustration of attempted removal of the pancreaticoduodenectomy specimen from the mesenteric vessels without mobilization of the SMPV confluence and direct identification of the SMA. This maneuver should not be performed, as it is associated with two potential complications: iatrogenic injury to the SMA and inadequate control of the inferior pancreaticoduodenal arteries due to their mass ligation with adjacent soft tissue. The failure to identify directly and ligate individually the inferior pancreaticoduodenal arteries is the major cause of postoperative hemorrhage. SMA injury and postoperative retroperitoneal hemorrhage are avoidable complications if the SMA is routinely exposed for identification. This technique also facilitates a complete retroperitoneal dissection minimizing the risk of the operation resulting in a margin positive resection.

uncinate process), travels posterior to the SMA, and enters the medial (proximal) aspect of the jejunal mesentery (Fig. 18.13). This first jejunal branch usually has two or three venous tributaries draining the uncinate process; these tributaries need to be divided. If tumor involvement of the SMV at the level of the first jejunal branch prevents dissection of the uncinate process from the SMV, the first jejunal branch should be divided. Division of the first jejunal branch is per-

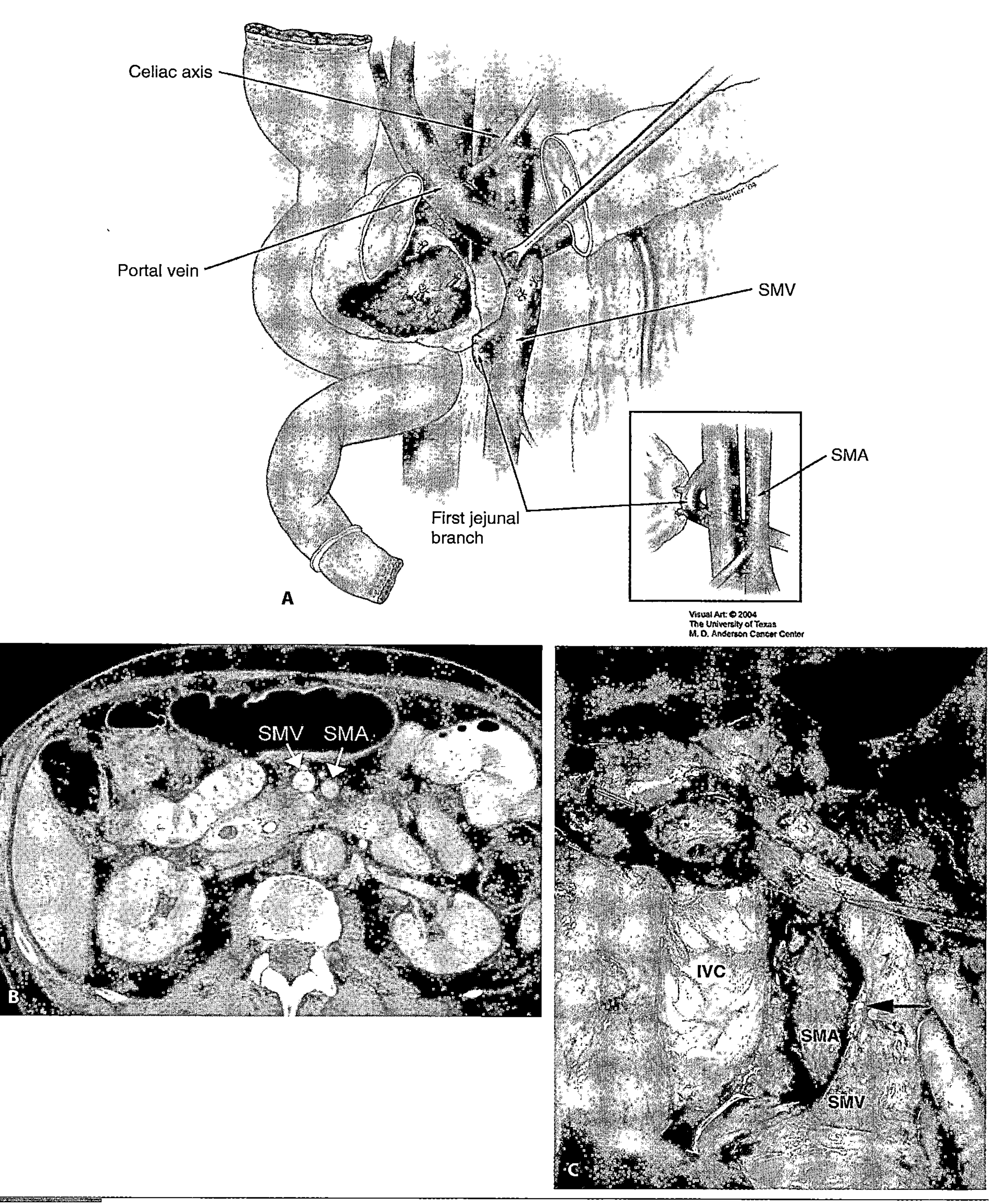

Figure 18.13

(A) An illustration of the important surgical anatomy of the SMV at the level of the uncinate process. The first jejunal branch of the SMV drains the proximal jejunum, travels posterior to the SMA, and enters the SMV along its posterolateral wall. The first jejunal branch usually has a few venous tributaries that drain the uncinate process *(inset).* If necessary, the first jejunal branch can be divided. The most feared complication during this part of the operation is a tangential laceration of the first jejunal branch extending posterior to the SMA. In an attempt to control such an injury, poorly placed sutures may result in an injury to the SMA. Very rarely, the first jejunal branch will travel anterior to the SMA. **(B)** A multidetector CT scan demonstrating tumor extension to the first jejunal branch of the SMV. **(C)** An intraoperative photograph showing how it was operatively managed. The first jejunal branch was divided proximal to the site of tumor involvement and again at the level of the SMV. The resulting venotomy in the SMV was repaired with a saphenous vein patch *(marked with the arrow).*

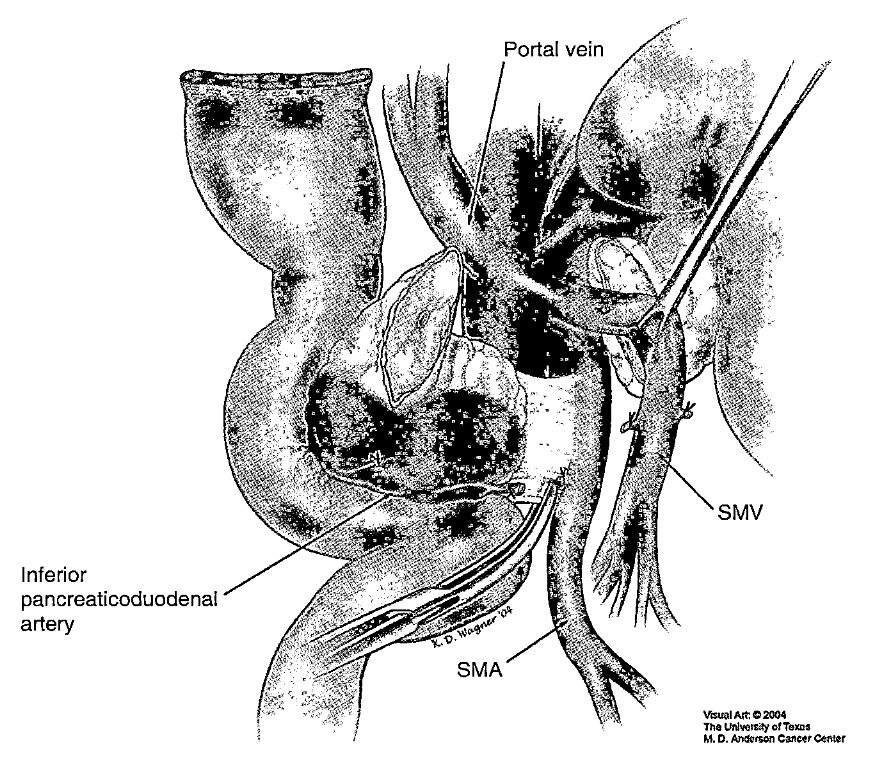

Figure 18.14
An illustration of the continuation of Step 6, and the final step in resection of the pancreaticoduodenectomy specimen. Medial retraction of the SMPV confluence facilitates dissection of the soft tissues adjacent to the lateral wall of the proximal SMA; this site represents the retroperitoneal margin. The inferior pancreaticoduodenal artery (or arteries) is identified at its origin from the SMA and is ligated and divided.

formed by exposing the SMA medial to the SMV and dividing the mesenteric soft tissue between these vessels in a posterior direction until the first jejunal branch is identified proximal to its junction with the SMV where it can then be ligated. Injury to the distal SMV at the level of the first jejunal branch or a tangential laceration in its first jejunal branch as it courses posterior to the SMA is hard to control and probably represents the most frequent cause of iatrogenic SMA injury as one attempts to suture a venous injury before full exposure of the SMA.

Once the uncinate process is separated from the distal SMV, medial retraction of the SMPV confluence allows identification of the SMA lateral to the SMPV confluence and facilitates dissection of the pancreatic head and associated soft tissues off of the right lateral wall of the proximal SMA (Fig. 18.14). Most patients have one or two pancreaticoduodenal arteries that are identified and ligated in continuity at their origins from the SMA. Failure to identify accurately and ligate these vessels may be a common cause of early postoperative bleeding. A representative intraoperative photograph of the resected pancreatic bed is illustrated in Fig. 18.15.

The soft tissue adjacent to the right lateral border of the proximal 3–4 cm of the SMA represents the retroperitoneal margin, also termed the "mesenteric margin" or the "uncinate margin".[53] Close attention must be paid to this margin given the high incidence of local recurrence after standard pancreaticoduodenectomy. A grossly positive (R2) retroperitoneal margin should not be found if high-quality preoperative imaging is performed. A microscopically positive (R1) retroperitoneal margin will occur in 10%–20% of cases.[21] An R1 resection may occur despite a gross complete resection due to perineural invasion along the mesenteric plexus at the SMA origin and tumor cell infiltration of lymphatic vessels and connective tissue that extends microscopically beyond the confines of the palpable tumor.[54,55]

Pathologic Assessment of Pancreaticoduodenectomy Specimens

Frozen-section evaluation of the pancreaticoduodenectomy specimen is limited to analysis of the common hepatic duct and pancreatic transection margins. In general, positive resection margins on the biliary or pancreatic duct are an indication for further resection until clear margins are achieved. However, changes caused by pancreatitis should not be confused with margin positivity. Pancreatitis usually involves the pancreatic body and tail distal to the tumor and may result in dysplastic cells at the pancreatic transection margin on frozen-section evaluation. Further resection of the pancreas should be performed only if there is histologic evidence on frozen-section analysis of invasive carcinoma at the margin. Dysplasia (low-grade) in the absence of invasive carcinoma or carcinoma in situ (high-grade dysplasia) is usually not an indication for further pancreatic resection. Invasive carcinoma extending along the main pancreatic duct is uncommon.

Complete permanent-section analysis of the pancreaticoduodenectomy specimen involves evaluation of the retroperitoneal margin on permanent sections by inking the margin and sectioning the tumor perpendicular to the margin (Fig. 18.16). It is critical that the surgeon identify this margin at the time of resection because it cannot be assessed retrospectively and many pathologists cannot accurately identify the retroperitoneal margin on a pancreaticoduodenectomy specimen. The differentiation between a microscopically negative margin (RO) and a microscopically positive

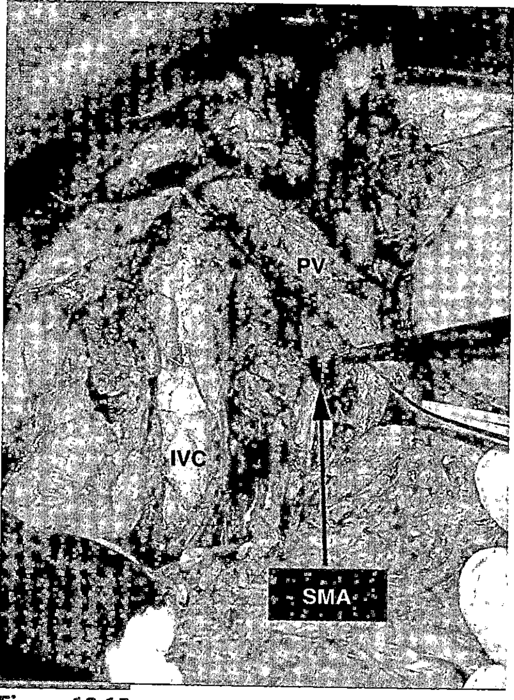

Figure 18.15
An intraoperative photograph of the right upper quadrant following pancreaticoduodenectomy. The relationship between the SMV, SMA, and retroperitoneal margin is clearly illustrated. IVC = inferior vena cava.

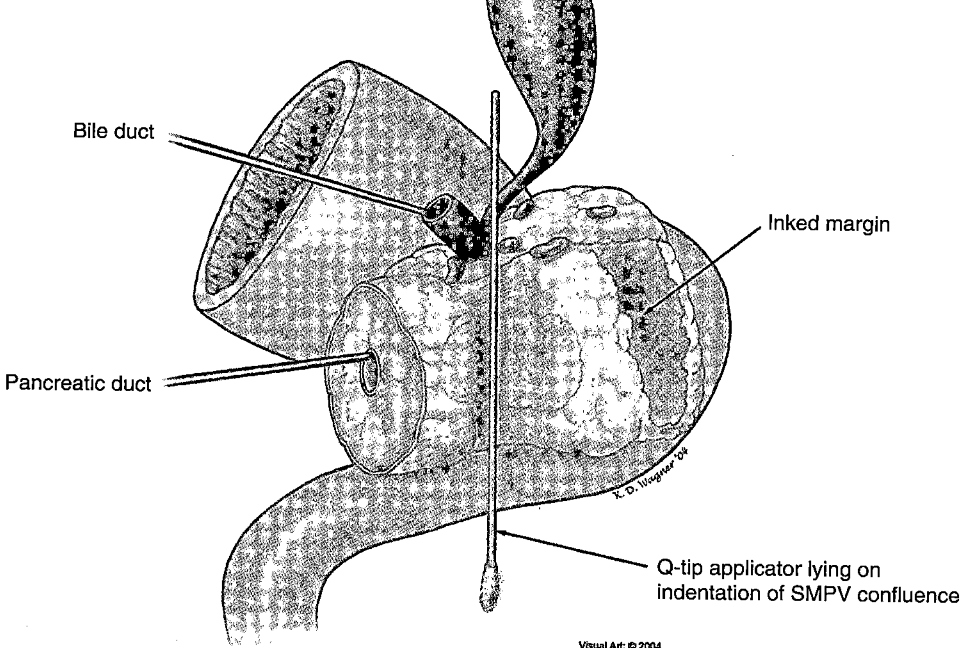

Figure 18.16
An illustration of a pancreaticoduodenectomy specimen. The retroperitoneal margin (also termed "mesenteric margin" or "uncinate margin") is the tissue adjacent to the SMA and should be inked for evaluation of margin status. For orientation, a small probe is in the bile duct and the pancreatic duct. A Q-tip applicator stick lies over the indentation from the SMPV confluence. Complete permanent-section analysis of the pancreaticoduodenectomy specimen requires that it be oriented to enable the pathologist to assess accurately the retroperitoneal margin and to determine the adequacy of resection (R status).

margin (RI) cannot be made if the retroperitoneal margin is not assessed histologically. Because we advocate removal of all tissue to the right of the SMA, further resection at the retroperitoneal margin is not possible. Most importantly, this margin should be classified by the surgeon and pathologist after integrating the operative findings and the histologic assessment of this margin. All pancreatic resections should be classified according to margin or residual disease status (RO, R1, or R2) as previously defined. The pathologist cannot usually differentiate an R1 (microscopically positive) from an R2 (grossly positive) retroperitoneal margin in the absence of information regarding the retroperitoneal dissection, which should be included in the operative note. The R designation should appear in the final pathology report and should be consistent with the dictated operative note. For example, if the surgeon states that gross tumor was encountered when completing the retroperitoneal dissection, a positive histologic margin should result in the R2 designation in the final pathology report. In the absence of this information being included in the operative report, the proper R designation cannot be determined. The difficulty in differentiating R1 from R2 resections has significant implications for the conduct of clinical trials examining the potential survival advantage of nonsurgical therapies.

Pancreatic, Biliary, and Gastrointestinal Reconstruction

Reconstruction after pancreaticoduodenectomy involves completion of the pancreatic, biliary, and gastric (duodenal) anastomoses. To facilitate construction of the pancreaticojejunostomy, the pancreatic remnant is mobilized from the retroperitoneum and splenic vein for a distance of 2–3 cm. Failure to mobilize the pancreatic remnant adequately may result in poor suture placement at the pancreaticojejunal anastomosis. However, overly extensive mobilization of the remaining pancreas may devascularize the pancreatic neck and may increase the risks for anastomotic failure. The transected jejunum is brought through a generous incision in the transverse mesocolon to the left of the middle colic vessels. We prefer to bring the jejunum retrocolic rather than retroperitoneal (posterior to the mesenteric vessels in the bed of the resected

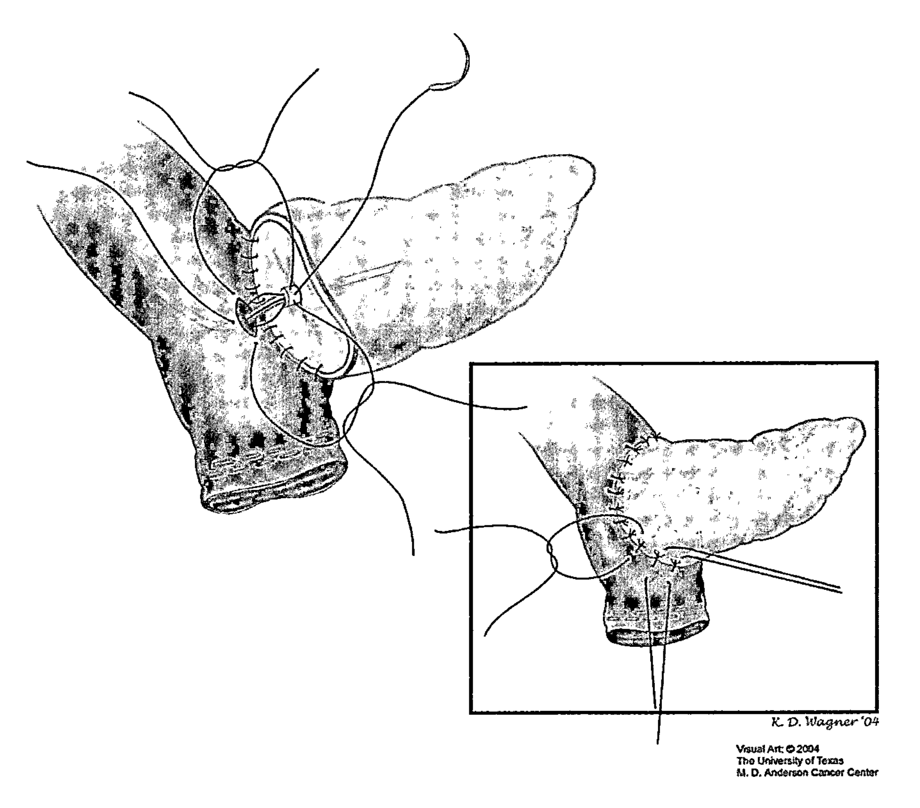

Figure 18.17
An illustration of pancreaticojejunostomy. A two-layer, end-to-side, duct-to-mucosa retrocolic pancreaticojejunostomy is performed with (when the pancreatic duct is not dilated) or without a small stent. When used, the stent (4–5 cm long) is sewn to the pancreatic duct with a single absorbable monofilament suture.

duodenum). A two-layer, end-to-side, duct-to-mucosa pancreaticojejunostomy is performed, and a small silastic ureteral stent is placed in the pancreatic duct when the pancreatic duct is not dilated (Fig. 18.17). After completion of the posterior row of interrupted 4–0 seromuscular monofilament sutures, a small, full-thickness opening in the bowel is made. The anastomosis between the pancreatic duct and the small bowel mucosa is completed with 4–0 or 5–0 monofilament sutures. Each stitch incorporates a generous bite of the pancreatic duct and a full-thickness bite of the jejunum. The posterior knot(s) is tied on the inside and the lateral and anterior knots on the outside. If a stent is used, it is placed across the anastomosis before securing the anterior surface so that it extends into the pancreatic duct and small bowel for a distance of approximately 2–3 cm. The anastomosis is completed with the placement of an anterior row of 4–0 seromuscular monofilament sutures. If the pancreatic duct is not suitable for a duct-to-mucosa anastomosis, a two-layer anastomosis that invaginates the cut end of the pancreas into the jejunum can be performed.

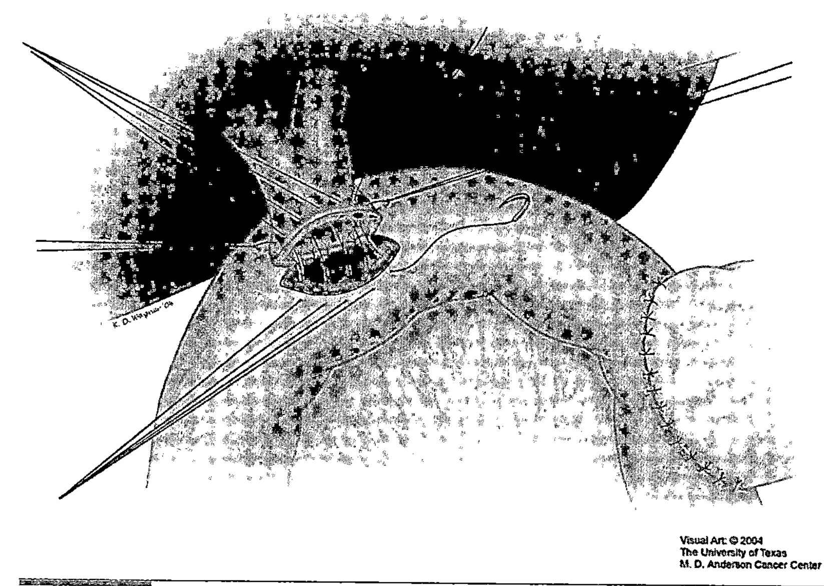

Figure 18.18
An illustration of hepaticojejunostomy. A one-layer, end-to-side hepaticojejunostomy is performed, with 4–0 or 5–0 absorbable monofilament sutures, distal to the pancreaticojejunostomy. A stent is rarely placed in this anastomosis. Care is taken to allow enough distance between the pancreatic and biliary anastomoses so that the falciform ligament can be placed anterior to the hepatic artery and posterior to the jejunal limb.

Distal to the pancreaticojejunostomy, a single-layer biliary anastomosis is performed using interrupted 4–0 absorbable monofilament sutures (Fig. 18.18). It is important to align the jejunum with the bile duct to avoid tension on the pancreatic and biliary anastomoses. A stent is not used in the construction of the hepaticojejunostomy. Approximately 40–50 cm from the hepaticojejunostomy, an antecolic, end-to-side gastrojejunostomy is constructed in two layers. Starting from the greater curvature, a length of 6–8 cm of the gastric staple line is removed. A posterior row of 3–0 silk sutures is placed, followed by a full-thickness inner layer of running monofilament suture. An anterior row of silk sutures completes the anastomosis. When the pylorus is preserved, the duodenojejunostomy is created in an end-to-side fashion with a single-layer technique using monofilament absorbable sutures. The distance between the biliary and gastric anastomoses should be at least 50 cm, thereby allowing the jejunum to assume its antecolic position (for the gastrojejunostomy) without tension and also preventing bile reflux cholangitis. We prefer an antecolic gastrojejunostomy to prevent possible outlet obstruction caused by the colonic mesentery. Finally, the jejunal limb should be aligned so that the efferent limb is adjacent to the greater curvature of the stomach. A 10-Fr feeding jejunostomy tube may be placed distal to the gastrojejunostomy. We rarely use a gastrostomy tube for postoperative gastric decompression.

Before abdominal closure, the abdomen is carefully irrigated in all four quadrants. In patients with a previous indwelling endobiliary stent, the bile is contaminated and often has had free access to at least the right upper quadrant of the abdomen despite placement of a bulldog clamp on the transected bile duct (Step 3). Careful irrigation may prevent postoperative infectious complications. Next, one closed suction drain may be placed in the right upper quadrant; we rarely drain the pancreatic anastomosis. Finally, we place the mobilized falciform ligament (carefully preserved when the abdomen was opened) between the CHA, at the level of the GDA stump, and the afferent jejunal limb to cover the GDA stump. This is one simple strategy to minimize the risk for pseudoaneurysm formation at the site of the GDA stump, in the event of a pancreatic anastomotic leak and resulting abscess formation (Fig. 18.19).

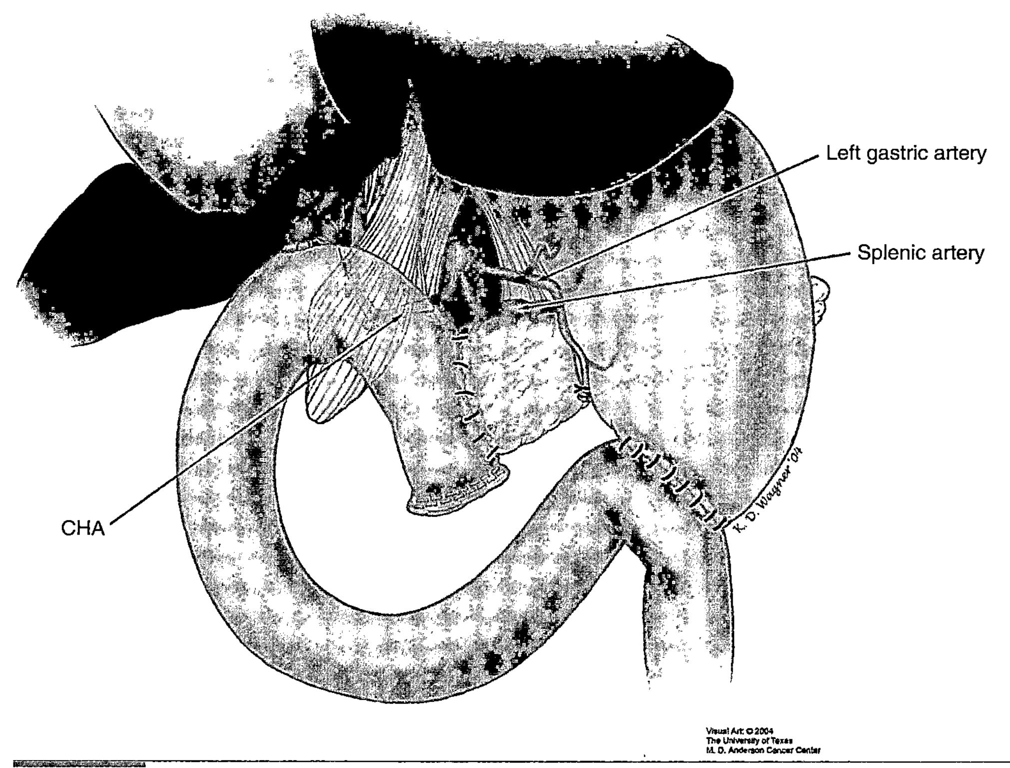

Figure 18.19
An illustration of the completed reconstruction after pancreaticoduodenectomy. The falciform ligament, mobilized on opening the abdomen, is placed over the hepatic artery to cover the stump of the gastroduodenal artery (GDA), thereby separating the hepatic artery from the afferent jejunal limb. CHA = common hepatic artery.

Perioperative Complications

As with all complex surgery, a good outcome after pancreaticoduodenectomy depends on meticulous perioperative care.[56] A clinical pathway is used and orders revised by a multidisciplinary group of clinicians every 12 to 18 months to insure the optimal perioperative and postoperative care of the pancreatic surgery patient.[56] We prefer combined general and epidural anesthesia during surgery, with the epidural catheter usually remaining in place for 72 hours. All postoperative patients are managed initially in the intensive care unit or in the recovery room and transferred to the floor on postoperative day 1.

Postoperative fevers are common in pancreatectomy patients. However, fevers occurring after postoperative days 3 to 4 demand careful evaluation. Potential sources of fever include those common to all major abdominal surgery: pneumonia, deep vein thrombosis, central line sepsis, urinary tract infection, and wound infection. Patients who undergo pancreaticojejunostomy are at particular risk of developing an intra-abdominal abscess as a result of leakage from the pancreatic anastomosis. Because leaks from either the biliary or gastric anastomoses are uncommon, intra-abdominal sepsis is considered to be due to a pancreatic anastomotic leak until proven otherwise. Clinically, these patients present with fever, abdominal distention, ileus, and leukocytosis. The study of choice for evaluating presumed intra-abdominal sepsis is CT of the abdomen and pelvis with oral and intravenous administration of contrast material. The finding of a localized fluid collection in the region of the pancreaticojejunostomy with or without an air–fluid level requires consideration for CT-guided aspiration. Percutaneous catheter drainage is indicated if the fluid appears infected grossly or on Gram stain, as discussed in Chapter 24. Careful clinical judgment is needed to determine which peripancreatic fluid collections are aspirated and drained, as this practice is not routinely performed in all situations. As discussed later here and in more detail in Chapter 24, percutaneous catheters are not without complications, most notably, erosion into the hepatic or splenic artery. In addition, it is common to identify nonloculated ascitic fluid on postoperative CT scans in pancreatectomy patients. However, this finding rarely represents infection or anastomotic leak and does not demand aspiration or drainage unless clinical signs of sepsis persist and another source of infection has not been identified. Pancreaticojejunostomy anastomotic leaks generally close once adequate drainage has been established. We commonly use octreotide to treat established pancreatic anastomotic leaks that have required percutaneous drainage.

The culture results and antibiotic sensitivities of the operative cultures of the common hepatic duct bile can be used to guide antibiotic selection when postoperative intra-abdominal or wound infections require antibiotic treatment. Reports have demonstrated high rates of concordance between isolates obtained from bile and those obtained from subsequent cultures from wound or intra-abdominal sources.[44]

Postoperative gastrointestinal or drain tract bleeding should prompt immediate evaluation with arteriography. Although uncommon, an arterial–enteric fistula occasionally occurs in the postoperative setting, but rarely before postoperative days 7 to 10. The most common cause is a pancreatic anastomotic leak with surrounding inflammation and infection that results in a blowout of the ligated GDA stump. Gastrointestinal or drain tract bleeding represents a true emergency, as the only patients likely to survive are those in whom the diagnosis is made immediately. Although experience with this complication is anecdotal, we would proceed with stenting or embolization of the hepatic artery at the time of diagnostic arteriography. Surgical control of hemorrhage from the stump of the GDA is exceedingly difficult in a postoperative pancreaticoduodenectomy patient and in our opinion carries a mortality rate higher than that associated with hepatic artery embolization.

Delayed gastric emptying is common after standard pancreaticoduodenectomy and may occur more frequently with pylorus preservation.[4,57] Unless secondary to intra-abdominal infection, this complication is largely related to denervation of the upper gastrointestinal tract during resection of the pancreatic head and attached soft tissues and nerves to the right of the SMA. Delayed gastric emptying causes nausea, vomiting, and postprandial fullness; however, these symptoms resolve in 4–12 weeks in virtually all patients. The nutritional consequences of delayed gastric emptying are most significant in those patients with some degree of nutritional depletion preoperatively and in older patients with significant medical comorbid conditions. In such patients, we may place a gastrostomy tube at the time of surgery in the hope of avoiding patient morbidity due to temporary gastric emptying dysfunction. Similarly, a feeding jejunostomy tube may prevent the high cost and inconvenience of intravenous hyperalimentation, even though it may be needed in only a minority of patients. Patients can then be discharged from the hospital while they are still receiving enteral feeding via the jejunostomy tube and allowed to advance their oral diet as tolerated.

Conclusion

In summary, accurate preoperative imaging and proper surgical technique will maximize the chance for a safe and uncomplicated pancreaticoduodenectomy and potentially minimize local tumor recurrence. Because the goal of therapies directed at the primary tumor is to maximize local–regional tumor control and thereby enhance the quality of life and length of patient survival, pancreaticoduodenectomy should be performed only when complete removal of the tumor can be achieved. In addition, the relatively low cure rate and modest median survival after potentially curative pancreaticoduodenectomy mandate efforts to minimize treatment-related morbidity and death by using standardized surgical techniques and postoperative care on a clinical pathway. Finally, given the recent data demonstrating a linear relationship between surgical volume and outcome after pancreatic resection, it seems reasonable that patients be given the option of having surgery at a high-volume center by experienced surgeons to further minimize operative morbidity and mortality.

References

1. Whipple AO, Parsons WB, Mullins CR. Treatment of carcinoma of the ampulla of Vater. *Ann Surg.* 1935;102:763–779.
2. Whipple AO. The rationale of radical surgery for cancer of the pancreas and ampullary region. *Ann Surg.* 1941;114:612.
3. Waugh JM, Claggett OT. Resection of the duodenum and head of the pancreas for carcinoma. *Surgery.* 1946;20:224.
4. Balcom JH 4th, Rattner DW, Warshaw AL, et al. Ten-year experience with 733 pancreatic resections: changing indications, older patients, and decreasing length of hospitalization. *Arch Surg.* 2001;136:391–398.
5. Martignoni ME, Wagner M, Krahenbuhl L, et al. Effect of preoperative biliary drainage on surgical outcome after pancreatoduodenectomy. *Am J Surg.* 2001;181:52–59.
6. Pisters PW, Hudec WA, Hess KR, et al. Effect of preoperative biliary decompression on pancreaticoduodenectomy-associated morbidity in 300 consecutive patients. *Ann Surg.* 2001;234:47–55.
7. Sewnath ME, Birjmohun RS, Rauws EA, et al. The effect of preoperative biliary drainage on postoperative complications after pancreaticoduodenectomy. *J Am Coll Surg.* 2001; 192:726–734.

8. Sohn TA, Yeo CJ, Cameron JL, et al. Resected adenocarcinoma of the pancreas: 616 patients: results, outcomes, and prognostic indicators. *J Gastrointest Surg.* 2000;4:567–579.
9. Povoski SP, Karpeh MS Jr, Conlon KC, et al. Association of preoperative biliary drainage with postoperative outcome following pancreaticoduodenectomy. *Ann Surg.* 1999;230: 131–142.
10. Yeo CJ, Cameron JL, Sohn TA, et al. Six hundred fifty consecutive pancreaticoduodenectomies in the 1990s: pathology, complications, and outcomes. *Ann Surg.* 1997;226: 248–260.
11. Doerr RJ, Yildiz I, Flint LM. Pancreaticoduodenectomy: university experience and resident education. *Arch Surg.* 1990;125:463–465.
12. Edge SB, Schmieg RE Jr, Rosenlof LK, Wilhelm MC. Pancreas cancer resection outcome in American University centers in 1989–1990. *Cancer.* 1993;71:3502–3508.
13. Wade TP, Kraybill WG, Virgo KS, Johnson FE. Pancreatic cancer treatment in the U.S. veteran from 1987 to 1991: effect of tumor stage on survival. *J Surg Oncol.* 1995;58:104–111.
14. Billingsley KG, Hur K, Henderson WG, et al. Outcome after pancreaticoduodenectomy for periampullary cancer: an analysis from the Veterans Affairs National Surgical Quality Improvement Program. *J Gastrointest Surg.* 2003;7: 484–491.
15. Birkmeyer JD, Finlayson SR, Tosteson AN, et al. Effect of hospital volume on in-hospital mortality with pancreaticoduodenectomy. *Surgery.* 1999;125:250–256.
16. Birkmeyer JD, Warshaw AL, Finlayson SR, et al. Relationship between hospital volume and late survival after pancreaticoduodenectomy. *Surgery.* 1999;126:178–183.
17. Birkmeyer JD, Siewers AE, Finlayson EV, et al. Hospital volume and surgical mortality in the United States. *N Engl J Med.* 2002;346:1128–1137.
18. Finlayson EV, Goodney PP, Birkmeyer JD. Hospital volume and operative mortality in cancer surgery: a national study. *Arch Surg.* 2003;138:721–725.
19. Birkmeyer JD, Stukel TA, Siewers AE, et al. Surgeon volume and operative mortality in the United States. *N Engl J Med.* 2003;349:2117–2127.
20. Evans DB, Abbruzzese JL, Willett CG. Cancer of the pancreas. In: DeVita VT, Hellman S, Rosenberg SA, eds. *Cancer: Principles and Practice of Oncology.* 6th ed. Philadelphia: Lippincott Williams and Wilkins; 2001:1126–1161.
21. Breslin TM, Hess KR, Harbison DB, et al. Neoadjuvant chemoradiotherapy for adenocarcinoma of the pancreas: treatment variables and survival duration. *Ann Surg Oncol.* 2001;8:123–132.
22. Nitecki SS, Sarr MG, Colby TV, van Heerden JA. Long-term survival after resection for ductal adenocarcinoma of the pancreas. Is it really improving? *Ann Surg.* 1995; 221:59–66.
23. Geer RJ, Brennan MF. Prognostic indicators for survival after resection of pancreatic adenocarcinoma. *Am J Surg.* 1993;165:68–73.
24. Foo ML, Gunderson LL, Nagorney DM, et al. Patterns of failure in grossly resected pancreatic ductal adenocarcinoma treated with adjuvant irradiation ±5-fluorouracil. *Int J Radiat Oncol Biol Phys.* 1993;26:483–489.
25. Griffin JF, Smalley SR, Jewell W, et al. Patterns of failure after curative resection of pancreatic carcinoma. *Cancer.* 1990;66:56–61.
26. Johnstone PA, Sindelar WF. Patterns of disease recurrence following definitive therapy of adenocarcinoma of the pancreas using surgery and adjuvant radiotherapy: correlations of a clinical trial. *Int J Radiat Oncol Biol Phys.* 1993;27:831–834.
27. Westerdahl J, Andrén-Sandeberg Å, Ihse I. Recurrence of exocrine pancreatic cancer: local or hepatic? *Hepatogastroenterology.* 1993;40:384–387.
28. Willett CG, Lewandrowski K, Warshaw AL, et al. Resection margins in carcinoma of the head of the pancreas. Implications for radiation therapy. *Ann Surg.* 1993;217:144–148.
29. Wolff RA, Abbruzzese JL, Evans DB. Neoplasms of the exocrine pancreas. In: Kufe DW, Pollock RE, Weichselbaum RR, et al., eds. *Holland-Frei Cancer Medicine.* 6th ed. Ontario: BC Decker; 2003:1585–1614.
30. Pisters PW, Abbruzzese JL, Janjan NA, et al. Rapid-fractionation preoperative chemoradiation, pancreaticoduodenectomy, and intraoperative radiation therapy for resectable pancreatic adenocarcinoma. *J Clin Oncol.* 1998;16:3843–3850.
31. Lillemoe KD, Sauter PK, Pitt HA, et al. Current status of surgical palliation of periampullary carcinoma. *Surg Gynecol Obstet.* 1993;176:1–10.
32. Kelsen DP, Portenoy R, Thaler H, et al. Pain as a predictor of outcome in patients with operable pancreatic carcinoma. *Surgery.* 1997;122:53–59.
33. de Rooij PD, Rogatko A, Brennan MF. Evaluation of palliative surgical procedures in unresectable pancreatic cancer. *Br J Surg.* 1991;78:1053–1058.
34. Neoptolemos JP, Stocken DD, Dunn JA, et al. Influence of resection margins on survival for patients with pancreatic cancer treated by adjuvant chemoradiation and/or chemotherapy in the ESPAC-1 randomized controlled trial. *Ann Surg.* 2001;234:758–768.
35. Millikan KW, Deziel DJ, Silverstein JC, et al. Prognostic factors associated with resectable adenocarcinoma of the head of the pancreas. *Am Surg.* 1999;65:618–624.
36. Nishimura Y, Hosotani R, Shibamoto Y, et al. External and intraoperative radiotherapy for resectable and unresectable pancreatic cancer: analysis of survival rates and complications. *Int J Radiat Oncol Biol Phys.* 1997;39:39–49.
37. Sperti C, Pasquali C, Piccoli A, Pedrazzoli S. Survival after resection for ductal adenocarcinoma of the pancreas. *Br J Surg.* 1996;83:625–631.
38. A multi-institutional comparative trial of radiation therapy alone and in combination with 5-fluorouracil for locally unresectable pancreatic carcinoma: the Gastrointestinal Tumor Study Group. *Ann Surg.* 1979;189:205–208.
39. Whittington R, Neuberg D, Tester WJ, et al. Protracted intravenous fluorouracil infusion with radiation therapy in the management of localized pancreaticobiliary carcinoma: a phase I Eastern Cooperative Oncology Group Trial. *J Clin Oncol.* 1995;13:227–232.
40. O'Malley ME, Boland GW, Wood BJ, et al. Adenocarcinoma of the head of the pancreas: determination of surgical unresectability with thin-section pancreatic-phase helical CT. *AJR Am J Roentgenol.* 1999;173:1513–1518.

41. Yeung RS, Weese JL, Hoffman JP, et al. Neoadjuvant chemoradiation in pancreatic and duodenal carcinoma: a phase II Study. *Cancer.* 1993;72:2124–2133.
42. Warshaw AL, Gu ZY, Wittenberg J, Waltman AC. Preoperative staging and assessment of resectability of pancreatic cancer. *Arch Surg.* 1990;125:230–233.
43. Raut CP, Grau AM, Staerkel GA, et al. Diagnostic accuracy of endoscopic ultrasound-guided fine-needle aspiration in patients with presumed pancreatic cancer. *J Gastrointestinal Surg.* 2003;7:118–128.
44. Povoski SP, Karpeh MS Jr, Conlon KC, et al. Preoperative biliary drainage: impact on intraoperative bile cultures and infectious morbidity and mortality after pancreaticoduodenectomy. *J Gastrointest Surg.* 1999;3:496–505.
45. Sohn TA, Yeo CJ, Cameron JL, et al. Do preoperative biliary stents increase postpancreaticoduodenectomy complications? *J Gastrointest Surg.* 2000;4:258–268.
46. Pisters PW, Hudec WA, Lee JE, et al. Preoperative chemoradiation for patients with pancreatic cancer: toxicity of endobiliary stents. *J Clin Oncol.* 2000;18:860–867.
47. Staley CA, Lee JE, Cleary KR, et al. Preoperative chemoradiation, pancreaticoduodenectomy, and intraoperative radiation therapy for adenocarcinoma of the pancreatic head. *Am J Surg.* 1996;171:118–125.
48. Robinson EK, Lee JE, Lowy AM, et al. Reoperative pancreaticoduodenectomy for periampullary carcinoma. *Am J Surg.* 1996;172:432–438.
49. Tyler DS, Evans DB. Reoperative pancreaticoduodenectomy. *Ann Surg.* 1994;219:211–221.
50. Evans DB, Lee JE, Pisters PWT. Pancreaticoduodenectomy (Whipple Operation) and total pancreatectomy for cancer. In: Baker RJ, Fischer JE, eds. *Mastery of Surgery.* 4th ed. Philadelphia: Lippincott Williams & Wilkins; 2001:1299–1318.
51. Bold RJ, Charnsangavej C, Cleary KR, et al. Major vascular resection as part of pancreaticoduodenectomy for cancer: radiologic, intraoperative, and pathologic analysis. *J Gastrointest Surg.* 1999;3:233–243.
52. Cattell RB, Braasch JW. A technique for the exposure of the third and fourth portions of the duodenum. *Surg Gynecol Obstet.* 1960;111:378–381.
53. Greene FL, Page DL, Fleming ID, et al., eds. *AJCC Cancer Staging Manual.* 6th ed. New York: Springer-Verlag; 2002.
54. Nagakawa T, Kayahara M, Ohta T, et al. Patterns of neural and plexus invasion of human pancreatic cancer and experimental cancer. *Int J Pancreatol.* 1991;10:113–119.
55. Nagakawa T, Mori K, Nakano T, et al. Perineural invasion of carcinoma of the pancreas and biliary tract. *Br J Surg.* 1993;80:619–621.
56. Porter GA, Pisters PW, Mansyur C, et al. Cost and utilization impact of a clinical pathway for patients undergoing pancreaticoduodenectomy. *Ann Surg Oncol.* 2000;7:484–489.
57. Warshaw AL, Torchiana DL. Delayed gastric emptying after pylorus-preserving pancreaticoduodenectomy. *Surg Gynecol Obstet.* 1985;160:1–4.

CHAPTER 19

The Role of Total Pancreatectomy in the Treatment of Pancreatic Cancer

John D. Christein, MD
Michael B. Farnell, MD

Although the role of total pancreatectomy in the treatment of ductal adenocarcinoma of the pancreas may currently be characterized as limited, this has not always been the case. In the 1940s and 1950s, surgeons were discouraged both by the high operative mortality rate of subtotal pancreatectomy and by the dismal long-term survival in patients who recovered from the operation. As early as the 1960s, investigators began to focus on improving the surgical treatment of ductal adenocarcinoma of the pancreas, and many became keenly interested in total pancreatectomy.

The factors that prompted interest in total pancreatectomy were both technical and oncologic. The operative mortality for pancreatoduodenectomy was reported to be greater than 25% and was thought to be primarily related to leakage from the pancreatoenteric anastomosis. Further, it was believed that transecting the pancreatic duct led to spillage of tumor cells.[1] At about this same time, the multicentricity of pancreatic adenocarcinoma was reported.[2] It seemed rational, therefore, to consider total pancreatectomy to prevent the need for a pancreatoenteric anastomosis, prevent tumor spillage, address possible multicentricity, and perform a more radical operation by including nodes in the region of the body and tail of the pancreas. This trend was embraced by surgeons at Mayo Clinic, who reported on a series of 64 total pancreatectomies for ductal carcinoma of the pancreas from 1942 to 1973.[3] Unfortunately, as these and other series matured,[3-11] survival following total pancreatectomy was no better than that for Whipple resection, and the brittle diabetes of the apancreatic state was difficult to manage. These observations, coupled with substantial improvement in the morbidity and mortality of Whipple resection and reports suggesting that the rate of multicentric disease is very low, have allowed the pendulum to swing in favor of subtotal pancreatectomy for the vast majority of patients with resectable adenocarcinoma of the pancreas.[12-16]

Presently, although limited, the role of total pancreatectomy remains secure in a select subset of patients. Total pancreatectomy is commonly required for patients with intraductal papillary mucinous neoplasm, which is addressed in Chapter 53. This chapter addresses patient selection, technique, and outcome of total pancreatectomy for ductal adenocarcinoma of the pancreas. Diagnosis and staging are reviewed in detail in Chapters 12 through 17.

Indications for Operation

For most patients who present with probable localized pancreatic ductal adenocarcinoma, either a proximal (Whipple) or a distal subtotal pancreatectomy is generally preferred. However, certain factors determined both before and during surgery may dictate consideration for total pancreatectomy. Tumor size and location, presence of marked atrophy of the body and tail, and presence of endocrine and exocrine pancreatic insufficiency should lead to the consideration of total pancreatectomy.

If the lesion is located in the neck of the pancreas and is generous in size, it may be difficult to obtain negative margins with either head resection or extended distal pancreatectomy. If the body and tail are atrophic, particularly if preoperative pancreatic insufficiency is present such that safe anastomosis is problematic, total pancreatectomy should be considered from the onset.

Occasionally, because of obstructive chronic pancreatitis, tumor extent within the gland is not obvious, either on preoperative imaging or at exploration. The margin of the transected neck is routinely assessed on frozen section. If the results are positive in spite of reresection, consideration should be given to completion pancreatectomy. The anastomosis becomes more difficult the further it is to the patient's left, because of a smaller duct and the unfavorable shape of the gland. Furthermore, as more gland is resected in order to obtain a negative margin, preservation of pancreatic function is problematic.

On rare occasions, the senior author has opted for total pancreatectomy because the remnant pancreatic body and tail were so soft and unforgiving that the risk of pancreatic leak was thought to be prohibitive. This is most unusual in recent years because we have refined our techniques for mucosa-to-mucosa pancreaticojejunostomy with the use of magnification.

Lastly, two-stage or completion pancreatectomy may be required after Whipple resection for anastomotic dehiscence resulting in sepsis or bleeding.

Preoperative Evaluation

Before pancreatoduodenectomy or total pancreatectomy, the patient should undergo routine cardiovascular and respiratory evaluation and receive indicated interventions. Often, a jaundiced patient has little hepatic functional reserve secondary to longstanding obstructive jaundice. In these situations, when operation is to be delayed because of comorbid medical conditions or necessity for further diagnostic testing, biliary stenting not only relieves pruritus but also allows for hepatic recovery. In patients with obstructive jaundice, parenteral vitamin K is also recommended. A relative coagulopathic state is created by vitamin K deficiency secondary to decreased absorption of fat-soluble vitamins and the resultant inability to process dependent aspects of the coagulation cascade, namely factors II, V, VII, and IX.[17] All patients should undergo mechanical bowel preparation.

Technical Aspects of Total Pancreatectomy

A right subcostal or upper midline incision is used to gain access to the peritoneal cavity. A thorough exploration is performed, including careful bimanual palpation of the liver, both hemidiaphragms, all peritoneal surfaces, and pelvis, the latter in order to look for drop metastasis. The mesenteries and retroperitoneum should also be carefully evaluated for nodal disease outside of the field of resection. Nodal disease within the field to be resected is not a contraindication to resection and typically does not undergo biopsy. Once metastatic disease is excluded, if a subcostal incision is used, it is extended bilaterally and fixed retractors are applied. Maximum exposure is further gained by securing the lower abdominal incisional flap with heavy suture inferiorly to the abdominal wall. After metastatic disease is excluded, the next step is to assess the pancreas and determine whether criteria for local resectability are met.

For tumors of the head or neck of the pancreas, local resectability is determined by the relationship of the tumor to adjacent vasculature, including the celiac axis, superior mesenteric artery (SMA), and portal vein/superior mesenteric vein (PV-SMV) confluence. Although this information is provided by preoperative imaging, it is ultimately confirmed by exploration, ensuring lack of involvement of the aforementioned vessels. To assess the head of the pancreas and exclude retroperitoneal extension, an extensive Kocher maneuver is performed (Fig. 19.1). By incising the peritoneum over the lateral edge of the duodenum, the head of the pancreas can be palpated (Fig. 19.2). This dissection should be carried to the left side of the aorta, which allows for palpation of the SMA for gross tumor extension from the uncinate process. Mobilization and release inferiorly of the hepatic flexure of the colon aid in this exposure.

The greater omentum is mobilized from the transverse colon in an avascular manner (Fig. 19.3). The lesser sac is

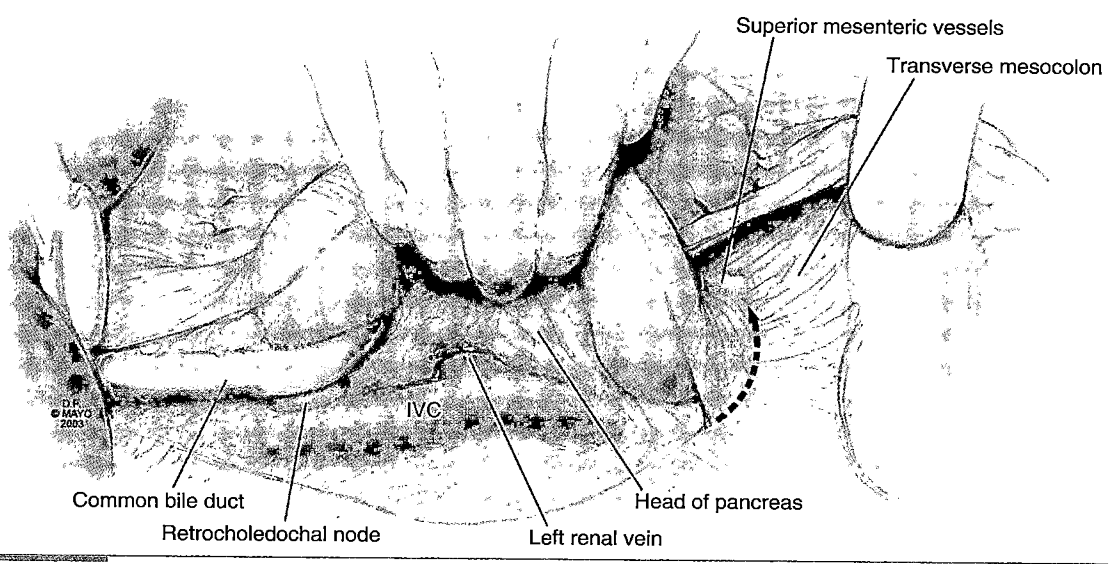

Figure 19.1
The hepatic flexure of the right colon is released inferiorly to aid in performing a Kocher maneuver, which elevates the duodenum and the head of the pancreas (view from right lateral side of the patient). IVC, inferior vena cava.

entered and the superior aspect of the right transverse mesocolon is exposed, which aids in the identification of the superior mesenteric vein. The middle colic vein, within the transverse mesocolon, is followed centrally to its junction with the SMV. For optimal exposure and to prevent avulsion injury, division of this vessel may be necessary. Also, the gastrocolic venous trunk is routinely divided to ensure optimal exposure of the neck of the pancreas and access to the anterior surface of the SMV (Fig. 19.4A). To assess the relationship between the posterior surface of the neck of the pancreas and the anterior surface of the PV-SMV confluence, careful dissection of the anterior surface is performed and confirmed by the insinuation of a blunt clamp into this plane (Fig. 19.4B). To further develop this plane, the superior edge of the pancreas is examined. This exposure is best gained by dividing the gastrohepatic

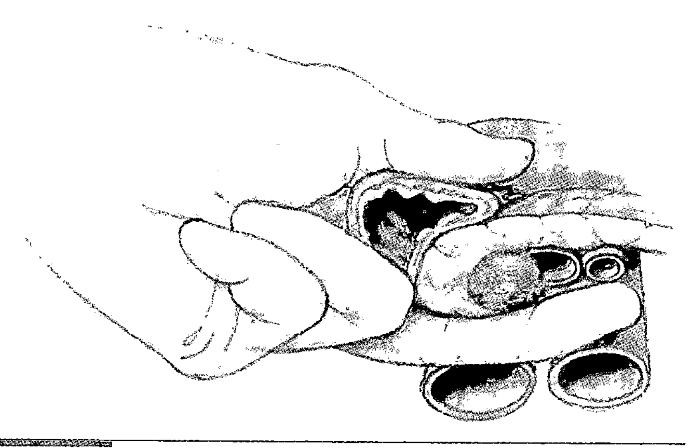

Figure 19.2
The head of the pancreas is palpated with the left hand, assessing both for a discrete mass and evidence of extension to the superior mesenteric artery.

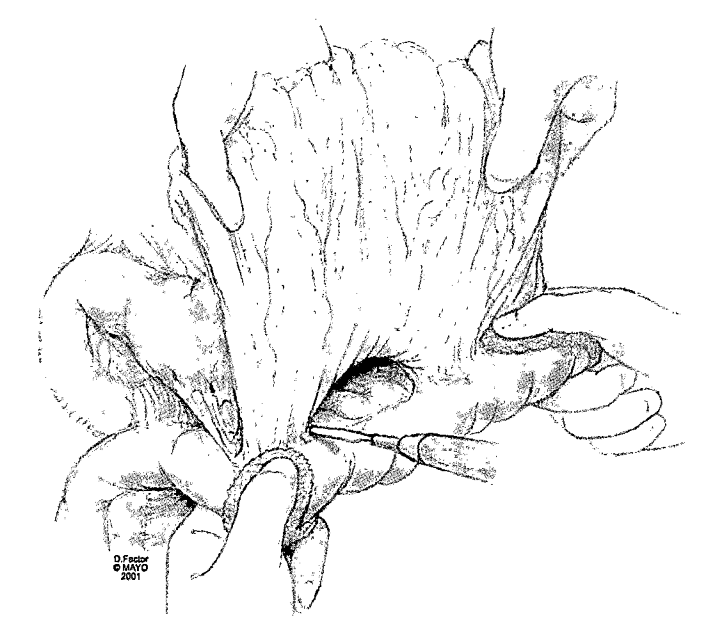

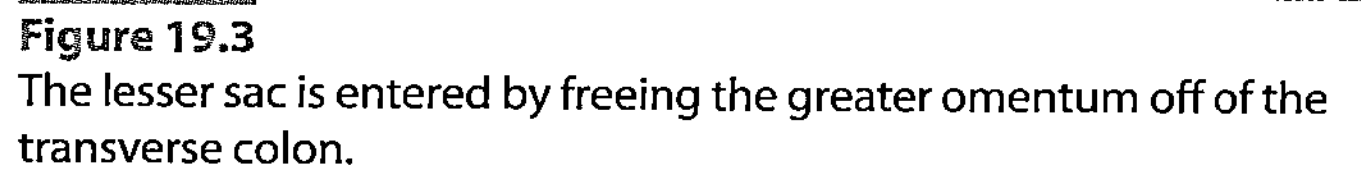

Figure 19.3
The lesser sac is entered by freeing the greater omentum off of the transverse colon.

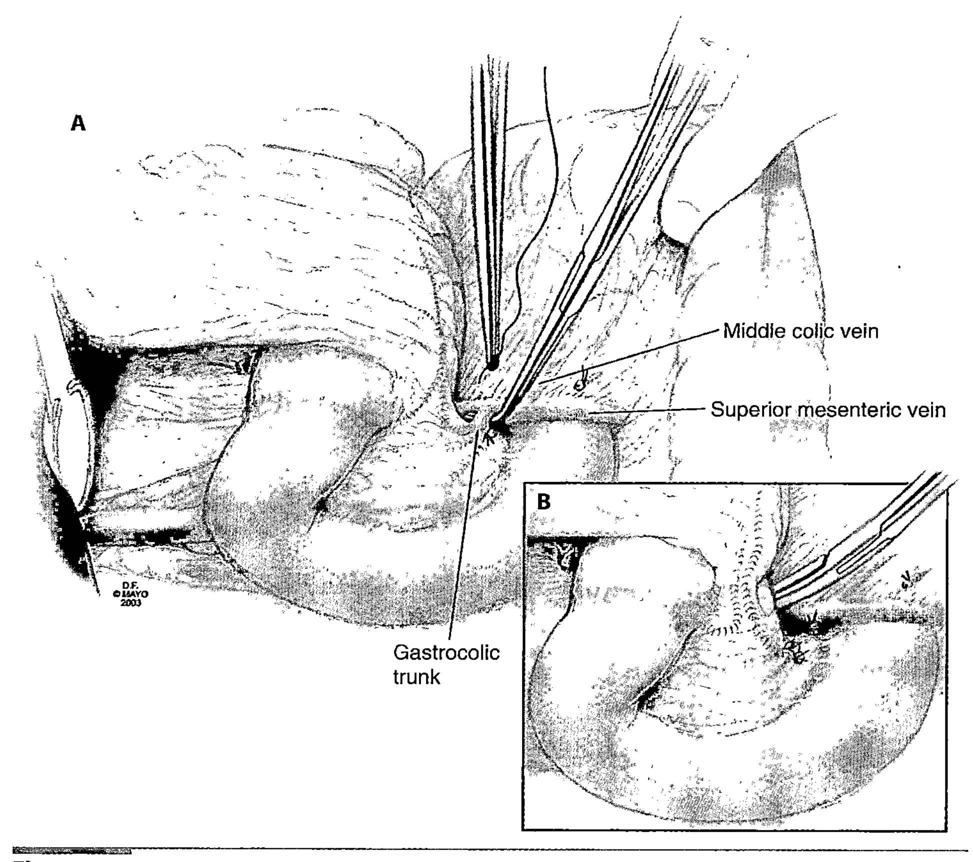

Figure 19.4
(A) The anterior and lateral exposure to the superior mesenteric vein is facilitated by ligation of the gastrocolic venous trunk. **(B)** Careful dissection with a blunt clamp anterior to the superior mesenteric vein/portal vein confluence aids in assessing the relationship of the neck of the pancreas to the vein (view from right lateral side of the patient).

omentum, then exposing the inferior aspect of the common hepatic artery. The right gastric and gastroduodenal arteries are identified, ligated, and divided at this time (Figs. 19.5A and B). Once this step is complete, the portal vein superior to the neck of the pancreas can carefully be dissected, with the aim of completing the plane posterior to the pancreas (Figs. 19.5C and D). By developing this plane, the right lateral portion of the PV-SMV is also assessed for involvement. If venous involvement is encountered, one should be prepared to perform a venous resection en bloc with the pancreatectomy specimen. Options include tangential excision and a transverse lateral venorrhaphy or segmental resection. In the latter situation, reconstruction consists of an end-to-end anastomosis or an interposition graft using autogenous vein or polytetrafluoroethylene as conduit and is dependent on the length of PV-SMV that requires resection. The technique of en bloc resection of PV-SMV is addressed in Chapter 22.

After resectability relative to the PV-SMV confluence is assessed, the body and tail of the pancreas are approached through the lesser sac. Access to the left portion of the lesser sac is gained through mobilization of the omentum off of the left transverse colon through an avascular plane (Fig. 19.3). Care must be taken to remain in this avascular plane, thereby avoiding injury to the middle colic vessels. Once the anterior surface of the pancreas has been identified, further mobilization is achieved by dividing avascular attachments between the posterior wall of the stomach and the pancreas.

Once the pancreas is exposed, the dissection continues to the left by incising the peritoneum along the inferior border of the pancreas (Fig. 19.6). By doing so, access is gained to a plane posterior to the pancreas. The splenic flexure of the colon is mobilized and released inferiorly, which facilitates mobilization of the spleen and tail of the pancreas. Sequential division of the left gastroepiploic and short gastric vessels free the spleen from the stomach (Figs. 19.7A and B) and retraction of the spleen medially allow division of the lateral and posterior peritoneal attachments (Fig. 19.7C).

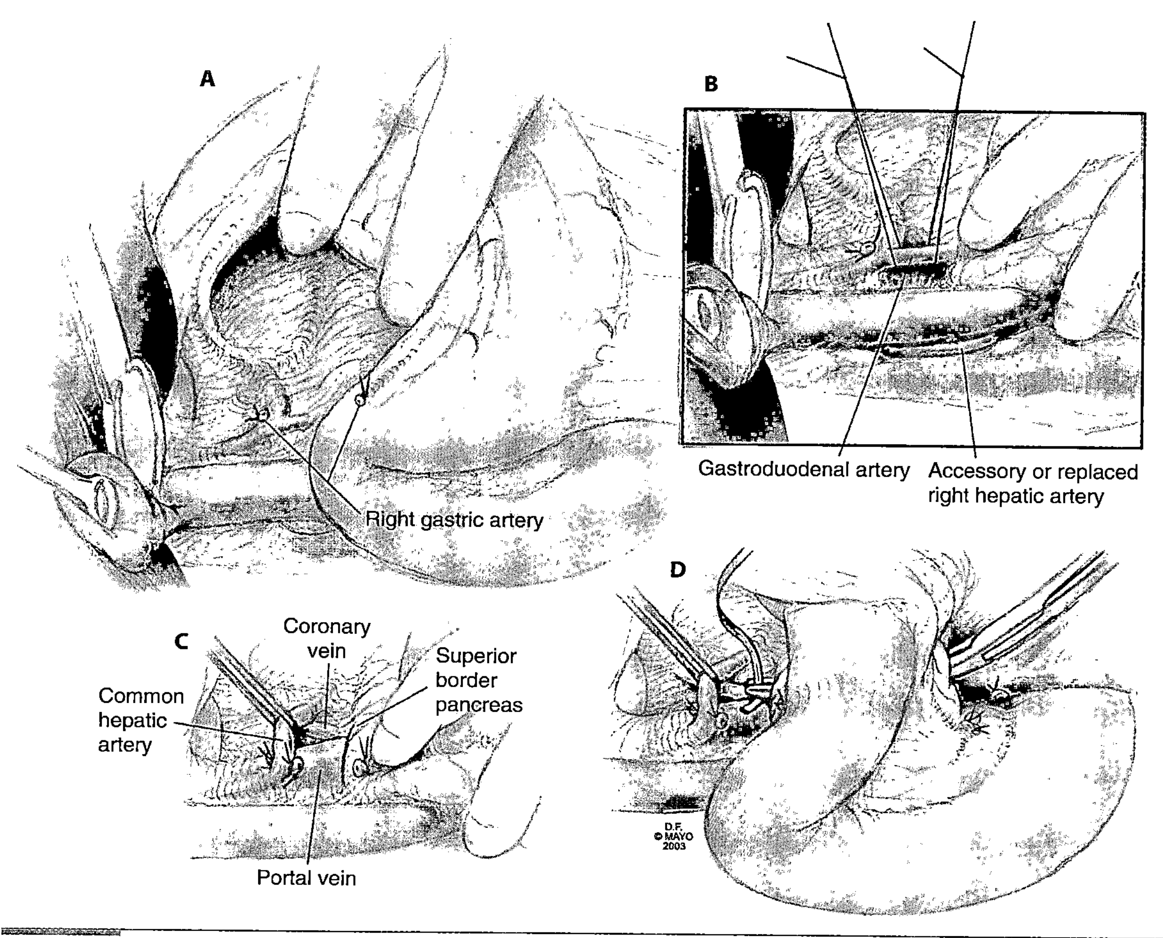

Figure 19.5
(A) Placement of inferior traction on the lesser curvature of the stomach allows incision of the gastrohepatic ligament and exposure and ligation of the right gastric artery. **(B)** Inferior traction on the neck of the pancreas allows for optimal dissection and ligation of the gastroduodenal artery. An accessory or replaced right hepatic artery can be seen or palpated posterior to the common bile duct. **(C)** Superior retraction of the common hepatic artery allows exposure of the anterior surface of the portal vein as well as identification of the coronary vein. **(D)** A tape is passed around the neck of the pancreas (view from right lateral side of patient).

By performing these steps, the stomach and omentum are completely freed from the pancreas and spleen. A dissection plane is then developed between the pancreas anteriorly and the left kidney and adrenal gland posteriorly. Now the spleen and pancreas complex can be lifted out of its bed and the posterior pancreatic attachments can further be divided, ultimately exposing the splenic artery and the junction of the splenic and superior mesenteric veins. The splenic artery and vein can be optimally visualized with the tail of the pancreas retracted anteriorly and to the right. The splenic artery should be divided near its origin and secured with a transfixing suture. The splenic vein is exposed in a similar manner. The confluence of the inferior mesenteric vein and the splenic vein should be identified, and if technically feasible, the splenic vein should be suture-ligated proximal to this juncture. If this is not feasible, the splenic vein should be ligated and divided flush with the lateral aspect of portal vein. During this delicate dissection, the coronary vein is identified and preserved. Once this mobilization is accomplished, the entire specimen is retracted to the right, which allows dissection of the uncinate process from both the PV-SMV and the SMA (Fig. 19.8).

Now that resectability has been confirmed relative to the SMV, the spleen, body and tail of the pancreas have been mobilized, and the splenic artery and vein have been ligated, the duodenum should be dissected from the superior portion of the pancreas and prepared for division approximately 3 cm distal to the pylorus. This is facilitated by dividing the right gastroepiploic artery and vein (Fig. 19.9A). Although our preference

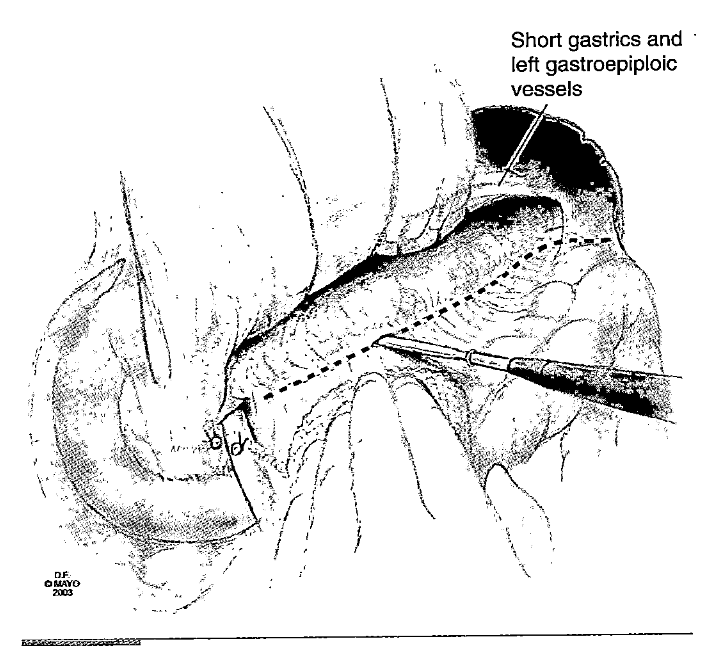

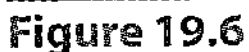

Figure 19.6
The transverse mesocolon is retracted in an inferior direction as the peritoneum at the inferior border of the pancreas is incised. The inferior mesenteric vein is identified and at this stage preserved.

is for pylorus-preserving total pancreatectomy, any concern regarding inadequate blood supply to the distal stomach or tumor encroachment on the antrum or pylorus warrants distal gastrectomy. Attention is directed to the biliary system. The gallbladder is dissected from the liver, and the cystic duct is followed to its junction with the common bile duct. During this careful exposure of the common duct, one should be prepared to identify an accessory or aberrant right hepatic artery, which usually lies posterior and lateral to the common bile duct within the hepatoduodenal ligament (Fig. 19.5B). At this time, the common hepatic duct is encircled and divided sharply (Fig. 19.9B).

Next, the ligament of Treitz is mobilized, and the jejunum, about 10 cm distal to the ligament of Treitz, is prepared for division. Transillumination of the jejunal mesentery may aid in a clean and efficient dissection of the mesenteric window. A stapler is used to divide the jejunum. The jejunal mesenteric vessels are divided and ligated, progressing toward the fourth portion of the duodenum. This technique continues until the uncinate process of the pancreas is encountered. The proximal je-

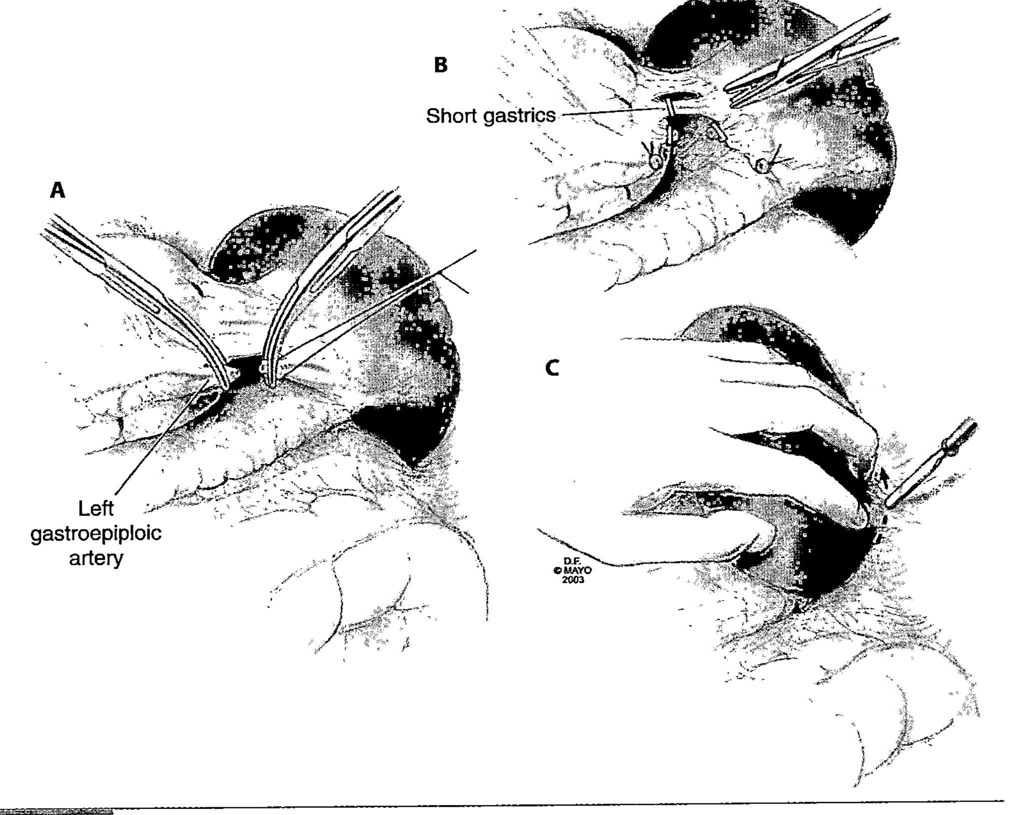

Figure 19.7
(A) Ligation of left gastroepiploic vessels allows access to the gastrosplenic ligament in anticipation of dissecting the short gastric vessels. **(B)** Ligation of short gastric vessels. **(C)** Retraction of the spleen to the right allows incision of the lateral and superior peritoneal attachments.

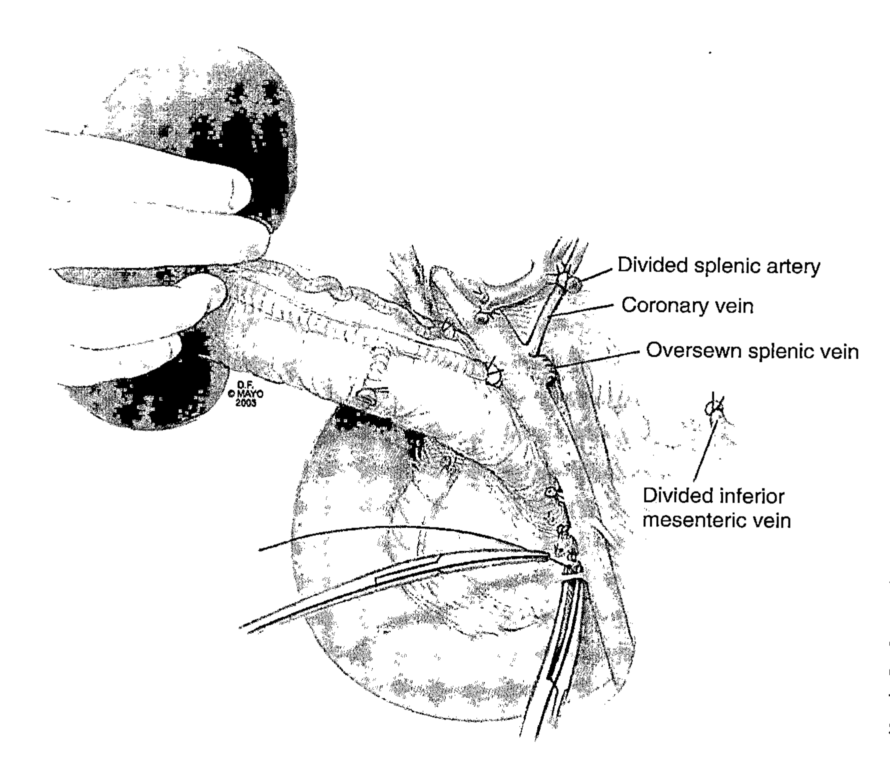

Figure 19.8
After the spleen is mobilized from its bed, the plane posterior to the pancreas is dissected to allow for proximal ligation of the splenic artery and vein. The splenic artery and vein are individually ligated with transfixing sutures. Careful dissection of the splenic vein/portal vein confluence prevents injury to the coronary vein. If the inferior mesenteric vein enters the splenic vein remote from the portal vein, the inferior mesenteric vein is clamped, divided, and ligated. Venous branches draining the uncinate are ligated in continuity and divided. This enables leftward traction of the portal vein/superior mesenteric vein to expose the superior mesenteric artery.

junum is then passed beneath the superior mesenteric vessels into the right supramesocolic compartment. It is recommended that the defect created with this mobilization be closed in order to prevent internal herniation and subsequent bowel obstruction.

As the dissection continues along the portal vein groove at the caudal aspect, it is necessary to identify the highest jejunal and uncinate venous branches. Division of these venous branches affords sufficient mobility to allow retraction of the PV-SMV and exposure of the SMA. It is important to carefully ligate these delicate vessels in order to prevent traction injury (Fig. 19.10A). The dissection continues along the posterior surface of the portal vein; identification and preservation of the coronary

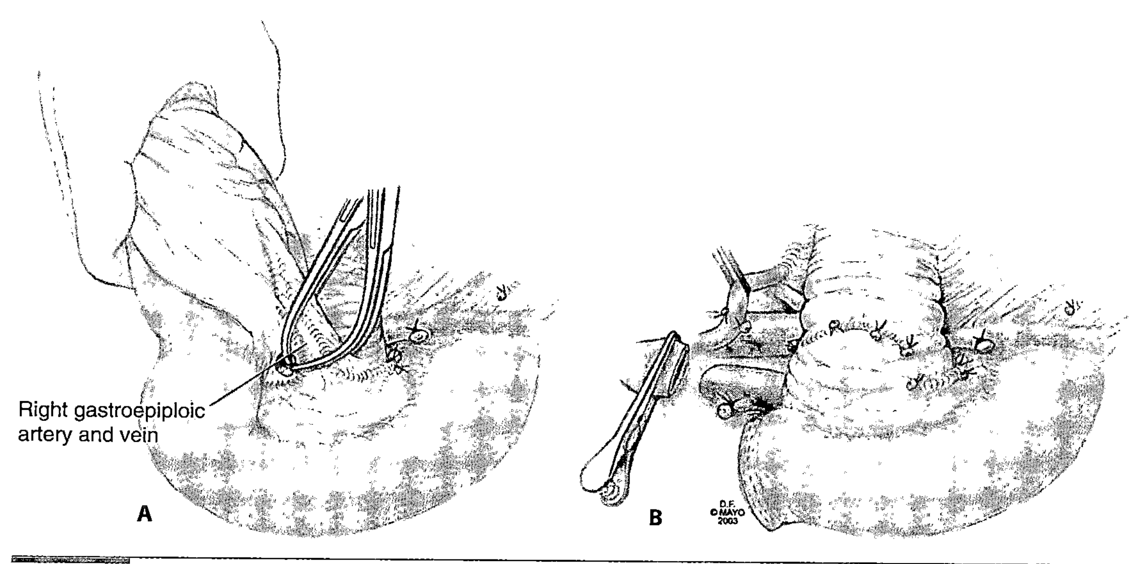

Figure 19.9
(A) Before division, the proximal duodenum is skeletonized on its inferior border by clamping, dividing, and ligating the right gastroepiploic vessels. **(B)** After the gallbladder is mobilized from its bed, the common hepatic duct is transected proximal to the cystic duct. Control is achieved with a bulldog clamp (view from right lateral side of patient).

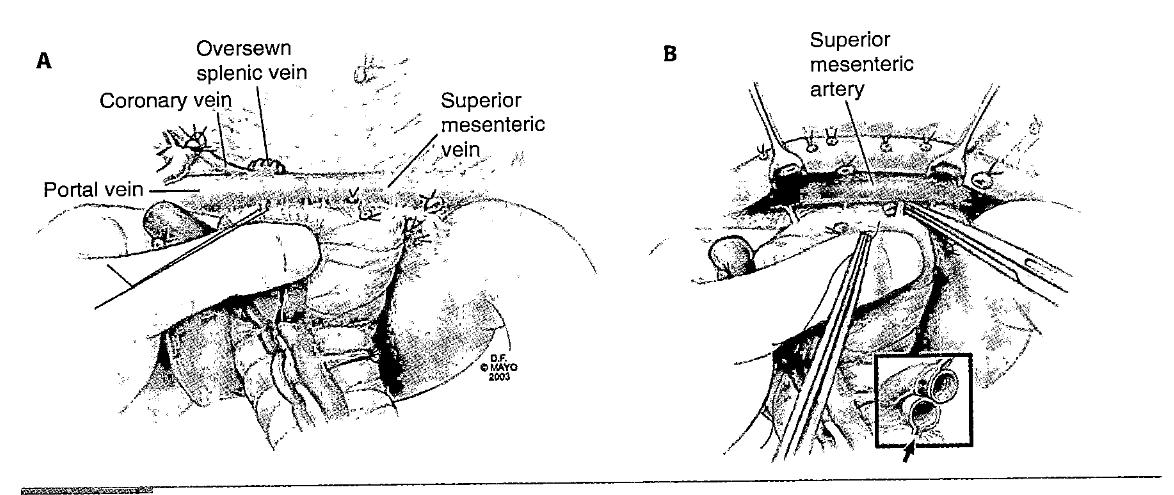

Figure 19.10
(A) The spleen and tail of the pancreas are retracted to the patient's right as the portal vein/superior mesenteric vein confluence is retracted to the left. Venous branches from the head and uncinate process are dissected and ligated. Careful dissection safely exposes the superior mesenteric artery and its branches. **(B)** Once the vein is mobilized, further traction anterior and to the patient's left allows for dissection and individual ligation of the branches of the superior mesenteric artery branches to the uncinate process. Care is taken to identify and, if possible, preserve the highest jejunal arterial branches. The arterial branches originating from the posterolateral aspect of the SMA are very friable, are easily partially avulsed, and may cause troublesome hemorrhage (*inset*) (view from right lateral side of the patient).

vein are necessary to ensure adequate venous drainage of the stomach after the short gastric vessels and the right gastric vessels have been divided.

Once the portal vein dissection is complete, the focus should be placed on the SMA. Retracting the specimen to the patient's right while gentle traction with vein retractors displaces the portal vein to the left facilitates this dissection. Retroperitoneal soft tissue posterior to the pancreas is divided to skeletonize the SMA and its branches coursing into the pancreas and duodenum. This important step ensures that the maximal retroperitoneal/uncinate margin may be obtained (Fig. 19.10B).

Margins are reviewed during surgery by frozen section analysis. Particular attention is paid to the biliary and duodenal margins. If either of these margins shows tumor infiltration, further resection is mandatory until a negative margin is obtained. The retroperitoneal/uncinate margin is of staging benefit, but if the original dissection has completely skeletonized the SMA, no further tissue is available to resect. Although en bloc venous resection is used as necessary, we do not advocate en bloc arterial resection and reconstruction.

Now that extirpation is complete, reconstruction begins. This stepwise process involves restoring biliary and gastrointestinal continuity. The authors' preference is to bring the jejunal limb in a retrocolic fashion to the right of the middle colic vessels, as opposed to the left in the native retromesenteric configuration. The hepaticojejunostomy is completed in an end-to-side orientation with a single layer of continuous or interrupted absorbable suture. The continuous technique is used for a large-caliber bile duct, and interrupted sutures are used for small or thin-walled bile ducts. The authors have discontinued routine bilioenteric anastomotic stenting.[18] The jejunum is then fixed to the mesocolon in a tension-free manner. The antecolic end-to-side duodenojejunostomy is completed in two layers (Fig. 19.11). A surgical drain is routinely placed in Morrison's pouch. Gastrostomy and jejunostomy tubes are used only on a selective basis.

Postoperative Care

The perioperative care of a patient undergoing a major pancreatic resection is essential to obtaining a good outcome. Although arrangement for postoperative intensive care admission is not routine, provisions need to be made for continuous infusion of insulin and hourly glucose checks.[19] Prophylactic antibiotics and antacids are used routinely. Antibiotics are given to maintain adequate tissue levels during surgery, and after surgery, they are discontinued within 24 hours. Cholangitis secondary to preoperative biliary stenting may be present, and in this case, appropriate antibiotic coverage should continue. Closed-suction intraperitoneal drainage accompanies total pancreatectomy. Subhepatic drainage is continued un-

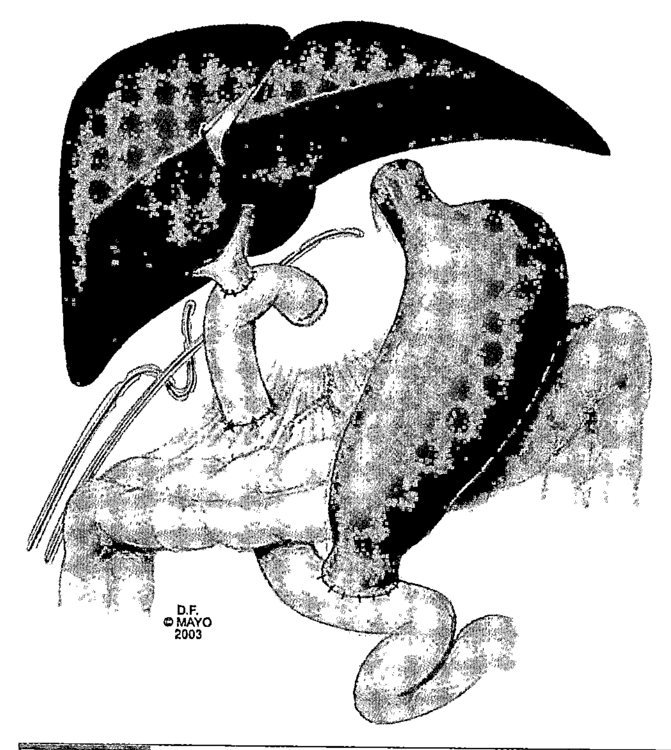

Figure 19.11
The proximal jejunum is passed through the transverse mesocolon to the right of the middle colic vessels, and an end-to-side hepaticojejunostomy is performed with a single layer of interrupted or continuous absorbable suture. An antecolic end-to-side duodenojejunostomy is performed in two layers. Surgical drains are routinely placed behind the hepaticojejunostomy and in the subhepatic space.

til the output volume is low, less than 30 mL/day, and serous in nature. Nasogastric decompression is maintained for less than 24 hours. Liquid diet is started with the onset of bowel function, and advancement to diabetic diet occurs as tolerated.

During total pancreatectomy, attention is focused on blood glucose levels immediately as the specimen is removed. Communication between the operating and anesthesiology teams should occur. Continuous insulin infusion may be necessary in the operating room and for the immediate postoperative period. Reflectance meter glucose (RMG) monitoring is performed every hour until glucose levels stabilize in the target range (100–200 mg/dL). Once glucose levels have stabilized, the frequency of (RMG) monitoring is decreased, and transition is made from continuous infusion to intermittent percutaneous injection. With resumption of oral intake, the home-going insulin regimen can be determined. Diabetic management and oral pancreatic enzyme supplementation are taught to the patient and caretakers.

In contrast to proximal Whipple pancreatoduodenectomy, a pancreatoenteric leak is not an issue in the postoperative period. Other complications, such as delayed gastric emptying, biliary leak, intra-abdominal sepsis, hemorrhage, and wound infection, are managed similarly to those encountered after Whipple pancreatoduodenectomy.

Because the spleen is removed in total pancreatectomy, the patient should be vaccinated against common encapsulated bacterial pathogens and educated regarding the entity of postsplenectomy sepsis.[20,21]

Total pancreatectomy results in loss of the acid-neutralizing effects of pancreatic bicarbonate secretion within the bowel lumen. Although we have found that the incidence of marginal ulceration at the gastrojejunostomy was greater after total pancreatectomy than after Whipple resection (11% vs 5%),[22] these data were accrued before the development of the H_2-receptor antagonists or proton-pump inhibitors.

Surgical Outcome

Complications and operative mortality following pancreatoduodenectomy for ductal adenocarcinoma have been extensively analyzed in large, contemporary series of patients.[12-16] These reports confirm that at centers of excellence, operative mortality is less than 5%, and although morbidity remains substantial (40%), most complications are managed without surgery and are not life threatening. Interventional radiologic techniques have greatly enhanced the postoperative management of these cases. The literature regarding morbidity and mortality for total pancreatectomy for ductal adenocarcinoma is not nearly as refined and is, in many respects, outdated. For example, Pliam and ReMine[3] reported on 64 total pancreatectomies (1942–1973) and carefully catalogued postoperative complications, but the patients were treated in an era that preceded modern imaging, interventional radiologic techniques, surgical intensive care concepts, and intravenous hyperalimentation. The operative mortality in this series was 14% and the morbidity 56%; however, this may not be relevant to current practice for the reasons previously mentioned. On the other hand, Pliam and ReMine's observations regarding the brittle diabetes occurring in these apancreatic patients is relevant to contemporary surgical practice. Twenty percent of patients had ketoacidosis or hypoglycemia requiring rehospitalization.

The results for total pancreatectomy for ductal adenocarcinoma performed at Mayo Clinic were updated by Sarr et al.[7] and reported in 1993. Between 1955 and 1990,

99 total pancreatectomies were performed for ductal adenocarcinoma. The operative mortality was 6%, but postoperative morbidity was not reported.

More contemporary reports addressing total pancreatectomy for ductal adenocarcinoma reflect the evolution in thought regarding the indications for total gland extirpation. More recent series reflect the current trend in selection of patients, with more extensive tumors being treated with total pancreatectomy rather than wide application of the technique, as was practiced in the earlier era. Because total pancreatectomy is now primarily undertaken for more extensive tumors, it can be anticipated that both the morbidity and the mortality will be higher than that reported after Whipple resection.

The most contemporary series of total pancreatectomy patients for ductal adenocarcinoma of the pancreas was reported by Karpoff et al.[11] in 2001. Twenty-eight patients underwent total pancreatectomy from 1983 to 1998. Their report reflects the selective use of total pancreatectomy for extensive tumors. The median blood loss was 2800 mL, 61% developed postoperative complications, and the median length of stay was 32 days. Fifty-four percent required rehospitalization, with a median stay of 22 days. These surgeons have extensive experience with pancreatic resection and have reported superb results for Whipple resection.[23]

These data underscore the selection that occurs for patients who undergo total pancreatectomy and the fact that series of Whipple resections and total pancreatectomy are not strictly comparable. Most surgeons now limit total pancreatectomy for adenocarcinoma to a very small percentage of patients. In the series by Karpoff et al.,[11] 409 patients underwent Whipple resection for adenocarcinoma during the study interval, whereas 28 underwent total pancreatectomy. The in-hospital mortality in their series was 8.6%.[11]

Of 166 patients undergoing pancreatoduodenectomy for ductal adenocarcinoma of the pancreatic head performed by the senior author from 1981 to 2001, one-stage total pancreatectomy was performed in only six patients (3.6%). Moreover, in only one patient was this decision made before surgery. The patient had been treated at an outside hospital with external drainage of an obstructive pseudocyst in the tail of the pancreas. The presence of a ductal carcinoma in the head of the pancreas resulted in a chronic pancreaticocutaneous fistula. A planned total pancreatectomy was performed. In the remaining five patients, the decision to perform total pancreatectomy was made during surgery. In two cases, positive pancreatic neck margins prompted conversion from partial to total pancreatectomy. Another two were converted to total pancreatectomy based on marked atrophy of the chronically obstructed body and tail. In one patient, the pancreatic remnant was extremely soft and held suture poorly, and attempts to perform pancreaticojejunostomy were abandoned and completion pancreatectomy was performed. Two-stage or completion pancreatectomy was required in two patients in the early postoperative period; both had anastomotic dehiscence, causing peritonitis in one and hemorrhage in the other.

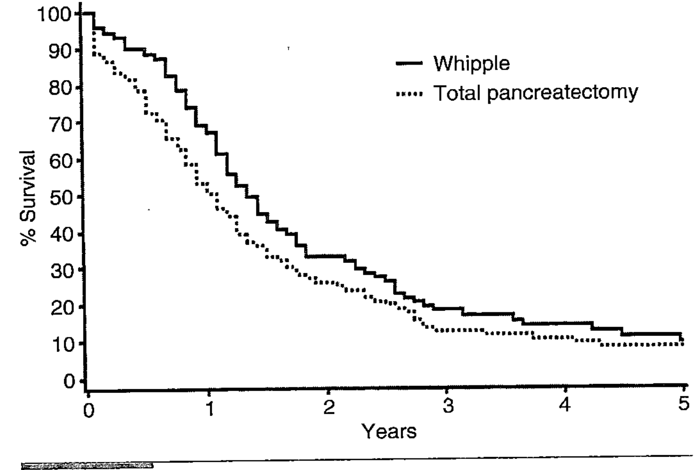

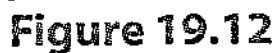

Figure 19.12
Kaplan-Meier survival curves of 203 patients treated at Mayo Clinic with either total pancreatectomy (1955–1990, $N = 99$) or Whipple resection (1980–1990, $N = 104$) for ductal adenocarcinoma of the pancreas. (From Sarr et al.[7]; with permission.)

Total pancreatectomy was more widely applied in an earlier era, when it was suggested that the procedure was more oncologically sound than subtotal pancreatectomy. The advantages of total pancreatectomy have not been borne out by an improvement in long-term survival. In our most recent report, the survival after total pancreatectomy for 99 patients was no better than that of 104 patients undergoing Whipple resection for ductal adenocarcinoma of the pancreas from 1980 to 1990 (Fig. 19.12).[7] Although Whipple resection and total pancreatectomy are not comparable statistically for reasons already alluded to, it is clear that total pancreatectomy does not afford a survival advantage for patients with ductal adenocarcinoma of the pancreas. Our data are consistent with that reported by other investigators in the field. The operative mortality and long-term survival for total pancreatectomy for ductal adenocarcinoma of the pancreas for collected series are summarized in Table 19.1.[3-11]

Table 19.1. Operative Mortality and Long-Term Survival After Total Pancreatectomy for Ductal Adenocarcinoma of the Pancreas

Author (Date of Publication)	Study Interval(s)	Patients, No.	30-Day Mortality, %	5-Year Survival, %
Pliam and ReMine[3] (1975)	1942–1969	36	17	8.3
	1969–1973	28	11	8.3
van Heerden et al.[4] (1988)	1951–1985	89	10	7
	1980–1985	32	6.2	
Fortner[5] (1984)	1979–1983	20	10	N/A
Brooks et al.[6] (1989)	1970–1976	48	8	14
Sarr et al.[7] (1993)	1955–1990	99	6	10
Trede[8] (1993)	1972–1984	44	7	11
Launois et al.[9] (1993)	1968–1986	47	13	8
Edge et al.[10] (1993)	1989–1990	11	1	N/A
Karpoff et al.[11] (2001)	1983–1998	35	3	11

Conclusion

Whipple resection remains the procedure of choice for the vast majority of patients with ductal adenocarcinoma of the pancreatic head. Prior surgical investigators touted total pancreatectomy as a superior procedure for both oncologic and technical considerations. Total pancreatectomy addressed both multicentricity and removed additional lymph nodes and soft tissue. Moreover, the need for a pancreaticoenterostomy was eliminated. The rate of multicentric ductal cancer is now known to be minimal. Leak from the pancreaticojejunostomy does not have the serious implications once attributed to it; the apancreatic state may result in brittle diabetes, and long-term survival after total pancreatectomy is no better than with Whipple resection. For these reasons, total pancreatectomy should be used only selectively in patients with ductal carcinoma of the pancreas. The extent of tumor in the pancreas or the inability to perform a safe pancreaticoenterostomy are the main indications. In the senior author's experience, fewer than 5% of patients with ductal carcinoma of the pancreatic head require total pancreatectomy.

If total pancreatectomy is performed, risk of operation may be increased because of selection of patients with more extensive tumors. Long-term survival is no better than that observed after Whipple resection. Immediate postoperative management is similar to that after Whipple resection, combined with the need for intensive glucose monitoring and continuous insulin infusion. Long-term survivors require both education and ongoing management of the apancreatic and asplenic states.

References

1. Ross DE. Cancer of the pancreas: a plea for total pancreatectomy. *Am J Surg*. 1954;87:20–33.
2. Brooks JR. The case of total pancreatectomy. In: Delaney JP, Vargo RL, eds. *Controversies in Surgery*. Philadelphia: WB Saunders; 1983:327–335.
3. Pliam MB, ReMine WH. Further evaluation of total pancreatectomy. *Arch Surg*. 1975;110:506–512.
4. van Heerden JA, McIlrath DC, Ilstrup DM, Weiland LH. Total pancreatectomy for ductal adenocarcinoma of the pancreas: an update. *World J Surg*. 1988;12:658–662.
5. Fortner JG. Regional pancreatectomy for cancer of the pancreas, ampulla and other related sites: tumor staging and results. *Ann Surg*. 1984;199:418–425.
6. Brooks JR, Brooks DC, Levine JD. Total pancreatectomy for ductal cell carcinoma of the pancreas: an update. *Ann Surg*. 1989;209:405–410.
7. Sarr MG, Behrns KE, van Heerden JA. Total pancreatectomy: an objective analysis of its use in pancreatic cancer. *Hepatogastroenterology*. 1993;40:418–421.
8. Trede M. The surgical options. In: Trede M, Carter DC, eds. *Surgery of the Pancreas*. New York: Churchill Livingstone; 1993:433–443.
9. Launois B, Franci J, Bardaxoglou E, et al. Total pancreatectomy for ductal adenocarcinoma of the pancreas with special reference to resection of portal vein and multicentric cancer. *World J Surg*. 1993;17:122–127.

10. Edge SB, Schmieg Jr RE, Rosenlof LK, et al. Pancreas cancer resection outcome in American university centers in 1989–1990. *Cancer*. 1993;71:3502–3508.
11. Karpoff HM, Klimstra DS, Brennan MF, Conlon KC. Results of total pancreatectomy for adenocarcinoma of the pancreas. *Arch Surg*. 2001;136:44–48.
12. Michelassi F, Erroi F, Dawson PJ, et al. Experience with 647 consecutive tumors of the duodenum, ampulla, head of pancreas, and distal common bile duct. *Ann Surg*. 1989;210:544–556.
13. Aranha GV, Hodul PJ, Creech S, Jacobs W. Zero mortality after 152 consecutive pancreaticoduodenectomies with pancreaticogastrostomy. *J Am Coll Surg*. 2003;197:223–231.
14. Yeo CJ, Cameron JL, Sohn TA, et al. 650 consecutive pancreaticoduodenectomies in the 1990's: pathology, complications, and outcomes. *Ann Surg*. 1997;226:248–260.
15. Miedema SS, Sarr MG, van Heerden JA, et al. Complications following pancreaticoduodenectomy: current management. *Arch Surg*. 1992;127:945–950.
16. Millikan KW, Dexiel DJ, Silverstein JC, et al. Prognostic factors associated with resectable adenocarcinoma of the head of the pancreas. *Am Surg*. 1999;65:618–624.
17. Armas-Loughran B, Kalra R, Carson JL. Evaluation and management of anemia and bleeding disorders in surgical patients. *Med Clin North Am*. 2003;87:229–242.
18. Fallick JS, Farley DR, Farnell MB, et al. Venting intraluminal drains in pancreaticoduodenectomy. *J Gastrointest Surg*. 1999;3:156–161.
19. Trede M. Treatment of pancreatic, ampullary and periampullary neoplasms. In: Braasch JW, Tompkins RK, eds. *Surgical Disease of the Biliary Tract and Pancreas*. St. Louis: Mosby; 1994:540–564.
20. Brigden ML. Detection, education and management of the asplenic or hyposplenic patient. *Am Fam Physician*. 2001;63:499–506.
21. Pate JW, Peters TG, Andrews CR. Postsplenectomy complications. *Am Surg*. 1985;51:437–441.
22. Grant CS, van Heerden JA. Anastomotic ulceration following subtotal and total pancreatectomy. *Ann Surg*. 1979;190:1–5.
23. Conlon KC, Klimsta DS, Brennan MF. Long-term survival after curative resection for pancreatic ductal adenocarcinoma: clinicopathologic analysis of 5-year survivors. *Ann Surg*. 1996;223:273–279.

CHAPTER

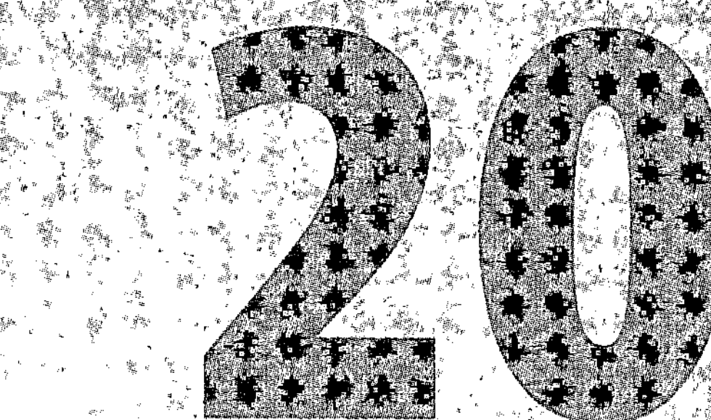

Distal Pancreatectomy

Scott F. Gallagher, MD
Emmanuel E. Zervos, MD
Michel M. Murr, MD

Distal pancreatectomy was first completed by Billroth in 1884 as reported by Finney[1] and has remained essentially unchanged for a century with only minor technical innovations. Clearly, the most critical consideration regarding cancer in the body and tail of the pancreas is the high likelihood of unresectability. Although distal pancreatectomy, like pancreaticoduodenectomy, has increased in frequency over the past decade, a smaller percentage of tumors (7%–10% vs 15%) are resectable at presentation. This is directly attributable to the absence of obstructive jaundice and subsequent delayed presentation associated with lesions in the body and tail, as compared with the classic, and thus earlier, presentation of periampullary lesions.[2,3]

Distal pancreatectomy as depicted herein remains the standard operation for tumors of the body and tail of the pancreas. Variations (extent of resection, lymphadenectomy, minimally invasive access, and splenic preservation) are based primarily on the histology and location of individual lesions. Although laparoscopic pancreatic resections are currently evolving, experience is limited to few centers with a small cohort of patients. However, laparoscopic staging has become integral in determining resectability and avoiding unnecessary laparotomy, especially in body and tail lesions.[4] Nevertheless, an aggressive approach for open resection of distal pancreatic tumors should be maintained. Resection not only offers the only chance for long-term survival but also represents the best palliative modality currently available.[5]

This chapter outlines a practical approach, including a treatment decision algorithm for operative treatment of tumors in the body and tail of the pancreas. The utility of diagnostic testing as well as other imaging modalities, although especially important to distal pancreas tumors, is thoroughly discussed in other chapters.

Clinical Presentation

Primary neoplastic lesions of the pancreas are often asymptomatic and may be found during the evaluation of pancreatitis or vague abdominal symptoms.[6] Pain is one of the most common symptoms and tends to be a poor prognostic indicator as a marker of advanced disease and unresectability, particularly back pain associated with adenocarcinoma or other noncystic neoplasms. Additionally, patients often complain of vague epigastric pain, which can at times be relieved by hunching and accentuated by lying supine. Therefore, the importance of the liberal use of multimechanism analgesia as well as a multidisciplinary approach during the course of both diagnostic and therapeutic interventions cannot be overemphasized.[7]

Additional signs and symptoms associated with tumors in the body and tail of the pancreas are usually nonspecific: anorexia, malaise, decreased endurance, early satiety, weight loss, abdominal fullness, or a palpable abdominal mass. Unlike the association of painless jaundice and periampullary tumors, there is no such association with an early marker of disease for tumors in the distal pancreas; in fact, painless jaundice rarely exists at presentation. Although not pathognomonic, the closest similar association is the onset of glucose intolerance in an elderly patient, especially if nonobese, with vague gastrointestinal complaints; this association should alert the physician to the possibility of pancreatic cancer in general.[7]

In addition to symptoms, four physical findings are associated with disseminated cancer: supraclavicular lymphadenopathy (Virchow's node), periumbilical lymphadenopathy (Sister Mary Joseph's node), a palpable pelvic shelf on rectal examination (Blumer's shelf), and ascites. As indicators of metastatic disease and therefore unresectability, the presence of any of these signs portends the same poor prognosis associated with unresectability of any other foregut malignancy.[7-9]

Staging Modalities

A detailed description of imaging and diagnostic modalities is the subject of many earlier chapters in this textbook (see Chapters 12 through 17). Imaging modalities are used liberally; triple-phase helical computed tomography (CT) with three-dimensional reconstruction as well as oral and intravenous contrast is our preferred modality for staging tumors of the body and tail. As a second tier when vascular involvement cannot be otherwise determined, magnetic resonance imaging, angiography, or endoscopic ultrasound are incorporated, the latter particularly important when tissue diagnosis would be necessary to guide neoadjuvant therapy.

The role of laparoscopy as an additional staging modality (see Chapter 14) is more useful for tumors in the body and tail of the pancreas than for tumors in the head of the pancreas because most of the former are metastatic at presentation. Staging laparoscopy is used selectively to determine local-regional involvement or to detect distant metastases and avoid an unnecessary laparotomy, because previously unrecognized metastatic disease is present in one third of all patients with pancreatic cancer who had undergone routine preoperative imaging studies (CT, magnetic resonance imaging, and angiography), regardless of tumor location.[7,10,11] Table 20.1 summarizes the

Table 20.1 Impact of Laparoscopy on Staging Tumors in the Head (H), Body (B), and Tail (T) of the Pancreas

Author	Institution	Year	*N*	Location	Up-staged	Comments
Pisters et al.[11]	MDACC	2001	594	NR [review]	4%–15%	Must have high-quality CT; would be spared celiotomy
Kwon et al.[15]	Kansai	2002	52	75% H 25% B/T	35%	10% up-staged with LUS
Hochwald et al.[43]	UF	2001	48	56% H 44% B/T	41%	All nonfunctioning islet cell tumors
Jimenez et al.[44]	MGH	2000	125	62% H 38% B/T	38%	7% up-staged with peritoneal washings
Minnard et al.[16]	MSKCC	1998	90	72% H 21% B 3% T	54%	8% up-staged with LUS
Conlon et al.[45]	MSKCC	1996	115	64% H 18% B 7% T	43.5%	Extensive diagnostic laparoscopy
Fernandez-del Castillo et al.[46]	MGH	1995	114	78% H 22% B/T	18% H 44% B/T 8% other	14% positive peritoneal washings; 8% without other visible metastases

Abbreviations: MDACC, M D Anderson Cancer Center; NR, not reported; CT, computed tomography; UF, University of Florida; MGH, Massachusetts General Hospital; MSKCC, Memorial Sloan-Kettering Cancer Center; LUS, laparoscopic ultrasound.

studies of patients with pancreatic cancer who were upstaged with staging laparoscopy.[11,12]

The Mayo Clinic reviewed all pancreatic resections in patients who were preoperatively predicted to have clinically resectable pancreatic cancer that was ultimately deemed unresectable during surgery, in order to infer those who would benefit from staging laparoscopy. Patients with metastasis to the liver or peritoneum had a significantly shorter median survival (<7 months); therefore, laparoscopic staging would have eliminated the need for celiotomy in these patients, who either would not have benefited from resection or were otherwise palliated endoscopically.[10]

Use of ultrasound (endoscopic and intraoperative) is increasing. Endoscopic ultrasound is specifically useful for detection, diagnosis, and staging.[13] Ultrasound facilitates examining the tumor's relationship to the superior mesenteric artery and vein, the splenic artery and vein, and the portal vein. Additionally, ultrasound is helpful for visualizing the main pancreatic duct and for localizing small, neuroendocrine tumors as well as for obtaining tissue for histologic confirmation in order to be eligible for neoadjuvant protocols.[13,15,16] Several studies have established the utility of laparoscopic ultrasound to overcome the limitations of laparoscopy, particularly when the findings at laparoscopy are equivocal, while improving assessment and staging of pancreatic cancer.[15,16]

Although resection is the only chance of significantly improving survival, prudence is of paramount importance because patients with unresectable, pancreatic neoplasms have a mean survival ranging from 4 to 11 months. Consequently, all diagnostic and minimally invasive modalities are exploited to avoid unnecessary laparotomy and the subsequent convalescence, if possible, especially because palliation for obstruction (biliary or gastric outlet) is rarely necessary for tumors in the body and tail of the pancreas.

Resection: Treatment and Technique

Indications

The most common indications for distal pancreatectomy are chronic pancreatitis and pseudocysts that masquerade as tumors, cystic neoplasms, adenocarcinoma, intraductal papillary mucinous neoplasms (IPMNs), and neuroendocrine tumors.[2,17,18] Unlike adenocarcinoma, cystic lesions (benign or malignant) are more likely to be resectable than solid lesions. In fact, all patients with complex cystic neoplasms, in particular cystadenocarcinoma, without obvious metastatic disease should undergo planned resection.[3,6] Similarly when disease is limited to the pancreas, patients with nonfunctioning neuroendocrine tumors or ductal adenocarcinoma should undergo curative resection.[3] An aggressive approach is preferred for locally advanced neuroendocrine tumors, including resection of adjacent organs (i.e., stomach, spleen, liver, colon, adrenal, kidney) for debulking.[14,17]

Preoperative Preparation

Vaccines are administered before surgery for pneumococcus, meningococcus, and *Haemophilus influenzae*, in anticipation of splenectomy. A full, mechanical bowel preparation, including oral antibiotics, is also prescribed. This not only decompresses the colon while facilitating exposure but it also anticipates the possibility of colectomy—specifically, the transverse colon, should the bowel or its mesentery demonstrate local tumor involvement. Although rarely required, the groin should be prepared, anticipating possible vein graft reconstruction during the course of an operation for tumors in the neck or the proximal body of the pancreas.

Anatomic Considerations

While pancreatic resections are planned and conducted, as with other oncologic operations, there are two goals of resection for adenocarcinoma.[19] The first is to confirm the diagnosis histologically. The second includes complete tumor resection with adequate margins and resection of regional lymph nodes for accurate staging (Fig. 20.1). Additionally, it is important to conduct an exhaustive, preoperative, and intraoperative search for extrapancreatic disease because resection may be contraindicated in patients with involved extrapancreatic lymph nodes or evidence of distant metastatic disease.[3]

For patients suspected of having locally advanced tumors, laparoscopy is used to examine the liver and peritoneal surfaces to exclude extrapancreatic spread that would otherwise preclude resection. When the tumor is confined to the pancreas, then celiotomy is indicated. The choice of incision is surgeon dependent; however, a transverse abdominal incision or a midline incision is preferred. If there has been a prior celiotomy, attempts are made to incorporate an existing abdominal incision. Although left subcostal incision or extension to a chevron incision is acceptable, the choice should be individualized to each patient, tumor, and body habitus.

A thorough abdominal exploration includes palpation of all peritoneal surfaces, the liver, and the lesser sac. Within the lesser sac, attention should be directed

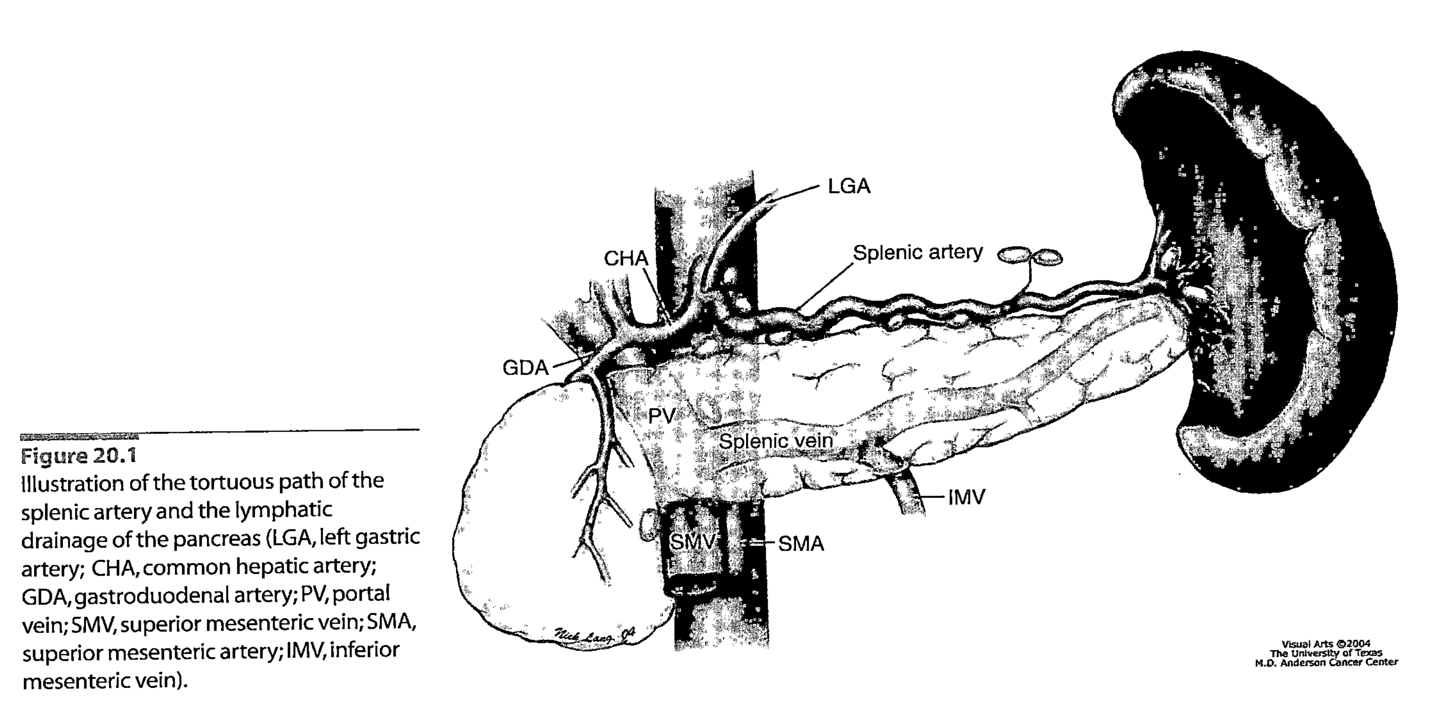

Figure 20.1
Illustration of the tortuous path of the splenic artery and the lymphatic drainage of the pancreas (LGA, left gastric artery; CHA, common hepatic artery; GDA, gastroduodenal artery; PV, portal vein; SMV, superior mesenteric vein; SMA, superior mesenteric artery; IMV, inferior mesenteric vein).

at the posterior stomach along the lesser curvature, the splenic hilum, the root of the mesentery, the celiac axis, and the greater curvature along the gastrocolic omentum (Figs. 20.1 and 20.2).

Distal Pancreatectomy with Splenectomy

In the absence of extrapancreatic metastasis, the operation proceeds by dissecting the gastrocolic ligament from the colon along the avascular plane adjacent to the colon and proceeding from left to right, beginning at the splenocolic ligament. The remaining avascular splenic attachments (phrenosplenic, splenorenal, and splenocolic ligaments) are divided. All short gastric vessels are divided near the stomach between clamps and ligated; alternatively, the ultrasonic dissector or the electrothermal bipolar vessel sealer can be used to expedite this dissection. Once the lesser sac is entered, the stomach is retracted cephalad and the transverse colon is retracted caudad, exposing the anterior surface of the pancreas and spleen (Fig. 20.2).

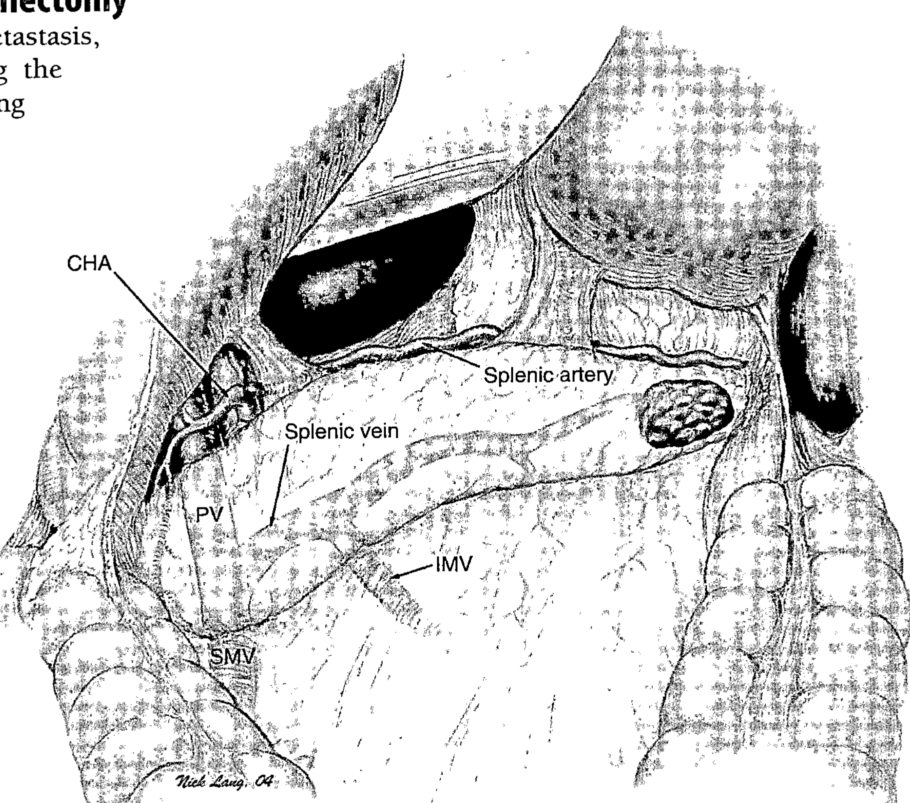

Figure 20.2
Exposure within the lesser sac once the gastrocolic omentum has been completely dissected off of the colon. The stomach is retracted cephalad, while the colon is retracted caudad (CHA, common hepatic artery; PV, portal vein; SMV, superior mesenteric; IMV, interior mesenteric vein).

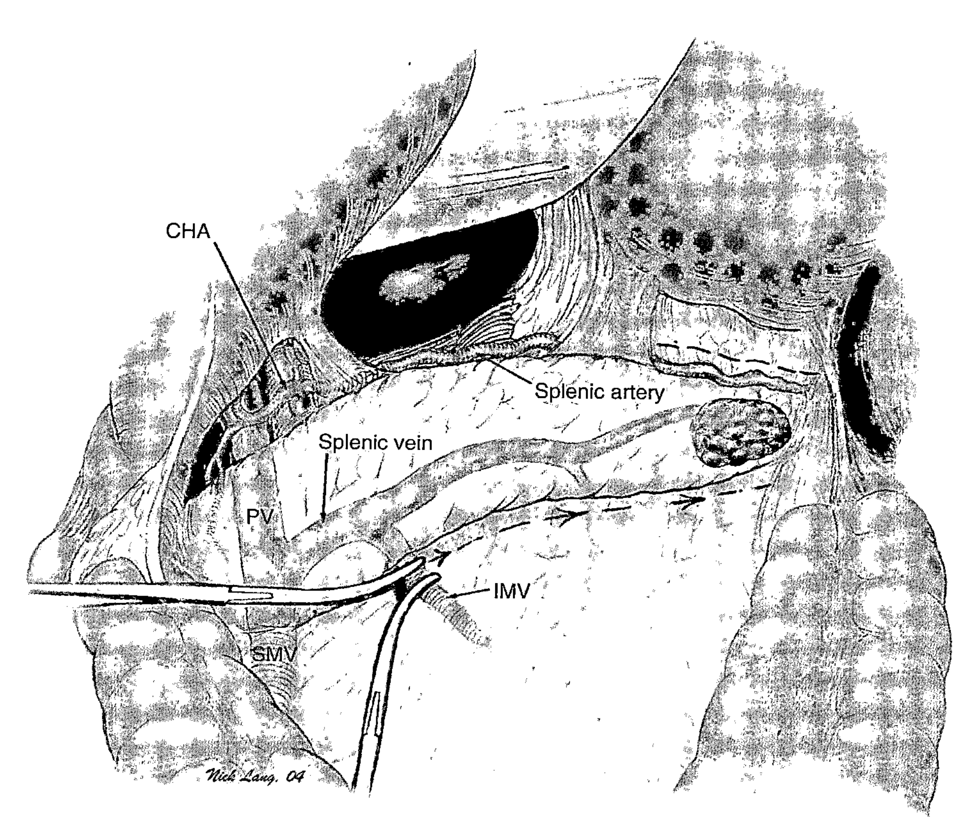

Figure 20.3
The plane for dissecting the inferior border of the pancreas is illustrated. The initial dissection proceeds from medial to lateral along the inferior border of the pancreas. (CHA, common hepatic artery; PV, portal vein; SMV, superior mesenteric; IMV, interior mesenteric vein.)

The splenic artery is identified at its origin from the celiac axis; the artery may be doubly ligated and divided when possible, before the posterior dissection, thereby minimizing blood loss during the course of the operation (Fig. 20.2). The proximal splenic artery is optimal for splenic inflow control should inadvertent splenic laceration or avulsion occur. The inferior border of the distal pancreas is then mobilized; dissection of the retroperitoneal attachments begins in an avascular retroperitoneal plane, starting medially and going from the superior mesenteric vein to the splenic hilum (Fig. 20.3).

The next step is to determine the posterior extent of the dissection and resection. As a rule, it is advisable to stay anterior to the adrenal gland unless it is to be included in the resection. The pancreas and the spleen are retracted anteriorly and to the patient's right as the pancreas is mobilized out of the retroperitoneum (Fig. 20.4), thereby allowing visualization of the splenic artery and the confluence of the splenic vein with the superior mesenteric vein. The inferior mesenteric vein may be ligated or preserved, depending on whether the inferior mesenteric vein enters the splenic vein or the superior mesenteric vein. Our preference is to ligate the splenic artery before ligating the splenic vein and after the full extent of the tumor has been clearly identified. The splenic vein is then ligated with a suture ligature, with care being taken to avoid narrowing of the superior mesenteric vein or the portal vein.

A retropancreatic tunnel is created for tumors in the neck or proximal body requiring resection of the pancreas over or to the left of the portal vein. The pancreas is dissected off of the superior mesenteric vein and portal vein confluence, first on the anterior aspect, and then, if necessary depending on the location of the tumor, off of the right/lateral aspect of the portal vein. Meticulous attention and care are required during dissection of the many small, thin-walled, venous tributaries, which drain directly into the superior mesenteric vein or portal vein and hemorrhage profusely when torn. Combinations of blunt instruments (i.e., a right-angled clamp, a Kelly clamp, and a hemostat) are used while careful dissection is completed adjacent to the portal vein.

If concomitant lymphadenectomy is to be performed, the right gastric artery is divided to facilitate lymphatic dissection along the porta hepatis and common hepatic artery. Celiac node dissection can be undertaken at this juncture for staging purposes; however, previous in-

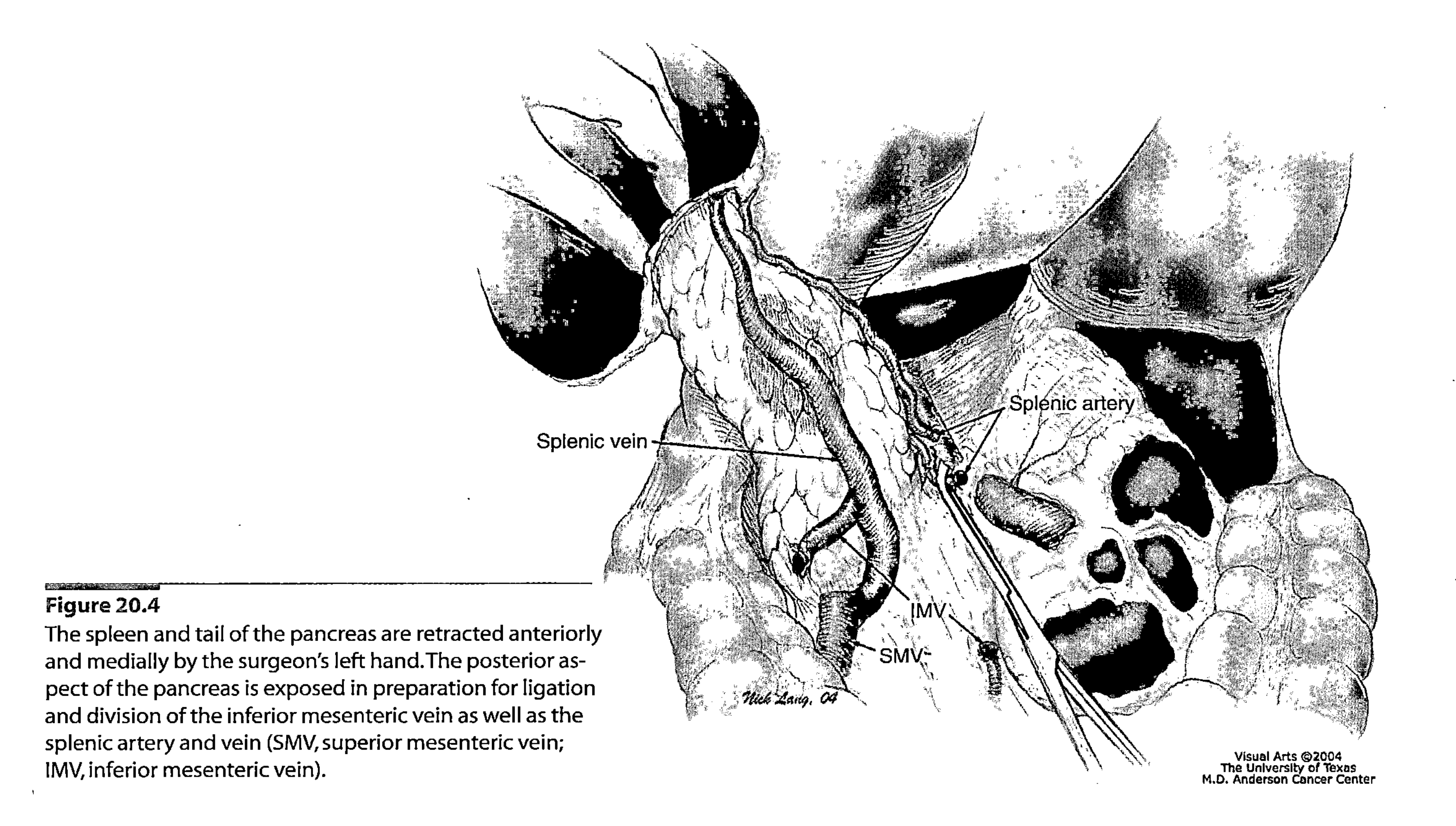

Figure 20.4
The spleen and tail of the pancreas are retracted anteriorly and medially by the surgeon's left hand. The posterior aspect of the pancreas is exposed in preparation for ligation and division of the inferior mesenteric vein as well as the splenic artery and vein (SMV, superior mesenteric vein; IMV, inferior mesenteric vein).

vestigators have shown that extended lymphadenectomy does not improve survival after distal pancreatectomy or pancreaticoduodenectomy, and its routine use has been abandoned by many.[8,19,20]

It is critically important to not divide the pancreas until the feasibility of tumor resection including all gross disease has been confirmed. Once the extent of resection has been clearly defined, 3-0 silk sutures are placed along the superior and inferior borders of the pancreas on both sides of the planned level of pancreas transection for hemostasis as well as retraction. These sutures purposely include the inferior and superior pancreaticoduodenal arcades. The pancreas can be divided with electrocautery, mechanical stapling devices, or a scalpel. If the tumor is near the margin or if the suspected histopathology predicts either ductal involvement or diffuse, parenchymal infiltration, the scalpel is the best method to preserve tissue along the resection margin. It minimizes tissue artifact, which facilitates identification of the pancreatic duct for subsequent ligation and affords the pathologist the best opportunity for accurate frozen section interpretation. The advantages of dividing the pancreas with electrocautery or a stapler are most apparent when wide margins exist between the tumor and the resection margin, because hemostasis with those devices is nearly instantaneous.

Subsequently, the main pancreatic duct is identified and ligated with nonabsorbable suture (Fig. 20.5). Direct identification and ligation of the main pancreatic duct significantly reduces pancreatic duct leaks.[18,21] The end of the pancreatic remnant is oversewn with interlocking, nonabsorbable horizontal-mattress sutures for hemostasis and to minimize the chance of pancreatic fistula (Fig. 20.5).

Soft, closed suction drains are often placed in a dependent position. It is our preference to leave at least one drain extending from deep in the splenic bed up through the pancreatic bed.

Splenic Preservation

Splenic preservation during distal pancreatectomy was first described by Mallet-Guy and Vachon in 1943.[22] Subsequently, the safety and experience with splenic preservation during this procedure has been documented without any increase in complication rate, operative time, or length of stay.[23-25] Splenic preservation is recommended when distal pancreatectomy is completed for either benign disease or small, symptomatic lesions, which are also likely

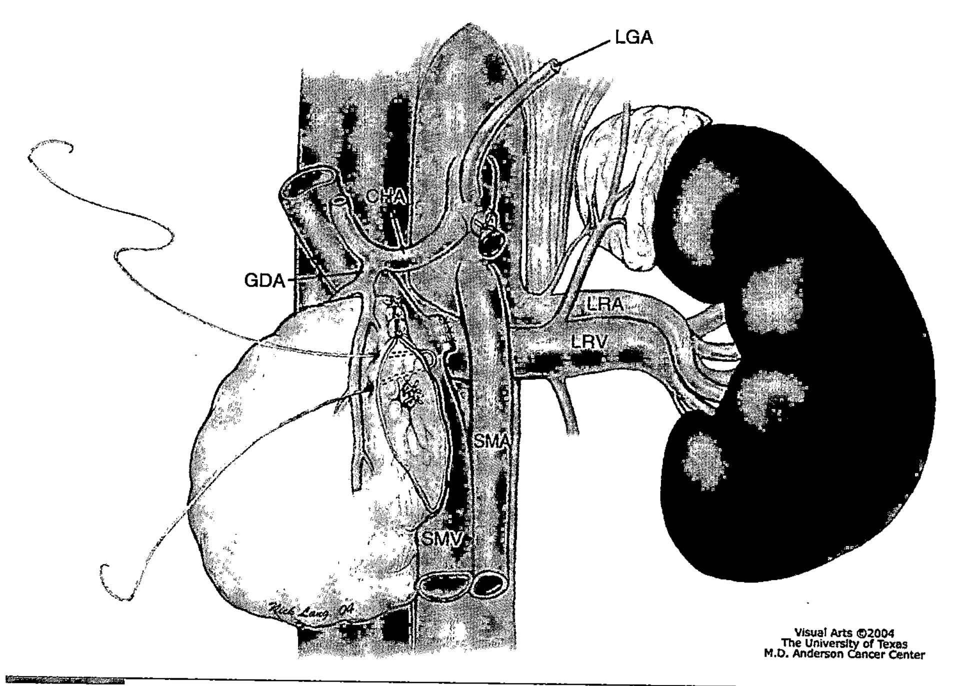

Figure 20.5
The tail of the pancreas has been resected. The main pancreatic duct in the transected edge of the remaining pancreas is identified and ligated. Interlocking, horizontal mattress sutures are placed in the cut edge for hemostasis and occlusion of small ducts (LGA, left gastric artery; CHA, common hepatic artery; GDA, gastroduodenal artery; SMV, superior mesenteric vein; SMA, superior mesenteric artery; LRV, left renal vein; LRA, left renal artery).

benign (Fig. 20.6). Neuroendocrine tumors that are not amenable to enucleation and meet the aforementioned criteria are also candidates for splenic preservation (Fig. 20.7). When performing distal pancreatectomy, one should consider splenic preservation selectively based on the anatomic relationship of the surrounding structures, the presence or absence of splenic vein involvement, and the extent of resection necessary, as determined by the underlying pathology.[2]

The salient features of splenic preservation are the relationship of the tail of the pancreas to the splenic hilum and the tumor location relative to the splenic vessels. Both must be anatomically distinct, as shown in Figs. 20.6 and 20.7, to permit splenic preservation. If these criteria are met, the lesser sac is entered as described earlier, and the distance between the tail of the pancreas and the splenic hilum is inspected to determine whether dissection of the tail is feasible. Subsequently, the tail of the pancreas is dissected with particular attention being paid to avoiding injury to the splenic vein or small venous tributaries to the tail of the pancreas. The peritoneum is opened along the inferior border of the pancreas starting medially and proceeding laterally to aid in the subsequent dissection of the tail from the splenic vein. Dissection proceeds medially until an adequate margin is achieved. Small vessels are controlled by sutures rather than electrocautery and may be aided by using magnifying loops.

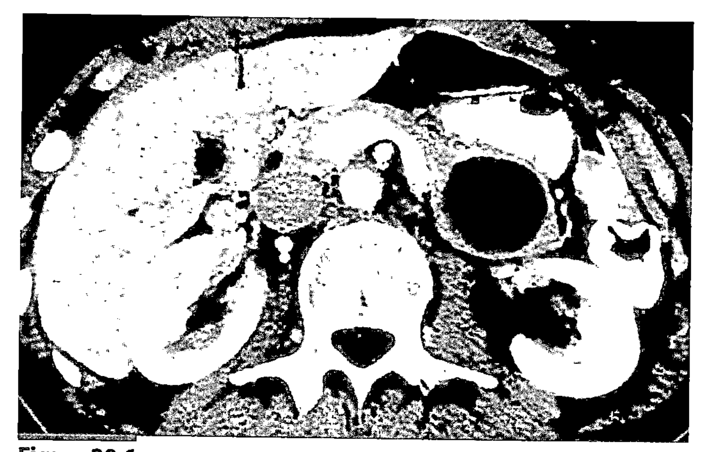

Figure 20.6
Computed tomography of a solitary, cystic lesion in the tail of the pancreas.

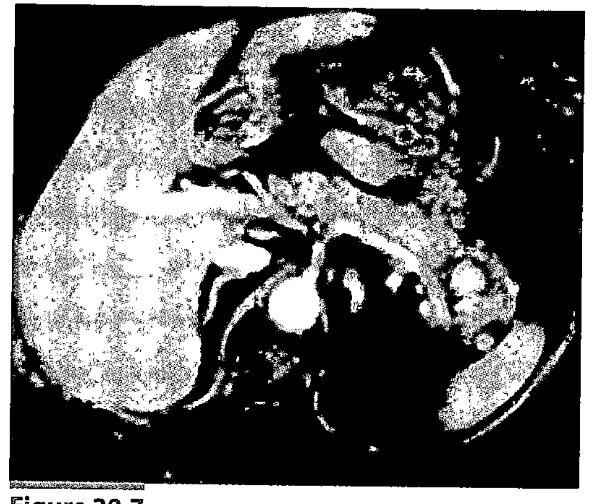

Figure 20.7
Computed tomography demonstrating the classic, early enhancement of a well-encapsulated insulinoma in the tail of the pancreas.

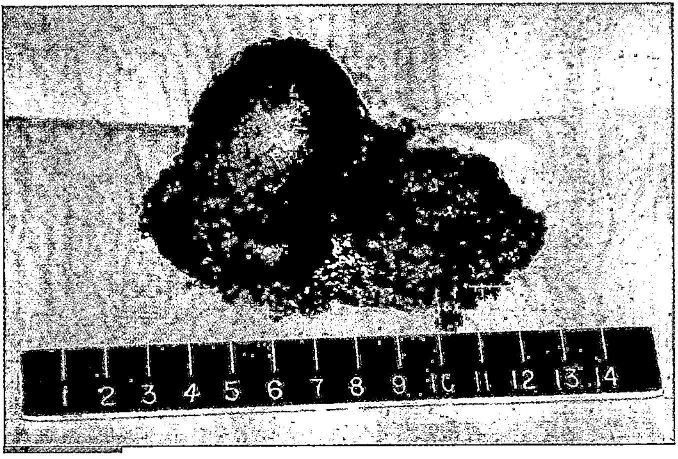

Figure 20.8
Photograph of the specimen resected during a distal pancreatectomy with splenic preservation. The circumscribed insulinoma in the tail of the pancreas involves the main pancreatic duct and could therefore not be enucleated.

The pancreas is divided, and the stump is handled as previously described; the resected distal pancreas with tumor is shown in Fig. 20.8.

Middle-Segment Pancreatectomy

Middle-segment pancreatectomy is specifically advantageous for the rare neck and proximal, midbody pancreatic tumors, which are small and suboptimally managed by pancreaticoduodenectomy or distal pancreatectomy, yet are amenable to limited pancreatic resection. The closer the tumor is to the neck, the less pancreas would remain from an anatomic proximal or distal resection; hence, the significant waste of normal pancreas and the unnecessary risk of endocrine and exocrine insufficiency (as well as splenectomy when extended distal pancreatectomy is performed).[26] Specifically, small cystic neoplasms and neuroendocrine tumors with close proximity to the main pancreatic duct are suitable for middle-segment pancreatectomy, which has been well-described and illustrated by Warshaw et al.[26]

Briefly, the operation begins with exposure as described earlier. The body and neck of the pancreas are dissected from its retroperitoneal attachments while a retroperitoneal tunnel anterior to the superior mesenteric vein is developed for tumors in the neck of the gland. Stay sutures are then placed in the superior and inferior borders of the pancreas on both sides of the tumor. The tumor is resected with adequate margins. The pancreatic stump on the proximal pancreatic remnant is handled in the same manner as a distal pancreatectomy margin where the pancreatic duct is identified and ligated; the cut edge of the pancreas is controlled with interlocking mattress sutures.[21,22,26] The pancreatic stump on the distal pancreatic remnant (tail of the pancreas) is managed identically to pancreaticoduodenectomy (i.e., using Roux-en-Y pancreaticojejunostomy). A duct-to-mucosa pancreaticojejunostomy is ideal, with the use of monofilament 4-0 and 5-0 sutures as well as a second layer approximating the edge of the pancreas to the serosa of the jejunum. In pancreata with small ducts and soft texture, the pancreatic stump is invaginated into the open end of the jejunum and secured with a purse-string suture in addition to interrupted sutures.[27]

Laparoscopic Resections

The principles of anatomic, oncologic resections should not be compromised by the feasibility of minimal access. Laparoscopic procedures have been completed safely in select patients. Small, neuroendocrine or islet cell tumors and cystic tail lesions are particularly amenable to laparoscopic resections (Figs. 20.6 and 20.7), but such patients have largely been the subject of case reports, such as the first-reported laparoscopic distal pancreatectomy and splenectomy for symptomatic serous oligocystic adenoma.[28] Little long-term data exist regarding the outcomes and efficacy of laparoscopic pancreatic resection for cancer.[4,29] Prospective, randomized trials must be undertaken before embracing laparoscopic resection as the standard of care.

Management of Postoperative Complications

Common complications after distal pancreatic resection are summarized in Table 20.2.

Pancreatic Stump Fistula

Pancreatic leak is one of the most dreaded complications after distal pancreatectomy and can be significantly reduced when the pancreatic duct is identified and directly ligated.[21] Although the use of octreotide remains controversial for soft glands and small ducts, the most significant, adequately powered, prospective, randomized,

Table 20.2 Complications Following Distal Pancreatectomy and Middle-Segment Pancreatectomy

	Author Year					
	Bilimoria et al.[21] 2003	Lillemoe et al.[2] 1999	Fabre et al.[47] 1996	Fernandez-del Castillo et al.[18] 1995	Dalton et al.[3] 1992	Warshaw et al.[26] 1998
Institution or location	MDACC	JH	France	MGH	Mayo	MGH
N	126	235	128	71	44	12
Overall morbidity	NR	31%	42% early	20%	27%	25%
Mortality	3%	1%	1%	1%	2%	0%
Pancreatic fistula	10%	5%	17%	10%	4%	17%
Endocrine insufficiency	NR	8%	3%	NR	NR	0%
Exocrine insufficiency	NR	NR	11%	NR	NR	0%
Abscess	4%	4%	8%	4%	4%	0%
Bowel obstruction	0%	4%	5%	NR	NR	0%
Hemorrhage	1%	4%	6%	0%	2%	0%
Pneumonia	1%	2%	NR	4%	2%	0%
Wound infection	8%	NR	3%	1%	NR	0%
Sepsis	2%	NR	NR	3%	NR	0%
Reoperation	2%	6%	27%	1%	NR	0%
Median LOS (days)	13	15	8	10	13	8
Mean age (years)	57	51	59	54	NR	59
Comments	34% pancreatic fistula if duct not identified and ligated.		Multiple centers, retrospective review			Middle-segment pancreas resection

Abbreviations: LOS, length of stay; MDACC, MD Anderson Cancer Center; JH, Johns Hopkins; MGH, Massachusetts General Hospital; NR, not reported.

blinded, multicenter trial, in which we and many contributors to this book participated, failed to show any benefit from the routine, perioperative, prophylactic use of vapreotide to prevent pancreatic fistula.[30]

The mainstay of treatment for any pancreatic leak is the diligent maintenance of surgically placed drains. Percutaneous drainage is another option if drains have become dislodged and removed or were simply not placed at the time of the initial operation. For any patient with sustained fevers, leukocytosis, persistent ileus, abdominal pain, or failure to thrive in the immediate postoperative period, CT with oral and intravenous contrast is performed to eliminate the possibility of an intra-abdominal abscess or undrained fluid collection.

Hemorrhage

Hemorrhage is usually secondary to a pancreatic duct leak associated with the development of a pseudoaneurysm in the splenic artery or erosion through sutures into the splenic vein or other vessel stump. Less commonly hemorrhage may be from the cut edge of the pancreas. In hemodynamically stable patients, angiography with embolization of the bleeding vessel with the use of Gelfoam or coils is nearly always effective.

Endocrine Insufficiency

Routine monitoring of serum glucose level and aggressive correction with insulin during postoperative hospitalization is essential to prevent sequelae of hyperglycemia and ketoacidosis.

Special Considerations: Microscopically Positive Pancreatic Margins

Mucinous cystic neoplasms as well as other cystic tumors and IPMNs are thoroughly discussed in Chapters 51–53. Routine preoperative use of endoscopic retrograde cholangiopancreatography is advocated for IPMNs, with intraoperative verification of margins by frozen section; a total pancreatectomy for positive margins is reserved for a very select group of patients.[6]

Positive margins at the neck, regardless of histopathology, dictate extending the resection as far as the gastroduodenal artery. However, total pancreatectomy is rarely performed, and proper planning with intraoperative assessment of tumor location should occur before the surgeon commits to a specific resection. Likewise, it important to consider the usual sites of positive margins and the propensity of some tumors for neural plexus invasion along the medial border of the uncinate process.[12,31]

Distal Pancreatectomy for Metastatic Tumors

Solitary metastases to the pancreas account for 1%–3% of all pancreatic tumors and have been reported with renal cell carcinoma as well as lung, colon, breast, endometrial, and transitional cell carcinoma. They have also been reported with melanoma, sarcoma, and malignant fibrous histiocytoma. However, meaningful survival has only been observed with isolated, renal cell carcinoma.[32-38] Unfortunately, these lesions are often misdiagnosed as primary metasteses from pancreatic tumors.[33] We and other high-volume centers uniformly pursue aggressive treatment with resection for solitary metastatic lesions when possible, in order to offer palliation and possibly even long-term survival.[2,33-35]

The most commonly described resectable metastatic tumor to the pancreas is renal cell carcinoma. This is due to the relatively favorable prognosis associated with good histopathology in a solitary, pancreatic metastasis after a long, disease-free interval. In fact, the subset of patients with metastatic renal cell carcinoma may experience long disease-free intervals and enjoy long-term survival after pancreatic metastasectomy.[33,39] Although it has been determined that tumor stage is the single most accurate predictor of overall survival, the only significant prognostic factor identified by a review of patients from the Mayo Clinic was an increased histologic tumor grade of the metastatic lesion relative to the original tumor was associated with a worse prognosis.[34,40,41]

We and others concur that an aggressive approach to resection should be advocated in selected solitary metastases to the pancreas.[33-39] The extent of pancreatectomy should be governed by metastasis location balanced with the need for adequate resection margins while retaining enough pancreatic tissue to preserve normal endocrine as well as exocrine function.[38]

Future Directions in the Diagnosis and Treatment of Pancreatic Tumors

As technology continues to progress in both imaging and molecular techniques, the future will most certainly herald more accurate diagnosis and targeted therapies for pancreatic tumors. Endoscopic ultrasound now provides a means to visualize and obtain tissue (either transduodenal or transgastric) from lesions at any location within the pancreas without significant risk of needle tract seeding or pancreatic fistula.[13] Large-gauge core needle biopsy of solid tumors can provide enough tissue to undertake sophisticated molecular assays (i.e., gene chip or microarray). Incorporating these modern, "high throughput" techniques, the relative expression of thousands of genetic markers can now be simultaneously assayed. Universal expression of a gene implicated in carcinogenesis provides justification for further investigation and preclinical studies using pharmacologic or molecular inhibitors of the gene, protein, or protein synthesis pathway.[42] Examples of potential targets discovered or validated by such techniques are listed in Table 20.3.

At our institution, we harvest tissue from all resected pancreatic tumors to determine gene expression profiles for various pancreatic tumor types. We anticipate that establishing a genetic classifier for pancreatic tumors will ultimately prove to be as valuable as conventional histology in offering diagnostic and prognostic data while avoiding the morbidity of a major pancreatic resection. In addition, we expect to elucidate new therapeutic targets based on those markers that differentiate the various types of pancreatic tumors. Finally, we hope that adding molecular markers to the diagnostic profile of pancreatic tumors may further help clarify the clinical dilemma of differentiating pancreatic cancer from chronic pancreatitis, a diagnostic conundrum that has plagued surgeons for years. Table 20.4 lists novel potential targets in neuroendocrine tumors and pancreatic carcinoma that have

Table 20.3. Potential Molecular Targets in Pancreatic Cancer

Target	Novel Agents
K-*ras*	Farnesyl transferase inhibitors
Cyclooxygenase	Cox-2 inhibitors
Her-2/neu	Trastuzumab (Herceptin)
EGF receptor	Erlotinib (Tarceva), IMC225 (Erbitux)
Immune system	Vaccine therapy
Cachexia	Eicosapentaenoic acid
Topoisomerase	CPT-11 (irinotecan)
Angiogenesis factors	Angiostatin
Matrix metalloproteinases	Marimastat, Bay 12-9566

Abbreviations: EGF, epidermal growth factor; IMC, ImClone; CPT-11, Camptothecin-11

Table 20.4. Potential Novel Therapeutic Targets Identified in Pancreatic Adenocarcinoma and Neuroendocrine Tumors

Adenocarcinoma	Neuroendocrine Tumors
Apolipoprotein A-IV	Angiopoietin 2
Trefoil factor	*NPDC* gene (neural proliferation, differentiation, and control)
14-3-3 sigma (stratifin)	Wnt inhibitory factor 1
S100-A6 calcium binding protein	Calcitonin receptor

been identified with the use of microarray with normal pancreas as the reference standard.

Conclusion

Distal pancreatectomy is relatively safe and can be undertaken with low morbidity and rare mortality. The algorithm in Fig. 20.9 demonstrates the crucial points in the decision-making process for patients with tumors in the body and tail of the pancreas.

All patients are preoperatively staged with high-quality CT. If the tumor appears resectable at imaging, staging laparoscopy is indicated. If metastatic disease or a locally advanced tumor is confirmed at laparoscopy, tissue is obtained for diagnosis, if a cytologic or histologic diagnosis has not already been determined. If no metastatic disease is discovered, the surgeon should proceed to celiotomy for resection.

As a rule, pancreatic ductal adenocarcinoma in the body and tail of the pancreas has a poor prognosis because of the late occurrence of nonspecific symptoms. However, stage for stage, the prognosis for tumors in the distal pancreas is no worse than that for similar tumors in the head of the pancreas.

Therefore, it is our practice and recommendation in the spirit of evidence-based medicine that selected, good-risk patients with carcinoma of the distal pancreas without locally advanced or metastatic disease are candidates for curative resection, which is supported by the benchmark reports for distal pancreatectomy.[2,3,18,41,42] Similarly, primary cystic neoplasms as well as solitary metastatic lesions with favorable histology should be resected. Our

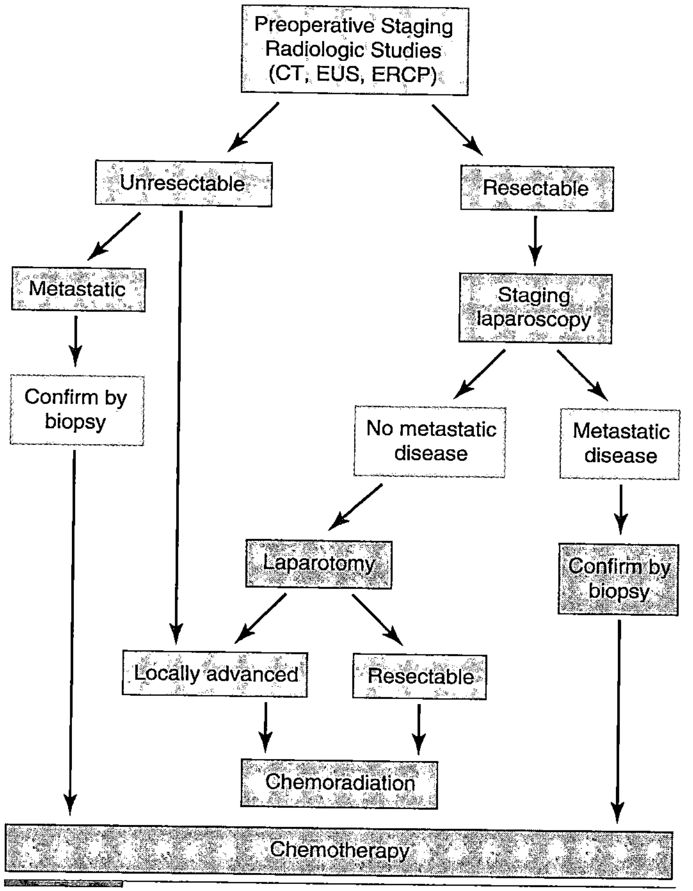

Figure 20.9
Decision-making algorithm for managing, evaluating, and treating tumors in the body and tail (*distal/left*) of the pancreas. CT, computed tomography; EUS, endoscopic ultrasound; ERCP, endoscopic retrograde cholangiopancreatography.

understanding of IPMN and its treatment by resection continues to evolve. Minimal access surgery will have broader applications in the resection of tumors in the body and tail of the pancreas with further refinement of current technology and anticipated improvements in our technologies for early diagnosis.

References

1. Finney JMT. Resection of the pancreas: report of a case. *Trans Am Surg Assoc.* 1910;28:315–330.
2. Lillemoe KD, Kaushal S, Cameron JL, et al. Distal pancreatectomy: indications and outcomes in 235 patients. *Ann Surg.* 1999;229:693;discussion 698–700.
3. Dalton RR, Sarr MG, van Heerden JA, Colby TV. Carcinoma of the body and tail of the pancreas: is curative resection justified? *Surgery.* 1992;111:489–494.
4. Melvin WS. Minimally invasive pancreatic surgery. *Am J Surg.* 2003;186:274–278.
5. Conlon KC, Klimstra DS, Brennan MF. Long-term survival after curative resection for pancreatic ductal adenocarcinoma: clinicopathologic analysis of 5-year survivors. *Ann Surg.* 1996;223:273–279.
6. Sarr MG, Murr MM, Smyrk TC, et al. Primary cystic neoplasms of the pancreas: Neoplastic disorders of emerging importance: current state-of-the-art and unanswered questions [review]. *J Gastrointest Surg.* 2003;7:417–428.
7. Murr MM, Sarr MG, Oishi AJ, van Heerden JA. Pancreatic cancer. *Cancer.* 1994;44:304–318.
8. Farnell MB, Nagorney DM, Sarr MG. The Mayo Clinic approach to the surgical treatment of adenocarcinoma of the pancreas. *Surg Clin North Am.* 2001;81:611–623.
9. Luque-de Leon E, Tsiotos GG, Balsiger B, et al. Staging laparoscopy for pancreatic cancer should be used to select the best means of palliation and not only to maximize the resectability rate. *J Gastrointest Surg.* 1999;3:111–117; discussion 117–118.
10. Warshaw AL, Tepper JE, Shipley WU. Laparoscopy in the staging and planning of therapy for pancreatic cancer. *Am J Surg.* 1986;151:76–80.
11. Pisters PW, Lee JE, Vauthey JN, et al. Laparoscopy in the staging of pancreatic cancer [review]. *Br J Surg.* 2001;88:325–337.
12. Espat NJ, Brennan MF, Conlon KC. Patients with laparoscopically staged unresectable pancreatic adenocarcinoma do not require subsequent surgical biliary bypass or gastric bypass. *J Am Coll Surg.* 1999;188:649–655; invited commentary 655–657.
13. Sandhu IS, Bhutani MS. Gastrointestinal endoscopic ultrasonography. *Med Clin North Am.* 2002;86:1289–1317.
14. Sarmiento JM, Que FG, Grant CS, et al. Concurrent resections of pancreatic islet cell cancers with synchronous hepatic metastases: outcomes of an aggressive approach. *Surgery.* 2002;132:976–983.
15. Kwon AH, Inui H, Kamiyama Y. Preoperative laparoscopic examination using surgical manipulation and ultrasonography for pancreatic lesions. *Endoscopy.* 2002;34:464–468.
16. Minnard EA, Conlon KC, Hoos A, et al. Laparoscopic ultrasound enhances standard laparoscopy in the staging of pancreatic cancer. *Ann Surg.* 1998;228:182–187.
17. Norton JA, Kirlen M, Li M, et al. Morbidity and mortality of aggressive resection in patients with advanced neuroendocrine tumors. *Arch Surg.* 2003;138:859–866.
18. Fernandez-del Castillo C, Rattner DW, Warshaw AL. Standards for pancreatic resection in the 1990s. *Arch Surg.* 1995;130:295–299; discussion 299–300.
19. Strasberg SM, Drebin JA, Linehan D. Radical antegrade modular pancreatosplenectomy, *Surgery.* 2003;133:521–527.
20. Yeo CJ, Cameron JL Sohn TA, et al. Pancreaticoduodenectomy with or without extended retroperitoneal lymphadenectomy for periampullary adenocarcinoma: comparison of morbidity and mortality and short-term outcome. *Ann Surg.* 1999;229:613–622.
21. Bilimoria MM, Cormier JN, Mun Y, et al. Pancreatic leak after left pancreatectomy is reduced following main pancreatic duct ligation. *Br J Surg.* 2003;90:190–196.
22. Mallet-Guy P, Vachon A. *Pancreatities Chroniques Gauches.* Paris: Masson; 1943.
23. Aldridge MC, Williamson RC. Distal pancreatectomy with and without splenectomy. *Br J Surg.* 1991;78:976–979.
24. Warshaw AL. Conservation of the spleen with distal pancreatectomy. *Arch Surg.* 1988;123:550–553.
25. Richardson DQ, Scott-Conner CE. Distal pancreatectomy with and without splenectomy: a comparative study. *Am Surg.* 1989;55:21–25.
26. Warshaw AL, Rattner DW, Fernandez-del-Castillo C, Z'graggen K. Middle segment pancreatectomy: a novel technique for conserving pancreatic tissue. *Arch Surg.* 1998;113:327–331.
27. Murr MM, Nagorney DM. An end-to-end pancreaticojejunostomy using a mechanical purse-string device. *Am J Surg.* 1999;177:340–341.
28. Obermeyer RJ, Fisher WE, Sweeney JF, et al. Laparoscopic distal pancreatectomy for serous oligocystic adenoma. *Surg Rounds.* 2003;26:423–426.
29. Gagner M, Pomp A. Laparoscopic pancreatic resection: is it worthwhile? *J Gastrointest Surg.* 1997;1:20–26.
30. Sarr MG and the Pancreatic Surgery Group. The potent analogue vapreotide does not decrease pancreas-specific complications after elective pancreatectomy: a prospective, double-blind, randomized, placebo-controlled trial. *J Am Coll Surg.* 2003;196:556–564.
31. Nakao A, Harada A, Nonami T, et al. Clinical significance of carcinoma invasion of the extrapancreatic nerve plexus in pancreatic cancer. *Pancreas.* 1996;12:357–361.
32. Robbins EG 2nd, Franceschi D, Barkin JS. Solitary metastatic tumors to the pancreas: a case report and review of the literature. *Am J Gastroenterol.* 1996;91:2414–2417.
33. Z'graggen K, Fernandez-del Castillo C, Rattner DW, et al. Metastases to the pancreas and their surgical extirpation. *Arch Surg.* 1998;113:413–417; discussion 418–419.

34. Kierney PC, van Heerden JA, Segura JW, Weaver AL. Surgeon's role in the management of solitary renal cell carcinoma metastases occurring subsequent to initial curative nephrectomy: an institutional review. *Ann Surg Oncol*. 1994;1:345–352.
35. Sohn TA, Yeo CJ, Cameron JL, et al. Renal cell carcinoma metastatic to the pancreas: results of surgical management. *J Gastrointest Surg*. 2001;5:346–351.
36. Kassabian A, Stein J, Jabbour N, et al. Renal cell carcinoma metastases to pancreas: a single-institution series and review of the literature. *Urology*. 2000;56:211–215.
37. Faure J, Tuech J, Richer J, et al. Pancreatic metastases of renal cell carcinoma: presentation, treatment and survival. *J Urol*. 2001;165:20–22.
38. Stankard CE, Karl RC. The treatment of isolated pancreatic metastases from renal cell carcinoma: a surgical review. *Am J Gastroenterol*. 1992;87:1658–1660.
39. Hiotis SP, Klimstra DS, Conlon KC, Brennan MF. Results after pancreatic resection for metastatic lesions. *Ann Surg Oncol*. 2002;9:675–679.
40. Yeo CJ, Cameron JL, Sohn TA, et al. Six hundred fifty consecutive pancreaticoduodenectomies in the 1990s: pathology, complications, and outcomes. *Ann Surg*. 1997;226: 248–257, discussion 257–260.
41. Brennan MF, Moccia RD, Klimstra D. Management of adenocarcinoma of the body and tail of the pancreas. *Ann Surg*. 1996;223:506–511, discussion 511–512.
42. Cowgill SM, Muscarella P. The genetics of pancreatic cancer. *Am J Surg*. 2003;186:279–286.
43. Hochwald SN, Weiser MR, Colleoni R, et al. Laparoscopy predicts metastatic disease and spares laparotomy in selected patients with pancreatic nonfunctioning islet cell tumors. *Ann Surg Oncol*. 2001;8:249–253.
44. Jimenez RE, Warshaw AL, Rattner DW, et al. Impact of laparoscopic staging in the treatment of pancreatic cancer. *Arch Surg*. 2000;135:409–415.
45. Conlon KC, Dougherty E, Klimstra DS, et al. The value of minimal access surgery in the staging of patients with potentially resectable peripancreatic malignancy. *Ann Surg*. 1996;223:134–140.
46. Fernandez-del Castillo C, Rattner DW, Warshaw AL. Further experience with laparoscopy and peritoneal cytology in the staging of pancreatic cancer. *Br J Surg*. 1995;82: 1127–1129.
47. Fabre JM, Houry S, Manderscheid JC, et al. Surgery for left-sided pancreatic cancer. *Br J Surg*. 1996;83:1065–1070.

CHAPTER 21

Pylorus Preservation Versus Standard Pancreaticoduodenectomy

Taylor S. Riall, MD
Charles J. Yeo, MD

In the United States, pancreatic adenocarcinoma occurs with an incidence of nine cases per 100,000 population. Pancreatic adenocarcinoma accounts for more than 75% of primary malignancies of the pancreas and periampullary region. It is an aggressive tumor with an overall 5-year survival rate of less than 3% and a death-to-incidence ratio approaching one.[1]

Unfortunately, at the time of presentation, less than 20% of patients have disease amenable to surgical resection; most patients have advanced-stage disease, and their disease is unresectable secondary either to widespread metastatic disease or to locally advanced disease involving the visceral vessels. Current chemotherapeutic regimens are largely ineffective and do not offer cure. Therefore, surgical resection remains the only hope for long-term survival in patients with pancreatic adenocarcinoma. Pancreaticoduodenectomy remains the gold standard for resection of pancreatic adenocarcinoma arising in the pancreatic head, neck, or uncinate process, with this operation being performed with increasing frequency at many institutions over the past several decades.[2-8]

Several controversies exist regarding the technical aspects of pancreaticoduodenectomy. This chapter focuses on the debate surrounding the issue of pylorus preservation (retention of entire stomach [Fig. 21.1]) versus standard pancreaticoduodenectomy (which includes a distal gastrectomy [Fig. 21.2]).

History of Pancreaticoduodenal Resection and Pylorus Preservation

Halsted[9] performed the first successful local resection of a periampullary adenocarcinoma in 1898. In the early 20th century, Codivilla performed the first en bloc resection of the head of the pancreas and duodenum, but this patient did not survive the immediate postoperative period.[10] The first successful en bloc resection was performed by Kausch[11] in 1912. This operation was performed in two stages, with delayed reconstruction. In the 1930s, Whipple and colleagues[12] popularized pancreaticoduodenal resection after presenting three cases at the American Surgical Association meeting. This, too, was initially a two-stage procedure, but it evolved to a one-stage procedure in the 1940s and 1950s. High morbidity rates and mortality rates approaching 25% in the 1960s and 1970s led authors to suggest that the procedure be abandoned.[13,14] In the 1980s and 1990s, improvements in surgical technique and postoperative care led to many centers reporting mortality rates of less than 5%.[2-8] With

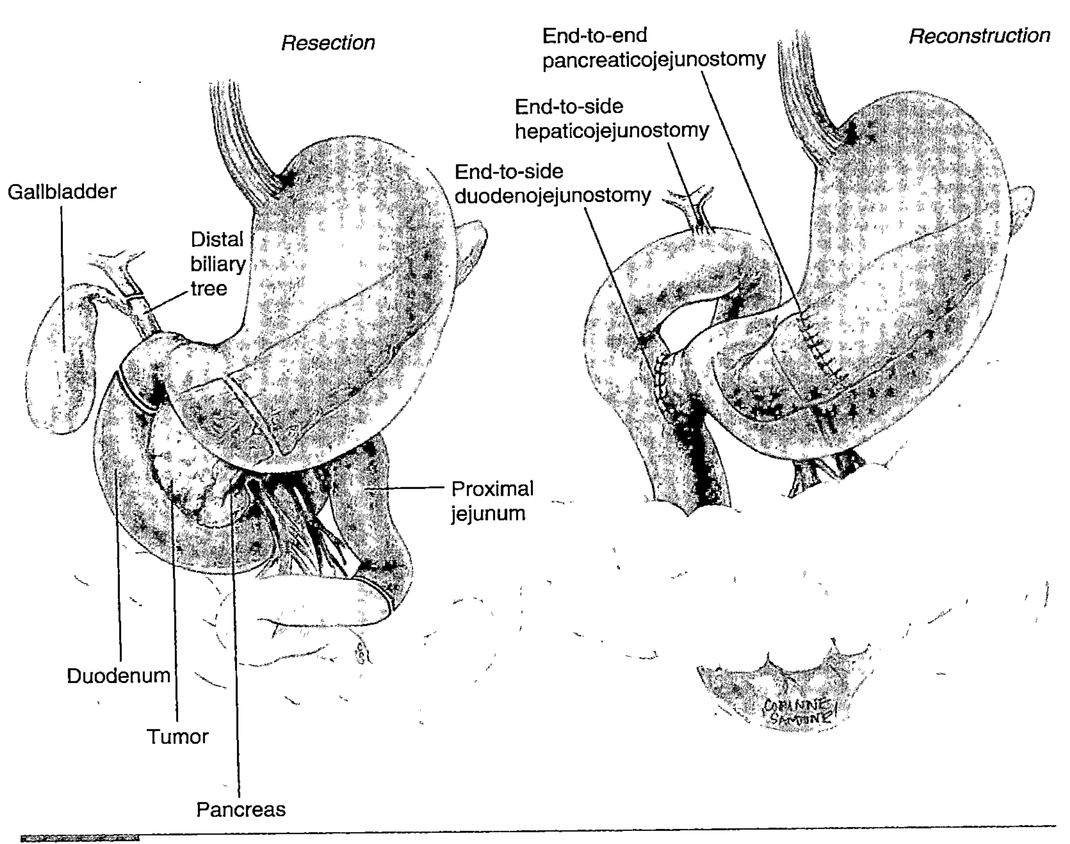

Figure 21.1
Pylorus-preserving pancreaticoduodenectomy. The image on the left demonstrates a pancreatic cancer in the head of the gland (tumor). Double black lines demonstrate the extent of resection, with division of the common hepatic duct, duodenum just distal to pylorus, neck of the pancreas, and proximal jejunum. The right-sided image shows one reconstruction option after pylorus-preserving pancreaticoduodenectomy with an end-to-end pancreaticojejunostomy, end-to-side hepaticojejunostomy, and end-to-side duodenojejunostomy. (Cameron JL. *Atlas of Surgery*. Toronto, Canada: Ed. Decker, Inc; 1990:407, images HH and II; with permission).

this reduction in mortality, many centers began performing pancreaticoduodenectomy with increasing frequency for both benign and malignant diseases of the right side of the pancreas.

The earliest reports by Kausch[11] and Whipple[12] described pancreaticoduodenal resections that saved the pylorus, thus retaining the entire stomach. However, in the 1950s, 1960s, and 1970s, most pancreaticoduodenal resections included a distal gastric resection. The performance of a distal gastric resection was based on three beliefs: (1) the fact that distal gastrectomy led to better oncologic therapy, with obligate resection of the peripyloric and perigastric lymph nodes, (2) the need to resect the duodenum and proximal stomach because of close tumor proximity, and (3) the reduction of marginal ulceration at the site of gastrojejunostomy by performing an antrectomy, thereby decreasing circulating gastrin levels and reducing acid secretion.

In the late 1970s, Traverso and Longmire[15] again introduced the concept of pylorus preservation (Fig. 21.1). They suggested that preserving antral and pyloric function might avoid some of the long-term nutritional sequelae of standard pancreaticoduodenal resection, which includes a distal gastrectomy. Pylorus preservation preserves the entire gastric reservoir, maintains the pyloric sphincter mechanism, and may shorten the operative time.

Pylorus Preservation: Physiologic Effects and Long-Term Survival

Delayed gastric emptying (DGE) remains a leading cause of morbidity after pancreaticoduodenectomy. The etiology of DGE after pancreaticoduodenectomy is thought to be multifactorial, with contributing factors including ischemia of the antropyloric muscle layer, peritonitis or intra-

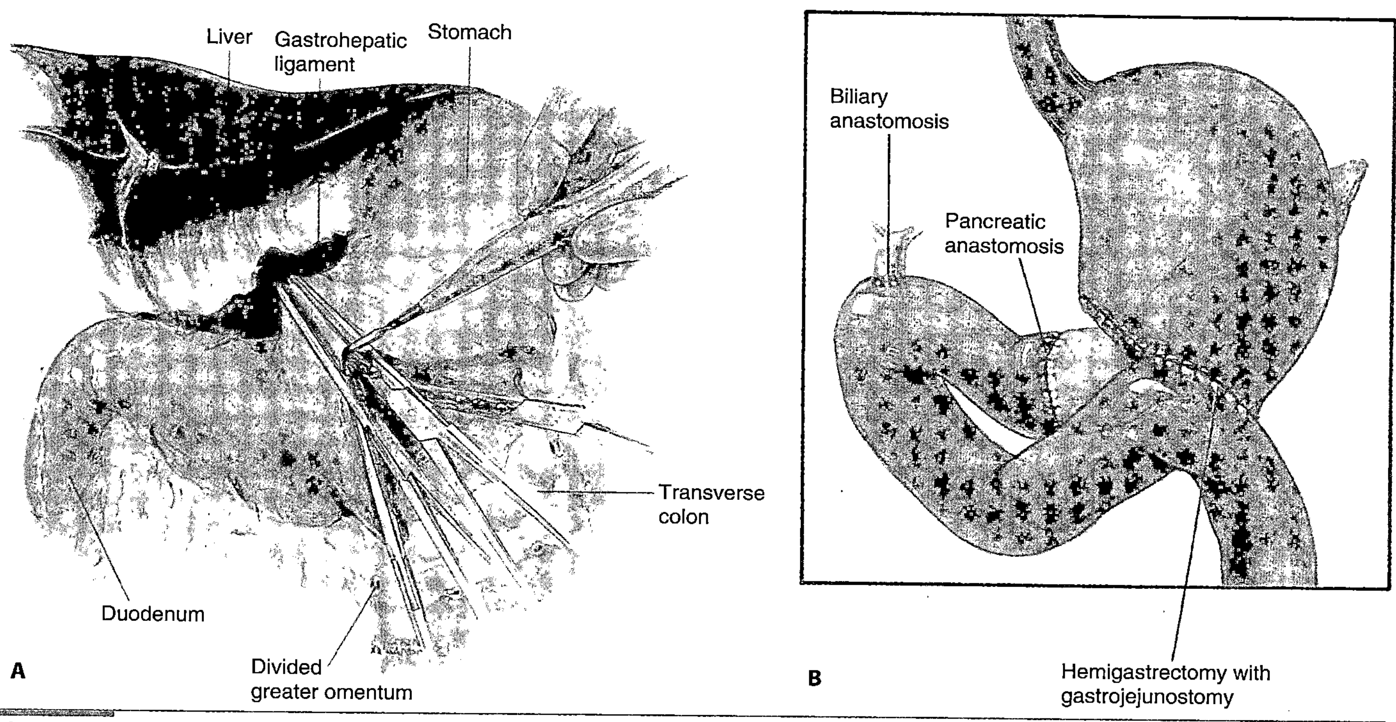

Figure 21.2
(A) This figure demonstrates the performance of a distal gastrectomy as part of a standard (classic) pancreaticoduodenectomy. Typically, a 30%–40% distal gastrectomy is performed. (Cameron JL. *Atlas of Surgery*. Toronto, Canada: Ed. Decker, Inc; 1990:411, image QQ; with permission). **(B)** One method of reconstruction after standard pancreaticoduodenectomy including distal gastrectomy. The pancreaticojejunostomy and hepaticojejunostomy are identical to those diagrammed for the pylorus-preserving procedure. A gastrojejunostomy restores intestinal continuity. (Cameron JL. *Atlas of Surgery*. Toronto, Canada: Ed. Decker, Inc; 1990:413, Inset; with permission).

abdominal infection secondary to anastomotic leaks, gastric atony as a result of resection of the duodenal pacemaker and division of the gastroduodenal innervation, and gastric atony secondary to reduction in circulating motilin levels. Initial studies reported a 30%–50% incidence of DGE in patients undergoing pylorus preservation[16,17]; however, more recent studies have noted a decrease in the incidence of DGE.[6,7,18] This reduction is likely multifactorial, including changes in operative technique with care to preserve the antropyloric blood supply, maintenance of a 2- to 3-cm duodenal cuff, and optimization of anastomotic techniques, thereby reducing leaks.[19]

In addition, the use of the prokinetic agent erythromycin, a motilin agonist, has been shown to accelerate gastric emptying in a randomized, controlled trial.[20] Motilin is a 22-amino-acid peptide found primarily in the enterochromaffin cells of the duodenum and proximal small intestine. It acts on receptors located in the antrum and upper duodenum. One hundred and eighteen patients who underwent both pylorus-preserving and classic pancreaticoduodenectomy were randomly assigned to receive either erythromycin 200 mg intravenously every six hours from day three to day 10 or placebo on the same schedule. On day 10, a radionuclide gastric-emptying study was performed. Patients receiving erythromycin had (1) a reduction in the radiographic incidence of DGE, (2) a reduction in the need for nasogastric tube reinsertion, and (3) a reduction in the percent retention of solids and liquids. Based on these data, erythromycin is used routinely after pancreaticoduodenectomy at our institution.

Many studies have examined the long-term physiologic effects of pylorus preservation during pancreaticoduodenectomy. Traverso and Longmire[21] reported a follow-up to their original study, describing 18 patients who had undergone pylorus-preserving resections. All patients were studied by upper gastrointestinal fluoroscopy, nuclear medicine gastric emptying, and small bowel absorption studies. In most cases, these results were normal and patients reported normal bowel habits. Fink and colleagues[22] compared six patients who underwent pylorus-preserving pancreaticoduodenectomy with six patients who underwent classic pancreaticoduodenectomy. Patients who underwent pylorus preservation had a liquid gastric emptying half-life of 37 minutes, compared with

9 minutes in those who underwent standard resection, at a mean follow-up of 4 years. Williamson et al.[23] compared 24 patients who underwent pylorus-preserving resections with 12 patients who underwent classic resection. They demonstrated no prolongation of liquid or solid emptying in the pylorus-preserving group. Patti et al.[24] also demonstrated normal emptying of solids after pylorus-preserving resection in six of 10 patients studied.

To the contrary, Warshaw and Torchiana[25] compared eight patients who underwent pylorus preservation with eight who underwent classic resection. In the early postoperative period, six of eight patients who underwent classic resection, but only one of eight patients who underwent pylorus-preserving resection, were able to tolerate regular diet within 10 days of surgery. As a result, the average postoperative length of stay was 7 days longer in their pylorus-preserving group.

In a 1997 report, Mosca et al.[26] compared long-term survival in 221 patients who underwent either pylorus-preserving or classic pancreaticoduodenectomy for periampullary adenocarcinoma. Morbidity and mortality rates were similar between the two groups. Univariate analysis did not demonstrate any differences in survival for patients with adenocarcinoma of the pancreas or other periampullary adenocarcinomas.

In 1999, Di Carlo and colleagues[27] reported on a series of 113 patients, 39 who underwent classic pancreaticoduodenectomy and 74 who underwent pylorus preservation. All resections were performed for adenocarcinoma of the pancreas, and the two groups were similar with regard to tumor characteristics and adjuvant treatment. There were no significant differences in the two groups with regard to mortality, morbidity, gastric emptying, resumption of food intake, and length of hospital stay. Nutritional outcomes in both groups were similar; however, in the subset of patients who underwent adjuvant chemotherapy, the nutritional recovery was improved with preservation of the pylorus/stomach. In addition, both multivariate and univariate survival analyses showed no difference in survival between the two groups.

Lin and Lin[28] reported on the results of a randomized trial comparing standard ($N = 15$) to pylorus-preserving pancreaticoduodenectomy ($N = 16$). Operative time, blood loss, and pancreatic fistula formation were similar between the two groups. Delayed gastric emptying occurred in one of 15 patients undergoing standard resection and six of 16 patients who underwent pylorus preservation.

In a randomized, prospective trial reported in 2000, Seiler and colleagues[29] compared the mortality, morbidity, intraoperative course, and long-term survival of patients who underwent pylorus-preserving and classic pancreaticoduodenectomy. They accrued 118 patients in a 3-year time period who were randomly assigned to either pylorus-preserving pancreaticoduodenectomy or classic pancreaticoduodenectomy. Seventy-seven patients were included in the final analysis (40 classic, 37 pylorus preserving). Patients who underwent pylorus preservation had shorter operative times, reduced blood loss, and fewer blood transfusions. There were fewer complications in the pylorus-preserving group and no differences in mortality between the two groups. The incidence of DGE was similar between the two groups. Long-term survival was analyzed in 61 patients with histologically proven periampullary adenocarcinoma, with no differences noted.

In two separate reports, Yeo and colleagues,[30,31] from Johns Hopkins Hospital, described the results of a randomized clinical trial comparing pancreaticoduodenectomy with or without extended retroperitoneal lymphadenectomy for periampullary adenocarcinoma. Two hundred ninety-four patients were analyzed (148 with extended retroperitoneal lymphadenectomy, 146 without) and included in the final data. In this study, all patients who underwent extended retroperitoneal lymphadenectomy had concomitant distal gastrectomy (classic pancreaticoduodenectomy, [Fig. 21.3A]) and retroperitoneal lymphadenectomy in an attempt to maximize lymph node clearance (Fig. 21.3B). Eighty-six percent of patients in the group that did not undergo extended lymphadenectomy underwent pylorus-preserving procedures. The operative time was significantly longer in the group who underwent distal gastrectomy and extended retroperitoneal lymphadenectomy. The overall complication rate was also significantly higher in this group, as was the incidence of DGE (16% vs 6% [Table 21.1]). This is contrary to most series, in which the incidence of DGE is higher with pylorus preservation. This is likely partially related to the increased complication rate (including pancreatic fistula) in the extended-resection group.

In only one patient was there histologic evidence of metastatic adenocarcinoma in a perigastric lymph node, without lymph node metastases being identified in the pancreaticoduodenectomy specimen. Importantly, survival was similar between the two groups (Fig. 21.4). These data further support the contention that there is no survival difference between standard and pylorus-preserving pancreaticoduodenectomy.

Quality-of-Life Analysis

An additional study from Johns Hopkins Hospital evaluated quality of life in the same cohort of patients, comparing those who underwent pylorus-preserving pancreaticoduodenectomy with those who underwent

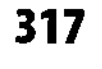

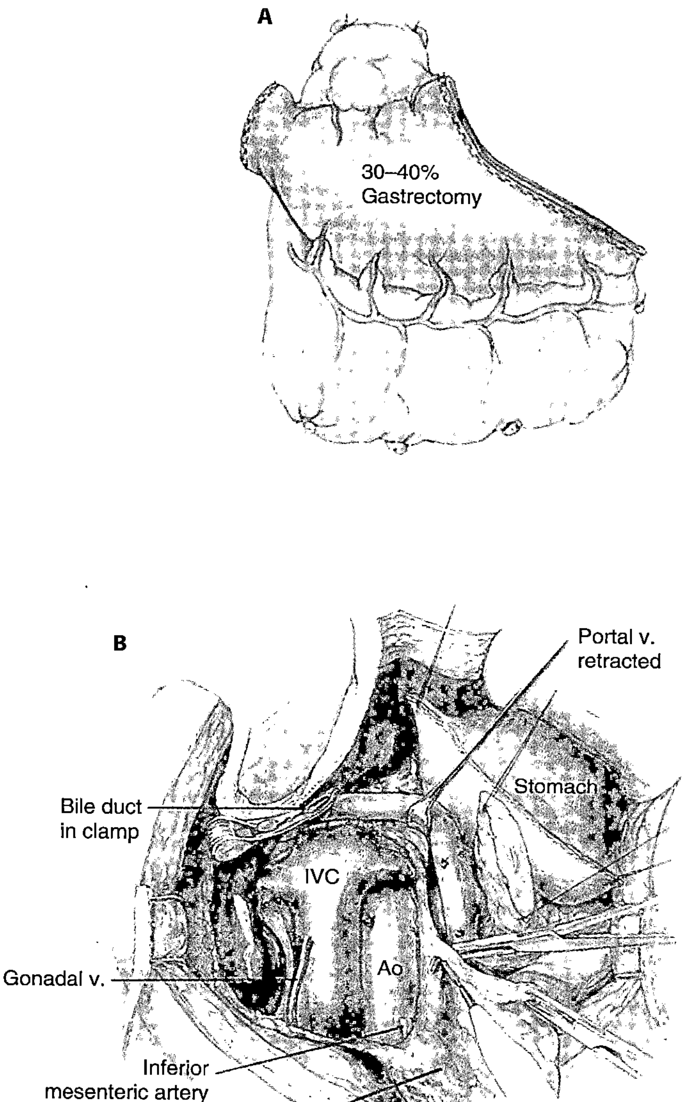

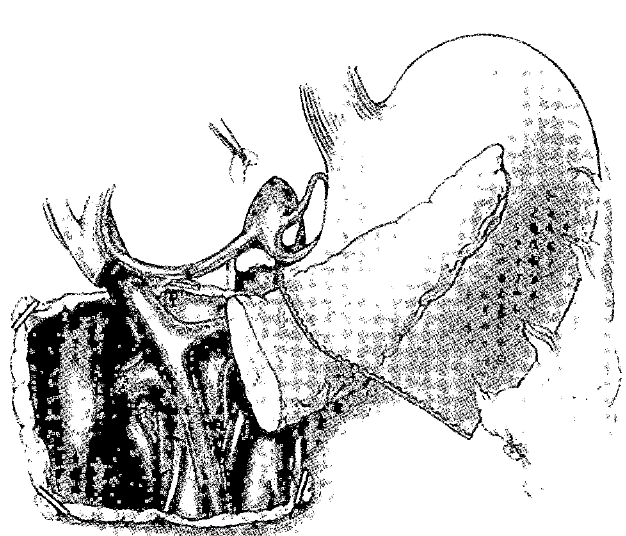

Figure 21.3
(A) Components of extended pancreaticoduodenectomy, with distal gastrectomy and retroperitoneal lymphadenectomy. At the left side is the 30%–40% distal gastrectomy specimen that includes the pylorus and a 1- to 2-cm cuff of duodenum. At the right is the retained stomach, the pancreatic body and tail, and an overview of the retroperitoneal dissection. A celiac node is shown being removed for histologic analysis. **(B)** Detailed view of the retroperitoneal lymphadenectomy. The retroperitoneum is dissected from the hilum of the right kidney to the left lateral border of the aorta (Ao) in the horizontal axis, exposing the left renal vein. In the vertical axis, the dissection extends from the level of the portal vein to below the level of the third portion of the duodenum. Shown here, the pancreatic remnant and gastric staple line are being retracted toward the upper right. The inferior vena cava (IVC) and aorta are fully exposed, and the right gonadal vein has been preserved. A curved vascular clamp gently occludes the inferior aspect of the common hepatic duct. The retroperitoneal fat and lymph nodes are being resected en bloc (*bottom right*). IMA = Inferior mesenteric artery (from Yeo et al.[30]; with permission).

Table 21.1 Postoperative Complications and Hospital Course After Pancreaticoduodenectomy: Comparing Pancreaticoduodenectomy With (Radical) or Without (Standard) Distal Gastrectomy and Retroperitoneal Lymphadenectomy

Complication	Standard (N = 146)	Radical (N = 148)	P Value
Perioperative mortality	6 (4%)	3 (2%)	0.30
Overall complications	42 (29%)	64 (43%)	0.01
Delayed gastric emptying	9 (6%)	24 (16%)	0.006
Pancreatic fistula	9 (6%)	19 (13%)	0.05
Wound infection	7 (5%)	16 (11%)	0.06
Intraabdominal abscess	5 (3%)	6 (4%)	0.77
Postoperative length of stay	11.3 days	14.3 days	0.003

Modified from Yeo et al.[31]; with permission.

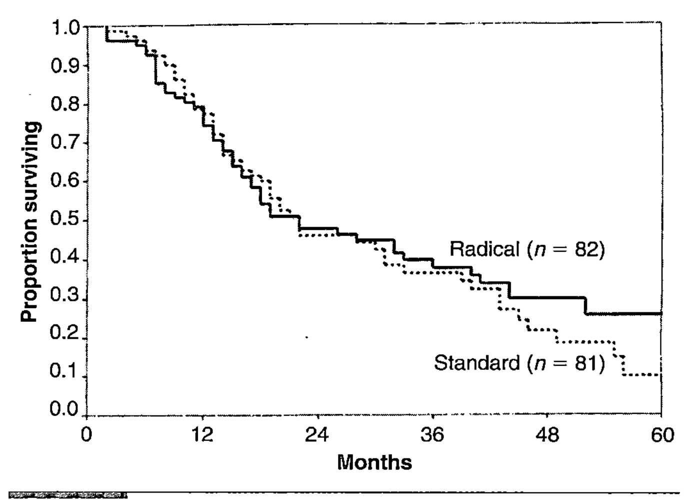

Figure 21.4
The actuarial survival curves for 163 patients with pancreatic adenocarcinoma who survived the immediate postoperative period, comparing the standard pylorus-preserving pancreaticoduodenectomy group ($N = 81$; dashed line) with the radical pancreaticoduodenectomy with distal gastrectomy and retroperitoneal lymphadenectomy group ($N = 82$; straight line). The 1-, 3-, and 5-year survival rates are 77%, 36%, and 10%, respectively, for the first group and 74%, 38%, and 25% for the second group, respectively ($P = 0.57$). There are no significant differences in survival between the two groups and no differences in median survival (20–21 months). (From Yeo et al.[31]; with permission.)

the more radical operation, including distal gastrectomy and retroperitoneal lymphadenectomy.[32] A standard Functional Assessment of Cancer Therapy-Hepatobiliary (FACT-Hep) quality-of-life survey designed for hepatobiliary cancer was sent to 150 patients surviving after pancreaticoduodenectomy for periampullary adenocarcinoma. One hundred and five surveys (70%) were returned. As part of this study, these patients were randomly assigned to either pylorus-preserving pancreaticoduodenectomy or to pancreaticoduodenectomy with distal gastrectomy and retroperitoneal lymphadenectomy. There were no differences in the physical, social, emotional, and functional well-being domains between the two groups. A subgroup of 45 patients completed preoperative and postoperative questionnaires asking about weight loss, pancreatic enzyme usage, and bowel habits. Patients in both groups reported significant weight loss both before surgery and at 6 months after surgery. However, there were no differences in quality of life between the two groups (Table 21.2). In addition, there was no difference in pancreatic enzyme usage or number of bowel movements per day.

Conclusion

A recent review of an evidence-based approach to the surgical management of resectable pancreatic adenocarcinoma discusses the issue of pylorus preservation.[33] The authors concluded that the current evidence for or against pylorus preservation demonstrates no long-term sequelae or differences in survival when comparing pylorus preservation with standard pancreaticoduodenectomy. They cautioned that this conclusion was based on data derived from underpowered studies, some of which were discussed in this

Table 21.2 Overall Quality of Life Assessment: Comparing Pancreaticoduodenectomy With (Radical) or Without (Standard) Distal Gastrectomy and Retroperitoneal Lymphadenectomy

FACT-G Scales* (possible range)	Standard ($N = 5$)	Radical ($N = 50$)	P Value
Physical well-being subscale (0–28)	22.1 ± 6.4	23.3 ± 5.8	0.32
Social/family well-being subscale (0–28)	24.5 ± 3.8	24.4 ± 3.7	0.96
Emotional well-being subscale (0–24)	19.2 ± 5.0	19.6 ± 4.7	0.65
Functional well-being subscale (0–28)	20.6 ± 7.4	22.4 ± 6.0	0.19
Total FACT-G scores (0–108)	86.4 ± 18.4	89.7 ± 15.4	0.32
FACT-Hep subscale† (0–72)	57.1 ± 10.9	57.6 ± 11.2	0.83
Total FACT-Hep score‡ (0–180)	143.5 ± 28.3	147.3 ± 22.5	0.45

*Highest possible scores for the FACT-G physical, social, and functional subscales are all 28. The highest possible score for the FACT-G emotional subscale is 24. This yields a highest possible FACT-G score of 108.
†The highest possible score for the FACT-Hep subscale is 72.
‡The highest possible score for the total FACT-Hep score is 180.
Abbreviations: FACT-G, Functional Assessment of Cancer Therapy-General; FACT-Hep, Functional Assessment of Cancer Therapy-Hepatobiliary.
From Nguyen et al.[32]; with permission.

chapter. Nonetheless, the currently available data do favor the performance of pylorus-preserving pancreaticoduodenectomy for patients with resectable cancers in the head, neck, or uncinate process of the pancreas.

After considering the data that compare classic pancreaticoduodenectomy to the pylorus-preserving modification, it has been our practice at The Johns Hopkins Hospital to favor pylorus preservation in patients undergoing right-sided pancreatic resection for adenocarcinoma of the pancreas. Pylorus preservation is favored because it preserves the entire gastric reservoir, maintains the pyloric sphincter mechanism, and shortens the operative time. The concern regarding an increased incidence of DGE with pylorus preservation has not been borne out by recent randomized data. In addition, the DGE occasionally observed is an early phenomenon and almost uniformly resolves in the first few weeks following pancreaticoduodenectomy, with no apparent adverse late sequelae. Although experts in this field originally expressed concern that pylorus preservation might compromise anticancer therapy, this has not been demonstrated in multiple prospective and retrospective trials.[6-7,18,26-27,29-31]

Pylorus preservation is achieved in approximately 85% of patients at Johns Hopkins Hospital. In some situations, this is not possible. The most common reasons for performing a classic resection (including distal gastrectomy) are (1) tumor involvement of the first portion of duodenum or pylorus found at the time of exploration, (2) ischemia of the duodenal cuff secondary to sacrifice of branches of the right gastric artery or an incomplete gastroepiploic arcade, or (3) prior surgery involving the distal stomach or proximal duodenum (i.e., prior distal gastrectomy).

References

1. Greenlee RT, Hill-Harmon MB, Murray T, Thun M. Cancer statistics, 2001. *CA Cancer J Clin.* 2001;51:15–36.
2. Crist DL, Sitzmann JV, Cameron JL. Improved hospital morbidity, mortality and survival after the Whipple procedure. *Ann Surg.* 1987;206:358–365.
3. Geer RJ, Brennan MF. Prognostic indicators for survival after resection of pancreatic adenocarcinoma. *Am J Surg.* 1993;217:43–49.
4. Trede M, Schwall G, Saeger H-D. Survival after pancreaticoduodenectomy: 118 consecutive resections without a mortality. *Ann Surg.* 1990;211:447–458.
5. Cameron JL, Pitt HA, Yeo CJ, et al. One hundred and forty five consecutive pancreaticoduodenectomies without mortality. *Ann Surg.* 1993;217:430–438.
6. Yeo CJ, Cameron JL, Sohn TA, et al. Six hundred fifty consecutive pancreaticoduodenectomies in the 1990s: pathology, complications, outcomes. *Ann Surg.* 1997;226:248–260.
7. Sohn TA, Yeo CJ, Cameron JL, et al. Resected adenocarcinoma of the pancreas: 616 patients: results, outcomes, and prognostic indicators. *J Gastrointest Surg.* 2000;4: 567–579.
8. Sohn TA, Yeo CJ, Cameron JL, et al. Intraductal papillary mucinous neoplasms of the pancreas: an increasingly recognized clinicopathological entity. *Ann Surg.* 2001;234:313–321.
9. Halsted WS. Contributions to the surgery of the bile passages, especially of the common bile duct. *Boston Med Surg J.* 1899;141:645–654.
10. Sauve L. Des pancreatectomies et specialement de la pancreatectomie cephalique. *Rev Chir.* 1908;37:335–385.
11. Kausch W. Das carcinom der papilla duodeni und seine radikale entfeinung. *Beitr Klin Chir.* 1912;78:439–486.
12. Whipple AO, Parson WB, Mullins CR. Treatment of carcinoma of the ampulla of Vater. *Ann Surg.* 1935;102:763–779.
13. Crile G Jr. The advantages of bypass over radical pancreaticoduodenectomy in the treatment of pancreatic carcinoma. *Surg Gynecol Obstet.* 1970;130:1049–1053.
14. Shapiro TM. Adenocarcinoma of the pancreas: a statistical analysis of bypass vs. Whipple resection in good risk patients. *Ann Surg.* 1975;182:715–721.
15. Traverso LW, Longmire WP. Preservation of the pylorus in pancreaticoduodenectomy. *Surg Gynecol Obstet.* 1978;146: 959–972.
16. Braasch JW, Rossi RL, Watkins E, et al. Pyloric and gastric preserving pancreatic resection: experience with 87 patients. *Ann Surg.* 1986;204:411–418.
17. Itani KMF, Coleman RE, Akwari OE, et al. Pylorus-preserving pancreaticoduodenectomy: a clinical and physiological appraisal. *Ann Surg.* 1986;204:655–664.
18. Yeo CJ, Cameron JL, Lillemoe KD, et al. Pancreaticoduodenectomy for cancer of the head of the pancreas: 201 patients. *Ann Surg.* 1995;221:721–733.
19. Yeo CJ. Management of complications following pancreaticoduodenectomy. *Surg Clin North Am.* 1995;75:913–924.
20. Yeo CJ, Barry MK, Sauter PK, et al. Erythromycin accelerates gastric emptying following pancreaticoduodenectomy: a prospective, randomized placebo controlled trial. *Ann Surg.* 1993;218:229–238.
21. Traverso LW, Longmire WP. Preservation of the pylorus in pancreaticoduodenectomy: a follow-up evaluation. *Ann Surg.* 1980;192:305–310.
22. Fink AS, DeSouza LR, Mayer EA, et al. Long-term evaluation of pylorus preservation during pancreaticoduodenectomy. *World J Surg.* 1988;12:663–670.
23. Williamson RCN, Bliouras N, Cooper MJ, et al. Gastric emptying and enterogastric reflux after conservative and conventional pancreaticoduodenectomy. *Surgery.* 1993;114:82–86.
24. Patti MG, Pellegrini CA, Way LW. Gastric emptying and small bowel transit of solid food after pylorus-preserving pancreaticoduodenectomy. *Arch Surg.* 1987;122:528–532.
25. Warshaw AL, Torchiana DL. Delayed gastric emptying after pylorus-preserving pancreaticoduodenectomy. *Surg Gynecol Obstet.* 1985;160:1–4.
26. Mosca F, Guilianotti PC, Balestracci T, et al. Long-term survival in pancreatic cancer: pylorus-preserving versus Whipple pancreaticoduodenectomy. *Surgery.* 1997;122:553–556.

27. DiCarlo V, Zerbi A, Balzano G, et al. Pylorus-preserving pancreaticoduodenectomy vs. conventional Whipple operation. *World J Surg*. 1999;23:920–925.
28. Lin PW, Lin YJ. Prospective randomized comparison between pylorus-preserving and standard pancreaticoduodenectomy. *Br J Surg*. 1999;86:603–607.
29. Seiler CA, Wagner M, Sadowski C, et al. Randomized prospective trial of pylorus-preserving vs. classic duodenopancreatectomy (Whipple procedure): initial clinical results. *J Gastrointest Surg*. 2000;4:443–452.
30. Yeo CJ, Cameron JL, Sohn TA, et al. Pancreaticoduodenectomy with or without extended retroperitoneal lymphadenectomy for periampullary adenocarcinoma: comparison of morbidity and mortality and short-term outcome. *Ann Surg*. 1999;229:613–624.
31. Yeo CJ, Cameron JL, Sohn TA, et al. Pancreaticoduodenectomy with or without distal gastrectomy and extended retroperitoneal lymphadenectomy for periampullary adenocarcinoma, part 2. Randomized controlled trial evaluating survival, morbidity, and mortality. *Ann Surg*. 2002; 236:355–368.
32. Nguyen TC, Sohn TA, Cameron JL, et al. Standard vs. radical pancreaticoduodenectomy for periampullary adenocarcinoma: a prospective, randomized trial evaluating quality of life in pancreaticoduodenectomy survivors. *J Gastrointest Surg*. 2003;7:1–11.
33. Stojadinovic A, Brooks A, Hoos A, et al. An evidenced-based approach to the surgical management of resectable pancreatic adenocarcinoma. *J Am Coll Surg*. 2003; 196:954–964.

CHAPTER 22

Pancreaticoduodenectomy with en bloc Vascular Resection and Reconstruction for Localized Carcinoma of the Pancreas

Charles R. Scoggins, MD
Jeffrey E. Lee, MD
Douglas B. Evans, MD

Many malignant pancreatic tumors are not successfully resected because of unsuspected vascular involvement or extrapancreatic spread by tumor.[1] Patients in whom a complete resection (R0, R1) cannot be performed have a short survival, similar to that for patients treated nonoperatively with chemoradiation for presumed locally advanced disease.[2-6] Therefore, various attempts have been made to expand the subset of patients that can undergo successful pancreaticoduodenectomy (PD). Several centers have evaluated en bloc resection of the superior mesenteric-portal vein (SMPV) confluence at the time of PD in selected patients who exhibit evidence of venous involvement on preoperative imaging or at the time of intraoperative assessment of resectability. In contrast to resection of the superior mesenteric artery (SMA) or celiac axis (CA), resection of the superior mesenteric vein (SMV), portal vein (PV), or SMPV confluence can be safely performed with similar rates of perioperative morbidity and mortality.[7,8] In addition, there is general consensus that tumor involvement of the SMA or CA represents unresectable disease; these arteries are sheathed by a mesenteric neural plexus that becomes diffusely involved by malignant cells, thus precluding a complete resection in most patients.[9-11] The soft-tissue margin along the SMA is termed the retroperitoneal margin (see Chapter 18), and evaluation of this margin is necessary to insure that a complete resection has been performed. Indeed, the 6th edition of the *American Joint Committee on Cancer (AJCC) Staging Manual* reflects the fundamental anatomic difference between the CA, SMA, and SMPV confluence; tumor involvement of the SMA or CA is considered locally advanced (T4), Stage III unresectable disease.[12]

Anatomy of the Peripancreatic Mesenteric Vasculature

The intimate relationship of the pancreatic head and uncinate process to the mesenteric vasculature places these vessels at risk, and complete tumor extirpation will often require vascular resection and reconstruction. The SMV drains the mid gut, courses posterior to the neck of the pancreas, and joins the splenic vein to form the PV. The inferior mesenteric vein most commonly drains into the splenic vein; however, it may also drain into either the proximal SMV or a common confluence with the SMV and splenic vein. The middle colic vein and right gastroepiploic vein are early tributaries of the SMV and share a common trunk in 27% of patients.[13] The first jejunal branch (FJV)

Table 22.1 Hepatic Arterial Variations*

Type	Incidence	Description
Type I	55%	RHA, MHA, and LHA arise from the CA
Type II	10%	RHA, MHA from CA; replaced LHA from LGA
Type III	11%	MHA, LHA from CA; RRHA from SMA
Type IV	1%	MHA from CA; RRHA from SMA; replaced LHA from LGA
Type V	1%	RHA, MHA, and LHA from CA; accessory LHA from LGA
Type VI	7%	RHA, MHA, and LHA from CA; accessory RHA from SMA
Type VII	1%	RHA, MHA, and LHA from CA, accessory LHA from LGA; accessory RHA from SMA
Type VIII	2%	RRHA and accessory LHA, or replaced LHA and accessory RHA
Type IX	4.5%	Absent celiac HA; entire hepatic trunk from SMA
Type X	0.5%	Absent celiac HA; entire hepatic trunk from LGA
Type X (variant)	NA	Double celiac HA (no common HA)

* Adapted from Spitz et al.[43]

Abbreviations: CA, celiac artery; HA, hepatic artery; LGA, left gastric artery; LHA, left hepatic artery; MHA, middle hepatic artery; RHA, right hepatic artery; SMA, superior mesenteric artery; RRHA, replaced right hepatic artery; NA, not available.

of the SMV enters the posterior–medial aspect of the SMV after coursing behind the SMA as it drains the proximal jejunum. This vein may be particularly troublesome, as infiltrative tumors of the uncinate process that involve the SMV at the junction of the FJV may prevent separation of the SMV from the uncinate process. Injury to the FJV may lead to excessive hemorrhage caused by a posterior tear in the FJV and limited exposure for repair. Attempted suture repair of the FJV at that level may result in SMA injury if the SMA has not been exposed. Therefore, exposure of the SMA (medial to the SMV) should always be considered before excessive dissection of the SMV. The FJV can then be approached from the left (medial) of the SMV by transecting the root of the small-bowel mesentery between the SMA and SMV. This permits direct ligation of the FJV proximal to its junction with the SMV.

The SMA provides blood supply to the pancreatic head, duodenum, small bowel, and proximal colon. It arises from the aorta and courses caudally posterior to the pancreas. Early branches of the SMA include the inferior pancreaticoduodenal arteries and tributaries to the uncinate process. Several centimeters distal to its origin, the SMA gives off the jejunal branches and the middle colic artery. The SMA maintains a relatively constant posteromedial relationship to the SMV. It is uncommon for the SMA to be involved by a pancreatic head tumor without concomitant SMV involvement, although this can occur. It is a mistake to assume that if one is able to separate a pancreatic head tumor from the SMPV confluence that it will be free of the SMA. Although infrequent, a posteriorly located tumor arising from the uncinate process will encase the SMA with no involvement of the SMV—such a finding should be apparent on preoperative computed tomography (CT) imaging. Similarly, it is rare to have an uninvolved SMA in cases where the tumor has caused complete occlusion of the SMPV confluence because of the close proximity of the SMA to the SMV. As previously discussed, the SMA is ensheathed by autonomic nerves and lymphatic tissue that extends to the celiac ganglia.[14] Even when the surgeon performs a complete gross resection of a pancreatic head tumor, a microscopically positive margin may result because of tumor cell infiltration of the perineural plexus surrounding the SMA.[15,16]

Locally invasive pancreatic carcinoma may also involve the hepatic artery. The common hepatic artery (CHA) is typically a branch of the CA; however, multiple anatomic variants of the hepatic arterial tree have been described (Table 22.1). Pancreatic tumors arising in the cephalad aspect of the pancreatic head may involve the CHA distal to its takeoff from the CA; such limited, isolated hepatic artery involvement is not considered a contraindication to resection in the absence of tumor extension to the CA.[17] An aberrant hepatic artery arising from the SMA courses posterior to, or through, the pancreatic head and is thus at risk for tumor invasion. An accessory right hepatic artery (RHA) may be simply ligated if involved by tumor, as the blood supply to the biliary anastomosis would remain intact via the native RHA. In contrast, a replaced RHA (RRHA) involved by tumor may require reconstruction, usually by means of a reversed saphenous vein graft.[17] In such cases, we assess back bleeding in the resected artery and have a low threshold for reconstruction to maintain adequate arterial flow to the proximal bile duct and right liver. A replaced CHA arising from the SMA (type IX hepatic arterial variant) man-

Table 22.2 Accuracy of CT in Detecting Superior Mesenteric/Portal Venous Involvement by Pancreatic Cancer

Author	N	Criteria	%				
			Sensitivity	Specificity	PPV	NPV	Accuracy
Gmeinwieser et al.[21]	29	Occluded PV/SMV, semicircular encasement	91	94	91	94	93
Lu et al.[19]	28	Tumor contiguous with one fourth to one half of the vessel wall	84	98	95	93	NA
Furukawa et al.[22]	27	PV involvement >90° vein circumference	83	100	100	75	89
Loyer et al.[18]	22	Presence of fat plane or pancreatic tissue between tumor and PV	95	100	100	95	NA
Saldinger et al.[23]	52	Presence of fat plane around vessels	95	100	NA	NA	NA
Prokesch et al.[24]	20	>50% circumference and/or occlusion	77	97	86	74	NA
Lepanto et al.[20]	36	Vessel stenosis, occlusion, >50% circumference	NA	NA	86	95	92

Abbreviations: NA, not available; NPV, negative predictive value; PPV, positive predictive value; PV, portal vein; SMV, superior mesenteric vein.

dates reconstruction (usually with a reversed saphenous vein graft) when resected en bloc during PD in order to avoid potentially life-threatening hepatic necrosis.[17]

Indications for PD with en bloc Vascular Resection

All patients with suspected or biopsy-proven pancreatic carcinoma should undergo radiographic staging as discussed in Chapter 12. Multidetector CT imaging has emerged as the most commonly used staging modality because of its superb anatomic definition of tumor–vessel relationships. The accuracy of CT in demonstrating venous invasion by pancreatic cancer has been reported to be between 89%–93% (Table 22.2).[18-24] In the authors' experience, 84% of patients with evidence of venous involvement by tumor on preoperative CT required en bloc venous resection at the time of PD.[17] Objective anatomic criteria for resectability used by the authors and based on contrast-enhanced CT include (1) absence of extrapancreatic disease; (2) absence of tumor extension to the SMA or CA, as evidenced by an intact fat plane between the tumor and these arteries (Fig. 22.1); and (3) a patent SMPV confluence.[25] A CT-based classification system to describe and thus predict vascular involvement by pancreatic cancer has been developed (Table 22.3).[18] Venous resection is rarely required with types A (intact perivascular fat plane)

Table 22.3 Loyer Classification of Vascular Involvement

Group	CT Image Findings	Resectability Rate (% VR)*
Type A	The fat plane separates the tumor and/or the normal pancreatic parenchyma from adjacent vessels.	100 (0)
Type B	Normal parenchyma separates the hypodense tumor from adjacent vessels.	100 (5)
Type C	Hypodense tumor is inseparable from adjacent vessels, and the points of contact form a convexity against the vessels.	89 (33)
Type D	Hypodense tumor is inseparable from adjacent vessels; the points of contact form a concavity against the vessels or partially encircle the vessels.	47 (93)
Type E	Hypodense tumor encircles adjacent vessels, and no fat plane is identifiable between the tumor and the vessels.	0
Type F	Tumor occludes the vessels.	0

*The percentage of resected patients in whom an en bloc venous resection was required to achieve an R0 resection appears in parentheses.
Adapted from Loyer et al.[18]
Abbreviation: VR, venous resection.

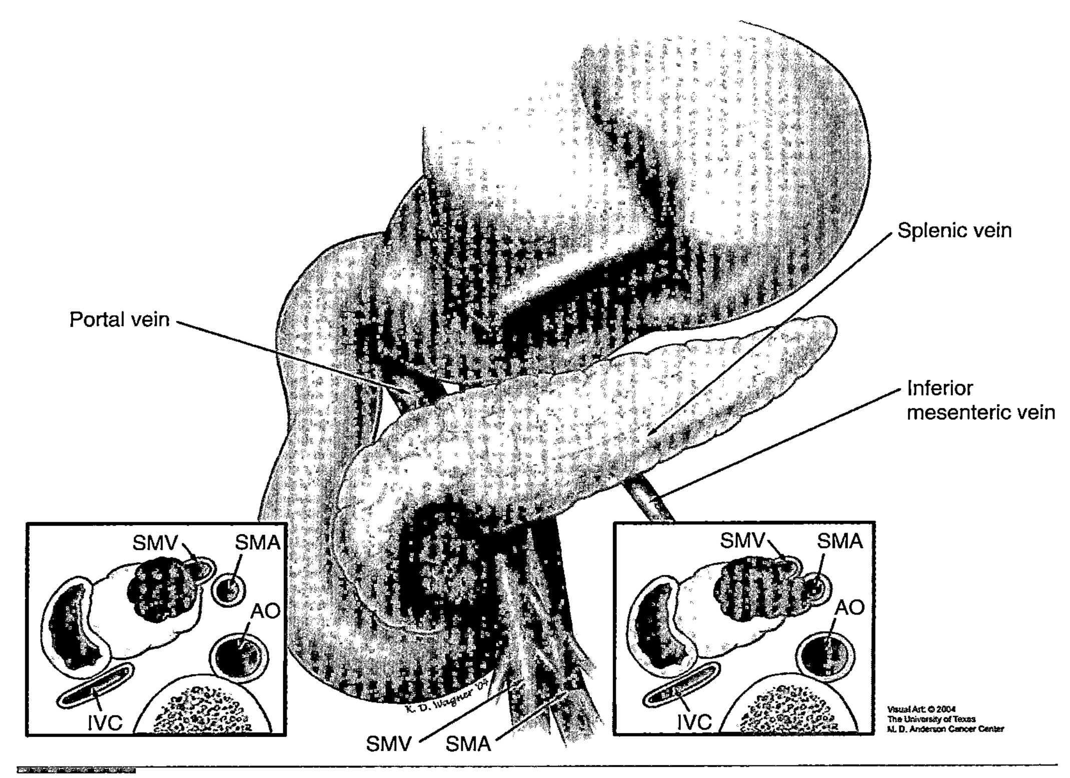

Figure 22.1
Illustration of the fundamental anatomic difference between a potentially resectable pancreatic head cancer (*left insert*) and one that is locally advanced (*right insert*). The authors consider PD with venous resection only when there is venous involvement in the absence of tumor extension to the SMA or CA. The extent of tumor growth into the small-bowel mesentery with respect to the SMA and SMV should be assessed preoperatively on high-quality CT images; intraoperative assessment is difficult or impossible until the surgeon has divided the stomach and pancreas, thereby committing to resection. Many reports of venous resection and reconstruction at the time of PD contain patients in whom the need for vascular resection was not planned, often complicated by iatrogenic venous injury and excessive blood loss; such cases probably resemble the right insert and underwent incomplete resection due to tumor extension to the SMA. The key to extended PD to include vascular resection and reconstruction is proper patient selection based on preoperative imaging as discussed in Chapter 12. AO = aorta; IVC = inferior vena cava; SMA = superior mesenteric artery; SMV = superior mesenteric vein.

and B (normal parenchyma separating the tumor and vessel) vascular anatomy.[18] When the tumor contact points with the vessel result in a convexity on CT (type C), one third of the patients who underwent PD required en bloc vascular resection.[18] Ishikawa et al.[26] described a similar angiography-based classification system and demonstrated that patients with angiographic evidence of bilateral invasion of the SMPV confluence had short survival times that were similar to patients treated nonoperatively; these patients probably had arterial involvement, as evidenced by tumor extension to the left of the SMV, and likely underwent a grossly incomplete (R2) resection. These results were corroborated by Nakao et al.[14] and Suzuki et al.,[27] who demonstrated short survival for patients with angiographic evidence of arterial involvement—it is no surprise that there is little place for debulking (incomplete resection) procedures in the treatment of pancreatic adenocarcinoma.

Regional Pancreatectomy Is Not PD with en bloc Vascular Resection

The Japanese experience with regional and extended pancreatectomy is quite extensive, including resection of the SMPV confluence. They have clearly demonstrated that failure to achieve a grossly complete (R0 or R1) resection, despite more radical surgery, results in early tumor recurrence and short survival.[15,16] Takahashi et al.[16] evaluated patients in whom they had performed combined

Table 22.4 Reports of Venous Resection during PD

Reference	No. of Patients	Mortality Rate (%)	Median Survival (Months)	For or against Venous Resection	Positive Retroperitoneal Margin (%)
Capussotti et al.[44]	24	0	NA	For	83
Howard et al.[45]	13	8	13	For	25
van Geenen et al.[30]	34	0	14	For	59[a]
Bachellier et al.[31]	21	3.2	12	For	38[b]
Bold et al.[17]	66	1.6	NA	For	13[b]
Roder et al.[28]	22	0	8	Against	68[b]
Harrison et al.[8]	50	6	13	For	24[b]
Yeo et al.[46]	10	NA	NA[c]	For	NA
Launois et al.[47]	9	0	6.1 (mean)	Against	NA
Trede et al.[4]	12	0	NA	For	NA
Sindelar[48]	20	20	12	Against	NA

[a] This includes all positive margins; 44 positive PV/SMV or SMA margins were noted.
[b] This includes all positive margins.
[c] The 3-year survival is 13%.
Abbreviation: NA, not available.

pancreatectomy and resection of mesenteric vessels. Patients with en bloc venous resection and negative (R0) margins had similar survival times compared with patients not requiring venous resection.[16] There were no long-term survivors after combined venous and arterial resection demonstrating the anatomic difference between tumor involvement of the SMPV confluence and tumor involvement of the SMA or CA.[16] Despite arterial resection and reconstruction, gross residual disease is usually present after PD once the tumor gains access to the autonomic ganglia at the origin of the CA or SMA.

Survival data from retrospective studies comparing patients receiving standard PD with those requiring venous resection are difficult to interpret because of the failure of most authors to assess the adequacy of resection. For example, Roder et al.[28] demonstrated a median survival after venous resection of only 8 months; however, the rate of margin positivity was exceedingly high (68%), suggesting that most of these patients had locally advanced, unresectable disease and thus were poor candidates for PD. Table 22.4 lists the survival after PD with en bloc venous resection; the median survival for patients who required venous resection ranged from 8–14 months.[8,16,28-34] However, many patients underwent a grossly positive margin resection or did not have the completeness of resection recorded. In the absence of information on the prospective evaluation of the retroperitoneal margin, reports of venous resection during PD are impossible to interpret. When venous involvement is an unexpected finding at the time of PD, surgeons will often attempt to separate the SMPV confluence from the pancreatic head. When unsuccessful, the surgeon is left either with a grossly positive margin or an inadvertent venotomy. Venous injury often results in uncontrolled hemorrhage and the necessity for rapid removal of the tumor without the necessary attention paid to the SMA dissection; such cases often also result in an incomplete (R2) resection. Therefore, studies that retrospectively examine the presence or absence of vascular resection as a prognostic factor for survival should include only those patients who have undergone a complete gross resection (R0 or R1). Patients who undergo a grossly incomplete resection have a predictable course; local and eventually distant recurrence will limit survival duration. It is inappropriate to include such patients in an analysis of prognostic factors predictive of survival duration under the assumption that they have undergone complete tumor removal in the form of PD.

Operative Technique

Venous Resection

A six-step systematic approach to PD for carcinoma of the pancreatic head has been previously described by the authors and is detailed in Chapter 18. This systematic approach allows for optimal exposure of the mesenteric vasculature, thus facilitating extended resection when necessary.[17] Patient preparation and positioning are similar to that for standard PD, with the addition of exposing the left side of the neck and one proximal thigh for potential internal jugular and saphenous vein harvest, respectively.

Step 1. Step 1 is performed as outlined in Chapter 18 and involves mobilizing the right colon and incising the visceral peritoneum of the small bowel mesentery up to the ligament of Treitz. This is necessary to release the mesenteric attachments of the small bowel, thus allowing maximal mobility of the SMV. In fact, some authors have described using this form of mesenteric release to allow primary anastomosis in all cases of segmental resection of the SMV or SMPV confluence, regardless of the length of vein resected. We do not agree with this practice and prefer to avoid any possible tension on the anastomotic reconstruction of the SMV or the SMPV confluence. We reconstruct the SMV with an autologous interposition graft in any patient in whom a primary anastomosis would be under tension. The infrapancreatic SMV is then identified, and the middle colic vein is usually ligated at its junction with the SMV to prevent traction injury and to expose the SMV widely in preparation for further dissection during Step 6.

Steps 2–5. These are completed as in standard PD and are described in detail in Chapter 18.

Step 6. The pancreas is transected along the anterior surface of the SMPV confluence. It may be necessary to transect the pancreas further to the patient's left based on the medial extent of the tumor. If this is necessary, division of the pancreatic substance must be done carefully so as to avoid injury to the underlying splenic vein. Only after complete pancreatic transection can accurate intraoperative assessment of the tumor–vessel relationship be made, thus emphasizing the importance of accurate preoperative assessment. The extent of venous resection to be performed is dictated by the extent of tumor adherence with reference to venous anatomy. We consider venous resection and reconstruction only when the SMV, PV, or SMPV confluence cannot be dissected off of the tumor. This is based on good surgical judgment and experience. If the tumor cannot be separated from these venous structures, the options are to perform a controlled resection and reconstruction of the involved venous segment or to leave gross tumor behind. Continued dissection of the tumor from the involved venous segment in an area of obvious tumor adherence will likely result in venous injury. Tumors of the pancreatic head and uncinate process typically involve the right lateral and posterior walls of the SMV and/or PV; it is uncommon for the anterior surface of the SMPV confluence to be involved in the absence of a locally advanced tumor of the pancreatic neck.

Before segmental resection of the SMPV confluence and tumor removal, the right colon is returned to its normal anatomic position, removing the clockwise twist in the mesentery that often occurs during the retroperitoneal dissection. Tumor adherence to the lateral wall of the SMPV confluence prevents dissection of the SMV and PV off of the pancreatic head and uncinate process, thereby inhibiting medial retraction of the SMPV confluence (and lateral retraction of the specimen). Therefore, the standard technique for segmental venous resection involves transection of the splenic vein (Fig. 22.2). Division of the splenic vein allows complete exposure of the SMA medial to the SMV and provides increased SMV and PV length (as they are no longer tethered by the splenic vein) for a primary venous anastomosis after segmental vein resection. The retroperitoneal dissection is completed by sharply dividing the soft tissues anterior to the aorta and to the right of the exposed SMA; the specimen is then attached only by the SMPV confluence. Vascular clamps are placed 2 to 3 cm proximal (on the PV) and distal (on the SMV) to the involved venous segment, and the vein is transected, allowing tumor removal. A generous 2- to 3-cm segment of SMPV confluence can be resected without the need for interposition grafting if the splenic vein is divided. Venous resection is always performed with inflow occlusion of the SMA to prevent small-bowel edema, which makes pancreatic and biliary reconstruction more difficult. Systemic heparinization is employed before occluding the SMA. The free ends of the vein are reapproximated using interrupted sutures of 6–0 Prolene; some surgeons prefer a running anastomosis (Fig. 22.3). Great care must be taken to avoid a twist in performing the venous reconstruction. We typically mark the SMV and PV at the 3 o'clock and 9 o'clock positions before dividing the SMV and PV and removing the specimen. This ensures that an inadvertent twist will not occur after reconstruction.

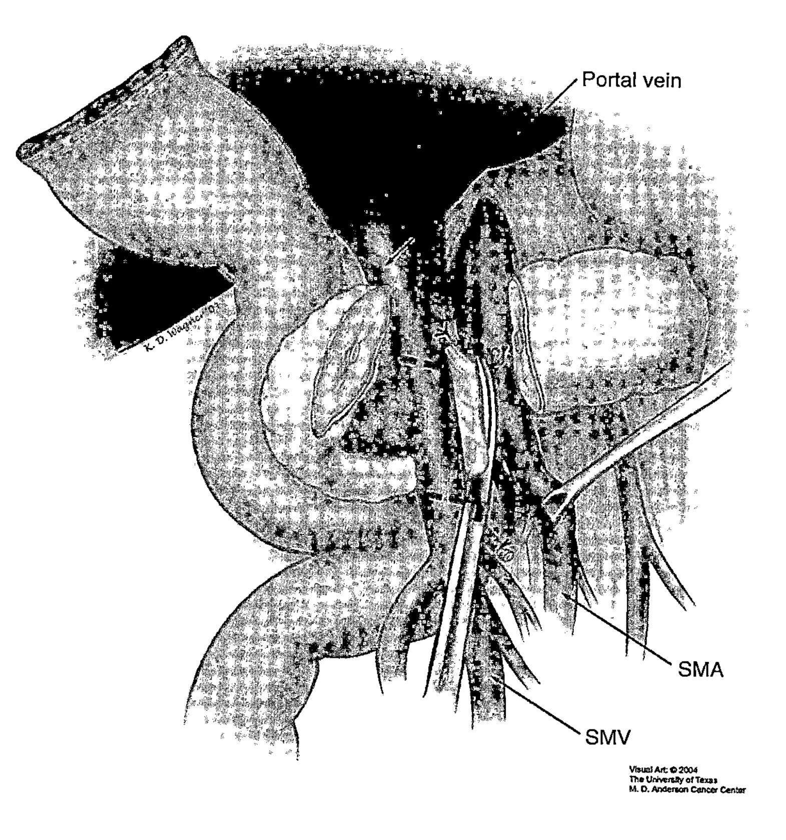

Figure 22.2
Illustration of the final step (Step 6) in PD when segmental venous resection is required and the decision is made to divide the splenic vein. In the early experience with resection and reconstruction of the superior mesenteric vein (SMV)-portal vein (PV) confluence, splenic vein ligation was routine. Currently, we ligate the splenic vein only when the tumor involves the splenic vein confluence. By dividing the splenic vein, the superior mesenteric artery (SMA), which is identified medial to the SMV, can be exposed to its origin from the aorta and the pancreatic head removed from the right lateral border of the SMA. This dissection is considerably more difficult when the splenic vein-SMV-PV confluence is intact. The tumor is then attached only by the SMPV confluence, which can be divided proximal and distal to the involved venous segment.

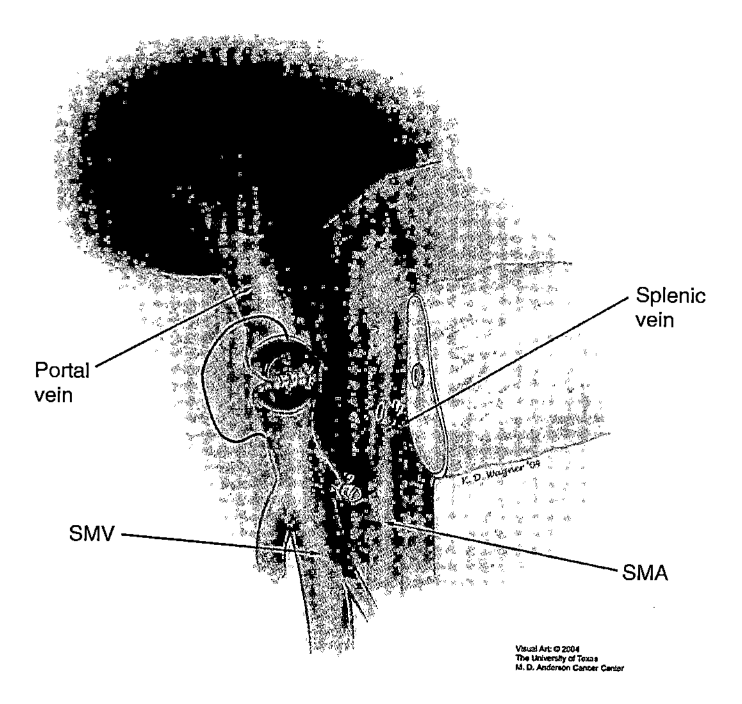

Figure 22.3
Illustration of a primary anastomosis of the superior mesenteric vein (SMV) and the portal vein (PV) after segmental resection of the SMPV confluence with splenic vein ligation. By ligating the splenic vein, the PV is quite mobile, allowing a generous segment of SMV-PV to be resected without the need for interposition grafting. After systemic heparinization and inflow occlusion on the SMA, reconstruction is performed by an end-to-end anastomosis of the PV and the SMV with 6–0 Prolene sutures. The anastomosis can be run or interrupted; the authors frequently interrupt the anastomosis, especially when there is a size discrepancy between the PV and the SMV.

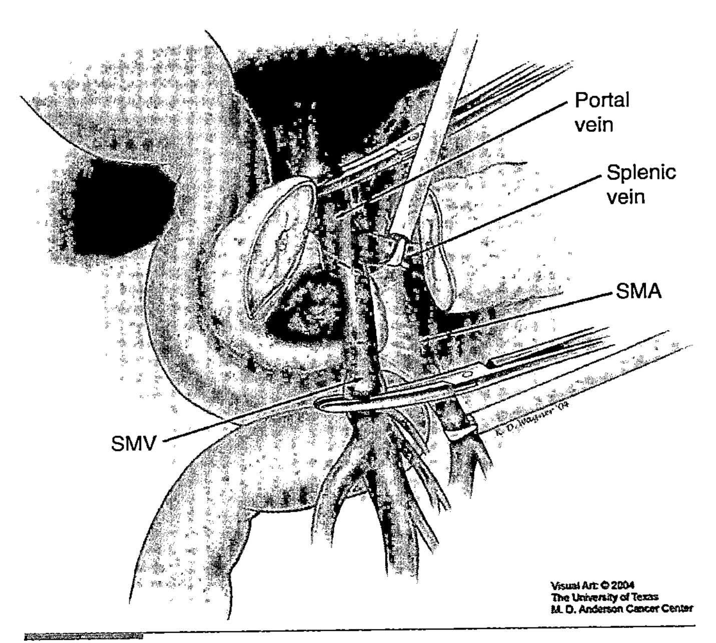

Figure 22.4
An illustration of resection of the superior mesenteric vein (SMV) with splenic vein preservation. The intact splenic vein tethers the portal vein (PV), making a primary anastomosis impossible in most cases. With the splenic vein intact, one cannot complete the dissection of the specimen from the right lateral border of the superior mesenteric artery (SMA) to the origin of this vessel in standard fashion. Therefore, options include either placing the graft prior to specimen removal (as shown here where inflow occlusion is established on the SMA) or separation of the pancreatic head from the SMA by medial rotation of the specimen as described by Leach et al.[35] Segmental resection of the SMV with splenic vein preservation adds significant complexity to this operation but prevents the complication of hypersplenism, which may result in mild to significant thrombocytopenia, thereby complicating (or preventing) the delivery of cytotoxic chemotherapy.

In contrast to previously published reports, we have seen upper gastrointestinal hemorrhage caused by sinistral portal hypertension after splenic vein ligation. Therefore, we currently preserve the splenic vein–SMPV confluence whenever possible. Splenic vein preservation is possible only when tumor invasion of the SMV or PV does not involve the splenic vein confluence (Fig. 22.4). Preservation of the splenic vein–SMPV confluence significantly limits the mobilization of the PV and prevents primary anastomosis of the SMV (after segmental SMV resection) unless segmental resection is limited to 2 cm or less. As discussed previously here, the mesenteric release performed in Step 1 of PD may fool the surgeon into thinking that a primary anastomosis is possible, only to result in an anastomosis under excessive tension after reconstruction. Therefore, in our practice, an interposition graft is used in most patients who undergo SMV resection with splenic vein preservation. Our preferred conduit for interposition grafting is the internal jugular vein (Figs. 22.5 to 22.7). Preservation of the splenic vein adds significant complexity to venous resection because it prevents direct access to the most proximal 3 to 4 cm of the SMA (medial to the SMV). Venous resection and reconstruction can be performed either before the specimen has been separated from the right lateral wall of the SMA or after complete mesenteric dissection by separating the specimen first from the SMA (Figs. 22.8 and 22.9).[35] This later technique as initially described by Leach et al. is preferred by the authors.

There are several choices of conduit for reconstruction of the SMPV confluence, including synthetic materials and autologous vein. PTFE has been used; however, there is a high rate of postoperative thrombosis as initially described by Symbas et al.[36] when first studied in a canine model.[17] An autologous vein has several advantages over a synthetic conduit, including a higher rate of long-term patency and the avoidance of possible graft infection, which can be associated with prosthetic materials. The internal jugular vein is ideally suited for interposition grafting in the SMPV confluence; it provides an optimal size match, both in terms of length and diameter, and may be harvested with no clinically significant sequelae. Tangential resections of the SMV or PV may be reconstructed with an on-lay patch of saphenous vein. The saphenous vein has been widely used in both arterial and venous reconstructions and provides excellent patency rates and a low incidence of harvest-site complications.[37-39] The retroperitoneal (RP) margin is evaluated as described in the 6th edition of the *AJCC Cancer Staging Manual*[12] and is illustrated in Fig. 22.10.

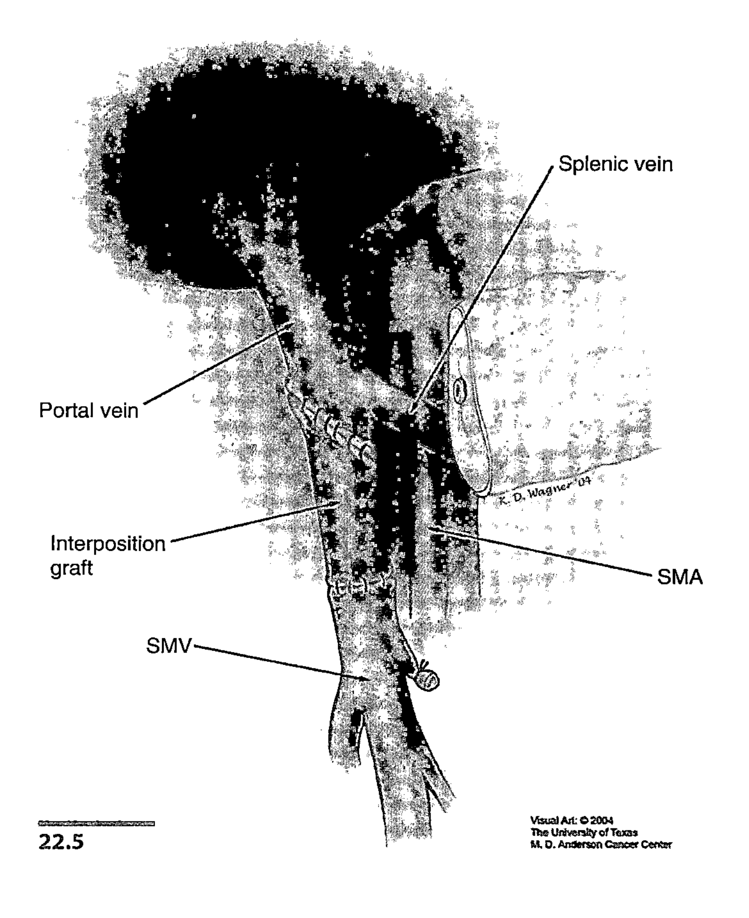

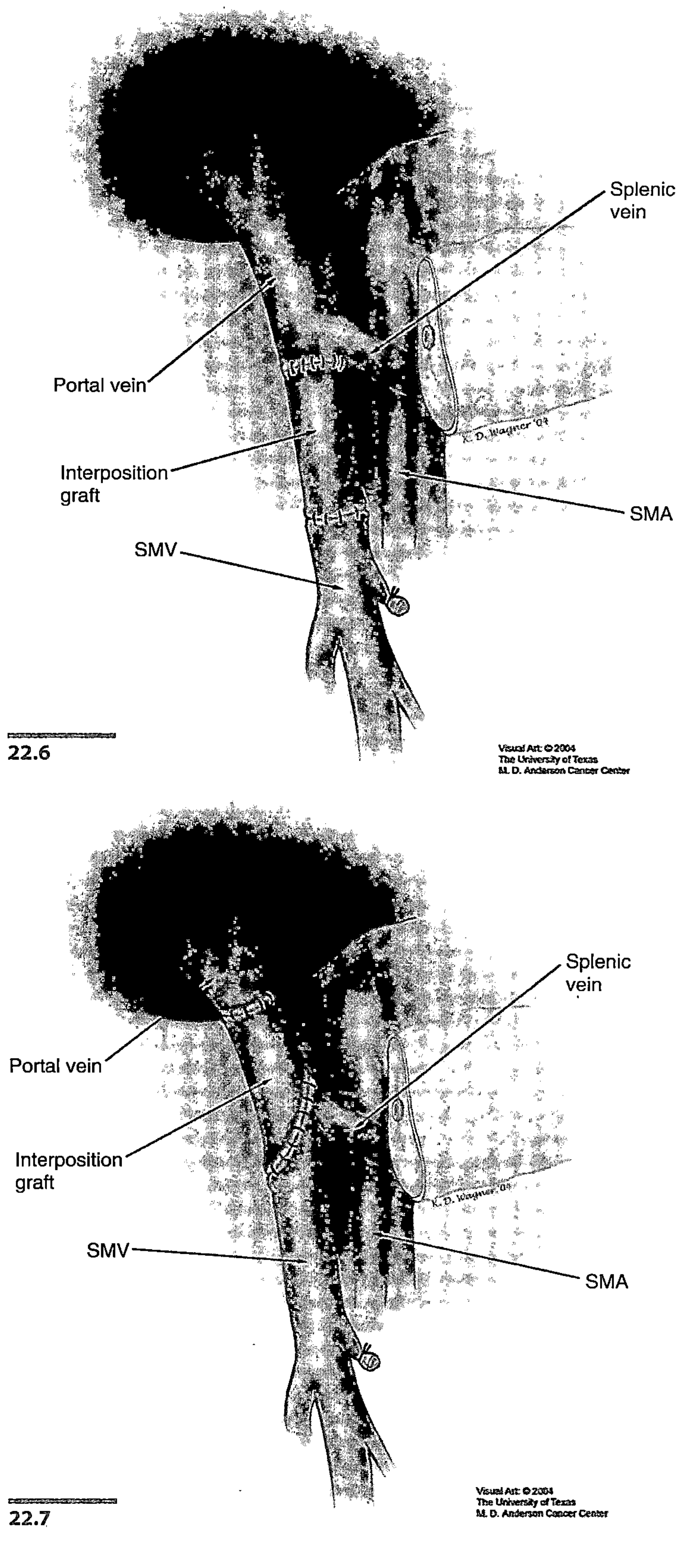

Figures 22.5, 22.6, 22.7
Our preferred method of reconstruction of the superior mesenteric vein (SMV) (22.5, *top left,* and 22.6, *top right*) or portal vein (PV) (22.7, *bottom right*) when the splenic vein is preserved is to use an internal jugular vein interposition graft. As previously stated, when the SMV-PV is occluded for reconstruction, the patient is systemically heparinized and inflow occlusion is obtained on the superior mesenteric artery (SMA). This prevents small-bowel edema from complicating the pancreatic and biliary reconstruction. The anastomoses are usually performed with interrupted 6–0 Prolene sutures.

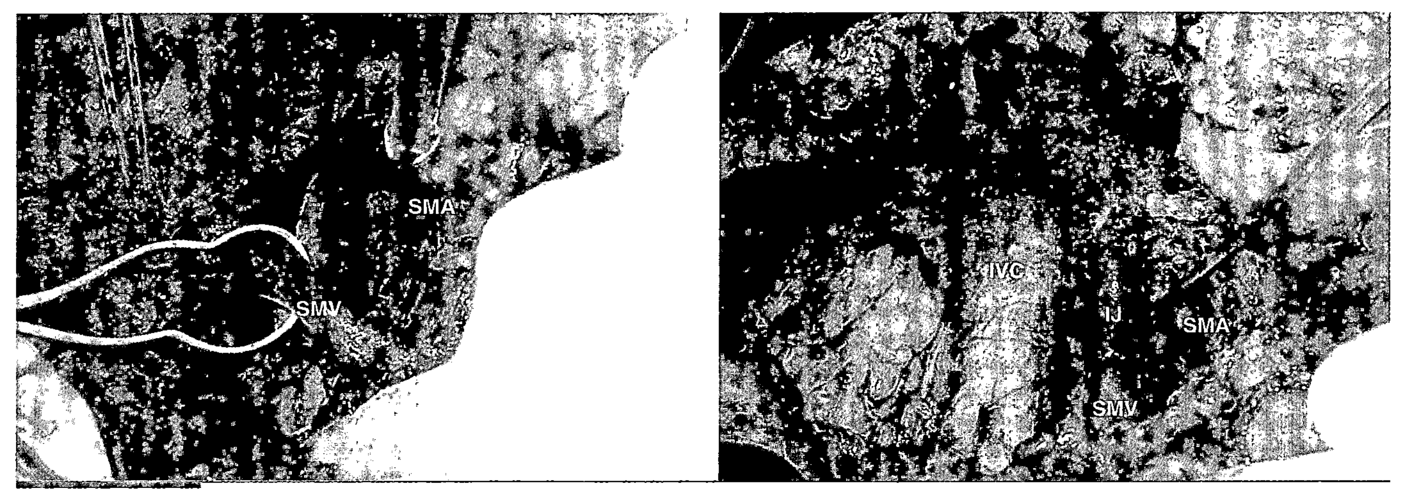

Figures 22.8, 22.9
Intraoperative photographs of venous resection and reconstruction with splenic vein preservation using an autologous internal jugular vein (IJ) interposition graft. The specimen is first removed from the superior mesenteric artery (SMA) (using the technique described in Leach et al.[35]) as shown in 22.8, *left*, where the suction tip identifies the SMA. The internal jugular vein interposition graft is an excellent size match, as shown in 22.9, *right*, (umbilical tape remains around the SMA). IVC = inferior vena cava; SMV = superior mesenteric vein.

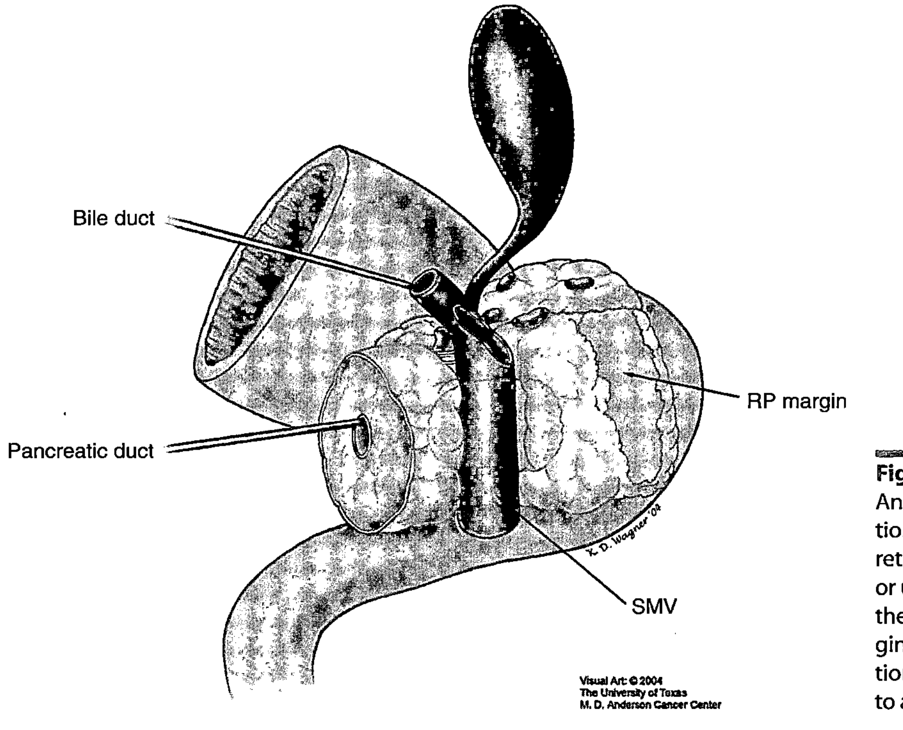

Figure 22.10
An illustration of a PD specimen with en bloc resection of the superior mesenteric vein (SMV). The retroperitoneal (RP) margin (also termed mesenteric or uncinate margin) represents the tissue adjacent to the SMA. This margin is inked for evaluation of margin status exactly as performed when venous resection is not required (Chapter 18). This is the only way to assess the completeness of resection objectively.

Arterial Resection and Reconstruction

The CA, CHA, and SMA all reside in close proximity to the pancreatic head and uncinate process, thus placing them at risk for tumor involvement. As discussed previously, tumor encasement of the proximal CA and SMA defines a locally advanced unresectable primary tumor. However, limited involvement of the distal CHA, at the gastroduodenal artery origin, and a RRHA arising from the SMA coursing posterior to the head of the pancreas may be resected and reconstructed to achieve a margin-negative PD. The hepatic artery may be reconstructed with either a primary anastomosis or a reversed saphenous vein interposition graft (Figs. 22.11 and 22.12).[17]

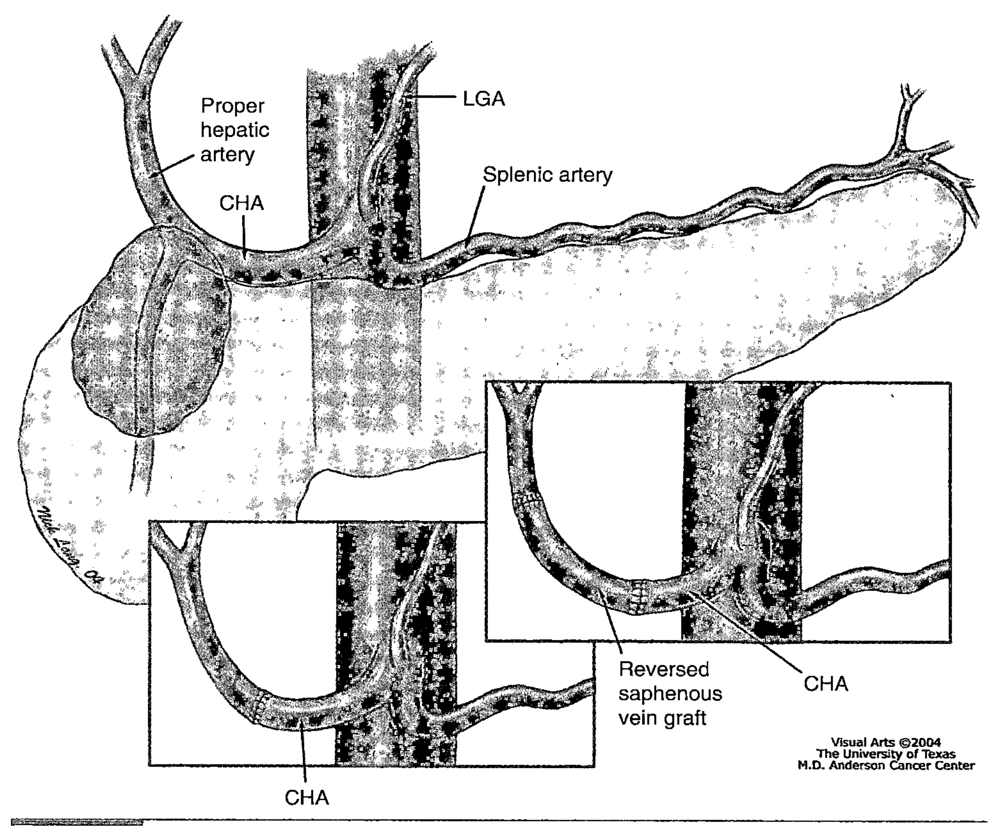

Figure 22.11
An illustration of the most common arterial reconstruction required during PD. Cephalad extent of tumor growth may result in limited involvement of the hepatic artery at the origin of the gastroduodenal artery. In such cases, this may represent the only barrier to a complete margin negative (RO) resection. In such cases, persistent attempts to control the origin of the gastroduodenal artery are ill advised, as this may result in injury to the hepatic artery possibly resulting in a dissection of this vessel. Frequently, the hepatic artery is redundant, and a primary anastomosis can be performed (*lower left insert*); if not, an interposition graft can be used (*upper right insert*). CHA = common hepatic artery; LGA = left gastric artery.

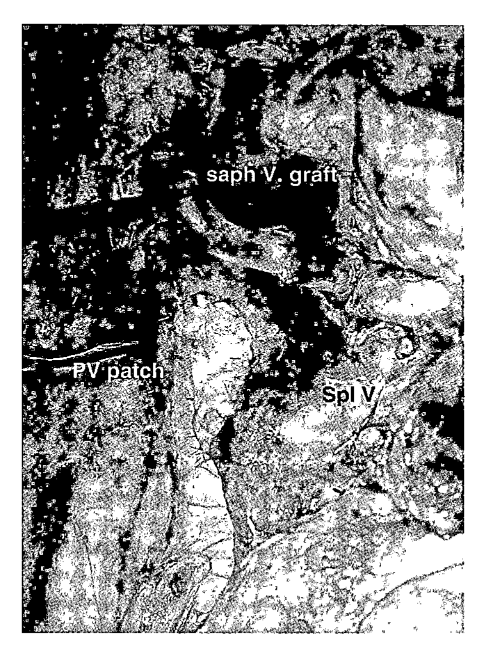

Figure 22.12
An intraoperative photograph of a reversed saphenous vein graft (*anterior to the forceps*) replacing a short segment of the hepatic artery at the origin of the gastroduodenal artery, combined with a saphenous vein patch on the portal vein (PV). Spl V = splenic vein.

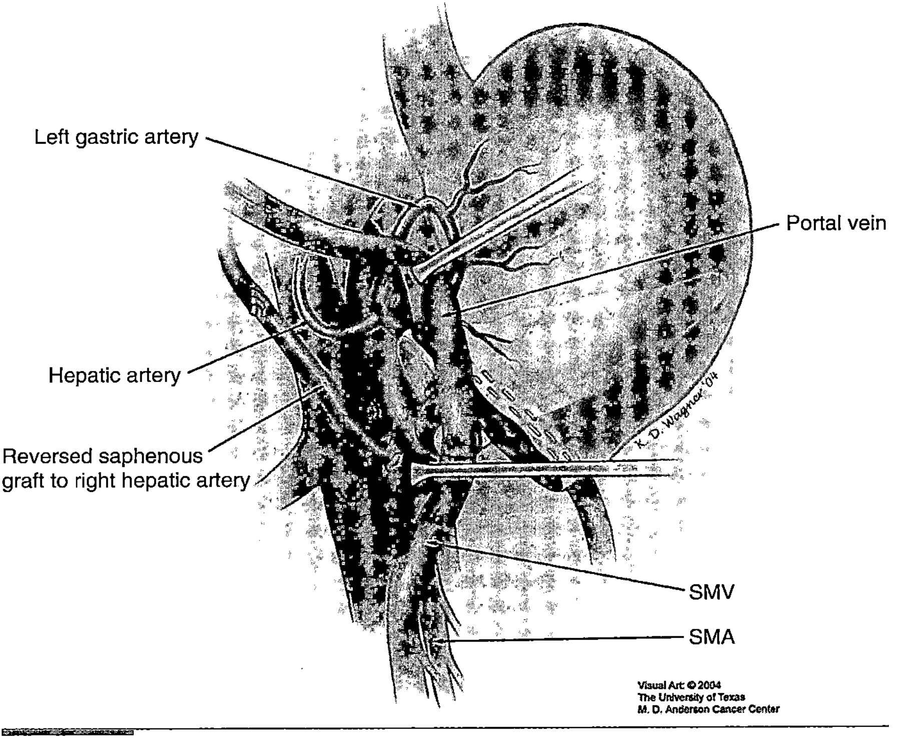

Figure 22.13
An illustration of reconstruction of a replaced right hepatic artery (RRHA) using a reversed saphenous vein interposition graft from the aorta. Occasionally, the proximal aspect of the RRHA can be used for the proximal anastomosis. SMA = superior mesenteric artery; SMV = superior mesenteric vein.

The authors consider arterial resection and reconstruction only in the setting of limited arterial involvement with no evidence of tumor extension to the CA or SMA. A RRHA is also reconstructed, when necessary, with a reversed saphenous vein interposition graft (Fig. 22.13).[17] This reconstruction is especially important when there is poor reversed flow in the resected vessel because the proximal bile duct receives nearly all of its blood supply from the RHA after division of the gastroduodenal artery. In reoperative cases, a RRHA may be difficult to locate if the foramen of Winslow is obliterated due to adhesions. We are always careful to reestablish the foramen of Winslow when completing Step 2 (Kocher maneuver) to allow careful palpation of the porta hepatis in an effort to detect an aberrant RHA.

A rare indication for arterial reconstruction in conjunction with PD is celiac stenosis. Celiac stenosis may be caused by atherosclerotic disease at the origin of the CA or by compression from the median arcuate ligament. This results in compensatory retrograde blood flow to the hepatic artery via the gastroduodenal artery. Celiac stenosis is therefore clinically silent because of this collateral pathway. For this reason, routine preoperative angiography was advocated before the current era of high-quality CT imaging, which allows for three-dimensional visceral anatomic reconstructions.[40,41] In the event of hemodynamically significant celiac stenosis, interruption of the collateral blood flow during portal dissection by ligation of the gastroduodenal artery may result in hepatic ischemia.[41] This could result in breakdown of the hepaticojejunostomy resulting in a bile fistula. The quality of the CHA pulse is easily assessed after ligation of the gastroduodenal artery, and in cases of significant diminution of the CHA pulse, the CA may be dissected to its origin and the median arcuate ligament divided. Failure to restore the CHA pulse after division of the median arcuate ligament mandates arterial revascularization with a reversed saphenous vein graft taken usually from the aorta to the CHA or stump of the gastroduodenal artery.

Complications

The addition of vascular resection and reconstruction to PD has not resulted in a significant increase in perioperative morbidity or mortality when compared with standard PD.[7,8] When performed by experienced pancreatic surgeons, resection of the SMV and/or PV does not result in increased mortality rates.[7,8,17,34,42] The types of complications after en bloc venous resection are identical to those seen after standard PD,[8,17] suggesting that complications relating specifically to the vascular reconstructions are infrequent. Postoperative occlusion of the reconstructed vascular segment is an obvious concern. Clinically evident early postoperative mesenteric venous thrombosis has not been seen in the authors' experience. Leach et al.[32] noted that 7 of 31 patients (23%) appeared to have an occluded segment of the reconstructed SMV or SMPV confluence on follow-up outpatient CT imaging. The venous occlusion was asymptomatic in all patients whose reconstruction was with autologous saphenous or internal jugular vein. Antiplatelet therapy (aspirin) has been recommended in an attempt to minimize late thrombosis.[32] Operative time and blood loss have been greater in patients who required vascular resection attesting to the increased complexity, which is required when this additional procedure is added to an already large operation.[8,32]

Conclusion

Isolated pancreatic tumor involvement of the SMPV confluence and selected segments of visceral arteries does not preclude curative PD. The survival of patients treated with en bloc vascular resection is no different than that of patients who undergo standard PD; however, by considering these patients as potentially resectable, a greater number of patients may be offered potentially curative surgery. This is in contrast to SMA or CA involvement, which defines locally advanced, unresectable disease caused by the inability to achieve a complete gross resection in the setting of proximal arterial encasement. The extension of standard PD with the addition of en bloc SMPV confluence resection should be a planned event based on high-quality preoperative contrast-enhanced CT imaging. Isolated venous involvement should not be a cause for local tumor unresectability.

References

1. Evans DB, Abbruzzese JL, Willett CG. Cancer of the pancreas. In: DeVita VT, Hellman S, Rosenberg SA, eds. *Cancer: Principles and Practice of Oncology*. Philadelphia: Lippincott Williams and Wilkins; 2001:1126–1161.
2. Klempnauer J, Ridder GJ, Bektas H, Pichlmayr R. Surgery for exocrine pancreatic cancer: who are the 5- and 10-year survivors? *Oncology*. 1995;52:353–359.
3. Nitecki SS, Sar MG, Colby TV, vanHerden JA. Long-term survival after resection for ductal adenocarcinoma of the pancreas: is it really improving? *Ann Surg*. 1995;221:59.
4. Trede M, Schwall G, Saeger HD. Survival after pancreatoduodenectomy: 118 consecutive resections without an operative mortality. *Ann Surg*. 1990;211:447–458.
5. Willett CG, Lewandrowski K, Warshaw AL, et al. Resection margins in carcinoma of the head of the pancreas: implications for radiation therapy. *Ann Surg*. 1993;217:144.
6. Yeo CJ, Cameron JL, Lillemore KD, et al. Pancreaticoduodenectomy for cancer of the head of the pancreas: 201 patients. *Ann Surg*. 1995;221:721–731.
7. Fuhrman GM, Leach SD, Staley CA, et al. Rationale for en bloc vein resection in the treatment of pancreatic adenocarcinoma adherent to the superior mesenteric-portal vein confluence: Pancreatic Tumor Study Group. *Ann Surg*. 1996;223:154–162.
8. Harrison LE, Klimstra DS, Brennan MF. Isolated portal vein involvement in pancreatic adenocarcinoma: a contraindication for resection? *Ann Surg*. 1996;224:342–347; discussion 347–349.
9. Kayahara M, Nagakawa T, Konishi I, Ueno K, Ohta T, Miyazaki I. Clinicopathological study of pancreatic carcinoma with particular reference to the invasion of the extrapancreatic neural plexus. *Int J Pancreatol*. 1991;10:105–111.
10. Nagakawa T, Kayahara M, Ohta T, et al. Patterns of neural and plexus invasion of human pancreatic cancer and experimental cancer. *Int J Pancreatol*. 1991;10:113–119.
11. Nagakawa T, Mori K, Nakano T, et al. Perineural invasion of carcinoma of the pancreas and biliary tract. *Br J Surg*. 1993;80:619–621.
12. Greene FL, Fleming ID, Fritz AG, Balch CM, Haller DG, Morrow M, eds. *AJCC Cancer Staging Manual*. New York: Springer; 2002.
13. Scoggins CR, Leach SD, Pearson AS. Vascular resection and reconstruction for localized pancreatic cancer. In: Evans DB, Abbruzzese JL, eds. *Pancreatic Cancer*. New York, NY: Springer-Verlag; 2002:161–169.
14. Nakao A, Harada A, Nonami T, Kaneko T, Takagi H. Clinical significance of carcinoma invasion of the extrapancreatic nerve plexus in pancreatic cancer. *Pancreas*. 1996;12:357–361.
15. Nagakawa T, Konishi I, Ueno K, et al. The results and problems of extensive radical surgery for carcinoma of the head of the pancreas. *Jpn J Surg*. 1991;21:262–267.
16. Takahashi S, Ogata Y, Tsuzuki T. Combined resection of the pancreas and portal vein for pancreatic cancer. *Br J Surg*. 1994;81:1190–1193.
17. Bold RJ, Charnsangavej C, Cleary KR, et al. Major vascular resection as part of pancreaticoduodenectomy for cancer: radiologic, intraoperative, and pathologic analysis. *J Gastrointest Surg*. 1999;3:233–243.
18. Loyer EM, David CL, Dubrow RA, Evans DB, Charnsangavej C. Vascular involvement in pancreatic adenocarcinoma: reassessment by thin-section CT. *Abdom Imaging*. 1996;21:202–206.
19. Lu DS, Reber HA, Krasny RM, Kadell BM, Sayre J. Local staging of pancreatic cancer: criteria for unresectability of major vessels as revealed by pancreatic-phase, thin-section helical CT. *AJR Am J Roentgenol*. 1997;168:1439–1443.

20. Lepanto L, Arzoumanian Y, Gianfelice D, et al. Helical CT with CT angiography in assessing periampullary neoplasms: identification of vascular invasion. *Radiology.* 2002;222: 347–352.
21. Gmeinwieser J, Feuerbach S, Hohenberger W, et al. Spiral-CT in diagnosis of vascular involvement in pancreatic cancer. *Hepatogastroenterology.* 1995;42:418–422.
22. Furukawa H, Kosuge T, Mukai K, et al. Helical computed tomography in the diagnosis of portal vein invasion by pancreatic head carcinoma: usefulness for selecting surgical procedures and predicting the outcome. *Arch Surg.* 1998;133:61–65.
23. Saldinger PF, Reilly M, Reynolds K, et al. Is CT angiography sufficient for prediction of resectability of periampullary neoplasms? *J Gastrointest Surg.* 2000;4:233–237; discussion 238–239.
24. Prokesch RW, Chow LC, Beaulieu CF, et al. Local staging of pancreatic carcinoma with multi-detector row CT: use of curved planar reformations initial experience. *Radiology.* 2002;225:759–765.
25. Evans DB, Rich TA. Cancer of the Pancreas. In: De Vita VT, Rosenberg SA, eds. *Cancer: Principles and Practice of Oncology.* 5th ed. Philadelphia: JB Lippincott; 1997:1054–1087.
26. Ishikawa O, Ohigashi H, Imaoka S, et al. Preoperative indications for extended pancreatectomy for locally advanced pancreas cancer involving the portal vein. *Ann Surg.* 1992;215:231–236.
27. Suzuki T, Kawabe K, Imamura M, Honjo I. Survival of patients with cancer of the pancreas in relation to findings on arteriography. *Ann Surg.* 1972;176:37–41.
28. Roder JD, Stein HJ, Siewert JR. Carcinoma of the periampullary region: who benefits from portal vein resection? *Am J Surg.* 1996;171:170–174; discussion 174–175.
29. Richter A, Niedergethmann M, Sturm JW, Lorenz D, Post S, Trede M. Long-term results of partial pancreaticoduodenectomy for ductal adenocarcinoma of the pancreatic head: 25-year experience. *World J Surg.* 2003;27:324–329.
30. van Geenen RC, ten Kate FJ, de Wit LT, van Gulik TM, Obertop H, Gouma DJ. Segmental resection and wedge excision of the portal or superior mesenteric vein during pancreatoduodenectomy. *Surgery.* 2001;129:158–163.
31. Bachellier P, Nakano H, Oussoultzoglou PD, et al. Is pancreaticoduodenectomy with mesentericoportal venous resection safe and worthwhile? *Am J Surg.* 2001;182:120–129.
32. Leach SD, Lee JE, Charnsangavej C, et al. Survival following pancreaticoduodenectomy with resection of the superior mesenteric-portal vein confluence for adenocarcinoma of the pancreatic head. *Br J Surg.* 1998;85:611–617.
33. Yeo CJ, Abrams RA, Grochow LB, et al. Pancreaticoduodenectomy for pancreatic adenocarcinoma: postoperative adjuvant chemoradiation improves survival. *Ann Surg.* 1997;225:621–636.
34. Allema JH, Reinders ME, van Gulik TM, et al. Portal vein resection in patients undergoing pancreaticoduodenectomy for carcinoma of the pancreatic head. *Br J Surg.* 1994;81: 1642–1646.
35. Leach SD, Davidson BS, Ames FC, Evans DB. Alternative method for exposure of the retropancreatic mesenteric vasculature during total pancreatectomy. *J Surg Oncol.* 1996;61:163–165.
36. Symbas PN, Foster JH, Scott HW, Jr. Experimental vein grafting in the portal venous system. *Surgery.* 1961;50:97–106.
37. Hagino RT, Bengtson TD, Fosdick DA, Valentine RJ, Clagett GP. Venous reconstructions using the superficial femoral–popliteal vein. *J Vasc Surg.* 1997;26:829–837.
38. Wells JK, Hagino RT, Bargmann KM, et al. Venous morbidity after superficial femoral–popliteal vein harvest. *J Vasc Surg.* 1999;29:282–289; discussion 289–291.
39. Modrall JG, Sadjadi J, Joiner DR, et al. Comparison of superficial femoral vein and saphenous vein as conduits for mesenteric arterial bypass. *J Vasc Surg.* 2003;37:362–366.
40. Biehl TR, Traverso LW, Hauptmann E, Ryan JA, Jr. Preoperative visceral angiography alters intraoperative strategy during the Whipple procedure. *Am J Surg.* 1993;165:607–612.
41. Thompson NW, Eckhauser FE, Talpos G, Cho KJ. Pancreaticoduodenectomy and celiac occlusive disease. *Ann Surg.* 1981;193:399–406.
42. Tyler DS, Evans DB. Reoperative pancreaticoduodenectomy. *Ann Surg.* 1994;2:211–221.
43. Spitz FR, Yahanda AM. Hepatobiliary Cancers. In: Feig BW BD, Fuhrman GM, eds. *The M.D. Anderson Surgical Oncology Handbook.* 2nd ed. Philadelphia: Lippincott Williams and Wilkins; 1999:223–255.
44. Capussotti L, Massucco P, Ribero D, Vigano L, Muratore A, Calgaro M. Extended lymphadenectomy and vein resection for pancreatic head cancer: outcomes and implications for therapy. *Arch Surg.* 2003;138:1316–1322.
45. Howard TJ, Villanustre N, Moore SA, et al. Efficacy of venous reconstruction in patients with adenocarcinoma of the pancreatic head. *J Gastrointest Surg.* 2003;7:1089–1095.
46. Yeo CJ, Cameron JL, Lillemoe KD, et al. Pancreaticoduodenectomy for cancer of the head of the pancreas. 201 patients. *Ann Surg.* 1995;221:721–731.
47. Launois B, Franci J, Bardaxoglou E, et al. Total pancreatectomy for ductal adenocarcinoma of the pancreas with special reference to resection of the portal vein and multicentric cancer. *World J Surg.* 1993;17:122–126; discussion 126–127.
48. Sindelar WF. Clinical experience with regional pancreatectomy for adenocarcinoma of the pancreas. *Arch Surg.* 1989;124:127–132.

CHAPTER 23

Reducing the Risks of Pancreaticoduodenectomy

Laura A. Lambert, MD
John D. Birkmeyer, MD

Since Whipple's first description of his two-staged procedure for en bloc resection of the pancreatic head and duodenum, outcomes for pancreaticoduodenectomy have improved substantially.[1] Previously, operative mortality rates as high as 20% (higher than the 5-year survival rates after resection) were not uncommon. Furthermore, some studies suggested that patients with resectable pancreatic cancer who underwent palliative bypass did as well as, if not better than, patients who underwent pancreaticoduodenectomy. Such observations led many to question the value of pancreaticoduodenectomy in the treatment of even early-stage pancreatic cancer.[2-4]

Significantly better results for pancreaticoduodenectomy have been reported in recent times, with operative mortality rates of less than 5% at many large academic centers (Table 23.1).[5-23] Reasons for the lower operative mortality rates are likely multifactorial, including refinements in operative techniques and improvements in perioperative care. However, population-based studies suggest that mortality rates for pancreaticoduodenectomy remain quite high at many smaller hospitals. Thus, the therapeutic margin for pancreaticoduodenectomy—the difference between its risks and benefits—remains quite low in many settings.

Strategies for improving the safety of pancreaticoduodenectomy could take two basic approaches. First, patients undergoing this procedure could be referred to hospitals likely to achieve the best results—so-called evidence-based referral. Driven by reports of improved outcomes with increasing volume of pancreatic resection, interest in evidence-based referral is growing. For example, the Leapfrog Group, a coalition of public and private healthcare purchasers, is using a variety of incentives to concentrate pancreatic resections in high-volume hospitals. Second, efforts could be made to improve the quality of surgical care at all hospitals. Although there are currently no such initiatives underway for pancreatic resection, several states have implemented successful quality improvement initiatives targeting cardiac surgery.[24,25] In addition, the National Surgical Quality Improvement Program of the Department of Veterans Affairs is widely cited for its efforts in measuring and improving the quality of other procedures.[26]

This chapter reviews the relative merits of evidence-based referral strategies in pancreatic resection. After describing the current evidence linking hospital volume to outcomes for this procedure, we consider the policy implications of evidence-based referral, including some of its potential downsides. We then consider strategies for improving care at all hospitals, even low-volume ones.

Table 23.1 Mortality from Pancreaticoduodenectomy Reported in Case Series with over 100 Patients

Author	Years	Patients (n)	Mortality (%)
Smith[17]	1943–1969	224	7
Herter et al.[13]	1945–1973	102	15
Su et al.[18]	1965–1995	132	14
Yeo et al.[22]	1974–1994	201	5
Andersen et al.[6]	1976–1990	117	8
Tsao et al.[21]	1980–1992	101	2
Nitecki et al.[16]	1981–1991	186	3
Allema et al.[5]	1983–1992	176	5
Bakkevold and Kambestad[7]	1984–1987	108	11
Gordon et al.*[12]	1985–1990	271	2
Bottger and Junginger[8]	1985–1997	221	3
Swope et al.[19]	1987–1991	299	8
Cameron et al.*[9]	1988–1991	145	0
Yeo et al.*[23]	1990–1996	650	1
Castillo et al.[10]	1991–1994	231	0

* Overlapping series from same institution; thus, some patients reported likely more than once.

Evidence-Based Referral

Interest in evidence-based referral strategies for high-risk surgical procedures is growing. By far the most visible effort is being led by the Leapfrog Group, a coalition of large employers, including General Motors, General Electric, and the U.S. Office of Personnel Management, which collectively employ over 40 million people. The basic premise of the Leapfrog Group is so-called value-based purchasing—using the leverage of large payers to encourage improvements in healthcare quality. The use of higher quality hospitals is encouraged through public recognition and reimbursement premiums for hospitals meeting Leapfrog criteria. The use of lower quality hospitals is discouraged by higher patient co-payments and, in some instances, removal of hospitals from health plans.

To meet Leapfrog criteria fully, hospitals must have computerized order entry systems for inpatient care and intensive care units (ICUs) staffed by full-time, board-certified intensivists. The Leapfrog Group has also set evidence-based criteria for referral for selected surgical procedures. For some procedures, including coronary artery bypass, percutaneous coronary intervention, and elective abdominal aortic aneurysm repair, the 2003 Leapfrog standards involve a composite of quality indicators, such as procedure volume, process measures (e.g., use of perioperative β-blockers), and risk-adjusted mortality rates. For pancreatic resection, however, criteria for evidence-based hospital referral are based on minimum hospital volume standards alone. The small number of pancreatic resections performed annually in the United States severely limits the ability to measure mortality rates accurately at individual hospitals (particularly low-volume hospitals). Moreover, hospital pancreatic resection volume is a particularly strong determinant of operative mortality rate, as discussed later in this chapter.

Volume–Outcome Relationships for Pancreatic Resection

Surgical volume–outcome relationships have been recognized for decades.[27] In recent years, the volume–outcome literature has expanded dramatically. Although early studies focused primarily on cardiovascular surgery, a growing number of studies have targeted cancer surgery, including pancreatic resection.

As part of a report for the Institute of Medicine, Halm et al.[28] systematically reviewed 20 community- or population-based studies that evaluated volume as an independent variable with regard to outcomes of cancer surgery. The authors used 10 explicit criteria for judging the quality of each study, including the generalizability of the patient population, the sample size, and the source of the data (administrative vs clinical). Of the 20 cancer studies meeting the inclusion criteria for this review, 11 focused on pancreatectomy. These studies were very heterogeneous. Study quality scores varied from 3–10 (a maximum score of 18); sample sizes ranged from 130 to 7,229 patients and from 39 to 1,772 hospitals, and the data sources ranged from state and regional databases to national databases from Medicare or the Department of Defense. The criteria used to define low-volume hospitals also varied widely, from less than one to less than nine procedures per year. Except for one study that included SEER (Surveillance, Epidemiology, and End Results) data, all studies were based on administrative data.

Ten of the 11 studies reviewed described a significant relationship between volume and operative mortality rate for pancreatic resection.[28] Only one study failed to detect a significant volume–outcome relationship,[29] and that study had the lowest quality score because of its small sample size, nonrepresentative study population (Department of Defense patients), and lack of risk adjustment. On the other hand, in the study with the highest quality score, the risk-adjusted mortality rate for pancreatic resection was more than 10% lower at high-volume hospitals (3.5%) than at low-volume hospitals (14%).[30] In addition, volume-related differences in mortality rates were larger for pancreatic resection than for any other surgical procedure assessed in the remaining nine studies, in both absolute and relative terms. Similar to the review by Halm et al.,[28] a systematic review by Dudley et al.[31] also concluded that published studies strongly support the presence of a volume–outcome relationship for pancreatic resection.

Since completion of these reviews, a large national study has further confirmed the importance of hospital volume for pancreatic resection. Birkmeyer et al.[32] evaluated the outcomes in 2.5 million Medicare patients undergoing 1 of 14 different cardiovascular procedures or cancer resections between 1994 and 1999. For each procedure, hospitals were ranked in order of increasing total hospital volume and then divided into five volume groups of equal size (quintiles). After adjustment for case mix, hospital volume was inversely related to operative mortality for all 14 procedures ($P < 0.001$ for all trends). The importance of hospital volume varied according to the type of procedure. As in the review by Halm et al.,[28] the greatest volume-related differences in mortality rates were observed for pancreatic resection, with adjusted mortality rates at very low-volume hospitals of 16.3% versus 3.8% at very high-volume hospitals (an absolute difference of 12.5%).[32]

Although most volume–outcome studies have focused on operative mortality, volume has also been linked to other outcomes, including long-term survival rates after cancer surgery.[33-36] Birkmeyer et al.[33] were the first to assess the relationship between hospital volume and long-term survival rates after pancreaticoduodenectomy on a population-based level. In a retrospective cohort study of 7,229 Medicare patients who underwent pancreaticoduodenectomy from 1992 to 1995, the authors found that the 3-year survival rate was higher at high-volume centers (37%) than at medium-volume (29%), low-volume (26%), and very low-volume hospitals (25%) ($P < 0.01$). In another study, Finlayson and Birkmeyer[37] performed a decision analysis to estimate the cumulative effect of volume-related differences in operative and long-term mortality rates for patients undergoing pancreatic, lung, or colon resections for cancer. They found that patients gained 20.8 months of life expectancy after pancreatic resection at a very high-volume hospital as compared with a very low-volume hospital.

Criticisms of Volume-Based Referral Strategies

The potential of volume-based referral strategies to avert unnecessary surgical deaths is clear.[38] By one estimate, limiting pancreatic resection to high-volume hospitals would save 100–200 lives per year in the United States. However, hospital procedure volume-based referral is widely criticized on other grounds. It is worth considering the common criticisms of volume-based referral in the context of pancreatic resection.

"Volume doesn't reflect quality at my hospital." It is true that observed volume–outcome relationships reflect only average mortality rates. Furthermore, it has been shown that some low-volume hospitals have excellent outcomes for pancreatic resection.[39] Unfortunately, it is impossible to predict accurately which low-volume hospitals will have the best outcomes. Although successful models for measuring risk-adjusted mortality rates have been developed for coronary artery bypass grafting,[24,25] sample size and precision issues preclude similarly meaningful outcome measurements for uncommon procedures such as pancreatic resection. Even with standardized, detailed, and reliable reports of provider quality, little meaningful information about pancreatic resection mortality rates could be gleaned from hospitals performing two (the U.S. median) or fewer procedures each year. Consequently, surrogate markers of quality, like procedure volume, become even more important predictors of patient outcomes for procedures such as pancreaticoduodenectomy.

"Patients will have to travel too far." Increased travel burden is a common criticism of plans for regionalization of surgical care, particularly for people in rural areas. However, a recent study by Birkmeyer et al.[40] showed that if

Table 23.2 Distribution of Travel Times for Medicare Patients Undergoing Pancreatic Resection in the Status Quo (1994–1999) and If All Patients Were Required to Undergo These Procedures in Hospitals Exceeding a Minimum Volume Standard

	Distribution of Patients by Travel Time in Minutes, No. (%)			
	<30	30–60	60–120	≥120
Pancreatic resection (n = 9,825) status quo	5,969 (61)	1,523 (16)	1,376 (14)	957 (10)
With minimum volume standard (procedure/year)				
Low (≥1)	5,580 (57)	1,700 (17)	1,549 (16)	996 (10)
Medium (≥3)	4,549 (46)	1,852 (19)	2,068 (21)	1,356 (14)
High (≥6)	3,395 (35)	1,728 (18)	2,325 (24)	2,377 (24)
Very high (≥17)	1,992 (20)	1,276 (13)	1,965 (20)	4,592 (47)

the hospital procedure volume bar is not set too high, regionalization of care could be implemented for select surgical procedures without imposing unreasonable travel burdens on patients and their families. Using Medicare claims and U.S. road network data, the authors simulated a volume–standard trial and estimated the impact on patient travel. All hospitals in the continental United States that performed esophagectomy and pancreatic resections were included, and the additional travel time needed for 15,796 patients undergoing either of these two procedures to reach a higher volume center was measured. Although the authors found that overall travel times would increase if minimum volume standards were implemented, the magnitude of the change depended on the volume cut point. For pancreatectomy, under the status quo, 61% of patients travel less than 30 minutes and 24% travel more than 1 hour to receive their care. With minimum volume standards, 57% of patients would travel less than 30 minutes, and 26% would travel more than 1 hour to reach a low-volume center (≥1 per year). To reach a medium-volume center (≥3 per year), 46% would still travel less than 30 minutes, and 36% would have to travel over 1 hour. To reach a high-volume center (≥6 per year) or very high-volume center (≥17 per year), 48% and 67% of patients would have to travel more than 1 hour, respectively (Table 23.2). With low-volume standards, only 15% of patients would need to change hospitals, and 74% would need to travel less than 30 additional minutes. Furthermore, only 11% would increase their travel time by more than 1 hour, and only 3% would increase by more than 2 hours. Some patients already living closer to a high-volume center (25%) could even see shorter travel times.

"Volume standards could lead to unnecessary surgery." Some have argued that the implementation of volume standards may create incentives to perform unnecessary surgery, particularly for centers with current volumes near the minimum threshold. For discretionary procedures such as coronary artery bypass grafting or carotid endarterectomy whose loss might indeed impose an economic hardship on a low-volume center, this may pose a potential problem. However, with respect to pancreatic resection, because low-volume hospitals perform fewer than one or two a year on average, volume standards for pancreatectomy will not threaten the financial well-being of low-volume surgeons or hospitals. Furthermore, given the high-risk nature of the procedure, it is extremely unlikely that implementation of volume standards would create incentives to perform unnecessary pancreatic resections.

Other concerns about regionalization of certain surgical procedures include potential negative effects on the quality of urgent or related procedures at low-volume hospitals. For example, hospitals no longer performing elective repair of abdominal aortic aneurysms may become less proficient at dealing with patients who present with a ruptured aneurysm. Furthermore, if regionalization creates economic hardships for low-volume surgeons and hospitals, reduced patient access to basic surgical care may be compromised if those hospitals are unable to recruit and retain general surgeons. Again, although these arguments against regionalization may be valid for more common procedures, they are less persuasive for pancreatic resection, the loss of which is unlikely to inflict serious economic hardship on an already low-volume center.

Improving Care at All Hospitals

Although the case for volume-based referral is particularly strong for pancreatic resection, the ability of such a strategy to reduce the mortality rate for pancreatic resection is ultimately limited. First, the likelihood of moving all patients to high-volume hospitals is negligible. In the current climate, healthcare providers are unlikely to facilitate such policies and inform patients about the importance of procedure volume for some procedures. Even if fully informed, not all patients would choose to move. Second, even if all pancreatic resections were performed in high-volume centers, variations in performance and thus opportunity for improvement would still remain.

Another strategy is to improve quality at all hospitals, even at low-volume ones. Some options for reducing the risks of pancreatic resection are discussed later in this chapter. Some of these options pertain to the setting in which surgery is performed or to the surgeon doing these operations. Others relate to specific processes of care associated with better patient outcomes—with high-risk procedures in general or pancreatic resection specifically.

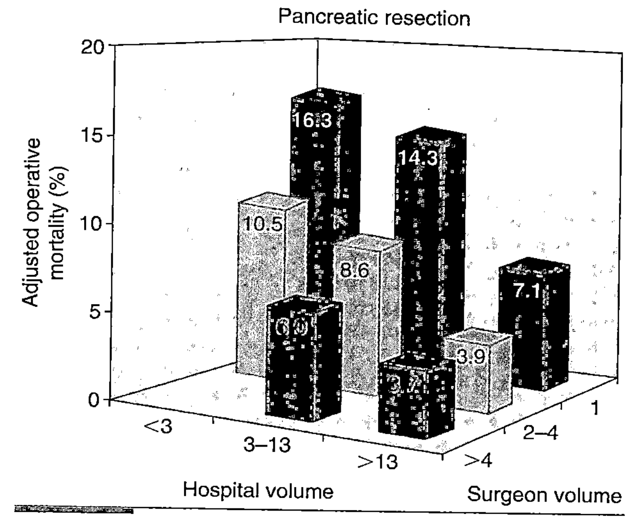

Figure 23.1
Adjusted operative mortality among Medicare patients undergoing pancreatic resection in 1998 and 1999, according to surgeon–volume stratum. Reprinted with permission from *N Engl J Med.* 2003;349:2127 (Copyright 2003, Massachusetts Medical Society; all rights reserved).

Restriction of Pancreatic Resection to a Limited Number of Surgeons at Each Hospital

The relationship between surgeon volume and outcome is less well studied than that between hospital volume and outcome. However, a recent study by Birkmeyer et al.[41] suggested that surgeon volume may account for a large proportion of apparent hospital volume effects. Using the national Medicare claims database (1998–1999), the authors examined mortality in 474,400 patients undergoing one of eight cardiovascular or cancer surgeries, including pancreatic resection. They found that surgeon volume was inversely related to operative mortality for all eight procedures, with the adjusted odds ratio of death (low- vs high-volume surgeons) varying from 1.2 for lung resection to 3.6 for pancreatic resection. When the authors adjusted for hospital volume, the strength of the surgeon volume–outcome relationship weakened, but surgeon volume remained statistically significant for seven of the eight procedures, including pancreatic resection. Furthermore, even within the high-volume hospital stratum, patients who received care from low-volume surgeons had considerably higher mortality rates from several procedures, including pancreatic resection, than those who were treated by high-volume surgeons (Fig. 23.1).

Optimization of Care in the ICU

Postoperative complications are a well-known risk of pancreatic resection. Whereas avoiding all complications would have the greatest impact on mortality, a significant difference can also be made by effectively treating complications once they happen. Most patients who die after pancreatic resection usually do so after a prolonged hospital and ICU stay. For these patients, optimizing care in the ICU is important. It has been shown that the use of an intensivist-model staff organization can significantly decrease ICU mortality rates. Seventeen studies assessing mortality at hospitals with so-called low-intensity ICU physician staffing (either no intensivist or elective intensivist consultation) versus those with high-intensity staffing (mandatory intensivist consultation or "closed" ICU with all care directed by an intensivist) were reviewed by Pronovost et al.[42] Sixteen of the 17 studies showed both a lower hospital mortality rate and lower in-ICU mortality rate with high-intensity ICU staffing. Although these studies were heterogeneous and observational in nature, their findings were remarkably consistent. In fact, the Leapfrog Group has adopted intensivist-staffed ICUs as one of their evidence-based hospital referral standards.

Implementation of Critical Pathways with "Best Practices"

Another avenue toward quality improvement for patients undergoing high-risk, complex procedures involves identification and implementation of beneficial procedure-specific processes of care. Identifying and incorporating "best practice" processes into critical pathways has been shown to reduce the length of hospital stay, the cost, or both for several common surgical procedures.[43,44] Furthermore, resource use and patient satisfaction also appear to be improved with the implementation of such pathways, which are gaining in popularity throughout the medical industry.[45] Despite the complexity of the surgery, similar benefits of critical pathways for pancreatic resection have also been demonstrated.[46,47]

In 2001, Balcom et al.[46] published a retrospective case series of 733 consecutive patients undergoing pancreatic resection from 1990 to 2000; during this period, case management and clinical pathways were implemented (1995 and 1998, respectively). Many variables were compared across three periods (1990–1995, precase management; 1995–1998, preclinical pathway; and 1998–2000). No detrimental effects of implementation of the clinical pathway were appreciated. On the other hand, a major finding of the study was that the mean length of hospital stay for patients undergoing pancreaticoduodenectomy decreased from 16.1 days in the first period to 12.2 days in the second period to 9.5 days in the third period ($P < 0.001$). Using multivariate analysis, the time period was identified as an independent predictor of decreased length of stay. The authors attributed this decrease to the implementation of case management and clinical pathways.

In another study, Porter et al.[47] evaluated the cost and use impact of a clinical pathway for patients undergoing pancreaticoduodenectomy at the University of Texas M.D. Anderson Cancer Center. One hundred forty-eight consecutive patients undergoing pancreaticoduodenectomy or total pancreatectomy from 1996 to 1998 were reviewed. Sixty-eight patients underwent surgery in the 18 months preceding implementation of the pathway, and 80 were treated in the 18 months after pathway implementation. The pathway components included preoperative care (inpatient and outpatient) and all components of postoperative care until discharge. Preprinted orders were created for all aspects of inpatient care, except intraoperative management. Specifically, the pathway included management of all drains and tubes, medications, and criteria for their discontinuation, diet, enteral feeding, and laboratory and radiologic tests. For the evaluation, an independent department determined total costs for each patient, in a blinded review. There were no significant differences before and after the pathway implementation in perioperative mortality (3% vs 1%), readmission to the hospital within 1 month of discharge (15% vs 11%), or mean number of clinic visits within 90 days of discharge (3.3 vs 3.4). However, both the mean total costs and mean length of hospital stay were significantly reduced in the postpathway patients (\$36,627 vs. \$47,515, $P = 0.003$; 13.5 vs 16.4 days, $P = 0.001$). The differences in total cost could not be attributed solely to the differences in cost of room and board.

Optimization of Preoperative Staging: Dynamic CT ± Diagnostic Laparoscopy

Despite improvements in diagnosis, only 10%–15% of pancreatic cancer patients present with resectable tumors. Because complete surgical resection offers the only chance for cure, identification of the subgroup of patients who have truly resectable disease is critical. Equally important is the identification before laparotomy of patients who will not benefit from surgical intervention. Currently, dynamic, contrast-enhanced computed tomography (CT) scanning is the imaging study of choice for the preoperative evaluation of pancreatic malignancies. Unfortunately, initial CT scans obtained in patients with pancreatic cancer are often suboptimal with respect to proper contrast agent administration or technical attention to the anatomic region. In addition, because of a lack of clear, objective radiographic criteria for resectability, published resectability rates based on CT scans alone have varied from 55%–80%. This has led some to recommend diagnostic laparoscopy as part of the staging work-up.

The literature evaluating the use of staging laparoscopy is difficult to interpret for a number of reasons. Within the literature, there has been inconsistent use of high-quality CT, a lack of definition of the term "resectable," a comparison of inhomogeneous patient populations, and inconsistent reporting of margin status. A 2001 review by Pisters et al.[48] concluded that when high-quality, dynamic CT scanning protocols are used with objective, anatomy-based CT criteria to define potentially resectable pancreatic cancer, the accuracy of prediction of resectability increases to 75%–89%. Employing this type of CT method, the authors estimated that the use of routine laparoscopy would benefit only 4%–13% of patients, making its use as a routine staging procedure unjustifiable. However, selective use of laparoscopy, at the time of laparotomy, in patients at higher risk for occult M1 disease (large primary lesion, lesion not in the head of the pancreas, equivocal radiographic findings, or subtle clinical or laboratory findings) may be appropriate and more cost-effective. Rigorous studies are needed to settle the questions about the ultimate role for laparoscopy.

Preoperative Management of Hyperbilirubinemia

Pancreatic cancer patients who present with hyperbilirubinemia are known to be at higher risk during pancreaticoduodenectomy.[49,50] The question remains as to whether this risk can be reduced by preoperative biliary drainage (PBD). No significant difference in mortality rates with PBD has been identified in at least six prospective studies and numerous retrospective analyses.[6,7,51-58] In Sewnath et al.'s[59] recent meta-analysis evaluating the efficacy of PBD for tumors causing obstructive jaundice, the mortality and complication rates for patients undergoing pancreatic surgery with or without PBD were compared. Five relevant randomized studies and 18 nonrandomized studies were identified. This analysis found no significant difference in the overall death rate between patients who had surgery with PBD and those who had surgery without PBD. The overall complication rate was significantly higher with PBD than without PBD (57.3% vs 41.9%; odds ratio, 1.99; 95% confidence interval, 1.25–3.16), but the postoperative complication rate was significantly lower in patients who underwent PBD than in those who did not (29.9% vs 41.9%; odds ratio, 0.59; 95% confidence interval, 0.37–0.94). Findings were similar in the evaluation of the nonrandomized studies, except no difference was seen in the postoperative complication rate.

Although this review of the literature was thorough, characteristics of the individual studies must be considered when weighing the results of the meta-analysis. It has been argued that broad eligibility criteria, small sample sizes, and variations in interventions and procedures make it hard to draw meaningful conclusions.[60] Furthermore, the results must be applied in the context of how patients are actually treated. For example, the majority of patients with symptomatic obstructive jaundice present for surgical evaluation with pre-existing biliary decompression. In addition, patients with malignant biliary obstruction require significant preoperative assessment. Although patients with obstructive jaundice who present to a high-volume center may benefit from immediate surgery, for the majority of patients, a policy of endobiliary stent placement and referral to a tertiary care center is reasonable.

Prevention of Pancreatic Fistulas

Pancreatic fistulas—usually resulting from anastomotic leaks from the pancreaticojejunostomy—are an important cause of both morbidity and mortality after pancreaticoduodenectomy. Prophylactic administration of octreotide (a somatostatin analogue) perioperatively has been advocated by some to reduce the incidence of postoperative pancreatic fistulas by inhibiting pancreatic exocrine function.

The effectiveness of perioperative octreotide after pancreatic resection has been evaluated in four prospective, randomized, double-blind, placebo-controlled, multicenter trials.[61-64] All four trials demonstrated a significant reduction in the postoperative complication rate in patients who received octreotide. Overall, 21.5% of patients in the octreotide group (103 of 480) experienced complications, as compared with 37.5% (181 of 483) receiving placebos. None of the trials found a significant difference in mortality rates.

Of note, these trials enrolled patients with both neoplastic disease and chronic pancreatitis, who received a variety of pancreatic resections, and all trials had pancreatic fistula rates of greater than 19% in the placebo groups. On the other hand, two prospective, randomized trials—each performed at a single referral center—evaluated the use of perioperative octreotide specifically in patients undergoing pancreaticoduodenectomy for malignancy. Like previous trials, mortality rates in both studies were similar for patients receiving octreotide and those receiving placebo. In contrast to the other trials, however, these studies did not find a significant reduction in morbidity rates in patients receiving octreotide, leaving the question of routine octreotide use open to debate.[65,66]

Use of Neoadjuvant Chemoradiation

Finally, as discussed elsewhere in this text, the role of neoadjuvant chemoradiation is still being delineated. Because of high disease recurrence rates and low survival rates after pancreaticoduodenectomy for pancreatic cancer, interest in adjuvant chemoradiation is growing. There is also increasing awareness of the advantages of neoadjuvant chemoradiation over postoperative therapy. Chemoradiation may be more efficacious before surgical devascularization of the tumor bed. There are also practical advantages to preoperative therapy. Prolonged recovery times after pancreaticoduodenectomy are common and prevent many patients from receiving postoperative chemoradiation. Furthermore, there is no evidence to date that neoadjuvant chemoradiation increases morbidity or mortality after pancreaticoduodenectomy. Although no randomized clinical trials have assessed this issue, several case series have described outcomes of patients undergoing pancreaticoduodenectomy after neoadjuvant or intraoperative therapy.[67-72] Among a total of 160 patients in these series, there were only two deaths (1.3% mortality). Moreover, two studies suggested that preoperative chemoradiation may reduce the incidence of pancreatic anastomotic leak, an important source of morbidity and mortality after pancreaticoduodenectomy.[73,74] Long-term survival data are awaited.

Summary

The outcomes for pancreaticoduodenectomy have improved significantly over time. Currently there is little doubt that, in general, high-volume hospitals and surgeons have lower operative mortality rates, fewer complications, and better survival outcomes with this procedure. Despite this recognition, most patients still undergo pancreatic resection at low-volume hospitals, often facing double-digit mortality rates, unlike patients at higher volume hospitals. This chapter reviewed two basic approaches to improving the outcome of pancreatic resection: evidence-based referrals and quality improvement. Because of the lack of direct tracking of individual hospital and surgeon risk-adjusted morbidity and mortality rates, surrogate measures of quality are needed. Procedure volume is the most recognized measure of quality in the outcomes literature. With increasing demands for accountability in medicine as well as the current economic environment of "value-based purchasing" in healthcare, policies such as volume-based referrals are already being implemented. Equally important for a high-risk procedure like pancreatic resection are procedure-specific processes of care that can provide a significant reduction in both morbidity and mortality. Ultimately, some combination of these two approaches will likely provide the greatest benefit to pancreatic cancer patients.

References

1. Whipple A, Parsons W, Mullins C. Treatment of carcinoma of the ampulla of Vater. *Ann Surg.* 1935;102:763–776.
2. Crile G, Jr. The advantages of bypass operations over radical pancreaticoduodenectomy in the treatment of pancreatic carcinoma. *Surg Gynecol Obstet.* 1970;130:1049–1053.
3. Gudjonsson B. Cancer of the pancreas: 50 years of surgery. *Cancer.* 1987;60:2284–2303.
4. Shapiro TM. Adenocarcinoma of the pancreas: a statistical analysis of biliary bypass vs Whipple resection in good risk patients. *Ann Surg.* 1975;182:715–721.
5. Allema JH, Reinders ME, van Gulik TM, et al. Prognostic factors for survival after pancreaticoduodenectomy for patients with carcinoma of the pancreatic head region. *Cancer.* 1995;75:2069–2076.
6. Andersen HB, Baden H, Brahe NE, Burcharth F. Pancreaticoduodenectomy for periampullary adenocarcinoma. *J Am Coll Surg.* 1994;179:545–552.
7. Bakkevold KE, Kambestad B. Morbidity and mortality after radical and palliative pancreatic cancer surgery: risk factors influencing the short-term results. *Ann Surg.* 1993;217:356–368.
8. Bottger TC, Junginger T. Factors influencing morbidity and mortality after pancreaticoduodenectomy: critical analysis of 221 resections. *World J Surg.* 1999;23:164–171; discussion 171–172.
9. Cameron JL, Pitt HA, Yeo CJ, Lillemoe KD, Kaufman HS, Coleman J. One hundred and forty-five consecutive pancreaticoduodenectomies without mortality. *Ann Surg.* 1993;217:430–435; discussion 435–438.
10. Fernandez-del Castillo C, Rattner DW, Warshaw AL. Standards for pancreatic resection in the 1990s. *Arch Surg.* 1995;130:295–299; discussion 299–300.
11. Geer RJ, Brennan MF. Prognostic indicators for survival after resection of pancreatic adenocarcinoma. *Am J Surg.* 1993;165:68–72; discussion 72–63.
12. Gordon TA, Bowman HM, Tielsch JM, Bass EB, Burleyson GP, Cameron JL. Statewide regionalization of pancreaticoduodenectomy and its effect on in-hospital mortality. *Ann Surg.* 1998;228:71–78.
13. Herter FP, Cooperman AM, Ahlborn TN, Antinori C. Surgical experience with pancreatic and periampullary cancer. *Ann Surg.* 1982;195:274–281.
14. Kayahara M, Nagakawa T, Ueno K, Ohta T, Takeda T, Miyazaki I. Pancreatic resection for periampullary carcinoma in the elderly. *Surg Today.* 1994;24:229–233.
15. Nakase A, Matsumoto Y, Uchida K, Honjo I. Surgical treatment of cancer of the pancreas and the periampullary region: cumulative results in 57 institutions in Japan. *Ann Surg.* 1977;185:52–57.
16. Nitecki SS, Sarr MG, Colby TV, van Heerden JA. Long-term survival after resection for ductal adenocarcinoma of the pancreas: is it really improving? *Ann Surg.* 1995;221:59–66.
17. Smith R. Progress in the surgical treatment of pancreatic disease. *Am J Surg.* 1973;125:143–153.
18. Su CH, Shyr YM, Lui WY, P'Eng FK. Factors affecting morbidity, mortality and survival after pancreaticoduodenectomy for carcinoma of the ampulla of Vater. *Hepatogastroenterology.* 1999;46:1973–1979.
19. Swope TJ, Wade TP, Neuberger TJ, Virgo KS, Johnson FE. A reappraisal of total pancreatectomy for pancreatic cancer: results from U.S. Veterans Affairs hospitals, 1987–1991. *Am J Surg.* 1994;168:582–585; discussion 585–586.
20. Trede M, Schwall G, Saeger HD. Survival after pancreaticoduodenectomy: 118 consecutive resections without an operative mortality. *Ann Surg.* 1990;211:447–458.
21. Tsao JI, Rossi RL, Lowell JA. Pylorus-preserving pancreaticoduodenectomy: is it an adequate cancer operation. *Arch Surg.* 1994;129:405–412.

22. Yeo CJ, Cameron JL, Maher MM, et al. A prospective randomized trial of pancreaticogastrostomy versus pancreaticojejunostomy after pancreaticoduodenectomy. *Ann Surg.* 1995;222:580–588; discussion 588–592.
23. Yeo CJ, Cameron JL, Sohn TA, et al. Six hundred fifty consecutive pancreaticoduodenectomies in the 1990s: pathology, complications, and outcomes. *Ann Surg.* 1997;226: 248–257; discussion 257–260.
24. Hannan EL, Kilburn H, Jr, Racz M, Shields E, Chassin MR. Improving the outcomes of coronary artery bypass surgery in New York State. *JAMA.* 1994;271:761–766.
25. O'Connor GT, Plume SK, Olmstead EM, et al. A regional intervention to improve the hospital mortality associated with coronary artery bypass graft surgery: the Northern New England Cardiovascular Disease Study Group. *JAMA.* 1996;275:841–846.
26. Khuri SF, Daley J, Henderson W, et al. The Department of Veterans Affairs' NSQIP: the first national, validated, outcome-based, risk-adjusted, and peer-controlled program for the measurement and enhancement of the quality of surgical care: National VA Surgical Quality Improvement Program. *Ann Surg.* 1998;228:491–507.
27. Luft HS, Bunker JP, Enthoven AC. Should operations be regionalized? The empirical relation between surgical volume and mortality. *N Engl J Med.* 1979;301:1364–1369.
28. Halm E, Lee C, Chassin MR. *Appendix A: Volume and Outcome in Cancer Surgery: Excerpted from "How is volume related to quality in health care? A systematic review of the research literature."* National Academies Press, Washington, D.C. 2000.
29. Wade TP, Halaby IA, Stapleton DR, Virgo KS, Johnson FE. Population-based analysis of treatment of pancreatic cancer and Whipple resection: Department of Defense hospitals, 1989–1994. *Surgery.* 1996;120:680–685; discussion 686–687.
30. Glasgow RE, Showstack JA, Katz PP, Corvera CU, Warren RS, Mulvihill SJ. The relationship between hospital volume and outcomes of hepatic resection for hepatocellular carcinoma. *Arch Surg.* 1999;134:30–35.
31. Dudley RA, Johansen KL, Brand R, Rennie DJ, Milstein A. Selective referral to high-volume hospitals: estimating potentially avoidable deaths. *JAMA.* 2000;283:1159–1166.
32. Birkmeyer JD, Siewers AE, Finlayson EV, et al. Hospital volume and surgical mortality in the United States. *N Engl J Med.* 2002;346:1128–1137.
33. Birkmeyer JD, Warshaw AL, Finlayson SR, Grove MR, Tosteson AN. Relationship between hospital volume and late survival after pancreaticoduodenectomy. *Surgery.* 1999;126:178–183.
34. Bach PB, Cramer LD, Schrag D, Downey RJ, Gelfand SE, Begg CB. The influence of hospital volume on survival after resection for lung cancer. *N Engl J Med.* 2001;345:181–188.
35. Roohan PJ, Bickell NA, Baptiste MS, Therriault GD, Ferrara EP, Siu AL. Hospital volume differences and five-year survival from breast cancer. *Am J Public Health.* 1998;88: 454–457.
36. Schrag D, Cramer LD, Bach PB, Cohen AM, Warren JL, Begg CB. Influence of hospital procedure volume on outcomes following surgery for colon cancer. *JAMA.* 2000;284: 3028–3035.
37. Finlayson EV, Birkmeyer JD. Effects of hospital volume on life expectancy after selected cancer operations in older adults: a decision analysis. *J Am Coll Surg.* 2003;196: 410–417.
38. Birkmeyer JD, Finlayson EV, Birkmeyer CM. Volume standards for high-risk surgical procedures: potential benefits of the Leapfrog initiative. *Surgery.* 2001;130:415–422.
39. Kotwall CA, Maxwell JG, Brinker CC, Koch GG, Covington DL. National estimates of mortality rates for radical pancreaticoduodenectomy in 25,000 patients. *Ann Surg Oncol.* 2002;9:847–854.
40. Birkmeyer JD, Siewers AE, Marth NJ, Goodman DC. Regionalization of high-risk surgery and implications for patient travel times. *JAMA.* 2003;290:2703–2708.
41. Birkmeyer JD, Stukel TA, Siewers AE, Goodney PP, Wennberg DE, Lucas FL. Surgeon volume and operative mortality in the United States. *N Engl J Med.* 2003;349:2117–2127.
42. Pronovost PJ, Jenckes MW, Dorman T, et al. Organizational characteristics of intensive care units related to outcomes of abdominal aortic surgery. *JAMA.* 1999;281:1310–1317.
43. Horne M. Involving physicians in clinical pathways: an example for perioperative knee arthroplasty. *Jt Comm J Qual Improv.* 1996;22:115–124.
44. Pearson SD, Goulart-Fisher D, Lee TH. Critical pathways as a strategy for improving care: problems and potential. *Ann Intern Med.* 1995;123:941–948.
45. Renholm M, Leino-Kilpi H, Suominen T. Critical pathways: a systematic review. *J Nurs Adm.* 2002;32:196–202.
46. Balcom JH, Rattner DW, Warshaw AL, Chang Y, Fernandez-del Castillo C. Ten-year experience with 733 pancreatic resections: changing indications, older patients, and decreasing length of hospitalization. *Arch Surg.* 2001;136:391–398.
47. Porter GA, Pisters PW, Mansyur C, et al. Cost and utilization impact of a clinical pathway for patients undergoing pancreaticoduodenectomy. *Ann Surg Oncol.* 2000;7:484–489.
48. Pisters PW, Lee JE, Vauthey JN, Charnsangavej C, Evans DB. Laparoscopy in the staging of pancreatic cancer. *Br J Surg.* 2001;88:325–337.
49. Braasch JW, Gray BN. Considerations that lower pancreaticoduodenectomy mortality. *Am J Surg.* 1977;133:480–484.
50. Andren-Sandberg A, Ihse I. Factors influencing survival after total pancreatectomy in patients with pancreatic cancer. *Ann Surg.* 1983;198:605–610.
51. Lygidakis NJ, van der Heyde MN, Lubbers MJ. Evaluation of preoperative biliary drainage in the surgical management of pancreatic head carcinoma. *Acta Chir Scand.* 1987;153:665–668.
52. Snellen JP, Obertop H, Bruining HA, et al. The influence of preoperative jaundice, biliary drainage and age on postoperative morbidity and mortality after pancreaticoduodenectomy and total pancreatectomy. *Neth J Surg.* 1985;37:83–86.
53. Hatfield AR, Tobias R, Terblanche J, et al. Preoperative external biliary drainage in obstructive jaundice: a prospective controlled clinical trial. *Lancet.* 1982;2:896–899.
54. Heslin MJ, Brooks AD, Hochwald SN, Harrison LE, Blumgart LH, Brennan MF. A preoperative biliary stent is associated with increased complications after pancreaticoduodenectomy. *Arch Surg.* 1998;133:149–154.

55. McPherson GA, Benjamin IS, Hodgson HJ, Bowley NB, Allison DJ, Blumgart LH. Pre-operative percutaneous transhepatic biliary drainage: the results of a controlled trial. *Br J Surg*. 1984;71:371–375.
56. Pitt HA, Gomes AS, Lois JF, Mann LL, Deutsch LS, Longmire WP, Jr. Does preoperative percutaneous biliary drainage reduce operative risk or increase hospital cost? *Ann Surg*. 1985;201:545–553.
57. Povoski SP, Karpeh MS, Jr, Conlon KC, Blumgart LH, Brennan MF. Association of preoperative biliary drainage with postoperative outcome following pancreaticoduodenectomy. *Ann Surg*. 1999;230:131–142.
58. Thomas JH, Connor CS, Pierce GE, MacArthur RI, Iliopoulos JI, Hermreck AS. Effect of biliary decompression on morbidity and mortality of pancreaticoduodenectomy. *Am J Surg*. 1984;148:727–731.
59. Sewnath ME, Karsten TM, Prins MH, Rauws EJ, Obertop H, Gouma DJ. A meta-analysis on the efficacy of preoperative biliary drainage for tumors causing obstructive jaundice. *Ann Surg*. 2002;236:17–27.
60. Pisters PW, Lee JE, Vauthey JN, Evans DB. Comment and perspective on Sewnath and colleagues' recent meta-analysis of the efficacy of preoperative biliary drainage for tumors causing obstructive jaundice. *Ann Surg*. 2003;237: 594–595; author reply 595–596.
61. Buchler M, Friess H, Klempa I, et al. Role of octreotide in the prevention of postoperative complications following pancreatic resection. *Am J Surg*. 1992;163:125–130; discussion 130–131.
62. Friess H, Beger HG, Sulkowski U, et al. Randomized controlled multicentre study of the prevention of complications by octreotide in patients undergoing surgery for chronic pancreatitis. *Br J Surg*. 1995;82:1270–1273.
63. Pederzoli P, Bassi C, Falconi M, Camboni MG. Efficacy of octreotide in the prevention of complications of elective pancreatic surgery: Italian Study Group. *Br J Surg*. 1994;81:265–269.
64. Montorsi M, Zago M, Mosca F, et al. Efficacy of octreotide in the prevention of pancreatic fistula after elective pancreatic resections: a prospective, controlled, randomized clinical trial. *Surgery*. 1995;117:26–31.
65. Lowy AM, Lee JE, Pisters PW, et al. Prospective, randomized trial of octreotide to prevent pancreatic fistula after pancreaticoduodenectomy for malignant disease. *Ann Surg*. 1997;226:632–641.
66. Yeo CJ, Cameron JL, Lillemoe KD, et al. Does prophylactic octreotide decrease the rates of pancreatic fistula and other complications after pancreaticoduodenectomy? Results of a prospective randomized placebo-controlled trial. *Ann Surg*. 2000;232:419–429.
67. Yeo CJ, Abrams RA, Grochow LB, et al. Pancreaticoduodenectomy for pancreatic adenocarcinoma: postoperative adjuvant chemoradiation improves survival: a prospective, single-institution experience. *Ann Surg*. 1997;225:621–633; discussion 633–636.
68. Staley CA, Lee JE, Cleary KR, et al. Preoperative chemoradiation, pancreaticoduodenectomy, and intraoperative radiation therapy for adenocarcinoma of the pancreatic head. *Am J Surg*. 1996;171:118–124; discussion 124–115.
69. Spitz FR, Abbruzzese JL, Lee JE, et al. Preoperative and postoperative chemoradiation strategies in patients treated with pancreaticoduodenectomy for adenocarcinoma of the pancreas. *J Clin Oncol*. 1997;15:928–937.
70. Pisters PW, Abbruzzese JL, Janjan NA, et al. Rapid-fractionation preoperative chemoradiation, pancreaticoduodenectomy, and intraoperative radiation therapy for resectable pancreatic adenocarcinoma. *J Clin Oncol*. 1998;16: 3843–3850.
71. Hoffman JP, Weese JL, Solin LJ, et al. A pilot study of preoperative chemoradiation for patients with localized adenocarcinoma of the pancreas. *Am J Surg*. 1995;169:71–77; discussion 77–78.
72. Evans DB, Termuhlen PM, Byrd DR, Ames FC, Ochran TG, Rich TA. Intraoperative radiation therapy following pancreaticoduodenectomy. *Ann Surg*. 1993;218:54–60.
73. Evans DB, Rich TA, Byrd DR, et al. Preoperative chemoradiation and pancreaticoduodenectomy for adenocarcinoma of the pancreas. *Arch Surg*. 1992;127:1335–1339.
74. Avizonis VN, Sause WT, Noyes RD. Morbidity and mortality associated with intraoperative radiotherapy. *J Surg Oncol*. 1989;41:240–245.

CHAPTER 24

Interventional Radiology in the Management of Postoperative Complications

Michael J. Wallace, MD
Stephen McRae, MD

Over the past 2 decades, the role of interventional radiology in the management of cancer has shifted from diagnosis to therapy. The interventional radiologist uses those standard imaging techniques that best define the target organ or lesion to guide minimally invasive vascular and nonvascular procedures. These procedures are adapted from standard surgical approaches to establish a diagnosis, initiate therapeutic management, or provide palliative care for patients with cancer. Compared with their surgical alternatives, minimally invasive approaches are often safer, less traumatic, and less painful but are equally therapeutic and more cost effective. This diverse group of procedures includes imaging-guided biopsy and drainage (gastrostomy, nephrostomy, abscess, and biliary), arterial interventions (infusion, embolization, chemoembolization, balloon angioplasty, stent/stent-graft placement), and venous interventions (insertion and repositioning of long-term central venous access devices, stents, inferior vena caval filters, foreign body retrieval, and thrombolysis), among others. Percutaneous biliary drainage (PBD) and percutaneous aspiration/drainage of intraabdominal abscesses, bilomas, bile ascites, or pancreatic leaks are more commonly used in the management of pancreatic cancer. Vascular interventions are used predominantly for the diagnosis and transvascular treatment of arterial hemorrhage. State-of-the-art imaging modalities, including fluoroscopy, ultrasound, computed tomography (CT), are used to guide the placement of needles, catheters, and devices directly to the target sites. These procedures are often performed under local anesthesia and intravenous sedation and typically do not require general anesthesia.

Pancreatic surgery has become a safe method of treating patients with malignant and benign pancreatic diseases. However, despite a mortality rate of less than 3%,[1-3] the rate of major complications requiring intervention can be as high as 40%.[1-3] Interventional radiologists play a critical role in the management of these postoperative complications by shortening hospital stays, speeding recovery times, avoiding reoperation at times, and minimizing morbidity.[4]

Nonvascular Interventions

A major contribution of the interventional radiologist to the care of patients with cancer is percutaneous catheter drainage, especially in the perioperative setting. Catheters are inserted into an obstructed or leaking biliary system (including bilomas and the gallbladder), as well as into intraabdominal fluid collections (abscesses, bile ascites, and peripancreatic leaks) under radiologic guidance by using the Seldinger technique. This technique makes use of a needle, guidewire, and catheter. In a review of 1061 patients who had post-pancreaticoduodenectomy complications, Sohn et al.[4] found that 129 of 1061 patients (12%) required postoperative procedures performed by interventional radiology.

Percutaneous Drainage of Intraabdominal Fluid Collections

Fever due to sepsis is common in the perioperative oncologic setting and is often the result of abscess formation within the abdomen. A septic episode is often accompanied by leukocytosis; cyclic or constant temperature elevation; and renal, pulmonary, or cardiovascular failure.[5] When left untreated, intraabdominal abscesses have a mortality rate of nearly 100%.[6] Thirty-six percent of intraabdominal abscesses are located within the peritoneal cavity, 38% within the retroperitoneum, and 26% within the viscera.[7] Over the past 2 decades, percutaneous drainage has largely replaced surgical drainage as the treatment of choice for abscesses and other abnormal fluid collections, such as bilomas, bile ascites, pseudocysts, and lymphoceles.[8-10] Fig. 24.1 demonstrates the effectiveness of imaging-guided drainage of bile ascites after hepaticojejunostomy. Percutaneous drainage is less invasive than surgical drainage, better maintains the integrity of surrounding structures and overlying skin, and can be performed at the time of initial diagnosis, thus saving time and expense. In addition, most percutaneous drainage procedures are performed with sedation induced by intravenous agents (e.g., midazolam and fentanyl), eliminating the need for general anesthesia. Percutaneous drainage also makes nursing care easier because drainage systems are closed, so there is no extensive surgical wound that requires frequent dressing changes.

Imaging, primarily by ultrasound and CT, is essential for both diagnosis and intervention. The advantages of ultrasound are that it can be used to guide needle placement in real time and can be performed at the bedside of patients in the intensive care unit that are not able to travel to the radiology department, especially when the abscess is superficial.[9] Limitations include image degradation in the presence of intraabdominal air or gas (e.g., postoperative intraperitoneal free air or intestinal air secondary to postoperative ileus), in obese patients, and in patients with overlying surgical dressings.

CT has emerged as the imaging modality of choice for the evaluation of patients with intraabdominal sepsis.[9] The availability of rapid-acquisition multislice CT scanners now allows for adequate diagnostic examinations, even in critically ill patients who are unable to hold their breath. CT is better at determining the depth of an abscess, the site of cutaneous entry, and the best angle of approach for avoiding adjacent vital structures, such as the bowel, organs, or major vessels. As in ultrasound, however, the appearance of fluid collections on CT scans is nonspecific; thus, sterile collections cannot be differentiated from infected ones. Criteria used to identify an abscess include intracavitary gas, thick or irregular walls, heterogenous internal debris, and contrast enhancement. Many studies report that CT is more accurate than ultrasound for identifying intraabdominal fluid collections and abscesses, with a sensitivity of 90%–100% for CT versus 80%–85% for ultrasound.[9,11-15]

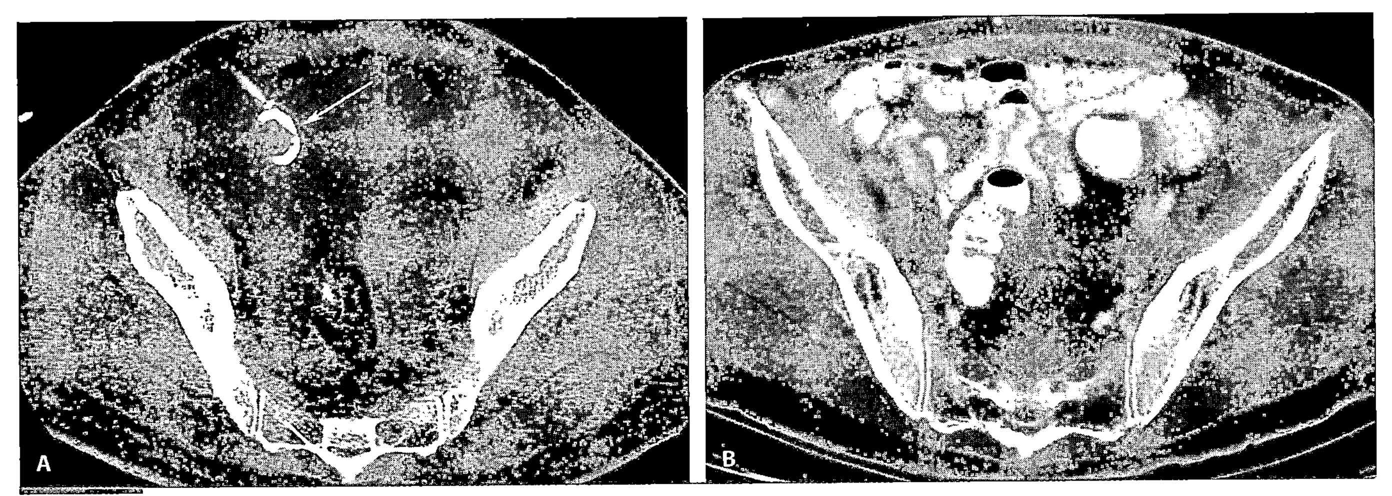

Figure 24.1
Treatment of a patient with bile leak and bile ascites after hepaticojejunostomy. Computed tomography performed immediately after 10-Fr Cope loop drain (*white arrow*) placement **(A)** and 2 months after drain removal **(B)** demonstrates resolution of bile ascites.

The most important step in any percutaneous drainage procedure is planning the access route.[10] This is performed after review of all pertinent imaging studies. In general, the shortest, straightest approach is the best. Care must be taken to avoid adjacent bowel, pleura, and major blood vessels. Diagnostic aspiration can be performed initially with an 18- to 22-gauge needle, whose positioning is confirmed by either ultrasound or CT. Fluid is aspirated for culture, Gram staining, and other pertinent laboratory studies. If frank pus is aspirated, the fluid can be drained immediately by inserting a 10- to 20-Fr catheter into the collection. The choice of an appropriately sized drainage catheter is based on the type and the viscosity of fluid obtained at the initial aspiration.

Percutaneous drainage is most successful when the fluid collection is well defined, unilocular, and free flowing, characteristics that apply to more than 90% of intraabdominal collections.[16] Postoperative abscesses have the best outcomes, with a success rate of 90%.[17] More complex collections (e.g., abscesses that communicate with bowel) have a lesser cure rate of between 80% and 90%. Pancreatic collections, abscesses infected with yeast, and tumors in which an abscess or phlegmon intermingles with an area of necrosis have cure rates as low as 30%–50%.[10,17,18] Nevertheless, percutaneous drainage may still be helpful in less favorable situations (e.g., multilocular collection, necrotic debris), particularly when the risk of surgical complications is high. In these less optimal circumstances, percutaneous drainage may improve the patient's condition so that a more definitive surgical drainage can be performed at a later time.[17]

In the pancreaticoduodenectomy series reported by Sohn et al.,[4] 84 of 1061 patients (8%) required imaging-guided percutaneous aspiration ($N = 4$) or catheter drainage ($N = 80$) for treatment of an intraabdominal abscess ($N = 65$), biloma ($N = 15$), or lymphocele ($N = 4$). Twenty-four required placement of two or more drains for adequate therapy. In the subgroup of patients with intraabdominal abscesses, the most common cause of abscess formation was an anastomotic leak. There were four deaths and 11 reexplorations in this subgroup. Four of the reexplorations were performed because the fluid collection was not amenable to drainage or because there was anastomotic dehiscence and widespread peritoneal contamination. Overall, percutaneous drainage of intraabdominal postoperative fluid collections was effective in 95% of cases.[4]

Peripancreatic fluid collections or abscesses that communicate with the pancreatic duct are more challenging and require prolonged percutaneous drainage. Fig. 24.2 demonstrates the sequence of percutaneous procedures used to resolve a fistulous communication between the pancreatic duct and a postoperative abscess in the left upper quadrant that developed after distal pancreatectomy. First, imaging was performed to identify the presence of a postoperative fluid collection (Fig. 24.2A) and followed by percutaneous drainage (Fig. 24.2B) to allow the cavity to decompress and heal (Fig. 24.2C). Then, the standard looped percutaneous radiologic drain was exchanged for a straight catheter, and its tip was positioned as close to the fistula tract as possible (Fig. 24.2D). Adjunctive endoscopic placement of a stent within the pancreatic duct was used to effectively decompress the pancreatic system (Fig. 24.2C, D). Next, the straight percutaneous drain was withdrawn slowly to allow the tract to heal, and follow-up imaging was used to document resolution of the leak (Fig. 24.2E). Communication with the pancreatic duct was documented throughout the course of therapy (Fig. 24.2C, D).

The only absolute contraindication to percutaneous drainage is the lack of a safe access route. This is rarely a problem when CT guidance is used. In very select cases in which fluid has collected deep within the pelvis, transrectal or transvaginal routes may be used under endocavitary ultrasound guidance.[19-21] The overall complication rate for percutaneous drainage is no more than 5%.[10] Minor complications include transient bacteremia, skin infection, and minor bleeding. Major complications include frank hemorrhage requiring transfusion, peritonitis, sepsis, and bowel perforation. The recurrence rate after percutaneous drainage is approximately 5%. Percutaneous drainage thus compares favorably with surgical alternatives, for which the mortality rates are 10%–20% and the recurrence rates are 15%–30%.

Percutaneous Biliary Drainage

In addition to being an important palliative adjunct in patients with inoperable cancer, PBD is used in the perioperative setting in patients with pancreatic disorders. Biliary drainage before pancreatic resection was once believed to reduce postoperative mortality in jaundiced patients.[22-27] Several recent studies have suggested that preoperative biliary decompression has no influence on postoperative morbidity and mortality.[28] Others have suggested that it has an unfavorable influence on morbidity.[29-31] These mixed findings regarding PBD have limited its current use to a smaller, select group of patients. PBD is more commonly used to treat acute suppurative cholangitis and failed biliary enteric bypass and to divert bile flow in cases of bile leaks (Fig. 24.2) and fistulas that form after pancreatic resection.

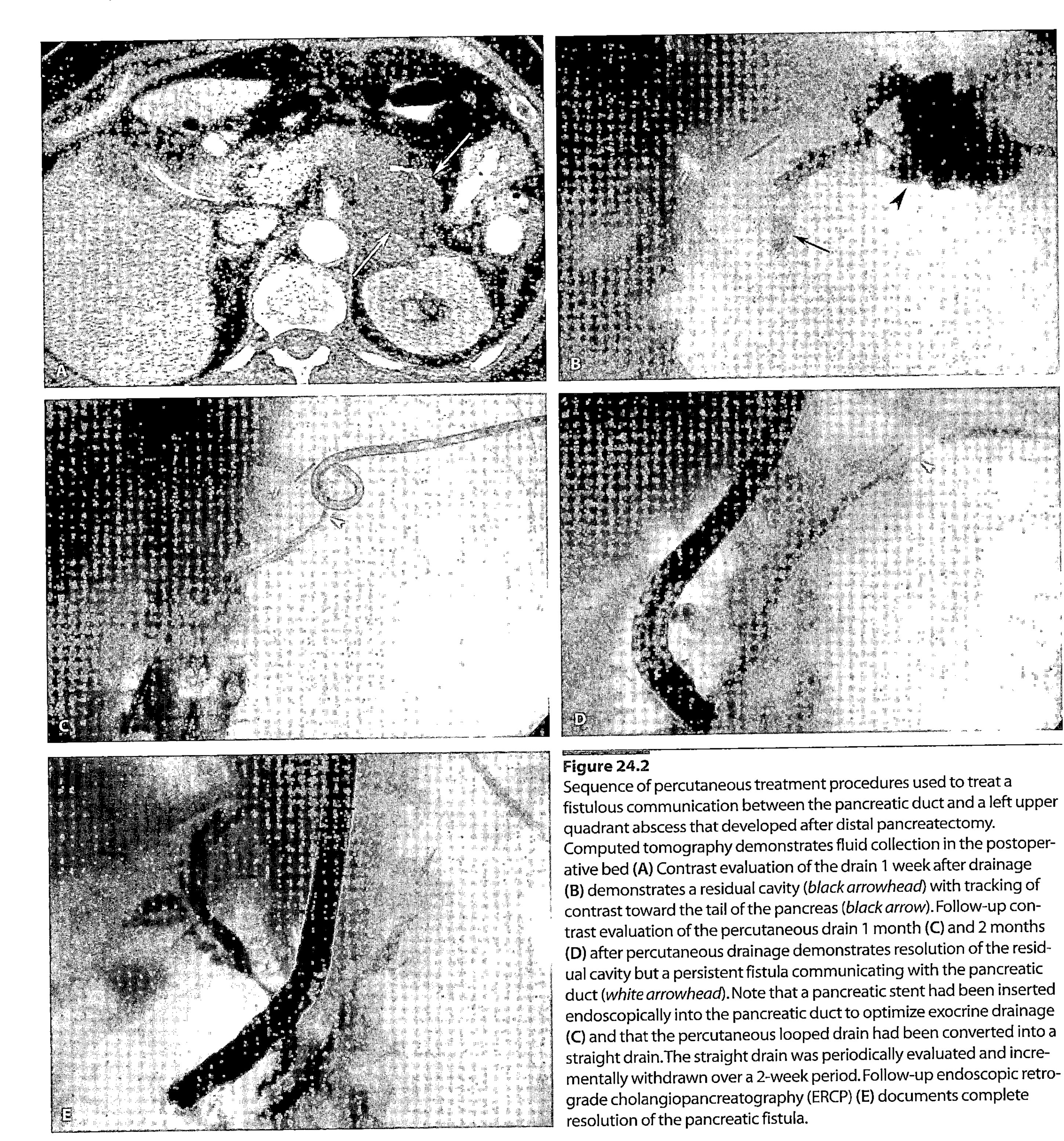

Figure 24.2
Sequence of percutaneous treatment procedures used to treat a fistulous communication between the pancreatic duct and a left upper quadrant abscess that developed after distal pancreatectomy. Computed tomography demonstrates fluid collection in the postoperative bed **(A)** Contrast evaluation of the drain 1 week after drainage **(B)** demonstrates a residual cavity (*black arrowhead*) with tracking of contrast toward the tail of the pancreas (*black arrow*). Follow-up contrast evaluation of the percutaneous drain 1 month **(C)** and 2 months **(D)** after percutaneous drainage demonstrates resolution of the residual cavity but a persistent fistula communicating with the pancreatic duct (*white arrowhead*). Note that a pancreatic stent had been inserted endoscopically into the pancreatic duct to optimize exocrine drainage **(C)** and that the percutaneous looped drain had been converted into a straight drain. The straight drain was periodically evaluated and incrementally withdrawn over a 2-week period. Follow-up endoscopic retrograde cholangiopancreatography (ERCP) **(E)** documents complete resolution of the pancreatic fistula.

There are three types of PBD: external, combined external-internal, and internal (through indwelling plastic or metallic stents).[32] External-drainage catheters completely divert bile to an external reservoir. Internal-external biliary catheters extend from the skin through the hepatic parenchyma into the biliary system and across the obstruction or leak, with the tip of the catheter being situated within the small bowel. Multiple side holes along the distal two thirds of the catheter (the functional portion) allow either external drainage of bile or internal flow of bile into the small bowel. Internal biliary drainage can be accomplished by placing plastic or metal percutaneously or endoscopically. The stents extend above and below the obstruction, allowing bile to flow in the normal direction into the small bowel. Although endoscopic retrograde cholangiopancreatography has essentially replaced PBD for the diagnosis and treatment of biliary disorders, PBD is more effective in patients who have undergone biliary bypass. Endoscopic retrograde cholangiopancreatography is less effective in this situation, because the anatomic distortion caused by surgery limits access to the hepaticoenterostomy.

The reported incidence of bile leaks (Fig. 24.3) after pancreatic resection is no more than 2% in several large series published over the past 5 years.[1,3,4] In the series reported by Sohn et al.,[4] 39 patients (4%) required immediate postoperative biliary intervention. Of these, 22 patients (2%) had a bile leak at the hepaticojejunostomy site, six had occluded T tubes, five had cholangitis due to an isolated left-sided ductal system, three had an aberrant right hepatic duct that was not incorporated into the hepaticojejunostomy, and three had dislodged T tubes. Seven patients in this subgroup of 39 patients required reexploration, and five died. None of the deaths or reexplorations resulted from complications, or the inadequacy of, percutaneous intervention.[4] In their experience with PBD as treatment for postoperative bile leaks in a series of 16 patients, Ernst et al.[33] found that healing occurred in 13 cases (81%) after PBD. Healing occurred after a mean of 78 days of percutaneous drainage.

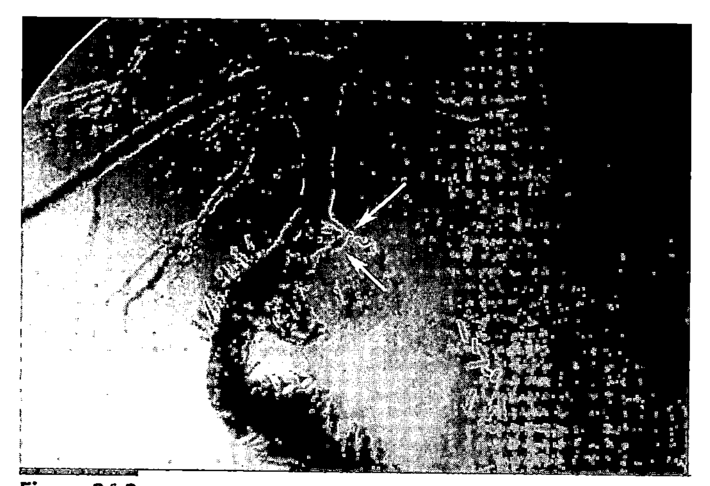

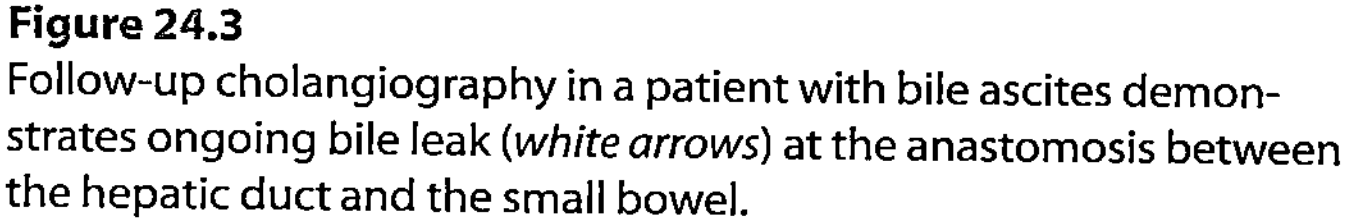

Figure 24.3
Follow-up cholangiography in a patient with bile ascites demonstrates ongoing bile leak (*white arrows*) at the anastomosis between the hepatic duct and the small bowel.

Biliary stricture after pancreatectomy is rare. Most cases occur in patients who have undergone liver transplantation (~10%)[34] and usually at or above the hepaticoenteric anastomosis. Regardless of etiology, surgical revision or intervention remains the therapy of choice for such strictures[35,36]; the 4-year success rate is 86%–88%.[35,37] However, biliary strictures that occur after surgery are often more difficult to manage, and the success rate for surgical repair declines with each successive surgical intervention.[38] Transhepatic balloon dilation and stent placement have been used with increasing frequency to treat postoperative biliary strictures.[34,39,40] In general, balloon dilation of benign strictures in liver transplantation patients produces poor results, although some series show better results for nonanastomotic strictures than for anastomotic strictures.[34,35] Zajko et al.[34] reported an optimistic success rate of 81% at 6 months that declined to 70% at 6 years. Their treatment regimen consisted of multiple balloon dilations per patient over a 1- to 2-week period. Each balloon inflation was performed with prolonged inflation times at high pressure and by means of sequential increases in balloon diameter. Unfortunately, most other series have had primary patency rates of less than 50% at 1–2 years.[39,41,42] Expandable metallic stents were once thought to be the solution for treating refractory biliary strictures.[43,44] In early series, initial technical success rates and short-term primary patency rates were nearly 85% at 6 months.[43,44] However, in subsequent series with longer follow-up, the primary patency rates fell to below 50% at 12–18 months[40,44] and to as low as 0% at 5 years.[40] In the series with the 0% primary patency rate,[40] the assisted primary and secondary patency rates were 88% at 5 years, but long-term patency was gained at the cost of repetitive interventions and increased complications, including death.

The rate of major PBD-associated complications ranges from 5% to 25%, and the incidence of procedure-related deaths ranges from 0% to 6%.[45] Major complications include hemobilia necessitating blood transfusion and cholangitis associated with hypotension. Hemobilia is the most common serious cause of postprocedural morbidity, occurring in 3%–10% of cases.

Complications of percutaneous transhepatic biliary stenting can be divided into short-term and long-term. Short-term complications include cholangitis (5%–7% of cases), hemobilia (2%), and bile leakage (2%).[46,47] The incidence of periprocedural cholangitis can be reduced by administering prophylactic intravenous antibiotics. Delayed cholangitis occurs in association with stent occlusion, which occurs more frequently in plastic stents than in metal stents.[48] Hemobilia is usually self-limiting and rarely necessitates blood transfusion. If bleeding persists and is severe, angiography and arterial embolization can be used.[49] Bile leakage is rarely significant, but when it does occur, it may signify stent occlusion. Because bile takes the path of least resistance, it flows in retrograde fashion and extravasates along the course of the catheter out to the skin surface or into the perihepatic space, where it can give rise to a subhepatic or subphrenic abscess. Long-term complications of the percutaneous placement of biliary stents include stent occlusion and migration and duodenal ulceration.

Vascular Interventions

The predominant endovascular therapy for iatrogenic arterial hemorrhage is embolization, which is the deliberate occlusion of the arterial supply to a site of hemorrhage or neoplasm. In the presence of hemorrhage, embolization effectively treats the arterial injury and avoids surgical intervention. Arterial occlusions can be performed at varying levels of the arterial system from large proximal vessels (e.g., hepatic or gastroduodenal artery) to small arterioles within the parenchyma. The embolic material is chosen for the required task. Large-vessel proximal occlusion is typically accomplished by intraarterial delivery of metallic coils and Gelfoam pieces. Small-vessel peripheral occlusion is typically accomplished by injection of particulate materials or liquid embolic agents. For tumor therapy, agents that result in small-vessel peripheral embolization are preferred over those that occlude larger central vessels. Central proximal occlusion of a vessel near its origin has an effect similar to that of surgical ligation, namely immediate formation of collateral circulation. The more proximal the occlusion, the more abundant the resulting collateral circulation. Proximal embolization is not, however, the best approach to direct intraarterial therapy from neoplasms, because it ultimately restricts the ability to re-treat the neoplasm via the same artery and necessitates the identification and catheterization of technically challenging collateral vessels for further therapy. For treatment of bleeding, the central embolic approach is desirable because the arterial pressure can be reduced at the bleeding site sufficiently to induce hemostasis. This approach has the added benefit of allowing development of a collateral arterial supply after embolization. Use of peripheral embolic agents would increase the risk of undesired tissue necrosis.

The delivery of therapeutic agents via the arterial system requires selective vascular catheterization, which is accomplished by tailoring the catheter configuration to the vascular anatomy. Current catheter technology now allows coaxial microcatheter systems ranging from 2 to 3 Fr in outer diameter to be delivered through standard 4 to 5 Fr angiographic catheters, thus easing the technical challenges posed by small-vessel catheterization. An additional advantage of these microcatheter systems is their potential for reducing the incidence of arterial injuries (e.g., dissection and perforation) that larger catheters can cause.

Hemorrhage after upper abdominal surgery is uncommon,[50,51] but when it occurs it can result in massive, life-threatening bleeding.[50,52] Vascular complications may occur as a result of intraoperative and preoperative arterial injury, anastomotic leakage, or localized infection.[50,52,53]

The frequency of hemorrhage-related complications after pancreatic surgery ranges from less than 2%[1,2,4] to 7.5%[53] in several large series published within the past decade. For two of these series,[4,53] the incidence, diagnosis, and management of postpancreatectomy hemorrhagic complications were determined. In a series of 1061 patients undergoing pancreaticoduodenectomy over a 5-year period between 1995 and 2000,[4] the postoperative hemorrhage rate was 1.6% (18/1061). Of the 18 patients who had postoperative bleeding, 12 underwent preoperative PBD, and the source of bleeding was attributed to the preoperative intervention in 11. Seven patients (0.7%) had hemorrhage related to the operative intervention.[4] In a series of 599 patients who underwent pancreatoduodenectomy in the 24-year period between 1972 and 1996,[53] the rate of bleeding was even higher (7.5%). The difference in bleeding rates between the two series may be due in part to the inclusion of patients from the early experience in the 1970s and to the smaller number of resections performed annually in one[53] and the inclusion of only patients from the last half decade of the 1990s in the other.[4] Although the overall mortality in the series by Rumstadt et al.[53] was 2.7%, the rate of postoperative bleeding was 7.5% (42/559). Postoperative bleeding included gastrointestinal hemorrhage in 22 patients and operative field bleeding in 20 patients. In 11 cases of operative field bleeding, hemorrhage resulted from erosive bleeding secondary to a leak at the pancreatojejunal anastomosis. In patients with jaundice ($N = 359$), there was no difference in postoperative bleeding between patients who underwent preoperative biliary drainage (8.7%) and those who did not (9.2%). The method of drainage (percutaneous vs endoscopic) was not noted in the report by Rumstadt et al.,[53] and thus the increase in the risk of postoperative hemorrhage reported by Sohn et al.[4] cannot be disputed.

Sites of arterial injury include the celiac artery, its distribution (gastroduodenal artery stump, hepatic artery), and the collateral supply from the inferior pancreaticoduodenal arcade arising from the superior mesenteric artery (Fig. 24.4). Angiographic findings can range from a focal pseudoaneurysm to gross extravasation of contrast. Although reexploration is a management option, the transarterial approach is a less invasive means of treating these difficult problems.

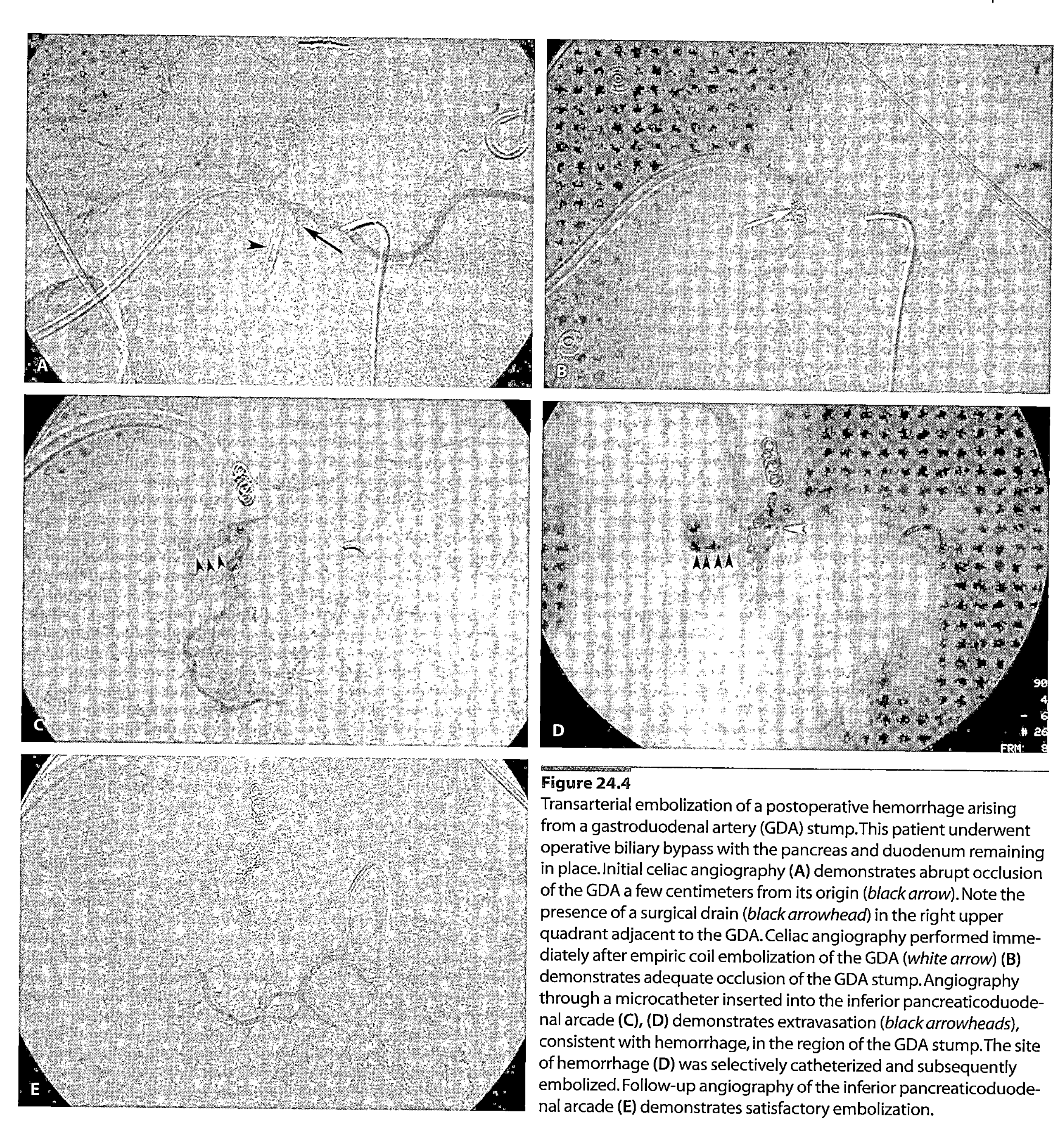

Figure 24.4
Transarterial embolization of a postoperative hemorrhage arising from a gastroduodenal artery (GDA) stump. This patient underwent operative biliary bypass with the pancreas and duodenum remaining in place. Initial celiac angiography **(A)** demonstrates abrupt occlusion of the GDA a few centimeters from its origin (*black arrow*). Note the presence of a surgical drain (*black arrowhead*) in the right upper quadrant adjacent to the GDA. Celiac angiography performed immediately after empiric coil embolization of the GDA (*white arrow*) **(B)** demonstrates adequate occlusion of the GDA stump. Angiography through a microcatheter inserted into the inferior pancreaticoduodenal arcade **(C)**, **(D)** demonstrates extravasation (*black arrowheads*), consistent with hemorrhage, in the region of the GDA stump. The site of hemorrhage **(D)** was selectively catheterized and subsequently embolized. Follow-up angiography of the inferior pancreaticoduodenal arcade **(E)** demonstrates satisfactory embolization.

Transarterial embolization (TAE) has been advocated by several authors as the first-line intervention for abdominal postoperative hemorrhage.[50,52,54] Several small series have demonstrated the efficacy of TAE in controlling all sources of upper gastrointestinal hemorrhage (80%–100%)[55-58] and postoperative abdominal hemorrhage (75%–100%)[4,50,52,54,59] from the splanchnic circulation. Sohn et al.[4] used embolization to treat postpancreatectomy bleeding in 16 of 18 patients and reported a success rate of 75% (12/16), thus negating the need for reexploration. As a result, hemorrhage-related mortality was 0.18%. In the series of Rumstadt et al,[53] three of 42 patients underwent angiography and successful embolization after re-laparotomy failed to stop the bleeding. Gastrointestinal hemorrhage was successfully managed endoscopically in 13 of 22 patients, and 29 patients underwent reexploration for bleeding. In addition to a higher overall mortality rate, the hemorrhage-related mortality in the series of Rumstadt et al.[53] was 1% (6/559), more than five times higher than in the series of Sohn et al.[4] This underscores the vital role that TAE plays in early intervention. Otah et al[59] used TAE successfully in five patients who underwent pancreatoduodenectomy, and Miyamoto et al.[54] used hepatic artery TAE successfully in eight of 10 patients who had postoperative abdominal hemorrhage arising from the celiac distribution. TAE has also been used effectively to treat nonoperative causes of bleeding related to pancreatic disorders. Dasgupta et al[60] reported on the successful use of TAE in five patients with haemosuccus pancreaticus.

Arterial embolization in the upper gastrointestinal tract is considered safe because of the tract's rich arterial collateral supply. Patients who have undergone visceral surgery or have severe atherosclerotic disease may be at higher risk of ischemic complications after embolotherapy. The complications that arise from embolization within the celiac or superior mesenteric artery distributions can be related to catheterization (e.g., pseudoaneurysm, arteriovenous fistula, dissection, thrombosis, perforation) or to intentional or unintentional occlusion of portions of the liver, spleen, pancreas, stomach, or small intestines (e.g., pain, ischemia/infarction, abscess). In a series reported by Hemingway and Allison,[61] representing a 10-year experience, 284 patients underwent 410 embolizations for a diverse group of disorders. Minor complications occurred in 16%, major complications in 6.6%, and death in 2%. Postembolization syndrome (i.e., fever, elevated white blood cell count, and discomfort) occurred after 42.7% of the procedures. The underlying abnormality and its location usually determined the nature and risk of complications.

Hepatic embolization can be accompanied by transient parenchymal ischemia or by more serious complications, including liver infarction, necrosis, potential abscess formation, and biliary complications (e.g., bile leak, stricture, fistula). In the series reported by Reber et al,[52] hepatic ischemia, evidenced by transient increases in transaminase levels, occurred in 2 of 6 patients who underwent TAE. In the series reported by Miyamoto et al,[54] transient ischemia ($N = 6$) and hepatic failure ($N = 2$) occurred in eight patients who underwent successful hepatic embolization. The presence or absence of angiographically identifiable collateral pathways was a key predictor of potential hepatic complications. Liver function returned to baseline levels in patients who had collateral pathways, and liver failure developed in two other patients who did not. All patients in this series had documented portal vein patency. Other case reports have described cases of pancreatic necrosis[57,62] and duodenal infarction.[57]

Alternative approaches to managing complex cases of postoperative arterial hemorrhage have been described. One such approach is direct percutaneous puncture of the pseudoaneurysm under ultrasound or computed tomographic guidance and occlusion of the cavity with coils,[63] thrombin,[64,65] or both (Fig. 24.5). This approach is usually reserved for situations in which the transarterial route is not feasible. An alternative endovascular approach is the exclusion of a gastroduodenal artery stump hemorrhage by placing a covered stent across the gastroduodenal artery origin.[66] This technique was used in a situation in which the gastroduodenal artery was too short for safe coil embolization and concomitant portal vein thrombosis increased the risk for hepatic failure should hepatic artery embolization be performed. Covered stent placement allowed both exclusion of the gastroduodenal artery and preservation of hepatic artery patency. This latter approach is technically more challenging with the currently available stent-graft devices but does offer an alternative for situations in which collateral hepatic arterial supply is insufficient or portal vein compromise is encountered.

Once the decision to proceed with angiography has been made, several considerations should be addressed. Multidisciplinary discussions should be carried out and a plan of action devised with regard to therapy should a source of bleeding be identified. Laboratory parameters should be evaluated and corrected when possible. For patients with coagulopathy (prothrombin time >16 seconds) or thrombocytopenia ($<70 \times 10^9$/L), transfusions of fresh frozen plasma, platelets, and other blood products can be initiated before and during angiography. For patients who are actively bleeding and hemodynamically unstable, angiography should proceed regardless of platelet count or coagulation parameters. A sheath can be left in place until these factors are corrected, because the life-saving potential of embolization outweighs the risk of procedure-related complications. For patients with elevated creatinine levels,

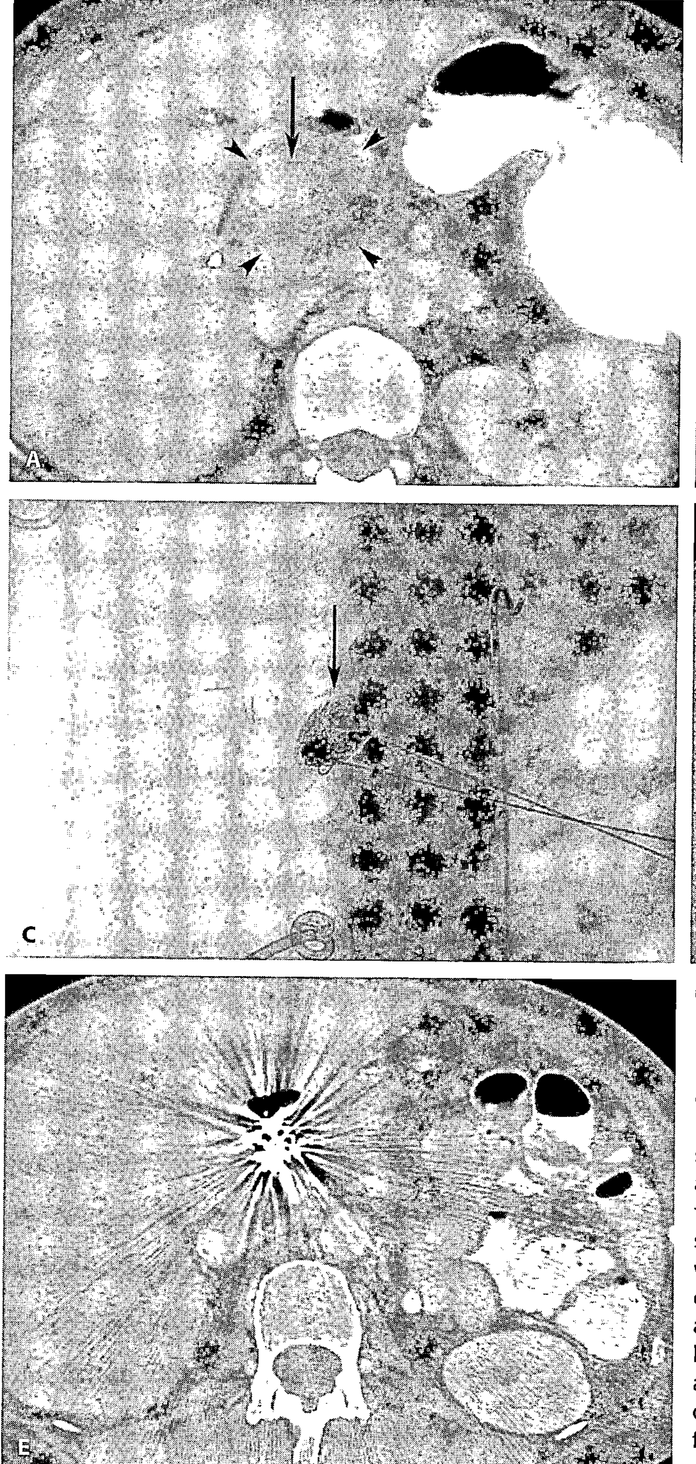

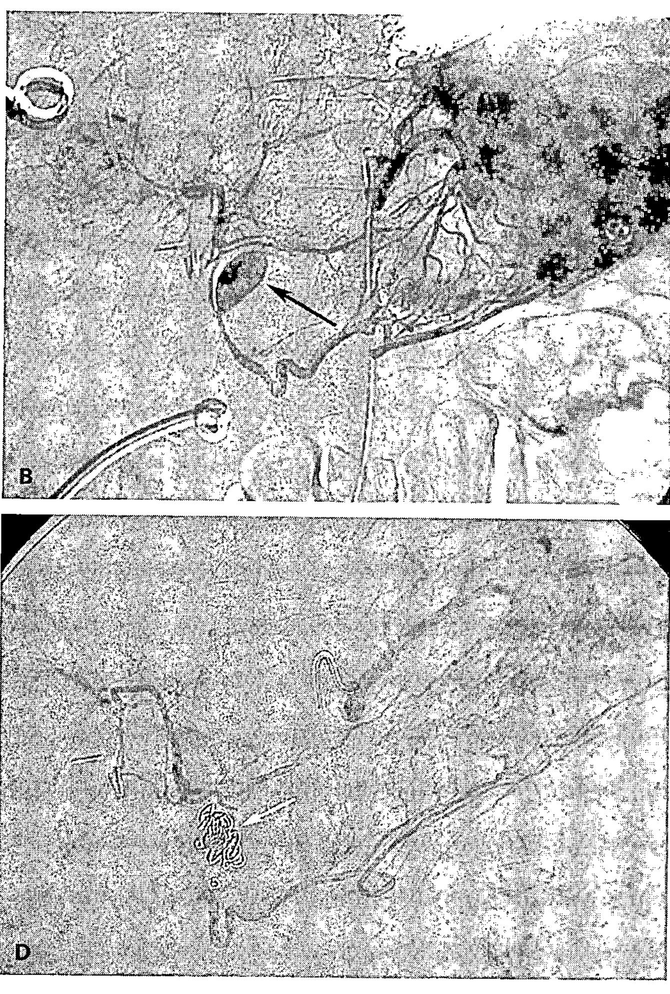

Figure 24.5
Diagnosis and management of a gastroduodenal artery hemorrhage. Intravenous contrast-enhanced computed tomography of the abdomen **(A)** demonstrates a large hematoma (*arrowheads*) in the right upper abdomen and a defined pseudoaneurysm (*black arrow*). Digital subtraction angiography **(B)** shows the pseudoaneurysm (*black arrow*) as it arises from the gastroduodenal artery before the origin of the gastroepiploic artery. The pseudoaneurysm could not be accessed via the standard transvascular approach, because the common hepatic artery was occluded and retrograde access via the inferior pancreaticoduodenal arcade was not feasible. The pseudoaneurysm was subsequently accessed by direct insertion of two 22-g needles and the lesion embolized by using a combination of coils and thrombin **(C)**. Follow-up angiography **(D)** and computed tomography **(E)** from the celiac artery demonstrate occlusion of the pseudoaneurysm but preservation of flow to the liver and resolution of the hematoma. Note the artifact caused by the nest of coils placed within the pseudoaneurysm.

every effort should be made to preserve renal function despite the requirements for contrast administration. In the acute setting, sufficient hydration of the patient may not be possible, but the use of fenoldopam has recently proved valuable in preserving renal function in this high-risk population.[67] Finally, the risk of renal failure must be weighed against the potential benefits of angiography and embolization.

References

1. Balcom JH 4th, Rattner DW, Warshaw AL, Chang Y, Fernandez-del Castillo C. Ten-year experience with 733 pancreatic resections: changing indications, older patients, and decreasing length of hospitalization. *Arch Surg*. 2001;136:391–398.
2. Yeo CJ, Cameron JL, Sohn TA, et al. Six hundred fifty consecutive pancreaticoduodenectomies in the 1990s: pathology, complications, and outcomes. *Ann Surg*. 1997;226: 248–257; discussion 257–260.
3. Sohn TA, Yeo CJ, Cameron JL, et al. Resected adenocarcinoma of the pancreas—616 patients: results, outcomes, and prognostic indicators. *J Gastrointest Surg*. 2000;4:567–579.
4. Sohn TA, Yeo CJ, Cameron JL, et al. Pancreaticoduodenectomy: role of interventional radiologists in managing patients and complications. *J Gastrointest Surg*. 2003;7:209–219.
5. Sirinek KR. Diagnosis and treatment of intra-abdominal abscesses. *Surg Infect (Larchmt)*. 2000;1:31–38.
6. Branum GD, Tyson GS, Branum MA, Meyers WC. Hepatic abscess: changes in etiology, diagnosis, and management. *Ann Surg*. 1990;212:655–662.
7. Altemeier WA, Culbertson WR, Fullen WD, Shook CD. Intra-abdominal abscesses. *Am J Surg*. 1973;125:70–79.
8. Men S, Akhan O, Koroglu M. Percutaneous drainage of abdominal abscess. *Eur J Radiol*. 2002;43:204–218.
9. Lee MJ. Non-traumatic abdominal emergencies: imaging and intervention in sepsis. *Eur Radiol*. 2002;12:2172–2179.
10. van Sonnenberg E, Wittich GR, Goodacre BW, Casola G, D'Agostino HB. Percutaneous abscess drainage: update. *World J Surg*. 2001;25:362–369; discussion 370–362.
11. Knochel JQ, Koehler PR, Lee TG, Welch DM. Diagnosis of abdominal abscesses with computed tomography, ultrasound, and leukocyte scans. *Radiology*. 1980;137:425–432.
12. Haaga JR, Alfidi RJ, Havrilla TR, et al. CT detection and aspiration of abdominal abscesses. *AJR Am J Roentgenol*. 1977;128:465–474.
13. Dobrin PB, Gully PH, Greenlee HB, et al. Radiologic diagnosis of an intra-abdominal abscess. Do multiple tests help? *Arch Surg*. 1986;121:41–46.
14. Roche J. Effectiveness of computed tomography in the diagnosis of intra-abdominal abscess: a review of 111 patients. *Med J Aust*. 1981;2:85–86, 87–88.
15. Carroll B, Silverman PM, Goodwin DA, McDougall IR. Ultrasonography and indium 111 white blood cell scanning for the detection of intraabdominal abscesses. *Radiology*. 1981;140:155–160.
16. Bernini A, Spencer MP, Wong WD, Rothenberger DA, Madoff RD. Computed tomography-guided percutaneous abscess drainage in intestinal disease: factors associated with outcome. *Dis Colon Rectum*. 1997;40:1009–1013.
17. Cinat ME, Wilson SE, Din AM. Determinants for successful percutaneous image-guided drainage of intra-abdominal abscess. *Arch Surg*. 2002;137:845–849.
18. Freeny PC, Hauptmann E, Althaus SJ, Traverso LW, Sinanan M. Percutaneous CT-guided catheter drainage of infected acute necrotizing pancreatitis: techniques and results. *AJR Am J Roentgenol*. 1998;170:969–975.
19. Alexander AA, Eschelman DJ, Nazarian LN, Bonn J. Transrectal sonographically guided drainage of deep pelvic abscesses. *AJR Am J Roentgenol*. 1994;162: 1227–1230; discussion 1231–1222.
20. Varghese JC, O'Neill MJ, Gervais DA, Boland GW, Mueller PR. Transvaginal catheter drainage of tuboovarian abscess using the trocar method: technique and literature review. *AJR Am J Roentgenol*. 2001;177:139–144.
21. van Sonnenberg E, D'Agostino HB, Casola G, Goodacre BW, Sanchez RB, Taylor B. US-guided transvaginal drainage of pelvic abscesses and fluid collections. *Radiology*. 1991; 181:53–56.
22. Gundry SR, Strodel WE, Knol JA, Eckhauser FE, Thompson NW. Efficacy of preoperative biliary tract decompression in patients with obstructive jaundice. *Arch Surg*. 1984; 119:703–708.
23. Hatfield AR, Tobias R, Terblanche J, et al. Preoperative external biliary drainage in obstructive jaundice: a prospective controlled clinical trial. *Lancet*. 1982;2: 896–899.
24. McPherson GA, Benjamin IS, Hodgson HJ, Bowley NB, Allison DJ, Blumgart LH. Pre-operative percutaneous transhepatic biliary drainage: the results of a controlled trial. *Br J Surg*. 1984;71:371–375.
25. Lygidakis NJ, van der Heyde MN, Lubbers MJ. Evaluation of preoperative biliary drainage in the surgical management of pancreatic head carcinoma. *Acta Chir Scand*. 1987; 153:665–668.
26. Lai EC, Mok FP, Fan ST, et al. Preoperative endoscopic drainage for malignant obstructive jaundice. *Br J Surg*. 1994;81:1195–1198.
27. Pitt HA, Gomes AS, Lois JF, Mann LL, Deutsch LS, Longmire WP, Jr. Does preoperative percutaneous biliary drainage reduce operative risk or increase hospital cost? *Ann Surg*. 1985;201:545–553.
28. Sewnath ME, Birjmohun RS, Rauws EA, Huibregtse K, Obertop H, Gouma DJ. The effect of preoperative biliary drainage on postoperative complications after pancreaticoduodenectomy. *J Am Coll Surg*. 2001;192:726–734.
29. Povoski SP, Karpeh MS, Jr., Conlon KC, Blumgart LH, Brennan MF. Association of preoperative biliary drainage with postoperative outcome following pancreaticoduodenectomy. *Ann Surg*. 1999;230:131–142.
30. Heslin MJ, Brooks AD, Hochwald SN, Harrison LE, Blumgart LH, Brennan MF. A preoperative biliary stent is associated with increased complications after pancreatoduodenectomy. *Arch Surg*. 1998;133:149–154.
31. Pisters PW, Hudec WA, Hess KR, et al. Effect of preoperative biliary decompression on pancreaticoduodenectomy-associated morbidity in 300 consecutive patients. *Ann Surg*. 2001;234:47–55.
32. Madoff DC, Wallace MJ. Palliative treatment of unresectable bile duct cancer: which stent? which approach? *Surg Oncol Clin N Am*. 2002;11(4):923–939.
33. Ernst O, Sergent G, Mizrahi D, Delemazure O, L'Hermine C. Biliary leaks: treatment by means of percutaneous transhepatic biliary drainage. *Radiology*. 1999;211:345–348.
34. Zajko AB, Sheng R, Zetti GM, Madariaga JR, Bron KM. Transhepatic balloon dilation of biliary strictures in liver transplant patients: a 10-year experience. *J Vasc Interv Radiol*. 1995;6:79–83.
35. Pitt HA, Kaufman SL, Coleman J, White RI, Cameron JL. Benign postoperative biliary strictures: operate or dilate? *Ann Surg*. 1989;210:417–425; discussion 426–417.

36. Lebeau G, Yanaga K, Marsh JW, et al. Analysis of surgical complications after 397 hepatic transplantations. *Surg Gynecol Obstet*. 1990;170:317–322.
37. McDonald ML, Farnell MB, Nagorney DM, Ilstrup DM, Kutch JM. Benign biliary strictures: repair and outcome with a contemporary approach. *Surgery*. 1995;118:582–590; discussion 590–581.
38. Pitt HA, Miyamoto T, Parapatis SK, Tompkins RK, Longmire WP, Jr. Factors influencing outcome in patients with postoperative biliary strictures. *Am J Surg*. 1982;144:14–21.
39. McDonald V, Matalon TA, Patel SK, et al. Biliary strictures in hepatic transplantation. *J Vasc Interv Radiol*. 1991;2:533–538.
40. Culp WC, McCowan TC, Lieberman RP, Goertzen TC, LeVeen RF, Heffron TG. Biliary strictures in liver transplant recipients: treatment with metal stents. *Radiology*. 1996; 199:339–346.
41. Ward EM, Kiely MJ, Maus TP, Wiesner RH, Krom RA. Hilar biliary strictures after liver transplantation: cholangiography and percutaneous treatment. *Radiology*. 1990;177:259–263.
42. Gomes AS. Diagnosis and radiologic treatment of biliary complications of liver transplantation. *Semin Intervent Radiol*. 1992;9:283–289.
43. Petersen BD, Maxfield SR, Ivancev K, Uchida BT, Rabkin JM, Rosch J. Biliary strictures in hepatic transplantation: treatment with self-expanding Z stents. *J Vasc Interv Radiol*. 1996;7:221–228.
44. Bonnel DH, Liguory CL, Lefebvre JF, Cornud FE. Placement of metallic stents for treatment of postoperative biliary strictures: long-term outcome in 25 patients. *AJR Am J Roentgenol*. 1997;169:1517–1522.
45. Venbrux AC, Osterman FA, (authors of chapter 11). Percutaneous transhepatic cholangiography and percutaneous biliary drainage: Step by step. Fairfax: The Society of Cardiovascular and Interventional Radiology; 1995. Laberge JM VA, ed. SCVIR Syllabus: Biliary Interventions.(this is a text and the title is Biliary interventions)
46. Adam A, Chetty N, Roddie M, Yeung E, Benjamin IS. Self-expandable stainless steel endoprostheses for treatment of malignant bile duct obstruction. *AJR Am J Roentgenol*. 1991;156:321–325.
47. Nicholson AA, Royston CM. Palliation of inoperable biliary obstruction with self-expanding metal endoprostheses: a review of 77 patients. *Clin Radiol*. 1993;47:245–250.
48. Knyrim K, Wagner HJ, Pausch J, Vakil N. A prospective, randomized, controlled trial of metal stents for malignant obstruction of the common bile duct. *Endoscopy*. 1993;25:207–212.
49. Cowling MG, Adam AN. Internal stenting in malignant biliary obstruction. *World J Surg*. 2001;25:355–359; discussion 359–361.
50. Okuno A, Miyazaki M, Ito H, et al. Nonsurgical management of ruptured pseudoaneurysm in patients with hepatobiliary pancreatic diseases. *Am J Gastroenterol*.2001; 96:1067–1071.
51. Cullen JJ, Sarr MG, Ilstrup DM. Pancreatic anastomotic leak after pancreaticoduodenectomy: incidence, significance, and management. *Am J Surg*. 1994;168:295–298.
52. Reber PU, Baer HU, Patel AG, Wildi S, Triller J, Buchler MW. Superselective microcoil embolization: treatment of choice in high-risk patients with extrahepatic pseudoaneurysms of the hepatic arteries. *J Am Coll Surg*. 1998; 186:325–330.
53. Rumstadt B, Schwab M, Korth P, Samman M, Trede M. Hemorrhage after pancreatoduodenectomy. *Ann Surg*. 1998;227:236–241.
54. Miyamoto N, Kodama Y, Endo H, Shimizu T, Miyasaka K. Hepatic artery embolization for postoperative hemorrhage in upper abdominal surgery. *Abdom Imaging*. 2003;28:347–353.
55. Ledermann HP, Schoch E, Jost R, Decurtins M, Zollikofer CL. Superselective coil embolization in acute gastrointestinal hemorrhage: personal experience in 10 patients and review of the literature. *J Vasc Interv Radiol*. 1998;9:753–760.
56. Okazaki M, Higashihara H, Koganemaru F, et al. Emergent embolization for control of massive hemorrhage from a splanchnic artery with a new coaxial catheter system. *Acta Radiol*. 1992;33:57–62.
57. Okazaki M, Higashihara H, Ono H, et al. Embolotherapy of massive duodenal hemorrhage. *Gastrointest Radiol*. 1992;17:319–323.
58. Toyoda H, Nakano S, Takeda I, et al. Transcatheter arterial embolization for massive bleeding from duodenal ulcers not controlled by endoscopic hemostasis. *Endoscopy*. 1995;27:304–307.
59. Otah E, Cushin BJ, Rozenblit GN, Neff R, Otah KE, Cooperman AM. Visceral artery pseudoaneurysms following pancreatoduodenectomy. *Arch Surg*. 2002;137:55–59.
60. Dasgupta R, Davies NJ, Williamson RC, Jackson JE. Haemosuccus pancreaticus: treatment by arterial embolization. *Clin Radiol*. 2002;57:1021–1027.
61. Hemingway AP, Allison DJ. Complications of embolization: analysis of 410 procedures. *Radiology*. 1988;166:669–672.
62. Bell SD, Lau KY, Sniderman KW. Synchronous embolization of the gastroduodenal artery and the inferior pancreaticoduodenal artery in patients with massive duodenal hemorrhage. *J Vasc Interv Radiol*. 1995;6:531–536.
63. Fann JI, Samuels S, Slonim S, Burdon TA, Dalman RL. Treatment of abdominal aortic anastomotic pseudoaneurysm with percutaneous coil embolization. *J Vasc Surg*. 2002;35:811–814.
64. Manazer JR, Monzon JR, Dietz PA, Moglia R, Gold M. Treatment of pancreatic pseudoaneurysm with percutaneous transabdominal thrombin injection. *J Vasc Surg*. 2003;38:600–602.
65. Patel JV, Weston MJ, Kessel DO, Prasad R, Toogood GJ, Robertson I. Hepatic artery pseudoaneurysm after liver transplantation: treatment with percutaneous thrombin injection. *Transplantation*. 2003;75:1755–1757.
66. Mansueto G, D'Onofrio M, Iacono C, Rozzanigo U, Serio G, Procacci C. Gastroduodenal artery stump haemorrhage following pylorus-sparing Whipple procedure: treatment with covered stents. *Dig Surg*. 2002;19:237–240.
67. Lepor NE. A review of contemporary prevention strategies for radiocontrast nephropathy: a focus on fenoldopam and N-acetylcysteine. *Rev Cardiovasc Med*. 2003;4[suppl 1]:S15–S20.

Commentary

Douglas B. Evans, MD

Because the majority of operable pancreatic cancers reside in the head and uncinate process, surgical extirpation requires not only removal of the appropriate amount of pancreas but also en bloc resection of the duodenum and distal bile duct. The routine need for multiorgan and occasionally vascular resection at the time of pancreatectomy is in contrast to surgery for tumors of the esophagus, stomach, liver, and rectum. In addition, only the most experienced surgeons will appreciate the complex anatomic relationship of the pancreas to the superior mesenteric artery, yet an understanding of this anatomy is critically important to insure a complete tumor resection. Finally, reconstruction requires anastomosis of the pancreas, bile duct, and stomach (or duodenum) to the jejunum. The need for such a complex reconstruction of the gastrointestinal tract is also unique to surgery of the pancreas. In fact, it was the high complication rate, including mortality, associated with the postresection reconstruction (namely, the pancreatic anastomosis) that was viewed as the major challenge in pancreatic surgery for malignancy in the 1980s and early 1990s. Over the past 2 decades, surgical controversies regarding the technical aspects of surgery and patient management have largely been resolved. Although many people are responsible for such progress, some deserve specific mention: Murray Brennan, John Cameron, Howard Reber, William Traverso, and Andrew Warshaw. These investigators demonstrated that pancreatic surgery could be performed safely by experienced surgeons with the routine use of critical pathways, that perioperative octreotide and surgical drains are often not necessary, that pylorus preservation may be advantageous in certain situations, that there is no significant benefit to extended regional lymph node dissection, and that adjuvant chemotherapy and irradiation after surgery may prolong survival and warrant further multi-institution phase II/III testing. The tremendous progress in pancreatic surgery (based on randomized trials and large-volume single-center experiences), anesthesia, and critical care medicine has now made pancreatic surgery for malignancy a routine procedure at many referral centers. Such progress has appropriately changed the focus of attention to oncologic and health policy areas of investigation.

Current and future challenges include, among others, these general areas of investigation: surgical and pathology quality control in clinical trial design, translational research and the importance of tumor banking, and healthcare policy with respect to regionalization of care. Although the chapters in this text discuss these and other important topics in detail, I wish to highlight selected areas of particular importance. The lack of phase II and phase III clinical trials since the completion of the Gastrointestinal Tumor Study Group trial in the mid-1980s has been answered by completion of the European Study Group for Pancreatic Cancer-1 trial in Europe and the Radiation Therapy Oncology Group 9704 trial in the United States.[1] Additional experience comes from the Eastern Cooperative Oncology Group and single institutions, including Johns Hopkins, Virginia Mason, and M. D. Anderson.[2-8] However, unlike surgical resections for other solid tumors, the completeness of resection is often not recorded by the surgeon or accurately assessed by the pathologist. The pancreaticoduodenectomy specimen is difficult to orient for many pathologists, and therefore, assessment of the retroperitoneal (mesenteric) margin of resection is either not done or not reported, thereby failing to identify this specific margin as positive or negative. Even more important, the pathologist cannot differentiate an R1 (microscopically positive) from an R2 (grossly positive) margin of excision in the absence of the surgeon noting (in his operative report) whether or not a complete resection was performed. Future clinical trials will need to incorporate a standardized system for surgical resection and the pathologic evaluation of the pancreaticoduodenectomy specimen to determine whether a complete (R0/R1) or incomplete (R2) resection was performed. In the presence of an incomplete resection, it is impossible to assess the impact of other potential prognostic variables (e.g., adjuvant therapy) on survival duration. Quality control will be equally important to determine whether investigators are in compliance with such requirements.

The emergence of targeted therapies such as bevacizumab (Avastin), cetuximab (C225), and others has renewed interest in the routine acquisition of human tissue specimens.[9-11] It is likely that the effectiveness of such targeted therapies will be determined by the molecular profile of the individual tumor, a finding that may vary between patients. In addition, human specimens are critical for the ongoing laboratory investigation of techniques for early diagnosis, signaling pathways, and pancreatic cancer model systems. Despite the increased regulatory requirements, it is important that surgeons (especially those without a laboratory research focus) appreciate the growing importance of tumor banking.

As discussed in detail in Chapter 23, there is a large body of literature on the relationship between volume and outcome, suggesting that patients who require major extirpative surgery for pancreatic adenocarcinoma be operated on by a surgeon at a center with a demonstrated interest and expertise in this disease. Advances in CT imaging and endobiliary stenting will allow patients to be radiographically staged and palliated with respect to biliary obstruction, thereby making possible their referral to a higher volume surgeon and institution. Such a policy will require that the higher volume institution be able to manage the increased demand. This is not as simple as it may appear. For example, it is likely that institutions wishing to refer patients thought to have potentially resectable disease will also wish to refer patients with more advanced disease. As their practice of "diagnose and refer" becomes more frequent, their overall experience in the care of patients with pancreatic cancer will decrease, possibly resulting in a limited ability to stage the disease accurately and to assess a patient's suitability (performance status, medical comorbidities, etc.) for surgery. The referral center will, therefore, receive not just the occasional patient who is an appropriate candidate for surgery, but more importantly, the large number of patients (the majority of those referred) who have locally advanced and metastatic disease in need of treatment planning. This latter group may contain some patients who are candidates for protocol-based therapy but will likely contain a majority who require very time-consuming treatment due to issues of pain management, anorexia, gastrointestinal or biliary obstruction, and often lengthy end-of-life discussions. Clearly, the referral of potentially resectable patients to a high-volume center is a complex policy that may have a much greater impact on the nonsurgeons (medical oncologists, radiation oncologists, support services) and infrastructure at the high-volume centers.

Finally, although the surgical chapters in this text focused on specific techniques, therapies, or programs, it is important to remember the surgeon's role in the global care of the cancer patient. As medicine becomes more subspecialized, reimbursement patterns continue to encourage procedure-oriented specialties, and as treatment options become more complex, we will see more patients in desperate need of a thoughtful review of their global oncologic problem not just a laundry list of possible treatments for the tumor that is apparent on their CT scan. Unfortunately, it is becoming less clear who should have this critically important responsibility. For example, I was recently called to see a patient late one evening (as the surgeon who was on call) who had a perforated cecal cancer with an abscess extending into his abdominal wall in the right lower quadrant. He had been initially referred to our institution for a colonoscopy, as his local hospital did not want to give him any sedation because of the magnitude of his chronic lung disease for which he required home oxygen. After a consultation with gastroenterology, he was seen by anesthesia and internal medicine. A CT scan was obtained that demonstrated the huge cecal cancer perforated into the abdominal wall and probable lung and bone metastases—findings also present on prereferral imaging. After notification of the CT scan results, the medical consultants instructed the patient to report to the emergency room and be seen by the emergency room physician who would then request a surgical consultation. I was therefore the sixth doctor to deal with this man's metastatic colon cancer (the referring physician followed by four doctors at our institution) yet was the first to inquire as to his performance status, family, home-living situation, and attitude toward end-of-life issues and aggressiveness of therapy; components that are critical to the decision-making process of whether or not to consider aggressive therapy versus hospice care at home. This discussion, even at midnight, took a minimum of 90 minutes with the patient and his family, undoubtedly part of the reason why previous physicians had not done it. As our technology brings greater complexity to the care of cancer patients, physicians will become less willing to inform a patient that there is no effective treatment for their disease. This may result in unnecessary testing, ill-advised surgery, and the occasional patient, such as the one described, who does not appreciate the magnitude of his problem. This man refused further therapy other than pain medication, completed his end-of-life documents to his wishes with his family, and died at home with the aid of the hospice program.

Surgeons will likely have a greater role in the multimodality care of the solid tumor patient despite the greater effectiveness of emerging systemic therapies. The complexity of integrating surgery into treatment programs involving cytotoxic chemotherapy, irradiation, and molecular-based targeted therapies (with intermediate and potentially long-term effects on healing, coagulation, etc.) will create a new set of challenges to replace the ones that we have already conquered.

References

1. Neoptolemos JP, Stocken DD, Friess H, et al. A randomized trial of chemoradiotherapy and chemotherapy after resection of pancreatic cancer. *N Engl J Med.* 2004;350:1200–1210.
2. Evans DB, Rich TA, Byrd DR, et al. Preoperative chemoradiation and pancreaticoduodenectomy for adenocarcinoma of the pancreas. *Arch Surg.* 1992;127:1335–1339.
3. Hoffman JP, Lipsitz S, Pisansky T, et al. Phase II trial of preoperative radiation therapy and chemotherapy for patients with localized, resectable adenocarcinoma of the pancreas: an Eastern Cooperative Oncology Group Study. *J Clin Oncol.* 1998;16:317–323.
4. Picozzi VJ, Kozarek R, Rieke JW, et al. Adjuvant combined modality therapy for resected, high-risk adenocarcinoma of the pancreas using cisplatin, 5-FU, and alpha-interferon as radiosensitizing agents: completion of a Phase II trial [abstract]. *Proc Am Soc Clin Oncol.* 2003;22:265a.
5. Pisters PWT, Abbruzzese JL, Janjan NA, et al. Rapid-fractionation preoperative chemoradiation, pancreaticoduodenectomy, and intraoperative radiation therapy for resectable pancreatic adenocarcinoma. *J Clin Oncol.* 1998;16:3843–3850.
6. Pisters PWT, Wolff RA, Janjan NA, et al. Preoperative paclitaxel and concurrent rapid-fractionation radiation for resectable pancreatic adenocarcinoma: toxicities, histologic response rates, and event-free outcome. *J Clin Oncol.* 2002;20:2537–2544.
7. Sohn TA, Yeo CJ, Cameron JL, et al. Resected adenocarcinoma of the pancreas—616 patients: results, outcomes, and prognostic indicators. *J Gastrointest Surg.* 2000;4:567–579.
8. Wolff RA, Evans DB, Crane CH, et al. Initial results of a preoperative gemcitabine (GEM)-based chemoradiation for resectable pancreatic adenocarcinoma [abstract]. *Proc Am Soc Clin Oncol.* 2002;21:130a.

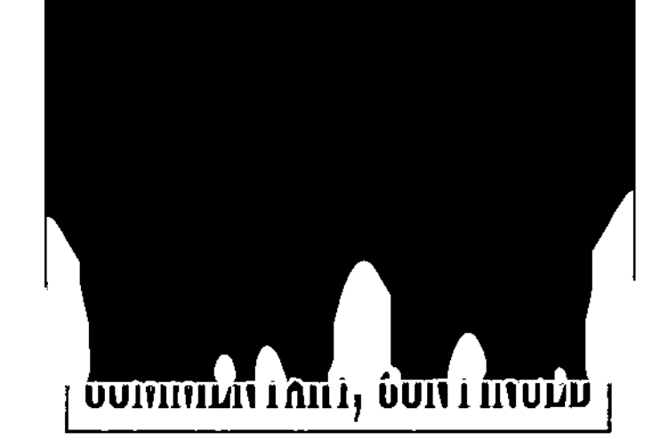

9. Abbruzzese JL, Rosenberg A, et al. Phase II study of anti-epidermal growth factor receptor (EGFR) antibody cetuximab (IMC-C225) in combination with gemcitabine in patients with advanced pancreatic cancer [abstract]. *Proc Am Soc Clin Oncol.* 2001; 20:130a.
10. Crane CH, Ellis LM, Xiong H, et al. *Preliminary Results of a Phase I Study of Rhumab VEGF (Bevacizumab) with Concurrent Radiotherapy (XRT) and Capecitabine* [abstract]. San Francisco: Proceedings of the Gastrointestinal Cancers Symposium (ASCO, AGA, ASTRO, SSO); January, 2004:84a.
11. Kindler HL, Friberg G, Stadler WM, et al. *Bevacizumab Plus Gemcitabine Is an Active Combination in Patients with Advanced Pancreatic Cancer: Interim Results of an Ongoing Phase II Trial from the University of Chicago Phase II Consortium* [abstract]. San Francisco: Proceedings of the Gastrointestinal Cancers Symposium (ASCO, AGA, ASTRO, SSO); January, 2004:84a.

CHAPTER

25

The Principles of Chemoradiation in Localized Pancreatic Cancer

Christopher H. Crane, MD

When the use of radiotherapy for pancreatic cancer is considered, it is important to appreciate several disease characteristics that differ greatly from those of most other malignancies. Even when local disease is controlled surgically, there is a strong force of disease-specific mortality due to distant metastases. Pancreatic cancers are typically resistant to the effects of chemotherapy and radiotherapy, the median survival is usually less than 1 year, and radiographic progression of local disease commonly occurs after chemoradiation treatment in patients who do not undergo curative resection. Most patients who present with pancreatic cancer have some combination of host-related factors, such as advanced age, poor performance status, and medical comorbidity, or tumor-related factors, such as anorexia and exocrine insufficiency, that make them relatively poor candidates for aggressive therapy. The challenge to clinical investigators as well as to clinicians who care for these patients is to develop and use therapies that address the pattern of disease recurrence without causing a significant negative impact on quality of life. The use of novel chemotherapeutic agents and molecular targeted therapies that selectively enhance the effects of radiotherapy and chemotherapy seems to be the most promising avenue of clinical research for this disease. Fortunately, investigators have placed more emphasis on pancreatic cancer in recent years than in the past, and clinical trials of novel treatments are ongoing. It is hoped that these efforts will lead to gradual improvements in outcome for patients with pancreatic cancer. In this chapter, the principles surrounding the dose and technique of radiotherapy as well as the use of radiosensitizers for pancreatic cancer are discussed.

Anatomy and Pattern of Disease Spread

The pancreas is drained by an abundant supply of lymphatics. Primary drainage occurs to the pancreaticoduodenal, suprapancreatic, pyloric, and pancreaticosplenic nodal regions, which all drain into the celiac and superior mesenteric lymph nodes and, especially in advanced disease, into the porta hepatis nodal region. These nodal areas are common regions of disease spread in patients with pancreatic cancer. The main pancreatic duct and the common bile duct are in proximity as they traverse the head of the pancreas on their way to the ampulla of Vater. Compressing or invading these ducts can produce symptoms of jaundice and pancreatic exocrine insufficiency.

Divisions of the vagus and splanchnic nerves form the celiac and superior mesenteric plexuses. Nerve fibers reach the pancreas and other abdominal organs by traveling along the celiac artery and the superior mesenteric artery and their branches. As a result of direct extension of tumor posteriorly to the first and second celiac ganglia, the patient experiences characteristic sharp pain, which is generally perceived as back pain.

Regardless of treatment, the pattern of failure includes both local and distant recurrence in both locally advanced and resected cases.[1-3] The most common sites of distant recurrence are the liver and peritoneum.[3] The lungs and bone are less commonly involved.

Diagnosis, Staging, and Initial Management of Pancreatic Cancer

The issues surrounding diagnosis, staging, and initial management of pancreatic cancer are addressed elsewhere in this book and so are only summarized here. The initial goals in the evaluation and treatment of symptomatic patients are to determine resectability, establish a histologic diagnosis, and reestablish biliary tract outflow. Pancreatic cancer is diagnosed, clinically evaluated, and managed differently from center to center in the United States, and the definition of resectability after clinical evaluation varies from surgeon to surgeon.

The various diagnostic approaches include preoperative imaging, laparoscopy, and laparotomy and attempted resection. Abdominal computed tomography (CT) is the most common diagnostic imaging technique used to reliably confirm and determine the stage of suspected pancreatic malignancies. In many centers, endoscopic ultrasonographically guided fine-needle biopsy of the pancreas is the procedure of choice for the diagnosis of pancreatic malignancies. Biliary outflow can be easily reestablished with the endoscopic placement of an endobiliary stent.

Determining resectability is the most important aspect of clinical staging. Changes in the most recent American Joint Committee on Cancer staging system for exocrine pancreatic cancer reflect a clinical definition of resectability based on computed tomographic assessment. The T-stage designation classifies T1 through T3 tumors as potentially resectable and T4 tumors as locally advanced (unresectable). Tumors with any involvement of the superior mesenteric artery or celiac artery are classified as T4; however, tumors that involve the superior mesenteric, splenic, or portal veins are classified as T3 because these veins can be resected and reconstructed, provided that they are patent.[4] Therefore, three criteria are necessary for resectability: (1) localized disease, (2) lack of involvement of the celiac axis or superior mesenteric artery, and (3) patency of the superior mesenteric/portal venous confluence.

Chemoradiation as a Component of Multidisciplinary Management

Chemoradiation appears to modestly improve median survival duration in both resectable and locally advanced disease. However, the impact of surgical resection, adjuvant locoregional therapy, and definitive nonsurgical local therapy is limited by the competing risk of distant metastatic disease in patients with pancreatic cancer. Chemoradiation is an important component of therapy for locally advanced disease, but even if chemoradiation were as effective as surgery for resectable disease, the development of distant metastatic disease would still undermine its impact on survival. In fact, studies that have attempted to increase the radiotherapeutic dose through novel means have improved local tumor control, have not made a lasting impact on the standard of care.[5,6] Therefore, the rationale for radiotherapy dose-intensification studies is less appealing than the investigation of strategies that include standard doses of radiotherapy with novel radiosensitizers that also address systemic disease spread. However, the importance of local disease control from chemoradiation in both resectable and locally advanced disease will be considerably greater if systemic therapies improve substantially because local disease would then become a greater component of the overall problem that it is currently.

Normal Tissue Constraints of Radiation Dose

Acute Effects of Radiotherapy

The acute effects of radiotherapy to the upper abdomen are most commonly caused by depletion of the rapidly dividing cells that make up the mucosal lining of the stomach or gastric remnant (in surgically treated patients). The common clinical manifestations of acute mucosal radiation injury in the upper abdomen are nausea, vomiting, anorexia, and, in severe cases, upper abdominal pain. Significant toxicity commonly results in dehydration and anorexia, which compounds the nutritional deficiency that patients with pancreatic cancer typically face. Severe acute radiation mucosal toxicity can lead to ulceration of the stomach or duodenum. Known as a *consequential reaction*, this type of radiation injury usually occurs within a few months of therapy. Nausea can also result from hepatic irradiation, but the volume of irradiated liver is rarely significant when appropriate treatment volumes are planned. Antiemetics can be used as needed initially, but if persistent nausea is observed, these agents should be used prophylactically. The use of proton pump inhibitors or H_2-blockers during radiotherapy may reduce the risk of significant mucosal injury. Diarrhea seldom results from pancreatic radiotherapy because typically only a relatively small volume of ileum and jejunum is within the radiation field. When diarrhea does occur, pancreatic exocrine insufficiency resulting from pancreatic duct obstruction is usually the cause.

Late Effects of Radiotherapy

The late effects of radiotherapy are permanent effects on tissues that limit the dose of radiation that can be safely given. The dose-limiting organs surrounding the pancreas include the stomach, duodenum, small bowel, kidneys, spinal cord, and liver. Each of these organs has known tolerances to late radiation injury. Because of the proximity of the pancreas to the gastric and duodenum, the dose of radiotherapy that can be safely given to pancreatic tumors is limited by these organs. The dose of conventional external-beam radiotherapy that can be safely used in the upper abdomen is generally limited by the gastric and duodenal mucosa's tolerance to late radiation injury. This dose has been clinically established in patients receiving radiotherapy alone[7-10] or in combination with 5-fluorouracil.[11-13] Given at 2 Gy per fraction, 50 Gy is well tolerated, even with large volumes of irradiated mucosa. However, doses between 55 and 60 Gy appear to cause chronic radiation injury if large volumes of the gastric and duodenal mucosa are treated. Conversely, doses up to 68 Gy can be safely delivered as long as only small volumes of mucosa are irradiated.[14] It is unlikely that doses higher than 60 Gy will be routinely delivered in pancreatic cancer patients because of the proximity of pancreatic head lesions to the duodenum and pancreatic body and tail lesions to the stomach. The most common late radiation injury is ulceration of the mucosal surface, and, in rare instances, perforation may occur. Usually, these complications can be managed medically.

With commonly used radiation techniques, the dose of radiation to the spinal cord, kidneys, and liver can easily be kept low enough to avoid late radiation injury. Even if an entire kidney is treated beyond the known tolerance (>26 Gy), overall kidney function is not affected in clinically relevant ways. Mean decreases in creatinine clearance of 10% and 24% have been observed in patients when 50% and 90%–100%, respectively, of a single kidney is irradiated beyond the known tolerance.[15] Clinically relevant kidney function compromise rarely develops as long as at least one kidney is spared from the radiation field.

Radiation-induced liver disease, often referred to as *radiation hepatitis*, is characterized by the development of anicteric ascites approximately 2 weeks to 4 months after hepatic irradiation.[16] The whole liver has been treated safely with doses of up to 20 Gy in patients with pancreatic cancer,[17] but whole-liver doses of more than 35 Gy have resulted in a significant risk of radiation-induced liver disease.[18] The risk can be predicted based on radiation dose and volume.[19,20] It is now clear that limited volumes of hepatic tissue can tolerate high doses of radiation.[14]

Adjuvant Chemoradiation in Potentially Resectable Disease

Chemoradiation is used to reduce the probability of local tumor recurrence in patients who undergo potentially curative resection of pancreatic cancer. Based on limited data,[21,22] chemoradiation is the standard adjuvant treatment in patients with resected pancreatic cancer in the United States. Neoadjuvant chemoradiation has also been investigated, has theoretical biologic advantages over postoperative chemoradiation, allows all patients access to adjuvant therapy, and provides an opportunity for identifying patients with rapidly progressive metastatic disease so that they may be spared nontherapeutic surgery.[23]

Postoperative Adjuvant Chemoradiation

The current standard of care for resected pancreatic cancer is in part based on a single randomized trial of postoperative adjuvant chemoradiation verses surgical resection alone conducted by the Gastrointestinal Tumor Study Group. Forty-three patients who had successfully recovered from pancreaticoduodenectomy were entered in the study over the course of 8 years. In the combined-modality arm, radiotherapy was delivered to the primary disease site and regional lymphatics in a split course of 40 Gy over 6 weeks with concurrent 5-fluorouracil (500 mg/m²/day IV bolus on days 1–3 each 2-week radiotherapy course). Weekly maintenance of 5-fluorouracil was then given for 2 years or until disease recurrence. The results in the combined-modality arm were statistically superior to those in the observation arm (43% vs 18% at 2 years, and 14% vs 5% at 5 years, $P < 0.05$).[24] An additional 30 patients were subsequently registered to the experimental treatment, and the results were duplicated.[22] Similar findings were reported by the European Organization for the Research and Treatment of Cancer.[25] Between 1987 and 1995, 218 patients who had undergone pancreaticoduodenectomy for adenocarcinoma of the pancreas or periampullary region were randomly assigned to receive either chemoradiation (40 Gy in a split course along with 5-fluorouracil given as a continuous infusion at a dose of 25 mg/kg/day during radiotherapy) or no further treatment. The median overall survival duration was 24.5 months for the group who received adjuvant therapy and 19 months for the group who received surgery alone ($P = 0.2$). The median overall survival duration was 17.1 months for patients with pancreatic cancer who received adjuvant therapy and 12.6 months for those who received surgery alone ($P = 0.099$). Twenty percent of 104 evaluable patients assigned to receive chemoradiation did not receive the intended therapy because of patient refusal, medical comorbidities, or rapid tumor progression. The low level of compliance and inadequate statistical power could explain the lack of a clear benefit. Both of these studies incorporated a suboptimal chemotherapy dose and schedule as well as an inadequate radiotherapy dose, equipment (supervoltage), and schedule (split course).

The standard postoperative chemoradiation regimen for pancreatic cancer in the United States is radiotherapy (50.4 Gy in 28 fractions) delivered to the operative bed and regional lymphatics with concurrent protracted venous infusion of 5-fluorouracil. There is typically a field reduction after 45 Gy in 25 fractions. The tumor bed, including the retroperitoneal margin, is then typically treated for an additional 5.4 Gy in three fractions. A multi-institutional assessment of treatment efficacy using modern doses, schedules, equipment, and techniques will be available when the results of the Radiation Therapy Oncology Group (RTOG)–led Gastrointestinal Intergroup Protocol 97-04 are reported. In that study, after undergoing pancreaticoduodenectomy, 538 patients were randomly assigned to receive either gemcitabine or protracted venous infusion of 5-fluorouracil (250 mg/m^2/day) before and after concurrent chemoradiation (50.4 Gy with protracted venous infusion of 5-fluorouracil at 250 mg/m^2/day). The chemoradiation component of the trial was not a randomized variable, but because locoregional control is one of the endpoints that will be evaluated, an assessment of the adequacy of current locoregional treatment will be possible.

The results of the European Study Group of Pancreatic Cancer (ESPAC-1) study raise questions about the benefit of radiotherapy in resected pancreatic cancer patients.[26] An analysis of all patients treated showed no benefit from postoperative chemoradiation but showed a survival benefit from adjuvant 5-fluorouracil and leucovorin chemotherapy without radiotherapy. Interpreting the data from this study is problematic, however, because of the lack of quality control, the use of off-study therapies in addition to the randomized therapy, and the use of an outdated chemoradiation dose and schedule. Nonetheless, this study contains the largest number of patients with resected pancreatic cancer who were randomly assigned to treatment with and treatment without chemoradiation.

Neoadjuvant Chemoradiation

Neoadjuvant chemoradiation has been used as a strategy to improve tumor control rates in patients who have resectable disease at the time of clinical evaluation. The rationale for the use of neoadjuvant therapy, as opposed to postoperative adjuvant therapy, has been discussed in detail elsewhere by investigators from the University of Texas M.D. Anderson Cancer Center.[23] The initial preoperative regimen at our institution was 50.4 Gy over 5.5 weeks (standard fractionation) with concurrent protracted venous infusion of 5-fluorouracil. In addition, intraoperative radiotherapy was used in selected cases. However, because of the significant acute toxicity seen,[27] that radiation dose was abandoned in favor of a short course of "rapid fractionation" radiotherapy (30 Gy in 10 fractions over 2 weeks), with a supplemental 10-Gy dose of intraoperative radiotherapy delivered at the time of surgical resection. The effective dose delivered to the tumor bed with the latter approach is comparable to that delivered with the former approach, as determined by linear quadratic modeling.[28] Initially, protracted venous infusion of 5-fluorouracil, subsequently paclitaxel,[29] and most recently gemcitabine[30] have been investigated in consecutive phase II studies of neoadjuvant chemoradiation. Further details of this neoadjuvant approach are discussed elsewhere in this book.

Radiotherapy Technique and Dose

Postoperative Radiotherapy

The standard dose of radiotherapy in the postoperative setting is typically 50.4 Gy in 28 fractions. Field reductions are often made after 45 Gy. A four-field technique using anterior, posterior, and opposed lateral fields allows critical tissues, such as the liver, kidneys, stomach, spinal cord, and small bowel, to be spared. Fields are weighted so that the dose contribution from the lateral fields is restricted to 20 Gy. This prevents the liver and kidney tissue in the lateral fields that are not also in the anterior and posterior fields from being treated beyond the known tolerance.

At the time of radiotherapy simulation, the patient is positioned supine with a treatment device that stabilizes the arms overhead. Barium is given at the time of simulation. After simulation films are taken, the preoperative tumor volume, duodenum, and kidneys are drawn on all films on the basis of the preoperative images. CT-based treatment planning with dose-volume histograms is helpful to verify the dose to the target and to limit the dose to critical structures.

For lesions located in the pancreatic head, the anterior and posterior fields typically cover the T11-L3 vertebral bodies. The celiac axis should be covered with a 2-cm margin superiorly. Inferiorly, the goal is to cover the tumor and duodenal bed with a 2-cm margin. The left border is located 2 cm to the left of the vertebral body edge, as long as there is adequate coverage of the preoperative tumor volume. The preoperative tumor volume and the preoperative location of the duodenum define the right field border and the anterior extent of the lateral fields as well. The porta hepatis should be identified on CT and included in all fields. This usually means that the upper right border of the anterior and posterior fields is located 4–5 cm to the right of the vertebral body edge, and the anterior aspect of the lateral field is 5–6 cm from the anterior vertebral body edge. Blocking is placed over the inferior pole of the right kidney in the anterior and posterior fields, bisecting the vertebral bodies in the lateral fields. Corner blocks are typically placed in the anterior aspect of the lateral fields as well. Care should be taken not to block the preoperative tumor volume or the porta hepatis.

For lesions of the pancreatic body and tail, similar fields are used, except that the splenic hilum is covered and the porta hepatis and duodenal bed are not covered. The right field border is typically located 2 cm from the right vertebral body edge. Similar fields are recommended for patients with an intact pancreas if the goal is neoadjuvant therapy with planned or likely surgical resection.

Radiotherapy Technique for Patients with Locally Advanced Disease

Because patients with locally advanced tumors probably do not benefit from regional nodal irradiation, radiotherapy fields should be confined to the gross tumor alone. This strategy reduces the gastrointestinal toxicity of chemoradiation. It is important therefore to identify the pancreatic tumor correctly. On contrast-enhanced CT, pancreatic tumors are typically hypodense compared with the surrounding pancreatic parenchyma. When there is doubt about the location of the primary tumor, the computed tomographic images should be reviewed with a diagnostic radiologist. Administration of an oral contrast agent at the time of simulation illuminates the duodenal "c-loop." Endobiliary biliary stents can also be visualized, which facilitates identifying the common bile duct.

The pancreas and duodenum move a median of 1 cm with respiratory excursion.[31] If the gross tumor alone is to be treated, respiratory motion must be either controlled or accounted for in radiotherapy planning. The most common way that this is accomplished is by simply adding an additional margin to the planned radiation fields in the cranial and caudal directions. However, because axial tumor motion is negligible, an additional margin for motion in the axial directions is not necessary. Radiation treatment that is gated to the respiratory cycle (respiratory gating)[32,33] is a necessary component of radiation dose escalation studies that seek to deliver >60 Gy to the primary tumor while sparing the duodenum. Thus, radiation fields designed to spare the duodenum that are tightly confined to the primary tumor without correction for organ motion could lead to underdosing of the tumor target, or "marginal miss." A four-field technique is recommended with equally weighted anterior, posterior, and opposed lateral fields. A 2-cm block margin is used in the radial directions, and a 3-cm margin is used in the cranial and caudal directions. The recommended radiation fields for locally advanced pancreatic cancer are found in Fig. 25.1.

The median survival in patients with locally advanced pancreatic cancer treated with concurrent protracted venous infusion of 5-fluorouracil and radiotherapy to a dose of 30 Gy in 10 fractions over 2 weeks is similar to that achieved with a dose of 50.4 Gy in 28 fractions over 5.5 weeks with the same chemotherapy (Wong et al,[33a] manuscript submitted). Although 50.4 Gy is more commonly prescribed, it probably does not significantly improve outcome and has a slightly higher risk of acute toxicity. However, patients with minimal arterial abutment ("marginally resectable" cases) should be treated with 50.4 Gy to maximize the possibility of surgical resection. Prospective studies that evaluate novel radiosensitizers should administer 50.4 Gy to maximize the opportunity for radiosensitization.

Three-Dimensional Conformal Radiotherapy

Three-dimensional conformal radiotherapy (3D-CRT) treatment planning and delivery have been a significant technical innovation in radiotherapy. The premise of this

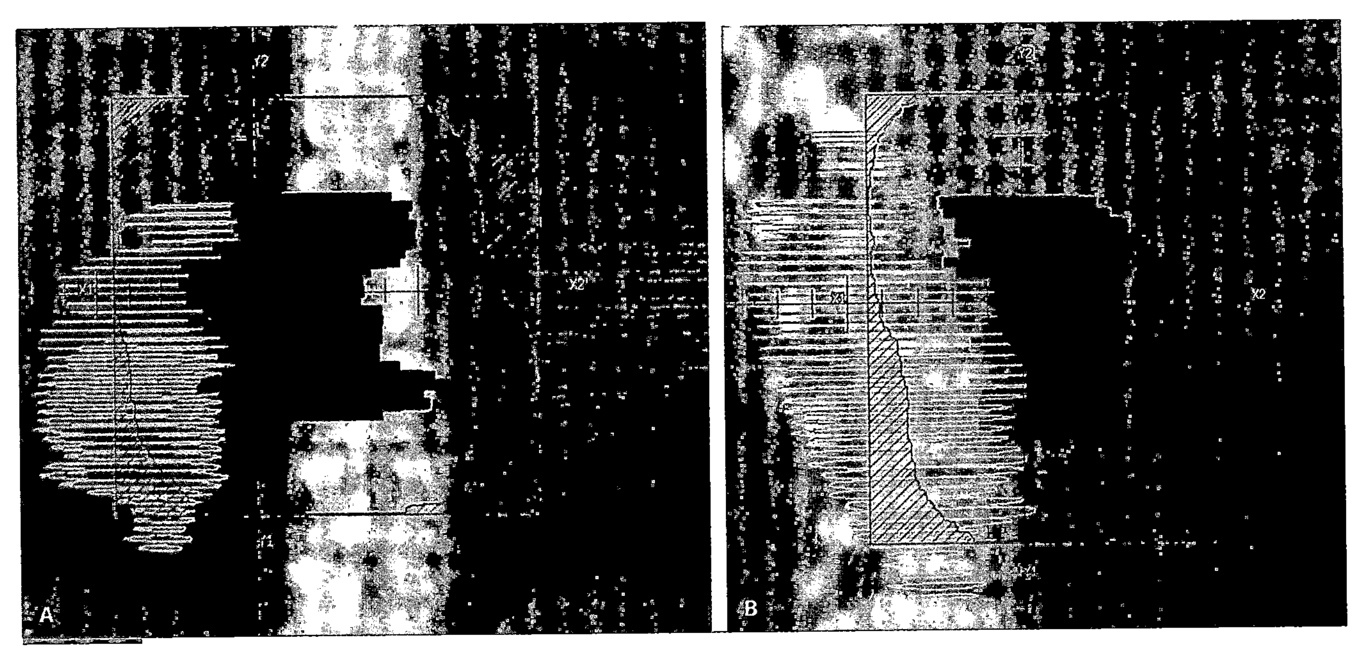

Figure 25.1
Typical radiation fields for locally advanced pancreatic cancer. The gross primary tumor (in red) and radiographically enlarged lymph nodes (none in this case) are treated. Uninvolved regional nodes are not specifically targeted. A four-field technique is recommended with equally weighted anterior **(A)**, posterior, and opposed lateral fields **(B)**. A 2-cm block margin is used in the radial directions and a 3-cm margin is used in the cranial and caudal directions. With this technique, the radiation dose to both the left kidney (in green) and the right kidney (in blue) can easily be kept within tolerance.

technology is to more accurately target the treatment volume while sparing the normal tissues as much as possible. In two randomized trials of patients treated with high-dose radiotherapy for prostate cancer,[34,35] this approach has been shown to reduce toxicity. Intensity-modulated radiotherapy (IMRT) is an advanced form of 3D-CRT made possible by improved computer technology as well as treatment delivery machine advances over the past 10–15 years. Investigators at Memorial Sloan-Kettering Cancer Center have reported reduced toxicity in prostate cancer patients with the use of this technology.[36] This improved therapeutic index has allowed safe escalation of radiation dose with a suggestion of improved biochemical disease-free survival.[37]

As discussed in the previous section, the most important aspect of radiotherapy technique in the treatment of locally advanced pancreatic cancer is that the treatment volumes be confined to the gross tumor and clinically enlarged lymph nodes. This can be accomplished with a standard four-field plan. In general, 3D-CRT options, such as specialized beam angles, weighting, and even beam-intensity modulation, do not meaningfully improve the clinical outcome or tolerability when moderate doses of radiation are used (30–50.4 Gy). Although data published in the medical physics literature have demonstrated that the dose distribution can be improved with advanced techniques,[38] there are no published clinical data demonstrating the clinical impact of improved dose distribution in pancreatic cancer. Clinically investigating and applying techniques such as IMRT with radiotherapy dose escalation to improve local disease control is not a priority at this time because of the challenges presented by organ motion and the limitation of treatment posed by distant disease recurrence.

It has been hypothesized that 3D-CRT or IMRT may improve tolerability of concurrent chemoradiation regimens. A phase I trial was designed and conducted at M.D. Anderson Cancer Center evaluating the ability of IMRT to reduce gastrointestinal toxicity in patients treated with a frequently toxic regimen of concurrent gemcitabine and radiotherapy. The attempt to reduce toxicity with IMRT was unsuccessful, possibly because of the trade-offs that are inherent in the technique and the problem of organ motion. Although the dose distribution at the target was better than that of standard conformal radiotherapy planning, more surrounding normal tissue was treated to a lower dose, possibly contributing to the hematologic and gastrointestinal toxicity that occurred.[39] Proof that advanced radiotherapy treatment planning and delivery can either improve outcome or reduce toxicity is lacking, and there is currently not a strong rationale for its continued investigation in patients with locally advanced pancreatic cancer. Priority should be given to investigating novel well-tolerated, tumor-specific radiosensitizers along with developing more effective systemic therapy.

Principles of Chemoradiation in Locally Advanced Disease

Although it has significant limitations, chemoradiation for locally advanced disease is considered a standard treatment. 5-Fluorouracil–based chemoradiation has led to better median survival than that afforded with either chemotherapy or radiotherapy alone[40,41] in randomized trials. Because the median survival in patients with locally advanced disease is generally less than 1 year and the benefit of treatment is limited, therapy should be well tolerated. Severe toxicity can usually be avoided, regardless of the radiosensitizing chemotherapy that is used if the radiation fields are confined to the gross primary tumor and clinically enlarged lymph nodes. Treating uninvolved regional lymph nodes with larger radiation fields is not likely to improve outcome; in fact, it may increase the risk of gastrointestinal toxicity.

All patients with locally advanced pancreatic cancer should be considered for protocol-based therapy. If they refuse or are ineligible, they are probably best served by a treatment strategy that takes advantage of the best available therapies. Patients should receive a well-tolerated chemoradiation regimen, either preceded or followed by systemic gemcitabine-based chemotherapy. A strategy that starts with 2–4 months of gemcitabine-based systemic therapy, followed by consolidation with chemoradiation, probably takes advantage of the best-available established therapies for this disease.

Radiotherapy Dose-Response Relationship in Locally Advanced Disease

Effective local tumor control in patients with locally advanced pancreatic cancer is important for symptom palliation and as a prerequisite to the development of curative therapy. Single-institutional studies have addressed the role of radiation dose escalation using novel techniques in improving local tumor control in patients with unresectable disease. Intraoperative electron-beam boost and brachytherapy implantation before or after external-beam radiotherapy have been explored in an attempt to intensify the radiation dose. Investigators have reported improvements in local tumor control and median survival with both intraoperative electron-beam boost[5,42-46] and brachytherapy implantation.[6,47] Both techniques have resulted in high local tumor control rates (35%–71%)[5,6,45] as well as a small percentage (7%)[5,6,45] of long-term survivors but significant perioperative and late treatment-related morbidity and mortality rates. Hepatic and peritoneal metastases have prevented a more meaningful improvement in median survival. If one assumes that improved local tumor control, rather than patient selection, led to an improvement in median survival, these studies illustrate the limitations of radiation dose-intensification strategies in locally advanced disease. In an effort to address systemic disease and enhance the effect of radiotherapy on local disease simultaneously, more recent studies have focused on the use of chemotherapeutic agents that have radiosensitizing properties in combination with standard doses of radiotherapy (50.4 Gy in 28 fractions).

Radiosensitization in Pancreatic Cancer and the Concept of Therapeutic Gain

Drugs that enhance the effects of radiotherapy are known as *radiosensitizers*. The ideal radiosensitizer would selectively enhance the effect of radiotherapy on the tumor such that the clinical outcome is increased local treatment effect with the same or less acute toxicity, resulting in therapeutic gain. If a radiosensitizer sensitizes both the tumor and normal tissue equally, then it may not result in therapeutic gain. The dose range of a particular treatment that produces a therapeutic effect without introducing unacceptable toxicity is known as the *therapeutic index*. Treatments that have significant acute toxicity may be acceptable if they are potentially curative, such as chemoradiation for anal cancer[48] and esophageal cancer.[49] However, if the efficacy of treatment is limited and the regimen is frequently toxic, then the addition of a radiosensitizer generally has not improved the therapeutic index. If increasing the dose of a radiosensitizer will predictably lead to severe toxicity, then that drug has a narrow therapeutic index.

Most conventional cytotoxic radiosensitizers, such as 5-fluorouracil and cisplatin, interact with DNA and RNA in various ways that increase cytotoxicity when compared with radiotherapy alone.[50] Newer cytotoxic radiosensitizers, such as gemcitabine, the taxanes, irinotecan, oxaliplatin, and capecitabine, are being investigated clinically for their radiosensitizing effect. In addition, novel molecularly targeted therapies are now being developed, such as inhibitors of the epidermal growth factor,[51] the cyclooxygenase-2 enzyme,[52] and angiogenic signaling,[53] that appear to more selectively enhance the effects of radiotherapy. They also appear to enhance the effects of chemotherapy. In locally advanced pancreatic cancer, curative nonsurgical therapies are clearly a long way from being developed. Therefore, it makes the most sense to build on the current chemoradiation strategies that are relatively well tolerated.

Paclitaxel-Based Chemoradiation

Paclitaxel is a chemotherapeutic agent that has radiosensitizing properties as well as systemic activity in pancreatic cancer. It has been combined with radiotherapy in a phase I study that included patients with locally advanced pancreatic cancer.[54] The dose-limiting toxicities were related to gastrointestinal effects in the radiation field: nausea, anorexia, and abdominal pain. At the dose recommended for further study, therapy was reported to be well tolerated. Subsequently, a phase II study was conducted by the RTOG. At a cost of significant but acceptable acute toxicity, patients achieved a median survival of 11.3 months, which compares favorably with that of historical control subjects.[55] In an effort to build on this regimen, gemcitabine was combined with paclitaxel in RTOG PA-0020, which has recently reached full accrual.[55] In a phase II study at M.D. Anderson Cancer Center of neoadjuvant chemoradiation in patients with potentially resectable tumors, the use of paclitaxel resulted in increased acute toxicity, but the histologic responses were similar to those in historical controls.[29] Because of this, paclitaxel was abandoned in favor of investigation of concurrent gemcitabine-based chemoradiation. Concurrent paclitaxel and radiotherapy can cause significant acute treatment-related morbidity. These studies all used radiation fields that targeted the regional lymph nodes. Treatment would likely be better tolerated if the gross tumor alone were treated.

Gemcitabine-Based Chemoradiation

The introduction of gemcitabine was a modest step forward in the treatment of pancreatic cancer. It prolongs median survival and leads to clinical benefit in patients with advanced disease.[56] The recognition of its radiosensitizing properties[57-61] stimulated the clinical investigation of concurrent gemcitabine and radiotherapy in patients with locally advanced pancreatic cancer. Initially, many different approaches were used to combine gemcitabine with radiotherapy in pancreatic cancer.[62] In a novel study, investigators at the University of Michigan combined full-dose gemcitabine with limited-field radiotherapy. They reported acceptable toxicity,[63] but other studies have reported more significant toxicity. Furthermore, concurrent gemcitabine as compared with 5-fluorouracil has not appeared to dramatically improve median survival in any study.[64] What is clear from studies of gemcitabine and radiotherapy studies is that the extent of mucosal irradiation correlates with gastrointestinal toxicity.[65] For this reason, radiation fields for all patients with locally advanced disease who are treated with concurrent gemcitabine should be confined to the gross tumor and any enlarged lymph nodes, sparing as much mucosa as possible.

In addition to the single-institutional studies, three multi-institutional studies have evaluated concurrent gemcitabine and radiotherapy in locally advanced pancreatic cancer. Of these, the only published randomized trial compared gemcitabine with an unconventional biweekly intravenous bolus of 5-fluorouracil, each given concurrently with radiotherapy to patients with locally advanced pancreatic cancer.[66] The results demonstrated that the toxicity was unacceptably high in both groups. Among all patients, a median of 25% of the patients' time alive was spent in the hospital, and only 75% of patients were able to complete the 50.4-Gy planned radiotherapy dose. Protracted venous infusion of 5-fluorouracil[64,67] or capecitabine[68] probably would have been much better tolerated by the control group and would likely have emphasized the significant toxicity of the gemcitabine arm. In addition, the median survival difference (14.5 months vs 6.7 months, $P = 0.027$) that was reported has to be interpreted with caution because of the poor results in the control group. Similarly, a phase II study conducted in patients with locally advanced pancreatic cancer by the Cancer and Leukemia Group B evaluated gemcitabine given at 40 mg/m^2 twice weekly. In that study, there were 35% and 50% grade 3 or 4 gastrointestinal and hematologic toxicities, respectively, and the median survival was only 8.5 months.[69] Not surprisingly, the Cancer and Leukemia Group B has abandoned this approach in locally advanced pancreatic cancer. Both of these studies used regional nodal fields that likely contributed to the significant gastrointestinal toxicity. In contrast, the approach that was developed at the University of Michigan delivers the manufacturer's recommended dose of gemcitabine (1 g/m^2) and a slightly lower radiotherapy dose (36 Gy in 15 fractions over 3 weeks), with conformal radiation fields encompassing the gross tumor volume alone. At that institution, the irradiation of a smaller volume of normal tissue was reported to be well tolerated.[63] Investigators have since embarked on a multi-institutional phase II study evaluating the same regimen. Preliminary results indicate that approximately 25% of patients experience grade 3 or 4 gastrointestinal toxicity (McGinn, Oral Presentation, European Cancer Conference, 2003[55a]).

Several points about gemcitabine-based chemoradiation are worth emphasizing. All chemoradiation regimens that have been studied in patients with locally advanced disease, including regimens that contain gemcitabine, have significant efficacy limitations. Similar to its value as a systemic agent,[56] gemcitabine is probably only modestly better than 5-fluorouracil when it is used with radiotherapy,[64,66] but it is not tolerated as well. The gastrointestinal toxicity reported in the three multi-institutional studies using gemcitabine calls into question whether the combination of gemcitabine and radiotherapy will be tolerated well enough for future studies that try to build on these experiences. Finally, compared with radiotherapy fields that target the gross tumor only,[63] elective regional nodal irradiation results in increased gastrointestinal toxicity.[62] Because currently available chemoradiation regimens cannot control the primary tumor, it is unlikely that irradiation of microscopic regional nodal metastases contributes anything positive to the outcome of patients with locally advanced pancreatic cancer, regardless of the concurrent chemotherapeutic agent used. Certainly, if gemcitabine is used in combination with irradiation of esophageal, gastric, or duodenal mucosa, the volume of mucosa being treated should be minimized or there will be a significant risk of severe acute toxicity.

The development of gemcitabine as a radiosensitizer is a good example of the potential pitfalls that can result from using a radiosensitizer with a narrow therapeutic index. In phase I studies that have used large radiation fields and concurrent gemcitabine, low doses of gemcitabine have been used to avoid severe toxicity.[64,70] Similarly, the combination of higher doses of gemcitabine (1 g/m^2) with radiotherapy (36 Gy) to the gross tumor alone appears to be well tolerated, but a slightly higher dose (42 Gy) resulted in four of six patients experiencing grade 4 acute or late toxicity.[63] Because combinations of gemcitabine with radiotherapy in locally advanced pancreatic cancer have the same efficacy limitations as any other treatment for pancreatic cancer,[63,64,66,69] more work needs to be performed in this area. In order to improve outcome in a meaningful way (i.e., prolong median survival), investigators will be challenged with the task of building on this strategy by adding novel chemotherapeutic or biologic agents without introducing additional toxicity. This may be a difficult task, given the narrow therapeutic index of gemcitabine-based chemoradiation. In contrast, protracted venous infusions of 5-fluorouracil are well tolerated with radiotherapy, have comparable efficacy, and produce a more favorable therapeutic index.[64] Concurrent capecitabine appears to be even better tolerated than 5-fluorouracil.[68]

Capecitabine-Based Chemoradiation as a Platform

Protracted venous infusion of 5-fluorouracil (225–300 mg/m^2/day) is well tolerated with radiotherapy. Acute gastrointestinal toxicity that results in hospitalization or a prolonged need for intravenous rehydration occurs in less than 10% of patients.[64] Capecitabine is an oral fluoropyrimidine that is converted to 5-fluorouracil more efficiently in tumors than in normal tissue because of the presence of increased thymidine phosphorylase activity in tumor cells.[71] Single-agent capecitabine has an increased response rate, equivalent progression-free and overall survival, and a more favorable toxicity profile than bolus 5-fluorouracil and leucovorin in metastatic colorectal cancer.[72] It also has a clinical benefit response similar to that of gemcitabine in patients with locally advanced or metastatic pancreatic cancer.[73] Furthermore, because capecitabine is administered orally, patients are not at risk for deep venous thrombosis and infections that occur with central venous lines. Additionally, the dose-limiting toxicity is hand and foot syndrome, which can serve as a signal to reduce the dose before gastrointestinal or hematologic toxicity occurs. At doses that are known to be systemically active, capecitabine is extremely well tolerated with radiotherapy. In a phase I study conducted in patients with rectal cancer, there were no grade 3 hematologic or gastrointestinal toxicities.[68] In contrast to gemcitabine or paclitaxel and radiotherapy, the favorable acute toxicity profile of capecitabine makes it an attractive platform upon which to build.

Future studies will combine molecular targeted therapies with capecitabine-based chemoradiation. For example, an ongoing phase I study at M.D. Anderson Cancer Center is evaluating capecitabine, bevacizumab (a monoclonal antibody against vascular endothelial growth factor), and radiotherapy in locally advanced pancreatic cancer. No hospitalizations have resulted from treatment-related toxicity, no grade 3 hematologic toxicity occurred, and only an 11% rate of grade 3 gastrointestinal toxicity has been reported.[74] This study is the basis of RTOG 04-11, a randomized, phase II study evaluating capecitabine-based chemoradiation in combination with either bevacizumab. The incorporation of molecularly targeted therapy with well-tolerated chemoradiation is a promising avenue of future investigation.

Down-Staging Patients with Locally Advanced Disease

The term "down-staging" is generally used to describe either the reduction of the clinical stage to a lower pathological stage than expected after neoadjuvant therapy and surgical resection or the conversion of an unresectable tumor to a resectable one with the use of cytotoxic therapy. In reference to pancreatic cancer, down-staging usually refers to the latter. The interpretation of whether true down-staging actually occurs is limited by inconsistent and subjective definitions of resectability and by inadequate preoperative radiologic assessments of resectability. Probably the most variable factor in determining resectability and thus interpreting whether down-staging has occurred is the meaning of vascular involvement. Although most surgeons would agree that tumor encasement of either the celiac artery or the superior mesenteric artery constitutes unresectable disease, opinions vary with regard to more limited arterial involvement. It is probably in this group of patients that, theoretically, active cytotoxic therapy could lead to down-staging. At M.D. Anderson Cancer Center, patients with locally advanced tumors who have undergone margin-negative resections have typically had very limited arterial involvement (<one third the circumference and <1 cm along the length of the artery) and tumors that have responded to chemoradiation.[65] These cases are sometimes referred to as "marginally resectable."

Another factor affecting the determination of resectability and of whether down-staging has occurred is the meaning of tumor involvement of the superior mesenteric/portal venous confluence. Tumor extension to a venous structure without occlusion is not an absolute contraindication to resection. As described elsewhere in this book, these veins can be successfully resected and reconstructed at the time of pancreaticoduodenectomy. However, many surgeons would consider this type of tumor extension, seen either during surgery or on preoperative imaging, as evidence of unresectability. Thus, the attribution of increased resectability to chemoradiation in some studies could simply be due to a difference in surgical opinion and practice. Thus, the existence of broader definitions of locally advanced pancreatic cancer gives the impression that down-staging occurs more commonly than it actually does. Another confounding variable in the interpretation of down-staging is often the lack of reproducible imaging before and after chemoradiation. Imaging that is not designed to address the issue of vascular involvement may not have resolution that is adequate for making an assessment. Thus, computed tomographic scans taken of the same patient at different times may result in different interpretations, even without therapy being administered.

Rigidly defined, true down-staging must include an objective definition of resectability as well as reproducible imaging before and after chemoradiation. Although many studies have reported that down-staging has occurred, very few fulfill these criteria. Even with nonrigid criteria, down-staging after 5-fluorouracil–based chemoradiation is uncommon. Review of the available literature suggests that a small number (8%–16%) of clinically unresectable cases treated with 5-fluorouracil–based chemoradiation have eventually undergone margin-negative resection.[75-81] The use of newer radiosensitizers, such as paclitaxel and gemcitabine, with radiotherapy could result in increased local tumor response and possibly increased resectability in patients with locally advanced disease, but this has not yet been clearly demonstrated. Ideally, all studies using novel chemoradiation regimens should adhere to a strict CT-based definition of locally advanced pancreatic cancer that includes arterial involvement (low-density tumor inseparable from the superior mesenteric artery or celiac axis on contrast-enhanced CT) or occlusion of the superior mesenteric/portal venous confluence when the issue of down-staging is addressed.

Conclusion

Improving the treatment of pancreatic cancer is a challenge. Whenever possible, patients should be enrolled in investigational studies that evaluate novel therapies. Outside of a clinical trial, postoperative chemoradiation is the current standard adjuvant treatment after pancreaticoduodenectomy. The results of RTOG 97-04 will provide information about the use of gemcitabine in the adjuvant setting compared with 5-fluorouracil. It will also provide multi-institutional data regarding the outcomes and patterns of failure with modern radiotherapy doses and techniques. For locally advanced disease, patients probably benefit from using gemcitabine-based chemotherapy as well as chemoradiation. A strategy that starts with gemcitabine-based systemic therapy for 2–4 months, followed by chemoradiation, probably takes advantage of the best-available established therapies. Radiation dose-intensification studies are probably of minimal value until distant disease is better controlled. The incorporation of molecularly targeted therapy with well-tolerated chemoradiation regimens is a promising approach that addresses the limitations of conventional therapy without introducing unacceptable toxicity. Fortunately, investigators have placed more emphasis on pancreatic cancer in recent years than in the past, and many more clinical trials evaluating novel treatments are available to patients. As clinicians caring for patients with pancreatic cancer, it our responsibility to enroll patients in these studies.

Acknowledgment

This work was supported in part by grants PO1 CA-06294, T32CA77050, and P30CA16672 awarded by the National Cancer Institute, United States Department of Health and Human Services.

References

1. Westerdahl J, Andren-Sandberg A, Ihse I. Recurrence of exocrine pancreatic cancer: local or hepatic? *Hepatogastroenterology*. 1993;40:384–387.
2. Willett CG, Lewandrowski K, Warshaw AL, et al. Resection margins in carcinoma of the head of the pancreas: implications for radiation therapy. *Ann Surg*. 1993;217:144–148.
3. Griffin JF, Smalley SR, Jewell W, et al. Patterns of failure after curative resection of pancreatic carcinoma. *Cancer*. 1990;66:56–61.
4. American Joint Committee on Cancer. Exocrine pancreas. In: Greene F, Page D, Irvin D, et al, eds. *AJCC Cancer Staging Manual*. 6th ed. New York: Springer; 2002:157–164
5. Garton GR, Gunderson LL, Nagorney DM, et al. High-dose preoperative external beam and intraoperative irradiation for locally advanced pancreatic cancer. *Int J Radiat Oncol Biol Phys*. 1993;27:1153–1157.
6. Mohiuddin M, Rosato F, Barbot D, et al. Long-term results of combined modality treatment with I-125 implantation for carcinoma of the pancreas. *Int J Radiat Oncol Biol Phys*. 1992;23:305–311.
7. Coia LR, Myerson RJ, Tepper JE. Late effects of radiation therapy on the gastrointestinal tract. *Int J Radiat Oncol Biol Phys*. 1995;31:1213–1236.
8. Goldgraber M, Rubin C, Palmer W, et al. The early gastric response to irradiation, a serial biopsy study. *Gastroenterology*. 1954;27:1–20.
9. Roswitt B, Malsky S, Reid C. Radiation tolerance of the gastrointestinal tract. *Front Radiat Ther Oncol*. 1971;5:160–180.
10. Hamilton F. Gastric ulcer following radiation. *Arch Surg*. 1947;55:394–399.
11. MacComb WS and Fletcher GH. Planned combination of surgery and radiation in treatment of advanced primary head and neck cancer. *Am J Roentgenol*. 1957;77:397–415.
12. Moertel CG, Frytak S, Hahn RG, et al. Therapy of locally unresectable pancreatic carcinoma: a randomized comparison of high dose (6000 rads) radiation alone, moderate dose radiation (4000 rads + 5-fluorouracil), and high dose radiation + 5-fluorouracil: The Gastrointestinal Tumor Study Group. *Cancer*. 1981;48:1705–1710.
13. Spitz FR, Abbruzzese JL, Lee JE, et al. Preoperative and postoperative chemoradiation strategies in patients treated with pancreaticoduodenectomy for adenocarcinoma of the pancreas. *J Clin Oncol*. 1997;15:928–937.
14. Dawson LA, McGinn CJ, Normolle D, et al. Escalated focal liver radiation and concurrent hepatic artery fluorodeoxyuridine for unresectable intrahepatic malignancies. *J Clin Oncol*. 2000;18:2210–2218.
15. Willett CG, Tepper JE, Orlow EL, et al. Renal complications secondary to radiation treatment of upper abdominal malignancies. *Int J Radiat Oncol Biol Phys*. 1986;12:1601–1604.
16. Lawrence TS, Robertson JM, Anscher MS, et al. Hepatic toxicity resulting from cancer treatment. *Int J Radiat Oncol Biol Phys*. 1995;31:1237–1248.
17. Komaki R, Wilson JF, Cox JD, et al. Carcinoma of the pancreas: results of irradiation for unresectable lesions. *Int J Radiat Oncol Biol Phys*. 1980;6:209–212.
18. Ingold J, Reed G, Kaplan H, et al. Radiation hepatitis. *Am J Roentgenol*. 1965;93:200–208.
19. Lawrence TS, Ten Haken RK, Kessler ML, et al. The use of 3-D dose volume analysis to predict radiation hepatitis. *Int J Radiat Oncol Biol Phys*. 1992;23:781–788.
20. McGinn CJ, Ten Haken RK, Ensminger WD, et al. Treatment of intrahepatic cancers with radiation doses based on a normal tissue complication probability model. *J Clin Oncol*. 1998;16:2246–2252.
21. Yeo CJ, Abrams RA, Grochow LB, et al. Pancreaticoduodenectomy for pancreatic adenocarcinoma: postoperative adjuvant chemoradiation improves survival: a prospective, single-institution experience. *Ann Surg*. 1997;225:621–633; discussion 633–636.
22. Anonymous, further evidence of effective adjuvant combined radiation and chemotherapy following curative resection of pancreatic cancer. Gastrointestinal Tumor Study Group. *Cancer*. 1987;59:2006–2010.
23. Wayne JD, Abdalla EK, Wolff RA, et al. Localized adenocarcinoma of the pancreas: the rationale for preoperative chemoradiation. *Oncologist*. 2002;7:34–45.
24. Kalser MH, Ellenberg SS. Pancreatic cancer: adjuvant combined radiation and chemotherapy following curative resection [published erratum appears in *Archives of Surgery*. 1986;121:1045]. *Archives of Surgery*. 1985;120:899–903.
25. Klinkenbijl JH, Jeekel J, Sahmoud T, et al. Adjuvant radiotherapy and 5-fluorouracil after curative resection of cancer of the pancreas and periampullary region: phase III trial of the EORTC gastrointestinal tract cancer cooperative group. *Ann Surg*. 1999;230:776–782; discussion 782–784.
26. Neoptolemos JP, Dunn JA, Stocken DD, et al. Adjuvant chemoradiotherapy and chemotherapy in resectable pancreatic cancer: a randomised controlled trial. *Lancet*. 2001;358:1576–1585.
27. Evans DB, Rich TA, Byrd DR, et al. Preoperative chemoradiation and pancreaticoduodenectomy for adenocarcinoma of the pancreas. *Arch Surg*. 1992;127:1335–1339.
28. Rich TA, Janjan NA, Abbruzzese JL, et al. Preoperative and postoperative chemoradiation strategies in patients treated with pancreaticoduodenectomy for adenocarcinoma of the pancreas [response]. *J Clin Oncol*. 1997;15:3292–3293.

29. Pisters P, Wolff R, Janjan N, et al. Preoperative paclitaxel and concurrent rapid-fractionation radiation for resectable pancreatic adenocarcinoma: toxicities, histologic response rates, and event-free outcome. *J Clin Oncol.* 2002;20: 2537–2544.
30. Wolff RA, Evans DB, Gravel DM, et al. Phase I trial of gemcitabine combined with radiation for the treatment of locally advanced pancreatic adenocarcinoma. *Clin Cancer Res.* 2001;7:2246–2253.
31. Bussels B, Goethals L, Feron M, et al. Respiration-induced movement of the upper abdominal organs: a pitfall for the three-dimensional conformal radiation treatment of pancreatic cancer. *Radiother Oncol.* 2003;68:69–74.
32. Ramsey CR, Scaperoth D, Arwood D, et al. Clinical efficacy of respiratory gated conformal radiation therapy. *Med Dosim.* 1999;24:115–119.
33. Balter JM, Lam KL, McGinn CJ, et al. Improvement of CT-based treatment-planning models of abdominal targets using static exhale imaging. *Int J Radiat Oncol Biol Phys.* 1998;41:939–943.
33a. Wong AA, Delclos ME, Wolff RA, et al. Radiation dose considerations in the palliative treatment of locally advanced adenocarcinoma of the pancreas. *Am J Clin Onc.* In Press 2004.
34. Koper PC, Stroom JC, van Putten WL, et al. Acute morbidity reduction using 3DCRT for prostate carcinoma: a randomized study. *Int J Radiat Oncol Biol Phys.* 1999;43: 727–734.
35. Dearnaley DP, Khoo VS, Norman AR, et al. Comparison of radiation side-effects of conformal and conventional radiotherapy in prostate cancer: a randomized trial. *Lancet.* 1999;353:267–272.
36. Zelefsky MJ, Cowen D, Fuks Z, et al. Long term tolerance of high dose three-dimensional conformal radiotherapy in patients with localized prostate carcinoma. *Cancer.* 1999;85:2460–2468.
37. Zelefsky MJ, Leibel SA, Gaudin PB, et al. Dose escalation with three-dimensional conformal radiation therapy affects the outcome in prostate cancer. *Int J Radiat Oncol Biol Phys.* 1998;41:491–500.
38. Higgins PD, Sohn JW, Fine RM, et al. Three-dimensional conformal pancreas treatment: comparison of four- to six-field techniques. *Int J Radiat Oncol Biol Phys.* 1995;31:605–609.
39. Crane CH, Antolak JA, Rosen, II, et al. Phase I study of concomitant gemcitabine and IMRT for patients with unresectable adenocarcinoma of the pancreatic head. *Int J Gastrointest Cancer.* 2001;30:123–132.
40. Anonymous. Treatment of locally unresectable carcinoma of the pancreas: comparison of combined-modality therapy (chemotherapy plus radiotherapy) to chemotherapy alone. Gastrointestinal Tumor Study Group. *J Natl Cancer Inst.* 1988;80:751–755.
41. Anonymous. A multi-institutional comparative trial of radiation therapy alone and in combination with 5-fluorouracil for locally unresectable pancreatic carcinoma. The Gastrointestinal Tumor Study Group. *Ann Surg.* 1979;189:205–208.
42. Raben A, Mychalczak B, Brennan MF, et al. Feasibility study of the treatment of primary unresectable carcinoma of the pancreas with 103Pd brachytherapy. *Int J Radiat Oncol Biol Phys.* 1996;35:351–356.
43. Roldan GE, Gunderson LL, Nagorney DM, et al. External beam versus intraoperative and external beam irradiation for locally advanced pancreatic cancer. *Cancer.* 1988; 61:1110–1116.
44. Gunderson LL, Martin JK, Kvols LK, et al. Intraoperative and external beam irradiation +/- 5-FU for locally advanced pancreatic cancer. *Int J Radiat Oncol Biol Phys.* 1987;13:319–329.
45. Mohiuddin M, Regine WF, Stevens J, et al. Combined intraoperative radiation and perioperative chemotherapy for unresectable cancers of the pancreas. *J Clin Oncol.* 1995;13:2764–2768.
46. Shipley WU, Tepper JE, Warshaw AL, et al. Intraoperative radiation therapy for patients with pancreatic carcinoma. *World J Surg.* 1984;8:929–934.
47. Shipley WU, Nardi GL, Cohen AM, et al. Iodine-125 implant and external beam irradiation in patients with localized pancreatic carcinoma: a comparative study to surgical resection. *Cancer.* 1980;45:709–714.
48. Flam M, John M, Pajak TF, et al. Role of mitomycin in combination with fluorouracil and radiotherapy, and of salvage chemoradiation in the definitive nonsurgical treatment of epidermoid carcinoma of the anal canal: results of a phase III randomized intergroup study. *J Clin Oncol.* 1996;14:2527–2539.
49. Herskovic A, Martz K, al-Sarraf M, et al. Combined chemotherapy and radiotherapy compared with radiotherapy alone in patients with cancer of the esophagus. *N Engl J Med.* 1992;326:1593–1598.
50. Lawrence TS, Blackstock AW, McGinn C. The mechanism of action of radiosensitization of conventional chemotherapeutic agents. *Semin Radiat Oncol.* 2003;13:13–21.
51. Nasu S, Ang KK, Fan Z, et al. C225 antiepidermal growth factor receptor antibody enhances tumor radiocurability. *Int J Radiat Oncol Biol Phys.* 2001;51:474–477.
52. Milas L, Kishi K, Hunter N, et al. Enhancement of tumor response to g-radiation by an inhibitor of cyclooxygenase-2 enzyme. *J Natl Cancer Inst.* 1999;91:1501–1504.
53. Gorski DH, Beckett MA, Jaskowiak NT, et al. Blockage of the vascular endothelial growth factor stress response increases the antitumor effects of ionizing radiation. *Cancer Res.* 1999;59:3374–3378.
54. Safran H, King TP, Choy H, et al. Paclitaxel and concurrent radiation for locally advanced pancreatic and gastric cancer: a phase I study. *J Clin Oncol.* 1997;15:901–907.
55. Willett CG, Safran H, Abrams RA, et al. Clinical research in pancreatic cancer: the Radiation Therapy Oncology Group trials. *Int J Radiat Oncol Biol Phys.* 2003;56:31–37.
55a. McGinn C, Talamont M, Small W, et al. A phase II trial of full-dose gemcitabine with concurrent radiation therapy in patients with resectable or unresectable non-metastatic pancreatic cancer. *Proc 2004 ASCO GI Symposium,* San Franciso, CA;89:Abst96, 2004.
56. Burris HA, 3rd, Moore MJ, Andersen J, et al. Improvements in survival and clinical benefit with gemcitabine as first-line therapy for patients with advanced pancreas cancer: a randomized trial. *J Clin Oncol.* 1997;15:2403–2413.

57. Mason KA, Milas L, Hunter NR, et al. Maximizing therapeutic gain with gemcitabine and franctionated radiation. *Int J Radiat Oncol Biol Phys.* 1999;44:1125–1135.
58. Milas L, Fujii T, Hunter N, et al. Enhancement of tumor radioresponse in vivo by gemcitabine. *Cancer Res.* 1999;59: 107–114.
59. Joschko M, Webster L, Groves J, et al. Radioenhancement by gemcitabine with accelerated fractionated radiotherapy in a human tumor xenograft model. *Radiat Oncol Invest.* 1997;5:62–71.
60. Lawrence TS, Chang EY, Hertel L, et al. Gemcitabine radiosensitizes human pancreas cancer cells. *Proc AACR.* 1994;35:A3855.
61. Lawrence T, Eisbruch A, Shewach D. Gemcitabine-mediated radiosensitization. *Semin Oncol.* 1997;24:S724–S728.
62. Crane CH, Wolff RA, Abbruzzese JL, et al. Combining gemcitabine with radiation in pancreatic cancer: understanding important variables influencing the therapeutic index. *Semin Oncol.* 2001;28:25–33.
63. McGinn CJ, Zalupski MM, Shureiqi I, et al. Phase I trial of radiation dose escalation with concurrent weekly full-dose gemcitabine in patients with advanced pancreatic cancer. *J Clin Oncol.* 2001;19:4202–4208.
64. Crane CH, Abbruzzese JL, Evans DB, et al. Is the therapeutic index better with gemcitabine-based chemoradiation than with 5-fluorouracil-based chemoradiation in locally advanced pancreatic cancer? *Int J Radiat Oncol Biol Phys.* 2002;52:1293–1302.
65. Crane C, Janjan N, Evans D, et al. Concurrent gemcitabine and rapid-fraction radiotherapy for unresectable pancreatic cancer: toxicity, local control and survival. *Int J Pancreatol.* 2001;29:59–68.
66. Li CP, Chao Y, Chi KH, et al. Concurrent chemoradiotherapy treatment of locally advanced pancreatic cancer: gemcitabine versus 5-fluorouracil, a randomized controlled study. *Int J Radiat Oncol Biol Phys.* 2003;57: 98–104.
67. Mehta VK, Poen JC, Ford JM, et al. Protracted venous infusion 5-fluorouracil with concomitant radiotherapy compared with bolus 5-fluorouracil for unresectable pancreatic cancer. *Am J Clin Oncol.* 2001;24:155–159.
68. Dunst J, Reese T, Sutter T, et al. Phase I trial evaluating the concurrent combination of radiotherapy and capecitabine in rectal cancer. *J Clin Oncol.* 2002;20:3983–3991.
69. Blackstock A, Tempero M, Niedwiecki D, et al. Cancer and Leukemia Group B (CALGB) 89805: phase II chemoradiation trial using gemcitabine in patients with locoregional adenocarcinoma of the pancreas [abstract 49]. *Int J Radiat Oncol Biol Phys.* 2001;51:31.
70. Blackstock AW, Bernard SA, Richards F, et al. Phase I trial of twice-weekly gemcitabine and concurrent radiation in patients with advanced pancreatic cancer. [comment]. *J Clin Oncol.* 1999;17:2208–2212.
71. Schuller J, Cassidy J, Dumont E, et al. Preferential activation of capecitabine in tumor following oral administration to colorectal cancer patients. *Cancer Chemother Pharmacol.* 2000;45:291–297.
72. Hoff PM, Ansari R, Batist G, et al. Comparison of oral capecitabine versus intravenous fluorouracil plus leucovorin as first-line treatment in 605 patients with metastatic colorectal cancer: results of a randomized phase III study. *J Clin Oncol.* 2001;19:2282–2292.
73. Cartwright TH, Cohn A, Varkey JA, et al. Phase II study of oral capecitabine in patients with advanced or metastatic pancreatic cancer. *J Clin Oncol.* 2002;20:160–164.
74. Crane C, Ellis L, Xiong H, et al. Preliminary results of a phase I study of rhuMAb VEGF (bevacizumab) with concurrent radiotherapy and capecitabine in locally advanced pancreatic cancer [abstract 980]. *Eur J Cancer.* 2003;1:S294.
75. Jeekel J, Treurniet-Donker AD. Treatment perspectives in locally advanced unresectable pancreatic cancer. *Br J Surg.* 1991;78:1332–1334.
76. Jessup JM, Steele G Jr, Mayer RJ, et al. Neoadjuvant therapy for unresectable pancreatic adenocarcinoma. *Arch Surg.* 1993;128:559–564.
77. Kallimanis GE, Gupta PK, al-Kawas FH, et al. Endoscopic ultrasound for staging esophageal cancer, with or without dilation, is clinically important and safe. *Gastrointest Endosc.* 1995;41:540–546.
78. White R, Lee C, Anscher M, et al. Preoperative chemoradiation for patients with locally advanced adenocarcinoma of the pancreas. *Ann Surg Oncol.* 1999;6:38–45.
79. Todd KE, Gloor B, Lane JS, et al. Resection of locally advanced pancreatic cancer after downstaging with continuous-infusion 5-fluorouracil, mitomycin-C, leucovorin, and dipyridamole. *J Gastrointest Surg.* 1998;2:159–166.
80. Bajetta E, Di Bartolomeo M, Stani SC, et al. Chemoradiotherapy as preoperative treatment in locally advanced unresectable pancreatic cancer patients: results of a feasibility study. *Int J Radiat Oncol Biol Phys.* 1999;45:285–289.
81. Kornek GV, Schratter-Sehn A, Marczell A, et al. Treatment of unresectable, locally advanced pancreatic adenocarcinoma with combined radiochemotherapy with 5-fluorouracil, leucovorin and cisplatin. *Br J Cancer.* 2000;82:98–103.

CHAPTER 26

Adjuvant and Neoadjuvant Therapies for Resectable Pancreatic Cancer

Robert A. Wolff, MD

Prolonged survival after pancreatic cancer can be achieved only in patients undergoing resection with curative intent, but fewer than 20% of these patients may be expected to live 5 years or longer.[1] Since the mid-1980s, efforts have been directed toward improving outcomes for patients with resected disease by delivering postoperative adjuvant therapy, but controversies persist regarding the role of chemotherapy and radiation in this setting. No major advances have been observed since then, and there is no consensus about the optimal management of resectable pancreatic cancer. More recently, preoperative or neoadjuvant strategies have been investigated as an alternative to adjuvant therapy. Thus far, however, preoperative approaches have not been shown to be superior to postoperative therapy, although single-institution trials have demonstrated some recent encouraging results.

Progress in the treatment of resectable disease has been hampered for a number of reasons. These include poor patient selection caused by insufficient use of modern imaging modalities, significant surgical morbidity precluding the enrollment of large numbers of patients on postoperative trials, and the lack of standardized criteria for evaluation of resection margins. Moreover, currently available cytotoxic therapy has minimal activity in this disease. With these issues in mind, this chapter reviews the rationale for adjuvant and neoadjuvant therapies for pancreatic cancer and the current data regarding their integration into management. Finally, suggestions regarding a logical approach to future investigations of both preoperative and postoperative modalities are discussed.

Rationale for Radiation in Resectable Pancreatic Cancer

Although pancreatic cancer has proven to be more resistant to modern treatments compared with other gastrointestinal (GI) tumors, the observed patterns of failure seen after surgical resection are not significantly different.[2-5] The pancreas, situated in the retroperitoneum, is surrounding by vital vascular structures to include the portal vein, the superior mesenteric vein, the celiac axis, and the superior mesenteric artery. Even when very small tumors are located in the head or neck of the pancreas, they are frequently in close proximity to these vessels, often rendering surgical margins measured in millimeters or microns. Thus, local failure is common after surgical intervention. Tepper et al.[6] performed a retrospective study of 31 patients undergoing curative pancreaticoduodenectomy at the Massachusetts General Hospital from 1963 to 1973. This analysis revealed that 50% of patients experienced local failure as a component of relapse. Failure was often determined using clinical grounds, and given the relatively crude imaging techniques available then, this is likely an underestimate of the true rate of local failure in that era. Supporting data come from an autopsy series in which postmortem examinations were performed on a group of patients who relapsed and died after undergoing surgery for pancreatic cancer.[7] Locoregional failure was noted in 80% of these patients. Other reports from single-institutional experience suggests that local failure occurs in 50%–80% of cases, and in 10%–19% of cases, isolated local failure without distant disease has been observed.[8-10] Factors predisposing to local recurrence have not been fully elucidated, but recent evidence implicates perineural invasion as an important mediating process.[11,12] Rich neural networks surround the pancreas and are intimately associated with the local vascular structures (Fig. 26.1). Invasion of nerve sheaths draping over the vessels may occur as a pervasive, superficial infiltration that cannot be appreciated intraoperatively, even by the most experienced surgeons. The molecular events leading to perineural invasion are beginning to be understood, and specific tumor mucins, such as MUC-1, may play an important role in tumor cell adhesion and invasion into surrounding tissues.[13] In addition, tumor cells may secrete neural growth factors, providing a permissive environment within the nerve sheaths for tumor cell invasion and growth.[14,15] Invasion into neural sheaths may explain not only the tendency toward local failure, but also the pain associated with it.[16]

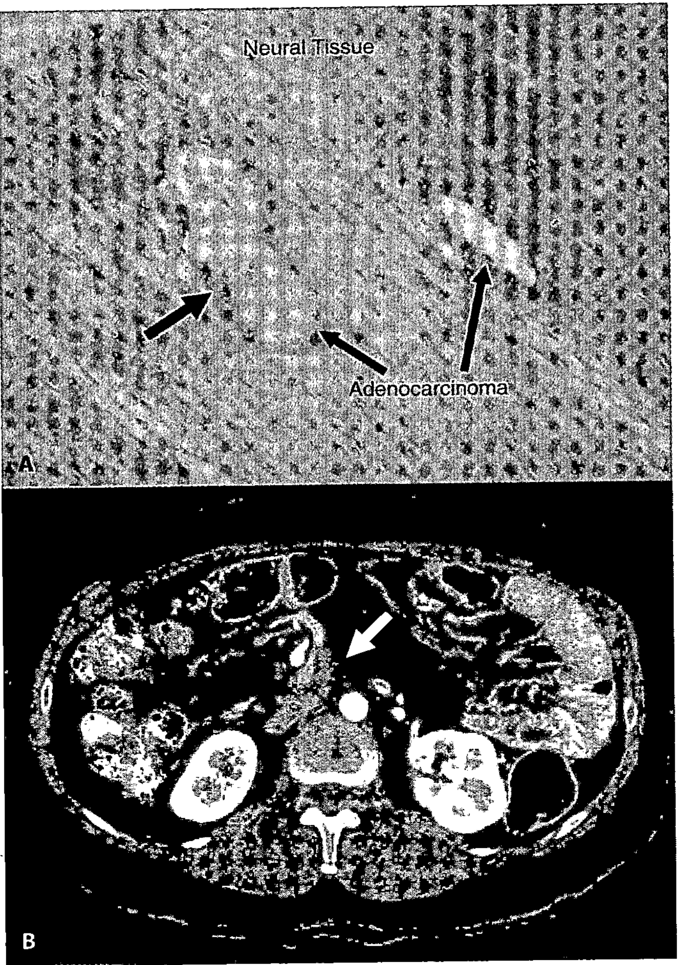

Figure 26.1
(A) Photomicrograph of high-power hematoxylin and eosin stain of pancreatic cancer specimen showing perineural invasion. The arrows demonstrate the nests of adenocarcinoma invading the neural tissue. **(B)** A CT image of a 57-year-old woman who underwent pancreaticoduodenectomy for adenocarcinoma of the pancreas (histology showed perineural invasion). The arrow depicts local tumor recurrence along the superior mesenteric artery.

Although local failure is common in pancreatic cancer, it is not unique to this disease; it is often observed in patients with other GI tumors and is commonly associated with morbidity. Efforts to reduce local failure rates have been well studied, most notably in rectal cancer, and radiotherapy has been proven to decrease the risk of local recurrence in this malignancy. In an often-cited study performed in the 1970s by the Gastrointestinal Tumor Study Group (GITSG), patients with surgically resected stage II or stage III rectal cancer were randomized to one of four arms.[17] Over 200 patients were randomized to undergo observation after surgery, radiation alone, chemotherapy alone, or a combination of chemotherapy and radiation. The results elegantly depict the role of these different modalities. Patients who underwent only surgery had the worst survival, whereas patients who received combined modality therapy enjoyed the best disease-free and overall survival.[18] Patients who received either radiation or chemotherapy had comparable outcomes, which were intermediate in relationship to the surgery-only group and the chemoradiation group. Importantly, those patients who received radiation had a lower incidence of local failure, whereas those who underwent surgery alone or surgery followed by chemotherapy had higher rates of local recurrence. In a subsequent trial performed by the National Surgical Adjuvant Breast and Bowel Project (NSABP), patients with stage II or stage III rectal cancer were randomized to receive chemotherapy alone or chemoradiation after

Table 26.1 Risk for Local Failure after Surgery with or without Adjuvant or Neoadjuvant Therapy

Author	No. of Patients	Adjuvant or Neoadjuvant Treatment	Percent Local Failure
Tepper et al.[6]	31	None	50
Kayahara et al.[7]	15	None	80
Whittington et al.[24]	33	None	85
Whittington et al.[24]	20	Adjuvant 5FU/EBRT	25
Morganti et al.[25]	17	Neoadjuvant EBRT or IORT/Postop EBRT	17.6
Foo et al.[26]	29	Adjuvant 5FU/EBRT	10
Spitz et al.[27]	26	Adjuvant 5FU/EBRT	26
Breslin et al.[28]	132	Neoadjuvant chemoradiation (5-FU, paclitaxel, gem) + EBRT	10

Abbreviations: EBRT, external beam radiotherapy; IORT, intraoperative radiotherapy; Gem, gemcitabine.

surgery.[19] Survival was not affected by treatment. However, as in the GITSG trial, the local failure rate was significantly lower in the cohort undergoing chemoradiation compared with the patients receiving chemotherapy alone (8% vs 13%). Although pancreatic cancer is not directly comparable to rectal cancer, important similarities exist. In the case of rectal cancer, it has been necessary to obtain adequate proximal and distal margins when the rectum is excised, as submucosal invasion may lead to a positive margin with subsequent recurrence at the anastomosis. However, given the anatomic constraints of surgery in the pelvis and the lack of a peritoneal surface, there has been growing appreciation for the radial (circumferential) resection margin in determining the risk of local failure.[20-22] Defining the radial margin and ensuring it is negative has been challenging. An analogous situation occurs in pancreatic cancer, where the bile duct margin, the gastric margin, or the pancreatic duct margin also may be involved with submusocal infiltration. Yet it is the retroperitoneal margin, defined by the tissue immediately adjacent to the right side of the superior mesenteric artery, that is commonly associated with a positive surgical margin and subsequent local failure.[23] Because it is hard to ensure and validate that a negative surgical margin has been achieved in both of these diseases and because radiation has been proven to reduce the risk of local failure in rectal cancer, it is logical to propose a role for radiation in the treatment of resectable pancreatic cancer. Recent publications of a single-institution experience suggest that local failure rates are lower when either postoperative or preoperative radiation is delivered (Table 26.1).[6,7,24-28] However, it is important to appreciate that when strategies to minimize local recurrence are employed, disseminated disease ultimately prevails and limits survival.[29] This paradigm holds true for other GI cancers, including those of the esophagus, stomach, extrahepatic bile duct, and possibly rectum.

Rationale for Chemotherapy in the Treatment of Resectable Pancreatic Cancer

Pancreatic cancer metastasizes early during its natural history, and despite surgical intervention with curative intent, most patients will ultimately die with disseminated disease. The majority of patients who present with potentially resectable tumors must therefore harbor occult metastatic cancer. The molecular mechanisms whereby pancreatic cancer cells spread are beyond the scope of this chapter but are thoroughly discussed elsewhere in this textbook. In recent years, adjuvant chemotherapy for cancers of the rectum, colon, and most recently stomach has proven that systemic therapy directed at microscopic tumor burden enhances the chances of disease-free and long-term survival for patients at high risk of relapse after surgery.[19,30-33] Thus, although pancreatic cancer is more resistant to currently available cytotoxic therapy, administering chemotherapy to patients who have undergone surgery has a sound foundation. Skeptics should be reminded that despite intensive investigation of adjuvant chemotherapy for colon cancer, it took approximately 30 years to establish its role.[34] Furthermore, progress in adjuvant therapy for colon cancer continues, and combination chemotherapy in the form of fluorouracil (5-FU), folinic acid (leucovorin), and oxaliplatin (which is a more active regimen compared with 5-FU and leucovorin in patients with metastatic colon cancer), has recently been shown to also improve 3-year disease-free survival for patients with stage III disease.[35] Although chemotherapy has quite modest benefits in the treatment of advanced pancreatic cancer, it continues to be incorporated into every recent trial of adjuvant and neoadjuvant therapy for resected pancreatic cancer.

Evidence Regarding 5-FU–Based Postoperative (Adjuvant) Therapy

Virtually all published trials of postoperative therapy for resected pancreatic cancer have been built on a foundation of 5-FU. For a review of the randomized trials of adjuvant therapy for pancreatic cancer, see Chapter 28. To summarize, the first randomized trial was performed by the GITSG and demonstrated a significant survival advantage with 5-FU–based chemoradiation compared with resection alone (20 vs 11 months).[36] In a subsequent, larger phase III study, the European Organization for Research and Treatment of Cancer (EORTC) randomized 218 patients with adenocarcinoma of the pancreas or periampullary region to receive either chemoradiation or no further treatment after pancreaticoduodenectomy.[37] In a subset analysis of the patients with pancreatic cancer, the median survival was 17.1 months for patients who received adjuvant therapy compared with only 12.6 months for those who had surgery alone ($p = 0.099$). Importantly, 21 of 104 evaluable patients (20%) assigned to receive chemoradiation did not receive intended therapy because of their refusal, medical contraindications, or rapid tumor progression. The survival of these untreated patients was included in the analysis of survival on the chemoradiation arm, based on intent-to-treat principles, and likely had a negative impact on the reported survival of the treatment group. Whether the results of the EORTC trial should be interpreted as a negative trial of adjuvant therapy, as concluded by the authors, or an underpowered positive study, as suggested by others, is still debated.[38,39] However, consistent with the GITSG result, the EORTC trial clearly demonstrates that survival for patients not receiving adjuvant therapy remains poor (10–12 months). Of further interest, the results from the GITSG trial and the EORTC trial are quite similar to the experience of the Johns Hopkins Medical Institutions (JHMI). In an analysis of 616 patients undergoing surgery for pancreatic cancer at that hospital from 1984 to 1999, data regarding the use of adjuvant therapy were available for 498 patients.[40] Of these, 366 (74%) received postoperative therapy, generally consisting of 5-FU–based chemoradiation, and 132 (26%) did not. Median survival for patients receiving adjuvant therapy was 19 months; those who did not had a median survival of only 11 months ($P = 0.003$). More nonrandomized data come from a population-based analysis performed by Lim et al.[41] from the Harvard School of Public Health. This study evaluated the outcomes of 396 Medicare-eligible patients residing in 1 of 11 Survival, Epidemiology, and End Results registries. The analysis found that adjuvant chemoradiation was associated with better survival compared with no adjuvant therapy (29 vs 12.5 months, $P = 0.0003$). These results are quite consistent when viewed in the context of the experience of the JHMI and the GITSG and EORTC trials. Another common finding from the JHMI, GITSG, and EORTC reports is the substantial proportion of patients who did not undergo adjuvant therapy or had a long delay before embarking on adjuvant therapy. These patients comprise 20%–26% of all resected patients. This likely represents a low estimate because in the database analysis performed by Lim et al.[41] adjuvant therapy was delivered less than half the time.

At odds with the experience of the JHMI and the findings of the EORTC and GITSG trials are the results from the largest and most recent randomized study of postoperative therapy for patients with resected pancreatic cancer. This study was conducted by the European Study Group for Pancreatic Cancer (ESPAC) and is referred to as the ESPAC-1 trial.[42] The study enrolled 541 patients who had undergone curative resection for adenocarcinoma of the pancreas. The study was conducted by 83 participating physicians in 61 hospital centers. Patients were assigned to treatment based on three separate randomizations. The majority of patients (285) were randomized using a 2×2 strategy, which assigned patients to observation, chemotherapy alone, chemoradiation, or chemoradiation followed by chemotherapy. In order to enhance patient accrual, an additional 256 patients were enrolled using alternative randomizations based on physician preference. The options included randomization to chemoradiation or no chemoradiation or to chemotherapy versus no chemotherapy. Surprisingly, physicians who enrolled patients outside the 2×2 design also had the option of delivering "background" chemotherapy or radiation before study entry. These background treatments were not standardized. Protocol therapy prescribed chemoradiation using bolus 5-FU and split-course radiation to a dose of 40 Gy. Chemotherapy consisted of bolus 5-FU (425 mg/m^2) and leucovorin (20 mg/m^2) given daily for 5 days on a 28-day cycle.

Pooled analysis of the ESPAC-1 trial demonstrated no survival advantage for patients receiving chemoradiation compared to those who did not (15.5 vs 16.1 months, $P = 0.24$). However, a statistically significant survival benefit was observed in patients who received chemotherapy compared with those who did not (19.7 vs 14.0 months, $P = 0.0005$). The results of ESPAC-1 were initially reported as a pooled analysis of patients randomized in the 2 × 2 portion of the trial combined with the outcomes of patients enrolled outside this mechanism. Recently, in another publication, a separate analysis of survival was reported only for those patients randomized in the 2 × 2 portion after further follow-up.[43] Again, the patients who received chemoradiation had an inferior survival compared with those patients who did not (15.9 vs 17.9 months, $P = 0.05$). Conversely, patients who received chemotherapy had an improved survival compared with those who did not receive it (20.1 vs 15.5 months, $P = 0.009$). Based on these two reports of the same study, the investigators have concluded there is no role for chemoradiation as part of adjuvant therapy for pancreatic cancer, but systemic chemotherapy in the form of bolus 5-FU offers a survival advantage. Patients who were assigned to observation had a median survival of 16.9 months, whereas patients who received chemoradiation as their only therapy did very poorly, with a median survival of only 13.9 months. Of note, patients who received chemoradiation and subsequent 5-FU with leucovorin did comparatively better, with a median survival of 19.9 months. Their survival was similar to the survival of patients who received chemotherapy alone (21.6 months). These findings suggest that chemoradiation alone is quite toxic and leads to early death compared with observation alone. However, chemoradiation followed by more chemotherapy appears to be protective and provides a survival advantage compared with observation alone. At face value, these results are incongruous.

Although the ESPAC-1 trial has been the largest and most ambitious randomized trial of adjuvant therapy to date, it has been criticized, not only for its fundamental design, but also for a lack of standardization of background therapies for patients enrolled outside the 2 × 2 design and lack of a central review of enrolled patients for quality-control purposes. Although there was an effort to review all pathology specimens, a full 25% of surgical specimens were not submitted for centralized review.[44] In addition, radiation treatment plans were not reviewed at the start of radiotherapy or at the completion of treatment.[45] This may explain in part the high local failure rates seen in the patients enrolled in the 2 × 2 portion of the trial. Of the 289 patients enrolled in that portion of the study, 158 patients had a known tumor recurrence pattern; 96 (61%) had local failure as a component of failure, similar to local recurrence rates seen in patients who do not receive any adjuvant therapy (see Table 26.1 for comparisons). This implies that neither chemotherapy nor radiation had much impact on local control, and by extension, the quality of the radiation delivery may have been substandard.

Table 26.2 Evidence Regarding Post-Operative 5-FU-Based Therapy

Study (Year)	No. of Patients	5-FU-Based Therapy MS (Months)	Observation MS (Months)	P-value
GITSG[36] 1985	49	ChemoXRT 21.0	10.9	0.005
EORTC[37] 1999	114	ChemoXRT 17.1	12.6	0.099
JHMI[40] 2000	366	ChemoXRT 19	11	0.005
ESPAC-1[42] 2001	541	Chemotherapy 19.7	NS	0.0005
ESPAC-1[43] 2004	289	Chemotherapy 21.6	16.9	NS

No matter how the ESPAC-1 results are interpreted, it is disappointing to note that there has been no significant change in the survival of patients undergoing adjuvant therapy after surgery in the form of 5-FU–based systemic therapy or chemoradiation from 1985 to the present time (Table 26.2).

Moving Beyond 5-FU–Based Postoperative Adjuvant Therapy

Despite 20 years of investigation, the role of adjuvant therapy for resected pancreatic cancer has remained controversial and not universally embraced. This may be explained by the reliance on 5-FU as both a systemic agent and radiosensitizer. In either role, bolus 5-FU does not appear to have sufficient activity in the setting of microscopic metastatic disease to have a major impact on patient survival after surgery. Supporting this is the minimal cytotoxicity observed with bolus 5-FU in advanced disease. For example, in the gemcitabine registration trial, which compared weekly bolus 5-FU with weekly gemcitabine, there were no objective responses observed in the 57 patients with measurable disease treated with bolus 5-FU.[46] In another trial reported by Rubin et al.,[47] a combination of bolus 5-FU with leucovorin given daily for 5 days yielded no objective responses among 31 patients.

Although there is no established role for bolus injections of 5-FU in the treatment of advanced pancreatic cancer, investigations of prolonged infusional 5-FU and orally bioavailable fluorinated pyrimidines delivered over extended time periods suggest modest activity. In a randomized trial comparing infusional 5-FU to infusional 5-FU with mitomycin-C, 105 patients were randomized to receive infusional 5-FU alone.[48] The response rate among these patients was 8.6% (confidence interval, 3.2%–13.7%), which is comparable to the response rate of gemcitabine as a single agent.[49,50] Likewise in a randomized study comparing infusional 5-FU and cisplatin to bolus single agent 5-FU, Ducreux et al.[51] demonstrated a higher response rate to the combination (12% vs 0%), with an improved 1-year progression-free survival but no clear improvement in overall survival. This study provides further evidence that bolus 5-FU has virtually no activity in the setting of advanced pancreatic cancer. However, similar to infusional 5-FU, the oral fluoropyrimidine capecitabine appears to have some modest activity in pancreatic cancer. Cartwright et al.[52] treated 42 patients with advanced disease (41 with measurable disease) and found an objective response rate of 7.3%, with 24% of these patients experiencing a clinical benefit with the drug. In summary, modern trials of 5-FU suggest that it is inactive in advanced disease when given as a bolus injection, but it appears to have some efficacy when given as a continuous infusion or in the form of capecitabine. As with rectal cancer, combining infusional 5-FU with modern radiotherapy may lead to better outcomes compared with bolus 5-FU, and it has been shown to be associated with greater dose intensity.[53,54] Infusional 5-FU as a radiosensitizer has been reported by investigators at Stanford University delivering 5-FU (200–250 mg/m²/day) and external beam radiation therapy (EBRT) to a total of 50.4 Gy in 52 patients undergoing pancreaticoduodenectomy for pancreatic adenocarcinoma.[55] Over one third of patients had positive surgical margins, and 59% had lymph node metastases. With a median follow-up of 24 months, the median survival is 32 months, with a 3-year survival rate of 39%. Although follow-up is early, this experience supports the recent trend in adjuvant trials being conducted: to move beyond 5-FU (particularly bolus 5-FU) and to investigate the incorporation of infusional 5-FU (alone or in combination with other drugs) or gemcitabine into adjuvant therapy (Table 26.3).

Because gemcitabine has shown superiority to 5-FU in advanced disease, current randomized trials of adjuvant therapy are testing it in the adjuvant setting. In Europe, where the role of radiotherapy has been predominantly dismissed on the basis of the EORTC and ESPAC-1 results, gemcitabine will be compared with bolus 5-FU and leucovorin. ESPAC-3 is a multicentered European trial that plans to enroll over 900 patients. Patients who recover adequately from surgery will be randomized to receive gemcitabine (1,000 mg/m² over 30 minutes, weekly ×3, every 28 days) for 6 months or bolus 5-FU and leucovorin (as administered in ESPAC-1) for 6 months.[42]

In the United States, where radiation is still considered an important component of adjuvant therapy, the role of gemcitabine is also being investigated. The Radiation Therapy Oncology Group (RTOG) conducted the first American phase III cooperative group study of postoperative adjuvant therapy for resected pancreatic adenocarcinoma (RTOG 9704) since the GITSG trial. In this study, which began in July 1998, patients have been randomly assigned to receive gemcitabine or infusional 5-FU to be given before and after 5-FU–based chemoradiation. The trial has reached its accrual goals, and preliminary survival results are anticipated in 2004. For details of this trial, see Chapter 28.

Other exploratory trials of adjuvant therapy are being conducted by the American College of Surgeons Oncology Group (ACoSOG) and the EORTC. ACoSOG-Z5006 has been designed on the basis of encouraging results from a single institution report of infusional 5-FU (200 mg/m²/day for 5 weeks), weekly cisplatin (30 mg/m²), and subcutaneous interferon-α (3 million international units, given subcutaneously every other day) combined with EBRT (50 Gy). Investigators at Virginia Mason University originally described this multiagent regimen.[56,57] The trial enrolled 43 patients over 7 years, with 84% of patients having node-positive tumors. Despite this high-risk population, the 3-year survival rate was 64%, and the 5-year rate was 55%; with a mean follow-up time of 31.7 months, median survival has not been reached. Although this regimen has been associated with significant toxicity (over one third of patients required hospitalization), no treatment-related deaths occurred. In addition to the ACoSOG trial, the EORTC is conducting a phase II/phase III two-arm trial of gemcitabine followed by gemcitabine in combination with radiation as adjuvant therapy versus observation. Given gemcitabine's modest activity in the setting of advanced disease and its potent radiosensitizing proper-

Table 26.3 Ongoing Adjuvant and Neoadjuvant Protocols for Localized Pancreatic Cancer

Study PI	Phase	Protocol Schema
Adjuvant Trials		
• RTOG 9704* Regine	III	Surgery → Register → Randomize → Gemcitabine weekly ×3 Inf. 5-FU/EBRT → Gem weekly 3 on 1 off ×3 cycles; ↘ Infusional 5-FU → Inf. 5-FU/EBRT → Inf. 5-FU × 3 months
• NCRI-ESPAC-3 Neoptolemos[42]	III	Surgery → Register → Randomize → Observation; ↘ Gemcitabine 3 weeks on, 1 week off × 6 months; ↘ 5-FU/Leucovorin daily × 5 q28 days × 6 months
• ACOSOG ZQ5031 Picozzi[57]	II	Surgery → Register → Infusional 5-FU, Weekly Cisplatin, Interferon-α MWF } + EBRT → Infusional 5-FU × two cycles
• UTMDACC 02-040 Pisters	II	Surgery → Register → Infusional 5-FU, Weekly cisplatin, Interferon-α MWF } + EBRT → Infusional 5-FU × two cycles
• EORTC 40013 Van Leathem	II	Surgery → Register → Randomize → Gem 3 weeks on, 1 week off × two cycles → Gem/EBRT; ↘ Observation
• JHMI J9988* Jaffee/Laheru	II	Surgery → Register → GVAX vaccine → 5-FU/EBRT+ chemotherapy → GVAX × four doses
Neoadjuvant Trials		
• ECOG- E1200 Hoffman	II	Preop staging and and evaluation → Register → Randomize → Gem + EBRT → Surgery → Gem; ↘ Gem/Cis/infusional 5-FU → Infusional 5-FU/EBRT → Surgery → Gem
• UTMDACC ID01-341 Evans/Wolff	II	Preop staging and evaluation → Register → Gem/Cis QOW × four doses → Gem/EBRT to 30 Gy → Surgery

* Elizabeth Jaffe and William Regine, personal communication. For details of other trials see www.cancer.gov.

Abbreviations: Inf, infusional; Gem, gemcitabine; Cis, cisplatin; Preop, preoperative; EBRT, external beam radiotherapy; GVAX, G-CSF transfected allogeneic pancreatic cancer cells for vaccination; QOW, every other week.

ties,[58] a number of studies of gemcitabine-based chemoradiation have been performed in patients with locally advanced pancreatic cancer.[59-61] A variety of doses and schedules for gemcitabine in combination with radiation have now been reported, with an emerging understanding of the factors associated with toxicity.[62] Although gemcitabine-based chemoradiation programs have been tested in patients with locally advanced disease and in patients with potentially resectable tumors, there is limited experience with adjuvant gemcitabine-based chemoradiation after pancreaticoduodenectomy. In a Belgian study involving 30 patients, weekly low-dose gemcitabine (300 mg/m^2) was delivered in combination with EBRT to a dose of 45 Gy. Toxicity was primarily hematologic, and dose reductions were required for half the patients. No bowel perforations were noted, and only 12% of patients developed grade 3 or grade 4 diarrhea.[63] In another European study, 22 patients with curatively resected pancreatic cancer were treated with full-dose gemcitabine (1000 mg/m^2, days 1 and 8, every 21 days) for three courses and then received a lower dose (300 mg/m^2) combined with a split course of EBRT to a dose of 40 Gy.[64] Only two patients did not complete all prescribed therapy. Grade 3 or grade 4 hematologic and nonhematologic toxicities were observed in 36% and 32% of patients, respectively. No late toxicities were observed. Follow-up is immature at this point. Finally, in a U.S. study, Blackstock et al.[65] reported preliminary results of gemcitabine-based chemoradiation as adjuvant therapy in 37 patients undergoing surgery for pancreatic cancer. Gemcitabine was delivered at a dose of 40 mg/m^2 twice weekly with standard fraction (180 cGy/fraction) EBRT to a total dose of 50.4 Gy. Toxicity was described as tolerable, but two patients experienced bowel perforation. Given the lack of consensus regarding the dose and schedule of gemcitabine to be combined with radiotherapy, caution will be needed as adjuvant gemcitabine-based chemoradiation programs are investigated.

Preoperative (Neoadjuvant) Therapy for Resectable Pancreatic Cancer

Sadly, there has been no significant progress in adjuvant therapy for resected pancreatic cancer since the GITSG study was first reported in 1985. More recent studies have been fairly consistent with the GITSG findings: The median survival for resected patients treated with postoperative therapy hovers around 20 months and remains at 12 months for patients undergoing surgery alone. Importantly, pancreaticoduodenectomy has been associated with significant morbidity and, in less experienced centers, mortality.[66,67] Of the patients who undergo potentially curative surgery for pancreatic cancer, at least 20%–25% do not recuperate adequately to embark on postoperative chemoradiation, or they require prolonged recovery in order to consider such treatment.[36,37,40] Moreover, rapid disease progression with early systemic relapse is not uncommon after surgery (Fig. 26.2). Therefore, neoadjuvant therapy followed by surgery offers some theoretical advantages over immediate surgery.

First, upfront surgery may preclude the delivery of postoperative treatment to some patients, whereas preoperative therapy allows all potential surgical candidates to receive neoadjuvant therapy. Second, patients who present with potentially resectable disease are generally physiologically fit and make attractive candidates for neoadjuvant therapy. (If not, they would not be considered surgical candidates.) In addition, tolerance to such treatment may be better before extensive intra-abdominal surgery than after. Third, preoperative therapy allows delivery of chemotherapy or chemoradiation to a relatively well-perfused tumor bed and provides early treatment to microscopic metastases. Fourth, positive surgical margins are commonly reported after resection, and this is associated with poor prognosis, suggesting that surgery alone provides inadequate local control.[40,68,69] Preoperative therapy may provide for sufficient tumor destruction, particularly at the periphery, to increase the chances of a margin negative resection. Fifth, preoperative therapy allows for observation of the tumor's underlying biology. Repeat staging computed tomography (CT) after chemoradiation reveals liver metastases in approximately 25% of patients who receive chemoradiation before planned pancreaticoduodenectomy.[70] If these patients had undergone pancreaticoduodenectomy at the time of diagnosis, the liver metastases would likely have gone undetected intraoperatively. Such patients would therefore have undergone a major surgical procedure only to have liver metastases found soon after surgery. In a series of trials performed at the University of Texas, M.D. Anderson Cancer Center (UTMDACC), patients who demonstrated disease progression after preoperative chemoradiation had a median survival of only 7 months.[28] Thus, many

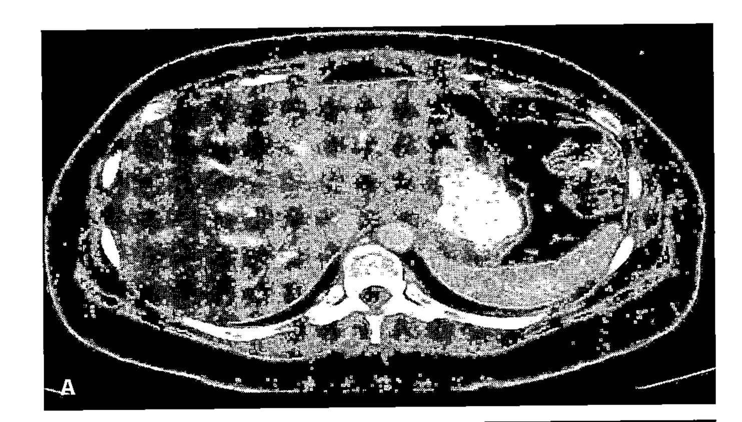

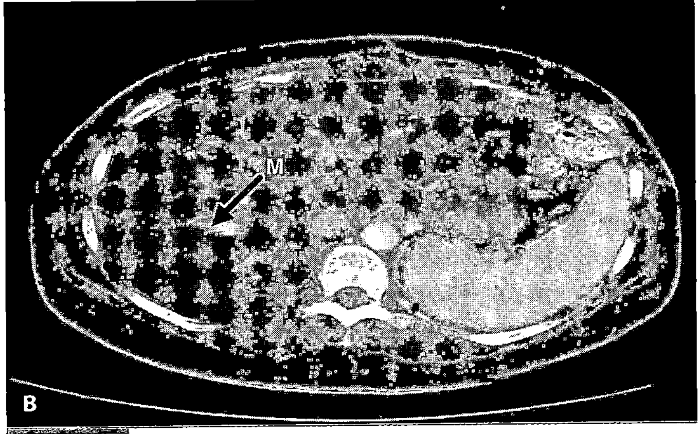

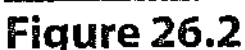

Figure 26.2
(A) Preoperative CT image of 45-year-old woman who underwent pancreaticoduodenectomy for adenocarcinoma of the pancreatic head. (B) Postoperative CT image from the same patient obtained 2.5 months after surgery revealing the interval development of a biopsy-proven hepatic metastasis *(M)*.

Table 26.4 Summary of Recent UTMDACC Trials of Preoperative Chemoradiation for Resectable Pancreatic Cancer

Study (Year)	No. of Patients	Regimen	Hospitalization Rate (%)	Resection Rate (%)	Path PR (%)	MS (Months)
Evans et al.[71] (1992)	28	5-FU/50.4 Gy	32	61	41	18
Pisters et al.[72] (1998)	35	5-FU/30 Gy	9	57	20	25
Pisters et al.[73] (2002)	35	Taxol/30 Gy	11	57	21	19
Wolff et al.[74] (2002)	86	Gem/30 Gy	43	74	58	36

Abbreviations: Path PR, pathological partial response (> 50% tumor kill); MS, median survival; Gem, gemcitabine.

institutions have begun to investigate the role of chemoradiation given preoperatively.

Since 1988, four prospective preoperative trials have been completed at UTMDACC (Table 26.4).[71-74] These trials, performed in sequence, have had nearly identical inclusion criteria, with a standardized surgical technique and assessment of resection margins. In addition, a pathologic grading system for tumor destruction after preoperative chemoradiation has also been developed to assess localized tumor response to therapy. This has maximized the number of variables held constant while varying only the chemoradiation regimens themselves. All eligible patients have been required to have biopsy-proven adenocarcinoma of the pancreatic head. Patients with neuroendocrine tumors or tumors located in the body or tail have been excluded. All patients have been required to undergo dual-phase, helical CT scan of the abdomen and pelvis and have a demonstrable tumor within the pancreatic head not involving the celiac axis or superior mesenteric artery. The superior mesenteric–portal venous confluence has had to be patent. Finally, patients with evidence of extrapancreatic disease such as liver metastases, lung metastases, or peritoneal disease have been excluded. The only exception to these criteria has evolved with the expanded use of endoscopic ultrasound as a diagnostic and staging modality. Since the late 1990s, patients with cytologically confirmed tumors only visible on endoscopic ultrasound have been eligible for preoperative treatment on protocol.

In the initial UTMDACC preoperative study performed by Evans et al.,[71] 28 patients received a course of continuous infusional 5-FU (300 mg/m^2/day) in combination with standard-fractionation external beam radiation (50.4 Gy; 180 cGy/fraction for 28 fractions over 5.5 weeks). The GI toxic effects (nausea, vomiting, and dehydration) were severe enough to require hospital admission in a third of patients. The resection rate among this group of patients was 60%, with 25% of patients having radiographic evidence of metastatic disease 4 to 5 weeks after completing preoperative therapy. Another 15% had intraoperative evidence of metastatic disease at laparotomy, and planned pancreaticoduodenectomy was aborted. The median survival for the patients undergoing resection with curative intent was 18 months, similar to that reported for patients undergoing postoperative 5-FU–based chemoradiation. The degree of tumor cell kill was graded using a standardized scoring system, and 40% of the resected specimens had a pathological partial response to therapy (>50% of the tumor cells were nonviable). Although the results from this initial trial of preoperative therapy for pancreatic cancer appeared equivalent to those seen with postoperative therapy, the toxicity and hospitalization rate were discouraging. These findings led to a change in the delivery of radiation therapy in all subsequent preoperative trials performed at UTMDACC. A rapid-fractionation program of chemoradiation was designed to avoid the GI toxicity associated with standard-fractionation chemoradiation delivered over 5.5 weeks, while maintaining the excellent local tumor control achieved with multimodality therapy. The revised regimen consisted of rapid-fractionation chemoradiation delivered over 2 weeks with 18-MeV photons using a four-field technique to a total dose of 30 Gy (3 Gy/fraction [10 fractions], 5 days/week). Sequentially performed preoperative chemoradiation trials have evaluated continuous infusion 5-FU, paclitaxel, and gemcitabine, all given as single agents.[72-74] Restaging with abdominopelvic CT and chest radiography has been performed 4 to 5 weeks after the completion of chemoradiation, in preparation for pancreaticoduodenectomy. In the UTMDACC study of rapid fractionation EBRT with infusional 5-FU, of the 35 patients enrolled, 27 were taken to surgery, and 20 (57%) underwent successful pancreaticoduodenectomy.[72] Local tumor control and patient survival were equal to the results with standard-fractionation (5.5 weeks) chemoradiation. Of note, only 2 of the 20 patients (10%)

who underwent resection developed local–regional recurrence, and the median survival for all 20 patients was 25 months.

Regrettably, because the rates of response to 5-FU–based systemic therapy are poor in patients with measurable metastatic disease, 5-FU–based preoperative chemoradiation regimens are unlikely to significantly impact the development of distant metastases. For example, in an ECOG study, 53 patients with potentially resectable tumors received chemoradiation with infusional 5-FU (300 mg/m^2/day, days 1–28) and mitomycin-C (10 mg/m^2 on day 1 only) and standard-fractionation EBRT to a total dose of 50.4 Gy.[75] Toxicity was substantial, with over 50% of patients requiring admission. There were two septic deaths, attributed to cholangitis before surgery. The resection rate and overall survival were disappointing, with 45% of enrolled patients ultimately undergoing resection with curative intent; their median survival was only 15 months. Therefore, more effective systemic agents are needed both to maximize local tumor destruction and to treat microscopic metastatic disease. Before the advent of gemcitabine, paclitaxel was investigated as a preoperative radiosensitizer in a group of patients with resectable pancreatic cancer at UTMDACC. Although the chemoradiaiton was well-tolerated, this agent did not appear to provide an incremental advantage over 5-FU-based chemoradiation programs in terms of resection rate, local treatment effect, or overall survival.[73]

Gemcitabine-Based Preoperative Chemoradiation for Pancreatic Cancer

As previously discussed, gemcitabine has potent radiosensitizing properties in vitro, and given its modest reproducible activity in advanced disease, it has been combined with radiation in a number of phase I and phase II trials. Before exploring preoperative gemcitabine-based chemoradiation for patients with resectable pancreatic cancer, a phase I study of gemcitabine in combination with EBRT was performed at UTMDACC in a group of patients with locally advanced disease.[60] This regimen was built on the previous UTMDACC radiation approach with rapid-fractionation EBRT. This was delivered in combination with weekly gemcitabine given over 7 weeks. The maximum tolerated dose of gemcitabine using this treatment schedule was 350 mg/m^2/week, roughly one third of the standard weekly dose. The dose-limiting toxic effects included fatigue, anorexia, nausea, vomiting, and dehydration; febrile neutropenia occurred in only one patient. The hospitalization rate in this phase I trial was significant, with 44% of patients being admitted during therapy. However, objective tumor regression was observed in 24% of patients, and one patient had dramatic radiographic evidence of tumor downstaging, justifying an attempt at surgical resection. The tumor, previously invading the portal vein, was resected with clear surgical margins and on pathologic assessment; 95% of the tumor specimen was nonviable. These results were sufficiently encouraging to proceed with a study of gemcitabine-based preoperative chemoradiation in a group of patients with potentially resectable disease as defined previously here. A total of 86 patients were enrolled in UTMDACC protocol ID 98-020 from July 1998 to October 2001.[74] Toxicities were similar to those observed in the initial phase I trial, and the hospitalization rate was nearly identical (40%). However, despite a longer elapsed time from enrollment to surgical intervention compared with previous trials (11–12 weeks rather than 7–9 weeks), 74% of patients underwent resection with curative intent. Furthermore, local treatment effect was more substantial, with 58% of the resected surgical specimens showing at least 50% tumor cell kill; two pathological complete responses were also observed. Importantly, with a median follow-up now extending beyond 3 years, the resected patients have a median survival of 36 months. This is clearly superior to survival seen in other preoperative trials performed at UTMDACC. The role of gemcitabine in combination with radiation for patients with potentially resectable tumors has also been investigated by others.[76,77] Hoffman et al.[77] have reported on a phase I study of preoperative standard-fractionation EBRT (50.4 Gy) and escalating weekly doses of gemcitabine (300, 400, and 500 mg/m^2) for potentially resectable pancreatic cancer. Eight of 15 patients (53%) required hospitalization after chemoradiation. Pancreaticoduodenectomy was completed in eight patients; the histologic response to the preoperative therapy was brisk, with fibrosis replacing 53%–78% of resected tumors. This study is useful in providing appropriate benchmarks for comparisons between various preoperative chemoradiation regimens, including hospitalization rate, resection rate, and treatment effect for patients undergoing surgery. Whether local treatment effect will become an important endpoint in future preoperative trials remains uncertain. In other GI tumors, such as rectal cancer and esophageal cancer, a complete pathological response to preoperative therapy has been associated with improved survival.[78-80] In the UTMDACC trial of gemcitabine-based chemoradiation, complete pathological responses were observed in two surgical specimens, and it has been observed sporadically in both gemcitabine-based and 5-FU–based neoadjuvant programs.[74,81,82] These observations are important, and

Table 26.5 Summary of Other Recent Trials of Neodjuvant Therapy for Patients with Resectable, Borderline Resectable, and Unresectable Pancreatic Cancer

Trial	No. of Patients	Tumor Status at Presentation			Treatment	Resection Rate	Survival of Resection Patients
		Resectable	Unresectable	Marginal			
ECOG[75]	53	53	—	—	5-FU/MITO 50.4 Gy	45%	15.7 Months
Duke[85]	111	53	58	—	5-FU/MITO +/– Cis 45 Gy	53% R 19% U	32% at 2 years
Stanford[86]	15	—	—	15	5-FU 50.4–56 Gy	60%	30 Months
Erlagen/Rostock[87]	27	—	27	—	5-FU/MITO 55 Gy	37%	11 Months
French[88]	41	41	—	—	5-FU/Cis 50 Gy	63%	NS
Wayne State[89]	20	—	20	—	5-FU/Cis/Ara-C/Caffeine 39.6 Gy/+8 Ngy	15%	67% at 2 years
Roger Williams[90]	14	—	14	—	5-FU/Cis 45 Gy	81%	16 Months
University of Michigan[76]	41 (32*)	12	20		Gem 36 Gy	75% R 10% U	NS
Fox Chase[91]	31+	10	17	—	5-FU/Mito 50.4 Gy	70% R 48% U	9 months (all patients) 14 months resected patients)
Brown/MGH/BU[92]	14		14		Paclitaxel 50 Gy	7%	NS
UCLA[93]	38	—	38	—	5-FU/MITO/ Dipyridamole	10%	28 months

* Depicts number of patients completing chemoradiation at the time of abstract submission.
+ Patients had either pancreatic cancer (27) or duodenal cancer. (4)
Abbreviations: MGH, Massachusetts General Hospital; BU, Boston University; MITO, mitomycin C; Cis, cisplatin; Ara-C, cytarabine; Pts, patients.

although preoperative chemoradiation has not been established as a standard approach, experience to date suggests it may increase the likelihood of a margin-negative resection. The literature has clearly demonstrated that grossly or microscopically positive surgical margins are associated with poor survival ranging from 6 to 12 months.[83] Even in experienced centers such as JHMI, positive surgical margins are identified in 30% of patients after pancreaticoduodenectomy or total pancreatectomy.[40] Using preoperative therapy, negative surgical margins are reported more frequently[84] and, although probably not sufficient to ensure cure, are likely to be necessary for extended survival.

Chemoradiation for Pancreatic Cancer: Is It Preoperative Therapy?

Unfortunately, many reports of neoadjuvant therapy for pancreatic cancer have included heterogeneous patient populations, enrolling patients with locally advanced, marginally resectable, and resectable pancreatic cancers (Table 26.5).[75,76,85-93] For example, investigators at Duke University reported on a group of 111 patients who underwent preoperative chemoradiation with infusional 5-FU and mitomycin-C and, in a subgroup of patients, cisplatin.[85] Some of the enrolled patients were considered to have potentially resectable disease,[53] whereas others were described as having locally advanced disease. Staging laparoscopy was performed in 58% of patients. Of the 53 resectable patients, 28 went on to have surgical resection (resection rate = 53%). Among the 58 patients with locally advanced disease (some of whom had tumors abutting but not encasing the critical vessels), radiographic evidence of downstaging occurred in 6 patients (10%). However, a total of 11 patients initially classified as having locally advanced disease were resected with curative intent after preoperative chemoradiation (19%).

In addition to the Duke data, which suggest some potential to downstage unresectable tumors, some of the early reports of gemcitabine-based chemoradiation reported on the same phenomenon.[60,61,94,95] These were usually phase I studies and were not specifically intended to be preoperative programs. In some of these studies, tumor downstaging was observed in a small subset of patients with locally advanced disease and ultimately led to attempts at surgical resection. However, careful review of the current evidence suggests that tumor downstaging occurs infrequently.[96] In a retrospective analysis of 163 patients with locally advanced pancreatic cancer seen at Memorial Sloan-Kettering Cancer Center in the period from 1993 to 1999, 87 received chemoradiation. Of this group, three (3.5%) had sufficient tumor downstaging to justify re-exploration with a view towards curative resection, but only one patient underwent such tumor removal; resection was aborted in the other two patients. Therefore, although tumor downstaging has been reported, it remains uncommon and dependent on varying definitions of unresectable disease. As the definition of locally advanced pancreatic cancer is relaxed, results of preoperative chemoradiation will appear more promising. In general, patients with locally advanced pancreatic cancer should not be included in studies of preoperative therapy because their inclusion confounds the reported resection rate and complicates comparisons to other studies. Whenever possible, patients with locally advanced pancreatic cancer should be enrolled in separate clinical trials and should be informed that tumor downstaging, although possible, is rarely sufficient to allow for surgical resection.

Preoperative Therapy for Borderline Resectable Pancreatic Cancer

As discussed previously here, current evidence suggests that downstaging locally advanced pancreatic cancer to the point of resectability is rare. However, high-quality preoperative imaging is now defining a distinct subgroup of patients with borderline (marginally) resectable tumors. These tumors may be defined by cuffing or abutment of a portion of a mesenteric vessel or celiac axis without complete encasement. Compression of the portal vein or superior mesenteric–portal venous confluence has also been considered a borderline resectable situation. Upfront surgery in these patients would be expected to lead to positive surgical margins in a significant proportion and should be discouraged. However, preoperative chemoradiation is an attractive alternative because it may cause sufficient killing in the tumor's periphery to render the patient surgically resectable with negative surgical margins. Identifying the small subset of patients with borderline resectable tumors using high-quality cross-sectional imaging and subsequently treating them with neoadjuvant therapy is a relatively new phenomenon (Fig. 26.3). Mehta et al.[86]

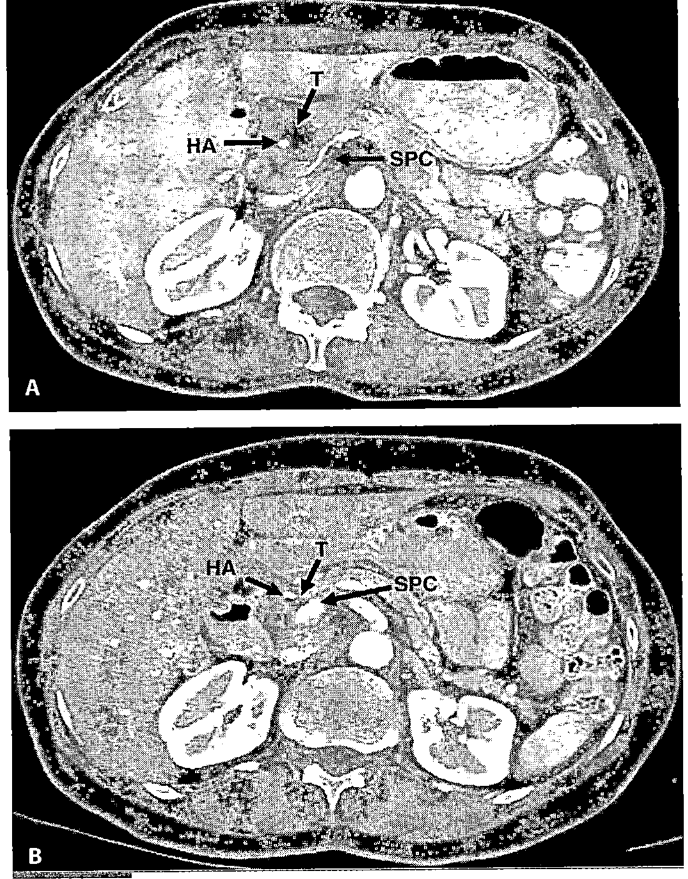

Figure 26.3
(A) Pretreatment CT image of a 51-year-old woman with borderline resectable pancreatic cancer (T) with encasement of the hepatic artery (HA) and narrowing of the splenoportal confluence (SPC). (B) Posttreatment CT image of the same patient demonstrating tumor reduction and decompression of the splenoportal confluence. The patient went on to have surgery with resection and reconstruction of a short segment of the HA. Surgical margins were negative; two lymph nodes were involved with metastatic disease.

has reported on the Stanford University experience using preoperative infusional 5-FU and EBRT in a group of patients with marginally resectable tumors. Fifteen patients received preoperative treatment, and nine (60%) underwent surgery with negative surgical margins; two patients had a complete pathologic response to treatment. Preoperative therapy for borderline resectable tumors is also part of the focus of an ECOG trial, which was activated in May 2003 (see Table 26.3). This study allows for the enrollment of patients determined to have borderline resectable tumors defined by the absence of 360° involvement of the hepatic artery, superior mesenteric artery, or celiac axis. Eligible patients will be randomized to a preoperative program of gemcitabine-based chemoradiation (500 mg/m^2 over 50 minutes weekly with 28 fractions of EBRT, 180 cGy/fraction; total dose of 50.4 Gy) or a regimen of gemcitabine, 5-FU, and cisplatin followed by 5-FU–based chemoradiation. Patients without evidence of disease progression after neoadjuvant therapy will undergo attempt at resection. Endpoints for the study will include the overall resection rate, the margin negative resection rate, extent of treatment-induced tumor fibrosis, and overall survival.

Special Issues in the Delivery of Neoadjuvant Therapy

Biliary Stenting and Neoadjuvant Therapy

Preoperative therapy for pancreatic cancer has usually involved the delivery of chemotherapy and radiation, followed by a rest period before surgery. This allows the patient to recover from myelosuppression or nonhematologic toxicities, including nausea, vomiting, and dehydration. Patients may also develop GI hemorrhage and radiation colitis or enteritis, which needs to resolve before surgical intervention. Thus, at least 2–4 months may elapse from initiation of therapy through recovery to subsequent surgery. Because obstructive jaundice is the most common presentation for patients with resectable pancreatic cancer, they require either operative biliary bypass or endobiliary stenting before preoperative therapy. Some centers have reported higher rates of postoperative infection in those patients who undergo endobiliary stenting before definitive surgery,[97] but these infections are not always serious.[98] For example, in a review of 300 patients undergoing pancreaticoduodenectomy at UTMDACC, the infection rate has been slightly higher in patients with biliary stents or operative biliary bypass compared with patients without biliary drainage before surgery (37% vs 31%).[99] However, most of these infections were wound infections without serious consequences, and no significant increase in postoperative morbidity or mortality.[99] Nevertheless, the observation that biliary stents lead to postoperative infections has generated resistance to neoadjuvant therapy. Moreover, endobiliary stents, in particular silastic stents, have a defined half-life and may occlude in the face of preoperative therapy. Stent occlusion during treatment can be a serious complication, leading to cholangitis and even biliary sepsis.[75] Therefore, in addition to the anticipated toxicities of chemotherapy and upper abdominal radiation, stent occlusion may also develop and lead to significant morbidity. Thus, safe preoperative therapy mandates the assembly of a dedicated multidisciplinary team comprised of surgeons, gastroenterologists, medical oncologists, and radiotherapists. Weekly evaluation with more than one team member is advised not only to assess the patient for toxicities related to chemoradiation, but also for early warning signs of impending stent occlusion, such as fevers and chills or elevations in transaminases. Recognition of these signs and symptoms can result in timely referral to a gastroenterologist with expertise in biliary drainage, for rapid stent exchange before the patient becomes seriously ill, necessitating a break from treatment.

Surgical Complications After Preoperative Chemoradiation

A common concern for clinicians considering preoperative therapy for any GI tumor is that such therapy may increase postoperative morbidity and mortality, and in the case of pancreatic cancer, the risk of pancreaticojejunal anastomotic leaks. These concerns have not been supported by experience with preoperative therapy for pancreatic cancer. In a randomized trial investigating the role of octreotide to prevent pancreatic fistula, there was no benefit to octreotide compared with placebo. Of note, the risk of a leak was reduced in patients who underwent preoperative chemoradiation compared with patients who did not undergo preoperative chemoradiation.[100] Furthermore, there is no evidence to suggest that any postoperative complications are increased after preoperative chemoradiation compared with upfront surgery.

Future Approaches to Resectable Pancreatic Cancer

Despite advances in cross-sectional imaging, modern surgical technique, and perioperative care, long-term survival for patients with resected pancreatic cancer remains dismal. Recent trials of adjuvant therapy have not led to significant improvements in survival compared with earlier programs, and most patients succumb with disseminated disease. Thus, improved systemic therapies must be developed in order to change the natural history of resectable pancreatic cancer. As recently demonstrated for patients with colon cancer, combination chemotherapy, which improves survival in advanced disease,[101] may also provide benefit to patients who require adjuvant therapy after surgery.[35] Thus, any treatment regimen demonstrating improved tumor control compared with standard therapy in advanced disease should be pursued as a component of therapy for resectable disease, whether delivered preoperatively or postoperatively. A few specific examples are outlined later here.

Conventional Chemotherapy Combinations

Several contemporary trials of systemic therapy for advanced pancreatic cancer have investigated the role of gemcitabine-based combinations. Phase II trials of gemcitabine combined with cisplatin, oxaliplatin, irinotecan, and 5-FU have often reported higher response rates compared with historical data of gemcitabine monotherapy.[102-105] Thus far, randomized trials of gemcitabine combinations have failed to demonstrate any significant survival advantage over single agent gemcitabine in advanced disease.[106,107] However, because patients with resectable disease have a lower metastatic tumor burden, combination systemic therapy using conventional cytotoxic agents may have greater impact on microscopic metastatic disease over gemcitabine alone and theoretically improve outcomes for patients with resectable pancreatic cancer. This rationale is the basis for ongoing trials of neoadjuvant therapy being conducted at UTMDACC and through ECOG. Currently, protocol patients with potentially resectable pancreatic cancer seen at UTMDACC are receiving systemic therapy using a combination of gemcitabine and cisplatin, followed by gemcitabine-based chemoradiation before attempted surgery. As previously described, one arm of ECOG 1200 will administer combination therapy with gemcitabine, cisplatin, and 5-FU, followed by 5-FU–based chemoradiation to patients with resectable or borderline resectable pancreatic cancer. If successful, such strategies may generate greater interest in more aggressive neoadjuvant or adjuvant chemotherapeutic regimens for this group of patients (see Table 26.3).

Exploiting Molecular Targets

Better outcomes may ultimately be observed in resectable patients undergoing multiagent cytotoxic chemotherapy, but any incremental improvements in survival are expected to be quite modest. Although the continued development of chemotherapy combinations is warranted, the investigation of novel biological agents should receive greater attention. As molecular events associated with pancreatic carcinogenesis and chemoresistance are elucidated and factors promoting angiogenesis and metastatic spread are identified, more targeted therapies are entering the clinic. (For a more detailed discussion of these molecular targets and agents, see Chapter ••.) Given the expanding availability of agents, which exploit molecular targets such as the epidermal growth factor receptor and vascular endothelial growth factor, exploratory trials have begun in patients with advanced pancreatic cancer. Thus far, gemcitabine-based combinations have yielded some provocative preliminary results when administered with cetuxumab (Erbitux), a monoclonal antibody to epidermal growth factor receptor, or bevacizumab (Avastin), a monoclonal antibody to vascular endothelial growth factor. Xiong et al. have submitted their results combining weekly gemcitabine (1,000 mg/m^2 over 30 minutes) and cetuxumab (400 mg/m^2 loading dose over 60 minutes; 250 mg/m^2 weekly maintenance dose) in 41 patients with advanced pancreatic cancer (H. Xiong, personal communication). Of note, over 80% of enrolled patients had measurable metastatic disease. Therapy was well tolerated, with rash, fatigue, and myelosuppression being the most common toxicities. The response rate to this combination was 12%, not a dramatic improvement over gemcitabine monotherapy. However, 1-year survival was 32%, far superior to the 1-year survival rate of 18% reported by Burris et al.[46] in a group of patients with advanced pancreatic cancer treated with gemcitabine alone; only 70% of whom had metastatic disease. Given these results, the Southwest Oncology Group is conducting a large randomized trial of gemcitabine with or without cetuxumab in patients with advanced pancreatic cancer.

Likewise, bevacizumab has been combined with gemcitabine in a group of 40 patients with metastatic pancreatic cancer. The response rate to this combination has been impressive, with 24% of patients achieving a confirmed partial response, and although follow-up data are immature, the estimated 1-year survival rate is 54%.[108] Therefore, a randomized trial comparing gemcitabine monotherapy to gemcitabine with bevacizumab is about to be launched through Cancer and Leukemia Group B.

Although the role of cetuxumab and bevacizumab in the treatment of pancreatic cancer is still being defined, these drugs have recently been approved by the Food and Drug Administration for use in patients with metastatic

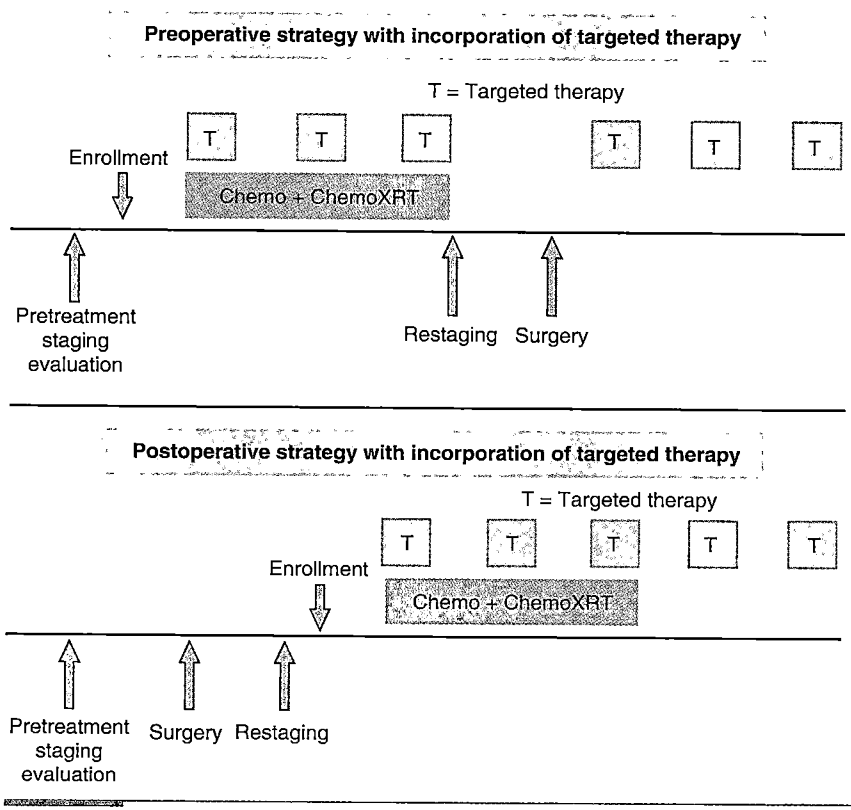

Figure 26.4
Proposed preoperative and postoperative treatment schemas incorporating targeted therapy.

colorectal cancer, and both are expected to be studied further as components of adjuvant therapy in patients with stage III colon cancer. Because the observed toxicities associated with these agents are generally manageable, with little evidence for added toxicity when combined with cytotoxic agents, intense interest in these and other molecular therapies is emerging for incorporation into neoadjuvant and adjuvant programs for pancreatic cancer (Fig. 26.4). In a phase I study, capecitabine and bevacizumab are being administered in combination with EBRT to a group of patients with locally advanced pancreatic cancer. Preliminary results reported by Crane et al.[109] from UTMDACC demonstrate that the regimen is generally well tolerated and leads to objective tumor regression.

Immunotherapy for Pancreatic Cancer

Patients with resectable pancreatic cancer harbor occult metastatic disease at the time of surgery and even with delivery of postoperative therapy remain at high risk for relapse with disseminated cancer. Therefore, strategies to augment immune surveillance and potentially eradicate small-volume metastatic disease through humoral or cell-mediated mechanisms are under investigation.[110]

Thus far, randomized trials of nonspecific immunotherapy for resected pancreatic cancer have been disappointing. For details of this studies, see Chapter 28. However, some pancreatic tumor antigens have been identified and are beginning to be exploited, such as mutated ras peptides, MUC-1, and heat shock proteins.[111-114] However, because pancreatic tumor cells express a wide array of potential immunogens that are as yet undefined, both autologous and allogeneic whole tumor cells have also been administered as vaccines. Of note, it has been well established that the immune response to solid tumors may be attenuated through a variety of mechanisms, including the downregulation of co-stimulatory cytokines. Therefore, genetically modified allogeneic tumor cells that express co-stimulatory cytokines, such as the granulocyte-macrophage colony stimulating factor, are being investigated as vaccines. This approach has been studied extensively by Jaffee et al.[115] of the JHMI and tested clinically. Early results indicate a significant immune response to vaccination with allogeneic tumor cells in a dose-dependent fashion. Other investigators have manipulated autologous dendritic cells, which are highly efficient antigen-presenting cells. Dendritic cells have been primed with both MUC-1 peptides and carcinoembryonic antigen mRNA. When dendritic cells are pulsed with MUC-1 fusion proteins and reinjected into patients with solid tumors, they produce an enhanced immune response to MUC-1.[116] Furthermore, ongoing work at Duke has shown that dendritic cells can also be loaded with carcinoembryonic antigen mRNA ex vivo and safely reinjected into patients who have undergone neoadjuvant chemoradiation and surgical resection for pancreatic cancer.[117]

Although immunotherapy for pancreatic cancer should be considered investigational, it is attractive to consider as a component of adjuvant therapy for patients with resectable disease. This is based on its relatively high specificity as a cytotoxic intervention with little associated toxicity. Moreover, given that immunotherapy would not be expected to worsen the morbidity from surgery, chemotherapy, or radiation therapy, it may be easily integrated into adjuvant therapy in combination with other modalities.

Clinical Trial Design for Resectable Pancreatic Cancer: The Need for Discipline

Although significant advances have been observed in the treatment of other solid tumors, little has been achieved for patients with pancreatic cancer. Presently, there is currently no consensus as to the standard management of resectable pancreatic cancer. Surgery remains the cornerstone of therapy but as a single modality leads to a median survival of only 10 to 12 months, with long-term survivors being rare. There are many factors hampering progress—some strategic, others technical, a few biological. As with many other malignancies, clinical trials of resectable pancreatic cancer have been performed in two distinct settings: the large, cooperative group, and in the single-institutional setting with expertise in the delivery of multidisciplinary care. There are obvious advantages and disadvantages to both, but it should be acknowledged that a certain degree of quality control is lost when multicentered trials, which include centers with suboptimal expertise in the multidisciplinary management of pancreatic cancer, are performed. For example, in the ECOG trial of neoadjuvant therapy, 53 patients were enrolled from eight sites. Patients were treated with infusional 5-FU, mitomycin-C, and radiation. The resection rate was 45%, lower than the results reported by other single-institutional groups; median survival was also disappointing at 15.7 months. The authors suggested that the overall poor outcomes reflected the advanced state of most resected cancers, with positive peritoneal cytology noted in 3 patients, close surgical margins in 13 patients, lymph node involvement in 4 patients, and the need for superior mesenteric vein resection in 4 others. Simply stated, patient selection may have been a significant factor leading to these discouraging results. In fact, part way through the protocol's completion, stricter criteria for resection were put in place, with the maximum diameter of a resectable tumor being defined as being no larger than 5 cm (initially, tumors up to 10 cm in maximum diameter were considered resectable).[75]

Logically, large multicentered studies should be designed with a view toward mimicking the expertise of high-volume centers. Strict, well-defined standards should be embedded into preoperative assessments of resectability, surgical and perioperative care, pathological assessment of the tumor and its relationship to the surgical margins, and the delivery of chemotherapy and radiation. In several recent trials of preoperative and postoperative therapy for resectable pancreatic cancer, little attention has been paid to these parameters, making interpretation and comparison of results challenging and outcomes disappointing. Progress will remain slow unless a more disciplined approach to clinical trial design, patient selection, and protocol implementation is used. A few recommendations are outlined later here.

1. Adequate preoperative assessment of resectability

   Despite clear evidence that high-quality, thin-cut, cross-sectional imaging predicts resectability accurately,[118,119] many patients undergo laparotomy for pancreatic cancer without adequate preoperative assessment. Some patients are found to have unresectable tumors intraoperatively when such a conclusion might have been possible before surgery. Conversely, because of a lack of adequate preoperative imaging and surgical expertise, many patients who are "resected with curative intent" have been left with gross residual disease not recognized by the surgeon intraoperatively. Thus, if the radiologist has not been sufficiently employed preoperatively and the surgeon has failed intraoperatively, the pathologist cannot be expected to distinguish between gross residual disease and microscopically positive margins (R2 versus R1 resection) postoperatively. It remains likely that patients enrolled in future postoperative trials of adjuvant therapy will be quite heterogeneous—some having completely excised tumors and others persistent disease, either microscopic or macroscopic. Under these circumstances, the task of assessing the added benefit of adjuvant therapy will not be particularly gratifying.

   Whether serum CA19-9 measurements should be assessed before surgery as an independent predictor of resectability is an open question. Most analyses have been performed retrospectively but suggest a high CA19-9 level (>300–600 U/mL), which implies more advanced disease not amenable to resection.[120,121] Recently, the UTMDACC group retrospectively analyzed pretreatment CA19-9 levels obtained from 79 patients enrolled in the trial of gemcitabine-based preoperative chemoradiation. All patients had radiographically defined, biopsy proven, resectable pancreatic cancer without any evidence of metastatic disease. Patients were eligible for protocol treatment irrespective of the serum CA19-9 level drawn at presentation. It was found that serum levels of greater than 668 U/mL predicted either the development of overt metastatic disease before surgery or early relapse after surgical resection.[122] If these findings are validated in a larger prospective study, low serum CA19-9 levels may be incorporated into future definitions of resectable disease. Alternatively, preoperative serum CA19-9 levels may become a parameter from which to base stratification in preoperative or postoperative regimens.

2. Adequate postoperative assessment of resected disease

Of the randomized trials of adjuvant therapy performed to date, there has been no consistent assessment of the postoperative tumor status before proceeding with adjuvant therapy. For instance, in the original GITSG study, the EORTC trial, and the ESPAC-1 trial, there were no reported requirements for a postoperative CT scan or other imaging to ensure the absence of persistent or metastatic disease.[36,37,42] Based on the experiences of several institutions investigating preoperative therapy in resectable pancreatic cancer, the onset of metastatic disease can be observed in at least 25% of patients within weeks of completion of preoperative therapy.[27,75,76] Rapid development of metastatic disease is likely to occur in a substantial subset of patients who undergo initial surgery. This is supported by the EORTC study in which 22% of patients randomized to adjuvant therapy did not receive it, based on a number of factors including medical contraindications, patient refusal (10 patients), or the interval development of metastatic disease (4 patients).[37] Although cost is an important variable to consider, obtaining new baseline imaging, perhaps 8–12 weeks postoperatively, would allow for the exclusion of patients with persistent disease or early relapse. Such patients will not benefit from adjuvant therapy and their enrollment in trials for advanced disease would be preferable.

As previously discussed, serum CA19-9 levels may also be considered an important variable, and a predetermined level could be required for study enrollment. For example, postoperative normalization of serum CA19-9 levels could be incorporated into inclusion criteria, as persistent elevation of this marker after surgery is associated with poor prognosis.[123]

3. Disciplined pathology assessment of the resected tumor

Another known prognostic factor in resected pancreatic cancer is the status of surgical margins. The large experience from JHMI exemplifies this. Patients with a positive surgical margin had a median survival of 12 months versus 19 months for those patients with negative margins.[40] However, given the complex anatomy and often distorted surgical specimen submitted for sectioning, accurate pathological assessment of resection margins grossly or microscopically is formidable. At UTMDACC, all submitted surgical specimens are inked at the retroperitoneal margin to assist the pathologist in their assessment. Unfortunately, in most studies of adjuvant therapy for pancreatic cancer, appraisal of margin status is not rigorously defined in the entry criteria and, given its importance as a prognostic variable, should receive greater attention. Stratification of patients based on margin status has been part of the RTOG 9704 trial, and it is hoped that future trials will incorporate this important variable into entry criteria in a clearly defined manner. Some investigators have separated patients with R1 resections (microscopically positive surgical margin) for postoperative treatment. Wilkowski et al.[124] has reported on a group of 30 patients undergoing R1 resection for pancreatic cancer. After recovery from surgery, they received four applications of gemcitabine 300 mg/m^2 and cisplatin (30 mg/m^2) with EBRT to 45–50 Gy. More gemcitabine and cisplatin were delivered thereafter (day 1 and day 15, every 28 days). The median survival for the cohort was 22.8 months, which is substantially longer than expected for this group. The authors therefore suggest comparative trials using this regimen for patients with pancreatic cancer undergoing R1 resections of their disease. Such studies can only be performed with strict criteria to determine the status of the surgical margins.

For patients undergoing preoperative therapy, local treatment effect may have some prognostic significance and, if assessed using a common grading system, would allow for some comparisons between differing regimens. At UTMDACC, treatment effect is graded based on the initial system proposed by Cleary and Evans (Table 26.6).[71] Broad use of this grading system could facilitate more rapid discovery of radiosensitizing drugs or combinational therapies, leading to better local tumor killing, accelerating advancement in the field.

4. Quality-control mechanisms for radiation therapy and chemotherapy

The importance of quality control in adjuvant trials cannot be overstated. The Southwest Oncology Group coordinated a large intergroup trial comparing the role of postoperative chemoradiotherapy after surgery to surgery alone in 556 patients who had undergone surgical resection for adenocarcinoma of the stomach or gastroesophageal junction.[33] Quality assurance for the radiotherapy treatment plan was performed by a radiation oncology coordinator before the start of radiation. Treatment fields, dosimetry, operative and pathology reports, and preoperative imaging all had to be submitted for review. Of note, 35% of treatment

Table 26.6 Grading System for Treatment Effect after Preoperative Chemoradiation

Grade	Histologic Appearance
I	Characteristic cytologic changes of malignancy are present, but little (<10%) or no tumor cell destruction is evident
II	In addition to characteristic cytologic changes of malignancy, 10% to 90% of tumor cells are destroyed
IIa	Destruction of 10% to 50% of tumor cells
IIb	Destruction of 51% to 90% of tumor cells
III	Few (<10%) viable-appearing tumor cells are present
IIIM	Sizable pools of mucin are present with few (<10%) viable tumor cells
IV	No viable tumor cells are present
IVM	Acellular pools of mucin are present

Adapted from Evans et al.[71]

plans were discovered to have either minor or major deviations from protocol-specified therapy and were modified before therapy began. On a final quality assurance review, deviations were found in only 6.5% of the treatment plans. Although the authors concluded that such therapy could be delivered safely, they noted that radiation oncologists had to be familiar with the proper techniques for the delivery of upper abdominal radiation in patients undergoing gastrectomy. Such a conclusion would certainly apply to the delivery of radiation to patients who have undergone a pancreaticoduodenectomy or other resections for pancreatic cancer. Critics have suggested that the lack of the central review of radiation treatment plans in the ESPAC-1 trial may in part explain the poor survival of patients randomized to chemoradiation compared with patients randomized to other arms of the study, including observation.[42,45]

Although quality assurance in large multi-institutional trials is challenging, centralized data review and individualized treatment proposals are feasible. Moreover, limited data suggest that patient outcome is improved when high-quality treatment planning is used in diseases such as medulloblastoma and pediatric Hodgkin's disease.[125,126] Such findings are probably true in the delivery of chemotherapy as well, where cooperative group efforts have shown benefits in decreasing protocol deviations and increased quality data collection.[127]

Conclusion

Drawing conclusions about the standard treatment for resectable pancreatic cancer has been perplexing and not necessarily aided by the results of recent large randomized trials of adjuvant therapy or smaller single-institution trials of preoperative therapy. Currently, adjuvant therapy in the form of 5-FU–based chemotherapy or carefully delivered 5-FU–based chemoradiation is reasonable for patients with adequate recovery from surgical intervention. Preoperative therapy remains investigational but has a sound clinical basis and remains a reasonable alternative to upfront surgery. This is particularly true for patients with marginally resectable tumors. Whenever possible, enrollment of patients into ongoing clinical trials of pre- or postoperative therapy should be seriously considered. However, these therapies should be offered only to those patients with adequate performance status.

During the recent past, a better understanding of the variables associated with improved survival has emerged, and a more disciplined approach is needed to ensure that patients derive maximum benefit from currently available modalities. Although molecular therapies are beginning to change the standard of care in other solid tumors, their potential has yet to be realized for patients with resectable pancreatic cancer. No matter what promise these treatments hold, future clinical trials for resectable pancreatic cancer will only lead to progress if the principles of multidisciplinary cancer care and quality assurance are incorporated into study design and conduct.

References

1. Conlon KC, Klimstra DS, Brennan MF. Long-term survival after curative resection for pancreatic ductal adenocarcinoma: clinicopathologic analysis of 5-year survivors. *Ann Surg.* 1996;223:273–279.
2. Paulino AC. Resected pancreatic cancer treated with adjuvant radiotherapy with or without 5-fluorouracil: treatment results and patterns of failure. *Am J Clin Oncol.* 1999;22:489–494.
3. Sadahiro S, Suzuki T, Ishikawa K, et al. Recurrence patterns after curative resection of colorectal cancer in patients followed for a minimum of ten years. *Gastroenterology.* 2003;50:1362–1366.
4. Tepper JE, O'Connell M, Hollis D, et al. Analysis of surgical salvage after failure of primary therapy in rectal cancer: results from Intergroup Study 0114. *J Clin Oncol.* 2003;21:3623–3628.
5. Wu CW, Lo SS, Shen KH, et al. Incidence and factors associated with recurrence patterns after intended curative surgery for gastric cancer. *World J Surg.* 2003;27:153–158.

6. Tepper JE, Nardi G, Suit H. Carcinoma of the pancreas: review of MGH experience from 1963-1973: analysis of surgical failure and implications for radiation therapy. *Cancer.* 1976;37:1519–1525.
7. Kayahara M, Nagakawa T, Ueno K, et al. An evaluation of radical resection for pancreatic cancer based on the mode of recurrence as determined by autopsy and diagnostic imaging. *Cancer.* 1993;72:2118–2123.
8. Griffin JF, Smalley SR, Jewell W, et al. Patterns of failure after curative resection of pancreatic carcinoma. *Cancer.* 1990;66:56–61.
9. Willett CG, Lewandrowski K, Warshaw AL, et al. Resection margins in carcinoma of the head of the pancreas: implications for radiation therapy. *Ann Surg.* 1993;217:144–148.
10. Westerdahl J, Andrén-Sandeberg Å, Ihse I. Recurrence of exocrine pancreatic cancer: local or hepatic? *Hepatogastroenterology.* 1993;40:384–387.
11. Hirai I, Kimura W, Ozawa K, et al. Perineural invasion in pancreatic cancer. *Pancreas.* 2002;24:15–25.
12. Takahashi T, Ishikura H, Motohara T. Perineural invasion by ductal adenocarcinoma of the pancreas. *J Surg Oncol.* 1997;65:164–170.
13. Kohlgraf KG, Gawron AJ, Higashi M, et al. Contribution of the MUC1 tandem repeat and cytoplasmic tail to invasive and metastatic properties of a pancreatic cancer cell line. *Cancer Res.* 2003;63:5011–5020.
14. Zhu Z, Kleeff J, Kayed H, et al. Nerve growth factor and enhancement of proliferation, invasion, and tumorigenicity of pancreatic cancer cells. *Mol Carcinog.* 2002;35:138–147.
15. Miknyoczki SJ, Lang D, Huang L, et al. Neurotrophin and Trk receptors in human pancreatic ductal adenocarcinoma: expression patterns and effects on in vitro invasive behavior. *Int J Cancer.* 1999;81:417–427.
16. Zhu Z, Friess H, diMola FF, et al. Nerve growth factor expression correlates with perineural invasion and pain in human pancreatic cancer. *J Clin Oncol.* 1999;17:2419–2428.
17. Gastrointestinal Tumor Study Group. Prolongation of disease-free interval in surgically treated rectal carcinoma. *N Engl J Med.* 1985;312:1465–1472.
18. Douglass HO, Moertel CG, Mayer RJ, et al. Survival after post-operative combination treatment of rectal cancer [letter]. *N Engl J Med.* 1986;315:1294–1295.
19. Wolmark N, Wieand HS, Hyams DM, et al. Randomized trial of postoperative adjuvant chemotherapy with or without radiotherapy for carcinoma of the rectum: National Surgical Adjuvant Breast and Bowel Project Protocol R-02. *J Natl Cancer Inst.* 2000;92:388–396.
20. Wibe A, Rendedal PR, Svensson E, et al. Prognostic significance of the circumferential resection margin following total mesorectal excision for rectal cancer. *Br J Surg.* 2002;89:327–334.
21. Birbeck KF, Macklin CP, Tiffin NJ, et al. Rates of circumferential resection margin involvement vary between surgeons and predict outcomes in rectal cancer surgery. *Ann Surg.* 2002;235:449–457.
22. Nagtegaal ID, van de Velde CJ, van der WE, et al. Macroscopic evaluation of rectal cancer resection specimen: clinical significance of the pathologist in quality control. *J Clin Oncol.* 2002;20:1729–1734.
23. Luttges J, Vogel I, Menke M, et al. The retroperitoneal resection margin and vessel involvement are important factors determining survival after pancreaticoduodenectomy for ductal adenocarcinoma of the head of the pancreas. *Virchows Arch.* 1998;433:237–242.
24. Whittington R, Bryer MP, Haller DG, et al. Adjuvant therapy of resected adenocarcinoma of the pancreas. *Int J Radiat Oncol Biol Phys.* 1991;21:1137–1143.
25. Morganti AG, Valentini V, Macchia G, et al. Adjuvant radiotherapy in resectable pancreatic carcinoma. *Eur J Surg Oncol.* 2002;28:523–530.
26. Foo ML, Gunderson LL, Nagorney DM, et al. Patterns of failure in grossly resected pancreatic ductal adenocarcinoma treated with adjuvant irradiation ± 5-fluorouracil. *Int J Radiat Oncol Biol Phys.* 1993;26:483–489.
27. Spitz FR, Abbruzzese JL, Lee JE, et al. Preoperative and postoperative chemoradiation strategies in patients treated with pancreaticoduodenectomy for adenocarcinoma of the pancreas. *J Clin Oncol.* 1997;15:928–937.
28. Breslin TM, Hess KR, Harbison DB, et al. Neoadjuvant chemoradiotherapy for adenocarcinoma of the pancreas: treatment variables and survival duration. *Ann Surg Oncol.* 2001;8:123–132.
29. Staley CA, Lee JE, Cleary KA, et al. Preoperative chemoradiation, pancreaticoduodenectomy, and intraoperative radiation therapy for adenocarcinoma of the pancreatic head. *Am J Surg.* 1996;171:118–125.
30. Krook JE, Moertel CG, Gunderson LL, et al. Effective surgical adjuvant therapy for high-risk rectal carcinoma. *N Engl J Med.* 1991;324:709–715.
31. Moertel CG, Fleming TR, Macdonald JS, et al. Fluorouracil plus levamisole as effective adjuvant therapy after resection of stage III colon carcinoma: a final report. *Ann Intern Med.* 1995;122:321–326.
32. Bleiberg H, Goffin JC, Dalesio O, et al. Adjuvant radiotherapy and chemotherapy in resectable gastric cancer: a randomized trial of the gastrointestinal tract cancer cooperative group of the EORTC. *Eur J Surg Oncol.* 1989;15:535–543.
33. MacDonald JS, Smalley SR, Benedetti J, et al. Chemoradiotherapy after surgery compared with surgery alone for adenocarcinoma of the stomach or gastroesophageal junction. *N Engl J Med.* 2001;345:725–730.
34. Moertel CG. Accomplishments in surgical adjuvant therapy for large bowel cancer. *Cancer.* 1992;70(Suppl. 5): S1364–S1371.
35. André T, Buni C, Murredj-Rerdal L, et al. Oxaliplatin, Flouroracil, and Leucovorin as adjuvant treatment for colon cancer. *N Eng J Med.* 2004;350:2343–2351.
36. Kalser MH, Ellenberg SS. Pancreatic cancer: adjuvant combined radiation and chemotherapy following curative resection. *Arch Surg.* 1985;120:899–903.
37. Klinkenbijl JH, Jeekel J, Sahmoud T, et al. Adjuvant radiotherapy and 5-fluorouracil after curative resection for the cancer of the pancreas and peri-ampullary region: phase III trial of the EORTC Gastrointestinal Tract Cancer Cooperative Group. *Ann Surg.* 1999;230:776–784.
38. Evans DB, Wolff RA, Hess KR. Adjuvant radiotherapy and 5-fluorouracil after curative resection of cancer of the pancreas and periampullary region [letter]. *Ann Surg.* 2000;232:727.

39. Regine WF, Abrams RA. Adjuvant therapy for pancreatic cancer: back to the future. *Int J Radiat Oncol Biol Phys.* 1998;42:59–63.
40. Sohn TA, Yeo CJ, Cameron JL, et al. Resected adenocarcinoma of the pancreas-616 patients: results, outcomes, and prognostic indicators. *J Gastrointest Surg.* 2000;4:567–579.
41. Lim JE, Chien MW, Earle CC. Prognostic factors following curative resection for pancreatic adenocarcinoma: a population-based, linked database analysis of 396 patients. *Ann Surg.* 2003;237:74–85.
42. Neoptolemos JP, Dunn JA, Stocken DD, et al. Adjuvant chemoradiotherapy and chemotherapy in resectable pancreatic cancer: a randomized controlled trial. *Lancet.* 2001;358:1576–1585.
43. Neoptolemos JP, Stocken DD, Friess H, et al. A randomized trial of chemoradiotherapy and chemotherapy after resection of pancreatic cancer. *N Engl J Med.* 2004;350: 1200–1210.
44. Evans DB, Hess KR, Pisters PW. ESPAC-1 trial of adjuvant therapy for resectable adenocarcinoma of the pancreas. *Ann Surg.* 2002;236:694.
45. Abrams RA, Lillemoe KD, Piantadosi S. Continuing controversy over adjuvant therapy of pancreatic cancer. *Lancet.* 2001;358:1565–1566.
46. Burris HA III, Moore MJ, Andersen J, et al. Improvements in survival and clinical benefit with gemcitabine as first-line therapy for patients with advanced pancreas cancer: a randomized trial. *J Clin Oncol.* 1997;15:2403–2413.
47. Rubin J, Gallagher JG, Schroeder G, et al. Phase II trials of 5-fluorouracil and leucovorin in patients with metastatic gastric or pancreatic carcinoma. *Cancer.* 1996;78:1888–1891.
48. Maisey N, Chau I, Cunningham D, et al. Multicenter randomized phase III trial comparing protracted venous infusion (PVI) fluorouracil (5-FU) with PVI 5-FU plus mitomycin in inoperable pancreatic cancer. *J Clin Oncol.* 2002;20:3130–3136.
49. Casper ES, Green MR, Kelsen DP, et al. Phase II trial of gemcitabine (2',2'-difluorodeoxycytidine) in patients with adenocarcinoma of the pancreas. *Invest New Drugs.* 1994;12:29–34.
50. Carmichael J, Fink U, Russell RC, et al. Phase II study of gemcitabine in patients with advanced pancreatic cancer. *Br J Cancer.* 1996;73:101–105.
51. Ducreux M, Rougier P, Pignon JP, et al. A randomised trial comparing 5-FU with 5-FU plus cisplatin in advanced pancreatic carcinoma. *Ann Oncol.* 2002;13:1185–1191.
52. Cartwright TH, Cohn A, Varkey JA, et al. Phase II study of oral capecitabine in patients with advanced or metastatic pancreatic cancer. *J Clin Oncol.* 2002;20:160–164.
53. O'Connell MJ, Martenson JA, Wieand HS, et al. Improving adjuvant therapy for rectal cancer by combining protracted-infusion fluorouracil with radiation therapy after curative surgery. *N Engl J Med.* 1994;331:502–507.
54. Mehta VK, Poen JC, Ford JM, et al. Protracted venous infusion 5-fluorouracil with concomitant radiotherapy compared with bolus 5-fluorouracil for unresectable pancreatic cancer. *Am J Clin Oncol.* 2001;24:155–159.
55. Mehta VK, Fisher GA, Ford JM, et al. Adjuvant radiotherapy and concomitant 5-fluorouracil by protracted venous infusion for resected pancreatic cancer. *Int J Radiat Oncol Biol Phys.* 2000;48:1483–1487.
56. Nukui Y, Picozzi VJ, Traverso LW. Interferon-based adjuvant chemoradiation therapy improves survival after pancreaticoduodenectomy for pancreatic adenocarcinoma. *Am J Surg.* 2000;179:367–371.
57. Picozzi VJ, Kozarek R, Rieke JW, et al. Adjuvant combined modality therapy for resected, high-risk adenocarcinoma of the pancreas using cisplatin, 5-FU, and alpha-interferon as radiosensitizing agents: completion of a phase II trial [abstract]. *Proc Am Soc Clin Oncol.* 2003;22:265a.
58. Lawrence TS, Chang EY, Hahn TM, et al. Radiosensitization of pancreatic cancer cells by 2',2'-difluoro-2'-deoxycytidine. *Int J Radiat Oncol Biol Phys.* 1996;34:867–872.
59. Blackstock AW, Bernard SA, Richards F, et al. Phase I trial of twice-weekly gemcitabine and concurrent radiation in patients with advanced pancreatic cancer. *J Clin Oncol.* 1999;17:2208–2212.
60. Wolff RA, Evans DB, Gravel DM, et al. Phase I trial of gemcitabine combined with radiation for the treatment of locally advanced pancreatic adenocarcinoma. *Clin Cancer Res.* 2001;7:2246–2253.
61. McGinn CJ, Zalupski MM, Shureiqi I, et al. Phase I trial of radiation dose escalation with concurrent weekly full-dose gemcitabine in patients with advanced pancreatic cancer. *J Clin Oncol.* 2001;19:4202–4208.
62. Crane CH, Wolff RA, Abbruzzese JL, et al. Combining gemcitabine with radiation in pancreatic cancer: understanding important variables influencing the therapeutic index. *Semin Oncol.* 2001;28(Suppl. 10)S1025–S1033.
63. Van Laethem JL, Demols A, Gay F, et al. Postoperative adjuvant gemcitabine and concurrent radiation after curative resection of pancreatic head carcinoma: a phase II study. *Int J Radiat Oncol Biol Phys.* 2003;56:974–980.
64. Anne D, Marc P, Marc P, et al. Adjuvant gemcitabine (GEM) and concurrent continuous radiation (45Gy) for resected pancreatic head carcinoma: a multicenter Belgian phase II study [abstract]. *Proc Am Soc Clin Oncol.* 2003;22:282a.
65. Blackstock AW, Tepper J, Kachnic L, et al. Adjuvant gemcitabine and concurrent radiation for resected pancreatic cancer: a phase II study [abstract]. *Proc Am Soc Clin Oncol.* 2003;22:266a.
66. Birkmeyer JD, Siewers AE, Finlayson EVA, et al. Hospital volume and surgical mortality in the United States. *N Engl J Med.* 2002;346:1128–1137.
67. Birkmeyer JD, Warshaw AL, Finlayson SR, et al. Relationship between hospital volume and late survival after pancreaticoduodenectomy. *Surgery.* 1999;126:178–183.
68. Neoptolemos JP, Stocken DD, Dunn JA, et al. Influence of resection margins on survival for patients with pancreatic cancer treated by adjuvant chemoradiation and/or chemotherapy in the ESPAC-1 randomized controlled trial. *Ann Surg.* 2001;234:758–768.
69. Millikan KW, Deziel DJ, Silverstein JC, et al. Prognostic factors associated with resectable adenocarcinoma of the head of the pancreas. *Am Surg.* 1999;65:618–624.
70. Wayne JD, Abdalla EK, Wolff RA, et al. Localized adenocarcinoma of the pancreas: the rationale for preoperative chemoradiation. *The Oncologist.* 2002;7:34–45.

71. Evans DB, Rich TA, Byrd DR, et al. Preoperative chemoradiation and pancreaticoduodenectomy for adenocarcinoma of the pancreas. *Arch Surg.* 1992;127:1335–1339.
72. Pisters PWT, Abbruzzese JL, Janjan NA, et al. Rapid-fractionation preoperative chemoradiation, pancreaticoduodenectomy, and intraoperative radiation therapy for resectable pancreatic adenocarcinoma. *J Clin Oncol.* 1998;16:3843–3850.
73. Pisters PWT, Wolff RA, Janjan NA, et al. Preoperative paclitaxel and concurrent rapid-fractionation radiation for resectable pancreatic adenocarcinoma: toxicities, histologic response rates, and event-free outcome. *J Clin Oncol.* 2002;20:2537–2544.
74. Wolff RA, Evans DB, Crane CH, et al. Initial results of a preoperative gemcitabine (GEM)-based chemoradiation for resectable pancreatic adenocarcinoma [abstract]. *Proc Am Soc Clin Oncol.* 2002;21:130a.
75. Hoffman JP, Lipsitz S, Pisansky T, et al. Phase II trial of preoperative radiation therapy and chemotherapy for patients with localized, resectable adenocarcinoma of the pancreas: an Eastern Cooperative Oncology Group Study. *J Clin Oncol.* 1998;16:317–323.
76. McGinn CJ, Talamonti MS, Small W, et al. A phase II trial of full-dose gemcitabine with concurrent radiation therapy in patients with resectable or unresectable non-metastatic pancreatic cancer [abstract]. San Francisco: Proceedings of Gastrointestinal Cancers Symposium (ASCO, AGA, ASTRO, SSO). January 2004:89a.
77. Hoffman JP, McGinn CJ, Szarka C, et al. A phase I study of preoperative gemcitabine with radiation therapy followed by postoperative gemcitabine for patients with resectable pancreatic adenocarcinoma [abstract]. *Proc Am Soc Clin Oncol.* 1998;19:283a.
78. Garcia-Aguilar J, Hernandez de Anda E, Sirivongs P, et al. A pathologic complete response to preoperative chemoradiation is associated with lower local recurrence and improved survival in rectal cancer patients treated by mesorectal excision. *Dis Colon Rectum.* 2003;46:298–304.
79. Ancona E, Ruol A, Santi S, at al. Only pathologic complete response to neoadjuvant chemotherapy improves significantly the long term survival of patients with resectable esophageal squamous cell carcinoma: final report of a randomized, controlled trial of preoperative chemotherapy versus surgery alone. *Cancer.* 2001;91:2165–2174.
80. Darnton SJ, Archer VR, Stocken DD, et al. Preoperative mitomycin, ifosfamide, and cisplatin followed by esophagectomy in squamous cell carcinoma of the esophagus: pathologic complete response induced by chemotherapy leads to long-term survival. *J Clin Oncol.* 2003;21:4009–4015.
81. White R, Lee C, Anscher M, et al. Preoperative chemoradiation for patients with locally advanced adenocarcinoma of the pancreas. *Ann Surg Oncol.* 1999;6:38–45.
82. Kamthan AG, Morris JC, Dalton J, et al. Combined modality therapy for stage II and stage III pancreatic carcinoma. *J Clin Oncol.* 1997;15:2920–2927.
83. Wolff RA, Abbruzzese J, Evans DB. Neoplasms of the exocrine pancreas. In: Holland JF, Frei E III, eds. *Cancer Medicine* (6th ed.). Hamilton: BC Decker Inc., 2003:1585–1614.
84. Pingpank JF, Hoffman JP, Ross EA, et al. Effect of preoperative chemoradiotherapy on surgical margin status of resected adenocarcinoma of the head of the pancreas. *J Gastrointest Surg.* 2001;5:121–130.
85. White RR, Hurwitz HI, Morse MA, et al. Neoadjuvant chemoradiation for localized adenocarcinoma of the pancreas. *Ann Surg Oncol.* 2001;8:758–765.
86. Mehta VK, Fisher G, Ford JA, et al. Preoperative chemoradiation for marginally resectable adenocarcinoma of the pancreas. *J Gastrointest Surg.* 2001;5:27–35.
87. Kastl S, Brunner T, Hermann O, et al. Neoadjuvant radiochemotherapy in the advanced primarily non-resectable carcinomas of the pancreas. *Eur J Surg Oncol.* 2000;26:578–582.
88. Mornex FM, Ychou M, Bossard N, et al. Preoperative concurrent chemoradiation in resectable pancreatic cancer: the French phase II FFCD9704-SFRO [abstract]. *Proc Am Soc Clin Oncol.* 2003;22:290a.
89. Al Sukhun S, Zalupski MM, Ben-Josef E, at al. Chemoradiotherapy in the treatment of regional pancreatic carcinoma: a phase II study. *Am J Clin Oncol.* 2003;26:543–549.
90. Wanebo HJ, Glicksman AS, Vezeridis MP, et al. Preoperative chemotherapy, radiotherapy, and surgical resection of locally advanced pancreatic cancer. *Arch Surg.* 2000;135:81–87.
91. Coia L, Hoffman J, Scher R, et al. Preoperative chemoradiation for adenocarcinoma of the pancreas and duodenum. *Int J Radiat Oncol Biol Phys.* 1994;30:161–167.
92. Safran H, King T, Choy H, et al. Paclitaxel and concurrent radiation for locally advanced pancreatic and gastric cancer: a phase I study. *J Clin Oncol.* 1997;15:901–907.
93. Todd KE, Gloor B, Lane JS, et al. Resection of locally advanced pancreatic cancer after downstaging with continuous-infusion 5-fluorouracil, mitomycin-C, leucovorin, and dipyridamole. *J Gastrointest Surg.* 1998;2:159–166.
94. Pipas JM, Mitchell SE, Barth RJ, et al. Phase I study of twice-weekly gemcitabine and concomitant external-beam radiotherapy in patients with adenocarcinoma of the pancreas. *Int J Radiat Oncol Biol Phys.* 2001;50:1317–1322.
95. Ammori JB, Colletti LM, Zalupski MM, et al. Surgical resection following radiotherapy with concurrent gemcitabine in patients with previously unresectable adenocarcinoma of the pancreas. *J Gastrointest Surg.* 2003;7:766–772.
96. Kim HJ, Czischke K, Brennan MF, Conlon KC. Does neoadjuvant chemoradiation downstage locally advanced pancreatic cancer? *J Gastrointest Surg.* 2002;6:763–769.
97. Povoski SP, Karpeh MS, Conlon KC, et al. Association of preoperative biliary drainage with postoperative outcome following pancreaticoduodenectomy. *Ann Surg.* 1999;230:131–142.
98. Pisters PW, Hudec WA, Lee JE, et al. Preoperative chemoradiation for patients with pancreatic cancer: toxicity of endobiliary stents. *J Clin Oncol.* 2000;18:860–867.
99. Pisters PWT, Hudec W, Hess KR, et al. Effect of preoperative biliary decompression on pancreaticoduodenectomy-associated morbidity in 300 consecutive patients. *Ann Surg.* 2001;234:47–55.
100. Lowy AM, Lee JE, Pisters PW, et al. Prospective randomized trial of octreotide to prevent pancreatic fistula after pancreaticoduodenectomy for malignant disease. *Ann Surg.* 1997;226:632–641.

101. Goldberg RM, Morton RF, Sargent, DJ, et al. N9741: oxaliplatin (Oxal) or CPT-11 + 5-fluorouracil (5FU)/leucovorin (LV) or oxal + CPT-11 in advanced colorectal cancer (CRC): updated efficacy and quality of life (QOL) data from an intergroup study. *Proc Am Soc Clin Oncol.* 2003;22:252.
102. Philip PA, Zalupski MM, Vaitkevicius VK, et al. Phase II study of gemcitabine and cisplatin in the treatment of patients with advanced pancreatic carcinoma. *Cancer.* 2001;92:569–577.
103. Louvet C, Andre T, Lledo G, et al. Gemcitabine combined with oxaliplatin in advanced pancreatic adenocarcinoma: final results of a GERCOR multicenter phase II study. *J Clin Oncol.* 2002;20:1512–1518.
104. Rocha Lima CM, Savarese D, Bruckner H, et al. Irinotecan plus gemcitabine induces both radiographic and CA 19-9 tumor marker responses in patients with previously untreated advanced pancreatic cancer. *J Clin Oncol.* 2002;20:1182–1191.
105. Hidalgo M, Castellano D, Paz-Ares L, et al. Phase I–II study of gemcitabine and fluorouracil as a continuous infusion in patients with pancreatic cancer. *J Clin Oncol.* 1999;17:585–592.
106. Colucci G, Giuliani F, Gebbia V, et al. Gemcitabine alone or with cisplatin for the treatment of patients with locally advanced and/or metastatic pancreatic carcinoma: a prospective, randomized phase III study of the Gruppo Oncologia dell'Italia Meridionale. *Cancer.* 2002;94:902–910.
107. Berlin JD, Catalono P, Thomas JP, et al. Phase III study of gemcitabine in combination with fluorouracil versus gemcitabine alone in patients with advanced pancreatic carcinoma: Eastern Cooperative Group Trial E2297. *J Clin Oncol.* 2002;20:3270–3275.
108. Kindler HL, Friberg G, Stadler WM, et al. Bevacizumab plus gemcitabine is an active combination in patients with advanced pancreatic cancer: interim results of an ongoing phase II trial from the University of Chicago Phase II Consortium [abstract]. San Francisco: Proceedings of Gastrointestinal Cancers Symposium (ASCO, AGA, ASTRO, SSO). January 2004:84a.
109. Crane CH, Ellis LM, Xiong H, et al. Preliminary results of a phase I study of rhuMab VEGF (bevacizumab) with concurrent radiotherapy (XRT) and capecitabine [abstract]. San Francisco: Proceedings of Gastrointestinal Cancers Symposium (ASCO, AGA, ASTRO, SSO). January 2004:84a.
110. Laheru D, Biedrzycki B, Jaffee EM. Immunologic approaches to the management of pancreatic cancer. *Cancer J.* 2001;7:324–337.
111. Gjertsen MK, Bakka A, Breivik J, et al. Vaccination with mutant ras peptides and induction of T-cell responsiveness in pancreatic carcinoma patients carrying the corresponding ras mutation. *Lancet.* 1995;346:1399–1400.
112. Finn OJ, Jerome KR, Henderson RA, et al. MUC-1 epithelial tumor mucin-based immunity and vaccines. *Immunol Rev.* 1995;145:61–89.
113. Ramanathan RK, Lee K, Mckolanis J, et al. Phase I study of a MUC-1 synthetic vaccine admixed with SB-AS2 adjuvant in resected and locally advanced pancreatic cancer [abstract]. *Proc Am Soc Clin Oncol.* 2000;19:45a.
114. Janetzki S, Palla D, Rosenhauer V, et al. Immunization of cancer patients with autologous cancer-derived heat shock protein gp96 preparations: a pilot study. *Int J Cancer.* 2000;88:232–238.
115. Jaffee EM, Hruban RH, Biedrzycki B, et al. Novel allogeneic granulocyte-macrophage colony-stimulating factor-secreting tumor vaccine for pancreatic cancer: a phase I trial of safety and immune activation. *J Clin Oncol.* 2001; 19:145–156.
116. Desai J, Mitchell P, Loveland B, et al. A phase I trial of dendritic cells pulsed with MUC-1 peptide in patients with solid tumors [abstract]. *Proc Am Soc Clin Oncol.* 2002; 21:15a.
117. Morse MA, Nair SK, Boczkowski D, et al. The feasibility and safety of immunotherapy with dendritic cells loaded with CEA mRNA following neoadjuvant chemoradiotherapy and resection of pancreatic cancer. *Int J Gastrointest Cancer.* 2002;32:1–6.
118. Tamm E, Charnsangavej C. Pancreatic cancer: current concepts in imaging for diagnosis and staging. *Cancer J.* 2001;7:298–311.
119. O'Malley ME, Boland GWL, Wood BJ, et al. Adenocarcinoma of the head of the pancreas: determination of surgical unresectability with thin-section pancreatic-phase helical CT. *AJR Am J Roentgenol.* 1999;173:1510–1518.
120. Forsmark CE, Lambiase L, Vogel SB. Diagnosis of pancreatic cancer and prediction of unresectability using the tumor-associated antigen CA19-9. *Pancreas.* 1994;9: 731–734.
121. Schlieman MG, Ho HS, Bold RJ. Utility of tumor markers in determining resectability of pancreatic cancer. *Arch Surg.* 2003;138:951–955.
122. Wolff RA, Ayers GD, Crane CH, et al. Serum CA19-9 levels in patients receiving preoperative gemcitabine-based chemoradiation for resectable pancreatic adenocarcinoma [abstract]. *Proc Am Soc Clin Oncol.* 2003:22:267a.
123. Safi S, Schlosser W, Falkenreck S, Berger HG. Prognostic value of CA 19-9 serum course in pancreatic cancer. *Hepatogastroenterology.* 1998;45:253–259.
124. Wilkowski R, Thoma M, Duhmke E, et al. Concurrent chemoradiotherapy with gemcitabine and cisplatin after incomplete (R1) resection of locally advanced pancreatic carcinoma. *Int J Radiat Oncol Biol Phys.* 2004;58: 768–772.
125. Grabenbauer GG, Beck JD, Erhardt J, et al. Postoperative radiotherapy of medulloblastoma. Impact of radiation quality on treatment outcome. *Am J Clin Oncol.* 1996;19:73–77.
126. Dieckmann K, Potter R, Wagner W, et al. Up-front centralized data review and individualized treatment proposals in a multicenter pediatric Hodgkin's disease trial with 71 participating hospitals: the experience of the German–Austrian pediatric multicenter trial DAL-HD-90. *Radiother Oncol.* 2002:62:191–200.
127. Verweij J, Nielsen OS, Therasse P, et al. The use of systemic therapy checklist improves quality of data acquisition and recording in multicentre trials: a study of the EORTC Soft Tissue and Bone Sarcoma Group. *Eur J Cancer.* 1997;33:1045–1049.

CHAPTER

27

Postoperative Adjuvant Therapy and the Rationale for the US Intergroup Trial

Young Kwok, MD
Michael C. Garofalo, MD
William F. Regine, MD

Despite the obvious evolution in our three major cancer treatment modalities—surgery, radiation, and chemotherapy—the overall prognosis of patients with pancreatic cancer remains dismal. In the United States, the annual age-adjusted pancreatic cancer death rate has been fairly steady over the last 30–40 years, with the estimated 30,700 new cases being nearly matched by the estimated 31,860 deaths in 2004.[1] Although this may be in part attributed to the limitations and the less than optimal integration of our current treatment modalities, it is in large part caused by the biologically aggressive nature of this malignancy. Only 10%–15% of patients with pancreatic cancer are able to undergo "potentially" curative resection, and despite this, the 5-year survival is usually less than 20%.[2-7] Even among the most favorable subset of patients—those with tumors measuring less than 3 cm, microscopically negative resection margins, and/or negative lymph node status—the 5-year survival is no more than 36%.[3,5-10] Studies by the Gastrointestinal Tumor Study Group (GITSG) have evaluated external beam radiation therapy with or without 5-fluorouracil (5-FU) in patients with locally unresectable disease. These studies have shown a definite survival advantage to the use of 5-FU in combination with radiation therapy. In addition, analyses of the patterns of failure after pancreatic resection suggest that both local and distant recurrences are frequent. Such failure patterns suggest a potential benefit to the addition of adjuvant chemoradiation.[11,12] The results of randomized trials, the evolving institutional and cooperative group experiences, and the future of postoperative adjuvant therapy for pancreatic cancer are presented in this chapter.

Adjuvant Randomized Trials: Immunotherapy

Randomized trials of immunotherapy in the adjuvant setting are rarely ever quoted, and all five were performed in Europe. The University of Ulm, Germany, reported the first published study of adjuvant immunotherapy. After resection, a total of 61 patients were randomized to intravenous murine monoclonal antibody 494/32 (an IgG1 antibody to human pancreatic cancer cells) or observation. The long-term prognosis was very poor in both groups, with the median survivals of the treatment and control arms being 14.1 and 12.7 months (no statistical difference), respectively.[13] Although the study was very safe and small, the authors concluded that the antibody was not helpful in the adjuvant setting of patients with pancreatic cancer.

In the 1990s, the group from Athens Medical Center conducted a series of four randomized trials of adjuvant locoregional chemoimmunotherapy for postoperative pancreatic cancer patients. The first study randomized 86 patients to locoregional chemoimmunotherapy versus observation. The treatment arm entailed locoregional delivery of interleukin (IL)-2, interferon-γ, mitomycin, cisplatin, 5-FU, and leucovorin via two arterial catheters, placed at the time of surgery in the superior mesenteric artery (SMA) and the splenic artery. The treatment arm had significantly longer survivals, with the median survival of the treatment and observation groups being 30 and 16.8 months ($P < 0.001$), respectively.[14]

The second trial published from the same group was a smaller study that randomized 26 patients to neoadjuvant and adjuvant locoregional chemoimmunotherapy versus observation. The treatment arm consisted of neoadjuvant IL-2, resection, and adjuvant locoregional carboplatin and docetaxel via catheters in the SMA and the splenic artery. The authors concluded that the study offered clear evidence to the benefit of this approach because 11 of the 14 treatment arm patients were alive without evidence of disease (range, 9–29 months).[15] The median and actuarial survival data were not reported.

The third trial reported by the Athens group randomized 512 patients after curative intent ($n = 274$) and palliative surgery ($n = 238$) to locoregional chemoimmunotherapy versus observation. The treatment arm consisted of locoregional delivery of gemcitabine, carboplatin, mitoxantrone, IL-2, and interferon-γ via splenic artery and SMA catheters. The regimen was given every 2 months for the first year and every 3 months thereafter. In the curative-intent arm, the treatment significantly improved the mean survival (32 vs 14 months), although the P value and the actuarial survival analysis were not reported.[16]

The latest study published by the same group randomized 128 postoperative patients to locoregional chemotherapy versus locoregional chemoimmunotherapy versus observation.[17] The chemotherapy arm ($n = 45$) consisted of locoregional delivery of gemcitabine, carboplatin, mitoxantrone, mitomycin, 5-FU, and folinic acid via a catheter into the SMA. The chemoimmunotherapy arm ($n = 43$) consisted of delivery of the previously mentioned chemotherapy agents as well as IL-2 via the SMA catheter. The toxicity was acceptable, and only six patients required removal of the catheters, four of which were replaced. The study was terminated early when interim analysis revealed significant differences in survival. The mean and 2- and 5-year survivals were as follows: 19 months, 29% and 0% for observation; 25 months, 53% and 0% for locoregional chemotherapy; and 31 months, 65% and 18% for locoregional chemoimmunotherapy. There were statistically significant differences in survival between all three groups ($P < 0.05$), with the best arm being the locoregional chemoimmunotherapy arm.

Although these studies are interesting, they have had limited impact because they can be viewed essentially as a single-institutional experience. The statistical analyses in the Athens studies were poor. Three of the studies did not report median survivals, whereas two of the studies did not report P values or actuarial survival analysis. Finally, the long-term prognosis in the best arm (i.e., locoregional chemoimmunotherapy) was still very poor, with a 5-year overall survival of 18%.

Adjuvant Randomized Trials: Chemotherapy

An infrequently quoted Norwegian trial, conducted from 1984–1987, demonstrated a statistically significant doubling in median survival for patients treated with adjuvant chemotherapy. Unfortunately, there was no associated significant improvement in long-term survival. The study compared adjuvant adriamycin, mitomycin, and 5-FU (AMF) chemotherapy ($n = 30$) to observation ($n = 31$). Therapy involved AMF given once every 3 weeks for six cycles. Overall, patients randomized to AMF had a median survival of 23 months as compared with 11 months in the control group ($P = 0.02$). However, this did not translate into a significant difference in long-term prognosis. The 2-, 3-, and 5-year survivals in the treatment group were 43%, 27%, and 4%, respectively, compared with 32%, 30%, and 8% in the observation group ($P = 0.6$ after 2 years).[18] Furthermore, the toxicity of combination chemotherapy was substantial. These included hematologic, cardiac, and renal toxicities that necessitated hospitalization in 73% of patients. As a result, less than one half of the patients were compliant with all treatment cycles.

The Japanese Study Group of Surgical Adjuvant Therapy for Carcinomas of the Pancreas and Biliary Tract has recently reported the results of a randomized trial of adjuvant chemotherapy for resected pancreaticobiliary carcinomas. Between 1986 and 1992, the trial randomized 508 patients with resected pancreaticobiliary carcinomas to mitomycin and 5-FU combination chemotherapy ($n = 232$) versus observation ($n = 204$). Therapy involved mitomycin given the day of surgery and 5-FU given during weeks 1 and 3 after surgery and then continuing with

Table 27.1 Randomized Chemotherapy Trials

		Survivals		
	n	Median (Months)	2-Year (%)	5-Year (%)
Norwegian				
Therapy	30	23.0	43	4
Observation	31	11.0	32	8
		$P = 0.02$		$P = 0.6$ (after 2 years)
Japanese*				
Therapy	81			11.5
Observation	77			18.0
				$P =$ NS

* Pancreatic carcinoma subgroup.

5-FU alone for 1 additional year beginning 5 weeks after surgery. Primary tumor sites included bile duct, gallbladder, and the ampulla of Vater; 158 patients (31%) had resected pancreatic carcinomas. Combination chemotherapy was well tolerated, with greater than 80% of patients receiving their planned doses. However, a significant improvement in 5-year survival with postoperative mitomycin, and 5-FU was limited only to the subgroup of patients with gallbladder carcinoma (26.0% vs. 14.4%, $P = 0.037$). Among the patients with pancreatic carcinoma, the 5-year survivals for the treatment and observation groups were 11.5% and 18.0%, respectively (no statistical difference).[19] A summary of the two chemotherapy trials is shown in Table 27.1.

Adjuvant Randomized Trials: Concurrent Chemoradiation

Among patients who have undergone a potentially curative resection, for nearly 20 years, phase III evaluation of postoperative adjuvant chemoradiation had been limited to a single trial. The GITSG trial (1974–1982), although terminated early because of poor patient accrual, showed a statistically significant doubling in median survival and modest improvement in 5-year survival for patients receiving adjuvant split-course chemoradiation. The trial randomized 43 patients with pancreatic adenocarcinoma who were felt to have undergone potentially curative resections with negative margins to chemoradiation versus observation. Therapy involved a split-course 40 Gy in 6 weeks with a 2-week break after the first 20 Gy, and 3-day infusions of 5-FU at the start of weeks 1 and 5, followed by weekly infusions of maintenance 5-FU for 2 years or until disease progression. Twenty-one patients randomized to adjuvant split-course chemoradiation had a median survival of 21 months, a 2-year survival of 43%, and a 5-year survival of 19% compared with 11 months, 18%, and 5%, respectively, for the observation group ($P = 0.03$). There were no life-threatening complications or deaths attributable to therapy.[20,21] These results were duplicated in an additional cohort of 30 patients treated on a nonrandomized basis achieving median and 2-year survivals of 18 months and 46%, respectively, and a 5-year survival of 17%, further substantiating the benefits of adjuvant chemoradiation.[21,22] Only 2 of the 51 treated patients (4%) in the GITSG study developed possible late treatment-related complications.

More recently, the European Organization for Research and Treatment of Cancer (EORTC) reported a phase III trial evaluating the same split-course chemoradiation regimen as in the GITSG trial but without maintenance therapy versus observation in patients after curative resection for cancer of the pancreatic head or periampullary region. Patients were stratified by tumor location. A total of 218 patients were randomized (110 to treatment and 108 to observation) from 1987–1995, of which 114 (52%) had pancreatic head lesions—60 to treatment and 54 to observation. Not surprisingly, therapy was well tolerated, with maximal World Health Organization toxicity being grade III and observed in only 7 patients; however, 21 patients in the treatment arm (20%) did not receive any treatment because of postoperative morbidity or patient refusal.

In the treatment arm, the median overall survival was 24.5 months, and the 2-year survival was 51% compared with 19 months and 41% for the observation group ($P = 0.208$). When analyzed by tumor location, the periampullary cancer group demonstrated median, 2-year, and 5-year survivals of 39.5 months, 70%, and 38% , respectively, for those randomized to treatment as compared with 40.1 months, 64%, and 36% for observation ($P = 0.737$). For pancreatic head tumors, the median, 2-year, 5-year survivals for those randomized to treatment were 17.1 months, 37%, and 20%, respectively as compared with 12.6 months, 23%, and 10% for those randomized to observation ($P = 0.099$).[23] The results of this trial cannot be considered definitive given the lack of use of maintenance therapy in the adjuvant regimen, the inclusion of patients with positive resection margins without stratification, the lack of radiation therapy quality assurance, and lack of statistical power. For example, to have had an 80% chance of detecting an increase in 2-year survival from 40%–55% would have required randomization of more than 300 patients, roughly three times the number of patients with pancreatic cancer actually entered.[24]

In 2001 the European Study Group of Pancreatic Cancer (ESPAC) reported a postoperative adjuvant trial, ESPAC-1. The trial accrued 541 eligible patients with pancreatic adenocarcinoma from 1994–2000. The design of the trial was complex, and the treating physician had an option to enter a patient into one of three randomization design arms: (1) chemotherapy versus no chemotherapy ($n = 188$), (2) chemoradiation versus no chemoradiation ($n = 68$), and (3) a 2×2 factorial design of observation versus chemotherapy versus chemoradiation versus chemoradiation with maintenance chemotherapy ($n = 285$). The therapy was very similar to the GITSG and EORTC trials with split-course radiotherapy of 40 Gy and 5-FU, but folinic acid was added. The results of the trial, based on pooled statistics of all three design arms in an intent-to-treat analysis, suggested a lack of benefit to chemoradiation versus no chemoradiation (15.5 vs 16.1 months, $P = 0.24$) and a survival benefit to chemotherapy versus no chemotherapy (19.7 vs 14.0 months, $P = 0.0005$). However, in the 2×2 factorial design arm, there were no differences in survival between chemotherapy versus no-chemotherapy patients (17.4 vs 15.9 months, $P = 0.19$), and there were no survival differences in any of the individual arms.[25] In the 2004 update report of the 2×2 factorial arm (median follow-up, 47 months), the analysis suggested now a detriment to chemoradiation versus no chemoradiation (15.9 vs 17.9 months, $P = 0.05$) and again the superiority of chemotherapy versus no chemotherapy (20.1 vs 15.5 months, $P = 0.009$), even though the study did not have the statistical power to compare these four groups directly.[26]

There have been a number of serious issues raised concerning the validity of this trial.[27] At its very essence, the trial cannot be considered a true randomized trial if the physician had a choice as to which design arm a patient is enrolled. This may have introduced serious biases that may not be readily apparent in the statistical analysis. For example, the median time to start of therapy after resection was 2 weeks longer for those assigned to the chemoradiation arm compared with the chemotherapy arm. Furthermore, the median survival in the chemoradiation arm (13.9 months) in the update report compares poorly with the older GITSG and EORTC reports (21.0 and 17.1 months, respectively). Rather, this trial should be thought of as three different trials being run simultaneously with the reporting of the pooled data analogous to a meta-analysis of the three trials. In addition, the physician had an option to give any "background therapy" before the patient entered the trial. Consequently, when the data were pooled from the three design arms, more than a third of the chemotherapy design arm (both yes and no arms) received "background therapy" that consisted of chemoradiation or chemotherapy. This could have significantly increased the median survival of the chemotherapy arm.

Furthermore, the adjuvant therapy used the split-course radiotherapy and bolus 5-FU and thus cannot be considered modern. Most patients in American academic centers are treated with dose-intensive 50.4–54 Gy via three-dimensional conformal radiotherapy without a planned break, whereas the chemotherapy is typically a continuous infusion (CI) of 5-FU. Finally, the quality assurance in this trial was less than ideal. There was no central radiation therapy quality-assurance monitoring of adequate dosimetry, physics support, or machine specifications. Because of these serious flaws, the results of ESPAC-1 have not changed practice in the United States, where concurrent chemoradiation continues to remain the standard of care. The ESPAC has taken the results of ESPAC-1 and eliminated radiotherapy from the design of the follow-up trial, ESPAC-3. This trial, now under accrual, randomizes patients to 5-FU plus folinic acid versus gemcitabine. Originally, an observation arm was included but was later closed when the final results of ESPAC-1 showed that the chemotherapy alone was the superior arm. A summary of the three chemoradiation trials is shown in Table 27.2.

The Evolution Toward Dose-Intensive Adjuvant Chemoradiation

Postoperative adjuvant therapy for pancreatic carcinoma and other gastrointestinal sites has evolved to higher dose, non-split course radiation and potentially more toxic chemoradiation regimens as compared with that used in the GITSG and EORTC/ESPAC trials.[27-30] Phase III evaluation of such an approach in rectal carcinoma, with use of radiation doses of 50.4–54 Gy in 6 weeks combined with CI 5-FU, has been associated with a significant improvement in survival when compared with a less dose-intensive postoperative chemoradiation regimen.[31] Whether similar improvements can be achieved without significant upper abdominal toxicity in patients with pancreatic carcinoma needs evaluation; however, phase II experiences have been promising.

Table 27.2 Randomized Chemoradiation Trials

		Survivals		
	n	Median (Months)	2-Year (%)	5-Year (%)
GITSG*				
Therapy	21	21.0	43	19
Observation	22	10.9	18	5
		$P = 0.03$		
EORTC†				
Therapy	60	17.1	37	20
Observation	54	12.6	23	10
		$P = 0.099$		
ESPAC-1				
Pooled Data (2001 Report)				
Chemotherapy	238	19.7		
No Chemotherapy	235	14.0 ($P = 0.0005$)		
ChemoRT	175	15.5		
No ChemoRT	178	16.1 ($P = 0.24$)		
2 × 2 Factorial Arm (2001 Report)				
Chemotherapy	146	17.4		
No Chemotherapy	139	15.9 ($P = 0.19$)		
ChemoRT	142	15.8		
No ChemoRT	143	17.8 ($P = 0.09$)		
2 × 2 Factorial Arm (2004 Update)				
Chemotherapy	147	20.1		
No Chemotherapy	142	15.5 ($P = 0.009$)		
ChemoRT	145	15.9	29	10
No ChemoRT	144	17.9 ($P = 0.05$)	41	20
Observation	69	16.9	11	
ChemoRT	73	13.9		7
Chemotherapy	75	21.6		29
ChemoRT + chemotherapy	72	19.9 ($P =$ NS)		13

*Original report.
†Pancreatic carcinoma subgroup.
Abbreviation: ChemoRT, chemoradiotherapy.

The Mayo Clinic experience among 29 patients treated with postoperative chemoradiation after potentially curative resection is reflective of an evolution toward dose-intensive adjuvant therapy. Nine patients were treated with split-course therapy, whereas the remainder was treated with continuous-course therapy. The median dose of radiation used was 54 Gy, with a range of 35–60 Gy. Twenty-seven of 29 patients also received concurrent bolus 5-FU chemotherapy. The median, 2-year, 3-year, and 5-year survivals for the group were 23 months, 48%, 24%, and 12%, respectively. Seventeen percent developed late treatment-related complications, whereas the rate of small bowel obstruction requiring operation among those receiving more than 45 Gy was 4.2%.[27]

The evolving Johns Hopkins Hospital experience with increasingly intensive chemoradiation after resection for adenocarcinoma of the pancreas was updated in 1997, with 173 patients undergoing three options of postoperative adjuvant therapy: (1) 99 patients receiving "standard" split-course or continuous-course radiation to doses of 40–45 Gy in conjunction with concurrent bolus 5-FU, (2) 21 patients receiving "intensive" therapy involving continuous-course radiation of 50.4–57.6 Gy to the tumor bed and prophylactic hepatic irradiation of 23.4–27 Gy with CI 5-FU plus leucovorin concurrently and as maintenance for 4 months, and (3) 53 patients having no therapy. The "intensive" therapy group experienced increased toxicity and had no survival benefit when compared with the "standard" therapy group. However, patients receiving adjuvant therapy had median and 2-year survivals of 19.5 months and 39% compared with 13.5 months and 30% for the patients who received no therapy ($P = 0.03$).[9,30]

The M.D. Anderson Cancer Center experience with postoperative adjuvant therapy among a cohort of 19 patients made use of infusional chemoradiation (50.4 Gy in 28 fractions over 5.5 weeks with CI 5-FU at 300 mg/m^2 per day) and intraoperative election-beam radiation therapy (10–15 Gy). The median, 2-year, and 3-year survivals for these patients were 22 months, 55%, and 39%, respectively.[32]

The Eastern Cooperative Oncology Group reported the results of a phase I trial evaluating the maximum tolerated dose of CI 5-FU with concurrent radiation in 25 patients with unresectable, residual, or recurrent carcinoma of the pancreas or bile duct.[33] Beginning at 200 mg/m^2 per day, CI 5-FU was given concurrently with radiation therapy (59.4 Gy in 33 fractions over 6–7 weeks). Chemotherapy began and continued through the entire course of treatment. After each cohort of five patients had been treated and observed, the daily dose was escalated in 25 mg/m^2 increments until dose-limiting toxicity was encountered. The dose-limiting toxicity was oral mucositis, and the maximum tolerated dose of 5-FU was found to be 250 mg/m^2 per day.

Although more dose-intensive chemoradiation regimens have become more prevalent, an associated improvement in patient outcome has, at most, been modest. In addition, the survival results achieved with 5-FU–based chemoradiation or combination chemotherapy regimens have reached a plateau, with median, 2-, 3-, and 5-year survivals of approximately 22 months, 45%, 30%, and less than 20%, respectively. Distant metastases continue to be a major cause of mortality in these patients; thus, the need for more effective systemic therapy is clear.

Gemcitabine, Background for Inclusion in the US Intergroup Trial

In 1996 the US Food and Drug Administration (FDA) approved gemcitabine for use in patients with pancreatic cancer. This was the first chemotherapeutic agent since 5-FU to be approved for use in patients with pancreatic cancer in 35 years. Gemcitabine is also unique in that the FDA approved the compound despite an objective response rate of 5.4%.[34] The FDA approved gemcitabine based on two registration trials in patients with symptomatic stage IV pancreatic cancer.[35,36] These trials introduced the concept of clinical benefit response. Pancreatic cancer patients almost always have devastating symptoms, including pain and weight loss, and experience declining performance status. Objective responses are also frequently difficult to assess noninvasively. Investigators combined changes in pain control, weight loss, and performance status to create clinical benefit response. The FDA accepted this patient-centered endpoint for the evaluation of gemcitabine in pancreatic cancer.

In the first trial, investigators randomized 126 stable symptomatic patients to one of two chemotherapy arms: (1) gemcitabine 1,000 mg/m^2 weekly for 7 weeks followed by a week's rest and then four cycles consisting of three weekly doses of gemcitabine at 1,000 mg/m^2 and 1 week rest[34] or (2) bolus 5-FU. The clinical benefit response was 24% for gemcitabine and 5% for 5-FU ($P = 0.0025$). In addition, patients achieving symptomatic relief did so within 6 weeks of initiating therapy. Symptomatic benefit lasted an average of 12 weeks. In addition to an improvement in clinical benefit, gemcitabine improved the median survival from 4.41 months with 5-FU to 5.65 months with gemcitabine ($P = 0.0025$). The average survival was 2% for patients receiving 5-FU and 18% for patients receiving gemcitabine. The second registration trial was a single-arm phase II trial in 63 patients who failed 5-FU.[35] Treatment was with gemcitabine at the same dose and schedule. The clinical benefit response was 27%, and the 1-year survival was 4%. The median survival was 3.9 months. Based on these two trials, the FDA approved gemcitabine in the treatment of advanced pancreatic cancer as both frontline and salvage therapy. The toxicity of gemcitabine was mild to moderate. Only 10% of patients discontinued therapy because of toxicity, and the most common toxicity was myelosuppression. Other toxicities included hepatitis, nausea, vomiting, hair loss, skin rash, and fever. Gemcitabine is now used in the primary therapy for metastatic pancreatic cancer. These results have also encouraged the use of gemcitabine in an adjuvant situation.

Postoperative Adjuvant Therapy: US Intergroup Trial

The Radiation Therapy Oncology Group completed a large randomized study of over 500 patients in July of 2002, and the results have yet to be reported. This US Intergroup trial (including the Eastern Cooperative On-

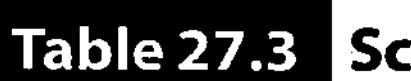

Table 27.3 Schema for US Intergroup Phase III Study of Prechemoradiation and Postchemoradiation 5-FU vs Prechemoradiation and Postchemoradiation Gemcitabine for Postoperative Adjuvant Treatment of Pancreatic Adenocarcinoma

STRATIFY		RANDOMIZE	Schema						
S T R	Surgical Margins 1. Negative 2. Positive 3. Unknown	R A N D	Arm 1:	Pre-CRT 5-FU	+	CRT (5-FU + RT)	+	Post-CRT 5-FU
A T	Tumor Diameter 1. < 3 cm 2. ≥ 3 cm	O M						
I F Y	Nodal Status 1. Negative 2. Positive	I Z E	Arm 2:	Pre-CRT Gemcitabine	+	CRT (5-FU + RT)	+	Post-CRT Gemcitabine

PRE-CRT CHEMOTHERAPY: Starting 3–8 weeks after definitive resection.
Arm 1: 3 weeks of CI 5-FU at 250 mg/m²/day.
Arm 2: 3 weeks of Gemcitabine at 1,000 mg/m²/day, once weekly.

CHEMORADIATION: Starting 1–2 weeks after completion of pre-CRT chemotherapy.
Arms 1 and 2: 50.4 Gy in 5.5 weeks at 1.8 Gy/fraction (field reduction after 45 Gy) concurrently with CI 5-FU at 250 mg/m²/d during radiation.

POST-CRT CHEMOTHERAPY: Starting 3–5 weeks after completing CRT.
Arm 1: Two cycles of CI 5-FU (one cycle = 4 weeks of CI 5-FU at 250 mg/m²/day ‡ 2 week rest) for a total duration of 3 months.
Arm 2: Three cycles of Gemcitabine (one cycle = 3 weeks of Gemcitabine at 1,000 mg/m²/d once weekly ‡ 1 week rest) for a total duration of 3 months.

Abbreviations: CRT, chemoradiation; CI, continuous infusion.

cology Group and the Southwest Oncology Group) tested prechemoradiation and postchemoradiation 5-FU versus prechemoradiation and postchemoradiation gemcitabine in the postoperative setting. The concurrent chemoradiation portion was identical in both treatment arms and consisted of concurrent 5-FU. This trial represents the first American phase III cooperative group study in nearly a quarter century (GITSG trial activated February 1974) evaluating adjuvant chemoradiation in patients with localized and resected adenocarcinoma of the pancreas. The schema of the trial is illustrated in Table 27.3.

The study incorporates modern therapeutic principles of chemoradiation and current developments in chemotherapy in pancreatic cancer. The study is the first of its kind to require prospective radiation therapy quality assurance. All radiation treatment fields, along with preoperative diagnostic information, are reviewed for compliance to protocol requirements before the start of chemoradiation. Examples of typical conventional anteroposterior "large fields" for pancreatic tumors of the head, body, and tail are shown in Figs. 27.1, 27.2, and 27.3, respectively. An example of a typical conventional lateral "large field" for pancreatic tumors is shown in Fig. 27.4. A companion biomolecular basic science study to the US Intergroup study is planned. This study is also the first to prospectively evaluate the ability of postresection CA 19-9 to predict outcome in pancreatic carcinoma.

Future Directions

Many questions remain to be answered in the adjuvant management of patients with pancreatic adenocarcinoma. Optimized integration of conventional treatment modalities of radiation, chemotherapy, and surgery still need to be established. Radiation dose, fractionation, and volume are critical issues that remain to be resolved, especially in conjunction with new cytotoxic agents that pose their own unique set of questions, including mode of drug delivery, combination of drugs, and dose intensification. The use of specialized programs such as intraoperative radiation, immunotherapy, and intensity-modulated radiation therapy has also not been fully explored. Evolving knowledge

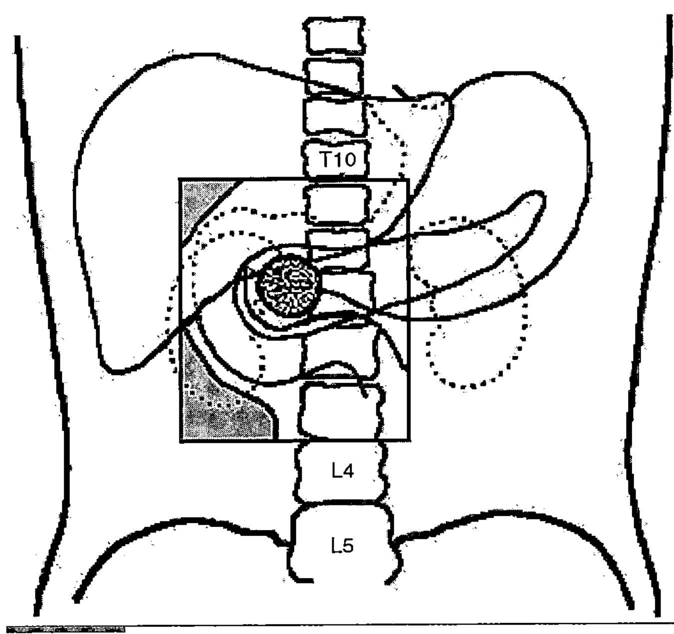

Figure 27.1
Field guidelines: head of the pancreas tumor.

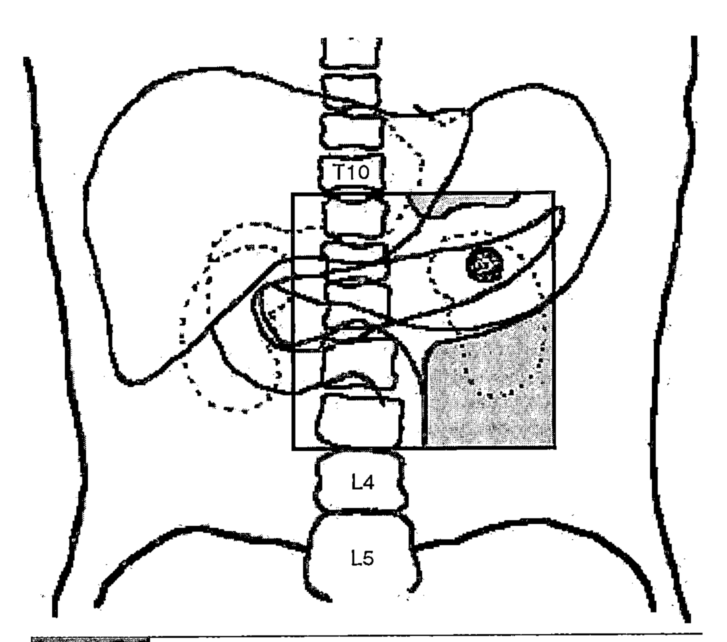

Figure 27.3
Field guidelines: tail of the pancreas tumor.

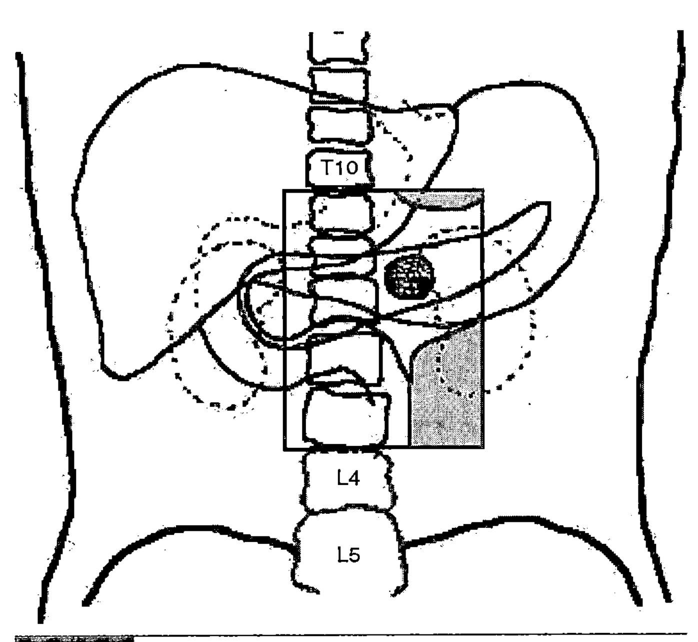

Figure 27.2
Field guidelines: body of the pancreas tumor.

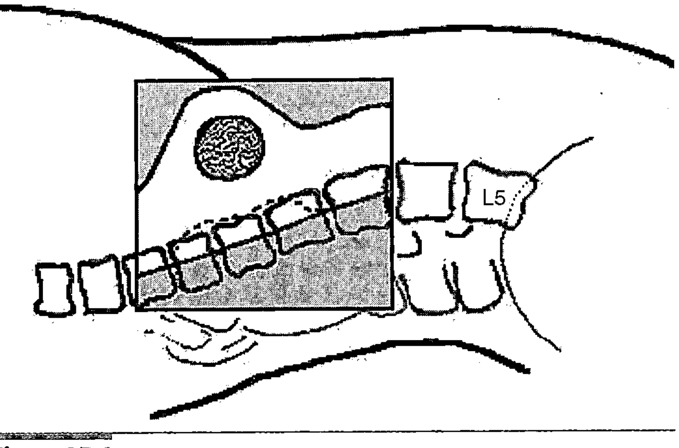

Figure 27.4
Field guidelines: lateral field.

in the biological behavior of these tumors based on genetic fingerprints could provide useful guides to designing customized treatment strategies. Mutations involving *p53*, *ras*, and *HER2/neu* have been implicated in conferring enhanced resistance to conventional adjuvant treatment strategies. Understanding the genetic profile of pancreatic cancers will be of immense value in shaping future treatment strategies. Future trials will have the opportunity to build upon modern, multi-institutional, quality-controlled, randomized trials that integrate and evaluate the potential of novel chemotherapy and radiotherapy combinations, basic science discovery, serum tumor markers, and quality-of-life issues.

References

1. Jemal A, Tiwari RC, Taylor M, et al. Cancer statistics, 2003. *Ca Cancer J Clin.* 2004;53:5–21.
2. Douglass H. Adjuvant therapy for pancreatic cancer. *World J Surg.* 1995:19:1701–1774.
3. Geer RJ, Brennan MF. Prognostic indicators for survival after resection of pancreatic adenocarcinoma. *Am J Surg.* 1993;165:68–73.
4. Shibamoto Y, Manabe T, Baba M. High dose, external beam and intraoperative radiotherapy in the treatment of resectable pancreatic cancer. *Int J Radiat Oncol Biol Phys.* 1990;19:605–611.
5. Nitecki SS, Sarr MG, Colby TV, Van Heerden JA. Long-term survival after resection for ductal adenocarcinoma of the pancreas: is it really improving? *Ann Surg.* 1995;221:59–66.
6. Piorkowski RJ, Believenicht SW, Lawrence W Jr. Pancreatic and periampullary carcinoma: experience with 200 patients over a 12-year period. *Am J Surg.* 1982;143:189–192.
7. Gudjonsson B. Cancer of the pancreas: 50 years of surgery. *Cancer.* 1987;60:2284–2303.
8. Trede M, Chir B, Schwall G, Saeger H-D. Survival after pancreaticoduodenectomy. *Ann Surg.* 1990;21:447–458.
9. Yeo CJ, Cameron JL, Lillemoe KD, et al. Pancreaticoduodenectomy for cancer of the head of the pancreas: two hundred and one patients. *Ann Surg.* 1995;221:721–731.
10. Gastrointestinal Tumor Study Group. Therapy of locally unresected pancreatic carcinoma: a randomized comparison of high dose (6000 rads) radiation alone, moderate dose radiation (4000 rads + 5-fluorouracil), and high dose radiation + 5-fluorouracil. *Cancer.* 1981;48:1705–1710.
11. Whittington R, Bryer MP, Haller DG, Solin LJ, Rosato EF. Adjuvant therapy of resected adenocarcinoma of the pancreas. *Int J Radiat Oncol Biol Phys.* 1991;21:1137–1143.
12. Tepper J, Nardi G, Suit H. Carcinoma of the pancreas: review of MGH experience from 1963 to 1973: analysis of surgical failure and implications for radiation therapy. *Cancer.* 1976;37:1519–1524.
13. Buchler M, Friess H, Schultheiss KH, et al. A randomized controlled trial of adjuvant immunotherapy (murine monoclonal antibody 494/32) in resectable pancreatic cancer. *Cancer.* 1991;68:1507–1512.
14. Lygidakis NJ, Stringaris K, Kokinis K, et al. Locoregional chemotherapy versus locoregional combined immunochemotherapy for patients with advanced metastatic liver disease of colorectal origin: a prospective randomized study. *Hepatogastroenterology.* 1996;43:212–220.
15. Lygidakis NJ, Spentzouris N, Theodoracopoulos M, et al. Pancreatic resection for pancreatic carcinoma combined with neo- and adjuvant locoregional targeting immunochemotherapy—a prospective randomized study. *Hepatogastroenterology.* 1998;45:396–403.
16. Lygidakis NJ, Berberabe AE, Spentzouris N, et al. A prospective randomized study using adjuvant locoregional chemoimmunotherapy in combination with surgery for pancreatic carcinoma. *Hepatogastroenterology.* 1998;45:2376–2381.
17. Lygidakis NJ, Sgourakis G, Georgia D, et al. Regional targeting chemoimmunotherapy in patients undergoing pancreatic resection in an advanced stage of their disease: a prospective randomized study. *Ann Surg.* 2002;236:806–813.
18. Bakkevold KE, Arnesjo B, Dahl O, Cambestad B. Adjuvant combination chemotherapy (AMF) following radical resection of carcinoma of the pancreas and papilla of vater: results of a controlled, prospective, randomized multicentre study. *Eur J Cancer.* 1993;29A:698–703.
19. Takada T, Amano H, Yasuda H, et al. Is postoperative adjuvant chemotherapy useful for gallbladder carcinoma? A phase III multicenter prospective randomized controlled trial in patients with resected pancreaticobiliary carcinoma. *Cancer.* 2002;95:1685–1695.
20. Kalser MH, Ellenberg SS. Pancreatic cancer: adjuvant combined radiation and chemotherapy following curative resection. *Arch Surg.* 1985;12:899–903.
21. Douglass HO, Strablein DM. Ten year follow-up of first generation surgical adjuvant studies of the Gastrointestinal Tumor Study Group. In: Salmon SE, ed. *Adjuvant Therapy of Cancer* (vol. 4). Philadelphia: WB Saunders; 1990:405–415.
22. Gastrointestinal Tumor Study Group. Further evidence of effective adjuvant combined radiation and chemotherapy following curative resection of pancreatic cancer. *Cancer.* 1987;59:2006–2010.
23. Klinkenbijl JHG, Jeekel J, Sahmoud T, et al. Adjuvant radiotherapy and 5-fluorouracil after curative resection of cancer of the pancreas and periampullary region: phase III trial of the EORTC gastrointestinal tract cancer cooperative group. *Ann Surg.* 1999;230:776–784.
24. Simon RMK. Design and analysis of clinic trials. In: DeVita VT, Hellman S, Rosenberg SA, eds. *Cancer: Principles and Practice of Oncology* (5th ed.). Philadelphia: Lippincott-Raven; 1997:513–528.
25. Neoptolemos JP, Dunn JA, Stocken DD, et al. Adjuvant chemoradiation and chemotherapy in resectable pancreatic cancer: a randomized controlled trial. *Lancet.* 2001;358:1576–1585.
26. Neoptolemos JP, Stocken DD, Friess H, et al. A randomized trial of chemoradiotherapy and chemotherapy after resection of pancreatic cancer. *N Engl J Med.* 2004;350:1200–1210.
27. Abrams RA, Lillemoe KD, Piantadosi S. Continuing controversy over adjuvant therapy of pancreatic cancer. *Lancet.* 2001;358:1565–1566.
28. Foo ML, Gunderson LL, Nagorney DM, et al. Patterns of failure in grossly resected pancreatic ductal adenocarcinoma treated with adjuvant irradiation + 5-fluorouracil. *Int J Radiat Oncol Biol Phys.* 1993;26:483–489.
29. Mohiuddin M, Rosato F, Schuricht A, Barbot D, Biermann W, Cantor R. Carcinoma of the pancreas: the Jefferson experience. 1975–1988. *Eur J Surg Oncol.* 1994;20:13–20.
30. Yeo CJ, Hruban RH, Kern SE, et al. Adenocarcinomas of the pancreas: factors influencing outcome after pancreaticoduodenectomy: the Johns Hopkins experience. *Cancer Bull.* 1994;46:504–510.
31. Yeo CJ, Abrams RA, Grochow LB, et al. Pancreaticoduodenectomy for pancreatic adenocarcinoma: postoperative adjuvant chemoradiation improves survival. *Ann Surg.* 1997;225:621–636.
32. Haller DG, Mayer RJ, Gunderson LL, et al. Improving adjuvant therapy for rectal cancer by combining protracted infusion fluorouracil with radiation therapy after curative surgery. *N Engl J Med.* 1994;331:502–507.

33. Spitz FR, Abbruzzese JL, Lee JE, et al. Preoperative and postoperative chemoradiation strategies in patients treated with pancreaticoduodenectomy for adenocarcinoma of the pancreas. *J Clin Oncol.* 1997;15:928–937.
34. Whittington R, Neuberg D, Tester WJ, Benson AB III, Haller DG. Protracted intravenous fluorouracil infusion with radiation therapy management of localized pancreaticobiliary carcinoma: a phase I Eastern Cooperative Group Trial. *J Clin Oncol.* 1995;13:227–232.
35. Burris HA, Moore MJ, Anderson J, et al. Improvements in survival and clinical benefit with gemcitabine as first-line therapy for patients with advanced pancreas cancer: a randomized trial. *J Clin Oncol.* 1997;15:2403–2413.
36. Rothenberg ML, Moore MJ, Cripps MC, et al. A phase II trial of gemcitabine in patients with 5-FU-refractory pancreas cancer. *Ann Oncol.* 1996;7:347–353.

CHAPTER

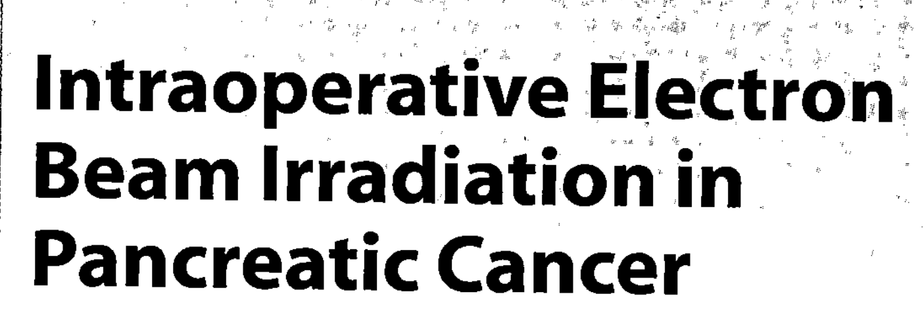

Intraoperative Electron Beam Irradiation in Pancreatic Cancer

Christopher G. Willett, MD
Peter J. Biggs, PhD
Carlos Fernández-del Castillo, MD

In the past 25 years, there has been substantial progress in the experimental and clinical application of intraoperative electron beam radiation therapy (IORT) as a treatment modality for head and neck, thoracic, abdominal, and pelvic neoplasms. Data regarding short- and long-term tolerances of normal tissues frequently irradiated with IORT have been established by canine experiments.[1-12] Clinically, numerous investigators have described treatment strategies and experience with IORT and have explored the potential value and limitations of this modality. More importantly, their efforts have identified disease sites in which IORT in combination with surgery and external beam radiation therapy (EBRT) may be of potential value. This chapter reviews the radiobiologic basis of IORT and technical aspects of treatment and summarizes the experience of this modality for patients with pancreatic cancer.

Experimental IORT Studies

The radiation tolerance of most normal tissues to conventional fractionated EBRT is well understood. Because it is always done during surgery, IORT is given as a single radiation fraction. IORT doses usually range from 20 to 40 Gy when given alone and from 10 to 20 Gy when given in combination with EBRT. The biologic effectiveness of this single fraction is incompletely understood; however, it is believed to be equivalent to that of a dose at least two times greater given by means of conventional fractionation. Data from canine experiments by Gillette et al.[6-12] indicate that the effectiveness of IORT may be as high as five times that of an equivalent dose given by means of conventional fractionation in certain normal tissues. Information about normal tissue tolerance after large single doses (>10 Gy) was first provided by canine experiments at the National Cancer Institute (Bethesda, MD).[1-5]

A series of experiments were done to evaluate the tolerance of normal retroperitoneal structures, including the aorta, vena cava, kidney, ureters, bile duct, and retroperitoneal soft tissues. In addition, attempts were made to define the tolerance of surgically manipulated tissues such as vascular and intestinal anastomosis. Animals were irradiated with doses of 20–50 Gy delivered in a single fraction with an 11-MeV electron beam. Does were selected as the animal model so that the size of the normal structures would be as close as possible to that in humans. Table 28.1 outlines the results of the experiments.[1-5]

To summarize those data, high doses of radiation are poorly tolerated by functioning organ systems, such as the liver and kidney, and by hollow viscus organs,

Table 28.1 Normal-Tissue Tolerance to IORT in Dogs

Tissue	Maximum Tolerated Dose (Gy)	Tissure Effect
Aorta, vena cava	50	Wall fibrosis at >30 Gy
Kidney	<20	Atrophy and fibrosis
Ureter	20	Fibrosis and stenosis
Bile duct	<20	Fibrosis and stenosis
Small intestine	<20	Ulceration, fibrosis, and stenosis at >20 Gy
Colon	15	Ulceration, fibrosis, and stenosis at >15 G

Data are from the National Cancer Institute.[1-5]

Table 28.2 Radiation Tolerance of Manipulated Tissue of Dogs to IORT

Tissue	Maximum Tolerated Dose (Gy)	Tissue Effect
Aortic anastomosis	20	Fibrosis and stenosis at >20 Gy, no anastomosis disruption at >45 Gy
Biliary anastomosis	< 20	Anatomic breakdown at >20 Gy
Defunctionalized small intestine	45	Fibrosis and stenosis at >20 Gy, no suture-line breakdown at >45 Gy

Data are from the National Cancer Institute.[9]

especially those with small diameter (ureter, bile duct, bowel), whereas the retroperitoneal soft tissues, vessels, and bones all appear to tolerate even the highest dose without significant complications. Additional studies were performed to determine the tolerance of surgically manipulated tissues because of the likelihood that manipulated bowel or blood vessels might often be in the radiation field when IORT is combined with resection. These studies, indicate the feasibility of combining IORT with extensive surgical resections, although there are areas in which significant toxicity can result (Table 28.2).[1-5]

Gillette et al.[6-12] have undertaken prospective long-term studies (2–5 years) of the response of normal tissues in a canine model to IORT, IORT with fractionated EBRT, and EBRT alone. Beagles were allocated to one of these three treatment arms: (1) IORT only, with single doses of 15–50 Gy, (2) 10–42.5 Gy IORT combined with 50 Gy EBRT in 2 Gy fractions or (3) ERBT alone, of 50, 60, 70 or 80 Gy given in 30 fractions of 2, 2.33, or 2.67 Gy over 6 weeks. These investigators performed detailed clinical, radiologic, physiologic, and pathologic analysis of irradiated aorta, branch arteries, ureter, bone, and peripheral nerves.

The results of these studies show the following: (1) The toxicity of combined IORT and EBRT is predominantly caused by the effect of IORT, not EBRT, on normal tissues. (2) IORT doses of 10–20 Gy, when combined with EBRT, are the maximum tolerable doses for blood vessels, ureter, bone, and peripheral nerve. (3) Previous experimental and clinical data have probably underestimated the long-term tolerance of normal tissues to IORT (Table 28.3).

Technical Aspects of IORT

At the Massachusetts General Hospital (MGH), there is a dedicated IORT suite within the operating room. This facility simplifies the integration of IORT with surgery and permits complete operating room capability as well as delivery of IORT. There is no requirement of a transport process from the operating room to a radiation therapy suite and operating room personnel (anesthesiologists, operating room nurses, and surgeons) remain in a familiar working environment.

The MGH facility employs the Siemen's ME accelerator, which provides electron energies ranging from 6 to 18 MeV. This system uses a "soft" dock system in which there is no physical contact between the cone and linear accelerator (Fig. 28.1). In the "soft" dock system, the cone is secured in the patient by a modified Bookwalter retraction system. There is no further movement of the cone in the patient after it has been immobilized. Once the patient is under the radiation therapy machine, geometric alignment of the treatment cone with the gantry head is achieved by a laser alignment system with appropriate couch movement and gantry rotation.

A large variety of applicators of different sizes and geometries are available to tailor the treatment to the individual anatomy and topography of the tumor bed. For treatment of the tumors that are commonly irradiated (rectal cancer with pelvic sidewall or sacral involvement, pancreas, bile duct, gastric bed, and abdominal or pelvic lymph node diseases), round cylinders are available at 5, 6, 7, 8, 9 and 10 cm, both with no bevel on the edge of the cylin-

Table 28.3 Tolerance of Canine Retroperitoneal Tissue to IORT/EBRT from Colorado State University

Tissue	Endpoint	Estimated Maximum Tolerated Dose: IORT + EBRT 30 Gy IORT
Aorta wall	Vascular Abnormalities: Branch Aneurysms,Thromboses, Narrowing	
Arteries	Same as above	20 Gy IORT + 50 Gy EBRT
Ureter	Radiographic abnormalities	25 Gy IORT
		17.5 Gy IORT + 50 Gy EBRT
Muscle	Muscle fibers decrease	20–25 Gy IORT + 50 Gy EBRT
	Vessel lesions	
Bone	Necrosis	15–20 Gy IORT + 50 Gy EBRT

Abbreviations: EBRT, external-beam radiation therapy; IORT, intraoperative (electron-beam) radiation therapy.[9-12]

der and with a 15 degree and a 30 degree bevel for each of the nominal cylinder diameters. Small-diameter cylinders of 3 and 4 cm are sometimes useful but have a more limited application. For treatment of some pancreatic tumors and for intra-abdominal tumors such as gastric carcinoma, retroperitoneal sarcomas, and colonic tumors, either rectangular or elliptical applicators should be available. Elliptical applicators of 12 × 7 cm and 11 × 6 cm have been very helpful and are easier to position than rectangular ones. An applicator called the "squircle," which has one circular end and one rectangular end, simplifies the problem of field abutment in patients who require more than one IORT field.

At the time of surgery, the tumor volume (tumor bed after resection or unresectable tumor) to be irradiated is defined by the surgeon and the radiation oncologist and marking sutures are placed around the perimeter of the lesion. An applicator is then selected that encompasses the tumor bed, usually with a 1-cm margin. A margin of at least 1 cm is optimal to allow for both dose and tumor variabilities. When the tumor or tumor bed is visualized through the cone, the marking sutures should be readily identified well within the perimeter of the cone, thus ensuring adequate coverage of the tumor volume.

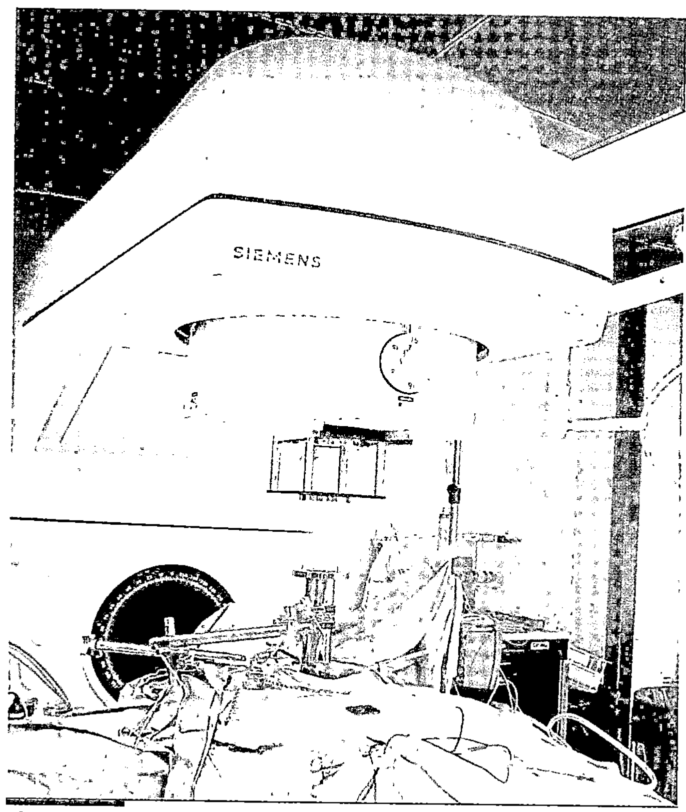

Figure 28.1
The Siemen's ME Accelerator.

Although the IORT cone can often function adequately as a normal tissue retractor to hold sensitive normal structures out of the IORT field, patient respiration or spontaneous movement of the bowel can allow normal tissues to move under the cone and insinuate themselves inside the intraoperative field. The cone must be observed to confirm that this is not occurring. If there is evidence that bowel or other normal tissues slip into the IORT field, surgical packing must be used to displace the tissues from the field. It is important that the packing itself does not enter into the field because this will decrease the electron beam penetration resulting in underdosage of a portion of the tumor volume.

There are certain situations in which normal tissues cannot be physically moved out of the radiation field. Thus, it is essential that a technique be available for secondary shielding. We have available standard lead sheets, which can be cut to the appropriate shape and an appropriate number used to attenuate 90% of the radiation beam. The lead is covered with saline-soaked gauze and placed over the normal tissues. Lead shielding is often essential if abutting IORT fields are to be used. Other methods for secondary collimation may be used, but we have found this method to be effective.

IORT is currently used as a component of a comprehensive treatment program of preoperative or postoperative external beam irradiation (45–54 Gy in 25–28 fractions), frequently with concurrent chemotherapy and surgery for a locally advanced malignancy. Because most patients have received a course of full-dose external beam irradiation, IORT doses usually are in the range of 7.5–20 Gy. The selection of dose as well as electron energy is dependent on the amount of residual tumor remaining after maximal resection. Guidelines are as follows: resection margin negative but narrow, – 7.5 to 10 Gy; margin microscopically positive or res(m), – 10 to 12.5 Gy; gross residual-res(g), 2 cm or less in largest diameter, –15 Gy; unresected or res(g) of 2 cm or greater, – 17.5 to 20 Gy. Doses of 20 Gy or higher are not used unless there have been limitations of delivery of external beam irradiation (EBRT).

Results of Clinical Studies Using Intraoperative Radiation Therapy for Pancreatic Cancer

Locally Advanced Pancreatic Cancer

Numerous institutions in Europe, Japan, and the United States have evaluated IORT in the treatment of patients with pancreatic cancer. European and Japanese investigators generally have used a large single dose of electron-beam IORT (20–40 Gy) without EBRT. At the MGH, the Mayo Clinic, and many other American institutions, IORT has been used as a boost treatment (10–20 Gy) in combination with EBRT and resection, when feasible.

Initial investigations during the 1970s and 1980s examined the feasibility, toxicity, and value of IORT in patients with locally advanced pancreatic tumors. This subset constitutes 40% of patients with pancreatic cancer.[13] Because these patients are unresectable by a Whipple procedure or distal pancreatectomy (mostly because of invasion of the portal or mesenteric vessels), treatment for these patients has usually been limited to combinations of EBRT and chemotherapy.

Conventional EBRT for unresectable pancreatic cancer improves the median survival when combined with 5-fluorouracil (5-FU) chemotherapy.[14] Because of the limited tolerance of normal tissue in the upper abdomen (liver, kidney, spinal cord, and bowel) to EBRT, total doses of only 45–54 Gy, in 25–30 fractions, have usually been given. For an unresectable lesion, this is an inadequate dose of irradiation, and treatment results from both prospective and retrospective studies reflect this, with high rates of tumor progression and poor survival. The Mayo Clinic reported a local failure rate of 72% for 122 patients with unresectable pancreatic cancer treated by 40–60 Gy EBRT.[15,16] In this setting of poor local control by conventional techniques, IORT is a logical means of increasing the effective radiation dose to the pancreatic tumor, with avoidance of normal-tissue treatment.

In the 1970s and 1980s, the treatment regimen at MGH was a combination of low-dose preoperative irradiation, IORT, and high-dose postoperative irradiation.[17-19] Patients with locally advanced unresectable disease without any evidence of distant metastases (by abdominal computed tomography [CT] scan and laparoscopy) received 10–15 Gy of preoperative irradiation to the pancreas and nodal tissue to prevent tumor seeding during surgery. The patients were then taken to the operating room, where an exploratory laparotomy was performed to determine whether any metastatic disease was present. If metastases were found, the patient was not eligible for the IORT. If a Whipple resection or distal pancreatectomy was possible, this was performed, and IORT was not delivered. If the tumor was thought to be locally unresectable (usually because of tumor adherence or fixation to the portal vein or superior mesenteric vessels, hepatic artery, or celiac axis), the patients were evaluated for IORT. Patients were acceptable for the IORT if an applicator could fully encompass the gross disease detectable at the time of surgery and if there was no evidence of metastatic disease beyond the regional nodes. Patients were treated with circular applicators measuring 6–9 cm. Electron energies were in the range of 15–23 MeV. This gave a 90% isodose line at the depth of 3.8–6.3 cm overall, with the depth chosen to conform to the measured thickness of the tumor mass at the time of exploration.

Patients received approximately 20 Gy in a single fraction calculated at the 90% isodose line. Biliary bypass was performed if biliary obstruction was present or imminent or if the bile duct was in the IORT field. Gastrojejunostomy was performed if there was a high risk of gastric-outlet obstruction or if any portion of the duodenum was in the IORT field. Generally, stomach and large and small bowel were excluded from the radiation field, except for a portion of the C-loop of the duodenum, which was irradiated.

After recovery from the surgery, the patients returned for postoperative irradiation, with an additional dose of

35–39.6 Gy being delivered by a four-field technique to the clipped pancreatic tumor. Postoperative irradiation was usually administered in coordination with intravenous 5-FU, generally on the first 3 days of postoperative irradiation. The median survival was 13 months for the first 68 patients who completed the entire protocol of preoperative irradiation, IORT, and postoperative irradiation. For 33 patients with tumors less than 5 cm in greater diameter, the 2-year actuarial survival and IORT control results were 20% and 56%, respectively, whereas for 35 patients with tumors greater than 5 cm, these results were 3% and 43%, respectively. Because the locoregional control rates were similar for lesions less than 5 cm and for those greater than 5 cm, the difference in survivals was likely due to the more rapid development of metastases in patients with lesions greater than 5 cm. Fifty-four of the 68 patients experienced distant metastases. Analysis of the sites of distant metastasis indicates that intra-abdominal locations (liver and peritoneal surfaces) were the most common sites, with 33 patients developing hepatic metastases and 12 patients with peritoneal spread. Local failure as an isolated failure pattern was less common, only 9 of 68 patients. It appears that abdominal metastases, predominantly liver, dominate the clinical course of these patients. The most frequent long-term normal-tissue morbidity was duodenal ulceration, which was usually satisfactorily managed by medical means.

Forty of the 68 patients had pain at presentation, requiring analgesics. Twenty-three of these 40 (58%) patients remained pain-free, without analgesics, until death. The early data from the MGH suggested better local control with the use of misonidazole as a hypoxic cell sensitizer than for an earlier group of patients treated with IORT but without the use of misonidazole.[18] However, this trend was not supported by follow-up data, which showed no advantage to the use of misonidazole. Median survival without misonidazole (15.7 months) was actually superior to that with misonidazole (12.5 months).[19]

The use of multiagent systemic chemotherapy in an attempt to control occult metastatic disease with pancreatic cancer has been disappointing, with most studies demonstrating no significant benefits from the use of chemotherapy alone.[20] Because of the high incidence of hepatic and peritoneal metastases and the poor results with standard chemotherapy, current and future therapeutic efforts now include evaluation of irradiation with new agents (taxol and gemcitabine). In our current phase I/II study, we are combining preoperative irradiation to the pancreas (50.4 Gy) with continuous-infusion 5-FU and weekly gemcitabine followed by restaging 3–4 weeks after completion of EBRT. If there is no evidence of distant metastases, IORT will be given to the primary pancreatic lesion. With this approach, we hope to improve locoregional control, as well as reducing the incidence of hepatic and peritoneal metastases.

The other major group studying IORT in unresectable pancreatic cancer has been the Mayo Clinic.[15,16] These investigators used IORT (20 Gy) first, followed by high-dose postoperative irradiation. Data from their initial studies revealed a highly significant advantage in local control with IORT and external irradiation, in comparison with external irradiation alone (40–60 Gy). The actuarial local control at 1 year for those who received IORT is 82% compared with 48% for those who did not. At 2 years, it was 66% and 20%, respectively ($P = 0.0005$). The significant improvement in local control did not translate into a survival advantage in the IORT group because of the high (>50%) incidence of abdominal failure in both groups. Median survival from the day of exploration was 12.6 months in the external irradiation alone group and 13.4 months in the IORT group, and the 2-year overall survivals were 16.5% and 12%, respectively.

The Mayo Clinic investigators have reported their results on using full-dose EBRT before IORT in an effort to improve patient selection for IORT.[22] This sequence allows restaging at 2–2.5 months after initiation of treatment. Of the initial 51 patients enrolled in this treatment schedule, 14 (27%) did not receive IORT (excluding three patients with recurrent disease and one patient with islet-cell tumor), the actuarial incidences of local control at 1 and 2 years were 86% and 68%, respectively. The median survival of 14.9 months in their current series compares favorably with survivals in other IORT and external-beam series. When compared with 56 patients treated during the same period at the Mayo Clinic with a different treatment sequence (IORT followed by high-dose EBRT), the median and overall 2- and 5-year survivals (calculated from the date of diagnosis) observed in the current series (full dose EBRT before IORT) were statistically higher (median, 14.9 months compared with 10.5 months; 2-year survival, 27% vs 6%; and 5-year survival, 7% vs 0%).

Survival improvements seen in the high-dose preoperative group of IORT patients probably reflect altered and improved patient selection, rather than treatment effect. These differences suggest that giving a full component of EBRT with 5-FU before exploration and IORT may be more appropriate than giving IORT as an initial component of treatment. The altered sequence did result in 27% of patients not receiving IORT as additional treatment because of already documented disease progression.

However, the alteration in treatment sequence did not appear to influence the incidence of abdominal-disease control. Actuarial local control at 1 year appeared to be better in the high-dose preoperative external-irradiation group (85% compared with 65%); however, this difference did not reach statistical significance.

Investigators at the National Cancer Institute reported results of IORT in the treatment of patients with unresectable pancreatic carcinoma.[23] Thirty-two patients with unresectable stage III (locally advanced, positive nodes) or stage IV (visceral or peritoneal metastases) pancreatic carcinoma underwent biliary and gastric bypasses and were randomly assigned to receive either IORT of 25 Gy and postoperative EBRT of 50 Gy to the upper abdomen or postoperative EBRT of 60 Gy without IORT. Both groups were treated with postoperative 5-FU. Median survival times for patients with stage III and stage IV disease were not different between the IORT and EBRT groups (8 months); however, for those with stage III disease, the median survival time and time to disease progression were superior in the IORT group. Complications in patients treated at the National Cancer Institute included late duodenal hemorrhage in three of 16 patients. They had one early death from respiratory failure in their IORT group.

In 1985, the Radiation Therapy Oncology Group began a study of IORT plus EBRT for patients with locally unresected nonmetastatic pancreatic cancer.[24] Patients were treated with a combination of 20 Gy of IORT and postoperative EBRT to 50.4 Gy, in combination with intravenous 5-FU (500 mg/m^2/day on the first 3 days of the EBRT). Eighty-six patients were entered in the study through June 1, 1988 and analyzed through April 1990. Fifty-one patients were fully analyzable. The median survival time of the 51 patients was 9 months, with an 18-month actuarial survival rate of 9%. Local control could not be adequately evaluated in this multi-institutional study. Major postoperative complications were not excessive and occurred in 12% of patients. Two patients had major late morbidity leading to death, one from duodenal bleeding and the second from biliary obstruction. Although this study does demonstrate the feasibility of IORT in a multi-institutional setting, it does not demonstrate any advantage of IORT over conventional therapy for this disease.

A more contemporary approach to the use of concurrent and maintenance chemotherapy was reported by investigators from Thomas Jefferson Medical Center. In this study, 49 patients with locally advanced pancreatic cancer received 10 to 20 Gy of IORT followed by postoperative irradiation with concurrent and maintenance 5-FU and leucovorin chemotherapy. Median survival was 16 months, with a 2-year survival rate of 22%, figures significantly better than historic control subjects. Local failure was seen in 31%. Early postsurgical morbidity was observed in 7 of 49 patients (14%) and late treatment related morbidity in 8 of 43 (19%) alive beyond 6 months.

Resectable Pancreatic Cancer

Local recurrence has been reported in 50%–90% of patients treated with pancreaticoduodenectomy for adenocarcinoma of the pancreas.[25] Efforts to improve local control have included the use of preoperative and postoperative irradiation with 5-FU. In the Gastrointestinal Tumor Study Group, 45 patients were randomized after resection to receive no further treatment or irradiation plus 5-FU.[26] A survival advantage was seen with the combined treatment, which had a 2-year survival rate of 42% and a 5-year survival rate of 14% over the control arm, which had a 2-year survival rate of 15% and a 5-year survival rate of 5%. The Gastrointestinal Tumor Study Group registered 30 additional patients in the treatment group and replicated and confirmed the improved survival.[27]

In the ESPAC I trial, a survival advantage was seen in patients receiving adjuvant 5-FU and leucovorin.[21]

Although overall survival has been improved by the use of EBRT and 5-FU, the incidence of tumor-bed recurrence has been reported to be as high as 60%, despite adjuvant treatment. This rate of failure is likely due to the high incidence of residual microscopic disease at the standard surgical–transection margins and in retroperitoneal soft tissues after pancreaticoduodenectomy and the inadequacy of 40–50 Gy of EBRT in controlling this level of tumor burden.[25]

IORT also has been added as a component of treatment for resectable disease, either at the time of initial surgical resection or after preoperative irradiation. Technically, IORT after pancreaticoduodectomy is delivered to the surgical tumor bed and includes, in the target area, large vessels and retroperitoneal tissues, whereas organ displacement protects the biliary duct, pancreatic remnant, right kidney upper pole, liver, stomach, transverse colon, and small bowel. The combination of tumor resection and high-dose radiation therapy (using well-designed IORT boosts) does generate the highest local control rates in pancreatic cancer, ranging from 80% to 90%. Reni et al.[28] have reported results with surgery alone in patients with resectable tumors or combined with IORT (10–17.5 Gy). In the 203 patients analyzed (127 boosted with IORT), there was no increased operative morbidity or mortality among the treatment groups. In early stages (I to II), local control was significantly superior for the IORT group (63% vs 40%, $P = 0.04$). There was also a significantly prolonged time to local failure (17.2 vs 12 months, $P = 0.003$), time to failure (17 vs 11.5 months, $P = 0.005$), as well as improved overall survival (18.5 vs 13 months, $P = 0.01$).

Summary

IORT is a technique in which a single high-dose fraction radiation treatment is administered at the time of surgery. With the use of IORT, the total radiation dose delivered to a tumor can be increased because sensitive normal tissues are removed from the radiation field during the surgical procedure. Furthermore, although the biologic effectiveness of this single fraction is incompletely understood, it is believed to be equivalent to that of a dose at least two times greater given by means of conventional fractionation. IORT may improve local tumor control in patients with resectable or locally advanced pancreatic cancer.

References

1. Tepper JE, Sindelar W. Summary of the workshop on intraoperative radiation therapy. *Cancer Treat Rep*. 1981; 65:911–918.
2. Sindelar W, Tepper JE, Travis EL. Tolerance of bile duct to intraoperative irradiation. *Surgery*. 1980;92:533–542.
3. Sindelar WF, Kinsella R, Tepper JE, Travis EL, Rosenberg SA, Glatstein E. Experimental and clinical studies with intraoperative radiotherapy. *Surg Gynecol Obstet*. 1983;157: 205–218.
4. Sindelar WF, Tepper JE, Travis EL, Terril RL. Tolerance of retroperitoneal structures to intraoperative radiation. *Ann Surg*. 1981;5:601–608.
5. Kinsella TJ, Sindelar WF, Deluea AM. Tolerance of peripheral nerve to IORT: clinical and experimental studies. *Int J Radiat Biol Oncol Phys*. 1985;11:1579–1585.
6. Ahmadu-Suka F, Gillette EL, Withrow SJ, Hasted PW, Nelson AW, Whiteman CE. Pathologic response of the pancreas and duodenum to experimental intraoperative irradiation. *Int J Radiat Oncol Biol Phys*. 1988;14: 1197–1204.
7. Gillette EL, Powers BE, McChesney SL, Withrow SJ. Aortic wall injury following intraoperative irradiation. *Int J Radiat Oncol Biol Phys*. 1988;15:1401–1406.
8. LeCouteur RA, Gillette EL, Powers BE, Child G, McChesney SL, Ingram JT. Peripheral neuropathies following experimental intraoperative radiation therapy (IORT). *Int J Radiat Oncol Biol Phys*. 1989;17:583–590.
9. Hoopes PJ, Gillette EL, Withrow SJ. Intraoperative irradiation of the canine abdominal aorta and vena cava. *Int J Radiat Oncol Biol Phys*. 1989;17:583–590.
10. McChesney Gillette SL, Gillette EL, Powers BE, Park RD, Withrow SJ. Ureteral injury following experimental intraoperative radiation therapy. *Int J Radiat Oncol Biol Phys*. 1989;17:791–798.
11. Powers BE, Gillette EL, McChesney Gillette SL, LeCoutcur RA, Withrow SJ. Bone necrosis and tumor induction following experimental intraoperative irradiation. *Int J Radial Oncol Biol Phys*. 1989;17:559–567.
12. Powers BE, Gillette EL, McChesney SL, LeCoutre RA, Withrow SJ. Muscle injury following experimental intraoperative irradiation. *Int J Radiat Oncol Biol Phys*. 1991;20:463–471.
13. Warshaw AL, Fernandez-Del Castillo C. Pancreatic carcinoma. *N Engl J Med*. 1992;326:455–464.
14. Moertel CG, Frytak S, Hahn RG, O'Connell MJ, Reitemeier RG, Rubin J. Gastrointestinal Tumor Study Group. Therapy of locally unresectable pancreatic cancer. *Cancer*. 1981;48:1705–1710.
15. Gunderson LL, Martin JK, Kvols LK, et al. Intraoperative and external beam irradiation ±5 FU for locally advanced pancreatic cancer. *Int J Radial Oncol Biol Phys*. 1986;13:319–329.
16. Roldan GE, Gunderson LL, Nagorney DM, et al. External beam vs intraoperative and external beam irradiation for locally advanced pancreatic cancer. *Cancer*. 1988;61:1110–1114.
17. Wood WC, Shipley WU, Gunderson LL, Cohen AL, Nardi GL. Intraoperative irradiation for unresectable pancreatic carcinoma. *Cancer*. 1982;49:1272–1275.
18. Shipley WU, Wood WC, Tepper JE, et al. Intraoperative electron beam irradiation for patients with unresectable pancreatic carcinoma. *Ann Surg*. 1984;200:289–296.
19. Tepper JE, Shipley WU, Warshaw AL, Nardi GL, Wood WC, Orlow EL. The role of misonidazole combined with intraoperative radiation therapy in the treatment of pancreatic carcinoma. *J Clin Oncol*. 1987;5:579–584.
20. Gastrointestinal Tumor Study Group. Treatment of locally unresectable carcinoma of the pancreas: comparison of combined modality therapy (chemotherapy plus radiotherapy) to chemotherapy alone. *J Natl Cancer Inst*. 1988;80:751–756.
21. Neoptolemos J, Stocker D, Friess H, et al. A randomized trial of chemoradiotherapy and chemotherapy after resection of pancreatic cancer. *N Engl J Med*. 2004;350: 1200–1210.
22. Garton GR, Gunderson LL, Nagomey DM, et al. High dose preoperative external beam and intraoperative irradiation for locally advanced pancreatic cancer. *Int J Radial Oncol Biol Phys*. 1993;27:1153–1157.
23. Sindelar WF, Kinsella TJ. Randomized trial of intraoperative radiotherapy in unresectable carcinoma of the pancreas. *Int J Radiat Oncol Biol Phys*. 1986;12(Suppl 1):S148–S149.
24. Tepper JE, Moyes D, Krall JM, et al. Intraoperative radiation therapy of pancreatic carcinoma: a report of RI'OG-8505. *Int J Radiat Oncol Biol Phys*. 1991;21:1145–1149.
25. Willet CG, Lewandrowski K, Warshaw AL, Efird J, Compton CC. Resection margins in carcinoma of the head of the pancreas. *Ann Surg*. 1992;217:144–148.
26. Kalser MAI, Ellenberg SS. Pancreatic cancer: adjuvant combined resection and chemotherapy following curative resection. *Arch Surg*. 1985;120:899–903.
27. Gastrointestinal Tumor Study Group. Further evidence of effective adjuvant combined radiation and chemotherapy following curative resection for pancreatic cancer. *Cancer*. 1987;59:2006–2010.
28. Reni M, Parucci M, Fesseti A, et al. Effect of local control and survival of electron beam intraoperative irradiation for resectable pancreas cancer. *Int J Radiat Oncol Biol Phys*. 2001;50:651–658.

CHAPTER 29

Systemic Therapy and Chemo-Radiotherapy

Ross A. Abrams, MD

Among patients with pancreatic adenocarcinoma, most (75%–80%) present with disease in the periampullary region of the pancreas (head, neck, uncinate process).[1] Unfortunately, 80% of patients with periampullary, pancreatic adenocarcinoma have a tumor that is not resectable for cure, either because of evidence of hepatic, peritoneal, or extra-abdominal dissemination, or, in the absence of such spread, inability to resect the tumor because of encasement of critical vascular structures.[2] These latter patients are designated as locoregionally unresectable or advanced, and their treatment is palliative, given the limitations of currently available, nonsurgical modalities. Consequently, this discussion relates predominantly to locoregionally unresectable adenocarcinoma of the periampullary pancreas.

Treatment of these patients presents many challenges. Some are technical, such as the need to use a meaningful dose of irradiation (if radiotherapy is to be a component of management) without exceeding renal, hepatic, gastric, duodenal, or spinal cord tolerance. Some are philosophical, such as finding the appropriate balance between treatment side-effect burden and limited treatment benefit in the presence of limited prognosis and minimally to moderately effective treatment options. Some involve issues of physician style and patient/family desire regarding communication, information sharing, and decision making in a threatening and anxiety-provoking clinical context.

This chapter attempts to bring clarity to the issues involved in treating these patients and to provide a review of the data available for rational decision making.

Nonmetastatic Presentations of Periampullary Pancreatic Adenocarcinoma: Resectable, Marginally Resectable, and Unresectable

Issues of clinical staging and pathology are presented elsewhere in this volume. Nevertheless, for this discussion, certain principles require emphasis.

The designation of a patient as having locoregionally unresectable pancreatic adenocarcinoma implies incurability and a limited prognosis. This is in contrast to the prognosis anticipated after successful resection, in which there is both expectation of possible cure and superior median survival.[3] This is also in contrast to expectations with locoregionally unresectable pancreatic malignancies that are not adenocarcinomas, such as nonfunctioning islet cell tumors or non-Hodgkin's lymphoma, in which there may be significantly increased expectation for survival (islet cell) or perhaps even opportunity for cure (lymphoma).[4-6]

Defining a case as locoregionally unresectable requires the collaborative input of a diagnostic radiologist experienced in interpreting appropriately obtained, contrast-enhanced, multiphased, helical computed tomographic scans of the abdomen and of an experienced pancreatic surgeon. The importance of surgical experience in these domains has been well documented because patients declared to be locally unresectable for cure at exploratory laparotomy by nonexpert pancreatic surgeons are frequently found to be resectable when explored by expert pancreatic surgeons at major referral centers.[7,8]

The features that define locoregionally unresectable status relate to tumor encasement of the superior mesenteric artery and vein, portal vein, and major branches of the celiac axis, especially the common and proper hepatic artery, in the absence of clinically evident hepatic, peritoneal, or extra-abdominal tumor. Between clearly resectable and clearly unresectable locoregional presentations, there is an intermediate presentation of relatively limited major vessel extension, variously called marginally or potentially resectable (Table 29.1).

Often, surgeons prefer to treat patients who have "potentially resectable features" with chemotherapy and radiotherapy combinations initially and reassess for surgery 6–8 weeks thereafter. This approach has the virtues of moving directly to active intervention, being the standard of care for clearly unresectablepatients, and not imposing the morbidity and treatment delay that would be associated with laparotomy without successful resection. Patients showing response to chemotherapy and radiotherapy may have an improved opportunity for resection (i.e., be less "marginal"), and patients showing tumor progression or dissemination have been spared surgical intervention that would likely have been futile. Patients successfully resected along this algorithm are often included in reports of conversion from unresectable to resectable[9-11] after chemoradiotherapy. Although this is a valid clinical paradigm that has the advantages of avoiding potentially futile operative interventions, the failure to distinguish *clearly unresectable* from *marginally or potentially resectable* presentations (Table 29.1) in describing this management has the potential to cause confusion and unrealistic expectations for truly unresectable patients, especially among patients, families, and physicians who are not expert in the management of periampullary, pancreatic adenocarcinoma. Patients who undergo exploratory surgery by expert surgeons and whose disease is found to be locoregionally unresectable are only extremely rarely found to have resectable disease after concurrent chemotherapy and radiotherapy. In the experience of Kim et al[12] at Memorial Sloan-Kettering, only one case of 87 was converted to resectability by chemotherapy and radiotherapy after determination of locally unresectable disease at exploration. Thus, there are varying operational definitions of unresectability, depending on whether the judgment was made by imaging, exploration by a nonexpert pancreatic surgeon, or exploration by an expert pancreatic surgeon. A special comment regarding the term *neoadjuvant* seems in order at this point. In the context of pancreatic adenocarcinoma, this term is probably best reserved for the use of chemotherapy and radiotherapy given before definitely anticipated surgery in patients presenting with *clearly resectable* imaging and clinical features who are directed toward the sequence of chemoradiotherapy followed by surgery because of institutional preference for this approach as the curative algorithm. A more hopeful use of the same term *neoadjuvant*, referring to chemotherapy and radiotherapy given to patients with marginally resectable features in the hope that this may be followed by surgery, is also understandable. However, using this term in patients whose disease is clearly unresectable serves only to confuse and obscure the realities and limitations of these latter, more ominous presentations.

The Eastern Cooperative Oncology Group (ECOG) is prospectively studying the ability to convert marginally resectable patients to resectability in trial E1200, in which patients are randomly assigned to either weekly

Table 29.1 Resectability Criteria

Structure	Potentially Resectable	Truly Unresectable
SMA	Tangential abutment	Encasement (i.e., ~360°)
SMV	Narrowing or occlusion <2 cm	Occlusion >2 cm
Portal vein	Tangential abutment—minimal	Occlusion or encasement
Metastases	None seen	Clinically visible
Celiac axis	Approximated	Encased or occluded
Chance for R_0, R_1 resection	Potentially present after posttreatment response	None

Abbreviations: R_0, R_1 resection, resection to histologically negative margins (R_0) or histologically positive, but grossly negative margins (R_1); SMA, superior mesenteric artery; SMV, superior mesenteric vein.

Modified from J. Hoffman, personal communication, 2003.

gemcitabine and radiotherapy (50.4 Gy) or gemcitabine, 5-fluorouracil (5-FU), and cisplatin followed by 5-FU and radiotherapy.

Locoregionally Advanced Presentations Are Prognostically Heterogeneous

Many factors have been identified as prognostically significant in patients with locoregionally unresectable and metastatic disease (Table 29.2).

In patients with unresectable pancreatic cancer, there is considerable overlap in the likely duration of survival between patients with locally advanced disease and those with overt evidence of more distant dissemination (metastatic disease); however, use of multivariate analysis that considers both performance status and extent of disease enables survival expectations to be significantly refined (Fig. 29.1).[13] Other factors that correlate with variation in survival for unresectable patients include surgical palliation of pain,[14] C-reactive protein level,[15-17] CA 19-9 levels,[17-19] and lactate dehydrogenase level.[20] This type of prognostic information has many potential uses, including surgical decisions regarding the pallia-

Table 29.2 Examples of Relevant Prognostic Factors: Unresectable Patients

Author(s)/Year	Factor	LRA or Met Disease	P Value	Median Survival w/o Adverse Factor	Median Survival w/Adverse Factor	Number of Cases Studied
Tas et al[20], 2001	LDH > nl	Met	0.00001	39 weeks	10 weeks	56
	PS ≥2	LRA	0.0009	30 weeks	6 weeks	55
Cubiella et al[13], 1999	PS >2	LRA	0.0001	5.6 months	1 month	63
	PS >2	Met	0.0001	2.0 months	1 month	71
Engelken et al[16], 2002	CRP ≥5 mg/dL	Not stated	0.0012	7.2 months	2.2 months	51

Abbreviations: LRA, locally regionally advanced disease; Met, metastatic disease; PS, Eastern Cooperative Oncology Group performance status; CRP, C-reactive protein.

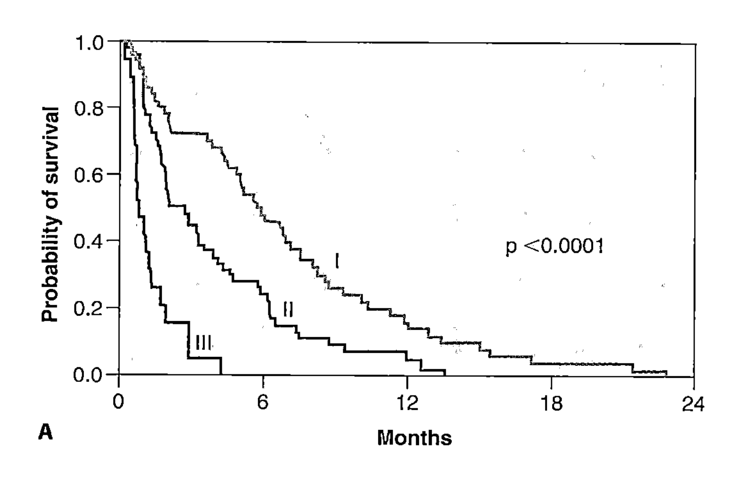

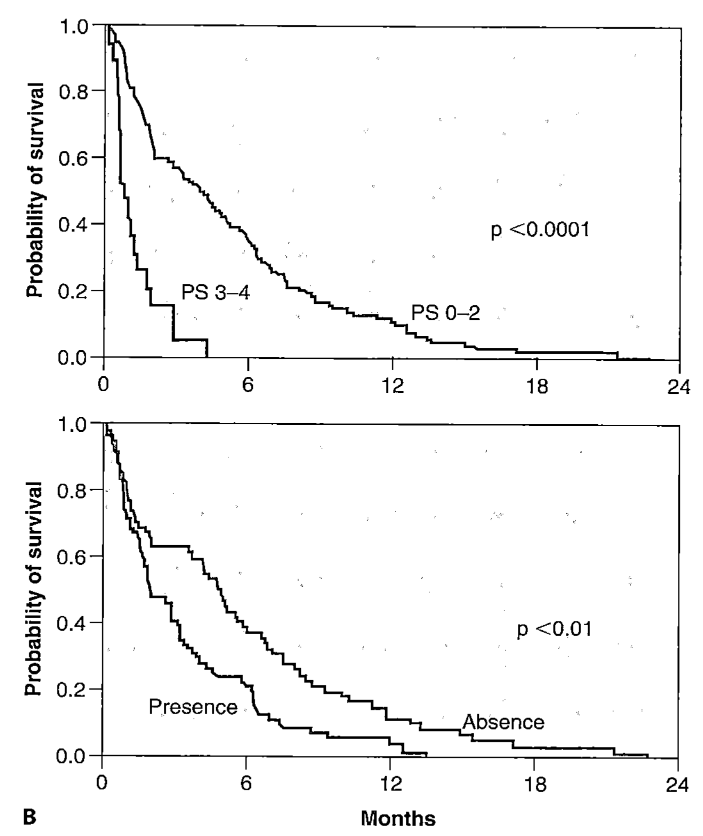

Figure 29.1
Effect of Eastern Cooperative Oncology Group (ECOG) performance status and extent of disease on survival among patients with unresectable pancreatic cancer. When considered concurrently, performance status and disease extent are better predictors of outcome (**A**) than either of these factors alone (**B**) (Modified from Cubiella et al.[13]) Abbreviations: I, no metastases, performance status (PS) 0–2; II, + metastases, PS 0–2; III, + metastases, PS 3–4.

tion of biliary and gastric obstruction,[21] and as potential stratification factors or factors about which data need to be collected to understand therapeutic effects in large clinical trials. The extent to which weight loss at presentation, a factor that intuitively would seem to correlate with poor prognosis, can be identified as an independent prognostic factor for pancreatic cancer is not completely clear. Loss of appetite[22] and loss of weight[23,24] have been associated with decreased survival in some reports, but not in others.[25] It may be that for patients with pancreatic cancer, weight loss is subsumed by performance status or that weight loss is more a predictor for intolerance to antineoplastic therapy rather than a direct predictor of survival.[26]

In summary, it is clear that there is substantial prognostic heterogeneity in patients presenting with unresectable presentations of periampullary pancreatic adenocarcinoma, and this variation is imperfectly appreciated by consideration only of the presence or absence of metastatic lesions beyond the region of the primary tumor and adjacent lymph nodes. The extent to which a more precise assessment of prognosis can be obtained by prospectively considering clinical factors (e.g., performance status, possibly extent of weight loss) and laboratory factors (C-reactive protein, lactate dehydrogenase, and CA19-9 levels) remains to be studied. It is possible that some observed variations in survival among clinical trials, especially single-institution trials, may be related to imbalance among these factors from trial to trial.

Table 29.3 Common Supportive Care Needs: Patients with Locally Advanced Pancreatic Cancer

Nausea
Weight loss
Malabsorption/pancreatic enzyme insufficiency/lactose intolerance
Duodenal obstruction
Hyperglycemia
Dehydration/electrolyte abnormalities
Pain
Depression
Jaundice
Anxiety
Constipation
Anemia

Management Options

Care delivered in the context of locoregionally unresectable, periampullary pancreatic cancer is expected to be palliative. As such, the treatment options available include best supportive care without specific antineoplastic intervention, single- and multi-agent chemotherapy regimens, or combinations of chemotherapy and radiotherapy. Selected chemotherapy or chemotherapy and radiotherapy regimens may either be "standard" or investigational.

Best Supportive Care

Issues of supportive care are addressed elsewhere in this volume. However, the supportive care needs of patients with locoregionally advanced, periampullary pancreatic cancer can be substantial (Table 29.3). Attention to the management of these significant medical issues forms the foundation of excellent palliation and care, regardless of whether intervention with antineoplastic therapy (chemotherapy with or without radiotherapy) is selected. Moreover, adequate attention to the medical optimization of these needs before and during antineoplastic therapy is essential for optimal intervention and opportunity for benefit. Weight loss correlates well with the inability to tolerate full-dose chemotherapy,[26] and patients are not well served when they receive systemic chemotherapy with unrelieved obstructive jaundice. Similarly, patients with incipient or fully expressed gastric outlet obstruction have difficulty tolerating intervention with irradiation to the upper abdomen because this is often associated with severe nausea, vomiting, and anorexia. Especially during the early phase of patient presentation and management, "best supportive care" should not be a euphemism for a passive medical stance of minimal involvement and attention.

Choosing Between Chemotherapy or Chemotherapy and Radiotherapy Combinations

The medical literature does not fully resolve whether patients with locoregionally advanced pancreatic cancer are best treated with palliative single-agent or combination chemotherapy on the one hand, or chemotherapy and concurrent radiotherapy combinations on the other. Patients with locally advanced disease are often included in reports of chemotherapy treatment regimens for "advanced pancreatic cancer," even though most patients in such reports have distant disease dissemination, and outcomes for the locoregionally advanced patients are generally not reported

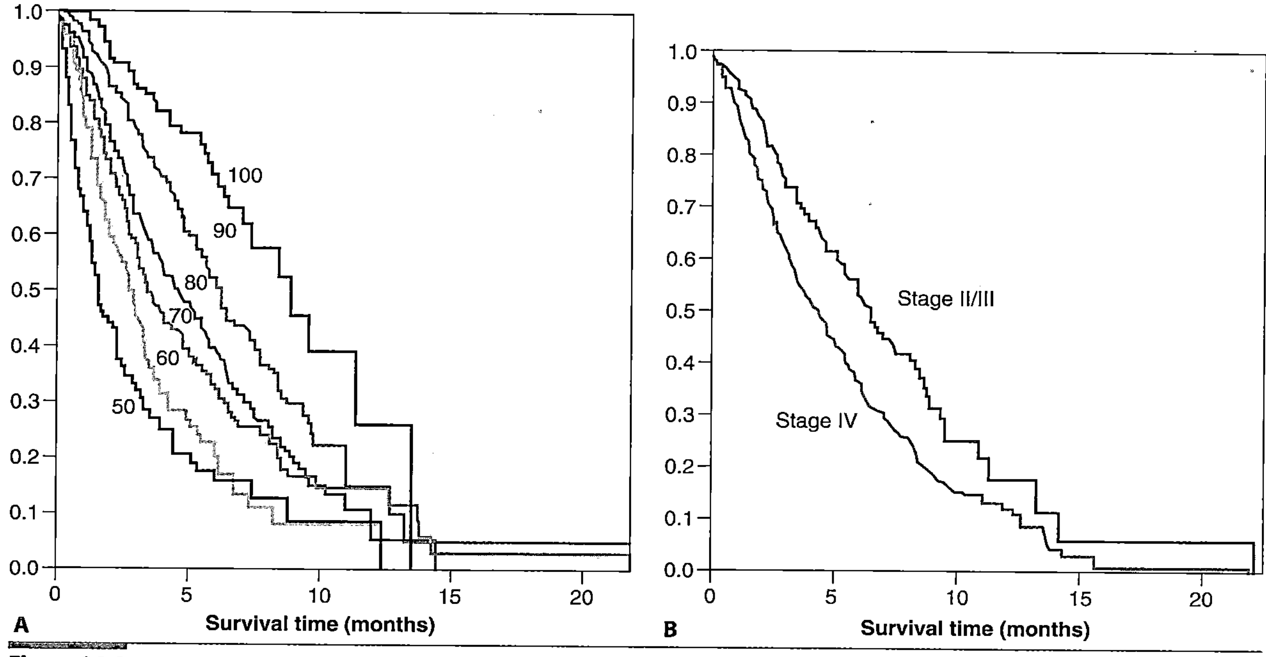

Figure 29.2
The extent to which performance status can be a dominant determinate of outcome (A) as compared with extent of disease (B) Data from approximately 2500 patients treated with single agent gemcitabine. (Modified from Storniolo et al.[31])

separately[27,28,29,30]. An important exception to this pattern is found in the report of Storniolo et al,[31] regarding single-agent gemcitabine, in which there were sufficient numbers of patients with stage II and III disease treated such that their data could be analyzed separately from that of patients with stage IV disease. In this report on approximately 2500 patients, of whom 20% had clinical stage II or III disease, the strongest correlation with outcome was noted with performance status (Fig. 29.2A). Moreover, the median survival of patients treated for locoregionally advanced (stages II and III unresectable) disease was 6.6 months, compared with 4.4 months for stage IV disease (Fig. 29.2B), a definite, but not clinically impressive, difference. These data may be significant in two ways. First, a median survival of 6.6 months (28–29 weeks) for patients with locoregionally advanced disease is less than that reported after combined chemotherapy and radiotherapy in available randomized trials (36–42 weeks) (vide infra). Second, in a prospective randomized trial of gemcitabine versus 5-FU, gemcitabine produced superior median and 1-year outcomes and is generally recognized as the standard of care for patients with pancreatic cancer with metastatic disease who desire chemotherapy.[32] Therefore, the limited survival of the patients with stage II and III disease does not reflect inferior chemotherapy by currently available standards. However, again because of the possible impact of factors other than therapy on outcome, it would be unwise to conclude that patients receiving chemotherapy without irradiation necessarily experience an inferior outcome. It may be that patients with relatively favorable prognostic factors were more likely to be selected for combined-modality chemotherapy and radiotherapy, whereas patients with less favorable factors were considered for chemotherapy alone. In fact, reports of chemotherapy alone that restricted accrual to patients with excellent performance status can be found with locoregionally advanced patients demonstrating survivals of 9–10 months.[33,34] In addition, data of Storniolo et al[31] appear to confirm the impression noted earlier that disease stage (metastatic versus non metastatic) is less of a prognostic factor for survival in unresectable patients than performance status (Fig. 29.2).

Two well-known trials from the Gastrointestinal Tumor Study Group strongly suggest a survival advantage for the use of concurrent chemotherapy and radiotherapy for locoregionally advanced pancreatic cancer as compared with radiotherapy alone (the first trial) and chemotherapy alone (the second trial). Both were prospective and randomized. The first trial, published initially in 1979, observed a median survival of 36–40 weeks with

5-FU and irradiation, compared with a median survival of 20 weeks with irradiation alone.[35,36] At 1 year, survival was 36%–38% for the 5-FU plus irradiation patients, compared with 11% for the radiotherapy-alone patients. The second Gastrointestinal Tumor Study Group trial compared survival using SMF (streptozotocin, mitomycin, 5-FU) chemotherapy with 5-FU plus irradiation followed by SMF for locally advanced pancreatic cancer and was published in 1988.[37] In this trial, chemotherapy alone produced median and 1-year survivals of 32 weeks and 19%, compared with median and 1-year survivals of 42 weeks and 41% with combined chemotherapy and irradiation. In contrast to these results, the ECOG found that 5-FU chemotherapy and radiotherapy increased toxicity without conferring survival benefit, compared with 5-FU alone.[38] Because of these disparate results, the issue of which therapy should be offered has never been fully resolved.

Krzyzanowska et al.[39] used the surveillance, epidemiology, and end-results Medicare database to analyze practice patterns and outcomes among Medicare-eligible patients with locally advanced pancreatic cancer in the United States. They identified 1696 patients with histologically proven pancreatic cancer who were treated between 1991 and 1996. Of these 1696 patients, 44% received cancer-directed therapy. In multivariate analysis, factors favoring the receipt of such therapy included younger age, increasing socioeconomic status, absence of comorbidities, treatment in a teaching hospital, and not living in the western United States. Patients receiving chemotherapy and radiotherapy (24% of patients) had a median survival of 47 weeks, patients receiving radiotherapy (13% of patients) or chemotherapy alone (7% of patients) had median survival of 29 and 27 weeks, respectively, and patients receiving no specific anticancer therapy (56% of patients) had median survival of 15 weeks. There was no apparent selection of more favorable patients toward combined-modality therapy as opposed to single-modality therapy. This nonrandomized, but statistically and methodologically rigorous, analysis of a large number of patients clearly confirms that patients who receive no specific anticancer therapy have reduced survival, but it does not answer whether this is due primarily to the selection factors identified or to the combination of these factors combined with the absence of therapeutic interventions. Equally important, this report again underscores the importance of understanding whether combined chemotherapy and radiotherapy produce a superior result to chemotherapy alone for locally advanced patients or whether observed differences simply reflect differences in patient selection.

Currently, ECOG is revisiting the question of whether chemotherapy or chemotherapy plus irradiation provide the best balance of efficacy and toxicity. ECOG protocol 4201 randomly assigned patients with locally unresectable cancer to receive either single-agent gemcitabine or radiotherapy concurrently with gemcitabine followed by single-agent gemcitabine. Given the improvements in supportive care and radiotherapy planning and administration that have occurred in the past 15–20 years, as well as the modest but definitely improved efficacy of gemcitabine as compared with that of 5-FU and the enhanced radiosensitizing properties of gemcitabine,[40-42] the results of this study should be helpful in clarifying these issues.

Phase II Trials of Chemotherapy and Irradiation

A substantial number of single-institution trials combining chemotherapy and radiotherapy can be found in the literature. These include 5-FU–based trials, taxane-based trials, and gemcitabine-based trials. Table 29.4 summarizes relevant data from published examples of such trials.[43-61]

The Radiation Therapy Oncology Group (RTOG) established the maximally tolerable dose for weekly Taxol (paclitaxel) and radiotherapy to 50.4 Gy in 28 fractions to be 50 mg/m^2 in RTOG 98-12.[54] Building on this information, RTOG PA0020, recently closed, combined weekly paclitaxel, 40 mg/m^2 and weekly gemcitabine, 75 mg/m^2 with 50.4 Gy in 28 fractions.

The current status of chemotherapy and radiotherapy for locally advanced pancreatic cancer can be summarized as follows. 5-FU-based combinations with irradiation are commonly accepted as standard treatment. Interest in combining radiotherapy with newer agents, especially gemcitabine is substantial. The optimal way of combining gemcitabine with irradiation for pancreatic cancer remains to be defined, and the MTDs for combining gemcitabine and irradiation with each other can vary considerably with the scheduling of the gemcitabine and the details of radiotherapy. With weekly gemcitabine and moderate-sized radiotherapy fields to 50 Gy,[57,58] the MTD for weekly gemcitabine is likely to be in the range of 500–600 mg/m^2, although it is disconcerting that a final report of this experience has yet to appear after initial abstract results were presented in 1998. With twice-weekly gemcitabine and moderate- to standard-sized radiotherapy fields at 1.8 Gy daily to 50.4 Gy, the MTD for gemcitabine is 40 mg/m^2.[56] With full-dose, weekly gemcitabine (1000 mg/m^2) and 15 fractions

Table 29.4 Radiotherapy and Chemotherapy Trials

Date	First Author	Chemotherapy	Radiotherapy Dose	Patient Numbers	Median Survival	Comment
5-FU–based trials						
1988	Komaki et al.[43]	5-FU (bolus)	61.2 Gy	15	60 weeks	23.4-Gy PHI
1988	Flickinger et al.[44]	5-FU (bolus), FAM	50–60 Gy	27	9 months	2.5-Gy fxs/ split course
1991	Boz et al.[45]	5-FU (bolus), cisplatin	60 Gy	22	7.5 months	Split course
1992	Komaki et al.[46]	5-FU (CI) 5 days	61.2 Gy	79	8.4 months	23.4-Gy PHI, RTOG study
1993	Bruckner et al.[47]	5-FU (CI), streptozocin, cisplatin	54 Gy	20	12 months	
1996	Luderhoff et al.[48]	5-FU (CI) 1,3 weeks	45–50 Gy	13	36 weeks	1.1 Gy t.i.d. (accelerated XRT)
1997	Ishii et al.[49]	5-FU (CI) 5.5 weeks	50.4 Gy	20	10.3 months	
1997	Prott et al.[50]	5-FU, leucovorin	44.8 Gy	32	12.7 months	1.6 Gy b.i.d. (accelerated XRT)
2000	Kornek et al.[51]	5-FU, leucovorin, cisplatin	55 Gy	38	14 months	
2002	Shinchi et al.[52]	5-FU (CI) 5.5 weeks	50.4 Gy	31	13.2 months	
Mean ± SD			53.9 Gy ± 5.7	30 ± 19	10.9 ± 2.5 months	4.3 weeks = 1 month
Taxane-based trials						
1997	Safran et al.[53]	Paclitaxel (Taxol) weekly	50 Gy	14	Not given	Phase I; paclitaxel MTD 50 mg/m²
2003	Willett et al.[54]	Paclitaxel weekly	50.4 Gy	122	11.9	RTOG 98-12; paclitaxel dose 50 mg/m²
2003	Ashamalla et al.[55]	Paclitaxel weekly	63.8 Gy	20	≥8 months	Paclitaxel MTD 60/m²; (accelerated XRT)
Gemcitabine-based trials						
1999	Blackstock et al.[56]	Gemcitabine twice weekly	50.4 Gy	19	Not stated	Phase I; 40-mg MTD
1998, 2003	McGinn et al.[57]; McGinn and Zalupski[58]	Gemcitabine weekly	50.4 Gy	>13	Not stated	Final report, details unpublished
2001	Crane et al.[59]	Gemcitabine 250–500 mg/m² weekly	30–33 Gy in 10–11 Fxs	51	11 months	24% severe toxicity
2001	McGinn et al.[60]	Gemcitabine 1000 mg/m² weekly	24–42 Gy in 15 Fxs	37	11.6 months	Phase I: Full-dose gemcitabine +15 fxs XRT
XRT MTD 36 Gy						
2002	Epelbaum et al.[61]	Gemcitabine 400 mg/m² weekly × 3	50.4 Gy	10	>8 months	IInduction gemcitabine; only CBR pts received gemcitabine + XRT
2002	Poggi et al.[62]	Gemcitabine 350–550 mg/m² weekly	54.0–55.8 Gy	19	39.0 weeks at MTD	MTD 440 mg/m²

Abbreviations: 5-FU, 5-fluorouracil; FAM, 5-fluorouracil, doxorubicin, mitomycin; PHI, prophylactic hepatic irradiation; XRT, radiotherapy; Fxs, fraction (treatment) dose; split course, planned interruption of treatment; CI, continuous infusion; b.i.d., twice a day; t.i.d., three times a day.

Table 29.5 Rationale and Limitations of IORT for Pancreatic Cancer

Theoretical Advantages	Limitations
Overlying and adjacent normal tissues (intestine, liver, stomach, kidney) surgically excluded from treatment area.	Subjacent nerves, major arteries, and spinal cord cannot be moved.
Use of electron beam limits dose to subjacent tissues due to reduced tissue penetration.	Most anterior subjacent tissues receive at least 50% of prescribed dose. Dose within and beyond bone difficult to assess.
Large, single fraction takes advantage of exponential increase in cell death with arithmetic increase in dose.	Local tumor control remains limited by hypoxia, tumor size, and dose constraints imposed by subjacent tissues.
IORT can be combined with external-beam chemoradiotherapy regimens.	Clinical realities of combining surgery and radiotherapy necessitate a significant interval between external-beam radiotherapy and IORT, during which tumor repopulation can occur.
IORT should enhance local control of primary tumor.	Propensity for hepatic and peritoneal spread may dilute or overwhelm benefit of enhanced local control.

Abbreviation: IORT, intraoperative (electron beam) radiotherapy.

of irradiation to small radiotherapy fields aimed at the gross tumor volume only, the radiotherapy MTD is 36 Gy.[60] This is in contrast to the experience of Crane et al,[59] in which an attempt to combine 30–33 Gy in 10–11 fractions with a modest dose of gemcitabine produced unacceptable toxicity.

Intraoperative Radiotherapy and Intraoperative Electron-Beam Radiotherapy

The motivation for using a single, relatively large, fraction of radiotherapy during an operative procedure (intraoperative radiotherapy, intraoperative electron-beam radiotherapy) derives from several considerations (Table 29.5). Over roughly 40 years of use, a substantial literature has developed on the use of this modality within the abdomen, especially for gastric, pancreatic, and colorectal adenocarcinomas and especially for large, adherent, difficult to resect tumor presentations. Intraoperative electron-beam radiotherapy may be used as the only radiotherapy modality or more commonly before or after a course of external-beam irradiation. Typical intraoperative radiotherapy doses have been between 10 and 20 Gy. Observed acute morbidity has included primarily acute nausea and rare anastomotic leak, and delayed complications have included fibrosis and intestinal ulceration.

Although numerous single-institution trials confirm the ability to incorporate intraoperative radiotherapy in the treatment of locally advanced patients, the marginal benefit obtained thereby is uncertain.[63-67]

Communicating About Treatment Options

The available treatments for this disease presentation are not as good as one would hope. This reality needs to be tactfully acknowledged in order for patients and families to make sense of the fact that their options range from support without specific antineoplastic intervention through chemotherapy alone to chemotherapy combined with irradiation. It is also important to acknowledge unresolved controversies and the limitations of available data. In fact, this acknowledgment can serve as a convenient point of connection to discussing available clinical trials. There can be considerable tension between the need to give patients and families enough information to allow them to be meaningful participants in selecting treatment and overwhelming them with more than they are prepared to handle. The challenges of this aspect of care and communication are discussed elsewhere.[68,69] Common pitfalls to be avoided include not finding out what the patient and family have already heard and understood, trying to set an agenda for the dialogue that the patient and family are not prepared for or are unwilling to engage in, imposing information that is unacceptably threatening or anxiety provoking, and moving the dialogue faster than the patient and family are able to accept.

Conclusion

The basic principles of palliative management for locally advanced periampullary adenocarcinoma of the pancreas include tissue diagnosis, attention to relief of metabolic and physiologic abnormalities caused by tumor, careful assessment of resectability status by an experienced surgeon, and distinguishing of marginally unresectable presentations from truly unresectable presentations. It is important to recognize the prognostic heterogeneity in these presentations, and this can be appreciated in part by considering performance status, possibly weight loss, and biochemical factors, such as CA19-9 and CRP levels. Available management options include active supportive care alone, gemcitabine-based chemotherapy regimens, and radiotherapy combined with gemcitabine, 5-FU, or paclitaxel chemotherapy. Data suggest that there may be somewhat longer median and 1-year survivals after chemotherapy and radiotherapy than after chemotherapy alone, and this possibility is being directly tested by ECOG (E4201).

References

1. Conlon KC, Brennan MF. Management of adenocarcinoma of the body and tail of the pancreas. In: Cameron JL, ed. *American Cancer Society Atlas of Clinical Oncology: Pancreatic Cancer*. Hamilton: BC Decker, Inc., 2001:255–263.
2. Brooks AD, Conlon KC. Pancreas cancer: staging systems and techniques. In: Kelsen DP, Daly JM, Kern SE, et al., eds. *Gastrointestinal Oncology: Principles and Practice*. Philadelphia: Lippincott, Williams & Wilkins, 2002:451–458.
3. Yeo CJ, Tempero M, Abrams RA. Pancreas cancer: clinical management. *Gastrointestinal Oncology: Principles and Practice*. Philadelphia: Lippincott, Williams & Wilkins, 2002: 477–512.
4. Phan GQ, Yeo CJ, Hruban RH, et al. Surgical experience with pancreatic and peripancreatic neuroendocrine tumors: review of 125 patients. *J Gastrointest Surg*. 1998;2:472–482.
5. Koniaris LG, Lillemoe KD, Yeo CJ, et al. Is there a role for surgical resection in the treatment of early-stage pancreatic lymphoma? *J Am Coll Surg*. 2000;190:319–330.
6. Bouvet M, Staerkel GA, Spitz FR, et al. Primary pancreatic lymphoma. *Surgery*. 1998;123:382–390.
7. Sohn TA, Lillemoe KD, Cameron JL, et al. Reexploration for periampullary carcinoma: resectability, perioperative results, pathology, and long-term outcome. *Ann Surg*. 1999;229:393–400.
8. Robinson EK, Lee JE, Lowy AM, et al. Reoperative pancreaticoduodenectomy for periampullary carcinoma. *Am J Surg*. 1996;172:432–437.
9. Brunner TB, Grabenbauer GG, Klein P, et al. Phase I trial of strictly time scheduled gemcitabine and cis-platin with concurrent radiotherapy in patients with locally advanced pancreatic cancer. *Int J Radiat Oncol Biol Phys*. 2003;55:144–153.
10. Aristu J, Canon R, Pardo F, et al. Surgical resection after preoperative chemoradiotherapy benefits selected patients with unresectable pancreatic cancer. *Am J Clin Oncol*. 2003; 26:30–36.
11. Ammori JB, Colletti LM, Zalupski MM, et al. Surgical resection following radiation therapy with concurrent gemcitabine in patients with previously unresectable adenocarcinoma of the pancreas. *J Gastrointest Surg*. 2003;7:766–772.
12. Kim HJ, Czischke K, Brennan M, Conlon KC. Does neoadjuvant chemoradiation downstage pancreatic cancer? *J Gastrointest Surg*. 2002;6:763–769.
13. Cubiella J, Castells A, Fondevilla C, et al. Prognostic factors in nonresectable pancreatic adenocarcinoma: a rationale to design therapeutic trials. *Am J Gastroenterol*. 1999;94: 1271–1278.
14. Lillemoe KD, Cameron JL, Kaufman HS, et al. Chemical splanchnicectomy in patients with unresectable pancreatic cancer: a prospective randomized trial. *Ann Surg*. 1993; 217:447–455.
15. Falconer JS, Fearon KC, Ross JA, et al. Acute-phase protein response and survival duration of patients with pancreatic cancer. *Cancer*. 1995;75:2077–2082.
16. Engelken FJF, Bettschart MQ, Rahman RW, et al. Prognostic factors in the palliation of pancreatic cancer. *Eur J Surg Oncol*. 2003;29:368–373.
17. Ueno H, Okada S, Okusaka T, Ikeda M. Prognostic factors in patients with metastatic pancreatic adenocarcinoma receiving systemic chemotherapy. *Oncology*. 2000;59:296–301.
18. Lundin J, Roberts PJ, Kuusela P, Haglund C. The prognostic value of preoperative serum levels of CA19-9 and CEA in patients with pancreatic cancer. *Br J Cancer*. 1994;69: 515–519.
19. Katz A, Hanlon A, Luciano R, et al. Prognostic values of CA19-9 level in patients with carcinoma of the pancreas treated with radiotherapy. *Int J Radiat Oncol Biol Phys*. 1998;41:393–396.
20. Tas F, Aykan F, Alici S, et al. Prognostic factors in pancreatic carcinoma: serum LDH levels predict survival in metastatic disease. *Am J Clin Oncol*. 2001;24:547–550.
21. Di Fronzo LA, Cymerman J, Egrari S, O'Connell T. Unresectable pancreatic carcinoma: correlating length of survival with choice of palliative bypass. *Am Surg*. 1999; 65:955–958.
22. Ridwelski K, Meyer F, Ebert M, et al. Prognostic parameters determining survival in pancreatic carcinoma and, in particular, after palliative treatment. *Dig Dis*. 2001;19:85–92.
23. Bakkevold KE, Kambestad B. Long-term survival following radical and palliative treatment of patients with carcinoma of the pancreas and papilla of Vater—the prognostic factors influencing the long-term results: a prospective multicentre study. *Eur J Surg Oncol*. 1993;19:147–161.
24. Terwee CB, Nieveen Van Dijkum EJ, Gouma DJ, et al. Pooling of prognostic studies in cancer of the pancreatic head and periampullary region: the Triple-P study. Triple-P study group. *Eur J Surg*. 2000;166:706–712.
25. Ikeda M, Okada S, Tokuuye K, et al. Prognostic factors in patients with locally advanced pancreatic cancer receiving chemoradiotherapy. *Cancer*. 2001;91:490–495.
26. Andreyev HJN, Norman AR, Oates J, Cunningham D. Why do patients with weight loss have a worse outcome when undergoing chemotherapy for gastrointestinal malignancies? *Eur J Cancer*. 1998;34:503–509.
27. Philip PA, Zalupski MM, Vaitkevicius VK, et al. Phase II study of gemcitabine and cis-platin in the treatment of patients with advanced pancreatic cancer. *Cancer*. 2001;92: 569–577.

28. Cascinu S, Labianca R, Catalano V, et al. Weekly gemcitabine and cisplatin chemotherapy: a well-tolerated but ineffective chemotherapeutic regimen in advanced pancreatic cancer patients. A report from the Italian Group for the Study of Digestive Tract Cancer (GISCAD). *Ann Oncol.* 2003;14:205–208.
29. Tempero M, Plunkett W, Ruiz van Haperen V, et al. Randomized phase II comparison of dose-intense gemcitabine: thirty-minute infusion and fixed dose rate infusion in patients with pancreatic adenocarcinoma. *J Clin Oncol.* 2003;21:3402–3408.
30. Petty RD, Nicolson MC, Skaria S, et al. A phase II study of mitomycin C, cisplatin, and protracted infusional 5-fluorouracil in advanced pancreatic carcinoma: efficacy and low toxicity. *Ann Oncol.* 2003;14:1100–1105.
31. Storniolo AM, Enas NH, Brown CA, et al. An investigational new drug treatment program for patients with gemcitabine: results for over 3000 patients with pancreatic carcinoma. *Cancer.* 1999;85:1261–1268.
32. Burris HA III, Moore MJ, Andersen J, et al. Improvements in survival and clinical benefit with gemcitabine as first line therapy for patients with advanced pancreatic cancer: a randomized trial. *J Clin Oncol.* 1997;15:2403–2413.
33. Rougier P, Adenis A, Ducreux M, et al. A phase II study: docetaxel as first line chemotherapy for advanced pancreatic adenocarcinoma. *Eur J Cancer.* 2000;36:1016–1025.
34. El-Rayes BF, Zalupski MM, Shields AF, et al. Phase II study of gemcitabine, cisplatin, and infusional fluorouracil in advanced pancreatic cancer. *J Clin Oncol.* 2003;21:2920–2925.
35. Gastrointestinal Tumor Study Group. Comparative therapeutic trial of radiation with or without chemotherapy in pancreatic cancer. *Int J Radiat Oncol Biol Phys.* 1979;5:1643–1647.
36. Moertel CG, Frytak S, Hahn RG, et al. Therapy of locally unresectable pancreatic carcinoma: a randomized comparison of high dose (6000 rads) radiation alone, moderate dose radiation (4000 rads + 5-fluorouracil), and high dose radiation + 5-fluorouracil. *Cancer.* 1981;48: 1705–1710.
37. Gastrointestinal Tumor Study Group. Treatment of locally unresectable carcinoma of the pancreas: comparison of combined-modality therapy (chemotherapy plus radiotherapy) to chemotherapy alone. *J Natl Cancer Inst.* 1988;80:751–755.
38. Klaasen DJ, MacIntyre JM, Catton GE, et al. Treatment of locally unresectable cancer of the stomach and pancreas: a randomized comparison of 5-fluorouracil alone with radiation plus concurrent and maintenance 5-fluorouracil—an Eastern Cooperative Oncology Group study. *J Clin Oncol.* 1985;3:373–378.
39. Krzyzanowska MK, Weeks JC, Earle CC. Treatment of locally advanced pancreatic cancer in the real world: population-based practices and effectiveness. *J Clin Oncol.* 2003;21: 3409–3414.
40. Abbruzzese JL. New applications of gemcitabine and future directions in the management of pancreatic cancer. *Cancer.* 2002;95:941–945.
41. Moore M. Activity of gemcitabine in patients with advanced pancreatic cancer. *Cancer.* 1996;78:633–638.
42. Kenny L, Peters L, Rodgers A, et al. Modern radiotherapy for modern surgeons: an update of radiation oncology. *ANZ J Surg.* 2002;72:131–136.
43. Komaki R, Hansen R, Cox JD, Wilson JF. Phase I-II study of prophylactic hepatic irradiation with local irradiation and systemic chemotherapy for adenocarcinoma of the pancreas. *Int J Radiat Oncol Biol Phys.* 1988;15:1447–1452.
44. Flickinger JC, Jawalekar K, Deutsch M, Webster J. Split course radiation therapy for adenocarcinoma of the pancreas. *Int J Radiat Oncol Biol Phys.* 1988;15:359–364.
45. Boz G, De Paoli A, Roncadin M, et al. Radiation therapy combined with chemotherapy for inoperable pancreatic carcinoma. *Tumori.* 1991;77:61–64.
46. Komaki R, Wadler S, Peters T, et al. High-dose local irradiation plus prophylactic hepatic irradiation and chemotherapy for inoperable adenocarcinoma of the pancreas. *Cancer.* 1992;69:2807–2812.
47. Bruckner HW, Kalnicki S, Dalton J, et al. Survival after combined modality therapy for pancreatic cancer. *J Clin Gastroenterol.* 1993;16:199–203.
48. Luderhoff EC, Gonzalez D, Bakker P. Pilot study in locally advanced unresectable pancreas carcinoma using a combination of accelerated radiotherapy and continuous infusion of 5-fluorouracil. *Radiother Oncol.* 1996;40:241–243.
49. Ishii H, Okada S, Tokuuye K, et al. Protracted 5-fluorouracil infusion with concurrent radiotherapy as a treatment for locally advanced pancreatic carcinoma. *Cancer.* 1997;79: 1516–1520.
50. Prott FJ, Schonekaes K, Preusser P, et al. Combined modality treatment with accelerated radiotherapy and chemotherapy in patients with locally advanced inoperable carcinoma of the pancreas: results of a feasibility study. *Br J Cancer.* 1997;75:597–601.
51. Kornek GV, Schratter-Sehn A, Marczell A, et al. Treatment of unresectable, locally advanced pancreatic adenocarcinoma with combined radiochemotherapy with 5-fluorouracil, leucovorin and cisplatin. *Br J Cancer.* 2000;82:96–103.
52. Shinchi H, Takao S, Noma H, et al. Length and quality of survival after external beam radiotherapy with concurrent continuous 5-fluorouracil infusion for locally unresectable pancreatic cancer. *Int J Radiat Oncol Biol Phys.* 2002;53:146–150.
53. Safran H, King TP, Choy H, et al. Paclitaxel and concurrent radiation for locally advanced pancreatic and gastric cancer. *J Clin Oncol.* 1997;15:901–907.
54. Willett CG, Safran H, Abrams RA, et al. Clinical research in pancreatic cancer: the radiation therapy oncology group trials. *Int J Radiat Oncol Biol Phys.* 2003;56[suppl]:S31–S37.
55. Ashamalla H, Zaki B, Mokhtar B, et al. Hyperfractionated radiotherapy and paclitaxel for locally advanced/unresectable pancreatic cancer. *Int J Radiat Oncol Biol Phys.* 2003;55:679–687.
56. Blackstock AW, Bernard SA, Richards F, et al. Phase I trial of twice-weekly gemcitabine and concurrent radiation in patients with advanced pancreatic cancer. 1999;17:2208–2212.
57. McGinn CJ, Smith DC, Szarka CE, et al. A phase I study of gemcitabine in combination with radiation therapy in patients with localized, unresectable pancreatic cancer [abstract]. *Proc ASCO.* 1998;17:264a.

58. McGinn CJ, Zalupski MM. Radiation therapy with weekly gemcitabine: current status of clinical trials. *Int J Radiat Oncol Biol Phys.* 2003;56[suppl]:S10–S15.
59. Crane CH, Antolak JA, Rosen II, et al. Phase I study of concomitant gemcitabine and IMRT for patients with unresectable adenocarcinoma of the pancreatic head. *Int J Gastrointest Cancer.* 2001;30:123–132.
60. McGinn CJ, Zalupski MM, Shureiqi I, et al. Phase I trial of radiation dose escalation with concurrent full dose gemcitabine in patients with advanced pancreatic cancer. *J Clin Oncol.* 2001;19:4202–4208.
61. Epelbaum R, Rosenblatt E, Nasrallah S, et al. Phase II study of gemcitabine combined with radiation therapy in patients with localized, unresectable pancreatic cancer. *J Surg Oncol.* 2002;81:138–143.
62. Poggi MM, Kroog GS, Russo A, et al. Phase I study of weekly gemcitabine as a radiation sensitizer for unresectable pancreatic cancer. *Int J Radiat Oncol Biol Phys.* 2002;54:670–676.
63. Willett CG, Warshaw AL. Intraoperative electron beam irradiation in pancreatic cancer. *Front Biosci.* 1998;3:207–213.
64. Calvo FA, Santos M, Azinovic I. Intraoperative radiotherapy: literature updating with an overview of results presented at the 6th international symposium on intraoperative radiotherapy. *Rays.* 1998;23:439–461.
65. Mohiuddin M, Cantor R, Biermann W, et al. Combined modality treatment of localized unresectable adenocarcinoma of the pancreas. *Int J Radiat Oncol Biol Phys.* 1988;14:79–84.
66. Furuse J, Kinoshita T, Kawashima M, et al. Intraoperative and conformal external beam radiation therapy with protracted 5-fluorouracil infusion in patients with locally advanced pancreatic carcinoma. *Cancer.* 2003;97:1346–1352.
67. Okamoto A, Tsuruta K, Karasawa K, et al. Resection versus palliation: treatment of stage III and IVA carcinomas of the pancreas employing intraoperative radiation. *World J Surg.* 2003;27:599–605.
68. Abrams RA. Communication. *Lancet.* 2002;359:1245.
69. Moryl N, Carver AC, Foley KM. Palliative care. In: Kufe DW, Pollock RE, Weichselbaum RR, et al. eds. *Cancer Medicine.* 6th ed. Hamilton: BC Decker, Inc., 2003:1113–1124.

CHAPTER 30

Endoscopic Palliation of Pancreatic Cancer

David Whitaker, MBBS
Benedict M. Devereaux, MBBS

The diagnosis is usually made in advanced stages, and as a result, metastatic or advanced disease is present in almost 90% of cases at the time of diagnosis.[1-2] The historical overall 5-year survival rate is 0.5%–2.0%, and only about 3% of patients who undergo a resection with curative intent survive 5 years with standard therapy.[3] Recent developments in neoadjuvant chemotherapy treatment have achieved improvements in survival.[3] This has potential impact on historical recommendations for planning therapy that have used survival estimates of less than 6 months.[4]

The contribution of therapeutic endoscopy to the management of pancreatic cancer dates back to 1979, with the first placement, at endoscopic retrograde cholangiopancreatography (ERCP), of a biliary stent for the palliation of malignant obstructive jaundice.[5] Today, the role of endoscopy in the treatment of patients with established pancreatic cancer incorporates preoperative relief of jaundice; palliation of jaundice in patients with unresectable disease; management of complications of pancreatic cancer, including gastric outlet obstruction; and management of associated pain.

Initial Biliary Decompression

The rationale for preoperative biliary drainage lies mainly in the relief of symptoms of biliary obstruction, including pruritus. The issue of whether ERCP is necessary for preoperative relief of jaundice has recently been extensively reviewed. Almost two decades ago, three prospective randomized trials did not show a significant benefit of preoperative biliary drainage.[6-8] Interpretability of these data is limited, however, because all drainage procedures were undertaken by the percutaneous transhepatic route. Most enrolled patients were also undergoing palliative surgery, rather than a pancreaticoduodenectomy with curative intent, and numbers were relatively small.

A recently published meta-analysis of randomized, controlled, and comparative cohort trials represents the most extensive review of this issue.[9] A second extensive meta-analysis of the effects of preoperative endoscopic stent placement on morbidity and mortality was also published in the same year.[10] Both of these reviews have shown that there is no benefit in preoperative biliary drainage with respect to perioperative mortality.

A total of five randomized, controlled trials have been conducted between 1982 and 1994.[7,8,11-13] Only one of these studies[13] demonstrated a benefit of endoscopic stenting. Only two trials used endoscopic drainage exclusively, and the other three used methods including percutaneous transhepatic drainage. Among the retrospective cohort series, most used a combination of techniques. Minor differences in complications between endoscopic drainage and transhepatic drainage have to be considered in the interpretation of these data.

Moreover, there is a lack of uniformity in the studies with obstruction due to malignancies other than pancreatic cancer included in the analyses, and a substantial difference exists in the approach to proximal obstruction when compared with distal obstruction. The other concern with the interpretation is variability in the type of surgery performed because rates of morbidity and mortality are different between pancreaticoduodenectomy and bypass procedures.

In view of concerns regarding the validity and interpretability of the results of the Sewnath et al.[9] meta-analysis, Pisters and colleagues[14] subsequently recommended that an experienced pancreaticobiliary surgeon should be involved in the decision-making process regarding initial biliary decompression for patients with obstructive jaundice. If this is not possible, they suggested a policy of endobiliary stent placement and tertiary-care referral.

More recently, an analysis was undertaken of 161 patients who underwent pancreaticoduodenectomy.[15] Seventy-eight percent of the patients had prior biliary instrumentation, of which 90% was via ERCP. Eighty percent of the patients underwent decompression with biliary drainage, and most of these had endoscopic sphincterotomy and stent placement. The group undergoing biliary instrumentation had significantly higher rates of positive biliary cultures. This group also had increased numbers of infectious complications, including intra-abdominal abscesses and wound infections and a statistically higher number of postoperative deaths. The authors concluded that preoperative biliary drainage was associated with higher morbidity due to biliary contamination.

In another retrospective analysis of 241 patients evaluated for the impact of preoperative biliary drainage, a significantly higher number of positive bile cultures were reported, but there was no overall difference in postoperative complications.[16]

Duration of stenting may also be influential on outcomes but has not been analyzed closely. The duration of stenting has ranged from 10 to 182 days in studies.[17] There is evidence from animal models that return of hepatic function after prolonged biliary obstruction takes several weeks after decompression.[18]

In summary, there is no evidence from published studies to support the routine use of preoperative biliary decompression. Nonetheless, a well-selected, high-risk subgroup of patients may benefit from the symptom relief afforded by biliary decompression, particularly if surgery is to be delayed.

Palliation of Jaundice

In patients with unresectable pancreatic cancer, obstructive jaundice is present in 70%–90%.[19] In these patients, palliation of jaundice and its associated symptoms is a primary therapeutic goal. Prolonged biliary obstruction is often associated with malabsorption and malnutrition. Patients generally feel unwell with malaise and may experience anorexia and nausea. Pruritus is also a common symptom and can be severe and debilitating. It is frequently refractory to medical therapy. Prolonged cholestasis can lead to hepatic dysfunction. Cholangitis may occur but with a frequency less than with biliary obstruction from other causes, such as choledocholithiasis. The relief of jaundice is usually associated with a dramatic albeit often short-term improvement in the patient's well being as well as having a positive psychological effect on the patient and family members.[20,21]

In pancreatic cancer, the level of biliary obstruction almost always occurs within the intrapancreatic portion of the distal common bile duct. Less frequently, obstruction can occur at the level of the proximal extrahepatic biliary tree due to compression from hilar lymphadenopathy. In both scenarios, biliary decompression is usually readily achievable because there is dilated common hepatic duct upstream from the stricture. Endoscopic biliary drainage is significantly more difficult if the stricture involves the bifurcation of the common hepatic duct because stents need to be positioned into both the right and left hepatic ducts. Preprocedure imaging with transabdominal ultrasound or computed tomography is beneficial in defining the primary lesion, its locoregional involvement, the level of biliary obstruction, and the presence of liver metastases. Multiple liver metastases may result in jaundice, and if multiple intrahepatic strictures are present, endoscopic biliary decompression is not achievable.

Method of Palliation

For patients with unresectable disease, relief of biliary obstruction can be achieved via surgical means or by stent insertion. Surgical methods include choledochoduodenostomy, choledochojejunostomy, and hepaticojejunostomy. The

Table 30.1. Endoscopic/Percutaneous Stenting Versus Surgical Bypass

Study (year)	Study Design	Number	Success Drainage (%)	Procedure-Related Mortality (%)	30-Day Mortality (%)	Mean Days in Hospital (range)	Complications (%)
Anderson et al.[24] (1989)	RCT	Stent $n = 25$	25 (100)	NS	5 (20)	26 (3–210)	9 (36)
		Surgery $n = 25$	NS	NS	6 (24)	27 (10–202)	5 (20)
							p = NS
Smith et al.[23] (1994)	RCT	Stent $n = 100$	92 (92)	3 (3)	8 (8)	19[a]	11 (11)
		Surgery $n = 101$	93 (92)	14 (14)	15 (15)	26	29 (29)
				$p = 0.006$	p = NS	(median)	$p = 0.02$
Shepherd et al.[25] (1998)	RCT	Stent $n = 23$	19 (82)	[b]	2 (9)	5 (2–16)	7 (30)
		Surgery $n = 25$	23 (93)	[b]	5 (20)	13 (8–49)	14 (56)
					p = NS	$p = 0.002$	p = NS

[a]Range not stated.
[b]Procedure-related mortality measured at 30-day survival.
Abbreviations: NS, not significant; RCT, randomized, controlled trial.

preferable bypass procedure is controversial, but the literature suggests that a choledochoenterostomy is preferable.[22] Access to the biliary tree for stent insertion can be achieved by either the endoscopic route or the percutaneous transhepatic route. These three modalities have been extensively compared over the past two decades.

Surgical Bypass Versus Stenting

Several randomized trials have compared surgical bypass procedures with biliary stenting.[23-25] Most patients in these studies had unresectable pancreatic cancer. The overall findings were that the surgical methods and stent insertion all provided adequate decompression of the biliary tree without any significant difference in success rates. Stent insertion was undertaken using percutaneous and endoscopic methods. The main differences appear to be related to early and late morbidity and mortality. In stented patients, there was a lower procedure-related mortality and a lower complication rate (Table 30.1). However, 30-day and 6-month mortality rates were comparable, and the stent group tended to undergo further procedures, often related to stent dysfunction. Stent dysfunction, although not clearly defined in these studies, is generally accepted as stent occlusion or migration, with or without associated cholangitis.

The major factors that determine the technique of biliary drainage are tumor stage and the patient's health status. The treating teams' personal preference and local expertise also dictates the approach in individual patients. Patients with few comorbid illnesses and relatively good operative risk may be more suitable for surgical bypass, whereas those with larger tumor burden or comorbid illness seem to be better candidates for endoscopic stenting. The authors recommend an initial endoscopic approach; surgical biliary bypass is reserved for patients in whom endoscopic biliary decompression is unsuccessful and for whom a percutaneous transhepatic choledochostomy is undesirable.

Patients with duodenal obstruction have traditionally been treated surgically. Smith et al.[23] studied patients who underwent surgical biliary bypass who also had prophylactic gastroenterostomy and found that this reduced the need for later surgery without having any impact on overall mortality. With the increased use of endoscopically placed self-expanding metal enteral stents, however, the endoscopic approach may be optimal for most patients (Table 30.1)

Endoscopic Versus Percutaneous Transhepatic Approach

Often, the levels of local expertise determine the preferred method of biliary stent placement. Relative contraindications to the percutaneous transhepatic approach include the presence of ascites, major intrahepatic metastases, and coagulopathy. There are no significant differences in success rates,[26] but currently, the endoscopic method predominates in most centers. When the inability to place a biliary stent is due to endoscopic failure to cannulate the common bile duct or traverse the biliary stricture, a combined percutaneous-endoscopic technique is very useful.

Table 30.2. Comparison of Patency of Plastic and Metal Stents in Malignant Biliary Obstruction

Author (year)	Study Design	Number (stent diameter)	Days Median Patency (range)	Length of Follow-Up	p value
Davids et al.[27] (1992)	RCT	Plastic (10 Fr) $n = 56$ Metal $n = 49$	126 (7–482) 273 (14–363)	40 months	*p = 0.006*
Knyrim et al.[28] (1993)	RCT	Plastic (11.5 Fr) $n = 31$ Metal $n = 31$	4.6 ± 0.7 months 6.2 ± 1.9 months	20 months	*p value not given*
Schmassmann et al.[29] (1996)	Retrospective	Plastic (10 and 12 Fr) $n = 70$ Metal $n = 95$	4 months 10 months	*Not given*	*p < 0.001*
Prat et al.[30] (1998)	RCT	Plastic (11.5 Fr) $n = 33$ Metal $n = 34$	3.2 months 4.8 months	12 months	*p value not given*
Kaassis et al.[31] (2003)	RCT	Plastic (10 Fr) $n = 59$ Metal $n = 59$	5 months Not reached	12 months	*p = 0.007*

Abbreviation: RCT, randomized, controlled trial.

During this so-called rendezvous procedure, an interventional radiologist passes a guide wire transhepatically into the bile duct, through the stricture and into the duodenum. The endoscopist then grasps the wire with the use of a snare or forceps and withdraws it through the duodenoscope to facilitate stent placement.

Choice of Stent

It is well established in the literature that metal stents, which expand to a maximum diameter of 30 Fr, remain patent longer and occlude less frequently than polyethylene stents[27-31] (Table 30.2). The important issue remains patient selection for the self-expanding metal stent (SEMS) and the cost-effectiveness of initial or subsequent biliary SEMS placement in the palliation of pancreatic cancer.

In inoperable cases, the objective of stenting the biliary system is not only to relieve jaundice and pruritus but also to improve the patient's general quality of life. Readmissions to the hospital with stent dysfunction, sometimes requiring repeated ERCP interventions, can adversely affect quality of life. Dysfunction of metal stents differs from that of polyethylene stents. In the latter, sludge and bacterial encrustation is the predominant cause of dysfunction, whereas metal stents fail usually because of tumor ingrowth through the mesh wall or tumor overgrowth of the ends of the stent.

Parameters influencing the choice of stent include the degree of diagnostic uncertainty as to the presence of a malignant lesion, the resectability of the lesion, and the relative cost of metal stents. In patients who have an inoperable tumor, there is evidence that initial insertion of a SEMS is both cost-effective and results in less patient morbidity in patients whose life expectancy is estimated to be greater than 3–6 months. In a randomized, controlled trial of 101 patients with malignant obstruction of the distal bile duct, most with pancreatic cancer, patients were randomly assigned to receive a 11.5 Fr polyethylene stent with expectant management, an 11.5 Fr polyethylene stent with 3-monthly exchange, or an initial uncovered Wallstent (Enteral Wallstent; Microvasive Endoscopy, Boston Scientific Corp., Natick, MA).[30] The Wallstent group had fewer symptomatic biliary complications, had a longer symptom-free survival, underwent fewer ERCPs, and spent less time in the hospital. The symptom-free survival of the polyethylene stent group undergoing 3-monthly exchange was similar to that of the metal stent group. Cost analysis found that for patients surviving 6 months or longer, it was more cost-effective to place an initial metal stent, and no difference was found between this group and the group undergoing frequent polyethylene stent changes. Yeoh et al.[32] found similar results using a decision analysis model and found that initial placement of a SEMS was economical if survival of greater than 4 months was predicted. The difficulty arises in predicting survival, and weight loss and tumor size have been identified as possible markers in univariate and multivariate analyses.[33] The presence of hepatic metastases has also been identified as predicting shorter median survival.[31]

Occlusion of metal stents is usually managed by insertion of a second stent, either a polyethylene stent or a metal stent. Insertion of a polyethylene stent through a metal stent has been shown to have longer patency than polyethylene stent exchange in patients with polyethylene stent dysfunction.[27,29] A possible mechanism is friction between the polyethylene and metal stents, allowing bile drainage around the polyethylene stent even when its lumen is occluded.

Comparisons of Wallstents with other commercially available metal stents, such as Ultraflex Diamond Stents (Microvasive) and Spiral Z-stents (Wilson-Cook Medical Inc., Winston-Salem, NC), have not shown any significant differences in technical success rates or occlusion rates.[34,35] Most cases of occlusion are not due to bile encrustation, as they are with polyethylene stents, but to tumor progression. Ensuring adequate length of the stent both proximally and distally to the tumor may prevent tumor overgrowth, but ingrowth through the mesh wires remains a problem. Partially covered Wallstents have been proposed as a solution to reduce the rates of metal stent occlusion secondary to tumor ingrowth.

Preliminary evaluation of covered metal stents was first undertaken in the early 1990s,[36] but surprisingly few published studies have evaluated their use. Occlusion of the orifices of the cystic duct and pancreatic duct are theoretical complications of a covered stent, although they do not appear to be prominent problems in the published literature. Stent migration of covered stents is also a potential problem, and partially covered stents have been designed to have approximately 10 mm of exposed mesh to allow anchoring to the biliary wall in an attempt to prevent migration. Stent migration of this design of stent has been reported previously[37] but was not found by Isayama et al.[38] in a recent evaluation of 21 patients treated with partially covered metal stents. In this study, low rates of occlusion were found (14%), compared with rates as high as 33% for uncovered stents (22%–39%) in other studies.[27,28,34] Median patient follow-up was similar in all studies (5–8 months).

Stent Dysfunction

Stent dysfunction is defined by migration of the stent, impaction of the stent orifice on the bile duct or duodenal wall, occlusion of the stent lumen, or the presence of cholangitis, whether the stent is patent or not. Stent dysfunction remains a significant issue and often leads to symptoms of recurrent biliary obstruction that can lead to cholangitis and sepsis. These complications require management with stent exchange and usually require hospitalization.

Biliary sludge, the material responsible for stent occlusion, is composed of an amorphous substance that is chemically distinct from the cholesterol-rich sludge implicated in the formation of western gallstones.[39] It is composed of protein and bacteria, calcium bilirubinate, and calcium palmitate.[40] Bacterial infection is thought to be the most important factor in the occlusion of stents[41]; however, current strategies to limit this have been disappointing. There is insufficient evidence available to conclude that antibiotic prophylaxis prolongs stent patency. This has been supported in a recent Cochrane review, which also assessed the use of ursodeoxycholic acid with or without antibiotics.[42] There is also potential for impregnation of stents with antineoplastic, anti-inflammatory, antiproliferative, and antimicrobial agents. Bioabsorbable stents are currently under development, however, these have not been extensively studied in human models.[43]

Animal studies have shown that placement of the stents above the intact ampulla reduces occlusion rates, but this has not been reproduced in a clinical trial.[44] There are clear problems with stent retrieval in this circumstance, and it may also not be feasible in pancreatic cancer with distal biliary obstruction.

Stent diameter remains the most widely accepted approach to limit the occlusion of plastic stents. There is a clear advantage of using stents of 10 Fr or greater over smaller stents,[45] although there appears to be no difference between 10 Fr and 11.5/12 Fr stents.[46,47] A 12 Fr stent is the maximal diameter that can be deployed via current duodenoscopes.

Gastric Outlet Obstruction/ Duodenal Stenosis

Pancreatic cancer is the most common cancer that obstructs the gastric outlet and occurs in approximately 17%–30% of patients with advanced disease.[48,49] The traditional approach to palliation consists of surgical gastrojejunostomy. Endoscopic management of gastric outlet obstruction consists of placement of one or more SEMS across the obstruction, and this is often performed in combination with biliary stenting. The most common SEMSs used for enteral placement have a narrow delivery system that can be passed down the working channel of therapeutic endoscopes or duodenoscopes, and the delivery system is similar to that of biliary Wallstents. The use of uncovered stents in the duodenum is recommended to avoid obstruction of the biliary or pancreatic ampullary orifices or preexisting biliary stent.

There are no controlled trials comparing surgical management of gastric outlet obstruction with endoscopic therapy. Traditionally, patients with adequate performance status would be offered surgical bypass, most commonly gastrojejunostomy, but there is growing experience with the use of SEMSs in gastric outlet obstruction. Their use was first reported in case reports dating back to 1993.[50] The advantage of endoscopic placement of these stents lies partly in better access to the stricture, as well as a mechanical advantage in being able to pass the stent through the working channel of the therapeutic endoscope.[51] Second stent deployment is also facilitated, and the adequacy of deployment can be assessed endoscopically.

The largest case series of endoscopic enteral stenting for gastric outlet obstruction consists of 36 patients from the Mayo Clinic.[52] In 19 of these patients, the primary cancer was pancreatic, and 16 of these patients also experienced biliary obstruction that required concomitant biliary stenting. Thirty-five of 36 patients were able to eat after stenting. Eight patients (22%) experienced recurrent obstruction, for which the causes consisted of overgrowth of the stent by tumor, tumor ingrowth of the stent, and stent migration (one case). The average time to reintervention in this group was 98.6 days (range, 2–307 days). In an earlier review of their experience with enteral stents, 19% of patients had recurrent obstructions, which were mainly due to tumor ingrowth and stent migration.[53]

Radiologic assessment is recommended before placement of an enteral stent. Abdominal computed tomography allows assessment of the primary lesion, the length of the duodenal stricture, and the level of the obstruction. It may also identify patients who are suboptimal candidates for enteral stenting, such as those with distal duodenal obstruction or multiple sites of obstruction.

Yim et al.[54] performed a retrospective analysis of 29 patients with enteral stent placement and compared them with a similar cohort with pancreatic cancer who had undergone surgical gastrojejunostomy. They found no differences in median or overall survival, but they did find significant differences with respect to cost (intervention and hospital stay: US$9,921 for enteral stent group compared with US$28,173 in the surgical gastrojejunostomy group), and length of hospital stay (4 vs 14 days enteral stent vs surgical group).

Endoscopic Management of Pain

Pain in pancreatic cancer occurs in 80%–85% of patients with advanced disease.[55] The main causes are believed to be tumor invasion of pancreatic and peripancreatic neural tissue, but also ductal hypertension due to obstruction of the main pancreatic duct. There is evidence that obstruction of the pancreatic duct and subsequent ductal hypertension results in pain, with most of the evidence arising from studies of patients with chronic pancreatitis.[56] Classically, "obstructive type" pain occurs after meals. Patients with morphologic features of ductal dilation in association with the obstructive type of pain are more likely to benefit from pancreatic duct stenting than those with chronic unremitting pain.[57]

Pancreatic Duct Stenting

The largest series of patients treated with pancreatic duct stents for malignant obstruction and pain is 10,[57] with only four reports in the literature totaling 23 patients. The patients in these series were all highly selected and had obstructive-type pain associated with a dilated pancreatic duct. Results have been variable, with success rates of pancreatic stenting ranging from 66%[58] to 100%[57] and clinically significant reductions in pain from 75% to 100%, measured by a reduction in pain scores and a reduction in narcotic usage. Explanations for poor symptom relief from stenting were causes for pain other than duct obstruction. Stent dysfunction from occlusion was not reported in any of the patients, although it is likely that clinically silent occlusion occurred in patients surviving longer than 2–3 months, given the data we have regarding rates of occlusion in pancreatic stents.[59]

A more recent series evaluated the use of SEMSs in the pancreatic duct in three patients. Pain was the indication in only one patient; duct disruption, and pancreatic fistula were the indications in the other two patients.[60]

Treatment was successful in the two patients with pancreatic duct fistulas. Two of these patients also underwent biliary stenting and one underwent enteral stenting, which is similar to earlier series, in which most patients also had biliary stents placed.[57,58] SEMSs were also used in two of 10 patients without complications in an earlier series, although survival was limited to 2 months.[57]

Endoscopic Ultrasound–Guided Celiac Plexus Neurolysis or Block

There has been only a single prospective study evaluating the use of endoscopic ultrasound–guided celiac plexus neurolysis for the management of pain in pancreatic cancer. This study found significant reduction in pain scores in 45 of 58 patients, all of whom had nonoperable pancreatic cancer.[61] There were no reported major complications, and minor complications included postural hypotension and diarrhea, which were transient. The benefit of the treatment seemed to diminish at 8–12 weeks, particularly if the patient was also not receiving adjuvant treatment with chemotherapy, radiotherapy, or both.

Although results have been promising, there is not enough evidence at present to make definitive conclusions regarding the safety and efficacy of endoscopic ultrasound–guided celiac plexus neurolysis in the management of pain from pancreatic cancer.[62]

Quality of Life Following Palliation of Jaundice

The main focus of biliary stent placement is relief of symptoms, improvement in well being, and it is hoped, improvement in functional status. It is well accepted that biliary stenting or bypass surgery relieves jaundice and pruritus, and these outcomes are easily measured. Anorexia is also accepted as a prominent symptom and has been evaluated in three series examining symptoms in patients with obstructive jaundice due to pancreatic cancer.[20,21,63] There have also been reports of improved appetite after stenting, and although there are several proposed theories, the mechanism is unknown.[20]

Weight loss and hyperbilirubinemia appear to be strong predictors of poor quality of life.[21,63] They are also predictors of decreased survival.[64] This group of patients had a symptomatically inferior improvement in social function scores (using the SF-36 measurement tool) after stenting than the group with lower levels of hyperbilirubinemia and no weight loss.[21]

References

1. Ries LAG, Eisner MP, Kosary CL, et al., eds. *SEER Cancer Statistics Review, 1973-1997*. Bethesda, MD: National Cancer Institute; 2000:378–391.
2. Malagelada J. Pancreatic cancer, an overview of epidemiology: clinical presentation and diagnosis. *Mayo Clin Proc.* 1979;54:459–467.
3. Bruckner H, Snady H, Cooperman A, Madeli J. Improvements in survival and clinical benefit for patients with metastatic pancreatic cancer. *Digestion.* 1998;59[suppl 3]:511.
4. Burris H, Moore M, Andersen J, et al. Improvements in survival and clinical benefit with gemcitabine as first-line therapy for patients with advanced pancreatic cancer: a randomised trial. *J Clin Oncol.* 1997;15:2403–2413.
5. Soehendra N, Reynders-Fredrix V. Palliative biliary duct drainage. A new method for endoscopic introduction of a new drain. *Dtsch Med Wochenshr.* 1979;104:206–207.
6. McPherson GA, Benjamin IS, Hodgson HJ, et al. Preoperative percutaneous biliary drainage: the results of a controlled trial. *Br J Surg.* 1984;71:371–375.
7. Hatfield AR, Tobias R, Terblanche J, et al. Preoperative external biliary drainage in obstructive jaundice: a prospective controlled clinical trial. *Lancet.* 1982;2:896–899.
8. Smith RC, Pooley M, George CR, et al. Preoperative percutaneous transhepatic internal drainage in obstructive jaundice: a randomized, controlled trial examining renal function. *Surgery.* 1985;97:641–648.
9. Sewnath ME, Karsten TM, Prins MH, Rauws EJA, Obertop H, Gouma DJ. A meta-analysis on the efficacy of preoperative biliary drainage for tumors causing obstructive jaundice. *Ann Surg.* 2002;236:17–27.
10. Saleh MMA, Norregaard P, Jorgensen HL, Anderson PK, Matzen P. Preoperative endoscopic stent placement before pancreaticoduodenectomy: a meta-analysis of the effect on morbidity and mortality. *Gastrointest Endosc.* 2002;56:529–534.
11. Pitt HA, Gomes AS, Lois JF, et al. Does preoperative percutaneous biliary drainage reduce operative risk or increase hospital cost? *Ann Surg.* 1985;201:545–553.
12. Lai EC, Mok FP, Fan ST, et al. Preoperative endoscopic drainage for malignant obstructive jaundice. *Br J Surg.* 1994;81:1195–1198.
13. Lygidakis NJ, van der Heyde MN, Lubbers MJ. Evaluation of preoperative biliary drainage in the surgical management of pancreatic head carcinoma. *Acta Chir Scand.* 1987;153:665–668.
14. Pisters PWT, Lee JE, Vauthey JN, Evans DB. Letter to the editor. *Ann Surg.* 2003;237:594–596.
15. Povoski SP, Karpeh MS, Conlon KC, Blumgart LH, Brennan MF. Association of preoperative biliary drainage with postoperative outcome following pancreaticoduodenectomy. *Ann Surg.* 1999;230:131–142.
16. Karsten TM, Allema JH, Reinders M, et al. Preoperative biliary drainage, colonisation of bile and postoperative complications in patients with tumours of the pancreatic head: a retrospective analysis of 241 consecutive patients. *Eur J Surg.* 1996;162:881–888.
17. Sewnath ME, Birjmohun RS, Rauws EA, Huibregtse K, Obertop H, Gouma DJ. The effect of preoperative biliary

drainage on postoperative complications after pancreaticoduodenectomy. *J Am Coll Surg*. 2001;192:726–734.

18. Aronsen DC, Chamuleau RA, Frederiks WM, et al. Reversibility of cholestatic changes following experimental common bile duct obstruction: fact of fantasy? *J Hepatol*. 1993;18:85–95.
19. Warshaw AL, Swanson RS. Pancreatic cancer in 1988: possibilities and probabilities. *Ann Surg*. 1988;208:541–553.
20. Ballinger AB, McHugh M, Catnach SM, Alstead EM, Clark ML. Symptom relief and quality of life after stenting for malignant bile duct obstruction. *Gut*. 1994;35:467–470.
21. Abraham NS, Barkun J.S, Barkun AN,. Palliation of malignant biliary obstruction: a prospective trial examining impact on quality of life. *Gastrointest Endosc*. 2002;56:835–841.
22. Wallanapa P, Williamson RN. Surgical palliation for pancreatic cancer. *Br J Surg*. 1992;79:8–20.
23. Smith AC, Dowsett JF, Russell RCG, Hatfield ARW, Cotton PB. Randomised trial of endoscopic stenting versus surgical bypass in malignant low bileduct obstruction. *Lancet*. 1994;344:1655–1660.
24. Anderson JR, Sorensen SM, Kruse A, Rokkjaer M. Randomised trial of endoscopic endoprosthesis versus operative bypass in malignant obstructive jaundice. *Gut*. 1989;30:1132–1135.
25. Shepherd HA, Royle G, Ross APR, Diba A, Arthur M, Colin-Jones D. Endoscopic biliary endoprosthesis in the palliation of malignant obstruction of the distal common bile duct: a randomized trial. *Br J Surg*. 1998;75:1166–1168.
26. Speer AG, Cotton PB, Russell RCG, Mason RR, Hatfield ARW, Leung JWC, et al. Randomised trial of endoscopic versus percutaneous stent insertion in malignant obstructive jaundice. *Lancet*. 1987;i:57–62.
27. Davids PHP, Groen AK, Rauws EA, Tytgat GN, Huibregtse K. Randomized trial of self-expanding metal stents versus polyethylene stents for distal malignant biliary obstruction. *Lancet*. 1992;340:1488–1492.
28. Knyrim K, Wagner HJ, Pausch J, Vakil N. A prospective, randomized, controlled trial of metal stents for malignant obstruction of the common bile duct. *Endoscopy*. 1993;25:207–212.
29. Schmassmann A, von Gunten E, Scheurer U, Fehr HF, Halter F. Wallstents versus polyethylene stents in malignant biliary obstruction: effects of stent patency of the first and second stent on patient compliance and survival. *Am J Gastroenterol*. 1996;91:654–659.
30. Prat F, Chapat O, Ducot B, Ponchon T, Pelletier G, Fritsch J, et al. A randomized trial of endoscopic drainage methods for inoperable malignant strictures of the common bile duct. *Gastrointest Endosc*. 1998;47:1–7.
31. Kaassis M, Boyer J, Dumas R, Ponchon T, Coumaros D, Delcenserie R, Canard J, et al. Plastic or metal stents for malignant strictures of the common bile duct? Results of a randomized prospective study. *Gastrointest Endosc*. 2003;57:178–182.
32. Yeoh KG, Zimmerman MJ, Cunningham JT, Cotton PB. Comparative costs of metal versus plastic biliary stent strategies for malignant obstructive jaundice by decision analysis. *Gastrointest Endosc*. 1999;49:466–471.
33. Prat F, Chapat O, Ducot B, et al. Predictive factors for survival of patients with inoperable malignant distal biliary strictures: a practical management guideline. *Gut*. 1998;42:76–80.
34. Dumonceau JM, Cremer MD, Auroux J, Delhaye M, Deviere JA. Comparison of Ultraflex Diamond stents and Wallstents for palliation of distal malignant biliary strictures. *Am J Gastroenterol*. 2000;95:670–676.
35. Shah RJ, Howell DA, Desilets DJ, et al. Multicenter randomized trial of Spiral Z-stent compared with the Wallstent for malignant biliary obstruction. *Gastrointest Endosc*. 2003;57:830–836.
36. Saito H, Sakurai Y, Takamura A, Horio K. Biliary endoprosthesis using Gore-Tex covered expandable metallic stents: preliminary clinical evaluation. *Nippon Acta Radiol*. 1994;54:180–182.
37. Wamsteker E, Elta GH. Migration of covered biliary self-expanding metallic stents in two patients with malignant biliary obstruction. *Gastrointest Endosc*. 2003;58:792–793.
38. Isayama H, Komatsu Y, Tsujino T, et al. Polyurethane-covered metal stent for management of distal malignant biliary obstruction. *Gastrointest Endosc*. 2002;55:366–370.
39. Libby E, Leung J. Prevention of biliary clogging: a clinical review. *Am J Gastroenterol*. 1996;91:1301–1307.
40. Moesch C, Santerrean D, Cessot F, et al. Physicochemical and bacteriological analysis of the contents of occluded biliary endoprostheses. *Hepatology*. 1991;14:1142–1146.
41. Leung JWC, Ling TKC, Kung JLS, et al. The role of bacteria in the blockage of biliary stents. *Gastrointest Endosc*. 1988;34:19–22.
42. Galandi D, Schwarzer G, Bassler D, Allgaier HP. Ursodeoxycholic acid and/or antibiotics for prevention of biliary stent occlusion. *Cochrane Database Syst Rev*. 2002;(3):CD003043.
43. Ginsberg G, Constantin C, Shah J, Martin T, Carty A, Habecker P, et al. In vivo evaluation of a new bioabsorbable self-expanding biliary stent. *Gastrointest Endosc*. 2003;58:777–784.
44. Geoghegan JG, Branch MS, Costerton JW, et al. Biliary stents occlude earlier if the distal tip is in the duodenum in dogs [abstract]. *Gastrointest Endosc*. 1991;37:257.
45. Speer AG, Cotton P, MacRea KD. Endoscopic management of malignant biliary obstruction: stents of 10 French gauge are preferable to stents of 8 French gauge. *Gastrointest Endosc*. 1988;34:412–417.
46. Kadakia SC, Starnes E. Comparison of 10 French gauge stent with 11.5 French gauge stent in patients with biliary tract diseases. *Gastrointest Endosc*. 1992;38:454–459.
47. Finnie IA, O'Toole PA, Rhodes JM, et al. A prospective randomised trial of 10 and 11.5 FG endoprostheses in malignant bile duct obstruction. *Gut*. 1994;35[suppl]:S50.
48. Sarr MG, Cameron JL. Surgical palliation of unresectable carcinoma of the pancreas. *World J Surg*. 1984;8:906–918.
49. Watanapa P, Williamson RC. Surgical palliation for pancreatic cancer: developments during the past two decades. *Br J Surg*. 1992;79:8–20.
50. Keymling M, Wagner JH, Vakil N, Krynim K. Relief of a malignant duodenal obstruction by percutaneous insertion of a metal stent. *Gastrointest Endosc*. 1993;39:439–441.

51. Baron TH, Harewood GC. Enteral self-expandable stents. *Gastrointest Endosc.* 2003;58:421–433.
52. Adler DG, Baron TH. Endoscopic palliation of malignant gastric outlet obstruction using self-expanding metal stents: experience in 36 patients. *Am J Gastroenterol.* 2002;97:72–78.
53. Mauro MA, Koehler RE, Baron TH. Advances in gastrointestinal intervention: the treatment of gastroduodenal and colorectal obstructions with metallic stents. *Radiology.* 2000;215:659–669.
54. Yim HB, Jacobsen BC, Saltzman JR, Johannes RS, Bounds BC, Lee JH, et al. Clinical outcome of the use of enteral stents for palliation of patients with malignant upper GI obstruction. *Gastrointest Endosc.* 2001;53:329–332.
55. Kaiser MH, Barkin J, MacIntyre JM. Pancreatic cancer: assessment of prognosis by clinical presentation. *Cancer.* 1985;56:397–402.
56. Carr-Locke DL. Endoscopic therapy of chronic pancreatitis. *Gastrointest Endosc.* 1999;49:s77–80.
57. Tham TCK, Lichtenstein DR, Vandervoort MD, Wong RCK, Slivka A, Banks A, et al. Pancreatic duct stents for "obstructive type" pain in pancreatic malignancy. *Am J Gastroenterol.* 2000;95:956–960.
58. Costamanga G, Gabbrielli A, Mutignani M, Perri V, Crucitti F. Treatment of "obstructive" pain by endoscopic drainage in patients with pancreatic head carcinoma. *Gastrointest Endosc.* 1993;39:774–777.
59. Ikenberry SO, Sherman S, Hawes RH, Smith M, Lehman GA. The occlusion rate of pancreatic stents. *Gastrointest Endosc.* 1994;40:611–613.
60. Keeley SP, Freeman ML. Placement of self-expanding metallic stents in the pancreatic duct for treatment of obstructive complications of pancreatic cancer. *Gastrointest Endosc.* 2003;57:756–759.
61. Gunaratnam NT, Sarma AV, Norton ID, Wiersema MJ. A prospective study of EUS-guided celiac plexus neurolysis for pancreatic cancer pain. *Gastrointest Endosc.* 2001;54:316–324.
62. Levy MJ, Wiersema MJ. EUS-guided celiac plexus neurolysis and celiac plexus block. *Gastrointest Endosc.* 2003;57:923–930.
63. Sherman S, Lehman G, Earle D, Lazaridis, Frakes J, Johanson J. Endoscopic palliation of malignant bile duct obstruction: improvement in quality of life [abstract]. *Gastrointest Endosc.* 1996;43:AB321.
64. Prat F, Chapat O, Ducot B, et al. Predictive factors for survival of patients with inoperable malignant distal biliary strictures: a practical management guideline. *Gut.* 1998;42:76–80.

31

Surgical Palliation of Pancreatic Cancer

Michael L. Kendrick, MD
Yun Shin Chun, MD
John D. Christein, MD
Michael G. Sarr, MD

Pancreatic cancer is the fourth most common cause of cancer-related death in the United States. Despite advances in diagnostic imaging and improved outcomes of pancreatic resection, the prognosis for this disease remains poor, with an overall 5-year survival of less than 5%. Of the 31,000 patients diagnosed with pancreatic cancer in the United States in 2003, more than 80% will have had locally advanced or metastatic disease that precludes resection with curative intent at the time of diagnosis.[1] Moreover, even though 20% of patients are clinically "resectable for cure," the 5-year survival rate after resection is at best 20%, and the absolute cure rate is even less. Therefore, we as physicians ultimately manage most patients with pancreatic cancer in a palliative manner. Palliation of symptoms to maximize quality of life thus becomes a central component of management in most of these cases. The major focus of palliation is aimed at three predominant complications of pancreatic cancer: obstructive jaundice, gastric/duodenal obstruction, and tumor-related pain.

Historically, the initial palliation was addressed predominantly by the surgeon. However, advances in endoscopic and percutaneous technical methodologies and improvements in preoperative staging have prompted enthusiasm about nonoperative and interventional approaches to palliation that avoid the need for a celiotomy. Each approach has its own benefits, with differences being in invasiveness, complications, and durability. The optimal treatment approach should be tailored to each patient in regard to expected survival, predominant symptoms, and operative risk.

The Problem

Pancreatic cancer is an intensely aggressive neoplasm both locally and systemically. By means of its unique tumor biology, it can metastasize early to lymph nodes, peritoneum, and liver, even when the primary lesion is less than 2 cm.[2] Moreover, by spreading locally along neural sheaths, it tends to involve intrapancreatic and extrapancreatic visceral afferent nerves, predisposing to the characteristic chronic, deep-seated visceral pain.[3] In addition, pancreatic cancer usually induces a local sclerosing reaction. Therefore, in combination with its aggressive, local neoplastic growth, this associated peritumoral fibrosis leads to the development of locoregional complications. When the primary neoplasm arises in the head of the pancreas (85% of patients), external compression and mechanical obstruction of nearby structures are early processes involving the intrapancreatic portion of the common bile duct (extrahepatic obstructive jaundice) and the portal and superior mesenteric vein confluence (splanchnic venous hypertension). Obstruction of the second portion of the duodenum (gastric outlet obstruction) occurs later in the disease. For primary neoplasms of the neck and proximal body of the gland, in addition to celiac plexus involvement (back pain), the splenic vein may become compressed, leading to sinistral portal hypertension and its consequences. For midbody and tail lesions, symptoms that lead to the diagnosis, such as significant local involvement (stomach, spleen, colon, adrenal), usually occur much later in the course of the disease after the disease has advanced locally, decreasing the likelihood of resectability. Duodenal obstruction may occur with midbody pancreatic cancers, but the duodenal obstruction does not occur in the second portion, but rather at the fourth portion of the duodenum as the tumor extends inferiorly through the mesocolon. Therefore, the problems that we as physicians need to address in these patients are primarily extrahepatic biliary obstruction, duodenal obstruction, and visceral pain.

Obstructive Jaundice

Because of the associated symptoms, relief of obstructive jaundice requires intervention in virtually everyone with biliary obstruction, even in those with advanced, unresectable pancreatic cancer. Justification for palliation of obstructive jaundice is centered on the morbidity and potential mortality of untreated biliary obstruction. Nausea and anorexia are frequent sequelae of obstructive jaundice and contribute to weight loss and malnutrition. The pruritus associated with biliary obstruction is often debilitating and seldom responds adequately to systemic or topical medications. Additionally, untreated chronic biliary obstruction induces progressive liver dysfunction, coagulopathy, and eventual liver failure (biliary cirrhosis) and death. Palliation is thus centered on internal (enteric) biliary decompression, redirection of serum bilirubin, and quality-of-life improvements. Relief of the jaundice results frequently in a dramatic improvement in appetite, abates pruritus, and improves sense of well-being. Sarr and Cameron,[4] in a review of more than 8000 patients, noted that surgical decompression was associated with a modest improvement in survival (5.4 months vs 3.5 months), but the real impact involved a substantive improvement in quality of life over diagnostic laparotomy alone without internal biliary drainage.

Therefore, the primary question facing the physician and surgeon caring for a patient with extrahepatic biliary obstruction secondary to an unresectable pancreatic cancer involves choosing the best overall approach *for that individual patient*: surgical internal drainage (open or laparoscopic approach) versus interventional internal drainage (endoscopic or percutaneous radiologic approach). Permanent external biliary drainage should be reserved for a very few selected individuals in whom internal (enteric) drainage is not possible. Each modality has its benefits and limitations, and the concept of quality of life *as defined by the patient* (not necessarily by long-term patency or the noninvasive nature of the intervention) should weigh into the ultimate decision.

Surgical Palliation of Obstructive Jaundice

Most pancreatic cancers occur in the head of the pancreas, where the proximity of the common bile duct and the proximal main pancreatic duct (the site of origin of most pancreatic cancers) results in the frequent development of progressive, external mechanical occlusion of the common bile duct. Currently, surgical palliation is usually provided for patients who, at the time of exploration for potential curative resection, are found to have unresectable disease or the unusual circumstance in which nonsurgical attempts at endoscopic or radiologic palliation have failed. The principle surgical options for palliation of obstructive jaundice include choledochojejunostomy or hepaticojejunostomy, cholecystojejunostomy, and choledochoduodenostomy.

The most widely accepted method of surgical biliary decompression is choledochojejunostomy or probably more appropriately termed *hepaticojejunostomy*. Several large series have demonstrated the effectiveness of this procedure in successful and durable biliary decompression.[5-7] This biliary-enteric bypass is constructed with either a jejunal loop or a Roux-en-Y limb. Neither construction has consistently shown superiority over the other; however, each has its advantages. Although the use of a jejunal loop may avoid an additional anastomosis (however, many surgeons add a Braun-type, side-to-side enteroenterostomy below the mesocolon), a Roux-en-Y limb improves mobility in reaching the hepatic hilum and makes anastomotic leaks easier to manage, because the Roux limb is a defunctionalized limb, should there be an anastomotic leak, only bile will extravasate and not also enteric chyme. Hepaticojejunostomy with a Roux-en-Y limb construction has been our preferred approach (Fig. 31.1). Although choledochojejunostomy may be technically possible, hepaticojejunostomy is especially advantageous in the setting of a "low" junction of the cystic and

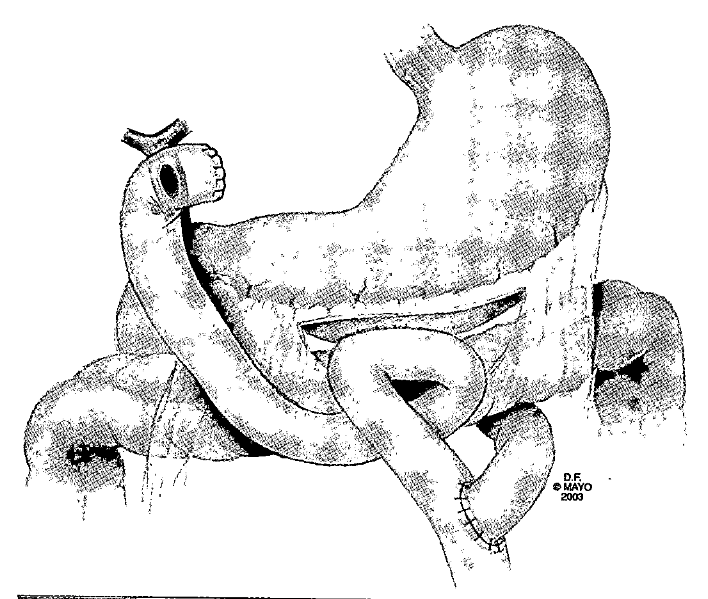

Figure 31.1
Side-to-side Roux-en-Y hepaticojejunostomy with loop gastrojejunostomy.

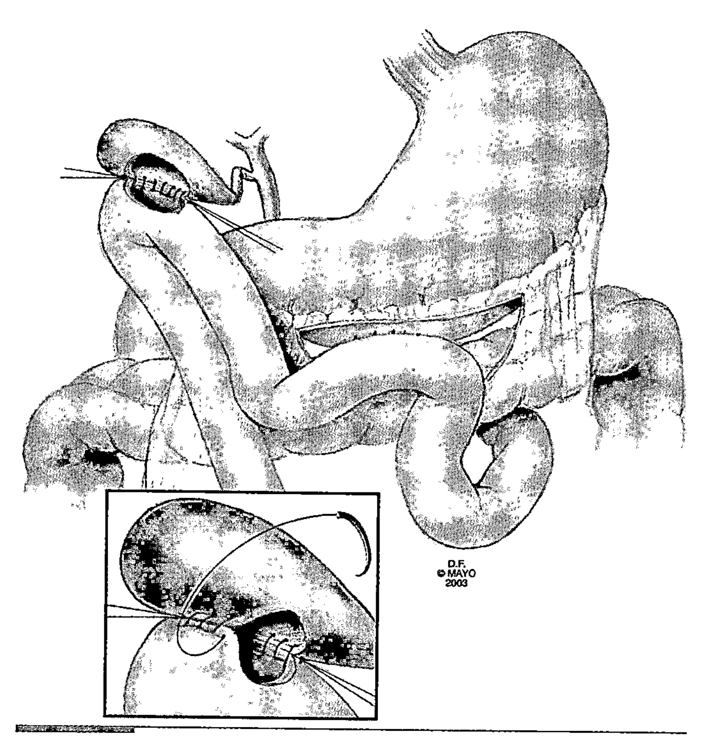

Figure 31.2
Cholecystojejunostomy. Requires patency of cystic duct with common hepatic duct.

hepatic duct, or when there is cephalad extension of the tumor into the hepatoduodenal ligament. Because pancreatic cancer tends to extend locally, hepaticojejunostomy, in conjunction with cholecystectomy, tends to be the procedure of choice by most pancreatic surgeons.[8] The technique involves either transection of the distal hepatic duct with an end-to-side anastomosis or a simple side-to-side anastomosis, as preferred by us (Fig. 31.1); the latter technique does not require circumferential dissection of the common hepatic duct or ligation of the distal common duct.

The use of cholecystojejunostomy has, in principle, several ostensible advantages over choledochojejunostomy and hepaticojejunostomy (Fig. 31.2). It is easier to perform and is more conducive to a laparoscopic approach. However, critics of cholecystojejunostomy have voiced concerns about recurrent jaundice as the pancreatic neoplasm invades the hepatoduodenal ligament encroaching on the junction of the cystic duct with the common hepatic duct. In one review of patients with obstructing periampullary malignancy, two thirds of patients had either cystic duct obstruction or tumor within 1 cm of this junction on endoscopic retrograde cholangiopancreatography.[9] Only one prospective, randomized trial has compared cholecystojejunostomy with choledochojejunostomy. In 31 patients, of whom only 71% had malignant biliary obstruction, Sarfeh and colleagues[5] concluded that cholecystojejunostomy was associated with decreased operative time and blood loss, but at the expense of increased postoperative complications and recurrent jaundice. Further, a meta-analysis of studies comparing cholecystojejunostomy with choledochojejunostomy found that cholecystojejunostomy resulted in less initial success (89% vs 97%) and was associated with an increased incidence of recurrent jaundice or cholangitis (20% vs 8%).[4,6] More recently, a population-based, retrospective, cohort study of 1919 patients older than 65 years who were undergoing biliary bypass for pancreatic cancer demonstrated that patients who underwent cholecystojejunostomy were about three times likelier to require additional biliary intervention than those who underwent hepaticojejunostomy.[7] In some situations, such as with uncinate cancer or a very scarred, inflamed hepatoduodenal ligament, cholecystojejunostomy may seem prudent to the surgeon. In these situations, if a cholecystojejunostomy is planned, the surgeon should ensure patency of the cystic duct into the distal biliary tree and should also ensure that the junction of the cystic duct is at least 2–3 cm above the tumor.[7,10] Preoperative endoscopic retrograde cholangiopancreatography, magnetic resonance cholangiopancreatography, or intraoperative cholangiography via a cholecystostomy is recommended and should determine these criteria. If, however, the surgeon is worried about the increased morbidity from a hepaticojejunostomy over that from a cholecystojejunostomy, then he or she probably should not be operating on these patients.

Choledochoduodenostomy or hepaticoduodenostomy has not been advocated widely for the treatment of obstructive jaundice in patients with pancreatic cancer by most pancreatic surgeons. Critics of this approach voice concerns regarding the proximity of the anastomosis to the cancer, the potential for associated duodenal obstruction distal to the anastomosis, and the theoretic risks of leakage of both bile and duodenal content. Moreover, these critics also cite reviews demonstrating an increased incidence of recurrent jaundice over that of choledochojejunostomy. Despite these concerns, Di Fronzo and colleagues[11] reported their experience using choledochoduodenostomy in 70 of 79 patients who underwent palliative biliary drainage for unresectable pancreatic cancer. Interestingly, none of these patients experienced recurrent jaundice during a mean survival of 13 months, and no biliary-enteric leaks occurred. Similar findings were reported by the Cleveland Clinic group.[12]

Laparoscopic Palliation of Biliary Obstruction

With the advent of advanced laparoscopic techniques, the ability to surgically palliate obstructive jaundice using a minimal access approach has come to fruition. Techniques to perform laparoscopic cholecystojejunostomy, choledochojejunostomy, and hepaticojejunostomy have all been described.[13-15] The potential advantages of these minimal access methods are the chance for a reduced procedural-related morbidity and the preservation of durability of palliation provided by a surgical approach. Although the precise role of laparoscopic staging is debated, the ability to perform palliation laparoscopically eliminates the need for a formal celiotomy and the subsequent convalescence of a celiotomy in patients who harbored unresectable disease at the time of laparoscopic staging or by preoperative imaging. In addition to demonstrating the feasibility of a laparoscopic biliary decompression either as a primary option or after failure of nonoperative palliation, initial results from centers with considerable laparoscopic expertise suggested a reduction in morbidity, mortality, and duration of hospital stay when compared with conventional palliation by open surgery.[13,15] Currently, the lack of widespread expertise in the advanced technical maneuvers required for laparoscopic palliation has limited its use, but the next generation of surgeons will be trained with these techniques. Although prospective, randomized trials are needed to substantiate these findings, laparoscopic palliation may fill the shortcomings of endoscopic and open surgical methods of palliation and should be evaluated in randomized trials. With the improved patency of newer endoscopic stents (improving failure rates) and the advantages of laparoscopic approaches (decreased morbidity and mortality compared to open surgery), these two modalities will likely compete as the most appropriate method of palliation in the next decade. This will be especially true if hepaticojejunostomy can be performed laparoscopically as opposed to the relatively simple cholecystojejunostomy.

Nonoperative Versus Operative Palliation of Obstructive Jaundice

Although controversy continues regarding the most appropriate method of palliation of jaundice in patients with malignant biliary obstruction, nonoperative methods are well established and should now be part of any center's therapeutic armamentarium. Several prospective, randomized studies have compared nonoperative with operative biliary decompression and have demonstrated no substantive difference in relief of obstructive jaundice (Table 31.1). The initial success rate of percutaneous transhepatic, endoscopic, and surgical decompression, in terms of relief of obstructive jaundice, varies between 75% and 100%. Surgical treatment is associated with an early, procedure-related increase in morbidity and mortality and a longer initial hospital stay. During the follow-up until death, however, nonoperative approaches were associated with recurrent jaundice or cholangitis requiring readmission and replacement of the endoprosthesis in up to 40% of patients. Another consideration is the potential development of duodenal obstruction requiring gastrojejunostomy in up to 15% of patients treated only with internal biliary drainage (without a duodenal bypass). In a meta-analysis of three randomized studies comparing endoscopic stenting and surgical bypass,[16-18] re-intervention because of recurrent jaundice was necessary in 36% of patients treated with biliary stents versus only 3% of patients treated with surgery.[19] Recurrent jaundice after stent placement is largely due to occlusion as a result of bacterial biofilm and biliary sludge that clogs the stent.[20] Newer stents designed to avoid this complication are currently under investigation.

Despite the less durable results afforded by endoscopic decompression, this nonoperative approach re-

Table 31.1 Randomized Trials Comparing Nonoperative and Operative Palliative Biliary Decompression

	First Author							
	Bornman[49]		Shepherd[16]		Andersen[17]		Smith[18]	
Parameters	Stent N = 25	Bypass N = 25	Stent N = 23	Bypass N = 25	Stent N = 25	Bypass N = 25	Stent N = 101	Bypass N = 100
Stent	Percutaneous		Endoscopic		Endoscopic		Endoscopic	
Success (%)	84	76	80	92	96	88	94	93
Morbidity (%)	28	32	30	56	36	20	30	58
Mortality (%)	8	20	9	20	20	24	8	15
Recurrent jaundice (%)	38	16	30	0	0	0	36	2
Survival (weeks)	19	15	22	18	12	14	21	26

mains the procedure of choice in most centers for patients with known, unresectable disease identified by preoperative staging and imaging. Indeed, at our institution, the use of operative biliary palliation has decreased markedly over the past two decades, and endoscopic decompression remains the procedure of choice unless other complications necessitate an operative approach (e.g., duodenal obstruction, patient preference, or the rare situation of a patient not living close to a center capable of interventional techniques). Although it is certainly attractive to avoid a major operation in these patients with such a limited life expectancy, it is also important to ensure that quality of life is not adversely affected by recurrent jaundice, cholangitis, and hospital readmission; few studies have adequately addressed this issue from a patient's perspective.

Duodenal Obstruction

Symptomatic duodenal obstruction occurs in 15%–30% of patients with pancreatic cancer, causing nausea and vomiting and subsequent electrolyte abnormalities and nutritional deterioration; which herald a significant decline in quality of life.

Similar to extrahepatic biliary obstruction, duodenal obstruction occurs secondary to extrinsic compression as the result of local neoplastic growth and associated peritumoral fibrosis. For pancreatic head and uncinate lesions, duodenal obstruction typically occurs in the second and occasionally the proximal third portion of the duodenum, whereas body and tail lesions more typically obstruct the fourth portion. Although up to 50% of patients with pancreatic cancer experience nausea and vomiting, many of these patients have symptoms that can be attributed to a functional gastroparesis believed to be caused by tumor invasion of retroperitoneal nerves[21-23]; thus, the cause of the obstruction (i.e., mechanical versus functional) should be determined when operative palliation is considered.

In the patient with symptoms attributable to mechanical duodenal obstruction, few dispute the value of a palliative gastrojejunostomy. However, prophylactic gastrojejunostomy in anticipation of potential duodenal obstruction remains a controversial topic.[4,22,24,25] Controversy surrounding duodenal bypass is centered on three central concepts: (1) the incidence of subsequent duodenal obstruction requiring intervention, (2) the efficacy of the procedure in preventing future symptoms of duodenal obstruction, and (3) the morbidity and mortality of the operative procedure.

The reported incidence of duodenal obstruction requiring intervention in patients with pancreatic cancer is from 2% to 30% in most large series.[22,25,26] This large range probably depends on the philosophy of the physician and to a lesser degree the patient. Undoubtedly, patients with an initially unresectable pancreatic cancer die with duodenal obstruction without further intervention, either because of advanced cachexia or a nihilistic philosophy regarding subsequent intervention. Ideally, the decision to perform a prophylactic gastrojejunostomy would be based on the factors predicting that symptomatic duodenal obstruction would occur before death. Although clear, indisputable predictive factors have yet to be determined, many experienced pancreatic surgeons offer prophylactic surgical palliation for "impending" (partial) obstruction of the duodenum. The likelihood of developing duodenal obstruction may best be related to the expected survival of the patient, because a decreased incidence of subsequent duodenal obstruction is observed in patients with a survival of less than 6 months,[11,27] suggesting that most patients, especially those with liver or peritoneal metastases, will not live long enough to develop duodenal obstruction.[27] Indeed, Di Fronzo et al.[28] reported a median survival of 5 months in patients with liver metastases or peritoneal disease, and none of these patients experienced duodenal obstruction. In contrast, patients with unresectability based on local extension with only major vessel involvement had a median survival of 12 months, and 20% of these patients experienced subsequent duodenal obstruction.

Gastrojejunostomy successfully abates symptoms of mechanical duodenal obstruction. A more difficult question, however, is the efficacy of *prophylactic* gastrojejunostomy in preventing future symptoms attributable to duodenal obstruction, given that many patients will experience symptoms (e.g., nausea, vomiting, bloating) from tumor-related gastroparesis. In a large review of surgically managed patients with unresectable pancreatic cancer, Sarr and Cameron[4] reported that 13% of patients who did not undergo gastric bypass at the initial surgical procedure developed subsequent duodenal obstruction requiring gastrojejunostomy, and another 20% of patients died with symptoms consistent with duodenal obstruction. Lillemoe and colleagues[25] conducted a prospective, randomized trial of prophylactic gastrojejunostomy or no gastrojejunostomy in 87 patients with unresectable periampullary cancer (>95% with pancreatic cancer) who were deemed by the surgeon to be at low risk for subsequent duodenal obstruction. Importantly, this study specifically excluded patients who had preoperative symptoms of functional gastric outlet obstruction (e.g., nausea, vomiting). Postoperative morbidity, duration of hospital stay, and mean survival were similar in the two groups. Among 43 patients randomly assigned to no gastrojejunostomy, eight (19%) experienced late gastric outlet obstruction requiring intervention after a median of 2 months. A very recently reported randomized, multicenter trial from Europe of prophylactic gastrojejunostomy in patients with unresectable periampullary cancer found very similar results.[29] There were no differences in duration of hospitalization, incidence of postoperative delayed gastric emptying, survival, or quality of life. However, gastrojejunostomy effectively prevented the future onset of duodenal obstruction requiring reoperation in 20% of patients who did not undergo gastrojejunostomy. Based on these data, the authors recommended routine prophylactic gastrojejunostomy. Table 31.2 compares studies evaluating the incidence of duodenal obstruction in patients who did not undergo prophylactic gastrojejunostomy after unresectability determined at operative exploration. Not only do these studies demonstrate a substantial incidence of subsequent duodenal obstruction necessitating gastrojejunostomy, these findings also underscore that this "delayed" procedure is associated with increased mortality when compared with that in patients whose prophylactic gastrojejunostomy was performed at the time of initial exploration.

In contrast to these studies, Espat et al.[22] from Memorial Sloan-Kettering Cancer Center reported a lower incidence of gastric outlet obstruction. They studied 155 patients with laparoscopically staged, unresectable pancreatic adenocarcinoma. After a median follow-up of 5.9 months, only 2% of patients had duodenal obstruction that required intervention. The investigators concluded that gastrojejunostomy was indicated only for patients with confirmed gastric outlet obstruction. Dif-

Table 31.2 Studies Evaluating Outcome of Patients Without Prophylactic Gastrojejunostomy

	First Author			
Parameters	Lillemoe[25] N = 43	Di Fronzo[11] N = 60	Sarr[4,a] N = 1800	Watanapa[6,a] N = 891
Required subsequent GJ (%)	19	12	13	17
Median time to obstruction (months)	5	14	-	9
30-day mortality after subsequent GJ (%)	12.5	33	16	22
Median survival after GJ (months)	5	9	-	2.5

[a]Collective review.
Abbreviation: GJ, Gastrojejunostomy.

ferences between these two studies can be attributed, in part, to the difference in expected incidence of duodenal obstruction. In the study by Espat and colleagues,[22] 35% of patients had lesions in the body or tail, whereas in the study by Lillemoe and colleagues,[25] all patients had tumors in the pancreatic head region. In summary, these findings suggest that patients who are most likely to benefit from prophylactic gastrojejunostomy are those with lesions in the head, neck, or uncinate process with unresectability secondary to local invasion or regional metastatic disease in whom a survival of greater than 6 months is expected. Indeed, a prophylactic gastrojejunostomy effectively prevents future gastric outlet obstruction.[25,26]

Critics of prophylactic gastrojejunostomy frequently cite the morbidity, and in some situations, the mortality associated with the gastrojejunostomy procedure. Weaver et al.[30] reported that of 36 patients with presumed mechanical duodenal obstruction who underwent gastrojejunostomy, 70% died within 30 days; the authors concluded that duodenal obstruction was a terminal event in pancreatic cancer. However, this study has been criticized, not only because of the inordinately high perioperative mortality (not representative of many other series) but also because the patients in this study were much later in the course of their disease than most patients considered for prophylactic gastrojejunostomy. Increased morbidity after gastrojejunostomy has been attributed largely to delayed gastric emptying, which has been reported to occur in up to 21% of patients after palliative gastrojejunostomy.[26] De Rooij and colleagues[31] evaluated 297 patients with unresectable pancreatic cancer who underwent surgical palliation. Morbidity rates were greater when duodenal bypass was accompanied biliary bypass (30%) than when biliary bypass alone was performed (18%), with the increased morbidity after gastrojejunostomy attributed primarily to delayed gastric emptying. Many of the patients in these two studies had preoperative symptoms of delayed gastric emptying, and many would argue that these patients would be expected to have delayed gastric emptying (or a persistent dysmotility?). Indeed, when such patients with mechanical or functional delayed gastric emptying were specifically excluded, Lillemoe and colleagues[25] reported no difference in postoperative morbidity or duration of postoperative stay in patients randomly assigned to biliary bypass either with or without gastrojejunostomy. Previous work by Doberneck and Berndt[32] and Sarr et al.[26] demonstrated similar results; among 57 patients with unresectable pancreatic carcinoma who underwent gastrojejunostomy with or without biliary bypass, 26% had delayed gastric emptying for an average of 16 days. The major predisposing factor for postoperative delayed gastric emptying was preoperative gastric outlet obstruction. Delayed gastric emptying occurred in 57% of patients with preoperative duodenal obstruction, compared with16% of patients without preoperative duodenal obstruction.

The causes of delayed gastric emptying are unknown. However, Weaver and colleagues[30] studied patients with an upper gastrointestinal series after gastrojejunostomy and found that in some patients, the stomach emptied preferentially through the duodenum, despite a patent gastrojejunostomy. Others have implicated (without solid, convincing data) that a recirculating limb is established, with the stomach emptying through the duodenum, and chyme traversing the ligament of Treitz and refluxing back into the stomach through the gastrojejunostomy. Weaver and colleagues[30] concluded that gastrojejunostomy was ineffective in patients with functional, rather than anatomic, gastric outlet obstruction. Lucas and colleagues[33] believe that the best means of avoiding problems with gastric emptying is to perform an antrectomy with gastrojejunostomy for palliation; this alternative approach has not received much support from surgeons throughout the world.

With improved preoperative determination of unresectability and successful endoscopic biliary bypass for the palliation of biliary obstruction, the surgeon is faced much less commonly with an intraoperative decision regarding prophylactic palliative gastrojejunostomy.[34] In our practice, we continue to perform prophylactic gastrojejunostomy in patients whose periampullary neoplasms are determined at operation to be unresectable.

Several issues may be of merit when the anatomic construction of the gastrojejunostomy is considered, including position relative to the colon, peristaltic orientation, and orientation of the limb with regard to biliary drainage if present. The antecolic gastrojejunostomy has been claimed to have the putative advantage of maximizing the anatomic distance of the anastomosis from areas of local tumor extension.[26] Although this is true for neoplasms of the body and tail of the pancreas, this is not true for cancer of the head of the gland. Lillemoe and colleagues[35] reported a higher rate of delayed gastric emptying after antecolic (17%) than after retrocolic (6%) gastrojejunostomy, but this finding was of questionable statistical significance. In contrast, Doberneck and Berndt[32] reported a lower incidence of delayed gastric emptying after antecolic (22%) than after retrocolic (42%) gastrojejunostomy, whereas data from our institution failed to demonstrate a relationship between antecolic or retrocolic gastrojejunostomy and the development of delayed gastric emptying.[26] Thus, this issue remains unresolved.

The question of the "peristaltic" orientation of the jejunum in the gastrojejunostomy (so-called isoperistaltic or antiperistaltic) was evaluated in a prospective randomized trial by Yilmaz and colleagues.[36] Measuring both preoperative and postoperative gastric emptying, they demonstrated that both anatomic constructions of the gastrojejunostomy decreased gastric emptying after surgery, but there were no significant differences between the two methods, as measured by delayed gastric emptying, overall morbidity, or duration of hospital stay. When one considers the physiology of gastric emptying via a gastroenterostomy (anterior vs posterior; antecolic vs retrocolic), at least in theory, neither orientation should make any difference. When the sphincteric mechanism (pylorus) is bypassed through a nonsphincteric stoma (gastroenterostomy), gastric emptying occurs by changes in pressure between the stomach and the jejunum and not by gravity or the antropyloric pump mechanism.[37]

If a biliary bypass is to be performed synchronously, some authors advise biliary bypass proximal to the gastrojejunostomy to alkalinize gastric juices and to lessen the chance of marginal ulcer and gastrointestinal bleeding.[36] Others recommend constructing the biliary bypass distal to the gastrojejunostomy to minimize the caustic effects of bile on the gastric mucosa (alkaline reflux gastritis),[32] or they add a Braun enteroenterostomy between different or efferent limbs of the jejunal loop. Our preference is to perform a prophylactic antecolic, isoperistaltic gastrojejunostomy, if possible distal to a Roux-en-Y hepaticojejunostomy (Fig. 31.1). However, the individual patient anatomy dictates whether it is antecolic or retrocolic, anterior or posterior, and isoperistaltic or antiperistaltic; there are no convincing data that one is superior to the other. In centers that perform routine laparoscopic staging, a laparoscopic gastrojejunostomy is a very reasonable alternative to open duodenal gastric bypass.[13,38,39] In a case-control study comparing laparoscopic with open palliation, the laparoscopic approach was associated with less morbidity, mortality, and duration of hospital stay.[13] Others have reported similar results with laparoscopic gastrojejunostomy for malignant duodenal obstruction. Nagy and colleagues[38] reported on 10 patients who underwent antecolic, stapled laparoscopic gastrojejunostomy for duodenal obstruction. Two patients required conversion to open surgery. Delayed gastric emptying occurred for an average of 10 days. Brune and colleagues[40] studied 16 patients who underwent laparoscopic gastrojejunostomy for malignant duodenal obstruction, seven of whom had pancreatic carcinoma and 11 of whom had undergone prior biliary stenting; only one required conversion to an open procedure. Median postoperative hospital stay was 7 days. Radiographically, about 20% had delayed gastric emptying, but clinically, all patients eventually tolerated an oral diet.

Intraluminal endoscopic stenting of the duodenum has been described predominantly for patients who have unresectable pancreatic cancer and are at high risk for any type of operative procedure. Typically, this procedure is performed with an expandable metal stent (Wallstent Enteral, Boston Scientific Mciroinvasive, Natick, MA), with stent diameters of 20–22 mm and lengths of 60–90 mm. Complications of duodenal stenting include erosions caused during the procedure or by the stent itself, stent obstruction from tumor ingrowth, and stent malposition.[41] The most serious complication is recognized or unrecognized duodenal perforation. Espinel and colleagues[42] reported on six patients with malignant duodenal obstruction treated with duodenal stenting. Food intake was started within 24 hours, and average postprocedure duration of stay was 2.5 days without complications. These patients were highly selected because median survival was only 9 weeks; however, no recurrent duodenal obstruction was reported. Similarly, Wong and colleagues[43] compared six patients who underwent endoscopic intraluminal stenting for duodenal obstruction with 17 patients who underwent operative gastrojejunostomy for pancreatic cancer-related duodenal obstruction. The median postprocedure duration of hospital stay was 4 days after stent, compared with 15 days after gastrojejunostomy. All patients with duodenal stenting tolerated a soft diet the day after stent placement; in contrast, nine patients in the gastrojejunostomy group had delayed gastric emptying. Although these studies suggest duodenal stenting to be an option for the palliation of duodenal obstruction, larger studies of comparable patients should be performed before this method of palliation is recommended for patients who are otherwise fit for surgical bypass, primarily because the durability (patency) of duodenal stents has yet to be determined.

Therefore, in patients with pancreatic cancer of the head of the pancreas in whom duodenal obstruction is determined by imaging, endoscopy, or intraoperative findings, palliative gastrojejunostomy seems indicated. Although the need for prophylactic gastrojejunostomy should be made on a patient-by-patient basis, we tend to favor both a biliary and a duodenal bypass in patients with obstructive jaundice found to be unresectable at exploration. In patients with unresectable disease at laparoscopic exploration, a prophylactic laparoscopic gastrojejunostomy should be considered in addition to some form of biliary decompression. The patient with duodenal obstruction and advanced disease in whom a short survival seems imminent may best be treated by an intraluminal stent.

"Palliative" Resection

Pancreatic resection for adenocarcinoma has been reserved for patients with the potential for curative resection. In about 20% of patients, however, positive microscopic (R_1) or gross margins (R_2) are found after attempted resection for cure. To address the role of palliative pancreatic resection, Lillemoe and colleagues[44] performed a retrospective review of patients with gross or microscopically positive margins after pancreaticoduodenectomy. Sixty-four such patients were compared with 62 patients with known unresectability who underwent surgical bypass only. These authors interpreted their data as showing improved survival and a lower incidence of hospital readmission (20% vs 11%) in the palliative resection group. However, the comparability of these two groups is questionable; those who underwent bypass had more apparent (i.e., locally advanced) disease. Moreover, patients who underwent a "palliative" resection were not really subjected to an *intended* palliative resection; indeed, the surgeons carried out the pancreatectomy with the impression that a curative resection was possible and learned that the resection was "palliative" only after the resection was completed. No one has presented a group of patients with known unresectable disease who have undergone resections that are known to be palliative. Thus, the term needs to be used appropriately, and the concept of palliative resection needs to be considered carefully if it is considered or suggested to be the appropriate intervention. The role of a palliative resection is not defined, is not standard practice, and at this time cannot be recommended in patients with a limited life expectancy.

Palliation of Tumor-Related Pain

Fifty percent to 90% of patients with unresectable pancreatic cancer will experience abdominal or back pain, often severe, during their limited survival. Multiple mechanisms have been proposed to account for the pain associated with pancreatic cancer; local, regional, and metastatic tumor-related mechanisms might all be involved. Direct perineural or neural invasion of autonomic and somatic nerves is a frequent histologic finding in pancreatic cancer specimens. This unique ability of pancreatic cancer cells to express and elaborate neurolytic enzymes that facilitate the spread into or along neural pathways may be responsible for most of the pain associated with pancreatic cancer.[45] Stretching or direct invasion of the peripancreatic and pancreatic nerves often occurs as tumor infiltration progresses, "sensitizing" visceral afferent nerves; as the disease becomes more advanced, further mechanical stimuli result in chronic pain.[46] Additionally, an obstructing lesion in the proximal pancreatic duct causes distal ductal dilation, stimulating afferent neural fibers. This long-standing ductal hypertension may lead to parenchymal fibrosis associated with nerve irritation and, consequently, pain. Pain attributed to pancreatic cancer may result less commonly from metastatic involvement of the hepatic capsule or the peritoneum and from biliary or duodenal obstruction.

The surgeon can and should serve an important role in the palliation of pain due to unresectable pancreatic cancer in certain situations. When operating either to palliate in a patient with known unresectable disease or when a neoplasm believed to be clinically resectable before surgery is found at exploration to be nonresectable, strong consideration should be given to performing an intraoperative chemical splanchnicectomy (commonly referred to as a *celiac plexus block*). This procedure is easy, fast, and effective.[47] When performed appropriately, it reduces the severity of pain and postoperative narcotic requirements. Furthermore, this procedure is performed with virtually no morbidity, having essentially no effect on postoperative complications, ability to tolerate a diet, or duration of hospital stay. In a prospective randomized trial, Lillemoe and colleagues[48] compared intraoperative chemical splanchnicectomy with placebo in patients with unresectable pancreatic cancer. They demonstrated no differences in morbidity, mortality, return to oral intake, or duration of hospital stay between the two groups. The mean pain scores were lower in the treatment group at all time points of follow-up. Further, chemical splanchnicectomy resulted in a delay in subsequent onset of pain in patients without preoperative pain and a reduction in existing pain in those with preoperative pain. Interestingly, patients with preexisting pain who underwent chemical splanchnicectomy also exhibited a trend toward improved survival when compared with control subjects.

Before an intraoperative celiac plexus block is performed, exposure to the retroperitoneal superior aspect of the pancreas and celiac axis must be gained.[47] The lesser omentum is incised, and the stomach is retracted inferiorly to expose the cephalad portion of the pancreatic body. The left hand of the surgeon provides caudad retraction, with the index and second finger placed on the right and left of the aorta, respectively, on the splenic and common hepatic arteries at the level of the celiac axis (superior to the midbody of the pancreas) (Fig. 31.3). Attention should be paid to leaving the peritoneal covering of the

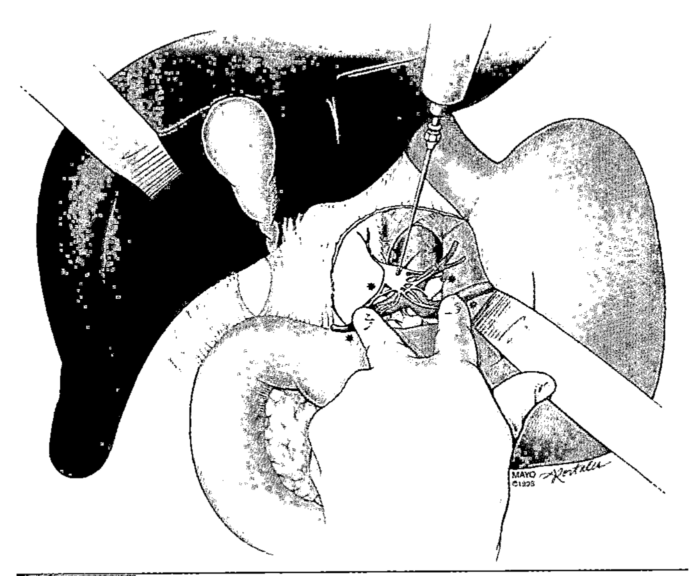

Figure 31.3
Intraoperative chemical splanchnicectomy (celiac plexus block). (Reprinted with permission from Mayo Foundation.)

retroperitoneal intact during this exposure to contain the neurolytic agent to be injected. A long needle, which is particularly useful in deep patients, is used to gain access to the area of the celiac plexus. For this maneuver, we have found that a 20-gauge spinal needle is ideal. Common neurolytic agents are 50% ethanol or 6% phenol. The right hand alone is used to steady and inject 20 mL on either side of the aorta around the celiac axis. These injections are divided into 10-mL increments injected just superior and just inferior to both the common hepatic and the splenic arteries. Routine practice should entail withdrawal on the syringe before injection to exclude intravascular installation of the neurolytic agent. The injected agent remains in the retroperitoneum if the peritoneal covering is left intact.

Side effects of the celiac plexus block are rare and usually self-limited. Unopposed parasympathetic tone to the viscera and the splanchnic circulation accounts for most of the adverse outcomes. Hypermotility causing diarrhea may occur as a result of the relative increase in parasympathetic input to the bowel, but this side effect is both rare and transient. Similarly, lack of sympathetic tone to the splanchnic vasculature may cause vasodilation and hypotension in 1%–2% of patients, but again, this effect, if present, is transient and lasts only 1 or 2 days. Any neurologic deficit is exceedingly rare.[46]

Despite the initial efficacy of chemical splanchnicectomy, the durability of pain relief is variable. Repeated splanchnicectomy (performed percutaneously or endoscopically) or alternative methods (oral narcotics) are required in many patients, because up to two thirds of patients who undergo palliative operation and intraoperative celiac plexus block, encounter recurrence of moderate-to-severe pain before death.[48] In addition to palliation of biliary and enteric obstruction for patients with unresectable pancreatic cancer, a chemical splanchnicectomy should be an integral part of the surgeon's armamentarium. By doing so, those patients without initial preoperative pain will benefit from delay in onset and perhaps even prevention of pain, and those with existing pain have clinically important pain relief after surgery.[46] When performed at the time of celiotomy, chemical splanchnicectomy eliminates the need for a separate percutaneous splanchnicectomy postoperatively.

Conclusion

With the advent and success of improved diagnostic imaging and nonoperative means of effective palliation, the role of surgical palliation in patients with unresectable pancreatic cancer has decreased. The optimal therapeutic approaches to palliation must be weighted against the patient's symptoms, overall health status, and projected survival, as well as specific procedure-related morbidity and mortality. Obstructive jaundice in a patient with known metastatic or locally unresectable disease is most appropriately treated with endoscopic stenting. However, patients without evidence of unresectability who are acceptable operative candidates should undergo exploration for curative resection. If exploration demonstrates unresectability, surgical palliation of established biliary obstruction, established or potential duodenal obstruction, and future abdominal/back pain is appropriate. Patients with documented gastric outlet obstruction who have acceptable operative risk should undergo gastrojejunostomy; endoscopic intraluminal duodenal stenting may also be considered.

The role of prophylactic gastrojejunostomy remains controversial. In a patient requiring palliative operative biliary bypass, a concomitant prophylactic gastrojejunostomy seems prudent, especially in patients with tumor locations that may lead to obstruction and in patients with an expected survival of greater than 6 months. Laparoscopic palliation reduces operative morbidity and will play an increasing role in the operative palliation of patients with unresectable pancreatic cancer. Palliation of pain continues to be a difficult problem in patients with pancreatic cancer. Intraoperative chemical splanchnicectomy is effective in reducing pain and may delay the onset of pain in patients without existing pain; these effects may be transient, requiring additional (percutaneous) chemical blocks.

A surgical approach to palliation in patients with unresectable pancreatic cancer provides the opportunity to simultaneously and effectively address all three of the major complications of pancreatic cancer—namely obstructive jaundice, duodenal obstruction, and tumor-related pain. In selected patients, any or all of these palliative procedures may be the optimal approach and should be considered in the context of the patient's overall condition and planned anticancer treatment.

Acknowledgment

The authors are grateful to Deborah Frank for her expert assistance in the preparation of this chapter.

References

1. Jemal A, Murray T, Samuels A, et al. Cancer statistics, 2003. *CA Cancer J Clin*. 2003;53:5-26.
2. Tsuchiya R, Noda T, Harada N, et al. Collective review of small carcinomas of the pancreas. *Ann Surg*. 1986;203: 77–81.
3. Kaneko T, Nakao A, Inoue S, et al. Extrapancreatic nerve plexus invasion by carcinoma of the head of the pancreas: diagnosis with intraportal endovascular ultrasonography. *Int J Pancreatol*. 1996;19:1–8.
4. Sarr MG, Cameron JL. Surgical management of unresectable carcinoma of the pancreas. *Surgery*. 1982;91:123–133.
5. Sarfeh JI, Rypins EB, Jakowatz JG, Juler GL. A prospective, randomized clinical investigation of cholecystoenterostomy and choledochoenterostomy. *Am J Surg*. 1988; 155:411–414.
6. Watanapa P, Williamson RCN. Surgical palliation for pancreatic cancer: developments during the past two decades. *Br J Surg*. 1992;79:8–20.
7. Urbach DR, Bell CM, Swanstrom LL, Hansen PD. Cohort study of surgical bypass to the gallbladder or bile duct for the palliation of jaundice due to pancreatic cancer. *Ann Surg*. 2003;1:86–93.
8. Van Wagensveld BA, Coene PPLO, van Gulik TM, et al. Outcome of palliative biliary and gastric bypass surgery for pancreatic head carcinoma in 126 patients. *Br J Surg*. 1997;84:1402–1406.
9. Tarnasky PR, England RE, Lail LM, et al. Cystic duct patency in malignant obstructive jaundice: an ERCP-based study relevant to the role of laparoscopic cholecystojejunostomy. *Ann Surg*. 1995;221:265–271.
10. Sohn TA, Lillemoe KD. Surgical palliation in pancreatic cancer. *Adv Surg*. 2000;34:237–248.
11. Di Fronzo LA, Egrari S, O'Connell TX. Choledochoduodenostomy for palliation in unresectable pancreatic cancer. *Arch Surg*. 1998;133:820–825.
12. Potts JR 3rd, Broughan TA, Hermann RE. Palliative operations for pancreatic carcinoma. *Am J Surg*. 1990;159:72–77.
13. Röthlin MA, Schöb O, Weber M. Laparoscopic gastro- and hepaticojejunostomy for palliation of pancreatic cancer. *Surg Endosc*. 1999;13:1065–1069.
14. Gentileschi P, Kini S, Gagner M. Palliative laparoscopic hepatico- and gastrojejunostomy for advanced pancreatic cancer. *JSLS*. 2002;6:331–338.
15. Rhodes M, Nathanson L, Fielding G. Laparoscopic biliary and gastric bypass: a useful adjunct in the treatment of carcinoma of the pancreas. *Gut*. 1995;36:778–780.
16. Shepherd HA, Royle G, Ross APR, et al. Endoscopic biliary endoprosthesis in the palliation of malignant obstruction of the distal common bile duct: a randomized trial. *Br J Surg*. 1988;75:1166–1168.
17. Andersen JR, Sorensen SM, Kruse A, et al. Randomised trial of endoscopic endoprosthesis versus operative bypass in malignant obstructive jaundice. *Gut*. 1989;30:1132–1135.
18. Smith AC, Dowsett JF, Russell RCG, et al. Randomised trial of endoscopic stenting versus surgical bypass in malignant low bile duct obstruction. *Lancet*. 1994;4:1655–1660.
19. Schwarz A, Beger HG. Biliary and gastric bypass or stenting in nonresectable periampullary cancer. *Int J Pancreatol*. 2000;1:51–58.
20. Speer A, Cotton PB, Rode J, et al. Biliary stent blockage with bacterial biofilm: a light and electron microscopy study. *Ann Intern Med*. 1988;34:19–22.
21. Andersson A, Bergdahl L. Carcinoma of the pancreas. *Am Surg*. 1976;42:173–177.
22. Espat NJ, Brennan MF, Conlon KC. Patients with laparoscopically staged unresectable pancreatic adenocarcinoma do not require subsequent surgical biliary or gastric bypass. *J Am Coll Surg*. 1999;188:649–657.
23. Singh SM, Reber HA. Surgical palliation for pancreatic cancer. *Surg Clin North Am*. 1989;69:599–611.
24. Egrari S, O'Connell TX. Role of prophylactic gastrojejunostomy for unresectable pancreatic carcinoma. *Am Surg*. 1995;61:862–864.
25. Lillemoe KD, Cameron JL, Hardacre JM, et al. Is prophylactic gastrojejunostomy indicated for unresectable periampullary cancer? *Ann Surg*. 1999;230:322–330.
26. Sarr MG, Gladen HE, Beart RW, Van Heerden JA. Role of gastroenterostomy in patients with unresectable carcinoma of the pancreas. *Surg Gynecol Obstet*. 1981;152:597–600.
27. Wade TP, Neuberger TJ, Swope TJ, et al. Pancreatic cancer palliation: using tumor stage to select appropriate operation. *Am J Surg*. 1994;167:208–213.
28. Di Fronzo LA, Cymerman J, Egrari S, O'Connell TX. Unresectable pancreatic carcinoma: correlating length of survival with choice of palliative bypass. *Am Surg*. 1999;65:955–958.
29. Van Heek NT, De Castro SMM, van Eijck CH, et al. The need for a prophylactic gastrojejunostomy for unresectable periampullary cancer: a prospective randomized multicenter trial with special focus on assessment of quality of life. *Ann Surg*. 2003;238:894–905.
30. Weaver DW, Wiencek RG, Bouwman DL, Walt AJ. Gastrojejunostomy: is it helpful for patients with pancreatic cancer? *Surgery*. 1987;102:608–613.
31. De Rooij PD, Rogatko A, Brennan MF. Evaluation of palliative surgical procedures in unresectable pancreatic cancer. *Br J Surg*. 1991;78:1053–1058.
32. Doberneck RC, Berndt GA. Delayed gastric emptying after palliative gastrojejunostomy for carcinoma of the pancreas. *Arch Surg*. 1987;122:827–829.

33. Lucas CE, Ledgerwood AM, Bender JS. Antrectomy with gastrojejunostomy for unresectable pancreatic cancer-causing duodenal obstruction. *Surgery*. 1991;110:583–590.
34. Molinari M, Helton WS, Espat NJ. Palliative strategies for locally advanced unresectable and metastatic pancreatic cancer. *Surg Clin North Am*. 2001;81:651–66.
35. Lillemoe KD, Sauter PK, Pitt HA, et al. Current status of surgical palliation of periampullary carcinoma. *Surg Gynecol Obstet*. 1993;176:1–10.
36. Yilmaz S, Kirimlioglu V, Katz DA, et al. Randomised clinical trial of two bypass operations for unresectable cancer of the pancreatic head. *Eur J Surg*. 2001;167:770–776.
37. Behrns KE, Sarr MG. Anticipating and avoiding postgastrectomy stasis problems. *Probl General Surg*. 1993;10:358–365.
38. Nagy A, Brosseuk D, Hemming A, et al. Laparoscopic gastroenterostomy for duodenal obstruction. *Am J Surg*. 1995;169:539–542.
39. Bergamaschi R, Marvik R, Thoresen JE, et al. Open versus laparoscopic gastrojejunostomy for palliation in advanced pancreatic cancer. *Surg Laparosc Endosc*. 1998;8:92–96.
40. Brune IB, Feussner H, Neuhaus H, et al. Laparoscopic gastrojejunostomy and endoscopic biliary stent placement for palliation of incurable gastric outlet obstruction with cholestasis. *Surg Endosc*. 1997;11: 834–837.
41. Carr-Locke DL. Role of endoscopic stenting in the duodenum. *Ann Oncol*. 1999;10:S261–S264.
42. Espinel J, Vivas S, Munoz F, et al. Palliative treatment of malignant obstruction of gastric outlet using an endoscopically placed enteral Wallstent. *Dig Dis Sci*. 2001;46: 2322–2324.
43. Wong YT, Brams DM, Munson L, et al. Gastric outlet obstruction secondary to pancreatic cancer. *Surg Endosc*. 2002;16:310–312.
44. Lillemoe KD, Cameron JL, Yeo CJ, et al. Pancreaticoduodenectomy: does it have a role in the palliation of pancreatic cancer? *Ann Surg*. 1996;223:718–728.
45. Kayahara M, Nagakawa T, Futagami F. Lymphatic flow and neural plexus invasion associated with carcinoma of the body and tail of the pancreas. *Cancer*. 1996;78:2485–2491.
46. Cameron JL. *American Cancer Society Atlas of Clinical Oncology: Pancreatic Cancer*. London: BC Decker Inc.; 2001:231–246.
47. Sakorafas GH, Tsiotou AG, Sarr MG. Intraoperative celiac plexus block in the surgical palliation for unresectable pancreatic cancer. *Eur J Surg Oncol*. 1999;25:427–431.
48. Lillemoe KD, Cameron JL, Kaufman HS, et al. Chemical splanchnicectomy in patients with unresectable pancreatic cancer: a prospective randomized trial. *Ann Surg*. 1993; 217:447–455.
49. Bornman PC, Harries-Jones EP, Tobias R, et al. Prospective controlled trial of transhepatic biliary endoprosthesis versus bypass surgery for incurable carcinoma of head of pancreas. *Lancet*. 1986;1:69–71.

CHAPTER 32

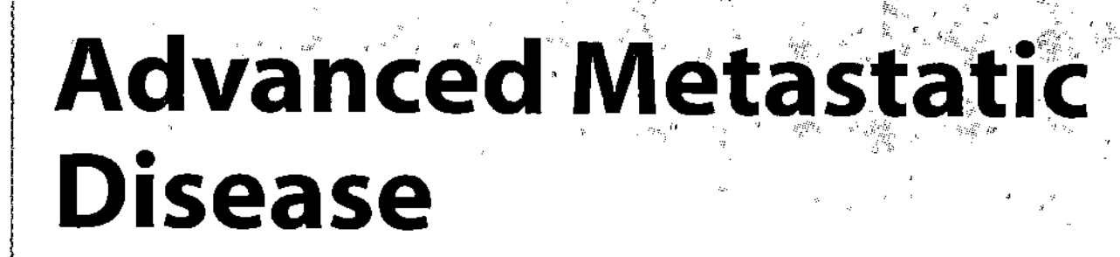

Advanced Metastatic Disease

Marcel Rozencweig, MD
Daniel D. Von Hoff, MD

Adenocarcinoma of the pancreas is an aggressive and rapidly fatal disease that has shown little sensitivity to currently available anti-cancer agents. The American Cancer Society estimates for 2004 in the United States anticipate 31,860 new cases of pancreas cancer and 31,270 deaths.[1] The vast majority of patients present with disease that is no longer suitable for surgical cure, and debilitating symptoms, including pain, emesis, weight loss, and weakness, are common features during the clinical course of the disease.[2] Large-scale chemotherapy trials have generally yielded marginal tumor response rates, and survival has been only minimally impacted.[3] Performance status and stage of disease are prominent prognostic factors in advanced disease. The median survival is 6–10 months for patients with locally advanced disease and 3–6 months for those with metastatic disease.[4]

This chapter reviews the randomized trials testing anti-cancer agents for locally advanced and metastatic pancreatic cancer. The review includes phase II and phase III trials. Most phase II trials were designed for screening purposes and focused on response rates based on tumor shrinkage. It has since been recognized, however, that low tumor response rates may be observed despite prolonged survival, emphasizing the need for other surrogate endpoints of efficacy. Response based on general symptom improvement has been recently proposed as a measure of efficacy for chemotherapeutic agents in pancreatic cancer. Whether this clinical benefit response will prove to be a more useful endpoint for screening new therapeutic approaches is still uncertain. Survival remains the most reliable endpoint in clinical trials for this disease, as long as study design is adequate and statistical power is commensurate with a small, but clinically significant improvement in outcome.

Randomized Trials Versus Best Supportive Care

Chemotherapy Trials

A number of randomized trials have compared combination chemotherapy with best supportive care in patients with advanced pancreatic cancer (Table 32.1). Although the results of these studies have been inconsistent, they did provide some support for the concept that chemotherapy can be beneficial in patients with metastatic cancer of the pancreas.

These studies accrued small numbers of patients. Most had less than 30 patients per treatment arm. Survival in

Table 32.1 Randomized Trials of Chemotherapy or Hormone Therapy Versus Best Supportive Care

Author(s)	Treatment	No. of Patients	Median Survival	*P* Value
Mallinson et al.[5]	Cyclophosphamide, 5-FU, Vincristine, Methotrexate	19	44 weeks	
	Control	21	9 weeks	0.00006
Palmer et al.[6]	5-FU, Doxorubicin, Mitomycin C	23	33 weeks	
	Control	20	15 weeks	<0.002
Glimelius et al.[7]	5-FU, Leucovorin, Etoposide	47	6 months	
	Control	43	2.5 months	<0.01
Andersen et al.[8]	5-FU, BCNU	20	13 weeks	
	Control	20	14 weeks	0.80
Frey et al.[9]	5-FU, CCNU	65	3 months	
	Control	87	3.9 months	0.17
Andren-Sandberg et al.[10]	5-FU, CCNU, vincristine	25	5 months	
	Control	22	4 months	NR
Bakkevold et al.[11]	Tamoxifen	92	115 days	
	Control	84	122 days	0.731
Keating et al.[12]	Tamoxifen	37	5.25 months	0.07 vs control
	Cyproterone acetate	32	4.25 months	0.50 vs control
	Control	39	3.0 months	
Greenway[13]	Flutamide	24	226 days	
	Control	25	120 days	0.001

Abbreviation: NR, not reported.

the control group ranged consistently between 2 and 5 months. Chemotherapy consisted of 5-fluorouracil (5-FU) combinations, and in the three chemotherapy trials reporting a survival benefit, these combinations were associated with a median survival of 6 to 10 months. In these trials, 5-FU was administered at 2- to 4-week intervals. The other three chemotherapy trials reported here used combination regimens of 5-FU and nitrosourea derivatives in cycles repeated every 6 to 8 weeks; all failed to show any difference in outcome, perhaps, in part, as a result of suboptimal 5-FU administration.

The first randomized study of combination chemotherapy versus best supportive care was published by Mallinson et al. in 1980.[5] A total of 40 patients with unresectable pancreatic cancer were randomized to receive no chemotherapy or an initiation course of 5-FU, methotrexate, vincristine, and cyclophosphamide followed after 4 weeks by a maintenance program with a combination of 5-FU and mitomycin C. Patients in the chemotherapy group had a median survival of 44 weeks, which was significantly longer than the median survival of 9 weeks in the group that did not receive chemotherapy ($P = 0.00006$). The difference in survival remained statistically significant among patients with histologically confirmed (n = 26) or unconfirmed diagnosis (n = 14), as well as those with local tumor only (n = 25) or those with hepatic metastases (n = 15). The favorable outcome in the chemotherapy group in this trial might have been amplified by the unusually short median survival in the control group.

The study of Palmer et al.[6] randomized 43 patients with unresectable pancreatic cancer. Histopathologic confirmation of the diagnosis was obtained in 31 of these patients. Chemotherapy consisted of the FAM regimen designed at Georgetown University. That regimen combines 5-FU 600 mg/m^2 on days 1, 8, 29, and 36; doxorubicin 30 mg/m^2 on days 1 and 29; and mitomycin C 10 mg/m^2 on day 1 with cycles repeated every 8 weeks. Compared with the control group that received no chemotherapy, the median survival in the FAM group was more than twice as long (33 vs 15 weeks, $P < 0.002$). Most chemotherapy-treated patients experienced toxicities, but these toxicities were usually mild and of short duration. There were only two instances of treatment delays because of neutropenia.

Another randomized study demonstrated that combination chemotherapy not only prolonged survival but also improved quality of life, as measured by the European Organization for Research and Treatment of Cancer Quality-of-Life Questionnaire-C30.[7] The trial randomized 93 patients with advanced pancreatic or biliary cancer to either chemotherapy in addition to best supportive care or to best supportive care alone. Chemotherapy was allowed in the latter group if satisfactory palliation could not be achieved with supportive measures. All patients had their diagnosis histologically verified. Randomization was stratified by primary tumor site (pancreatic and biliary) and participating hospital. Chemotherapy consisted of 5-FU, leucovorin, and etoposide. The older population and poor performance status patients received the same chemotherapy regimen without etoposide. Among patients with pancreatic cancer, overall survival was significantly longer for those randomized to chemotherapy than for those assigned to the best supportive care only treatment group (6 and 2.5 months, respectively, $P < 0.05$). Furthermore, 38% of patients in the chemotherapy group had a favorable quality-of-life outcome compared with only 13% of those in the control group.

Three other randomized studies failed to detect a benefit in survival or in quality of life (see Table 32.1). With a combination of 5-FU and carmustine, the median survival and 1-year survival were not significantly different than they were for control patients.[8] The median survival was 13 weeks in the treatment group versus 14 weeks for the control group ($P = 0.80$), and 1-year survival was 10% in both groups.

The Veterans Administration Surgical Adjuvant Cancer Chemotherapy Study Group compared the nitrosourea lomustine in combination with 5-FU to best supportive care in a randomized study of 152 patients with histologically proven inoperable pancreatic cancer.[9] The control subjects were to receive no chemotherapy. Both treatment groups were comparable in terms of age, weight loss, extent of metastases, and prior surgical procedure. Toxic effects for the most part were reportedly mild. There was no survival benefit associated with drug therapy. In fact, there was a trend suggesting a decrease in survival in the drug treatment group relative to the control group, but the difference (medians of 3.0 vs 3.9 months) did not reach statistical significance ($P = 0.17$).

A triple drug regimen consisting of vincristine 1 mg/m^2 intravenously on day 1, followed by oral lomustine 40 mg/m^2 on days 2 and 3 plus oral 5-FU 500 mg daily on days 2–5 was compared with the best supportive care in another randomized study involving 47 patients.[10] The median survival was 5 months in the treatment group and 4 months in the control group; that difference was not statistically significant. All patients randomized to chemotherapy in this study reported more or less marked gastrointestinal adverse events within days of each treatment cycle.

Hormone Therapy Trials

The concept that hormonal therapy might be useful in the treatment of pancreatic cancer is derived from the presence of estrogen and androgen receptors in pancreatic cancer cells. However, anti-estrogen treatment with tamoxifen has not proven to be an effective approach to improving survival in patients with pancreatic cancer. The median survival in a randomized trial comparing tamoxifen with placebo was 115 days for tamoxifen-treated patients compared with 122 days for patients in the placebo group.[11] Results were more encouraging in another trial where the median survival was longer for patients in the tamoxifen group than in the group receiving no active therapy (5.25 vs 3.0 months).[12] The difference was not statistically significant, but this was a small trial. The trial also included a third arm testing cyproterone acetate, an anti-androgen. No effect on survival was detected with this agent either versus the no active treatment arm.

Still, positive results from a more recent double-blind placebo controlled trial of flutamide suggest a possible role for androgen receptor antagonist in pancreatic cancer.[13] Patients were treated with flutamide 250 mg three times daily or placebo. This was a very small study (n = 49), and information on prognostic factors was missing. There was no apparent difference between treatment arms in terms of tumor regression, but an intent-to-treat analysis showed a significant prolongation of survival in the flutamide group (226 vs 120 days, $P = 0.01$). Flutamide treatment was well tolerated with minimal side effects. Further randomized trials are needed to evaluate the role of hormonal approaches in this disease.

Randomized Trials Versus 5-FU

5-FU was the reference standard to treat patients with advanced cancer of the pancreas for more than 2 decades. Its modest anti-tumor effect prompted large efforts aimed at identifying new active chemotherapeutic agents and more active combinations. Several groups used randomized trials to screen for new and promising approaches, with a focus on response rates in small numbers of patients with measurable disease. Many investigational agents were tested, mostly with disappointing results, in major research programs orchestrated by several cooperative groups, including the Gastrointestinal Tumor Study

Table 32.2 Randomized Trials of 5-FU Based Combination Regimens Versus 5-FU Alone

Author(s)	Treatment	No. of Patients	Median Survival	*P* Value
Kovach et al.[19]	5-FU, BCNU	30	NR	
	BCNU	21	NR	
	5-FU	31	NR	NR
Stolinsky et al.[20]	5-FU (oral)	16	53 days	
	5-FU (intravenous)	14	110 days	NR
Maisey et al.[21]	PVI 5-FU, Mitomycin C	92	5.1 months	
	PVI 5-FU	105	6.5 months	0.34
Cullinan et al.[22]	5-FU, Doxorubicin, Mitomycin C	50	NR	
	5-FU, Doxorubicin	44	NR	
	5-FU	50	NR	NS
Takada et al.[23]	5-FU, Doxorubicin, Mitomycin C	35	6.2 months	
	5-FU	36	6.0 months	0.67
Moertel et al.[26]	5-FU, Streptozotocin, Spironolactone	15	16 weeks	
	5-FU, Streptozotocin	19	18 weeks	
	5-FU, Spironolactone	16	15 weeks	
	5-FU	23	21 weeks	NR
Awrich et al.[28]	5-FU, Streptozotocin, Tubercidin	39	NR	
	5-FU	34	NR	NR
Ducreux et al.[32]	CI 5-FU, Cisplatin	104	112 days	
	5-FU	103	102 days	0.10
Cullinan et al.[34]	Mallinson Regimen	61	4.5 months	
	5-FU, Doxorubicin, Cisplatin	59	3.5 months	
	5-FU	64	3.5 months	0.68
Rougier et al.[35]	Oxaliplatin, 5-FU	28	8.5 months	
	Oxaliplatin	17	3.4 months	
	5-FU	14	2.4 months	NR
Burch et al.[36]	Octreotide	42	NR	
	5-FU with Leucovorin	22	NR	
	5-FU	22	NR	0.80*

Abbreviations: NR, not reported; NS, not significant; PVI, prolonged venous infusion; Mallinson regimen, induction with 5-FU, cyclophosphamide, methotrexate, and vincristine followed by maintenance with 5-FU, mitomycin C; CI, continuous infusion.

*There was no statistically significant difference between octreotide and the two 5-FU arms combined ($P = 0.80$) or between the two chemotherapy arms ($P = 0.08$).

Group,[14-16] the Southwest Oncology Group,[17] and the Eastern Cooperative Oncology Group.[18] Much of this work involved unfavorable patient selections, with prior chemotherapy, far-advanced disease, and median survival times often of 8-10 weeks.

5-FU has been combined with a number of agents, predominantly nitrosourea derivatives (BCNU, CCNU, MeCCNU, streptozotocin), mitomycin C, and doxorubicin. These 5-FU combination regimens have not demonstrated consistent and compelling superiority over single-agent 5-FU. The gains from combination therapy were modest, and there was no positive impact on survival. The risk of excess toxicity actually often diminished the feasibility of 5-FU–based combinations. The following section summarizes the long trail of randomized chemotherapy trials that compared a wide variety of 5-FU regimens with single-agent 5-FU therapy (Table 32.2).

An early trial of the Mayo Clinic compared 5-FU given intravenously (13.5 mg/kg/day × five repeated every 5 weeks) with BCNU and the combination of these two agents.[19] Of 82 patients evaluated in that trial, 49 had a primary pancreatic lesion established at surgery, and the remainder had a presumed diagnosis of pancreatic cancer based on histology of a metastatic lesion, negative barium roentgenologic studies, and a convincing clinical presentation. The response rates achieved with 5-FU alone

(16%, 5 of 31) or in combination (33%, 10 of 30) were significantly higher than with BCNU alone (0 of 21) ($P < 0.05$), but the combination was not significantly better than 5-FU alone, and there was no difference in survival among the three treatment options.

A randomized phase II trial compared oral versus intravenous administration of 5-FU given at 15 mg/kg/week in both arms.[20] No minimum performance status was required, but the median performance status at entry was 70 on the Karnofsky scale in both arms. Three responses were observed among 14 patients with intravenous therapy, whereas none of the 16 patients receiving oral 5-FU achieved a response. The corresponding median survival times were 110 and 53 days, respectively.

The potential value of mitomycin C was evaluated in combination with 5-FU relative to 5-FU alone.[21] Patients in both arms had protracted intravenous infusions of 5-FU at a daily dose of 300 mg/m^2. Those randomized to mitomycin C treatment also received a bolus of 7 mg/m^2 of mitomycin C on day 1. Treatment was repeated at 6-week intervals until four courses had been administered. Among evaluable patients, overall response rates favored the combination over the single agent (18.5% [n = 92] vs 8.6% [n = 105], $P = 0.04$). This statistically significant difference did not, however, translate into a significant difference in failure-free or overall survival. Both chemotherapy regimens were well tolerated.

A three-arm randomized trial compared single-agent 5-FU to a two-drug combination of 5-FU plus doxorubicin (FA) and a three-drug combination of 5-FU plus doxorubicin and mitomycin C (FAM).[22] Single-agent 5-FU was given at a dose of 500 mg/m^2 daily for 5 days and repeated every 4 weeks for two cycles and every 5 weeks thereafter. The FA regimen consisted of 5-FU given by a 4-day course at a daily dose of 400 mg/m^2 plus 40 mg/m^2 of doxorubicin on day 1 of a 4-week cycle. After two cycles, treatment was repeated every 5 weeks. The FAM regimen was comparable to the combination of 5-FU, doxorubicin, and mitomycin C that had demonstrated improved survival relative to best supportive care.[6]

A total of 144 patients with pancreatic cancer were randomized. The number of patients with measurable disease was too small for any meaningful comparison of response rates. However, survival curves and distribution of progression times between the three treatment arms were superimposable. Diarrhea and stomatitis occurred more frequently with single-agent 5-FU treatment, but the FAM regimen produced more nausea, vomiting, and myelosuppression.

A modified FAM regimen was also compared with 5-FU alone in a multicenter randomized trial carried out in Japan among 81 patients with nonresectable carcinoma of the pancreas or the biliary tract.[23] That trial also failed to detect a difference in time to progression or survival.

Streptozotocin is a nitrosourea derivative that underwent extensive testing in pancreatic cancer. Multiple combinations were tested, with mixed results, in several randomized trials. Bukowski et al.[24] evaluated the addition of streptozotocin to a regimen of 5-FU plus mitomycin C, with 5-FU given as a 24-hour intravenous infusion for 4 consecutive days every 4 weeks. The trial accrued 181 patients with inoperable pancreatic adenocarcinoma and no prior chemotherapy. Twenty percent of the patients were not evaluable and were excluded from the analysis of response and survival. Response rates were significantly higher (34% vs 8%) when streptozotocin was included in the regimen ($P = 0.009$). The median survival, however, was virtually the same (18 and 17 weeks) with and without streptozotocin, respectively.

Gastrointestinal toxicities were more frequent and more severe when streptozotocin was added. Mild and reversible renal toxicity was also associated with the use of streptozotocin. There were four treatment-related deaths in the 5-FU plus mitomycin arm and one in the SMF arm. All deaths were attributed to severe myelosuppression.

A different SMF combination was associated with prolonged survival in another randomized trial.[25] That trial compared the SMF regimen developed at Georgetown University to a regimen of cisplatin, cytosine arabinoside, and caffeine (CAC). SMF consisted of 8-week cycles with streptozotocin (1 g/m^2) and 5-FU (600 mg/m^2) given on days 1, 8, 29, and 36 and mitomycin C (10 mg/m^2) given on day 1. In the CAC arm, patients received a single dose of cisplatin 100 mg/m^2 and cytosine arabinoside 2 g/m^2, given as a 3-hour infusion for two doses, 12 hours apart, followed by caffeine administration. Caffeine was included because of its putative interference with DNA repair. Cycles were repeated every 4 weeks. Eligibility criteria included a Karnofsky performance status of 60 or better, a life expectancy of at least 8 weeks, and no prior chemotherapy. Only 4/39 (10.2%) patients receiving SMF and 2/36 (5.5%) patients receiving CAC had objective responses. Despite a negligible response rate, the median survival duration was twice as long in the SMF arm than in the CAC arm (10 vs 5 months, $P = 0.008$).

In contrast to these favorable results, several other randomized trials failed to substantiate a benefit for the streptozocin combinations; response rates were marginal, ranging from 7% to 12%, and there was no difference in survival.[17,18,26-28] These trials compared 5-FU versus 5-FU + streptozotocin (median survival, 18.4 vs 16.3 weeks),[26] 5-FU + streptozotocin versus 5-FU + cyclophosphamide (median survival, 13 vs 9 weeks),[27] 5-FU versus 5-FU + streptozotocin + tubercidin (median survival not reported),[28] 5-FU + MeCCNU versus 5-FU + MeCCNU + streptozotocin (median survival, 14 vs 12 weeks),[18] and investigational agents versus 5-FU + doxorubicin + mitomycin C + streptozotocin (FAM-S) (median survival, 3.4 vs 4.8 months).[17]

Finally, closing the loop around these 5-FU + mitomycin C combinations, the SMF regimen was found to be equivalent to the FAM regimen, which, in turn, had been shown to prolong survival versus best supportive care without, however, improving survival relative to 5-FU alone. A three-arm study conducted by the Gastrointestinal Tumor Study Group[29] compared the FAM regimen and the SMF regimen (SMF1), both from the Georgetown University group, and a modified SMF regimen (SMF2) that used daily administrations of bolus 5-FU for 5 days. A total of 130 patients with measurable disease were randomized, including 92 patients with no prior chemotherapy. Response rates for the three arms were virtually identical (13%, 15%, and 14% for FAM, SMF1, and SMF2, respectively), and the corresponding median survival times were 11.6, 17.7, and 13.3 weeks, respectively. Results were very similar when the analysis was restricted to patients with no prior chemotherapy. Severe leukopenia and stomatitis were more common with FAM, whereas emesis was more frequent with the SMF regimens.

The Cancer and Leukemia Group B also compared the FAM and the SMF regimens from Georgetown in a randomized trial involving 196 patients.[30] As in the previous study, there was no significant difference between FAM and SMF in terms of response rate (14% vs 4%) and overall survival (median survival, 26.4 vs 18.3 weeks).

Of note, the FEM regimen, substituting epirubicin for adriamycin, was evaluated versus epirubicin alone in a randomized trial involving 65 patients.[31] A survival advantage was suggested for the combination over single-agent therapy with a 1-year survival rate of 23.2% versus 15.4%, respectively. That difference was not significant, but the study was not powered for definitive statistical conclusions.

Platinum agents have not been extensively evaluated in randomized trials with 5-FU in pancreatic cancer. Three trials are reported here, and none showed an advantage in survival versus single-agent 5-FU therapy. Cisplatin was combined with 5-FU 1,000 mg/m^2/day given by continuous infusion over 5 days in a comparative trial in which the control was 5-FU 500 mg/m^2/day given by bolus injection for 5 days.[32] The role of cisplatin in that trial is difficult to assess considering that each arm used a different method of drug administration for 5-FU. Among patients with measurable disease, 10 of 98 (10%) experienced an objective tumor regression in the cisplatin arm versus 0 of 98 in the 5-FU–alone arm. Progression-free survival also favored the combination (median progression-free survival, 73 vs 59 days, $P < 0.0001$), but there was no difference in survival (Table 32.2). Of note, a screening randomized phase II trial in 36 patients failed to detect any suggested advantage of α-interferon added to a combination of cisplatin and continuous infusion of 5-FU.[33]

The following study was a randomized comparison of a combination of 5-FU plus doxorubicin plus cisplatin (FAP), the Mallison regimen, and 5-FU alone.[34] There was no significant difference among the three treatments with respect to survival (Table 32.2). As was the case with the FAM regimen, the Mallison regimen, which had demonstrated superiority over best supportive care in a previous study,[4] was ultimately found to have no advantage over single-agent 5-FU.

A possible role of oxaliplatin was suggested in a preliminary report from a randomized phase II trial that enrolled 65 patients with advanced cancer of the pancreas.[35] Patients were randomized to treatment with single-agent oxaliplatin 130 mg/m^2, single-agent 5-FU 1 g/m^2/day for 4 days, or a combination of these drugs at the same doses. All treatments were administered every 3 weeks. There were no responses in either of the single-agent arms and three responses (11%) in the combination arm. The median survival was longer in the combination arm (8.5 months compared with 3.4 and 2.4 months for single-agent oxaliplatin and single-agent 5-FU, respectively). These data would warrant further investigations if the results are confirmed in the final analysis.

Octreotide, a somatostatin analogue, yielded negative results versus 5-FU and 5-FU plus leucovorin.[36] In fact, time to progression was significantly shorter for octreotide (42 vs 105 days with chemotherapy, $P = 0.01$). There was, however, no difference in survival, possibly as the result of crossover therapy in octreotide failures. The data were in line with results of other randomized trials of somatostatin analogues in pancreatic cancer indicating a lack of activity when given as single agents versus untreated controls or when given in combination with 5-FU versus 5-FU alone.[36] The trial also compared 5-FU intravenous bolus 500 mg/m^2 for 5 consecutive days and 5-FU 425 mg/m^2 plus leucovorin 20 mg/m^2 daily for 5 consecutive days. Chemotherapy cycles were repeated every 5 weeks. No meaningful data were given for the comparison of these two 5-FU treatment options.

Table 32.3 Single-Agent Gemcitabine Randomized Trials

Author(s)	Treatment	No. of Patients	Median Survival	*P* Value
Burris et al.[37]	Gemcitabine	63	5.65 months	
	5-FU	63	4.41 months	0.0025
Moore et al.[38]	Gemcitabine	277 (Total)	6.4 months	
	BAY12-9566		3.2 months	0.0001
Tempero et al.[39]	Gemcitabine 30-minute infusion	49	5 months	
	Gemcitabine 10 mg/m^2/min	43	8 months	0.013
Smith and Gallagher[40]	Gemcitabine	25	109 days	
	ZD9331	30	152 days	NR
Lersch et al.[41]	Gemcitabine	30	4.4 months	
	SCH 66336	33	3.3 months	NR

Abbreviation: NR, not reported.

Randomized Trial of 5-FU Versus Gemcitabine

In the mid-1990s, gemcitabine replaced 5-FU as the reference standard treatment in randomized trials for patients with advanced pancreatic cancer. This occurred after a randomized comparison of gemcitabine to 5-FU in patients with a pathologic diagnosis of locally advanced or metastatic pancreatic cancer and no prior chemotherapy.[37] In that study, a minimum Karnofsky performance status and an estimated life expectancy of at least 12 weeks were required. Patients were assigned to treatment with gemcitabine 1,000 mg/m^2 once weekly for 7 weeks and then, after a 1-week rest period, weekly for 3 out of 4 weeks, or to treatment with bolus 5-FU 600 mg/m^2 weekly. Unlike previous trials in this setting, the primary efficacy endpoint was a measure of symptom improvement and palliation. The concept of clinical benefit response was developed as a method for assessing the effect of chemotherapy. Clinical benefit response was based on a composite of measurements of pain (analgesic consumption and pain intensity), Karnofsky performance status, and weight. Other efficacy endpoints in the study were response rate, survival, and time to progressive disease.

The trial accrued 63 patients in each arm. More than two thirds of the patients in each arm had a performance status of 50 to 70. The number of patients experiencing a clinical benefit response was significantly greater in the gemcitabine group than in the 5-FU group (15 of 63 [23.8%] vs 3 of 63 [4.8%], $P = 0.0022$). Only few objective tumor responses were seen, but there was a statistically significant advantage for gemcitabine in terms of time to progression and survival. Among patients with bidimensionally measurable disease at study entry, 3 of 56 (5.4%) achieved a partial response in the gemcitabine arm as compared with 0 of 57 in the 5-FU arm. Time to progression-free survival for gemcitabine was 9 weeks compared with 4 weeks for the 5-FU arm ($P = 0.0002$), and the corresponding median survival times were 5.65 months compared with 4.41 months ($P = 0.0025$) (Table 32.3).

Both treatments were generally well tolerated throughout the study, but there was more myelosuppression with gemcitabine then with 5-FU, especially in terms of grades 3–4 neutropenia (25.9% vs 4.9%) and grades 3–4 anemia (9.7% vs 0%). The gemcitabine arm was also associated with more fever (30.1% vs 16.1%), more rashes (23.8% vs 12.9%), and more severe emesis (12.7% vs 4.8%) than the 5-FU arm.

Randomized, Single-Agent Gemcitabine Trials

Randomized, single-agent gemcitabine trials were mostly designed to evaluate the relative role of new investigational agents while attempts at optimizing dose scheduling of gemcitabine were ongoing. The impact on survival of gemcitabine was confirmed in another randomized trial where single-agent gemcitabine was compared with the orally administered matrix metalloproteinase inhibitor, BAY12-9566 (see Table 32.3).[38] That trial was actually closed early after a planned interim analysis revealed a significant difference in overall survival between treatment groups. At the time of the analysis, a total of 277 patients had been accrued and 140 deaths had occurred. The median overall survival was 6.4 months for the gemcitabine arm and only 3.2 months for the BAY12-9566 arm (P = 0.0001). Progression-free survival also was longer in the gemcitabine arm, with corresponding median times of 3.5 months versus 1.7 month, respectively (P = 0.012).

Attempts at further optimizing dose scheduling of gemcitabine are ongoing. A randomized comparison of two gemcitabine regimens in 92 patients (1,500 mg/m^2 given intravenously at 10 mg/m^2 per minute versus a 30-minute intravenous infusion of 2,200 mg/m^2) appeared to favor the more prolonged infusion, with a median survival of 8 versus 5 months (p=0.013).[39] These observations were paralleled by greater hematologic toxicity and higher gemcitabine triphosphate levels in mononuclear cells.

ZD9331, an intravenously administered thymidylate synthase inhibitor, was compared with gemcitabine in patients with locally advanced or metastatic pancreatic cancer.[40] The study was stopped prematurely because of two drug-related deaths that occurred in the ZD9331 arm after the first cycle of treatment. Full assessment of the data available from 30 patients randomized to ZD9331 and 25 patients randomized to gemcitabine before the time the study was terminated showed median survival, 152 versus 109 days, and time to progression, 70 versus 58 days, favoring ZD9331. Tumor response and clinical benefit response rates were similar for both groups. More patients in the ZD9331 treatment group discontinued treatment because of toxicity, primarily myelosuppression, than did patients treated with gemcitabine. Gastrointestinal toxicities, including grade 3 nausea, vomiting, and diarrhea, were more common with ZD9331 treatment. The apparent improvement in median survival and time to progression observed with ZD9331 should be considered in the context of the toxicity associated with this treatment.

In a randomized phase II study, previously treated and chemotherapy-naïve patients were allocated to receive treatment with gemcitabine (n = 30) or SCH 66336 (n = 33), an orally administered farnesyl transferase inhibitor.[41] There was one partial response in the gemcitabine group, and there were two partial responses in the SCH 66336 group. The 3-month progression-free survival rate, the primary endpoint of the trial, favored the gemcitabine arm over SCH 66336 (31% vs 23%) and so were the median overall survival times (4.4 vs 3.3 months).

Randomized Trials of Gemcitabine-Based Combination Therapy

Several gemcitabine combinations were evaluated in randomized trials versus single-agent gemcitabine therapy (Table 32.4). Similar to what was observed when single-agent 5-FU was compared with 5-FU containing combination regimens, tumor response rates remained generally low. Some superiority in response rates was reported with cisplatin and irinotecan in combination with gemcitabine, and time to progression was improved with 5-FU and cisplatin combinations. However, with a single exception (NSC-631570), this series of studies did not identify a combination regimen that prolonged survival relative to gemcitabine alone.

The Eastern Oncology Cooperative Group (ECOG) compared gemcitabine 1000 mg/m^2 plus bolus 5-FU 600 mg/m^2 to the same dose of gemcitabine alone.[42] All drugs were given weekly for 3 of 4 weeks. Eligibility criteria included microscopically confirmed measurable or assessable disease and an ECOG performance status of 0–2. Of 327 patients enrolled, 322 were eligible. There were no complete responses in either of the treatment groups. The partial response rates were 6.9% and 5.6% for patients receiving gemcitabine plus 5-FU and single-agent gemcitabine, respectively. There was a statistically significant difference in progression-free survival favoring gemcitabine plus 5-FU (3.4 vs 2.2 months, P = 0.022). This difference, however, did not translate into a difference in survival, the primary endpoint for the study. The median overall survival was 6.7 months for the combination regimen and 5.4 months for gemcitabine alone. That difference did not reach the 0.05 level of significance, unless adjusted for an imbalance in baseline performance status (P = 0.037). The regression analysis suggested that survival results could have been different had patients been stratified by performance status, but this observation was felt unimportant in view of the minimal survival gain. Toxicities were also more common in the combination treatment group.

5-FU by continuous infusion in combination with gemcitabine did not result in any difference in response rate, progression-free, or overall survival as compared to gemcitabine alone.[43] The response rate for the combination was 13%, and it was 9% with single-agent gemcitabine. The median progression-free survival was 3 months in both arms, and the median overall survival was also the same in both arms at 6 months. There was somewhat more grade 3 to grade 4 toxicity with the combination than with single-agent therapy.

Three randomized phase III studies evaluated a combination of gemcitabine plus cisplatin compared with gemcitabine alone. The two largest trials showed a benefit in terms of time to progression, but not in terms of survival. These trials may have been inadequately powered to detect a small difference in survival.

A trial conducted in Italy used single-agent gemcitabine at a dose of 1000 mg/m^2 weekly for 7 consecutive weeks

Table 32.4 Randomized Trials of Gemcitabine-Based Combination Regimens Versus Gemcitabine Alone

Author(s)	Treatment	No. of Patients	Median Survival	*P* Value
Berlin et al.[42]	Gemcitabine, 5-FU	160	6.7 months	
	Gemcitabine	162	5.4 months	0.09
Di Costanzo et al.[43]	Gemcitabine, 5-FU (CI)	42	6.0 months	
	Gemcitabine	47	6.0 months	NR
Colucci et al.[44]	Gemcitabine, Cisplatin	53	30 weeks	
	Gemcitabine	54	20 weeks	0.43
Heinemann et al.[45]	Gemcitabine, Cisplatin	96	8.3 months	
	Gemcitabine	99	6.0 months	0.12
Wang et al.[46]	Gemcitabine, Cisplatin	20	217 days	
	Gemcitabine	22	273 days	NR
Scheithauer et al.[47]	Gemcitabine, Capecitabine	41	9.5 months	
	Gemcitabine	42	8.2 months	NR
Rocha Lima et al.[48]	Gemcitabine, Irinotecan	173	6.3 months	
	Gemcitabine	169	6.6 months	NS
Bramhall et al.[50]	Gemcitabine, Marimastat	120	165.5 days	
	Gemcitabine	119	164 days	0.95
Van Cutsem et al.[51]	Gemcitabine, tipifarnib	341	193 days	
	Gemcitabine	347	182 days	0.75
Gansauge et al.[53]	Gemcitabine, NSC-631570	30	10.4 months	
	NSC-631570	30	7.9 months	
	Gemcitabine	30	5.2 months	<0.01
Richards et al.[54]	Gemcitabine, permetrexed	283	6.2 months	
	Gemcitabine	282	6.3 months	0.84
Louvet et al.[55]	Gemcitabine, oxaliplatin	157	9.0 months	
	Gemcitabine	156	7.1 months	0.13

Abbreviations: NR, not reported; NS, not significant.

followed, after a 2-week rest, by drug administration on days 1, 8, and 15 of a 28-day cycle for two cycles.[44] In the combination arm, cisplatin was given at a weekly dose of 25 mg/m^2, and gemcitabine was given as in the single-agent arm. A total of 107 patients were entered; 53 were randomized to receive the gemcitabine plus cisplatin combination, and 54 were randomized to receive gemcitabine alone. That sample size had been selected to demonstrate a 30% improvement in time to progression. The overall response rate for the gemcitabine plus cisplatin arm was 26.4% compared with 9.2% for gemcitabine alone ($P = 0.02$). The median time to progression was 20 weeks for the combination and 8 weeks for single-agent gemcitabine ($P = 0.048$), whereas the median overall survival was 30 weeks for the combination arm and 20 weeks for single-agent gemcitabine arm ($P = 0.43$). There was no difference in clinical benefit derived from a composite assessment of pain, functional impairment, and weight loss. Toxicity was reportedly mild in both arms, but asthenia was more frequent with the combination.

Preliminary results from a larger study conducted in Germany also indicated a significant advantage in progression-free survival, but no significant superiority in terms of survival.[45] A total of 195 patients were enrolled. A combination of gemcitabine 1,000 mg/m^2 and cisplatin 50 mg/m^2 on days 1 and 15 of a 28-day cycle was compared with gemcitabine alone for 1000 mg/m^2 on days 1, 8, and 15 of a 28-day cycle. Progression-free survival markedly favored the combination over the single agent (5.4 vs 2.8 months, $P < 0.01$), but the advantage in survival (8.3 vs 6.0 months) was not significant ($P = 0.12$). Except for nausea and vomiting, 20.9% in the combination arm, and 6.4% in the single-agent arm, toxic effects were similar in both treatment groups.

Wang et al.[46] randomized 22 patients to treatment with a combination of gemcitabine plus cisplatin and 20 patients to treatment with gemcitabine alone. That small study did not show any difference in response rate or survival.

The oral 5-FU prodrug, capecitabine (1,250 mg/m^2 twice a day for 7 days), was given in combination with gemcitabine (2,200 mg/m^2 every 2 weeks) and compared with the same dose and schedule of gemcitabine alone in a randomized phase II trial.[47] Sample sizes were predetermined to detect an increase by 50% in time to progression at 5 months, relative to historical control subjects. A total of 83 patients were entered. The combination and single-agent treatment groups yielded similar results with respect to objective response (17% vs 14%), progression-free survival (5.1 vs 4.0 months), overall survival (9.5 vs 8.2 months), and clinical benefit response (48.4% vs 33%). Adverse reactions were more severe with the combination, especially with the addition of the capecitabine-related hand–foot syndrome, but dose reductions, treatment delays, or treatment discontinuations were fairly similar with both treatment options.

Irinotecan in combination with gemcitabine produced significantly better tumor response rates than gemcitabine alone, but this combination also failed to prolong significantly the time to progression or survival.[48] A total of 360 chemotherapy-naïve patients with locally advanced or metastatic pancreatic cancer were randomized after stratification by performance status, extent of disease, and prior radiotherapy to receive either gemcitabine 1,000 mg/m^2 immediately followed by irinotecan 100 mg/m^2 on days 1 and 8 of 3-week cycles or gemcitabine alone at a dose of 1,000 mg/m^2 weekly for 7 out of 8 consecutive weeks on cycle 1 and then 1,000 mg/m^2 on days 1, 8, and 15 of 4-week cycles. In a preliminary analysis, the overall response rate was 16.1% versus only 4.4% ($P < 0.001$). The median time to progression was 3.4 versus 3.0 months, and the median survival time was 6.3 versus 6.6 months. Combination chemotherapy was associated with more severe diarrhea than single-agent chemotherapy (18.5% vs. 1.8%).

Docetaxel has also been combined with gemcitabine. That combination was tested versus a combination of docetaxel and cisplatin in a randomized phase II trial that involved 96 patients.[49] No difference was found in terms of response rate, progression-free survival, or survival.

Gemcitabine was used in randomized trials in combination with a number of investigational agents, including marimastat,[50] tipifarnib,[51] and CI-994[52] (Table 32.4). In these three cases, a double-blind design was used to compare the two-drug regimens to gemcitabine and placebo. Adding marimastat, a matrix metalloproteinase inhibitor, did not result in any benefit in terms of response rate, progression-free survival, or overall survival, based on a trial that accrued 239 patients. The combination of tipifarnib, a farnesyltransferase inhibitor, with gemcitabine also failed to show an advantage in survival as compared with gemcitabine alone. There was, however, more severe neutropenia and more diarrhea with the combination. No published data are available, as yet, on the randomized phase II trial of CI-994, an oral histone deacetylase inhibitor, but the study was reported to show no difference in survival rates and perhaps an increase in toxicities.[52]

NSC-631570 (Ukrain) is a preparation derived from the Greater Celandine, a common herb, and thiotepa. It has been used in alternative medicine as an anticancer drug. It was tested alone or in combination with gemcitabine versus single-agent gemcitabine therapy in a three-arm phase II study performed at the University of Ulm in Germany.[53] A total of 90 patients were randomized. Limited details are available regarding study design, study execution, or statistical considerations. A significant survival advantage was reported with both investigational arms relative to gemcitabine alone ($P < 0.01$ in both comparisons), with no significant increase in toxicity. These findings were unexpected and make NSC-631570 worthy of further investigation.

Recent reports support a superiority of gemcitabine combined with permetrexed[54] or oxaliplatin[55] over gemcitabine alone in terms of response rate[54,55], and time to progression[54] or progression-free survival.[55] These combinations, however, failed to achieve a significant difference in survival. Both were associated with significantly more grade 3 and 4 toxicities.

The lithium salt of gamolenic acid, a highly unsaturated fatty acid, was also evaluated in a randomized trial that compared oral and intravenous administration at two doses. Results were comparable in all treatment groups. There was no known active control in that trial, but median survival times were reminiscent of historical controls treated with best supportive care.[56]

Randomized Second-Line Therapy Trials

The increased use of gemcitabine in first-line chemotherapy has now generated a new need for second-line treatment. Raltitrexed, a thymidilate synthase inhibitor, was evaluated in a randomized study as a single agent or in combination with irinotecan.[57] The trial accrued 38 patients with metastatic pancreatic adenocarcinoma, whose disease had progressed while receiving or within 6 months after discontinuation of palliative first-line chemotherapy with gemcitabine. The primary endpoint was response rate, and the study was terminated early because of a lack of tumor response in the single-agent raltitrexed arm (0%) compared

Table 32.5 Ongoing Randomized Trials in Advanced/Metastatic Pancreatic Cancer

Phase	Investigator (Group or Location)	Treatment
Phase II	Eastern Cooperative Oncology Group	Arm A: Irinotecan + Docetaxel + Cetuximab Arm B: Irinotecan + Docetaxel
Phase II	North Central Cancer Treatment Group	Arm A: Bortezomib Arm B: Gemcitabine + Bortezomib
Phase II	Cancer and Leukemia Group B	Arm A: Gemcitabine Arm B: Gemcitabine + Cisplatin Arm C: Gemcitabine + Docetaxel Arm D: Gemcitabine + Irinotecan
Phase II	Fox Chase	Arm A: Bevacizumab + Docetaxel Arm B: Bevacizumab
Phase III	Eastern Cooperative Oncology Group	Arm A: Gemcitabine 30-minute infusion Arm B: Gemcitabine 150-minute infusion Arm C: Gemcitabine 100-minute infusion + Oxaliplatin
Phase III	Swiss Institute for Applied Cancer Research/Central European Cooperative Oncology Group	Arm A: Gemcitabine + Capecitabine Arm B: Gemcitabine
Phase III	Cancer Research UK	Arm A: Gemcitabine + Capecitabine Arm B: Gemcitabine
Phase III	Wellstat Therapeutics	Arm A: 5-FU + Oral Triacetyl Uridine Arm B: Gemcitabine
Phase III	Lorus Therapeutics	Arm A: Gemcitabine + Virulizin Arm B: Gemcitabine
Phase III	Southwest Oncology Group	Arm A: Gemcitabine 30 minute infusion + Ce tuximab Arm B: Gemcitabine 30 minute infusion
Phase III	Cancer and Acute Leukemia Group B	Arm A: Gemcitabine 30 minute infusion + Bevacizumab Arm B: Gemcitabine 30 minute infusion

Arranged from National Cancer Institute Clinical Trials.[58]

with a 16% response in the combination arm. The clinical benefit response rate also favored the combination arm (29% vs 8%), as did median progression-free survival (4.0 vs 2.5 months) and median survival (6.5 vs 4.3 months).

Future Directions

Despite over 20 years of clinical investigations, the goal of producing meaningful prolongation of survival for patients with advanced pancreatic cancer remains elusive, and the prognosis for these patients remains extremely poor. Only a few agents have demonstrated anti-tumor activity in pancreatic cancer, including primarily 5-FU and gemcitabine. There are no randomized trials establishing an impact on survival with single-agent 5-FU therapy in this disease, but 5-FU combinations have been shown to prolong survival as compared with best supportive care, and comparisons of several combinations versus 5-FU alone have failed to demonstrate prolonged survival relative to 5-FU alone. Gemcitabine is another active agent that impacts on survival, as demonstrated in trials versus 5-FU and versus a matrix metalloproteinase inhibitor. A superiority over 5-FU has, however, been questioned, as both 5-FU and gemcitabine were possibly not compared at optimal dose schedules. The combination of 5-FU and gemcitabine has shown some benefit, but the advantage in survival versus gemcitabine alone was not pronounced enough to achieve strong statistical significance. Some agents, including flutamide and Ukrain, have unexpectedly been reported to prolong survival in relatively small-size randomized trials and confirmatory trials are needed for more definitive answers.

Elucidating molecular processes in cancer cells has identified a number of attractive targets. Although initial results from randomized studies using therapies targeted against matrix metalloproteinase, farnesyl transferase, or histone deacetylase have been disappointing, targeted therapies remain an active area of investigation (Table 32.5).[58] Ongoing randomized phase II trials are evaluating treatment options other than gemcitabine in chemotherapy-naïve patients with metastatic disease, including cetuximab, a monoclonal antibody that targets the epidermal growth factor receptor, and bortezomib, a proteasome inhibitor. The former has been incorporated in a regimen combining irinotecan and docetaxel. The latter is used as single-agent therapy and in combination with gemcitabine. Some phase II trials are also open to patients with prior exposure to chemotherapy. A number of two-drug combinations of gemcitabine with cisplatin, docetaxel, or irinotecan are being tested versus gemcitabine alone in patients who may have received prior 5-FU. Patients with prior exposure to gemcitabine are eligible for a trial of bevacizumab, a humanized monoclonal antibody directed against vascular endothelial growth factor.

All of the reported ongoing phase III trials use single-agent therapy with gemcitabine as a control. The issues that are being currently addressed concern the optimization of gemcitabine administration or the enhancement of the therapeutic index of single-agent gemcitabine with the addition of other agents. The role of capecitabine, oxaliplatin, irinotecan, and docetaxel is being further elucidated. Identifying new active agents from new classes of anti-cancer agents remains a high priority area for research in this disease.

References

1. Jemal A, Tiwari RC, Murray T, et al. Cancer Statistics, 2004. *CA Cancer J Clin.* 2004;54:8–29.
2. El Kamar FG, Grossbard ML, Kozuch PS. Metastatic pancreatic cancer: emerging strategies in chemotherapy and palliative care. *Oncologist.* 2003;8:18–34.
3. Abbruzzese JL. Past and present treatment of pancreatic adenocarcinoma: chemotherapy as a standard treatment modality. *Semin Oncol.* 2002;29(Suppl 20):S2–S8.
4. Haller DG. New perspectives in the management of pancreas cancer. *Semin Oncol.* 2003;30(Suppl 11):S3–S10.
5. Mallinson CN, Rake MO, Cocking JB, et al. Chemotherapy in pancreatic cancer: results of a controlled, prospective, randomised, multicentre trial. *Br Med J.* 1980;281:1589–1591.
6. Palmer KR, Kerr M, Knowles G, et al. Chemotherapy prolongs survival in inoperable pancreatic carcinoma. *Br J Surg.* 1994;81:882–885.
7. Glimelius B, Hoffman K, Sjödén P-O, et al. Chemotherapy improves survival and quality of life in advanced pancreatic and biliary cancer. *Ann Oncol.* 1996;7:593–600.
8. Andersen JR, Friis-Møller A, Hancke S, et al. A controlled trial of combination chemotherapy with 5-FU and BCNU in pancreatic cancer. *Scand J Gastroenterol.* 1981;16:973–975.
9. Frey C, Twomey P, Keehn R, et al. Randomized study of 5-FU and CCNU in pancreatic cancer: report of the Veterans Administration Surgical Adjuvant Cancer Chemotherapy Study Group. *Cancer.* 1981;47:27–31.
10. Andren-Sandberg A, Holmberg JT, Ihse I. Treatment of unresectable pancreatic carcinoma with 5-fluorouracil, vincristine and CCNU. *Scand J Gastroenterol.* 1983;18:609–612.
11. Bakkevold KE, Pettersen A, Arnesjo B, Espehaug B. Tamoxifen therapy in unresectable adenocarcinoma of the pancreas and the papilla of Vater. *Br J Surg.* 1990;77:725–730.
12. Keating JJ, Johnson PJ, Cochrane AMG, et al. A prospective randomised controlled trial of tamoxifen and cyproterone acetate in pancreatic carcinoma. *Br J Cancer.* 1989;60:789–792.
13. Greenway BA. Effect of flutamide on survival in patients with pancreatic cancer: results of a prospective, randomised, double blind, placebo controlled trial. *BMJ.* 1998;316:1935–1938.
14. Schein PS, Lavin PT, Moertel CG, et al. Randomized phase II clinical trial of adriamycin, methotrexate and actinomycin-D in advanced measurable pancreatic carcinoma: a Gastrointestinal Tumor Study Group Report. *Cancer.* 1978;42:19–22.
15. Gastrointestinal Tumor Study Group. Phase II trials of hexamethylmelamine, dianhydrogalactitol, razoxane, and β-2′-deoxythioguanosine as single agents against advanced measurable tumors of the pancreas. *Cancer Treat Rep.* 1985;69:713–716.
16. Gastrointestinal Tumor Study Group. Phase II trials of maytansine, low-dose chlorozotocin, and high-dose chlorozotocin as single agents against advanced measurable adenocarcinoma of the pancreas. *Cancer Treat Rep.* 1985;69:417–420.
17. Bukowski RM, Fleming TR, Macdonald JS, et al. Evaluation of combination chemotherapy and phase II agents in pancreatic adenocarcinoma. A Southwest Oncology Group Study. *Cancer.* 1993;71:322–325.
18. Horton J, Gelber RD, Engstrom P, et al. Trials of single-agent and combination chemotherapy for advanced cancer of the pancreas. *Cancer Treat Rep.* 1981;65:65–68.
19. Kovach JS, Moertel CG, Schutt AJ, et al. A controlled study of combined 1,3-BIS-(2-chloroethyl)-1-nitrosourea and 5-fluorouracil therapy for advanced gastric and pancreatic cancer. *Cancer.* 1974;33:563–567.
20. Stolinsky DC, Pugh RP, Bateman JR. 5-Fluorouracil (NSC-19893) therapy for pancreatic carcinoma: comparison of oral and intravenous routes. *Cancer Chemother Rep.* 1975;59:1031–1033.
21. Maisey N, Chau I, Cunningham D, et al. Multicenter randomized phase III trial comparing protracted venous infusion (PVI) fluorouracil (5-FU) with PVI 5-FU plus mitomycin in inoperable pancreatic cancer. *J Clin Oncol.* 2002;20:3130–3136.
22. Cullinan SA, Moertel CG, Fleming TR, et al. A comparison of three chemotherapeutic regimens in the treatment of advanced pancreatic and gastric carcinoma. Fluorouracil vs fluorouracil and doxorubicin vs fluorouracil, doxorubicin, and mitomycin. *JAMA.* 1985;253:2061–2067.
23. Takada T, Kato H, Matsushiro T, et al. Comparison of 5-fluorouracil, doxorubicin and mitomycin C with 5-fluorouracil alone in the treatment of pancreatic-biliary carcinomas. *Oncology.* 1994;51:396–400.
24. Bukowski RM, Balcerzak SP, O'Bryan RM, et al. Randomized trial of 5-fluorouracil and mitomycin C with or without streptozotocin for advanced pancreatic cancer: a Southwest Oncology Group Study. *Cancer.* 1983;52:1577–1582.

25. Kelsen D, Hudis C, Niedzwiecki D, et al. A phase III comparison trial of streptozotocin, mitomycin and 5-fluorouracil with cisplatin, cytosine arabinoside, and caffeine in patients with advanced pancreatic carcinoma. *Cancer.* 1991;68:965–969.
26. Moertel CG, Engstrom P, Lavin PT, et al. Chemotherapy of gastric and pancreatic carcinoma. *Surgery.* 1979;85:509–513.
27. Moertel CG, Douglas HO, Hanley J, Jr., Carbone PP. Treatment of advanced adenocarcinoma of the pancreas with combinations of streptozotocin plus 5-fluorouracil and streptozotocin plus cyclophosphamide. *Cancer.* 1977;40:605–608.
28. Awrich A, Fletcher WS, Klotz JH, et al. 5-FU versus combination therapy with tubercidin, streptozotocin, and 5-FU in the treatment of pancreatic carcinomas: COG protocol 7230. *J Surg Oncol.* 1979;12:267–273.
29. The Gastrointestinal Tumor Study Group. Phase II studies of drug combinations in advanced pancreatic carcinoma: fluorouracil plus doxorubicin plus mitomycin C and two regimens of streptozotocin plus mitomycin C plus fluorouracil. *J Clin Oncol.* 1986;4:1794–1798.
30. Oster MW, Gray R, Panasci L, Perry MC, for Cancer and Leukemia Group B. Chemotherapy for advanced pancreatic cancer: a comparison of 5-fluorouracil, adriamycin, and mitomycin (FAM) with 5-fluorouracil, streptozotocin and mitomycin (FSM). *Cancer.* 1986;57:29–33.
31. Topham C, Glees J, Rawson NSB, et al. Randomised trial of epirubicin alone versus 5-fluorouracil, epirubicin and mitomycin C in locally advanced and metastatic carcinoma of the pancreas. *Br J Cancer.* 1991;64:179–181.
32. Ducreux M, Rougier P, Pignon J-P, et al. A randomised trial comparing 5-FU with 5-FU plus cisplatin in advanced pancreatic carcinoma. *Ann Oncol.* 2002;13:1185–1191.
33. Wagener DJT, Wils JA, Kok TC, et al. Results of a randomised phase II study of cisplatin plus 5-fluorouracil versus cisplatin plus 5-fluorouracil with alpha-interferon in metastatic pancreatic cancer: an EORTC gastrointestinal tract cancer group trial. *Eur J Cancer.* 2002;38:648–653.
34. Cullinan S, Moertel CG, Wieand HS, et al. A phase III trial on the therapy of advanced pancreatic carcinoma: evaluations of the Mallinson regimen and combined 5-fluorouracil, doxorubicin, and cisplatin. *Cancer.* 1990;65:2207–2212.
35. Rougier P, Ducreux M, Ould Kaci M, et al. Randomized phase II study of oxaliplatin alone (OXA), 5-fluorouracil (5-FU) alone, and the two drugs combined (OXA-FU) in advanced or metastatic pancreatic adenocarcinoma (APC) [abstract 1018]. *Proc Am Soc Clin Oncol.* 2000;19:262a.
36. Burch PA, Block M, Schroeder G, et al. Phase III evaluation of octreotide versus chemotherapy with 5-fluorouracil or 5-fluorouracil plus leucovorin in advanced exocrine pancreatic cancer: a North Central Cancer Treatment Group Study. *Clin Cancer Res.* 2000;6:3486–3492.
37. Burris HA, Moore MJ, Andersen J, et al. Improvements in survival and clinical benefit with gemcitabine as first-line therapy for patients with advanced pancreas cancer: a randomized trial. *J Clin Oncol.* 1997;15:2403–2413.
38. Moore MJ, Hamm J, Eisenberg P, et al. A comparison between gemcitabine (GEM) and the matrix metalloproteinase (MMP) inhibitor BAY12-9566 (9566) in patients (pts) with advanced pancreatic cancer [abstract 930]. *Proc Am Soc Clin Oncol.* 2000;19:240a.
39. Tempero M, Plunkett W, Ruiz van Haperen V, et al. Randomized phase II comparison of dose intense gemcitabine: thirty-minute infusion and fixed dose rate infusion in patients with pancreatic adenocarcinoma. *J Clin Oncol.* 2003;21:3402–3408.
40. Smith D, Gallagher N. A phase II/III study comparing intravenous ZD 9331 with gemcitabine in patients with pancreatic cancer. *Eur J Cancer.* 2003;39:1377–1383.
41. Lersch C, Van Cutsem E, Amado R, et al. Randomized phase II study of SCH 66336 and gemcitabine in the treatment of metastatic adenocarcinoma of the pancreas [abstract 608]. *Proc Am Soc Clin Oncol.* 2001;20:153a.
42. Berlin JD, Catalano P, Thomas JP, et al. Phase III study of gemcitabine in combination with fluorouracil versus gemcitabine alone in patients with advanced pancreatic carcinoma: Eastern Cooperative Oncology Group Trial E2297. *J Clin Oncol.* 2002;20:3270–3275.
43. Di Costanzo F, Sdrobolini A, Carlini P, et al. Gemcitabine (GEM) alone or in combination with 5-FU continuous infusion (CI) in the treatment of advanced pancreatic cancer (APC): a GOIRC randomized phase II trial [abstract 612]. *Proc Am Soc Clin Oncol.* 2001;20:154a.
44. Colucci G, Giuliani F, Gebbia V, et al. Gemcitabine alone or with cisplatin for the treatment of patients with locally advanced and/or metastatic pancreatic carcinoma: a prospective, randomized phase III study of the Gruppo Oncologico dell'Italia Meridionale. *Cancer.* 2002;94:902–910.
45. Heinemann V, Quietzsch D, Gieseler F, et al. A phase III trial comparing gemcitabine plus cisplatin vs. gemcitabine alone in advanced pancreatic carcinoma [abstract 1003]. *Proc Am Soc Clin Oncol.* 2003;22:250.
46. Wang X, Ni Q, Jin M, et al. Gemcitabine or gemcitabine plus cisplatin for in 42 patients with locally advanced or metastatic pancreatic cancer. *Chin J Oncol.* 2002;24:404–407.
47. Scheithauer W, Schull B, Ulrich-Pur H, et al. Biweekly high-dose gemcitabine alone or in combination with capecitabine in patients with metastatic pancreatic adenocarcinoma: a randomized phase II trial. *Ann Oncol.* 2003;14:97–104.
48. Rocha Lima CMS, Rotche R, Jeffery M, et al. A randomized phase 3 study comparing efficacy and safety of gemcitabine (GEM) and irinotecan (I), to GEM alone in patients (pts) with locally advanced or metastatic pancreatic cancer who have not received prior systemic therapy [abstract 1005]. *Proc Am Soc Clin Oncol.* 2003;22:251.
49. Lutz MP, Ducreux M, Wagener T, et al. Docetaxel/gemcitabine or docetaxel/cisplatin in advanced pancreatic carcinoma: a randomized phase II study of the EORTC-GI group [abstract 498]. *Proc Am Soc Clin Oncol.* 2002;21:125a.
50. Bramhall SR, Schulz J, Nemunaitis J, et al. A double-blind placebo-controlled, randomised study comparing gemcitabine and marimastat with gemcitabine and placebo as first line therapy in patients with advanced pancreatic cancer. *Br J Cancer.* 2002;87:161–167.
51. Van Cutsem E, van de Velde H, Karasek P, et al. Phase III trial of gemcitabine plus tipifarnib compared to gemcitabine plus placebo in advanced pancreatic cancer. *J Clin Oncol.* 2004;22:1430–1438.

52. Richards DA, Waterhouse DM, Wagener DJT, et al. Randomized, double-blind, placebo controlled phase 2 study of the histone deacetylase inhibitor CI-994 plus gemcitabine (CI-994 + G) versus placebo plus gemcitabine (P + G) in the treatment of patients with advanced pancreatic cancer APC [abstract 644]. *Proc Am Soc Clin Oncol.* 2002;21:162a.
53. Gansauge F, Ramadani M, Pressmar J, et al. NSC-631570 (Ukrain) in the palliative treatment of pancreatic cancer: results of a phase II trial. *Arch Surg.* 2002;386: 570–574.
54. Richards DA, Kindler HL, Oettle RK, et al. A randomized phase III study comparing gemcitabine + pemetrexed versus gemcitabine in patients with locally advanced and metastatic pancreas cancer [abstract 4007]. *J Clin Oncol.* 2004;22:S14.
55. Louvet C, Labianca R, Hammel P, et al. GemOx (gemcitabine + oxaliplatin) versus Gem (gemcitabine) in non resectable pancreatic adenocarcinoma: final results of the GERCOR/GISCAD Intergroup phase III [abstract 4008]. *J Clin Oncol.* 2004;22:S14.
56. Johnson CD, Puntis M, Davidson N, et al. Randomized, dose-finding phase III study of lithium gamolenate in patients with advanced pancreatic adenocarcinoma. *Br J Surg.* 2001;88:662–668.
57. Ulrich-Pur H, Raderer M, Kornek GV, et al. Irinotecan plus raltitrexed vs raltitrexed alone in patients with gemcitabine-pretreated advanced pancreatic adenocarcinoma. *Br J Cancer.* 2003;88:1180–1184.
58. National Cancer Institute Clinical Trials. PDQ® Search-Stage IV Pancreas Cancer Randomized Phase II, III. Available at: http://cancer.gov. Accessed December 19, 2004.

CHAPTER 33

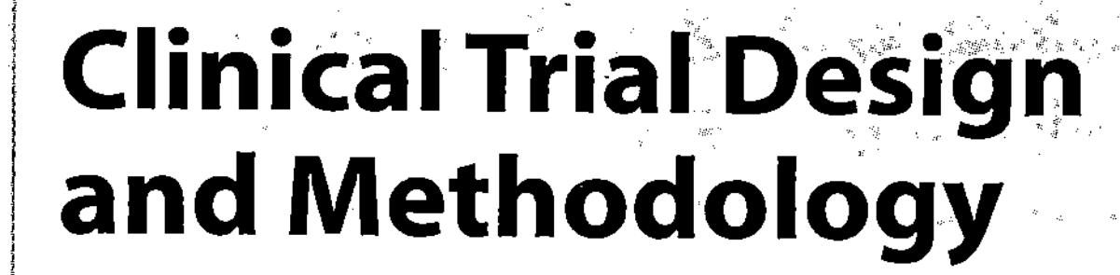

Jason A. Konner, MD
Eileen M. O'Reilly, MD

The design of clinical trials in oncology has become increasingly complex. The dual specters of rising health care costs and restricted budgeting have strained resources. An abundance of new biologically targeted agents is presenting unique challenges to the very structure of traditional trial design. Clinical research in pancreatic cancer (PC) is further burdened by limited numbers of eligible patients, and it is a cancer that remains difficult to diagnose, evaluate, and treat. These constraints demand an approach to trial design and methodology that emphasizes efficiency to maximize practicality, as well as scientific rigor to ensure interpretability.

History of Clinical Trials

Although large, multi-institutional, randomized, controlled studies represent the apogee of present-day clinical trials, this has not always been the case. The history of medicine has for the most part been motivated by empiricism and tradition and has been inhibited by cultural and religious forces. However, examples of medical trials can be gleaned from ancient texts. A biblical passage from the book of Daniel may represent the first clinical trial in recorded history.[1] "*Daniel said . . . 'Test your servants for ten days; let us be given vegetables to eat and water to drink. Then let our appearance and the appearance of the youths who eat the king's rich food be observed by you' . . . At the end of ten days it was seen that they were better in appearance and fatter in flesh than all the youths who ate the king's rich food.*" (Daniel 1:11–16)

In fairness, little is known of what clinical studies the Cro-Magnon medicine man, pictured in cave drawings at Ariège in France, might have designed. More is known of ancient Egyptian medicine men who, like the Cro-Magnon, ascribed disease to supernatural causes. It was priests to whom the sick would come for healing. Their experiences with disease and treatments were recorded on papyrus and became the first known medical texts. During the Third Dynasty 5000 years ago, King Zoser's high priest, known as Imhotep, or "he who comes in peace," was believed to be the man who was best in control of the evil spirits that brought disease and best able to engage the gods to aid the sick.[2] Posthumously, he was worshipped as a god of healing, and his teachings were influential.

Ancient Greek physicians, 2500 years ago, generated hypotheses on the basis of their understanding of natural physiology and disease. However, they did not establish a means of testing these hypotheses in a controlled, scientifically rigorous way, because the concepts of trial design had not been established. It was Hippocrates who best summarized the challenges the trialist would face: "Life is short, the Art is long, opportunity fleeting, experience delusive, judgment difficult."[3]

During the Roman Empire, the medical teachings of Galen, a Greek physician, remained dogmatic for a millennium, and medical progress largely stagnated until the doctors of the Muslim Empire picked up the torch. After the vast conquests of the Arabs, they were taught of the medical teachings of the Greeks and Romans by Byzantine priests.[2] Although evidence of human subjects' testing in this era is lacking, at least one trial involving surrogate tissue was performed. When the famed physician Rhazes (860–932) was to choose a location for a new hospital in Baghdad, he placed large pieces of meat throughout the city and chose the locale where the meat spoiled last.

The Common Era in Europe, influenced by religious and public condemnation of dissection or experimentation on humans, brought stagnation to the science of medicine up to the Renaissance.

In 1747, taking up the long-neglected reins of Daniel, James Lind undertook "the first deliberately planned controlled experiment . . . on human subjects."[4] Choosing 12 patients at sea with signs of scurvy—"putrid gums, the spots and lassitude, with weakness of their knees"—Lind randomly assigned two patients each to receive cider daily, vinegar three times daily, 25 "gutts of elixir vitriol" in acid gargle three times daily, sea water, or citrus fruits. The two sickest patients were not randomly assigned and instead were given nutmeg. This small, single-institution, randomized (after exclusion), multi-arm study succeeded in elucidating the cure for scurvy because it was carefully controlled.

The modern era of clinical trial design began in earnest fewer than 60 years ago. The first randomized therapeutic trial, conceived by Phillip D'Arcy Hart and designed by Sir Austin Bradford Hill, was carried out between 1946 and 1948.[5] Frustrated with a century of uncontrolled and uninterpretable studies on treatments for tuberculosis, Hart and Hill set out to test the efficacy of streptomycin, then in limited supply, in a scientifically meaningful way. They treated 50 patients randomly assigned to receive the drug or bed rest alone and then compared the consequences. The results not only established the efficacy of a tuberculosis drug for the first time as convincingly beneficial but also startlingly proved the power of carefully controlled prospective studies.[6]

It would be another decade before the first controlled trials in cancer treatment in the United States were conducted. This effort was spearheaded by Gordon Zubrod, whose mentor at the National Cancer Institute (NCI), Jerome Cornfield, was a strong advocate for organizing randomized studies using large populations. To this end, Zubrod, who had studied treatments for pneumonia and for malaria, now turned his attention to childhood leukemia. He proposed that academic centers around the country be organized into a group of regional cancer research groups that could pool their patients and coordinate their efforts to conduct large-scale clinical trials. Sidney Farber and Mary Lasker petitioned Congress for financial support. Sponsored by the NCI, Zubrod's group expanded into two cooperative groups: acute leukemia groups A and B. The latter group (later known as CALGB), led by Emil Frei and James Holland, published their first trial results in 1958.[7] In 1955, Zubrod and others also formed the Eastern Solid Tumor Group (later known as the Eastern Cooperative Oncology Group, or ECOG), whose first publication appeared in 1960.[5] The West, Mid-West, Southeast, and Southwest Oncology Groups also emerged from this effort, although only the Southwest Oncology Group (SWOG) remains. The CALGB, ECOG, and SWOG eventually decentralized from National Institutes of Health into their own central leadership roles.[8] Today, the NCI's Cancer Therapeutics Evaluation Program funds more than 150 cooperative agreements with a dozen major cooperative groups, whose annual federal funding remains just $90 million. The large, randomized, multi-institutional studies organized by these groups have contributed enormously to the continuing development of clinical oncology as a scientifically grounded, evidence-guided discipline.

For the field of PC, large, randomized studies have a short and mostly inglorious history. From 1899, when William Halsted performed the first successful resection of an ampullary cancer, development of pancreaticoduodenectomy represents a clear advance in surgical technique, with perioperative mortality declining from roughly 50%[9] in its early stages to 25% in the 1960s,[10] and recently to less than 5% in many centers.[11] A century later, the clinical benefit of this procedure remains in doubt. The surgical literature consists primarily of clinical series and retrospective reviews. A trial that can definitively answer the question of efficacy has not been performed.

Chemotherapeutic and radiation trials for PC shine with little more luster. In the 1980s, studies by the Gastrointestinal Study Group (GITSG) established the roles of 5-fluorouracil (5-FU) and radiotherapy as controversial standards of care for locally advanced[12] and resected[13] PC. The legacy and significance of the GITSG trials are plagued by poor accrual, poor quality control, outdated methodology, and lack of reproducibility. Later studies have struggled in the quest to confirm or deny the GITSG findings.[14,15] 5-FU also remained the cornerstone of palliative therapy for metastatic disease until a landmark trial in 1997 demonstrated a clinical benefit of gemcitabine over 5-FU for these patients.[16]

Currently, clinical trials in PC are addressing a number of important questions. What is the role of adjuvant or neoadjuvant therapy? What is the preferred regimen for perioperative therapy? Is gemcitabine a superior radiosensitizer to 5-FU? What are the optimal frequency, rate, and schedule of administration for gemcitabine both alone and in conjunction with radiation therapy? Can palliative treatment with gemcitabine be improved with combinations of agents? Will inhibitors of the epidermal growth factor receptor pathway, or of vascular endothelial growth factor play an important role in PC treatment? Which of the other emerging biologically targeted anticancer agents may be useful? Is it possible to identify and screen high-risk patients, and how should they be treated?

To address these and other important clinical questions, careful clinical trial design and methodology is crucial to optimize efficiency, potency of results, and use of limited resources.

Issues in Pancreatic Cancer Trial Design

PC differs from other malignancies in many ways, some of which facilitate clinical trials, and others that hamper them. These features must be taken into account when trials are planned.

A key limiting factor is the available study population. The relative infrequency of PC, as well as the poor functional status of many of its sufferers, makes accrual of large patient numbers inherently challenging. This is particularly true for trials involving resectable disease, where in the United States, the target population is only approximately 5000–6000 patients, not to mention long treatment delays that can follow pancreaticoduodenectomy. On the other hand, accrual for palliative treatment studies is relatively enhanced by the high frequency of unresectable disease and the eagerness of fit patients to seek an alternate to the largely disappointing standard therapeutic options.

As a result of anatomic and pathological issues, primary pancreatic tumors are difficult to assess by biopsy and to assess on serial radiologic imaging. Tissue samples are limited because the diagnosis is frequently made by fine-needle aspiration or liver biopsy, and with the exception of patients who undergo pancreaticoduodenectomy or palliative bypass, there is rarely an opportunity for obtaining additional tissue during the course of treatment. Seldom are there noninvasive options to do so.

Only a portion of the primary tumor mass itself consists of cancer cells; the rest is composed of a dense desmoplastic reaction with contributions from pancreatitis and a dilated pancreatic duct. This presents difficulties not only for molecular analysis but also for radiologic interpretation of tumor size, because bland fibrotic tissue, postradiation changes, and adjacent pancreatitis can make true tumor size difficult to reliably assess, even with modern imaging techniques.

The limited prognoses are unfortunate for patients but enhance opportunities for study. When sample size is calculated for a trial, a large number of adverse events can be expected for resected or unresected PC within a feasible time frame. This lessens the time (not the sample size) needed to conduct an adequately powered study. The rapidity of clinical deterioration to death in advanced disease often eliminates the need to use surrogate endpoints, when survival is the true endpoint of interest. Meaningful studies can thus be shorter and smaller. Additionally, the near-uniformly abysmal prognoses and paucity of effective therapies alter the risk-benefit balance in PC to ethically allow more risk than might be appropriate with other diseases and thus invite more flexibility in therapeutic plans, should a toxic treatment prove potentially efficacious. One must also be especially cautious about the potential for coercion to compromise the ethics of a study with these vulnerable patients, who face time pressure and may have decreased decision-making abilities.

At present, single-agent gemcitabine represents the standard of care for first-line treatment of metastatic PC and thus is the current control for trials with these patients. The standard treatment for resectable disease is still controversial, however, and what is an appropriate control for these studies remains a matter of some debate. It is important to note that from a regulatory perspective, randomized controlled trials are not an absolute requirement for approval of a new treatment, if convincing clinical benefit can be demonstrated without them. A demonstration of durable responses or improved quality of life (QoL) in patients with advanced disease might suffice for approval. A definitive comparative trial, answering a scientifically important question, may be performed in the postapproval setting.[17] A comparison with gemcitabine may not be required if a dramatic demonstration of efficacy in second-line treatment were demonstrated. PC, a disease that is frequently symptomatic, lends itself to use of symptomatic relief as an endpoint. Patients may be assessed for improvement from baseline in QoL, including measures such as pain, appetite, and performance.

Pitfalls and Promise of Past Trials

No area of study has been more contentious than the question of adjuvant therapy in PC. The discord has resulted in part from flawed trial designs and conduct that have characterized many of the large trials in PC. GITSG #9173[13] was the first major trial to compare chemoradiation (CRT) after resection with observation. This study established 5-FU–based CRT, followed by 5-FU, as the adjuvant standard of care in the United States. In this study, the treatment arm survived a median 20 months, versus 11 months for the control arm ($P = 0.03$), with a 5-year survival of 19% versus 5%. The credibility of these data has been burdened by sluggish accrual and poor quality control. Only 43 patients were enrolled over an 8-year period at 11 different institutions. A significant portion of patients had a poor performance status (44% ECOG 2–3), and roughly a quarter of patients did not receive the planned therapy. Additionally, the radiation was given in an outmoded, "split-course" fashion and encompassed large normal tissue volumes. Despite these criticisms, the result was quite striking and has resulted in adjuvant 5-FU–based CRT being adopted as a controversial standard of care.

A European study sponsored by the European Organization for Research and Treatment of Cancer (EORTC) attempted to confirm the findings of GITSG in a randomized study comparing the same two arms as in GITSG, with the exception that infusional 5-FU was used on the first and fifth weeks of radiation instead of bolus 5-FU and no additional 5-FU was given after CRT. The trial accrued patients with pancreatic, duodenal, ampullary, and distal common bile duct malignancies from 29 centers with 228 patients. In total, 104 patients with PC were accrued.[14] The treatment arm yielded a median survival of 17.1 months versus 12.6 months for the control arm, as well as a 2-year overall survival advantage, 34% versus 26%, but failed to reach statistical significance. These data can fuel arguments for or against adjuvant CRT. Although its result is negative, it is argued to have been underpowered to show a difference in survival and would have actually needed to accrue in excess of 300 patients for adequate power. Furthermore, there were no stratification by resection margins and no quality control for the administration of radiation therapy, which was the same out-moded, split-course protocol used in the GITSG trial.

The ESPAC-1, sponsored by the European Study Group for Pancreatic Cancer, was the largest randomized trial ever reported in PC. It had been intended to conclusively address the adjuvant therapy debate with an ambitious "2 × 2 factorial" design with four possible treatments of CRT, chemotherapy, radiation, or observation, following resection. There were 61 participating centers from 11 countries, which accrued 541 patients over 6 years. An intention to treat analysis with a primary survival endpoint yielded no benefit for CRT, although a probable benefit for chemotherapy alone. Radiation therapy was found to have a confounding negative effect.[15] This trial has been criticized for a plethora of violations of design and methodology.[18] Rather than the strict two-stage randomization required by 2 × 2 factorial designs, physicians and patients were allowed to select to be randomly assigned to different treatment arms. Additionally, nonrandomized radiation treatment modifications (split-course vs 60 Gy) occurred on an individual basis. There was no stratification by surgical margin status. Fifty patients dropped out after randomization.

In summary, more than 800 patients have been randomly assigned in three multicenter adjuvant PC trials over 25 years, yet the benefit of adjuvant CRT remains uncertain. A recently completed Radiation Therapy Oncology Group study of CRT with infusional 5-FU given before and after infusional 5-FU versus gemcitabine given before and after the same CRT with infusional 5-FU will not answer the question of the benefit of adjuvant therapy versus observation after surgery because of the absence of a no-treatment arm for accrual concerns. However, it may answer the question of whether administering gemcitabine versus 5-FU may be a better systemic adjuvant chemotherapy. Additional merits of the Radiation Therapy Oncology Group trial design include: (1) adequate power, with more than 500 patients having being accrued; (2) careful radiation quality control; and (3) appropriate stratification for known prognostic factors. An ongoing EORTC study of CRT with gemcitabine versus observation may, if executed properly, fill the void.

What these studies demonstrate is the preeminent importance of proper trial design and methodology in the conduct of clinical trials to ensure that meaningful conclusions can be drawn. Although the GITSG adjuvant PC trial is exemplary in its simplicity of design, it was a practical failure of accrual and eligibility. Conversely, the EORTC and ESPAC-1 trials demonstrated the feasibility of accruing larger numbers of resected patients but fell short on appropriate standards of quality control for randomization and treatment principles.

The clinical trials leading to the approval of gemcitabine for first-line treatment of metastatic PC were exemplary in their ingenuity in adapting trial design to fit the features particular to drug, patient, and disease.[16,19] The phase II trial defined a composite endpoint of a clinical benefit assessment, composed of pain level and analgesic consumption, dry weight gain, and performance status, which was used as a primary endpoint when gemcitabine was compared with 5-FU in a phase III trial, establishing a new standard of care for the field.[16,19]

Trials of novel therapies since the approval of gemcitabine have been somewhat disappointing. The farnesyl transferase inhibitors raised the hope that knowledge of a molecular feature of PC, namely the frequent occurrence of *ras* mutations, may translate into effective clinical treatment. These medicines proved to have higher toxicities than expected for a "cytostatic" drug and lacked efficacy.[20] Similarly disappointing have been the results from trials with matrix metalloproteinase inhibitors.[21] Although these drugs were also inspired by a strong scientific rationale and a well-defined molecular target, the clinical studies failed to demonstrate significant efficacy in PC or whether the molecular targets were even reached by appropriate concentrations of the drugs.[22] Trials using combinations of approved drugs—namely cisplatin and oxaliplatin—with gemcitabine have been more promising, although their clinical benefit has yet to be conclusively demonstrated.[23,24]

Clinical Trial Designs for Cytotoxic Chemotherapeutics

Contemporary clinical trials are organized in a progressive, stepwise fashion, into a series of phases, numbered I–IV, which have different goals and designs but build on and rely on each other. Phase I is primarily a dose and toxicity-seeking trial, and phase II evaluates safety and screens for efficacy in order to determine whether a treatment warrants further evaluation in a phase III trial, which is a large-scale effort to establish comparative treatment efficacy and may lead to a drug's approval by the US Food and Drug Administration (FDA). Once a treatment enters clinical use, phase IV, post-marketing, studies survey the treated patient population for rarer toxicities not detected during phases I–III but might be observed in wider-scale use of a drug.

Phase III randomized controlled trials are a cornerstone of clinical oncology and drug development and are considered a reference standard. They are also the largest, lengthiest, and costliest step in the process of drug development. With several hundred novel agents being considered for use in clinical oncology, it is neither ethical nor feasible to test them all in phase III.[25,26] Phase I and II trials are therefore critical not only in determining an appropriate dose, schedule, and target population for a treatment but also in guiding the selection of which treatments warrant the allocation of limited resources for further study. Additional benefits of phase II studies include the ability to assess toxicity and efficacy in a larger, more focused population than in phase I and to fine-tune schedules or doses approximated in phase I. In addition, phase II trials are viewed favorably by patients, who are less likely to receive suboptimal doses than in phase I, and because placebo controls are seldom used. On the other hand, if few useful data are anticipated from a given phase II trial, an alternate option that may expedite the process of drug development in certain circumstances is to perform an expanded phase I study, and then move directly to phase III.

Phase I

Phase I is the entry-level trial for a therapy previously studied only in experimental tumor models—a so-called "first in human" study—or in a novel schedule, dose, or route of administration, or in combination with another standard or novel agent. It is the portal through which all novel agents enter from the laboratory into the clinical realm. Careful trial design is critical early on in the drug development process; roughly 90% of new anti-cancer agents do not enter routine clinical use, in part as a result of neglect of preclinical information and inadequate trial design.[27]

Safety and efficacy Although the scientific goals of these trials are unrelated to efficacy, they carry a small potential for clinical benefit. Eligible patients frequently have advanced disease, and the likelihood of treatment effect with phase I drugs should parallel that of available agents. As such, a phase I trial is a standard of care in the appropriate setting.[28] If a phase I treatment is given as first-line therapy in PC, it should not interfere with the patients' potential to receive gemcitabine-based therapies at some point in their therapy, if they are eligible for them. The treatment plan, rationale, and alternatives must be explicit in the informed consent process.

Composite analyses of phase I trials have yielded insights into their typical features. An analysis of 187 phase I trials of 54 drugs in the 1970s revealed an overall response rate of 4.2%.[29] Most patients (90%) were pretreated and most had a good performance status. More than 60% received doses below those recommended for phase II studies, that is, they received potentially suboptimal therapy. A review analysis of 6639 patients in 211 phase I trials for

Table 33.1. Cytotoxic Drug Development in Pancreatic Cancer

	Phase I	Phase II	Phase III
Aims	Toxicity Maximum tolerated dose Pharmacokinetics	Response rate Toxicity	Response rate Survival Quality of life
Target population	Open	Pancreatic cancer	Pancreatic cancer
Principal endpoint	Toxicity	Response	Survival
Study design	Modified Fibonacci[a] Accelerated titration[b]	1–2 stage	Randomized ± placebo controlled

[a]Modified Fibonacci design: standard dose escalation schema using a modified Fibonacci sequence, e.g., 100%, 50%, 33%, 20%, dose increments, and so on.
[b]Accelerated titration design: trial designs to increase the efficiency and minimize the number of patients treated at subtherapeutic doses

87 drugs over 15 years (1972–1987) yielded an overall response of 4.5% and a toxic death rate of 0.5%.[30] In a similar study of 7960 patients in 228 trials over 14 years, a 6% response rate was seen.[31] Of note, in that analysis, no drug ultimately made it to market that had had no responses in phase I. Most responses occurred within 80%–120% of the phase II dose. Very similar response data were found in a survey of phase I studies in Japan.[32] In general, most responses in these trials occurred in hematologic cancers and chemosensitive solid tumors. One study demonstrated no decrement in QoL for participants in phase I trials.[33]

Standard design The entrance of a new agent into phase I follows extensive preclinical evaluation and is predicated on a reasonable expectation of some anti-tumor activity to be evident. For benign diseases, phase I typically involves administering subtherapeutic doses in healthy volunteers to assess toxicity; in oncology, however, phase I drugs are tested only in patients with cancer and have a potential therapeutic role.[28] The scientific goal of phase I trials is to identify toxicities and determine the dose for phase II and phase III settings. This dose is the maximum tolerated dose (MTD), which is the presumed optimal dose for cytotoxic chemotherapeutics. MTD is determined by the occurrence of dose-limiting toxicities encountered as doses increase in phase I trials. Dose-limiting toxicities are described in terms of adverse events, which are clinical or laboratory abnormalities, symptoms, or diseases temporally associated with treatment; these count against further dose escalation.[34] Several hundred adverse events are defined and ranked in severity (0–5 for none, mild, moderate, severe, life-threatening, or fatal, respectively) in the Common Toxicity Criteria for Adverse Events (CTCAE) (http://ctep.cancer.gov/forms/CTCAEv3.pdf). The CTCAE is published by the Cancer Therapy Evaluation Program of the NCI. The type and severity of adverse events, that which constitute a dose-limiting toxicity, must be predefined in the phase I clinical trial.

The dose at which 10% of animals die in preclinical experiments, known as LD_{10}, has been shown to correlate with MTD in humans.[35] One tenth of the murine (or most sensitive animal) LD_{10} is the typical starting dose for a phase I trial.[28,36,37] Although the area under the curve may be more accurately extrapolated between species, it can be very difficult to determine in mice.

Each dose tier consists of a group of three patients receiving the same dose. Doses are increased as per a modified Fibonacci sequence (e.g., incremental increases of 100%, then 50%, 33%, 20%, and so on) for successive tiers, and escalation may proceed until prespecified dose-limiting toxicities or unexpected toxicities are encountered.[38] Given the expected variation in bioavailability, incremental dose escalations of less than 20% are unlikely to be useful. The occurrence of grade 2 or 3 toxicity may prompt expansion of a tier to assess its frequency in a larger cohort. The phase II dose or MTD is generally chosen as the highest level associated with less than a 33% dose-limiting toxicity rate. Usually, at least six patients will have received this dose. Phase I studies may also be designed to clarify treatment mechanisms or to collect pharmacokinetic data.[28]

Alternate designs The standard design strategy outlined earlier is pervasive and considered safe, but it has been criticized for being inefficient, for exposing excessive numbers of patients to subtherapeutic doses, and for providing limited information about cumulative toxicities and interpatient differences.[39]

Although phase I trials remain an important, and generally safe, treatment option for patients with refractory cancers, it would be preferable to optimize the design of these trials to maximize patients' exposure to doses near the MTD by increasing efficiency of escalation, without significantly affecting safety. Applying some flexibility to escalation schemes can address this problem. For instance, if a therapy is not expected to produce significant toxicity, then smaller-tier groups of one or two patients may be acceptable. Intrapatient escalation may increase chance of benefit for participants and may enhance data collection at higher doses, although the risk of grade 4 toxicity may increase, and cumulative toxicity effects may be obscured. Simon et al.[40] described several possible strategies for accelerated dose titration, which may increase efficiency and yield of information, as well as provide more patients with an opportunity to receive therapeutic doses.[40] The continual reassessment method is an approach to safely maximize patient exposure to higher doses of a drug. Bayesian methods are applied to determine each successive dose level, based on information on dose and toxicity gleaned from all prior patients.[41,42] Although superior to accelerated dose titration, the continual reassessment method is also cumbersome and lengthy, and accelerated dose titration remains the standard of care. The adaptive dose–finding scheme is a two-stage design that incorporates features of standard escalation with continual reassessment method.[43] Escalation with overdose control designs aim to escalate rapidly to MTD in a manner akin to that of continuous reassessment method (CRM), but it is adaptive to avoid supratherapeutic doses.[44] Pharmacokinetically guided dose escalation designs use preclinical pharmacokinetic data to determine a target dose in patients based on plasma concentration.[45] Rapid escalation to a target plasma concentration, followed by more restrained escalation, is employed. Pharmacokinetically guided dose escalation is not useful for drugs with saturable kinetics.

One must be careful not to automatically discard a potentially efficacious agent because of dose-limiting toxicities until they are well understood. There are several examples of FDA-licensed chemotherapeutics—including doxorubicin, vincristine, paclitaxel, irinotecan, and cisplatin—whose development was halted because of severe toxicities but subsequently resumed development and were ultimately approved by the FDA, as a result of modifying treatment schedule or incorporating ancillary agents to ameliorate toxicities.[27] In early phase I trials, gemcitabine was given over 30 minutes for 5 consecutive days and yielded an MTD of 9 mg/m^2.[46] In other trials, gemcitabine was given over 30–240 minutes every 2 weeks, and the MTD was 3600 mg/m^2.[47]

Phase II

A crucial difference between phase I and phase II trials is that the latter are designed to demonstrate efficacy of a treatment in patients with a particular tumor type. The specific cancer may be chosen by a demonstration of efficacy (in even a single patient) in phase I, or it may be based on scientific rationale regarding the drug's mechanism of effect. The treatment can be a new drug, a new use, or a combination with an old drug. The patients selected for trial should be those who are most likely to respond. With relatively chemoresistant cancers, it is appropriate to offer patients a phase II treatment up front.[39] In advanced PC, the population treated would typically be untreated patients with good performance status, or the drug would be used as a second-line therapy in gemcitabine-refractory disease. The inclusion of heavily pretreated patients or of those too frail to tolerate otherwise manageable toxicities is seldom beneficial for the patient and may also result in an active agent being discarded. Other key functions of phase II trials are to evaluate toxicity and feasibility and to select out inactive treatments.[48] It is also an opportunity to implement dose modifications based on data from a larger, more narrowly defined population before phase III testing.[49]

Endpoints Ideally, all endpoints should be well defined, validated, reproducible, and uniform. Early efforts to define response were carried out at the NCI by the first cooperative groups.[50] In the 1970s, the World Health Organization proposed standardized response criteria.[51,52] In 2000, these criteria were revised by an international committee, yielding the Response Evaluation Criteria in Solid Tumors (RECIST).[53] These criteria employ unidimensional measurements of tumor lesions, in contrast to the more cumbersome bidimensional approach used in prior criteria.[54] This evolution in defining response, combined with advances in imaging technology, underscores the need to interpret historical data with caution, especially when response rates determined with different criteria are compared.[55]

When considering endpoints, one must take into account the natural history of the disease, the expected impact of treatment, and the efficacy of available treatments. For cytotoxic agents, response rate or frequency of at least 50% tumor shrinkage (partial response) is typically used, although survival and improved QoL are other options. Trials that assess response must limit eligibility to patients with measurable disease.

In order to define a level of response observed in a phase II trial that would warrant further investigation of the treatment, one must often rely on historical response data as a guide. This approach can be plagued by the common shortcomings of using historical data, namely selection bias, lack of standardization in data collection, and changes in response criteria.[56] These problems can be mitigated by using extremely well-matched patients, preferably from a single institution.[49] Alternatively, one can eliminate the need for comparison altogether by choosing an endpoint such as QoL, reflected by improvement in pain or performance status, which would not be anticipated in the absence of treatment.[19,49]

Although the ultimate goal is to convincingly demonstrate clinical benefit—improved quality or quantity of life—with acceptable toxicity in a phase III randomized, controlled trial, a phase II trial seldom gives conclusive evidence of clinical benefit and instead is designed with endpoints that serve as surrogates for this effect. A useful surrogate endpoint should not only correlate with a clinically meaningful outcome, but, ideally, changes in the surrogate should predict the effect on that outcome.[57] Unfortunately, there are few endpoints that strictly meet these requirements[58]; however, they remain an important component of phase II trials because clinical benefit is seldom demonstrated conclusively before a phase III randomized, controlled trial.

Overall survival is considered an endpoint of clear clinical significance. Improvements in overall survival in randomized controlled trials (RCT) typically change standards of care. It is easy, unambiguous, and inexpensive to assess, and it not influenced by intervals of evaluation. Its major limitations are the length of time required to reach the endpoint and the confounding effect of second-line therapies, especially in crossover studies.[25] However, these problems are diminished in PC because of the unfortunately short survival, the limited efficacy of second-line treatments, and the fact that crossover studies are seldom used in phase II trials. Censoring is a statistical technique that accounts for the situation in which a trial assessing overall survival ends before all patients enrolled have died.

Time to tumor progression (TTP) is an attractive surrogate endpoint, as postponing progression is of clear benefit in PC patients. TTP also is the endpoint that correlates best with tumor growth delay demonstrated preclinically by cytostatic drugs.[27,59] TTP is also the most expensive endpoint to assess. In comparison to a survival endpoint, it has the advantages of requiring less time and of not being confounded by crossover effect of second-line therapies.[25] On the other hand, the definition of progression is fraught with difficulty in interpretation. It can include death from disease or the appearance of new or larger tumors; however, it does not adequately account for increased symptoms, declining performance status, or increased tumor markers, which may influence a physician's assessment of progression.[60] The criteria for meeting this endpoint must be carefully defined and applied uniformly, as should the precise intervals of assessment and means of evaluation.[25] Trials assessing TTP require control groups and frequently must be randomized because historical data may be lacking.[61] An alternative would be to have patients act as their own controls, to see whether TTP is longer on the experimental treatment in second-line therapy than it was in first-line standard therapy. A ratio between TTP on second-line and TTP on first-line therapy, or a growth modulation index, can then be calculated as a measure of effect.[27] This approach is limited, however, by the need to enroll patients early on standard therapy, as well as by physician bias in declaring progression. Progression-free survival, similarly, can be highly subjective and also needs to be carefully controlled.[22] As a surrogate, however, it probably reflects benefit in PC, although this may not always be true in other, less aggressive malignancies.[62]

Time to treatment failure is a composite endpoint that may encompass disease progression, recurrence, or discontinuation of treatment due to toxicity. Because it does not distinguish efficacy from toxicity, however, its use may be best confined to the adjuvant setting.[17]

Disease-free survival is another endpoint that may be useful for adjuvant trials. Indeed, because recurrence of PC is frequently symptomatic and portends a poor outcome, an improvement in disease-free survival in PC may be considered sufficient evidence of clinical benefit to warrant FDA approval.[63]

QoL is an endpoint with the potential to play an increasingly important role in the development of novel therapeutics for PC. QoL is a multidimensional endpoint that represents a global sense of psychological and physical well-being, which may be represented by degree of tumor- or treatment-related symptoms, level of functional independence, reliance on medical support, or other, more specific, measures appropriate to the disease or treatment at hand. QoL is an endpoint that directly reflects a component of clinical benefit, and, in the analysis of risk-benefit relationship, QoL may alter the balance in favor of (or against) incorporating a new treatment. It is particularly relevant in PC for several reasons: the prevalence of debilitating symptoms from the disease; the lack of effective, durable palliation for these symptoms; and the unreliability of other surrogate endpoints, such as response rate, to predict clinical benefit. Indeed, the approval of gemcitabine in 1996 for the first-line treatment of PC was based on a modest survival benefit, in conjunction with an improvement as assessed by a "clinical benefit response" endpoint, incorporating pain, performance status, and weight gain.[63] Although this was established in a randomized, controlled trial, a comparative trial may not be absolutely necessary for regulatory approval, should an agent demonstrate a clear improvement in a QoL in PC.[17]

QoL can be assessed cross-sectionally, in a comparative trial, or longitudinally, in a single-arm study, using patients' baselines as controls. The latter may be appropriate for agents without significant side effects, which may confound interpretation of efficacy.[17] Comparative trials should be double-blinded to minimize bias, which is a major consideration for assessments that may be highly subjective.[25] Studies using QoL endpoints must use validated assessment tools and define prospectively exactly when and how they will be used. It is also critical to determine the type and the degree of benefit that is clinically and statistically significant. Many QoL assessments have been plagued by methodologic shortcomings, including missing data, unblended assessments, and poorly defined analytical plans.[63] To address the difficulty of obtaining useful data, the concept of clinically meaningful change has been developed.[64] Two methodologies are used to define clinically meaningful change. Anchor-based methods are used to define a change in a given measure over time for a particular study. Distribution-based methods define the variability in the measure and the magnitude of a meaningful change.[64]

Traditional design Regardless of the trial design used, prospective definition of the size and characteristics of the patient cohort is a critical element of proper conduct.[48] The size of a cohort is influenced by the competing constraints of having a large enough cohort to be statistically meaningful and yet constrained enough to limit the exposure of patients to inactive agents. In Fleming's one-sample, multiple-testing procedure, a minimum threshold of activity, below which the treatment is discarded, and a higher threshold, above which the treatment progresses in development is prospectively defined, along with a minimum sample size.[65] To further limit exposure to inactive agents, a two-stage design can be used. The first stage is used to eliminate treatments with unacceptably low response, although the second is used to better gauge response rates.[66] Accrual to the second stage does not begin until the first stage is fully accrued and responses assessed and proceeds unless insufficient activity is observed in the first. Simon's two-stage design is geared more toward eliminating inactive agents than determining response rates and thus further decreases cohort size.[67] The analysis of the first stage may include a multinomial stopping rule, in which early progression is taken into account when the decision is made about whether the treatment should proceed to the second stage.[68,69] The choice of design may be governed by the availability of alternate treatments. A stringent early stopping rule may be more critical, for example, in patients with advanced PC who have not received gemcitabine-based treatment than in those whose disease has progressed on standard therapy. In any case, eligible patients should fully understand the stopping rule as part of informed consent.[70]

Given the difficulty of accurately measuring primary pancreatic tumor masses, tumor response rates may not fully reflect clinical benefit in PC. This was well evidenced in the randomized controlled trial comparing gemcitabine and 5-FU, which did not demonstrate a statistically significant benefit for response rate but did show a symptom and survival advantage.[16] In fact, in both treatment arms, response rates were very low, 5% and 0% in the gemcitabine and 5-FU arms, respectively.

A phase II trial may be randomized. One possibility is to randomize against a placebo to reduce the reliance on historical data, but this runs the risk of limiting accrual. However, such a trial may lead directly into, and contribute data to, a phase III study. Alternatively, a treatment may be randomized against an alternate schedule or dose of the same medicine, especially in cases in which the phase I yields a range of possible doses.[71] This approach was used in determining the optimal dose of bevacizumab in advanced colorectal cancer.[72]

Phase III

Phase III trials are comparative trials that directly assess important, clinically relevant questions. They are the largest, lengthiest, and costliest trials and are a critical step in the development of new drugs and in new uses of approved drugs. A recent review of 409 active phase III trials found a median accrual goal of 481 patients and a median planned accrual period of 3.8 years.[26] Given the requisite expenditure of extensive resources and the importance of these studies to medical care, the adherence to proper trial design and conduct are critical. The objectives of these trials must be carefully conceived and clearly stated. Eligibility, treatment, and endpoints must be specified and must suit the stated objectives. The method of randomization, the type of stratification, and the size and duration of the trial need to be established prospectively. Assessment must be carried out in a uniform fashion at well-defined intervals, as best as possible. Every effort must be made to avoid bias into the trial design.

Sample size There are three important variables that contribute to sample size determination: type I error, type II error, and degree of difference one wishes to detect. The α level, known as type I error, relates to the *P* value and represents the likelihood of a false-positive result, which is usually 5%. The type II error of a study, denoted by β, is the likelihood of a false-negative result, and thus, $1 - \beta$ describes the likelihood that a true difference between arms will be detected (the power of the study), typically 90%. The degree of difference to be detected depends on the anticipated effect of the treatment under study. As the α or difference to be detected decreases, the required sample size increases accordingly. Trials are generally designed to have a sample population size, or *N*, that is just big enough so that the study is powered adequately to assess the defined endpoints. This is why subset analyses are generally underpowered to detect differences.[5] Trials should be sufficiently powered to detect the smallest difference that is clinically meaningful. An unrealistic degree of benefit may never be realized regardless of sample size. Type I error increases with the number of questions asked, as in multiarm trials. To avoid excessive false-positive rates, a global test can be performed to assess equality of arms before subsets are compared. Alternatively, the Bonferroni correction can be applied, whereby α is lowered, as a statistical compensation to account for this problem.[5]

Endpoints Regular approval of a new drug has been granted by the FDA for demonstration that a (safe) drug prolongs or improves life or a validated surrogate implies that it does. This doctrine was established by the Food, Drug, and Cosmetic Act of 1938, later amended in 1962 (http://vm.cfsan.fda.gov/~lrd/histor1a.html, http://vm.cfsan.fda.gov/~lrd/histor1b.html). In 1992, subpart H introduced accelerated approval, such that a drug could be approved based on "trials establishing that the drug product has an effect on a surrogate endpoint that is reasonably likely, based on epidemiologic, therapeutic, pathophysiologic, or other evidence, to predict clinical benefit..." (http://www.fda.gov/cder/rdmt/accappr1.htm). As a condition of accelerated approval, true clinical benefit must subsequently be demonstrated. Although improved survival remains the gold standard of clinical benefit, only 18 of 57 oncology drug regular approvals, and none of 14 accelerated approvals, between 1990 and 2002 were based on a survival benefit.[63] Response rate alone was the primary indication in 10 regular approvals and was used in conjunction with decreased symptoms in nine approvals and improved TTP in seven approvals. Disease-free survival was the primary indication only twice, on both occasions for breast cancer, in which its use in the adjuvant setting was appropriate because of the long interval between recurrence and death.[63] TTP was sufficient only for one breast cancer indication. None of the drugs receiving accelerated approvals have been taken off the market. Single-arm trials were the basis for 14 approvals (seven regular approvals, seven accelerated approvals), all of which were for refractory cancers.

Accrual Despite the best intentions of RCTs, accrual remains a ubiquitous difficulty. Only about 2%–4% of cancer patients per year in the United States participate in clinical trials.[73] Barriers include discomfort, among both patients and physicians, with the uncertainties of blinding and placebos, as well as the burden of cumbersome enrollment and monitoring requirements.[74] Lara et al.[73] also identified protocol eligibility requirements, as well as funding limitations as important barriers to accrual (Fig. 33.1). They suggest that strict eligibility criteria should be relaxed to increase access to trials by patients in reasonable physical condition. However, the need for adequate performance status cannot be substantially relaxed, as evidenced by the GITSG adjuvant PC study in which a quarter of patients on the treatment arm could not tolerate therapy.[13] Fuks et al.[75] showed that eligibility criteria can be limited without sacrificing quality and suggested that inclusion/exclusion criteria be abandoned, that the need for criteria that are used in each trial be continually reassessed, and that criteria that limit accrual in phase II RCTs be minimized.[75] Were these principles adopted, research on the effects of generalizability would be needed. Radical abandonment of cumbersome assessment methodologies has also been suggested.[76]

Sociodemographic analyses of accrual patterns have revealed that ethnic minorities, urban communities, the elderly, and the uninsured are underrepresented in clinical trials in the United States, and efforts need to be made to enable and enhance their participation.[77] A statistical approach, employing Bayesian techniques to incorporate data from related studies, can be applied when accrual barriers cannot be overcome.[78]

Accrual in PC is further burdened by a sense of therapeutic nihilism pervasive in the medical and patient communities, despite the clear, albeit modest, efficacy of currently available therapy.[16,23] The recent completion of accrual of more than 500 patients with PC to a national phase III study of adjuvant chemoradiotherapy nonetheless demonstrates the feasibility of accrual of large, well-organized PC trials.[79] This trial also demonstrates the statistical advantage of the high expected event rate for

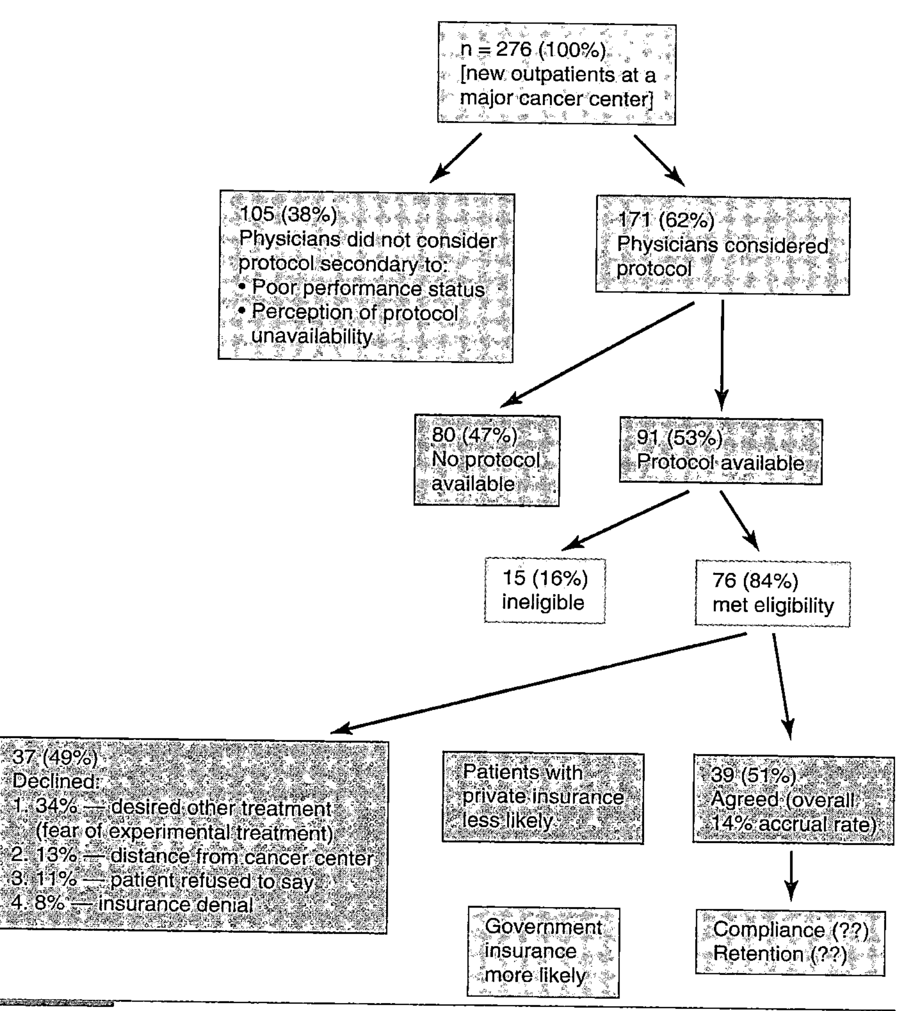

Figure 33.1
Summary of a prospective study of accrual. Oncologists at a center were asked to provide information regarding factors influencing decision making by doctors and patients on enrollment into clinical trials. (Adapted with permission from Lara et al.[73])

resected PC, which reduces the required sample size. The mean phase III adjuvant trial size is close to 1900 patients.[26]

Eligibility requirements must also balance the need for the population to be focused enough that treatment effects are likely to be seen, but not so narrow that the results cannot be extrapolated to a more general patient population. For example, studies involving patients with an excellent performance status are less likely to be reproducible, although those involving poor-function patients are less likely to demonstrate efficacy.

Design Randomization of treatment assignment is a sine qua non of meaningful RCTs because doctor and patient selection for participation inevitably creates immeasurable imbalances and introduces bias. Randomization must be unpredictable and must avoid introducing systemic bias. With conventional randomization, each successive patient has an equal chance of entrance into available arms. This simple method can be adjusted to apply to two-arm, multi-arm, or unequal-distribution randomizations. A minor modification is block randomization, which ensures equal distribution for a given number of patients. Alternatively, in cluster randomization, individual treatment centers in a multicenter trial may offer just one treatment. This has the practical benefit of simplifying trial conduct at individual locations, and it also avoids "contamination" resulting from patients in different arms interacting with each other.[5] Minimization is an allocation variant in which treatment for each patient depends on the balance of allocations for prior patients, thus minimizing imbalance. Although not technically random, this method is unpredictable and does avoid bias.

When definite independent risk variables for clinical outcome are well defined, it is reasonable to stratify randomization to ensure equal distribution of these factors between study arms.[39] For patients with resected PC, surgical margins, nodal status, and tumor size are reasonable variables for stratification. Adaptive stratification methods employ computers to account for multiple variables.[80]

Blinding is the process of concealing treatment arms from participants. It is useful to minimize bias, but it is often imperfect and is always cumbersome and expensive. In single-blind studies, the patient is unaware of the results of randomization. In double-blind studies, which are useful when clinical assessment is subjective, the physician is also unaware, and in triple-blind studies, those analyzing response data are also unaware. Blinding is difficult to achieve in most oncology trials because of obvious differences in scheduling and toxicities between treatment arms.

The number of treatment arms and the timing of randomization are critical variables.[5] The simplest design is the "parallel group" design. Willing, eligible patients from the desired population are enrolled and randomly assigned to the experimental arm or the control arm. Treatment results in both arms are assessed and compared. This design is powerful in its simplicity and has wide applicability. The number of arms is limited only in the number of available treatments of interest, the number of available patients, and the complexity of informed consent for multi-arm trials. The two-arm parallel design was used with success in the GITSG[13] and the gemcitabine versus 5-FU trials[16] and remains an important option for PC trials.

A potentially more efficient design for a trial with multiple arms is the 2 × 2 factorial design, in which a randomization is performed for each question asked. In a 2 × 2 factorial design, each patient would be randomly assigned twice, simultaneously—one randomization to either chemotherapy or no chemotherapy, and another randomization to either radiation therapy or no radiation therapy. Four arms result: observation, chemotherapy, radiation, and CRT. In the final analysis, the two chemotherapy arms are compared with the others, and the two radiation arms are compared with the others. In this manner, all patients, not just control subjects, are randomly assigned and compared twice and thus contribute to two questions.[5] For this design to work, the combination must be practically possible with regard to toxicity of the combined treatment. It also assumes an additive benefit for the two treatments, although deviations from this requirement may suggest antagonism or synergy between treatments. It is critical to note that this design differs from a four-arm parallel study in that it is powered to address both the efficacy of chemotherapy and the efficacy of radiation therapy. Any comparison of an individual arm with another treatment arm would be underpowered. The ESPAC-1 adjuvant PC trial employed a 2 × 2 factorial design, similar to that in the example. Its primary conclusion, that the study showed no survival benefit for adjuvant chemoradiotherapy but did suggest a benefit to adjuvant 5-FU and leucovorin chemotherapy alone,[15] has been criticized because among other methodologic problems, this is a question that the study was not designed to answer.[18]

Although factorial designs involve multiple simultaneous randomizations, one can also design sequential randomizations, either within a single study or as part of separate studies. These complex designs run the risk of introducing bias. For single studies, the impact of subsequent randomizations on outcome assessments of earlier randomizations must be considered. For sequential trials, the confounding impact of randomization in the first trial on entry into the second trial must be considered.[5]

Crossover trials can also require fewer patients (often 50% or less) than parallel trial designs. Crossover trials compare two treatments given sequentially to all patients, with the order of treatments for each patient being randomized. A washout period may be included between treatments to limit carryover effects of the first. Although this design may not be appropriate for most cytotoxic drugs, it is very useful for palliative treatments aimed at symptoms because each patient can act as his or her own control, thus limiting intrapatient variability and decreasing the sample size required to demonstrate efficacy.[5] One example of a crossover trial design in gastrointestinal oncology is the Tournigand et al.[81] trial in metastatic colon cancer, in which sequential administration of infusional 5-FU, leucovorin, and oxaliplatin (FOLFOX) is followed by infusional 5-FU, leucovorin, and irinotecan (FOLFIRI), or the reverse drug sequence, demonstrating no conclusive benefit with regard to overall survival for either drug sequence. Patients can also express a preference. This trial design may be appropriate for chronic conditions that are expected to remain stable over the study time period. Thus, the risk of death or cure during study should be low. A high dropout of patients before the second treatment would require the study to be analyzed as an underpowered parallel study. Duration of treatment effect should be limited to avoid carryover effects and the likelihood of dropout.

Clinical Trial Designs for Cytostatic Chemotherapeutics

Further, significant clinical trial design modifications are required for many novel agents. The traditional phase I design has been intended for drugs that target cellular machinery common to cancerous and healthy tissue. This design presumes a "more is better" relationship between dose and effect, as well as a narrow therapeutic window. Traditional chemotherapy drugs generally demonstrate both efficacy and dose-limiting toxicities (DLTs) in a dose-dependent manner. However, targeted biologic drugs are specific for perturbed biologic pathways and may not share these characteristics. Furthermore, they may demonstrate, in preclinical studies, inhibition or delay of tumor growth, rather than shrinkage of established tumors and are often referred to as *cytostatic* drugs, as opposed to classical, *cytotoxic* chemotherapeutics.[59]

Table 33.2 Cytostatic or Targeted Therapy Drug Development in Pancreatic Cancer

	Phase I	Phase II[a]	Phase III
Aims Pharmacokinetics	Toxicity Dose for chronic delivery	Activity Toxicity	Oncologic effect e.g., survival, clinical benefit quality of life
Target population	Open ± target present	Pancreas cancer ± target present	Pancreas cancer ± target present
Principal endpoint(s) Endpoint(s)	Toxicity Surrogate effect on target	Time to tumor progression (TTP) Response rate	Survival
Study design	Dose escalation Early combination with cytotoxic	Single-arm phase II Randomized phase II Randomized discontinuation	Randomized ± placebo controlled

[a]Phase II: Note, this step may be skipped in cytostatic/targeted-therapy drug development.

Similarly, cytostatic drugs may not be appreciably toxic to normal tissues and thus may not cause DLTs. This mandates that endpoints other than toxicity on normal tissue are needed for phase I trials of novel targeted treatments, and endpoints other than response rate may be appropriate for some phase II studies.

Phase I

A logical endpoint for molecularly targeted cytostatic agents is assessment of the intended biologic target in the patient. However, achieving this requires precise knowledge of the appropriate target and its tissue distribution, a reliable and reproducible assay for a relevant biologic effect that can be performed in real time, and accessibility of the target tissue or a surrogate.[25] It is critical that the target and appropriate assay be validated representatives of the intended drug effect. Assays may be correlative of biologic activity and may be used throughout drug development, or they may be predictive of clinical effect and can be tested only in randomized phase III studies.[22] One must be especially cautious when the drug mechanism of action is not completely understood because the choice of an inappropriate biologic parameter may result in an active drug being discarded. In addition, alternate, unmeasured redundant or interactive molecular pathways could negate the downstream effect of altering the target pathway. Enhanced communication between laboratory and clinical investigators is needed to ensure that an understanding of their mutual needs exists to assist this process.[27]

A phase I study should ask many relevant, practical questions simultaneously, including the drug's pharmacokinetic properties and relatedness to effect, tolerability, and toxicity, and whether a biologically active form of the drug is circulating. Various biologic assays can be examined simultaneously to validate and correlate them with pharmacokinetic data and toxicity.[22] These studies may not be relevant in drugs with zero-order kinetics or vaccines. Monoclonal antibody kinetics may depend on tumor burden.

When tumor tissue can be obtained, a phase I trial is a good opportunity to compare a biologic assay with tumor specimens. Because of the need for invasive procedures, routine sampling of PC is unrealistic, save for subcutaneous metastases, which are uncommon. Biologic assays would thus require a surrogate tissue, such as peripheral blood mononuclear cells, which are readily available, or the treatment dose may be established in patients with different tumor types, as is often the case with phase I studies.

Once a reliable biologic activity endpoint is established, a desired degree of effect must be defined. For instance, a phase I trial may be designed to distinguish between an activity rate of $<40\%$ (nonoptimal) and one of $\geq 90\%$ (acceptable).[49] The trial can then proceed much as a phase I, with escalations or de-escalations, guided by frequency of acceptable activity within dose tiers and aimed at achieving a rate of five or six acceptable levels of activity in a cohort of six patients receiving a dose that will be used in phase II.[34] Dose escalation may also be limited by a pharmacokinetic profile that suggests saturable absorption above a certain dose, or by practical considerations, such as cost or volume of infusate.[49] Intrapatient escalation is appropriate. The resultant dose would be considered the biologically effective dose, but the trial can also be designed to determine a dose-response curve, or the optimal biologic dose, which would usually require more patients.[82] When cytostatic drugs do produce DLTs, as if often the case,[83] then traditional phase I designs may be appropriate. However, a cytostatic drug that produces DLTs may nonetheless achieve biologic activity at a dose well below the MTD.[27] The 5 mg/m^2 dose of bevacizumab, for instance, may be more efficacious than 10 mg/m^2 in metastatic colorectal cancer.[72]

Phase II

The use of tumor response may not be an appropriate endpoint for cytostatic agents, which may function by preventing or delaying further tumor growth rather than causing tumor regression. Alternate endpoints must be used for such drugs. Unfortunately, none has yet been validated for general use in a later randomized controlled trial.[22] One possibility is to assess the intended biologic activity of the drug, as may have occurred in phase I. This approach is hampered by the need to use a surrogate tissue (because serial biopsies in PC are impractical and excessively invasive), the possibility that the drug could act through an unrecognized mechanism, and the likelihood that these data would not sufficiently or convincingly predict clinical benefit to justify progression to a randomized controlled trial.[49]

Changes in levels of tumor markers have also been proposed as a possible surrogate marker. Conceptually, use of tumor markers is appealing because of simplicity and ready availability of measurement. For some markers, percentage declines in their value may be a surrogate of biologic effect, such as that from prostate-specific antigen, CA-125. Although there are data to suggest that CA19-9 may indeed correlate to some degree with response to gemcitabine-based treatment,[85,86] this marker has not been validated as a reliable surrogate for activity in phase II studies.

Another approach to evaluating cytostatic agents is the use of variant clinical trial designs. One possibility is a randomized discontinuation design.[87] This is an example of an enrichment trial design, in which a defined subset of interest from the initial population, such as compliant patients with stable disease after an initial treatment period, are randomly assigned to continuation or discontinuation of the therapy, in an effort to assess whether the patients' stable disease was a result of the indolent activity of the cancer or of the effect of the cytostatic drug. This design has been promoted for diseases in which stable disease may be a clinically meaningful benefit and for those with limited patient population sizes. It has the potential benefits of comparing more homogeneous cohorts, of attracting patients to a randomized study who might otherwise avoid placebo trials (although phase II designs are generally single arm), and of avoiding the use of historical controls. Limitations include the possibilities of a carryover effect and of development of resistance during initial treatment.[88] However, a negative result may not justify the discarding of an agent. In addition, such designs may require sizeable accrual to ensure a sufficiently large population of patients with stable disease.[49] Determining the probability of stable disease and terminating the study at a predetermined checkpoint according to observed rates can limit accrual size in these studies.[87] However, this approach harkens back to a dependence on historical controls. Because patients with advanced PC have a fairly predictable progressive course, in contrast to, for example, renal cancer, which is frequently indolent and for which this design has been applied,[87] there appear to be few benefits to using this design in PC. One potential scenario would be in the assessment of using a novel agent after the completion of CRT for locally advanced, unresectable, stage III PC.

Randomized screening trials have been suggested as a means of excluding inactive agents during phase II.[49] The probability of declaring an inactive drug to be active is known as α error. The acceptable α of a phase III, randomized, controlled trial is typically 0.05, although 0.10 is often used for phase II evaluations of cytotoxic drugs. In a randomized screening trial, one might permit a larger α and thus require fewer patients. For example, to demonstrate an improvement in progression-free survival from 6 to 9 months, 228 patients would be required for an α of 0.05, but only 120 patients would be required for an α of 0.20. This design grants a lower threshold for advancement and thus decreases the likelihood of discarding an active agent prematurely. At the same time, it allows for smaller phase II trials and discards a portion of inactive agents.[49] Patients may be more hesitant to enroll in a placebo-controlled trial, so a crossover design may be appropriate. As a result, progression-free survival or TTP may be a better endpoint than overall survival to avoid confounding interpretation. This design, as a randomized, controlled trial, avoids bias and eliminates the need for historical data. It has the additional advantage that it can be prospectively planned to lead directly into a phase III, randomized, controlled trial.[22]

Conclusion

Pancreatic cancer is unique in the spectrum of solid organ malignancies in that it is a highly complex cancer with multiple genetic mutations and an inherent resistance to standard cytotoxic therapies, and in that the effects of any given treatment using standard response criteria assessment, such as RECIST, are difficult to reproduce. Because of the limitations of standard therapy and the short natural history of the disease, PC is appropriately seen as an excellent model for novel drug development.

Traditional cytotoxic drug development involves phase I studies, in which an MTD is established using, for example, a modified Fibonacci escalation scheme or (increasingly) using an accelerated titration design. The drug is then tested in a disease-specific phase II trial, intended to assess therapeutic efficacy and achieve a greater understanding of acute and chronic toxicity. A randomized phase III trial can then determine comparative efficacy against standard therapy. With the advent of the biologic and cytostatic drug era, in which aberrant biologic pathways, rather than fundamental cellular machinery, are targeted, the traditional clinical trial design approach may be less relevant. For example, phase II trials of cytostatic agents may serve a greater purpose if they are designed as randomized and dose ranging in their conception and if they use the endpoint of TTP. This is also a relevant consideration, if it is accepted that for many cytostatic-type agents we do not need to administer these drugs at the MTD for optimum biologic effect and that most phase I trials do not yield conclusive evidence about the optimal dose regardless. Validated biologic markers to serve as guides to dosing and efficacy are lacking, although their development is essential. Additionally, for cytostatic agents, long-term dosing and associated toxicities may be of greater consequence than the acute toxicity dosing information provided from traditional phase I studies.

Other considerations in clinical trial design include individualizing therapy, such as using pharmacogenetics and pharmacokinetic information to guide drug dosing. The use of functional imaging, such as perfusion computed tomography, positron emission tomographic/computed tomographic imaging, dynamic contrast-enhanced magnetic resonance imaging, and diffusion magnetic resonance imaging, are novel methodologies to augment an assessment of the biologic effect of targeted therapies. As biologic agents are added to conventional cytotoxic drugs, the trend is to proceed directly from phase I trials to randomized phase III trials using TTP or overall survival as the primary endpoints. In PC, a logical step to assess cytostatic-type agents is to examine their effect on TTP in the minimal residual disease setting, such as in an adjuvant patient population or after cytoreduction post-CRT for locally advanced unresectable PC.

In a disease such as PC, in which the anticipated morbidity from both disease and treatment can be substantial, the use of QoL endpoints has appeal. Nonetheless, the incorporation of QoL endpoints into clinical trials needs to be judicious because the instruments used to assess these endpoints are often not adequately validated, can greatly add to study complexity, and are time-consuming and resource intensive. Past efforts to use QoL endpoints have seldom altered the conclusion about therapeutic efficacy. As nonsurvival endpoints are increasingly used, QoL has the potential to complement the questions of clinical benefit left ambiguous by these surrogates. In general, their use should be limited to clearly asked and relevant QoL questions being assessed with the use of validated instruments.

The future is bright with regard to the multiplicity of new drugs for assessment in a disease such as PC. The challenges investigators face include, rigorous clinical trial design, incorporation of novel endpoints and methodologies of both drug and tumor assessment to maximize the quality of the information and the conclusions drawn from such studies. This will allow meaningful decisions to be made with regard to drug development, with an acceptance of the finite patient and dollar resources.

References

1. Fisher B. Winds of change in clinical trials: from Daniel to Charlie Brown. *Control Clin Trials*. 1983;4:65–73.
2. Haggard HW. *The Doctor in History*. New York: Dorset Press; 1989.
3. Nuland SB. *Doctors: The Biography of Medicine*. New York: Vintage Books; 1989.
4. Stuart CP, Guthrie DE. *Lind's treatise on scurvy*. Edinburgh, University Press; 1953.
5. Green S, Benedetti J, Crowley J. *Clinical Trials in Oncology*. 2nd ed. Boca Raton, FL: Chapman & Hall/CRC; 2003.
6. Gail MH. Statistics in action. *J Am Stat Assoc*. 1996;91:1–13.
7. Frei E 3rd, Holland JF, Schneiderman MA, et al. A comparative study of two regimens of combination chemotherapy in acute leukemia. *Blood*. 1958;13:1126–1148.
8. Catalano P, Finkelstein D. *The History of Cancer Clinical Trials at Harvard: Recollections of Marvin Zelen*. Cambridge, MA: Biotstat Connections; 1997.
9. Hunt VC, Budd JW. Transduodenal resection of the ampulla of Vater for carcinoma of the distal end of the common duct with restoration of continuity of the common and pancreatic ducts with the duodenum. *Surg Gynecol Obstet*. 1935;61:651-661.
10. Crile G Jr. The advantages of bypass operations over radical pancreatoduodenectomy in the treatment of pancreatic carcinoma. *Surg Gynecol Obstet*. 1970;130:1049–1053.
11. Yeo CJ, Cameron JL, Sohn TA, et al. Six hundred fifty consecutive pancreaticoduodenectomies in the 1990s: pathology, complications, and outcomes. *Ann Surg*. 1997; 226:248–257; discussion 257–260.
12. Moertel CG, Frytak S, Hahn RG, et al. Therapy of locally unresectable pancreatic carcinoma: a randomized comparison of high dose (6000 rads) radiation alone, moderate dose

radiation (4000 rads + 5-fluorouracil), and high dose radiation + 5-fluorouracil: the Gastrointestinal Tumor Study Group. *Cancer*. 1981;48:1705–1710.
13. Kalser MH, Ellenberg SS. Pancreatic cancer. Adjuvant combined radiation and chemotherapy following curative resection. *Arch Surg*. 1985;120:899–903.
14. Klinkenbijl JH, Jeekel J, Sahmoud T, et al. Adjuvant radiotherapy and 5-fluorouracil after curative resection of cancer of the pancreas and periampullary region: phase III trial of the EORTC gastrointestinal tract cancer cooperative group. *Ann Surg*. 1999;230:776–782; discussion 782–784.
15. Neoptolemos JP, Dunn JA, Stocken DD, et al. Adjuvant chemoradiotherapy and chemotherapy in resectable pancreatic cancer: a randomised controlled trial. *Lancet*. 2001;358:1576–1585.
16. Burris HA 3rd, Moore MJ, Andersen J, et al. Improvements in survival and clinical benefit with gemcitabine as first-line therapy for patients with advanced pancreas cancer: a randomized trial. *J Clin Oncol*. 1997;15:2403–2413.
17. O'Shaughnessy JA, Wittes RE, Burke G, et al. Commentary concerning demonstration of safety and efficacy of investigational anticancer agents in clinical trials. *J Clin Oncol*. 1991;9:2225–2232.
18. Abrams RA, Lillemoe KD, Piantadosi S. Continuing controversy over adjuvant therapy of pancreatic cancer. *Lancet*. 2001;358:1565–1566.
19. Casper ES, Green MR, Kelson DP, et al. Phase II trial of gemcitabine (2,2′-difluorodeoxycytidine) in patients with adenocarcinoma of the pancreas. *Invest New Drugs*. 1994;12:29–34.
20. Van Cutsem E, Karasek P, Oettle H, et al. Phase III trial comparing gemcitabine + R115777 (Zarnestra) versus gemcitabine + placebo in advanced pancreatic cancer (PC). *Proceedings of the American Society of Clinical Oncology Annual Meeting*, 2002, (Abs. #2002).
21. Moore MJ, Hamm J, Dancey J, et al. Comparison of gemcitabine versus the matrix metalloproteinase inhibitor BAY 12-9566 in patients with advanced or metastatic adenocarcinoma of the pancreas: a phase III trial of the National Cancer Institute of Canada Clinical Trials Group. *J Clin Oncol*. 2003;21:3296–3302.
22. Eckhardt SG, Eisenhauer E, Parulekar WR, et al. Developmental therapeutics: successes and failures of clinical trial designs of targeted compounds. In: Perry MC ed. *ASCO Educational Book 2003*. Alexandria, VA: ASCO; 2003:209–219.
23. Heinemann V, Quietzsch D, Gieseler F, et al. A phase III trial comparing gemcitabine plus cisplatin vs. gemcitabine alone in advanced pancreatic carcinoma. *Proceedings of the American Society of Clinical Oncology Annual Meeting*, 2003, (Abs. #250).
24. Louvet C, Labianca R, Hammel P, et al. Gemcitabine versus GEMOX (gemcitabine + oxaliplatin) in nonresectable pancreatic adenocarcinoma: interim results of the GERCOR/GISCAD Intergroup Phase III. *Proceedings of the American Society of Clinical Oncology Annual Meeting*, 2003, (Abs. #2003).
25. Schilsky RL. End points in cancer clinical trials and the drug approval process. *Clin Cancer Res*. 2002;8:935–938.
26. Roberts TG Jr, Lynch TJ Jr, Chabner BA. The phase III trial in the era of targeted therapy: unraveling the "go or no go" decision. *J Clin Oncol*. 2003;21:3683–3695.
27. Von Hoff DD. There are no bad anticancer agents, only bad clinical trial designs: Twenty-First Richard and Hinda Rosenthal Foundation Award Lecture. *Clin Cancer Res*. 1998;4:1079–1086.
28. Critical role of phase I clinical trials in cancer treatment: American Society of Clinical Oncology. *J Clin Oncol*. 1997;15:853–859.
29. Estey E, Hoth D, Simon R, et al. Therapeutic response in phase I trials of antineoplastic agents. *Cancer Treat Rep*. 70:1105–1115.
30. Decoster G, Stein G, Holdener EE. Responses and toxic deaths in phase I clinical trials. *Ann Oncol*. 1990;1:175–181.
31. Von Hoff DD, Turner J. Response rates, duration of response, and dose response effects in phase I studies of antineoplastics. *Invest New Drugs*. 1991;9:115–122.
32. Itoh K, Sasaki Y, Miyata Y, et al. Therapeutic response and potential pitfalls in phase I clinical trials of anticancer agents conducted in Japan. *Cancer Chemother Pharmacol*. 1994;34:451–454.
33. Melink TJ, Clark GM, Von Hoff DD: The impact of phase I clinical trials on the quality of life of patients with cancer. *Anticancer Drugs*. 1992;3:571–576.
34. Young D. Decision-Making in Phase I Trials in Oncology, 2002.
35. Freireich EJ, Gehan EA, Rall DP, et al. Quantitative comparison of toxicity of anticancer agents in mouse, rat, hamster, dog, monkey, and man. *Cancer Chemother Rep*. 1966;50:219–244.
36. Penta JS, Rozencweig M, Guarino AM, et al. Mouse and large-animal toxicology studies of twelve antitumor agents: relevance to starting dose for phase I clinical trials. *Cancer Chemother Pharmacol*. 1979;3:97–101.
37. Goldsmith MA, Slavik M, Carter SK. Quantitative prediction of drug toxicity in humans from toxicology in small and large animals. *Cancer Res*. 1975;35:1354–1364.
38. Dodion P, Kenis Y, Staquet M. Phase I trials of single agents in adult solid tumours: preclinical and clinical aspects. *Drugs Exp Clin Res*. 1986;12:23–30.
39. Simon R. Design and analysis of clinical trials. In: DeVita VT, Hellman S, Rosenberg SA, eds. *Cancer: Principles and Practice of Oncology*. 6th ed. Philadelphia: Lippincott Williams & Wilkins, 2001:521–538.
40. Simon R, Freidlin B, Rubinstein L, et al. Accelerated titration designs for phase I clinical trials in oncology. *J Natl Cancer Inst*. 1997;89:1138–1147.
41. Whitehead J, Zhou Y, Stallard N, et al. Learning from previous responses in phase I dose-escalation studies. *Br J Clin Pharmacol*. 2001;52:1–7.
42. O'Quigley J, Pepe M, Fisher L. Continual reassessment method: a practical design for phase 1 clinical trials in cancer. *Biometrics*. 1990;46:33–48.
43. Potter DM. Adaptive dose finding for phase I clinical trials of drugs used for chemotherapy of cancer. *Stat Med*. 2002;21:1805–1823.

44. Babb J, Rogatko A, Zacks S. Cancer phase I clinical trials: efficient dose escalation with overdose control. *Stat Med.* 1998;17:1103–1120.
45. Collins JM, Grieshaber CK, Chabner BA. Pharmacologically guided phase I clinical trials based upon preclinical drug development. *J Natl Cancer Inst.* 1990;82:1321–1326.
46. O'Rourke TJ, Brown TD, Havlin K, et al. Phase I clinical trial of gemcitabine given as an intravenous bolus on 5 consecutive days. *Eur J Cancer.* 1994;30A:417–418.
47. Brown T, O'Rourke T, Burris H, et al. A phase I trial of gemcitabine (LY188011) administered intravenously every two weeks. *Proceedings of the American Society of Clinical Oncology Annual Meeting*, 1991, (Abs. #115).
48. Girling DJ, Parmar MKB, Stenning SP, et al. *Clinical Trials in Cancer: Principles and Practice.* Oxford: Oxford University Press; 2003.
49. Korn EL, Arbuck SG, Pluda JM, et al. Clinical trial designs for cytostatic agents: are new approaches needed? *J Clin Oncol.* 2001;19:265–272.
50. Zubrod CG, Schneiderman SM, Frei EI, et al. Appraisal of methods for the study of chemotherapy of cancer in man: therapeutic trial of nitrogen mustard and thio phosphamide. *J Chronic Dis.* 1960;11:7–33.
51. Miller AB, Hoogstraten B, Staquet M, et al. Reporting results of cancer treatment. *Cancer.* 1981;47:207–214.
52. Gehan EA, Schneiderman MA. Historical and methodological developments in clinical trials at the National Cancer Institute. *Stat Med.* 1990;9:871–880; discussion 903–906.
53. Therasse P, Arbuck SG, Eisenhauer EA, et al. New guidelines to evaluate the response to treatment in solid tumors. European Organization for Research and Treatment of Cancer, National Cancer Institute of the United States, National Cancer Institute of Canada. *J Natl Cancer Inst.* 2000; 92:205–216.
54. James K, Eisenhauer E, Christian M, et al. Measuring response in solid tumors: unidimensional versus bidimensional measurement. *J Natl Cancer Inst.* 1999;91:523–528.
55. Gehan EA, Tefft MC. Will there be resistance to the RECIST (response evaluation criteria in solid tumors)? *J Natl Cancer Inst.* 2000;92:179–181.
56. Ratain MJ, Stadler WM. Clinical trial designs for cytostatic agents. *J Clin Oncol.* 2001;19:3154–3155.
57. Fleming TR, DeMets DL. Surrogate end points in clinical trials: are we being misled? *Ann Intern Med.* 1996;125:605–613.
58. Moertel CG. Improving the efficiency of clinical trials: a medical perspective. *Stat Med.* 1984;3:455–468.
59. Mick R, Crowley JJ, Carroll RJ. Phase II clinical trial design for noncytotoxic anticancer agents for which time to disease progression is the primary endpoint. *Control Clin Trials.* 2000;21:343–359.
60. Eisenhauer EA. Phase I and II trials of novel anti-cancer agents: endpoints, efficacy and existentialism: The Michel Clavel Lecture, held at the 10th NCI-EORTC Conference on New Drugs in Cancer Therapy, Amsterdam, 16-19 June 1998. *Ann Oncol.* 1998;9:1047–1052.
61. Fox E, Curt GA, Balis FM. Clinical trial design for target-based therapy. *Oncologist.* 2002;7:401–409.
62. Ozols RF. Maintenance therapy in advanced ovarian cancer: progression-free survival and clinical benefit. *J Clin Oncol.* 2003;21:2451–2453.
63. Johnson JR, Williams G, Pazdur R. End points and United States Food and Drug Administration approval of oncology drugs. *J Clin Oncol.* 2003;21:1404–1411.
64. Patrick-Miller LJ. Is there a role for the assessment of health-related quality of life in the clinical evaluation of novel cytostatic agents? Commentary re: P. M. LoRusso, Improvements in quality of life and disease-related symptoms in phase I trials of the selective oral epidermal growth factor receptor tyrosine kinase inhibitor ZD1839 in non-small cell lung cancer and other solid tumors. *Clin Cancer Res.* 2003;9:2040–2048.
65. Fleming TR. One-sample multiple testing procedure for phase II clinical trials. *Biometrics.* 1982;38:143–151.
66. Gehan EA. The determination of the number of patients required in a preliminary and a follow-up trial of a new chemotherapeutic agent. *J Chronic Dis.* 1961;13:346–353.
67. Simon R. Optimal two-stage designs for phase II clinical trials. *Control Clin Trials.* 1989;10:1–10.
68. Freidlin B, Dancey J, Korn EL, et al. Multinomial phase II trial designs. *J Clin Oncol.* 2002;20:599.
69. Dent S, Zee B, Dancey J, et al. Application of a new multinomial phase II stopping rule using response and early progression. *J Clin Oncol.* 2001;19:785–791.
70. Daugherty C, Goh B, Ratain MJ. The standard phase II trial design is NOT acceptable to most patients (Pts). *Proceedings of the American Society of Clinical Oncology Annual Meeting*, 2000, (abstract 811).
71. Simon R, Wittes RE, Ellenberg SS. Randomized phase II clinical trials. *Cancer Treat Rep.* 1985;69:1375–1381.
72. Kabbinavar F, Hurwitz HI, Fehrenbacher L, et al. Phase II, randomized trial comparing bevacizumab plus fluorouracil (FU)/leucovorin (LV) with FU/LV alone in patients with metastatic colorectal cancer. *J Clin Oncol.* 2003;21:60–65.
73. Lara PN Jr, Higdon R, Lim N, et al. Prospective evaluation of cancer clinical trial accrual patterns: identifying potential barriers to enrollment. *J Clin Oncol.* 2001;19:1728–1733.
74. Joseph RR. Viewpoints and concerns of a clinical trial participant. *Cancer.* 1994;74:2692–2693.
75. Fuks A, Weijer C, Freedman B, et al. A study in contrasts: eligibility criteria in a twenty-year sample of NSABP and POG clinical trials. National Surgical Adjuvant Breast and Bowel Program, Pediatric Oncology Group. *J Clin Epidemiol.* 1998;51:69–79.
76. Gray R. Better clinical trial design? A simple solution? *Ann Oncol.* 2000;11:6.
77. Sateren WB, Trimble EL, Abrams J, et al. How sociodemographics, presence of oncology specialists, and hospital cancer programs affect accrual to cancer treatment trials. *J Clin Oncol.* 2002;20:2109–2117.
78. Tan SB, Dear KB, Bruzzi P, et al. Strategy for randomised clinical trials in rare cancers. *BMJ.* 2003;327:47–49.
79. Willett CG, Safran H, Abrams RA, et al. Clinical research in pancreatic cancer: the Radiation Therapy Oncology Group trials. *Int J Radiat Oncol Biol Phys.* 2003;56:31–37.

80. Kalish LA, Begg CB. Treatment allocation methods in clinical trials: a review. *Stat Med.* 1985;4:129–144.
81. FOLFIRI followed by FOLFOX6 or the reverse sequence in advanced colorectal cancer: a randomized GERCOR study. Tournigand C, Andre T, Achille E, Lledo G, Flesh M, et al. *J Clin Oncol*. 2004;22:229–237.
82. Simon R. New statistical designs for clinical trials of immunomodulating agents. In: Kresina TF, ed. *Immune Modulating Agents*. New York: Marcel Dekker; 1998:539–550.
83. Marx GM, Steer CB, Harper P, et al. Unexpected serious toxicity with chemotherapy and antiangiogenic combinations: time to take stock! *J Clin Oncol*. 2002;20:1446–1448.
84. Rasmussen H, Rugg T, Brown P, et al. A 371 patient meta-analysis of studies of marimastat in patients with advanced cancer (meeting abstract). *ASCO*. 1997.
85. Ko A, Renshaw FG, Hwang J, et al. Prognostic value of CA 19-9 in patients with advanced pancreatic cancer receiving fixed-dose rate infusional gemcitabine. *Am Soc Clin Oncol*. 2003;259.
86. Rocha Lima C, Rotche R, Jeffrey M, et al. A randomized phase 3 study comparing efficacy and safety of gemcitabine and irinotecan to gem alone in patients with locally advanced or metastatic pancreatic cancer who have not received prior systemic therapy. *Am Soc Clin Oncol*. 2003;251.
87. Rosner GL, Stadler W, Ratain MJ. Randomized discontinuation design: application to cytostatic antineoplastic agents. *J Clin Oncol*. 2002;20:4478–4484.
88. Stadler WM, Ratain MJ. Development of target-based antineoplastic agents. *Invest New Drugs*. 2000;18:7–16.

CHAPTER 34

Supportive Care: Symptom Management

Suresh K. Reddy, MD
Ahmed Elsayem, MD
Rudranath Talukdar, MD

"Symptom control and palliative medicine is the management of patients with active, progressive, far-advanced disease for whom the prognosis is limited and the focus of care is the quality of life." The World Health Organization[1] has put forth a definition of palliative medicine: "Palliative care is an approach that improves the quality of life of patients and their families facing the problem associated with life-threatening illness, through the prevention and relief of suffering by means of early identification and impeccable assessment and treatment of pain and other problems, physical, psychosocial and spiritual." Many aspects of palliative care are also applicable earlier in the course of the illness in conjunction with anti-cancer treatment. Palliative medicine is total care of body, mind, and spirit. Subsequently, the traditional disease-focused medical model is slowly being replaced by patient- and family-focused interdisciplinary palliative care or the "bio–psychosocial–spiritual model" to address all aspects of patient and family needs.[2,3]

Patients with pancreatic cancer develop a number of devastating physical and psychosocial symptoms[4] that may occur during different phases and stages of cancer. These patients need optimal control of symptoms in order to continue receiving anti-cancer treatment, as well as to improve the quality of life in advanced stages. Symptoms include fatigue, pain, anorexia, nausea, dyspnea, constipation, anxiety, depression, and cachexia.

Principles of Symptom Control Include Assessment and Treatment

Assessment

A multidisciplinary assessment is the key to the successful management of symptoms in advanced cancer. The domains that needs to be assessed include the following:

1. Intensity of symptoms is on a 0–10 scale with a simple tool of Edmonton Symptom Assessment Scale (ESAS),[5] which provides a graphical display of all symptoms in real time and helps decision making on a day-to-day basis.
2. Psychosocial assessment includes questions pertaining to loss of autonomy, family conflicts, financial issues, social standing, fear of death, depression, and anxiety.
3. Spiritual assessment includes questions pertaining to meaning of life, connectedness to family, God, hope, and "why me."

Referral Date:						Referring Physician:						
Date:												
Pain (0–10)*												
Fatigue (0–10)*												
Nausea (0–10)*												
Depression (0–10)*												
Anxiety (0–10)*												
Drowsiness (0–10)*												
Shortness of Breath (0–10)*												
Appetite (0–10)*												
Sleep (0–10)*												
Feeling of Wellbeing (0–10)*												
Mini Mental State Score (0–30)												
Assessment from: Pt/SO/HCP (If SO or HCP – use red ink)												
Total Opioid MEDD: _____ mg/day												
Staff Initials (Signature and Title Below)												

* 0 = No Symptom/Best 10 = Worst Imaginable

Figure 34.1
Edmonton Symptom Assessment System (from Bruera et al.[5]).

Common Tools Employed

1. The ESAS[5] is employed to assess the intensity of different symptoms on a 0–10 scale, where 0 is the best possible intensity and 10 is the worst (Fig. 34.1).
2. The mini-mental state examination[6] is a screening tool that is used to evaluate cognitive function. It is a widely tested and well-accepted tool to test orientation, immediate recall, short-term memory, language, and the ability to perform constructive tasks.
3. The CAGE questionnaire[7] for alcoholism screening may reveal a patient's poor coping mechanisms at the time of stress. The CAGE comprises four questions, which together can help screen for alcohol addiction. The questions are as follows: Have you ever felt you should Cut down on your drinking? Have people Annoyed you by criticizing your drinking? Have you ever felt bad or Guilty about drinking? Have you ever had a drink in the morning (an Eye-opener) to steady your nerves or get rid of a hangover?

Principles of Treatment

1. Pharmacotherapy
2. Interventional management
3. Counseling
4. Behavioral management
5. Spiritual management
6. Bereavement care

Pain

Pain is one of the most common symptoms experienced by patients with pancreatic cancer and was the most common symptom (82%) among patients referred for palliative care service.[8] Pain may herald the diagnosis of cancer and may indicate the recurrence and spread of cancer. It can occur both during active treatment and in the advanced and terminal stages of cancer. Generally, in cancer, as many as 30%–50% of patients in active therapy and as many as 60%–90% of patients with advanced disease have pain.[9-13]

Pain in pancreatic cancer is mostly visceral, tends to be central abdominal or epigastric, and is described as deep with radiation to the back. Pain may be caused by direct invasion of the autonomic nerves by the tumor and by pancreatic ductal obstruction leading to ductal dilatation and pain. Also, invasion of the somatic nerves in advanced disease may result in somatic pain.[14]

Treatment of Pancreatic Cancer Pain

The treatment of pain should be preceded by a thorough assessment of pain and other associated symptoms, as pancreatic cancer is often associated with concomitant symptoms such as anorexia, nausea, vomiting, asthenia, cachexia, and psychologic distress, particularly depression.[15-17] Hence, a thorough multidisciplinary assessment should be done that includes physical as well as psychosocial components. Failure to treat pain in some patients with pancreatic cancer may be due to our inability to identify factors influencing pain. Some of the tools used in assessing pain and other symptoms include the ESAS, the mini-mental state examination, and the CAGE, as already mentioned. A thorough physical exam combined with a correlation of imaging studies will lead to a specific pain syndrome as well as a better understanding of other symptoms.

The treatment of the pancreatic cancer pain includes surgery, such as pancreaticoduodenectomy in operable cases, surgical neurectomy,[18] pharmacotherapy,[19] chemotherapy,[20] radiation therapy,[21-23] anesthetic interventions, including celiac/splanchnic neurolytic blocks,[24-26] and epidural and intrathecal therapy.[27-30]

General Pain-Management Principles

- Respect and accept the complaint of pain as real
- Treat pain appropriately
- Treat the underlying disorder(s)
- Address psychosocial issues
- Use a multidisciplinary approach

Pharmacotherapy

Principles of Pharmacotherapy

- Match the drug to the pain syndrome
- Have a low threshold to prescribe opioids
- Add adjunct medications where appropriate
- Use the oral as the route of choice
- Use the intravenous route for acute titration
- Treat side effects before switching opioids
- Perform sequential opioid trials (at least two to three strong opioids)
- Familiarize with equianalgesic dosing
- Familiarize with pharmacokinetics of opioids
- Differentiate between tolerance, physical dependence, and addiction
- Be aware of renal failure and analgesic drugs

Pharmacotherapy is the most simple and effective way to control cancer pain. The class of medications used includes opioids as well as nonopioids or adjuvant medications.

Opioid Medications

Opioid medications form the basis for the management of cancer pain regardless of the pathophysiology of pain. Opioids are drugs of choice for somatic pain, but evidence suggests that they are effective in neuropathic pain also, which is in contrast to the previous belief.[31,32]

Opioids are pharmacodynamically classified into pure agonists, mixed agonist–antagonists, and antagonists. As a rule in our practice, only pure agonists are used. Partial agonists and agonist–antagonists are not used because they exhibit a "ceiling effect" and have an unfavorable side-effect profile. Table 34.1 lists the most commonly used opioids in cancer pain with their equianalgesic dose ratios.

Low-Potency Opioid Agonists

This list includes codeine, propoxyphene, hydrocodone, and dihydrocodeine with a potency of about 1/4 to 1/10 that of morphine sulfate. Indications for drugs from this group include mild to moderate pain, not responsive to nonopioids. A good example is mild bone pain and an early visceral pain. They are also occasionally used for in-between breakthrough pain for patients with constant pain on sustained-release opioids. Some of the members of this group of drugs are formulated with acetaminophen. Hence, the dose escalation of these drugs is limited by the maximum allowable dose of acetaminophen. However, some pharmacies can prepare formulations without acetaminophen.

High-Potency Opioid Agonists

These classes of drugs are used for all pain types. Available as short- and long-acting, morphine is the standard drug; it is the most widely used and is the prototype drug of its class. It is converted to morphine-3-glucoronide and mophine-6-glucronide by glucuronyl transferase in the liver. Caution should be exercised in patients with renal impairment, as the kidney excretes these compounds. It is available in oral, rectal, intramuscular, intravenous, and sublingual use as well as intrathecal preparations. Other strong opioid class drugs include oxycodone, hydromorphone, and fentanyl. Methadone has recently re-emerged and is being used beneficially

Table 34.1 Opioid Analgesics and Equianalgesic Ratios

Drug	Usual Starting Dosages
Full opioid agonists	
Morphine*	15 to 30 mg orally every 3 to 4 hours
	30 to 60 mg orally every 8 to 12 hours
Hydromorphone (Dilaudid)	2 to 4 mg orally every 4 to 6 hours
Levorphanol (Levo-Dromoran)	2 to 4 mg orally every 4 to 6 hours
Fentanyl (Duragesic)	25 to 50 μg/hour transdermally every 3 days
Codeine	15 to 30 mg orally every 3 to 4 hours
Oxycodone (Percodan and others)	5 to 10 mg orally every 3 to 4 hours
Meperidine (Demoral hydrochloride)	75 to 100 mg intramuscularly every 3 to 4 hours
Methadone hydrochloride (Dolophine)	5 to 10 mg orally every 3 to 4 hours
Propoxyphene (Darvon and others)	100 mg orally every 4 to 6 hours
Partial agonists and mixed agonists/antagonists†	
Nalbuphine (Nubain)	10 mg intravenously every 3 to 4 hours
Butorphanol (Stadol)	0.5 to 2 mg intravenously every 3 to 4 hours
	1 to 2 mg sublingually three times a day
Dezocine (Dalgan)	10 mg intravenously every 3 to 4 hours
Pentazocine (Talwin)	50 mg orally every 4 to 6 hours

*Morphine can be given as an immediate-release formulation or as a sustained-release preparation. It is recommended that a relatively rapid onset, short-acting opioid preparation (such as immediate-release morphine) be given to patients who take sustained-release morphine to provide rescue medication for breakthrough pain.

† This class of drugs is *not* recommended for the management of chronic cancer pain because they will reverse analgesia when co-administered with full opioid agonists and precipitate withdrawal in physically dependent individuals.

Equianalgesic Dosing Table‡

Opioid	From Parenteral Opioid to Parental Opioid	From Same Parenteral Opioid to Oral Opioid	From Oral Opioid to Oral Morphine	From Oral Morphine to Oral Opioid
Morphine	1	2.5	1	1
Hydromorphone	5	2	5	0.2
Meperidine	0.13	4	0.1	10
Levorphanol	5	2	5	0.2
Codeine	NA	NA	0.15	7
Oxycodone	NA	NA	1.5	0.7
Hydrocodone	NA	NA	0.15	7

‡ (1) Take the total amount of opioid that effectively controls pain in 24 hours. (2) Multiply by conversion factor in table. Give 30% less of the new opioid to avoid partial cross-tolerance. (3) Divide by the number of doses per day.

Abbreviation: NA, Not applicable

METHADONE is 10 to 15 times more potent than morphine. Expertise is needed to use it.

Modified with permission from Elsayem A, Driver L, Bruera E, eds. *M.D. Anderson Palliative Care Handbook.* 2nd ed. Houston: M.D. Anderson; 2002.

to treat cancer pain. Recent updates[33] and research on the equianalgesic dosing[34,35] coupled with its lower cost, absence of active opioid metabolites, excellent bioavailability, and possible N-methyl D-aspartate antagonist action[36] enabled many to use methadone safely and to treat cancer pain effectively. The potency of methadone seems to be 10–15 times that of morphine. Hence, caution should be exercised when switching from an opioid to methadone. Meperidine (demerol) is another commonly used opioid analgesic, but chronic use is associated with the risk of accumulation of the metabolite normeperidine, produced by the liver. This compound may result in frank convulsions, especially in renally impaired and older patients.[37] Hence, the use of meperidine has been rapidly declining. Fentanyl is a semisynthetic opioid that is available in the parenteral as well as transdermal form. Its rapid onset and relatively short duration of action make it a good choice for the control of acute pain. A sustained-release, transdermal form has been developed and used successfully for stable pain. Each patch is changed every 72 hours and hence was found to be convenient in patients who have stable pain but have difficulties swallowing. Recently, an oral transmucosal fentanyl has been approved for use in breakthrough pain in cancer[38] and has been shown to be a useful medication to treat breakthrough or incident pain.[39]

Opioid medications exhibit a wide interindividual variation, possibly because of a difference in intrinsic activity and action at different receptors and subtypes.[40,41] Hence, opioid rotation is a worthwhile exercise when dose-limiting side effects are encountered. Some groups treat side effects of opioids before embarking on opioid rotation. The generally accepted method is to treat side effects before opioid switching. There is no general consensus as to the number of opioid rotations, but in the authors' experience, at least two to three opioid rotations, which should include methadone at some stage, are very successful.

The Adjuvant Medications

These groups of drugs are used mostly in conjunction with opioid medications in pancreatic cancer pain. The categories include nonsteroidal anti-inflammatories (NSAIDs), tricyclic antidepressants (TCAs), antiepileptic drugs (AEDs), and miscellaneous.

NSAIDs are essentially limited to the inhibitors of the enzyme cyclooxygenase (COX), thus inhibiting the synthesis of prostaglandins, the pain and inflammation mediators. This group is now subdivided into nonspecific COX inhibitors and selective COX-2 inhibitors. The nonselective inhibitors, which are also referred to as NSAIDs, are medications such as ibuprofen and naproxen. However, these drugs continue to cause concern with regard to the integrity of gastric mucosa and alteration in renal function.[42] These drugs which block the COX-2 enzyme with very little action on COX-1, thereby having minimal effect on the integrity of gastric mucosa and platelet aggregation. In clinical trials, these agents exhibited a safety profile that is comparable to a placebo compared with the nonselective group. However, the efficacy remains the same as conventional NSAIDs. The COX-2 inhibitor class of drugs offers significant advantages in patients with cancer who are undergoing chemotherapy.[43] Recently rofecoxib has been withdrawn due to higher incidence of heart attacks and strokes.

TCAs are the main group of antidepressants currently being used for the purpose of neuropathic pain syndromes.[44,45] They probably act by inhibiting reuptake of serotonin and norepinephrine at the nerve endings in the spinal cord as well as in the brain. TCAs are not universally tolerated, especially at the initiation of therapy, and often have to be discontinued or decreased because of dose-limiting side effects, most commonly the anticholinergic and sedative effects. Amitriptyline and nortriptyline are felt to be the most efficacious agents and are thus used more often.

AEDs are used commonly in neuropathic pain syndromes. Gabapentin, which is a class of AEDs, has been shown to be useful in neuropathic pain states.[46,47] With its wide therapeutic window and a comparable efficacy of other anticonvulsants, gabapentin is now widely used in neuropathic pain states. Sedation is a noted side effect that can be reduced by starting therapy at 100 mg three times a day and adding 100 mg to each dose every second or third day until the desired effect is acquired. If necessary, dose escalation up to 3,600 mg/day is recommended. Gabapentin is available in both tablet and elixir forms. Newer AEDs have been used recently with varying successes.[48] Some of the other AEDs include topiramate, felbamate, zonisamide, and oxcarbazepine.

Miscellaneous Group

In refractory pain situations, drugs from other classes have been tried—some with a good response and others with only a minimal response. They include psychotropic drugs,[49,50] benzodiazepines,[51] bisphosphonates,[52-54] steroids in spinal cord compression,[55] lidocaine, intravenous and patch,[56-58] ketamine,[59,60] capsaicin,[61] and radiopharmaceuticals (Strontium 89, Samarium).[62,63]

Nonpharmacologic treatment includes anesthetic procedures such as celiac/splanchnic nerve blocks and epidural/intrathecal management, but neurosurgical procedures are rarely indicated. Celiac plexus block has been shown to be very useful in many studies[24-26] and is often employed, preferably when the patient's general condition has not deteriorated. Debate exists about the efficacy of conservative treatment versus anesthetic interventions to treat pancreatic cancer pain. Some studies question the efficacy of celiac plexus block, whereas some favor it. In our experience, they are not mutually exclusive but should form the part of treatment algorithm to best deal with pain and other symptoms (Fig. 34.2).[64]

Other principles of symptom management are routinely employed, including counseling, psychotherapy, relaxation techniques, massage therapy, music therapy, address of psychosocial and spiritual needs, and bereavement counseling for family members.

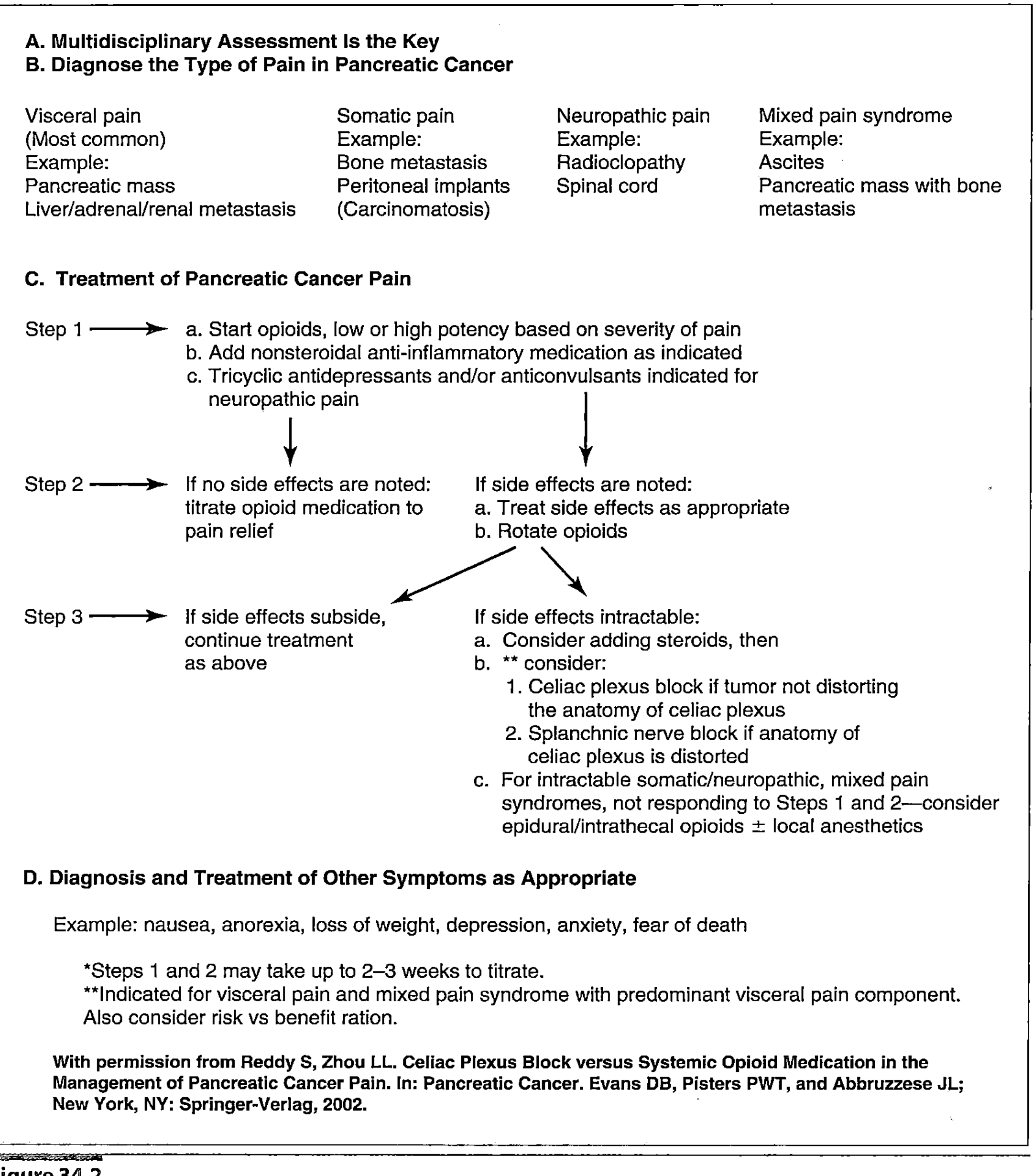

Figure 34.2
(A) Multidisciplinary assessment is the key. **(B)** Diagnose the type of pain in pancreatic cancer. **(C)** Treatment of pancreatic cancer pain. **(D)** Diagnosis and treatment of other symptoms as appropriate.

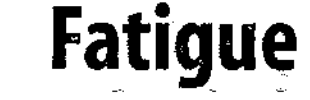

Fatigue

Fatigue is one of the most common symptoms in patients with cancer,[65] experienced by 70%-100% in patients receiving cancer treatment.[66] Fatigue refers to a subjective sense of decreased vitality in physical and/or mental functioning that usually occurs in the setting of medical disease. The physical dimension is usually described as a perception of muscle weakness or a tendency to fatigue rapidly. Physical activity is difficult to sustain, and in some cases, dyspnea accompanies minimal exertion. Rest or sleep does not return perceived strength or stamina to normal. The mental component is described as a lack of interest or motivation in objects or activities. Other symptoms include difficulty in concentrating or maintaining attention. Mood may be flat or depressed. Lethargy or a tendency to somnolence may be noted, but there is not a need for excessive sleep. Rest or sleep may improve symptoms, but not eliminate them. Fatigue is experienced during treatment as well as during terminal stages. For patients with advanced cancer, however, fatigue may be a severe symptom that either decreases their capacity for physical and mental work or renders them completely unable to function normally. Fatigue gets worse as the disease progresses toward the end stage. The presence of fatigue may also magnify other symptoms affecting the patient. The causes of fatigue are multifactorial and interrelated. These include problems related to the cancer itself, the treatment of side effects or toxicities, underlying systemic pathophysiologic disorders, and other causes (Fig. 34.3).

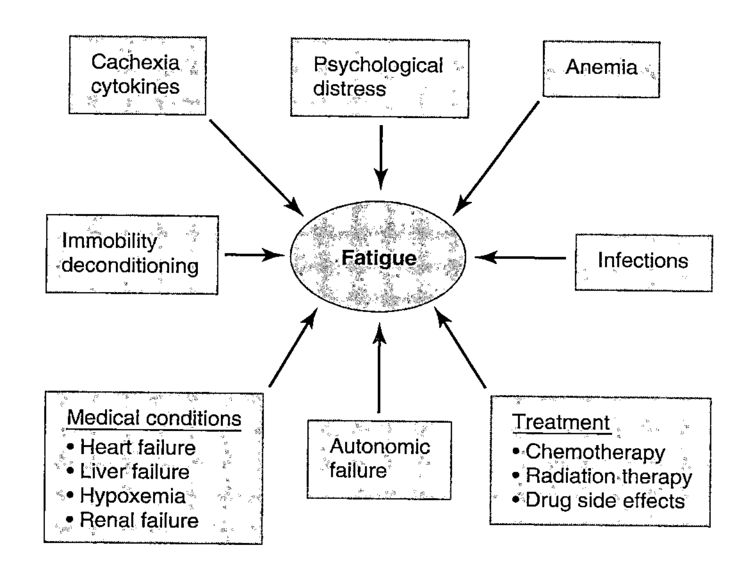

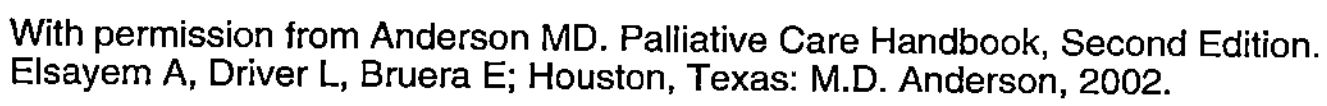
With permission from Anderson MD. Palliative Care Handbook, Second Edition. Elsayem A, Driver L, Bruera E; Houston, Texas: M.D. Anderson, 2002.

Figure 34.3
Causes of fatigue.

Assessment of Fatigue

The severity of fatigue can be measured on a scale of 0 to 10 (where 0 equals no fatigue and 10 equals the worst fatigue imaginable), as in ESAS, or by other numeric or verbal rating scales. Like other symptoms in cancer, the assessment of fatigue should focus on the multidimensional aspect. The impact of fatigue on activities, function, and the quality of life should be assessed. Laboratory investigations and imaging studies should be based on indications derived from the patient history and physical examination.

Management of Fatigue

As with other problematic symptoms in advanced cancer patients, the management of fatigue should address possible underlying etiologies as well as the patient's expression of symptoms.[67,68]

Treat underlying problems: pain, depression, anxiety, stress, or sleep disturbances. Dehydration should be corrected, and an attempt should be made to treat cachexia in appropriate cases. Simplify the medication regimes, and treat infections as well as anemia with transfusions where appropriate, administering epoetin-α 10,000 U subcutaneously three times weekly as indicated.[69] Low-dose steroids may alleviate some of the symptoms of fatigue in advanced cancer patients.[70,71] Psychostimulants, such as methylphenidate 5 to 10 mg in the morning and the same dose at noon, may be useful if the patient is experiencing concomitant problems such as depression, hypoactive delirium, or drowsiness caused by opioids.[72-74] Some antidepressants, such as serotonin-specific reuptake inhibitors, may improve energy levels in some fatigued patients, although their benefit is unproven. Recently, increasing evidence exists that patients with cancer and hypogonadism who are on chronic opioid therapy may suffer from fatigue.[75] Replacement therapy with testosterone may improve fatigue in these patients but needs to be studied in the future. Bruera et al.[76] showed that patient-controlled methylphenidate administration rapidly improved fatigue and other symptoms.

Dyspnea

Dyspnea is defined as the "uncomfortable awareness of breathing."[77] It is described in terms of air hunger, suffocation, choking, or heavy breathing. It is a subjective sensation, associated with and impacted by factors such as location and progression of the tumor, psychosocial phenomenon,[78] and pre-existing chronic lung pathology such as chronic obstructive airway disease, asthma, and congestive heart failure. The frequency and severity of dyspnea depend on the stage of the disease and increase in frequency when death is imminent.

Dyspnea as a lone symptom or in association with other parameters is a bad prognostic indicator of survival.[79,80] Dyspnea is a multidimensional symptom that is influenced by factors such as anxiety, tumor location, fatigue, and other factors. Dyspnea can be caused by a number of clinical conditions, but the cause mainly falls into two categories: (1) dyspnea with abnormal mechanics of ventilation (e.g., cachexia, asthenia, myesthenic syndrome, Eaton-Lambert syndrome) and dyspnea with the normal mechanics of ventilation (this category may be subdivided into a respiratory and nonrespiratory causes of dyspnea) (Table 34.2).

Table 34.2 Causes of Dyspnea in Cancer Patients

Dyspnea with Abnormal Mechanisms of Ventilation	Dyspnea with Normal Mechanisms of Ventilation
_Asthenia	Direct effect of the tumor
_Cachexia	_Primary or metastatic tumor
_Myasthenia gravis	_Pleural effusion/pericardial infusion
_Eaton-Lambert syndrome	_Superior vena cava syndrome
_Rib fracture	_Carcinomatous lymphangitis
_Chest wall deformity	_Atelectasis
_Neuromuscular disease (motor neuron disease)	_Phrenic nerve palsy
	_Tracheal obstruction
	_Tracheal–esophageal fistula
	_Carcinomatous infiltration of the chest wall (carcinoma en cuirasse)
	Effect of therapy
	_Postactinic fibrosis
	_Postpneumectomy
	_Mitomycin-vinca alkaloid (acute dyspnea syndrome)
	_Bleomycin-induced fibrosis
	_Adriamycin- and cyclophosphamide-induced cardiomyopathy
	Not directly related to the tumor or therapy
	_Anemia
	_Ascites
	_Metabolic acidosis
	_Fever
	_COPD
	_Asthma
	_Pulmonary embolism
	_Pneumonia
	_Pneumothorax
	_Heart failure
	_Obesity
	_Thyrotoxicosis
	_Psychosocial distress (i.e., anxiety, somatization)
	_Unknown

Assessment of Dyspnea

Dyspnea is a complex symptom that is caused by various factors, some not well understood. However, thorough history with physical examination and with appropriate laboratory and imaging studies should be undertaken to assess dyspnea. Some of the factors that contribute to dyspnea include anxiety, phobia, pain, and fatigue.

Treatment of Dyspnea

The aim of the dyspnea treatment is a subjective improvement in the patient's perception. Treatment involves treating the cause and the symptoms as well as managing psychosocial issues contributing to dyspnea.

Treatment of the Cause

Treating the underlying cause is attempted as an initial step: thoracentesis for pleural effusion, blood transfusion for anemia, corticosteroids for carcinomatosis lymphangitis, anticoagulants for pulmonary embolism, and antibiotics for pneumonia where appropriate.

Symptomatic Treatment

Oxygen therapy Long-term oxygen therapy has been shown to have beneficial effects on the outcome of patients with chronic obstructive pulmonary disease.[81,82] Studies in cancer dyspnea suggest beneficial effects of oxygen in patients with cancer in crossover trials.[83,84] Oxygen may be given by nasal cannula and may be humidified whenever feasible. Oxygen treatment toward the end of life may lead to anxiety among family members who sometimes interpret this as a way of prolonging life and suffering. Counseling of family members about this issue is of paramount importance.

Drug therapy A number of pharmacologic agents have been tried effectively to relieve the perception of dyspnea in terminal cancer patients. The major drugs are opioids, corticosteroids, and benzodiazepines. Many studies found that opioids of different types, doses, and routes of administration are capable of relieving dyspnea.[85,86] Nebulized opioids have also been shown to be effective in some studies.[87-91] Some conflicting studies exist about the use of nebulized opioids to treat dyspnea.[92] Opioids act possibly by reducing the subjective sensation of dyspnea without reducing the respiratory rate or oxygen saturation. They also possibly cause venodilation of pulmonary vessels, thereby reducing preload to the heart and improving breathing. Corticosteroids are useful only if dyspnea is caused by carcinomatosis lymphangitis or in superior vena caval syndrome. They also may play a role if associated with chronic obstructive pulmonary disease or asthma coexists in a patient.[93] Benzodiazepines have a limited role in dyspnea, except when anxiety and apprehension are the causes of dyspnea. Subsequently, they are commonly used medications for terminal dyspnea in hospice settings. Bronchodilators play a role if dyspnea is caused by bronchospasm. Both nebulized and oral agents are used. In a study by Congleton and Meurs,[94] bronchodilators provided significant relief of dyspnea in patients with lung carcinoma and airflow obstruction. Sometimes phenothiazines, such as chlorpromazine, may help in drying secretions and in reducing anxiety.[95]

General Supportive Measures

A number of measures can be implemented for the support of both the patient and the family. Relaxation techniques or guided imagery provides relief in patients with anticipatory or anxiety driven dyspnea. Assist devices can be used to minimize muscle effort. Maneuvers such as postural drainage and incentive spirometry can help in special situations.

Delirium

Delirium is defined as a transient organic brain syndrome that is characterized by the acute onset of disordered attention (arousal) and cognition, accompanied by disturbances of psychomotor behavior and perception.[96]

Table 34.3 Causes of Delirium in Cancer Patients

Tumor related
_Primary brain tumor or metastatic brain metastasis
_Leptomeningeal disease
_Paraneoplastic syndromes
_Seizure
Metabolic
_Electrolyte imbalance
_Metabolic encephalopathy secondary organ failure
_Hypercalcemia
Medications
_Chemotherapeutic agents (e.g., Ifosfamide)
_Opioid medications
_Benzodiazepines
_Antiemetics
_Steroids
_Anticholinergics
Infection
_Sepsis
_Pneumonia
Vascular
_Thromboembolic phenomenon
_Intracranial hemorrhage

Delirium is common with progressive disease and is common in patients with pancreatic cancer who are near death. It may signal a new and serious medical complication, markedly impair the function and comfort of the patient, and increase the family's distress.[97] The prevalence of delirium in hospitalized medical and surgical patients is approximately 10%, and the prevalence in hospitalized cancer patients ranges from 8%–40%.[98-100] Causes of delirium are listed in Table 34.3.

Clinical Features

The symptoms and signs of delirium fluctuate; therefore, careful attention should be paid to the mental status during an examination. The diagnosis is established by a new onset of cognitive dysfunction, accompanied by a disturbance of arousal or clouding of consciousness. Three clinical variants have been described based on the type of arousal disturbance: hypoalert–hypoactive, hyperalert–hyperactive, and mixed type.[101,102] The presenting features include memory impairment or confusion, dysphoria, hypomania, illusions, hallucinations, and altered arousal state. The DSM-IV American Psychiatric Association[103] criteria for delirium have been considered the gold standard for the diagnosis of delirium. These include impairment in responsiveness and alertness, as manifested by fluctuating inability to maintain or shift attention to external stimuli, cognitive dysfunction of recent onset, development of the disturbance over a short period of time, evidence from history, physical examination, or laboratory findings etiologically related to the disturbance.

Assessment

Delirium is a frequently missed diagnosis, and more frequently, it is misdiagnosed as insomnia, anxiety, or depression because the presenting symptoms may mimic any of these conditions. Understanding the patient's baseline and listening to the family members' and nurses' observations will help to pick up the diagnosis of delirium before the condition is florid and out of control. The cause of the delirium should be investigated if possible because the treatment will depend on correction of the cause. The history is of utmost importance, especially the acute onset of the condition. Medications, particularly opioids, benzodiazepines, some antiemetics, and corticosteroids, are frequent causes of delirium. Physical examination may reveal signs of dehydration or increased intracranial pressure. Laboratory examinations may show hypercalcemia, hyponatremia, and renal or hepatic failure.

Treatment of Delirium

If the diagnosis of delirium is suspected, the clinician should act immediately to establish the diagnosis and remove the inciting medication if this is the likely cause. Safety is of paramount importance, especially in the agitated (hyperactive) type, as patients may endanger themselves by removing intravenous lines, falling, or pacing about. Educating family members and nurses is important. The appropriate management includes identifying and treating the underlying causes. Other reversible causes should be identified and corrected. If opioids are the cause, dosage reduction or rotation to a different opioid should be attempted. Treating infection, hydrating a dehydrated patient, or correcting hypercalcemia may be all that is needed to treat the delirious patient. Symptomatic treatment to control agitation is achieved by the use of neuroleptics. Haloperidol remains the drug of choice for the treatment of delirium. It is a dopamine blocker with useful sedative effects and a low incidence of cardiovascular and anticholinergic side effects. Mostly haloperidol in the dose of 1–3 mg/day is effective in treating agitation paranoia and fear. A higher dose may be needed in special circumstances. Sometimes acute dystonias and extrapyramidal side effects are seen with haloperidol, in which case benztropine can be administered. Methotrimeprazine is sometimes used effectively to control agitation. It also has been shown to be an analgesic. Newer antipsychotics such as olanzapine[104] are as effective and may be more sedating in the control of agitated patients, but unfortunately, they are more expensive. Sometimes a combination of haloperidol with benzodiazepine is useful. In a study by Brietbart et al.,[105] lorazepam alone was ineffective in the treatment of delirium; in fact, it contributed to the worsening of delirium and increased cognitive impairment. In severe cases, a palliative care consultation is important, and if the condition proves to be refractory to antipsychotic in terminal cases, sedation should be considered.

Depression

Depression is a common and devastating problem for patients with cancer and other terminal diseases. Major depression can affect from 25%–35% of cancer patients.[106] This prevalence touches 77% in those with advanced disease.[107] Pancreatic cancer is more likely to be associated with depression. The depression seen in patients with pancreatic cancer will cause an even greater loss of appetite, weight loss, low energy, etc. Thus, it can be critically important to diagnose and treat depression early, thereby ameliorating some of the psychologic changes that are inevitable with advanced cancer. The cause of depression in pancreatic cancer is unclear. It may be caused by an indirect effect of cancer on the serotonergic function of the brain or may result from a psychologic reaction to cancer.[108] Pain has a close correspondence to psychiatric illness. It is twice as likely that patients reporting pain will have a psychiatric diagnosis as well.[109] The cardinal features of depression include a loss of interest or pleasure, impaired decision-making ability, changes in appetite, sleep, psychomotor activity, decreased energy, and feelings of guilt and/or worthlessness. Mild episodes may be masked by increased effort on the part of the individual.

Assessment of Depression

Diagnosis is confounded by the presence of normal sadness and grief and also by delirium. Anhedonia can be mistaken for the fatigue that occurs in cancer patients. Assessing depression quickly and accurately is important. No clear-cut guidelines exist on assessing depression in terminal cancer patients. A recent report by Fisch et al.[110] suggested the usefulness of a brief two-question assessment of depression in patients with advanced cancer with the primary objective being to measure the quality of life after intervention with fluoxetine and the secondary objective being to assess the reduction in depression. Other validated measures of assessing depression in the primary care setting include the WHO-5 Well being index,[111] the Patient health questionnaire screening test,[112] the Hamilton Rating Scale for Depression, and the Montgomery Asberg Depression Rating Scale. The patient should be evaluated for depressive episodes and substance abuse, family history of depression and suicide, concurrent life stressors, losses secondary to cancer, and the availability of social support.

Delirium, particularly in the early stages, is often misidentified as depression and is treated as such with poor effects.[113] The key is to diagnose the clinical problem accurately. In doubtful situations, a consultation with a palliative care physician or a psychiatrist should be obtained.

Treatment

A combination or a balanced approach of supportive psychotherapy and pharmacotherapy is key to the optimal treatment of depression. Individual or group counseling has been shown to be useful.[113] Other methods include relaxation techniques, guided imagery,[114] and music therapy.[115] Counseling both patients and their family is crucial to treat depression successfully. This helps to reduce anxiety and allows patients to express their fears and disappointments in a "safe" way and enhances well-being.

Pharmacotherapy

The mainstay of treatment of depression is pharmacotherapy. The agents commonly employed include newer selective serotonin reuptake inhibitors (SSRIs), TCAs, and psychostimulants. The SSRIs fluoxetine hydrochloride, sertraline hydrochloride, paroxetine hydrochloride, citalopram, and recently escitalopram have gained popularity because of fewer side-effect profiles compared with TCAs. For mild depression, SSRIs are very useful. They, however, take weeks to effect a change. Some, such as escitalopram, have a lower profile of side effects and work a little faster than the first-generation SSRIs such as fluoxetine. The side effects are generally mild and include problematic ones such as reduced appetite, nausea, and anxiety. They tend to be limited in duration and have not been a limiting factor in their application in cancer patients. Other problems arise from their mechanism of action and include diarrhea, fatigue, and sexual dysfunction. If a switch from a SSRI to another medication, especially a monoamine oxidase inhibitor, is considered, the washout period of various SSRIs will need to be taken into account. As such, it may be useful to have a patient take SSRIs such as sertraline or escitalopram, which have a shorter washout compared with older ones such as fluoxetine. Our experience has shown methylphenidate to be particularly useful, especially in patients with a limited life expectancy where a few weeks may be too much to ask.[116] Methylphenidate also helps to reduce the symptoms of fatigue, a common problem in patients with cancer; this makes it a potentially useful medication for a number of reasons.[76]

TCAs have been used and work faster than SSRIs; however, they have more side effects, some of which (such as the anticholinergic effects) can be a major problem for older patients with cancer. They do offer additional benefits for patients suffering from neuropathic pain. For that reason, these medications should be started at a low dose and slowly escalated as tolerated. Desipramine and nortriptyline are generally better tolerated in the older population as compared with amitriptyline and imipramine.

In a recent study, mirtazapine was found to be effective in ameliorating symptoms of depression in cancer patients.[117] Some additional benefits of mirtazapine may accrue from its beneficial effects on chemotherapy induced nausea/vomiting and insomnia.[118]

Constipation

Constipation is the infrequent and difficult passage of hard stool. It is a very common cause of morbidity in the palliative care setting and is thought to affect the overwhelming majority (>95%) of patients consuming opioids for cancer-related pain syndromes.[119,120] Constipation can be a difficult condition to assess and treat because of the wide variety of presenting symptoms. Patients may report a feeling of incomplete evacuation, bloating, decreased appetite, or generalized abdominal discomfort or pain. Because of the wide variability in normal bowel movement patterns in individual patients, the diagnosis of constipation can only be made in comparison with an individual's normal pattern.[121]

Causes

The most common causes of constipation include opioid medication and progressive disease. Other causes include anorexia/cachexia, bowel obstruction, immobility, hypercalcemia, and dehydration. In the palliative-care setting, careful attention must be given to the multifactorial nature of constipation. Common causes of constipation are outlined in Table 34.4.

Complications

Although constipation is often overlooked in the setting of other comorbid conditions, it is not necessarily a benign condition, and some of the complications of unrelieved constipation can indeed be life threatening.[122]

Table 34.4 Causes of Constipation in Advanced Cancer Patients

Causes
Structural abnormalities • Obstruction • Pelvic tumor mass • Radiation fibrosis • Painful anorectal conditions - Anal fissure, hemorrhoids, perianal abscess
Drugs • Opioids • Agents with anticholinergic actions - Anticholinergics - Antispasmodics - Antidepressants - Antipsychotics (e.g., phenothiazines, haloperidol) - Antacids (aluminum containing) - Antiemetics (e.g., ondansetron) • Diuretics • Anticonvulsants • Iron • Antihypertensive agents • Anticancer drugs (e.g., vinca alkaloids)
Metabolic disturbances • Dehydration (vomiting, fever, polyuria, poor fluid intake, diuretic use) • Hypercalcemia • Hypokalemia • Uremia • Diabetes • Hypothyroidism
Neurological disorders • Cerebral tumors • Spinal cord compression • Sacral nerve infiltration • Autonomic failure

Severe constipation can lead to bowel obstruction with attendant issues of severe morbidity. In patients who are neutropenic, severe constipation can lead to bacterial transfer across the colon with bacteremia and sepsis.

Diagnosis

The diagnosis of constipation begins with a careful history of the patient's recent bowel movements. Specific topics to be queried include the date of the last bowel movement, the characteristics of the stool (hard vs soft, loose vs formed, "ribbon-like" vs "pellet-like"), the degree of straining and pain involved, and whether the movement felt complete. Related questions include whether there was blood in the stool (possibly identifying tumor mass or a hemorrhoid) or an urge to defecate at all (suggesting colonic inertia).[119,121]

After the history, a careful physical examination should include an abdominal examination (distension, firmness, tenderness, and the presence or absence of bowel sounds) and a rectal examination. The rectal examination should assess the presence of hard stool in the vault and may reveal the presence of masses, hemorrhoids, fissures, or fistulae. Caution should be exercised in performing a rectal examination on anyone with neutropenia or thrombocytopenia.

In addition to the history and physical examination, a simple "constipation score"[123] may also be obtained. A flat abdominal radiograph of the abdomen is obtained, and the colon is divided into four quadrants (ascending, transverse, descending, and sigmoid) by drawing a large X with the umbilicus in the middle. Each quadrant is assigned a score from 0 to 3 based on the degree of stool in the lumen. A score of zero indicates no stool. A score of 1 indicates "less than 50%" occupancy. A score of 2 indicates "greater than 50% occupancy," and a score of 3 indicates complete occupancy of the lumen with stool. Scores may range from 0 to 12, and score of 7 (or greater) indicates severe constipation.

Prevention and Treatment

Prevention of constipation includes patient education on the various reasons for constipation, encouragement of adequate fluid intake, and prescription of stool softeners and laxatives. In addition, a high degree of vigilance should be maintained regarding the patient's other medications that may cause constipation.

Initial treatment of constipation includes starting the patient on a stool-softening agent (e.g., docusate 100–240 mg per os twice daily) with a laxative agent (e.g., senna, one to two tablets twice daily). Refractory constipation may be managed with lactulose 30-ml orally every 6 hours until a large bowel movement occurs. Intractable cases may require a bisacodyl suppository, milk-and-molasses enema, or Fleets enema. Proximal impaction may require magnesium citrate. In rare cases where hard stools are present in the vault, manual disimpaction may be necessary. In refractory cases, the opioid antagonist, naloxone given orally may result in laxation.[124-126] Mild opioid withdrawal may be seen with naloxone. Recently, methylnaltrexone given

Table 34.5 Causes of Nausea in Cancer Patients

Causes
Metabolic • Hypercalcemia • Renal failure • Adrenal failure
Increased intracranial pressure
General medical conditions • Peptic ulcer disease • Sepsis
Gastrointestinal • Constipation • Intestinal obstruction • Autonomic failure
Anxiety
Medications • Opioids • Anticholinergics • NSAIDs

parenterally is showing promising effects on opioid-induced constipation.[127,128]

Chronic Nausea

Nausea and vomiting are highly unpleasant symptoms that affect between 40% and 70% of patients in the palliative care setting.[129-131] In the cancer setting, nausea is prevalent in patients under the age of 65, in females, and in patients with breast, stomach, or gynecologic cancers. The etiology of chronic nausea is often multifactorial and could be caused by the underlying disease, its treatment, or a side effect of medications that treat cancer-related pain (e.g., opioids). The underlying cause of nausea should be ascertained, if possible, and the selection of the antiemetic agent should be tailored to maximize therapeutic value.[129] Table 34.5 lists the common causes of nausea in the cancer setting. Medication side effects and chronic constipation are the most common causes. As shown in the Fig. 34.4, the experience of nausea and vomiting is generated as a result of the complex interrelationship between the chemoreceptor trigger zone and the vomiting center. The chemoreceptor trigger zone could be affected directly by drugs, toxins, or metabolites or could receive afferent impulses from chemoreceptors and mechanoreceptors originating in the gastrointestinal tract, chest, or pelvis and could subsequently influence the vomiting center. The vomiting center also receives direct input from the cerebral cortex (Fig. 34.4).

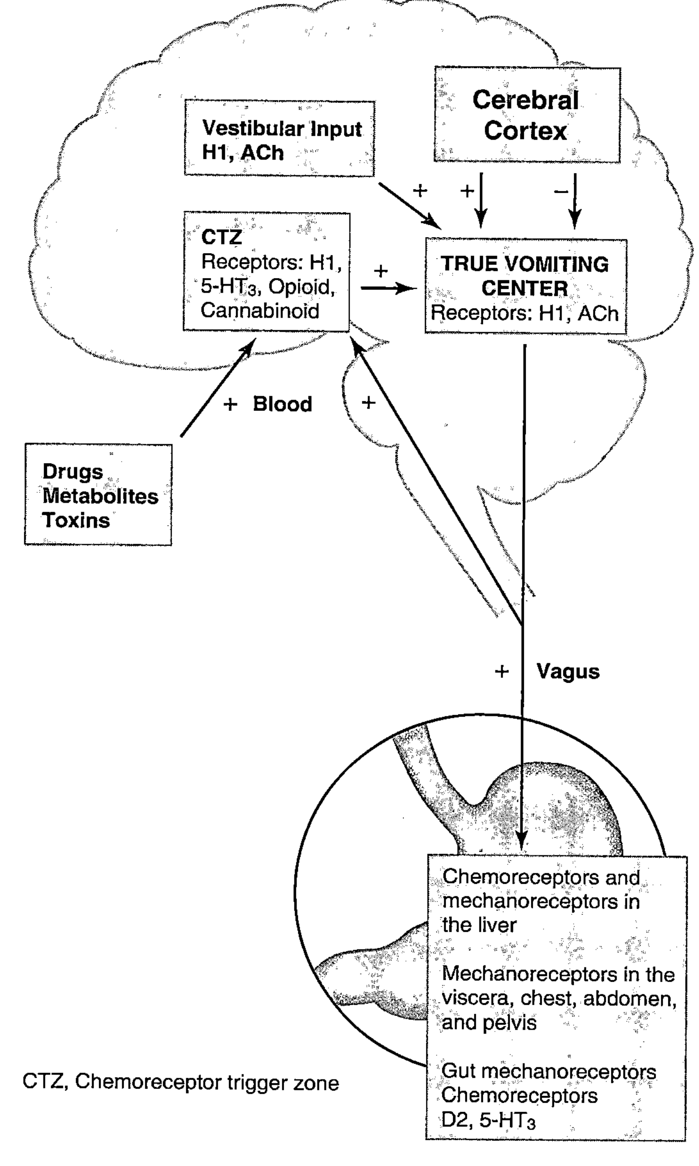

Modified with permission from M.D.Anderson Palliative Care Handbook. eds Elsayem A, Driver L, Bruera E. Second Editon, Houston, Texas. M.D. Anderson. 2002.

Figure 34.4
The vomiting cascade.

Assessment

The etiology of nausea should be determined if at all possible because proper management will depend on identifying and treating the underlying cause. The assessment

Table 34.6 ***Antiemetic Drugs:* Drugs and Doses Useful for the Treatment of Chronic Nausea**

Drug*	Main Receptor	Main Indication	Starting Oral Dose/Route	Side Effects
Metoclopramide	D2	Opioid induced; gastric stasis	10 mg every 4 hours (po, sc, iv)	EPS (akathisia, dystonia, dyskinesia)
Prochlorperazine	D2	Opioid induced	10 mg every 6 hours (po, iv)	Sedation, hypotension
Promethazine	H1	Vestibular, motion sickness, obstruction	12.5 mg every 4 hours (po, pr, iv)	Sedation
Haloperidol	D2	Opioid, chemical, metabolic	1–2 mg bid (po, iv, sc)	Rarely EPS
Ondansetron	5 HT_3	Chemotherapy	4–8 mg every 8 hours (po, iv, sc)	Headache, constipation
Diphenhydramine	H1, ACh	Intestinal obstruction, vestibular, ICP	25 mg every 6 hours (po, iv, sc)	Sedation, dry mouth, blurred vision
Hyoscine	ACh	Intestinal obstruction, colic, secretions	0.2–0.4 mg every 4 hours (sl, sc, td)	Dry mouth, blurred vision, urine retention, agitation

*Corticosteroids not included because of varied doses and limited indications (see text).

Abbreviations: ACh, acetylcholine; D2, dopamine; EPS, extra pyramidal symptoms; H1, histamine; ICP, intracranial pressure; pr, per rectum; sl, sublingual; td, transdermal

Modified with permission from Elsayem A, Driver L, Bruera E, eds. *M.D. Anderson Palliative Care Handbook.* 2nd ed. Houston: M.D. Anderson; 2002.

of the patient with nausea should be part of the multidimensional approach to assess multiple symptoms simultaneously. It begins by taking a detailed history, including the onset of the nausea, duration, frequency of episodes, and severity of the episode on a 0 to 10 scale of ESAS. In addition, because chronic constipation is one of the main causes of nausea, bowel function should also be assessed. The list of medications should be reviewed for possible medication side effects.

The examination of the patient should focus on life-threatening complications related to dehydration such as hypotension and tachycardia and, if present, should be corrected promptly. The abdominal exam, looking for signs of obstruction or constipation, the CNS exam to exclude raised intracranial pressure, and possibly even the cardiac exam to exclude initial symptoms to rule out a major cardiac event, should be done.

Diagnostic tests include serum evaluation of electrolytes, serum calcium, and liver and renal function. Abdominal X-rays may be obtained to gauge the degree of constipation (see the constipation section). Brain imaging may be considered if clinically appropriate.

Treatment

Correction of the underlying problem should be attempted if a cause could be found. Treating constipation or removing the inciting medication may relieve the nausea if it was caused by any of them. Steroids or radiation may help nausea caused by increased intracranial pressure. If opioids are the cause, adding an antiemetic may help, but rarely opioid rotation may be required. Pharmacologic therapy should be directed toward the underlying problem. Table 34.6 illustrates the most commonly used antiemetics. For most chronic, opioid-related nausea, a prokinetic agent such as metoclopramide (10 mg oral/intravenous/subcutaneous every 4–6 hours) is helpful. The antidopaminergic properties of haloperidol (1–2 mg oral/intravenous/subcutaneous every 4–8 hours) may help certain forms of refractory nausea. The 5HT3 antagonists (e.g., ondansetron 4–8 mg oral/intravenous/subcutaneous) may help chemotherapy-related nausea[129,130] but is less helpful in chronic nausea. Moreover, these agents are expensive and constipating. Octreotide, a somatostatin analogue that reduces gastric motility and secretions, is helpful in nausea caused by intestinal obstruction. Benzodiazepines and other H1 antagonists may help anxiety-provoked nausea. Finally, steroids have been shown to be helpful for nausea both with a direct effect (e.g., in certain chemotherapy or opioid-related problems with nausea) and an indirect effect (e.g., reducing intracranial pressure in patients with intracranial neoplasms).[131,132]

Small Bowel Obstruction

Pancreatic cancer is the second most common cause of gastroduodenal obstruction (gastric cancer is the most common).[133] Patients with pancreatic cancer present 6% of the time with upper bowel obstruction.[134] In one review, approximately 25% with unresectable disease developed gastroduodenal obstruction.[134] Pancreatic cancer frequently causes bowel obstruction by direct spread to the duodenum. Some patients may present with obstructive symptoms secondary to intestinal dysmobility or pseudo-obstruction. This condition may be caused by opioid medications, by denervation caused by celiac plexus infiltration, or by paraneoplastic syndrome.[135] The symptoms of bowel obstruction include abdominal pain, nausea, vomiting, and abdominal distension. Diagnosis is based on clinical suspicion as well as on abdominal radiography and ultrasonography, and in some cases, computed axial tomography offers the best diagnostic tool.[136]

Management of Bowel Obstruction

Initial stabilization should be done to restore major indices. It includes hydration, correcting electrolyte imbalances, and insertion of a nasogastric tube to relieve symptoms.[137]

Functional obstruction or pseudo-obstruction is usually dealt with by minimizing or discontinuing medications and by treating constipation aggressively. Sometimes a prokinetic agent such as metoclopramide is employed to resume bowel function.

Mechanical bowel obstruction can be dealt with by resection and anastomosis where indicated. In pancreatic cancer, a commonly employed procedure is gastrojejunostomy to provide palliative bypass to relieve obstruction. Occasionally, a self-expandable metal stent may be employed, where surgery is deemed not appropriate.[138] However, more commonly, a percutaneous endoscopic gastrostomy tube is employed to relieve obstructive symptoms for prolonged use. It avoids laparotomy, has a low morbidity, and can be employed at the bed side.[139,140]

Medical management is started when the diagnosis is made. It is continued in patients who are not surgical candidates. Pain is typically managed by opioid medications. Parenteral ketorolac for a short period of time may be a useful opioid-sparing anti-inflammatory medication. It does not interfere with bowel motility and is particularly useful in the opioid bowel syndrome.[141]

Antiemetics and medications that reduce gastrointestinal secretions are very useful to manage nausea and vomiting. Antiemetics, including prokinetics such metoclopramide, neuroleptics such as haloperidol, antihistamines such as cyclizine, and corticosteroids,[142,143] are sometimes very useful for nausea and vomiting. Drugs that decrease secretions include anticholinergics such as hyoscyamine butylbromide and glycopyrrolate, and somatostatin analogues such as octreotide are very useful to decrease copious secretions, indirectly helping with pain, nausea, and vomiting.[144,145] Octreotide modulates gastrointestinal function by reducing gastric acid secretion, slowing intestinal motility, decreasing bile flow, and reducing splanchnic blood flow. The effective dose of octreotide ranges from 0.2 to 0.9 mg daily, with a duration of action of 8–12 hours. In a randomized trial between octreotide and hyoscyamine, the octreotide group showed a significant improvement in nausea, vomiting, anorexia, and pain.[146,147] The role of total parenteral nutrition (TPN) is controversial.[148] In pancreatic cancer patients with advanced disease presenting with inoperable obstruction, TPN probably should not be employed, as it does not add to quality of life. However, simple hydration should be maintained to improve nausea and drowsiness and to prevent accumulation of opioid metabolites and associated delirium.[149]

Hydration

"To hydrate or not" is the topic that surfaces many times in a terminal situation by both the healthcare providers and patients and family members. The traditional medical model always supported the maintenance of intravenous fluids in patients who are terminal.[150,151] In a study at a tertiary-care teaching hospital, 73 of 106 patients died with an intravenous line running.[152] This practice was challenged by some palliative care providers.[153] The negative effect of hydration in terminal patients was based mostly on anecdotal evidence rather than on a scientifically tested data.[154-156] Other anecdotal evidence, however, pointed to the beneficial effect of hydration in terminal patients.[157] Dehydration could lead to delirium, exacerbate opioid side effects, and worsen other symptoms such as constipation, fatigue, and hypercalcemia. Although many patients die peacefully without parenteral fluids, there is some consensus on the need for individualized management.[158,159]

Assessment

Symptoms of dehydration may include fatigue, confusion/delirium, constipation, and dry mouth. The physical examination may reveal drowsiness or confusion, poor skin turgor, decreased jugular venous pressure, dry mucous membranes, decreased urinary sodium, elevated hematocrit reflecting hemoconcentration, hypernatremia, elevated blood urea nitrogen, and normal creatinine in early dehydration.

Management

The decision to hydrate a patient is based on individual patient assessment and clinical presentation. Principles include the following:

1. Considering a short therapeutic trial of hydration in cases like confusion
2. Considering maintenance hydration in patients with small bowel obstruction, especially when the overall quality of life is fair
3. Considering the disadvantages of hydration, like maintaining intravenous/subcutaneous lines, issues of care at home and in rural areas, cost, worsening of symptoms in pre-existing congestive heart failure, and discontinued hydration if the symptoms worsen

Methods of Hydration

The options to hydrate the patient depend on the ability of the patient to take fluids orally. Oral fluid intake is the preferred route because of the ease of administration, the low maintenance, and the cost involved. Terminal patients may be unable to take fluids by that route, especially if they are confused and drowsy. In that situation, fluids should be given by an intravenous route (if a pre-existing long intravenous line is already in place) or by a subcutaneous route, which is also known as hypodermoclysis or clysis and is considered the better option by many palliative care specialists.[160-162] Fluids may be administered via clysis either as a bolus or continuous infusion. Advantages of clysis include the following: easy site access, suitability for home administration, ease and safety, ability to use a single site for up to 7 days, and ease of disconnection for the patient's mobility. The method of administration includes normal saline at the rate of 70–100 ml/hour via continuous infusion for rehydration. For maintenance, 2/3 dextrose and 1/3 normal saline at the rate of 40–80 ml/hour or 1000 ml by gravity overnight or a 500-ml bolus twice a day, with each bolus infused over 1 hour can be given. On some occasions, hyaluronidase may facilitate fluid absorption.[163]

Symptom management in pancreatic cancer involves a true interdisciplinary approach because of the multitude of symptoms. Patients usually present in advanced stages, making symptom management a priority for improving and maintaining quality of life. A good symptom-management approach should incorporate appropriate principles to deal with complex symptoms, maintain an open dialogue with patients and families, discuss various options, including treatment options, prognosis, future course, possible symptoms during the treatment process, futility of treatment whenever applicable, and palliative care as a viable option. This can ideally be achieved by involving a palliative care team earlier in the disease trajectory rather than near the end of life.

References

1. World Health Organization. *Cancer Pain Relief and Palliative Care: Report of a WHO Expert Committee* (Technical Bulletin 804:11–12). Geneva, Switzerland: WHO; 1990.
2. Saunders JM, McCorkle R. Models of care for persons with progressive cancer. *Nurs Clin North Am.* 1985;20:365–377.
3. Cummings I. The interdisciplinary team. In: Doyle D, Hanks GWC, MacDonald N, eds. *Oxford Textbook of Palliative Medicine.* 2nd ed. Oxford, UK: Oxford University Press; 1998:20–30.
4. Sindelar WF, Kinsella TJ, Mayer RJ. Cancer of the pancreas. In: DeVita V, Hellman S, Rosenberg SA, eds. *Principles and Practice of Oncology.* Vol 2. Philadelphia: Lippincott; 1985:699.
5. Bruera E, Kuehn N, Miller MJ, Selmser P, MacMillan K. The Edmonton symptom assessment system: a simple method for the assessment of palliative care patients. *J Palliat Care.* 1991;7:6–9.
6. Folstein MF, Folstein S, McHugh PR. "Mini-mental state": a practical method for grading the cognitive state of patients for clinicians. *J Psychiatr Res.* 1975;12:189–198.
7. Mayfield D, McLeod B, Hall P. The CAGE questionnaire: validation of a new alcohol-screening instrument. *Am J Psychiatry.* 1994;131:1121–1123.
8. Krech RL, Walsh D. Symptoms of pancreatic cancer. *J Pain Symptom Manage.* 1991;6:360–367.
9. Foley KM. Pain syndromes in patients with cancer. In: Bonica JJ, Ventafridda V, eds. *Advances in Pain Research and Therapy.* New York: Raven Press; 1979:59–75.
10. Bonica JJ. Cancer pain. In: Bonica JJ, ed. *The Management of Pain.* Philadelphia: Lea & Febiger; 1990:400.
11. Twycross RG, Fairfield S. Pain in far-advanced cancer. *Pain.* 1982;14:303–310.
12. World Health Organization. *Cancer Pain Relief.* Geneva, Switzerland: World Health Organization; 1986.
13. Levin D, Cleeland CS, Dar R. Public attitudes toward cancer pain. *Cancer.* 1985;56:2337–2339.
14. Reber HA. Pancreatic cancer: presentation of the disease, diagnosis and surgical management. *J Pain Symptom Manage.* 1988;3:164–167.
15. Holland JC, Korzun AH, Tross S, et al. Comparative psychological disturbance in patients with pancreatic and gastric cancer. *Am J Psychiatry.* 1986;143:982–986.
16. Joffe RT, Adsett CA. Depression and carcinoma of the pancreas. *Can J Psychiatry.* 1985;30:117–118.
17. Shakin EJ, Holland J. Depression and pancreatic cancer. *J Pain Symptom Manage.* 1988;3:194–198.
18. De Takats G, Walter LE, Lasner J. Splanchnic nerve section for pancreatic pain. *Ann Surg.* 1950;131:44–57.

19. Jacox A, Carr DB, Payne R, et al. *Management of Cancer Pain.* Rockville, MD: U.S. Department of Health and Human Services, Agency for Health Care Policy and Research; 1994. Clinical Practice Guidelines No. 9, AHCPR Publication 94-0592.
20. Burris HA, III, Moore MJ, Andersen J, et al. Improvements in survival and clinical benefit with gemcitabine as first line therapy for patients with advanced pancreas cancer: a randomized trial. *J Clin Oncol.* 1997;15:2403-2413.
21. Whittington R, Dobelbower RR, Mohiuddin M, et al. Radiotherapy of unresectable pancreatic carcinoma: a six-year experience with 104 patients. *Int J Radiat Oncol Biol Phys.* 1981;7:1639–1644.
22. Sindelar WF, Kinsella TJ. Randomized trial of intraoperative radiotherapy in unresectable carcinoma of the pancreas. *Int J Radiat Oncol Biol Phys.* 1986;12:149.
23. Nishimura A, Nakano M, Otsu H, et al. Intraoperative radiotherapy for advanced carcinoma of the pancreas. *Cancer.* 1984;54:2375–2384.
24. Brown DL, Bulley CK, Quiel EL. Neurolytic celiac plexus block for pancreatic cancer pain. *Anesth Analg.* 1987;66: 869–873.
25. Lefkowitz M. Pain management of pancreatic cancer. *J Pain Symptom Manage.* 1989;36:360–367.
26. Eisenberg E, Carr DB, Chalmers TC. Neurolytic celiac plexus block for treatment of cancer pain: a meta-analysis. *Anesth Analg.* 1995;80:290–295.
27. Malone BT, Beye R, Walker J. Management of pain in the terminally ill by administration of epidural narcotics. *Cancer.* 1985;55:438–440.
28. Greenberg HS. Continuous spinal opioid infusion for intractable cancer pain. In: Foley KM, Inturrisi C, eds. *Advances in Pain Research and Therapy.* Vol 8. New York: Raven Press; 1986:351–359.
29. Krames ES, Gershow J, Glassberg A, et al. Continuous infusion of spinally administered narcotics for the relief of pain due to malignant disorders. *Cancer.* 1985;56:696–702.
30. Van Dongen RT, Crul BJ, DeBock M. Long term infusion of morphine and morphine/bupivacaine mixtures in the treatment of cancer pain: a retrospective analysis of 51 cases. *Pain.* 1993;55:119–123.
31. Raja SN, Haythornthwaite JA, Pappagallo M, et el. Opioids versus antidepressants in postherpetic neuralgia: a randomized, placebo-controlled trial. *Neurology.* 2002;59:1015–1021.
32. Rowbotham MC, Twilling L, Davies PS, Reisner L, Taylor K, Mohr D. Oral opioid therapy for chronic peripheral and central neuropathic pain. *N Engl J Med.* 2003;348: 1223–1232.
33. Davis MP, Walsh D. Methadone for relief of cancer pain: a review of pharmacokinetics, pharmacodynamics, drug interactions and protocols of administration. *Support Care Cancer.* 2001;9:63–83.
34. Ripamonti C, Groff L, Brunelli C, Polastri D, Stavrakis A, De Conno F. Switching from morphine to oral methadone in treating cancer pain: what is the equianalgesic dose ratio? *J Clin Oncol.* 1998;16:3216–3221.
35. Ripamonti C, de Conno F, Groff L, et al. Equianalgesic dose/ratio between methadone and other opioid agonists in cancer pain: comparison of two clinical experiences. *Ann Oncol.* 1998;9:79–83.
36. Gorman AL, Elliott KJ, Inturrisi CE. The d-and l-isomers of methadone bind to the non-competitive site on the N-methyl-D-aspartate (NMDA) receptor in rat forebrain and spinal cord. *Neurosci Lett.* 1997;223:5–8.
37. Szeto HH, Inturrisi CE, Houde R, Saal S, Cheigh J, Reidenberg MM. Accumulation of normeperidine, an active metabolite of meperidine, in patients with renal failure of cancer. *Ann Intern Med.* 1977;86:738–741.
38. Portenoy RK, Payne R, Coluzzi P, et al. Oral transmucosal fentanyl citrate (OTFC) for the treatment of breakthrough pain in cancer patients: a controlled dose titration study. *Pain.* 1999;79:303–312.
39. Tennant F, Hermann L. Self-treatment with oral transmucosal fentanyl citrate to prevent emergency room visits for pain crises: patient self-reports of efficacy and utility. *J Pain Palliat Care Pharmacother.* 2002;16:37–44.
40. Galer BS, Coyle N, Pasternak GW, Portenoy RK. Individual variation in the response to different opioids—report of five cases. *Pain.* 1992;49:87–91.
41. Hanks G, Forbes K. Opioid responsiveness. *Acta Anesthesiol Scand.* 1997;41:154–158.
42. Lane NE. Pain management in osteoarthritis: the role of COX-2 inhibitors. *J Rheumatol.* 1997;24:20–24.
43. Fine PG. The role of rofecoxib, a cyclooxygenase-2-specific inhibitor, for the treatment of non-cancer pain: a review. *J Pain.* 2002;3:272–283.
44. Magni G. The use of antidepressants in the treatment of chronic pain: a review of current evidence. *Drugs.* 1991; 42:730–748.
45. Kolke M, Hoffken K, Olbrich H, Schmidt CG. Antidepressants and anticonvulsants for the treatment of neuropathic pain syndromes in cancer patients. *Onkologie.* 1999;14:40–43.
46. Rowbotham M, Harden N, Stacey B, Bernstein P, Magnus-Miller L. Gabapentin for the treatment of postherpetic neuralgia: a randomized controlled trial. *JAMA.* 1998;280:1837–1842.
47. Backonja M, Beydoun A, Edwards KR, et al. Gabapentin for the symptomatic treatment of painful neuropathy in patients with diabetes mellitus: a randomized controlled trial. *JAMA.* 1998;280:1831–1836.
48. Zakrzewska JM, Chaudhry Z, Nurmikko TJ, Patton DW, Mullens EL. Lamotrigine (Lamictal) in refractory trigeminal neuralgia: results from a double-blind placebo controlled crossover trial. *Pain.* 1997;73:223–230.
49. Brietbart W. Psychotropic adjuvant analgesics for pain in cancer and AIDS. *Psychooncology.* 1998;7:333–345.
50. Patt R, Propper G, Reddy S. The neuroleptics as adjuvants analgesics. *J Pain Symptom Manage.* 1994;9:446–453.
51. Reddy S, Patt RB. The benzodiazepines as adjuvant analgesics. *J Pain Symptom Manage.* 1994;9:510–514.
52. Thiebaud D, Leyvarz S, von Fliedner V, et al. Treatment of bone metastases from breast cancer and myeloma with pamidronate. *Eur J Cancer.* 1991;27:37–41.
53. Berenson JR, Licherstein A, Porter L, et al. Efficacy of pamidronate in reducing skeletal events in patients with advanced multiple myeloma. *N Engl J Med.* 1996;334:488–493.

54. Grant R, Papadopoulos SM, Sandler HM, Greenberg HS. Metastatic epidural spinal cord compression: current concepts and treatment. *J Neurooncol.* 1994;19:79–92.
55. Hortobagyi GN, Theriault RL, Porter L, et al. Efficacy of pamidronate in reducing skeletal complications in patients with breast cancer and lytic bone metastases. *N Engl J Med.* 1996;335:1785–1791.
56. Nagaro T, Shimizu C, Inoue H, et al. The efficacy of intravenous lidocaine on various types of neuropathic pain. *Masui.* 1995;44:862–867.
57. Brose W, Cousins M. Subcutaneous lidocaine for the treatment of neuropathic cancer pain. *Pain.* 1991;45:145–148.
58. Galer BS, Rowbotham MC, Perander J, et al. Topical lidocaine patch relieves postherpetic neuralgia more effectively than a vehicle topical patch: results of an enriched enrollment study. *Pain.* 1999;80:533–538.
59. Mercadante S, Lodi F, Sapio M, et al. Long-term ketamine subcutaneous infusion in neuropathic cancer pain. *J Pain Symptom Manage.* 1995;10:564–568.
60. Yang CY, Wong CS, Chiang JY, Ho ST. Intrathecal ketamine reduces morphine requirements in patients with terminal cancer. *Can J Anaesth.* 1996;43:379–383.
61. Ellison N, Loprinzi CL, Kugler J, et al. Phase 3 placebo-controlled trial of capsaicin cream in the management of surgical neuropathic pain in cancer patients. *J Clin Oncol.* 1997;15:2974–2980.
62. Crawford ED, Kozlowski JM, Debruyne FM, et al. The use of strontium 89 for palliation of pain from bone metastasis associated with hormone-refractory prostate cancer. *Urology.* 1994;44:481–485.
63. Serafini AN, Houston SJ, Resche I, et al. Palliation of pain associated with metastatic bone cancer using samarium-153 lexidronam: a double blind placebo-controlled clinical trial. *J Clin Oncol.* 1998;16:1574–1581.
64. Reddy S, Zhou LL. Celiac plexus block versus systemic opioid medication in the management of pancreatic cancer pain. In: Evans DB, Pisters PWT, Abbruzzese JL, eds. *Pancreatic Cancer.* New York: Springer-Verlag; 2002.
65. Stone P, Richards M, Hardy J. Fatigue in patients with cancer. *Eur J Cancer.* 1998;34:1670–1676.
66. Jacobsen PB, Hann DM, Azzarello LM, et al. Fatigue in women receiving adjuvant chemotherapy for breast cancer: characteristics, course, and correlates. *J Pain Symptom Manage.* 1999;18:233–242.
67. Cella D, Peterman A, Passik S, et al. Progress toward guidelines for the management of fatigue. *Oncology.* 1998;12: 369–377.
68. Portenoy RK, Itri LM. Cancer-related fatigue: guidelines for evaluation and management. *Oncologist.* 1999;4:1–10.
69. Demetri GD, Kris M, Wade J, et al. Quality of life benefit in chemotherapy patients treated with epoetin alfa is independent of disease response or tumor type: results from a prospective community oncology study. *Oncology.* 1998;16:3412–3425.
70. Bruera E, Roca E, Cedaro L, et al. Action of oral methyl prednisolone in terminal cancer patients: a prospective randomized double-blind study. *Cancer Treat Rep.* 1985; 69:751–754.
71. Tannock I, Gospodarowicz M, Meakin W, et al. Treatment of metastatic prostate cancer with low dose prednisone: evaluation of pain and quality of life as pragmatic indices of response. *J Clin Oncol.* 1989;7:590–597.
72. Bruera E, Brenneis C, Paterson AH, Mac Donald RN. Use of methylphenidate as an adjuvant to narcotic analgesics in patients with advanced cancer. *J Pain Symp Manage.* 1989;4:3–6.
73. Breitbart W, Mermelstein H. An alternative psychostimulant for the management of depressive disorders in cancer patients. *Psychosomatics.* 1992;33:352–356.
74. Katon W, Raskind M. Treatment of depression in the medically ill elderly with methylphenidate. *Am J Psychiatry.* 1980;137:963–965.
75. Rajagopal A, Vassilopoulou-Sellin R, Palmer JL, Kaur G, Bruera E. Symptomatic hypogonadism in male survivors of cancer with chronic exposure to opioids. *Cancer.* 2004;100:851–858.
76. Bruera E, Driver L, Barnes EA, et al. Patient-controlled methylphenidate for the management of fatigue in patients with advanced cancer: a preliminary report. *J Clin Oncol.* 2003;23:4439–4443.
77. Wasserman K, Casaburi R. Dyspnea and physiological and athophysiological mechanisms. *Annu Rev Med.* 1988;39: 503–515.
78. Farncombe M. Dyspnea: assessment and treatment. *Support Care Cancer.* 1997;5:94–99.
79. Hardy JR, Turner R, Saunders M, A'Hern R. Prediction of survival in a hospital-based continuing care unit. *Eur J Cancer.* 1994;30:284–288.
80. Escalante CP, Martin CG, Elting LS, et al. Dyspnea in cancer patients: etiology, resource utilization, and survival. *Cancer.* 1996;78:1314–1319.
81. Anthonisen NR. Long-term oxygen therapy. *Ann Intern Med.* 1983;99:519–527.
82. Nocturnal Oxygen Therapy Trial Group. Continuous or nocturnal oxygen therapy in hypoxemic chronic obstructive lung disease. *Ann Intern Med.* 1980;93:391–398.
83. Bruera E, De Stoutz N, Velasco-Leiva, et al. The effects of oxygen on the intensity of dyspnea in hypoxemic terminal cancer patients. *Lancet.* 1993;342:13–14.
84. Bruera E, Scholler T, MacEachern T. Symptomatic benefit of supplemental oxygen in hypoxemic patients with terminal cancer: the use of the N of 1 randomized control trial. *J Pain Symptom Manage.* 1992;7:365–368.
85. Bruera E, MacEachern T, Ripamonti C, et al. Subcutaneous morphine for dyspnea in cancer patients. *Ann Intern Med.* 1993;119:906–907.
86. Bruera E, MacMillan K, Pither J, et al. The effects of morphine on the dyspnea of terminal cancer patients. *J Pain Symptom Manag.* 1990;5:341–344.
87. Cohen MH, Johnston Anderson A, Krasnow SH, et al. Continuous intravenous infusion of morphine for severe dyspnea. *South Med J.* 1991;84:229–234.
88. Davis CL, Hodder C, Love S, et al. Effect of nebulised morphine and morphine-6-glucuronide on exercise endurance in patients with chronic obstructive pulmonary disease. *Thorax.* 1994;49:393.
89. Farncombe M, Charter S, Gillin A. The use of nebulized opioids for breathlessness: a chart review. *Palliat Med.* 1994;8:306–312.
90. Farncombe M, Chater S. Clinical application of nebulized opioids for treatment of dyspnoea in patients with malignant disease. *Support Care Cancer.* 1994;2:184–187.

91. Zeppetella G. Nebulized morphine in the palliation of dyspnoea. *Palliat Med.* 1997;11:267–275.
92. Coyne PJ, Viswanathan R, Smith TJ. Nebulized fentanyl citrate improves patients' perception of breathing, respiratory rate, and oxygen saturation in dyspnea. *J Pain Symptom Manage.* 2002;23:157–160.
93. Weir DC, Gove RI, Robertson AS, et al. Corticosteroids trials in nonasthmatic chronic airflow obstruction: a comparison of oral prednisolone and inhaled beclomethasone dipropionate. *Thorax.* 1991;45:112–117.
94. Congleton J, Meurs MF. The incidence of airflow obstruction in bronchial carcinoma, its relation to breathlessness, and response to bronchodilator therapy. *Respir Med.* 1995;89:291–296.
95. Neil PA, Morton PB, Stark RD. Chlorpromazine: a special effect on breathlessness? *Br J Clin Pharmacol.* 1985;19: 793–797.
96. Lipowski ZJ. Delirium (acute confusional states). *JAMA.* 1987;258:1789–1792.
97. Rabins PV. Psychosocial and management aspects of delirium. *Int Psychogetriatr.* 1991;3:319–324.
98. Derogatis LR, Morrow GR, Fetting J, et al. The prevalence of psychiatric disorders among cancer patients. *JAMA.* 1983;249:751–757.
99. Levine PM, Silberfarb PM, Lipowski ZJ. Mental disorders in cancer patients: a study of 100 psychiatric referrals. *Cancer.* 1978;42:1385–1391.
100. Stiefel F, Finsinger R, Bruera E. Acute confusional states in patients with advanced cancer. *J Pain Symptom Manage.* 1992;7:94–98.
101. Lipowski ZJ. Delirium in the elderly patient. *N Engl J Med.* 1989;320:578–582.
102. Liptzin B, Levkoff SE. An empirical study of delirium subtypes. *Br J Psychiatry.* 1992;161:843–845.
103. American Psychiatric Association. *Diagnostic and Statistical Manual of Mental Disorders.* 4th ed. Washington, DC: American Psychiatric Association; 1994.
104. Voruganti L, Cortese L, et al. Switching from conventional to novel antipsychotic drugs: results of a prospective naturalistic study. *Schizophr Res.* 2002;57(2–3)201–208.
105. Brietbart W, Marotta R, Platt MM, et al. A double-blinded trial of haloperidol, chlorazepam, and lorazepam in the treatment of delirium in the hospitalized AIDS patients. *Am J Psychiatry.* 1996;153:231–237.
106. Derogatis LR, Marrow GR, Fettig J, et al. The prevalence of psychiatric disorders among cancer patients. *JAMA.* 1983;249:751–757.
107. Wilson KG, Chochinov HM, de Faye B, et al. Diagnosis and management of depression in palliative care. In: Chochinov HM, Breitbart W, eds. *Handbook of Psychiatry in Palliative Care.* Oxford, UK: Oxford University Press; 2000:25–49, 106.
108. Green AI, Austin PV. Psychopathology of pancreatic cancer: a psychobiologic probe. *Psychosomatics.* 1993;34:208.
109. Massie MJ, Holland J. The cancer patient with pain; psychiatric complications and their management. *Med Clin North Am.* 1987;71:243.
110. Fisch MJ, Loehrer PJ, Kristeller J, et al. Fluoxetine versus placebo in advanced cancer outpatients: a double-blinded trial of the Hoosier Oncology Group. *J Clin Oncol.* 2003;21:1937–1943.
111. Bonsignore M, Barkow K, Jessen F, Heun R. Validity of the five item WHO Well Being Index (WHO-5) in an elderly population. *Eur Arch Psychiatry Clin Neurosci.* 2001;251(Suppl 2):II27–II31.
112. Kroenke K, Spitzer RL, Williams JB. The PHQ-9: validity of a brief depression severity measure. *J Gen Intern Med.* 2001;16:606–613.
113. Massie MJ, Popkin MK. Depressive disorders. In: Holland JC, ed. *Psycho-Oncology.* New York: Oxford University Press; 1998:518–540.
114. Holland JC, Morrow G, Schmale A, et al. Reduction of anxiety and depression in cancer patients by alprazolam or by a behavioural technique [abstract]. *Proc Am Soc Clin Onco*l. 1988;6:A258.
115. Vickers AJ, Cassileth BR. Unconventional therapies for cancer and cancer-related symptoms. *Lancet Oncol.* 2001;2:226–232.
116. Pereira J, Bruera E. Depression with psychomotor retardation: diagnostic challenges and the use of psychostimulants. *J Palliat Med.* 2001;4:15–21.
117. Theobald DE, Kirsh KL, Holtsclaw E, Donaghy K, Passik SD. An open-label, crossover trial of mirtazapine (15 and 30 mg) in cancer patients with pain and other distressing symptoms. *J Pain Symptom Manage.* 2002;23:442–447.
118. Kast R. Mirtazapine may be useful in treating nausea and insomnia of cancer chemotherapy. *Support Care Cancer.* 2001;9:469–470.
119. Sykes NP. Constipation and diarrhoea. In: Doyle D, Hanks GWC, MacDonald N, eds. *Oxford Textbook of Palliative Medicine.* 2nd ed. Oxford, UK: Oxford University Press; 2001:513–526.
120. Mancini I, Bruera E. Constipation in advanced cancer patients. *Support Care Cancer.* 1998;6:356–364.
121. Mercadante S. Diarrhea, malabsorption and constipation. In: Berger AM, Portenoy RK, Weismann DE, eds. *Principles and Practice of Supportive Oncology.* Philadelphia: Lippincott-Raven; 1998:191–206.
122. Mercadante S, Casuccio A, Fulfaro F. The course of symptom frequency and intensity in advanced cancer patients followed at home. *J Pain Symptom Manage.* 2000;20:104–112.
123. Bruera E, Suarez-Almazor M, Velasco A, Bertolino M, MacDonald SM, Hanson J. The assessment of constipation in terminal cancer patients admitted to a palliative care unit: a retrospective review. *J Pain Symptom Manage.* 1994;9:515–519.
124. Sykes NP. An investigation of the ability of oral naloxone to correct opioid-related constipation in patients with advanced cancer. *Palliat Med.* 1996;10:135–144.
125. Latasch L, Zimmerman M, Eberhart B, et al. Oral naloxone antagonizes morphine-induced constipation. *Anesthetist.* 1997;46:191–194.
126. Meissner W, Schimdt U, Hartman M, et al. Oral naloxone reverses opioids-associated constipation. *Pain.* 2000;84: 105–109.
127. Yuan CS, Foss JF, O'Connor M, Osinski J, Karrison T, Moss J, Roizen MF. Methylnaltrexone for reversal of constipation due to chronic methadone use: a randomized controlled trial. *JAMA.* 2000;283:367–372.

128. Stephenson J. Methylnaltrexone reverses opioid-induced constipation. *Lancet Oncol.* 2002;3:202.
129. Mannix KA. Palliation of nausea and vomiting. In: Doyle D, Hanks GWC, MacDonald N, eds. *Oxford Textbook of Palliative Medicine.* 2nd ed. Oxford, UK: Oxford University Press; 2001:489–499.
130. Driver LC, Bruera E. *The M.D. Anderson Palliative Care Handbook.* Houston, Texas: M.D. Anderson Cancer Center, 2000.
131. Bruera ED, Roca E, Cedaro L, et al. Improved control of chemotherapy-induced emesis by the addition of dexamethasone to metoclopramide in patients resistant to metoclopramide. *Cancer Treat Rep.* 1983;67:381–383.
132. Mercadante S, Fulfaro F, Casuccio A. The use of corticosteroids in home palliative care. *Support Care Cancer.* 2001;9:386–389.
133. Shone DN, Nikoomanesh P, Smith-Meek MM, et al. Malignancy is the most common cause of gastric outlet obstruction in the era of H_2 blockers. *Am J Gastroenterol.* 1995;90:1769–1770.
134. Andersson A, Bergdahl L. Carcinoma of the pancreas. *Am Surg.* 1976;42:173–177.
135. Lautenbach E, Lichenstein GR. Retroperitoneal leiomyosarcoma and gastroparesis: a new association and review of tumor-associated intestinal pseudo-obstruction. *Am J Gastroenterol.* 1995;90:1338–1341.
136. Suri S, Gupta S, Sudhakar PJ, et al. Comparative evaluation of plain films, ultrasound and CT in the diagnosis of intestinal obstruction. *Acta Radiol.* 1999;40:422–428.
137. Baines MJ. The pathophysiology and management of malignant intestinal obstruction. In: Doyle D, Hanks GW, MacDonald N, eds. *Oxford Textbook of Palliative Medicine.* Oxford, UK: Oxford Medical Publications; 1999:526–533.
138. Singh S, Gagneja HK. Stents in the small intestine. *Curr Gastroenterol Rep.* 2002;4:383–391.
139. Malone JM, Koonce T, Larson DM, et al. Palliation of small bowel obstruction by percutaneous gastrostomy in patients with progressive ovarian carcinoma. *Obstet Gynecol.* 1986;68:431–433.
140. Campagnutta E, Cannizzaro R, Gallo A, et al. Palliative treatment of upper intestinal obstruction by gynecological malignancy: the usefulness of percutaneous endoscopic gastrostomy. *Gynecol Oncol.* 1996;62:103–105.
141. Joishy SK, Walsh D. The opioids-sparing effects of intravenous ketorolac as an adjuvant analgesic in cancer pain: application in bone metastases and the opioids bowel syndrome. *J Pain Symptom Manage.* 1998;16:334–339.
142. Feuer DJ, Broadley KE. Systematic review and meta-analysis of corticosteroids for the resolution of malignant bowel obstruction in advanced gynecological and gastrointestinal cancers. *Ann Oncol.* 1999;10:1035–1042.
143. Medecin LG, Girardier J, Lassauniere JM, et al. The use of steroids in the management of inoperable intestinal obstruction in terminal cancer patients: do they remove the obstruction? *Palliat Med.* 2000;14:3–10.
144. Davis M, Furst A. Glycopyrrolate: a useful drug in the palliation of mechanical bowel obstruction. *J Pain Symptom Manage.* 1999;13:153–154.
145. Ripamonti C, Mercadante S, Groff L. A role of octreotide, scopolamine butylbromide and hydration in symptom control of patients with inoperable bowel obstruction having a nasogastric tube: a prospective randomized clinical trial. *J Pain Symptom Manage.* 2000;19:23–34.
146. Mystakidou K, Tsilika E, Ourania K, et al. Comparison of octreotide administration vs. conservative treatment in the management of inoperable bowel obstruction in patients with far advanced cancer: a randomized, double-blind, controlled clinical trial. *Anticancer Res.* 2002; 22:1187–1192.
147. Ripamonti C, Panzeri C, Groff L, et al. The role of somatostatin and octreotide in bowel obstruction: pre-clinical and clinical results. *Tumori.* 2001;87:1–9.
148. Pasanisi F, Orban A, Scalfi L, et al. Predictors of survival in terminal-cancer patients with irreversible bowel obstruction receiving home parenteral nutrition. *Nutrition* 2001;17:581–584.
149. Fainsinger RL, Spachynski K, Hanson J, Bruera E. Symptom control in terminally ill patients with malignant bowel obstruction (MBO). *J Pain Symptom Manage.* 1994;9:12–18.
150. Micetich KC, Steinecker PH, Thomasma DC. Are intravenous fluids morally required for a dying patient? *Arch Intern Med.* 1983;143:975–978.
151. Siegler M, Weisbard AJ. Against the emerging stream: should fluids and nutritional support be discontinued? *Arch Intern Med.* 1985;145:129–131.
152. Hamdy RC, Braverman AM. Ethical conflicts in long-term care of the aged. *Br Med J.* 1980;280:717.
153. Burge FI. Dehydration and provision of fluids in palliative care: what is the evidence? *Can Fam Physician.* 1996;42:2383–2388.
154. Twycross RG. Symptom control: the problem areas. *Palliat Med.* 1993;7:1–8.
155. Andrews M, Bell ER, Smith SA, Tischler JF, Veglia JM. Dehydration in terminally ill patients: is it appropriate palliative care? *Postgrad Med.* 1993;93:201–208.
156. Sullivan RJ Jr. Accepting death without artificial nutrition or hydration. *J Gen Intern Med.* 1993;8:220–224.
157. Yan E, Bruera E. Parenteral hydration of terminally ill cancer patients. *J Palliat Care.* 1991;7:40–43.
158. Fainsinger R, Bruera E. The management of dehydration in terminally ill patients. *J Palliat Care.* 1994;10:55–59.
159. Berger EY. Nutrition by hypodermoclysis. *J Am Geriatr Soc.* 1984;32:199–203.
160. Bruera E, Legris MA, Kuehn N, Miller MJ. Hypodermoclysis for the administration of fluids and narcotic analgesics in patients with advanced cancer. *J Pain Symptom Manage.* 1990;5:218–220.
161. Hays H. Hypodermoclysis for symptom control in terminal cancer. *Can Fam Phys.* 1985;31:1253–1256.
162. Fainsinger RL, MacEachern T, Miller M J, et al. The use of hypodermoclysis for rehydration in terminally ill cancer patients. *J Pain Symptom Manage.* 1994;9:298–302.
163. Constans T, Dutertre JP, Froge E. Hypodermoclysis in dehydrated elderly patients: local effects with and without hyaluronidase. *J Palliat Care.* 1991;7:10–12.

CHAPTER

35

Supportive Care: Cachexia and Anorexia Syndrome

Michael J. Tisdale, PhD

Adenocarcinoma of the pancreas is responsible for about 5% of all cancer-related deaths in the western world.[1] The average survival time, in the absence of treatment, is only 4.2 months, and in patients with distant metastasis, the survival duration is generally less than 3 months. Even with treatment with the most effective therapy, which is with the nucleoside analogue gemcitabine, alone or combined with other chemotherapeutic agents, the average survival time is extended to only about 7 months.[2] The main problem is that most patients present with disease that is beyond the scope of surgical intervention. In addition, a high proportion (85%) experience cachexia,[3] a progressive wasting syndrome, involving loss of adipose tissue and skeletal muscle mass, although visceral protein appears to be preserved.[4] Loss of skeletal muscle reflects decreases in both cellular mass and intracellular potassium concentration, indicating a bioenergetic deficit.

Although anorexia and malabsorption are important factors contributing to the weight loss observed in patients with pancreatic cancer, the degree of wasting cannot be explained by the reduction in nutrient intake alone. Indeed, cachexia can occur in the absence of anorexia.[5] However, in patients with pancreatic cancer, there is a relationship between calorie intake and survival.[6] Thus, survival was found to be significantly longer for high- versus low-calorie intake groups (50 vs 32 days). This may also reflect the degree of involvement of the tumor and the extent of metastases.

Progressive changes in nutritional status have been investigated in a group of patients with pancreatic cancer from the time of diagnosis to a time point close to death.[7] Such patients had lost 15% of their pre-illness stable weight by the time of diagnosis, and this weight loss continued to progress with a median weight loss of 25% by the time of death. During this period, lean body mass fell from 43.4 to 40.1 kg and fat from 12.5 to 9.6 kg. Nutritional depletion is associated with reduced resistance to infection, muscle weakness, and impaired healing.[8,9] The morbidity and mortality associated with undernutrition has been related to loss of total body protein, and this is reflected by the high incidence of hypostatic pneumonia as the terminal event in starvation.[10]

Weight loss also accounts for the poor therapeutic response of pancreatic cancer to chemotherapy. A study of the outcomes of patients with or without weight loss and treated for locally advanced or metastatic tumors of numerous sites, including the pancreas, showed that although patients with weight loss received lower chemotherapy doses initially, they experienced more frequent and severe dose-limiting toxicity than patients who did not experience weight loss.[11] Thus, patients who had weight loss received on average of 1 month less treatment. In addition, weight loss correlated with shorter failure-free and overall survival, decreased response, quality of life and performance status. Patients who stopped losing weight had a better overall survival. Thus, knowledge of the mechanism of cachexia and anorexia syndrome may lead to effective therapeutic intervention with a consequent improvement in quality of life and survival time of patients with pancreatic cancer.

Anorexia and Cachexia

Although diminished dietary intake has been regularly noted in progressive cancer, there are few quantitative measurements of dietary intake and little evidence to support a role between anorexia and cachexia. Thus, a study of dietary intake of energy and macronutrients from a 4-day food record of 297 unselected cancer patients found that weight loss could not be accounted for by diminished dietary intake, because energy intake in absolute amounts was not different, and intake per kilogram body weight was greater in weight-losing patients than in weight-stable patients.[5] These results are similar to those seen in mice bearing an experimental cachexia-inducing tumor (MAC16), in which food intake per gram of body weight remained constant, despite loss of up to 30% of body weight[12] and suggests that food intake decreases to match the new body weight. In animal experiments, pair feeding does not lead either to the same extent of weight loss or to the metabolic abnormalities seen in tumor-bearing animals. Indeed, the changes in cachexia resemble those found in infection and injury rather than in starvation. In starvation, skeletal muscle is preserved, and the body utilizes fatty acids and ketone bodies as a source of energy. In anorexia nervosa, most of the weight loss arises from fat and only a small amount from muscle,[13] whereas in cachexia, there is approximately equal loss from each compartment[4] (Fig. 35.1).

Attempts to reverse wasting by nutritional supplementation have not produced a stable weight gain representing lean body mass, as also observed in patients with human immunodeficiency virus or sepsis. Any weight gain was transient and was composed of water and fat rather than lean body mass.[14] Attempts at pharmacologic manipulation of appetite have also been unsuccessful. Thus, medroxyprogesterone acetate given to patients with advanced malignant disease caused a significant improvement in appetite, but this did not result in weight gain or improved performance status (as determined by the Karnofsky index), energy levels, mood, or relief of pain.[15] Another progesterone and appetite stimulant, megestrol acetate, does improve body weight, at least in some subjects,[16] but as with nutritional supplementation, the gained weight was due to adipose tissue and water, with no significant effect on fat-free mass.[17] Other appetite stimulants, such as dronabinol, a cannabinoid,[18] and cyproheptadine, which increases serotonergic activity in the brain,[19] are also unable to reverse loss of body weight in cancer cachexia.

This effect suggests that anorexia and cachexia may be two separate phenomena requiring different therapeutic approaches. If weight loss in cancer is not due to a reduction in food intake, then other complex metabolic processes must be responsible.

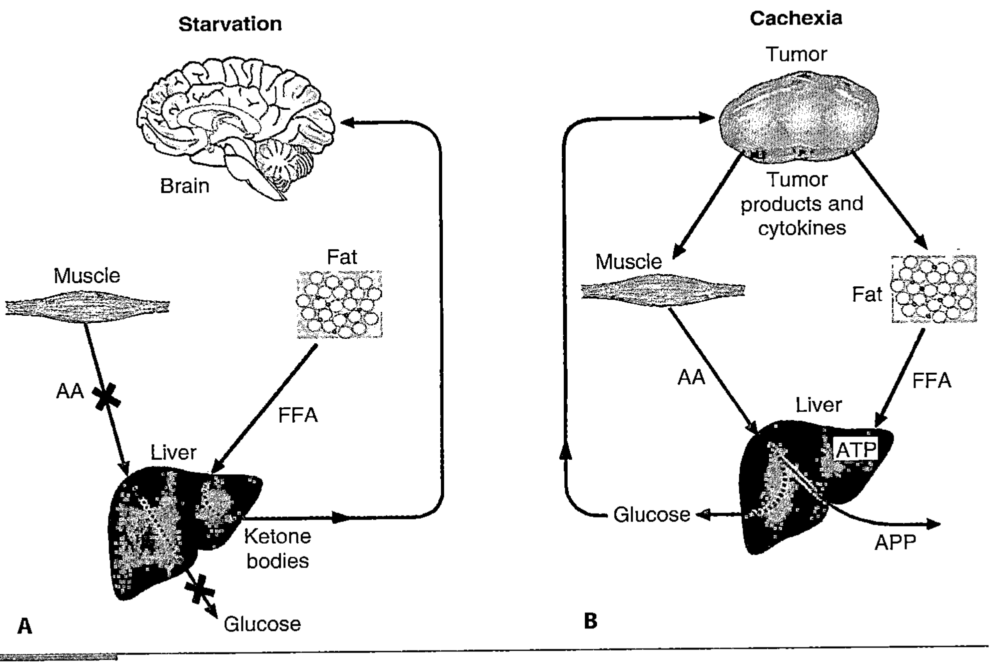

Figure 35.1
(A) In prolonged starvation, gluconeogenesis from amino acids is inhibited and the brain utilizes ketone bodies as a source of energy. **(B)** In cachexia, muscle protein degradation is not inhibited, and the amino acids (AA) provide a source of glucose for the tumor as well as for synthesis of acute-phase proteins (APP). Free fatty acids (FFAs) are used as a source of energy (ATP) by the liver to drive the extra metabolic reactions.

Energy Utilization

Body weight is the result of a balance between energy intake and energy expenditure. If energy intake is not directly responsible for the mass loss during cancer cachexia, then it might be expected that energy expenditure would be increased. In fact, an elevated resting energy expenditure (REE) has a much stronger association with weight loss than energy intake.[5] A major determinant of an increased energy expenditure appears to be tumor type because patients with lung[20] and pancreatic[21] cancer have a significantly greater REE than healthy control subjects, whereas patients with gastric and colorectal cancer showed no increase in REE.[20]

Increased glucose conversion to lactate by certain tumors promotes an increase in Cori cycle activity (lactate to glucose) in the liver, resulting in the consumption of 6 M of adenosine triphosphate for each mole of glucose formed, whereas only 2 M are formed in the conversion of glucose to lactate, which may account for the increase in REE[22] (Fig. 35.1). Although the Cori cycle normally accounts for 20% of glucose turnover, it was increased to 50% in patients with cachectic cancer.[22] It has been estimated that the Cori cycle may account for an additional loss of energy of 300 kcal/day in patients with cancer.[23] In addition to lactate, other substrates (e.g., glycerol) released from adipose tissue through increased lipolysis and certain amino acids released from skeletal muscle by increased proteolysis are important gluconeogenic substrates and contribute to increased hepatic glucose production.

Excess energy may also be dissipated as heat through the action of uncoupling proteins (UCPs), which increase proton transport across the inner mitochondrial membrane not coupled to adenosine triphosphate synthesis, thus constituting an energy sink. The main UCP is UCP1 found in brown adipose tissue (BAT) mitochondria. However, because adult humans contain little BAT, another UCP, UCP3, found in both BAT and skeletal muscle may play a more important role. UCP3 messenger RNA (mRNA) levels have been shown to be five times higher in the rectus abdominis muscle of cancer patients who had lost weight than that in muscle of control subjects and cancer patients who had not lost weight.[24] This increase in UCP3 may enhance energy expenditure and could contribute to tissue catabolism. Transgenic mice overexpressing UCP3 in skeletal muscle weighed less than their wild-type littermates, and there was a large reduction in adipose tissue mass, although they were hyperphagic.[25]

In patients with pancreatic cancer, REE was significantly greater in subjects with an acute-phase response (APR).[21] Increased levels of fibrinogen, an acute-phase reactant, were associated with shortened survival in patients with pancreatic cancer.[26] There is also an association between a chronic inflammatory response and the rate of loss of body mass in lung and gastrointestinal tumors.[27] The APR is a series of physiologic and metabolic changes in response to tissue injury, infection, or inflammation and is activated and modulated by cytokine production. Many cytokines, especially tumor necrosis factor-α (TNF-α), interleukins (IL)-1 and -6, interferon-γ (IFN-γ), Leptin, and leukemia inhibitory factor (LIF) have been considered to play a role in cancer cachexia from studies in animals. Their role, if any, in human cancer cachexia is still open to investigation.

Cytokines and Cachexia

TNF-α

TNF-α was first recognized as an agent capable of producing anorexia and weight loss from studies in trypanosome-infected rabbits, the macrophages of which produced a lipoprotein lipase (LPL)–inhibiting substance called cachectin, which was subsequently purified and shown to be homologous to TNF-α.[28] Although acute administration of TNF-α produced rapid weight loss, tachyphylaxis rapidly developed to subsequent treatment[29]; this could be alleviated by continuous exposure to lower doses of TNF-α by implantation of CHO cells transfected with the gene for human TNF-α.[30] TNF-α was suggested to produce effects on lipid metabolism through inhibition of LPL, thus preventing triglyceride re-synthesis in adipocytes, leading to hypertriglyceridemia. However, hypertriglyceridemia persisted even when animals were resistant to TNF-α–induced weight loss,[29] suggesting that other mechanisms may be operative. It now seems that TNF-α may directly stimulate lipolysis by activation of mitogen-activated protein kinase, extracellular signal-related kinase and elevation of intracellular cyclic AMP.[31] However, at least during the initial phase of weight loss after TNF-α administration in mice, no more weight was lost than that seen in pair-fed animals or those given a cytotoxic drug,[32] unlike the situation in cancer cachexia, in which the weight loss exceeds that seen in pair-fed animals. Interestingly, the effect of TNF-α on body weight loss in experimental animals appears to be dependent on the site of delivery. Thus, when CHO cells transfected with the gene for TNF-α were implanted intracerebrally, hypophagia and weight loss were observed, and the body composition was comparable to that seen in starvation, that is, a decrease of whole body lipid but a conservation of protein.[33] When the cells were transplanted intramuscularly, profound anorexia did not develop, but after a long period of tumor burden (50 days), cachexia developed with depletion of both protein and lipid.

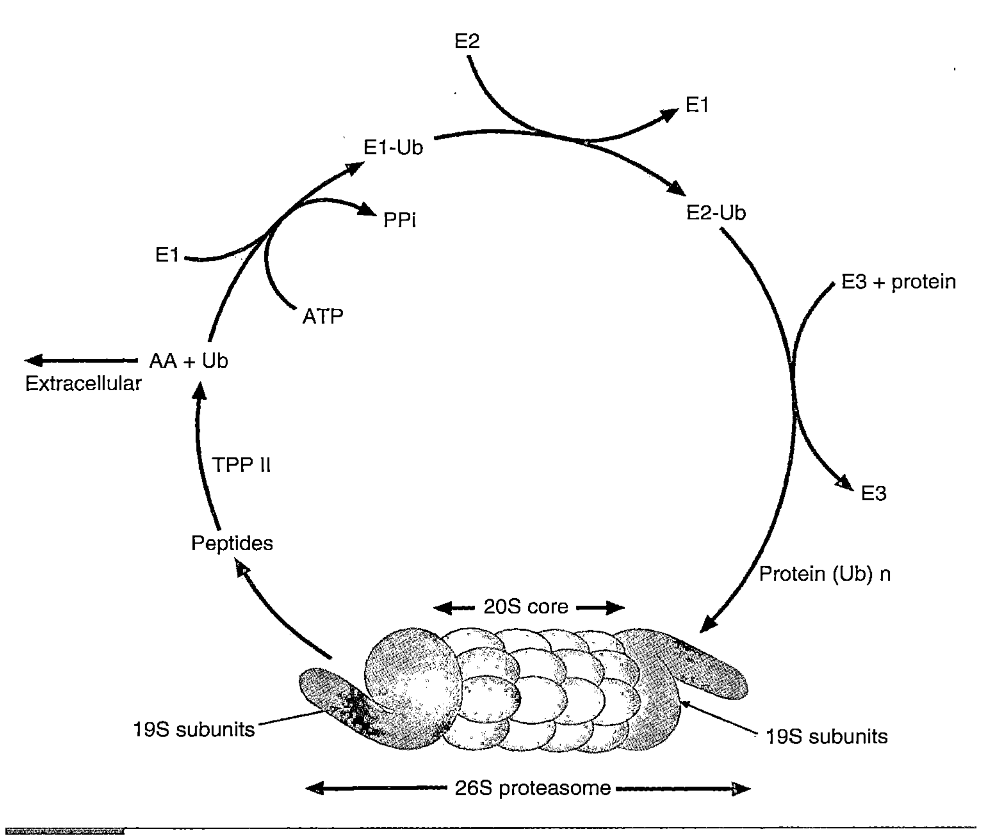

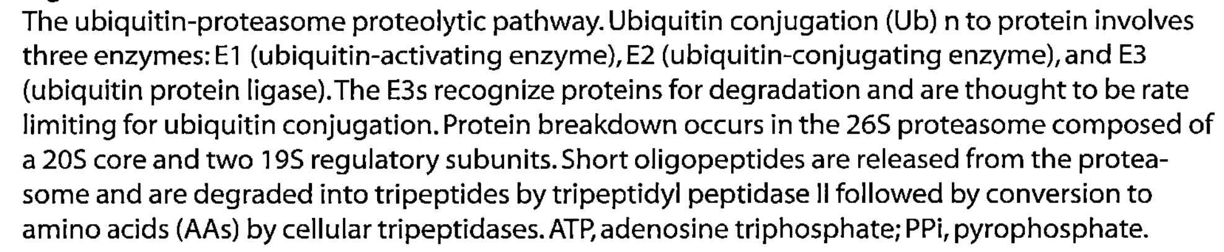
Figure 35.2
The ubiquitin-proteasome proteolytic pathway. Ubiquitin conjugation (Ub) n to protein involves three enzymes: E1 (ubiquitin-activating enzyme), E2 (ubiquitin-conjugating enzyme), and E3 (ubiquitin protein ligase). The E3s recognize proteins for degradation and are thought to be rate limiting for ubiquitin conjugation. Protein breakdown occurs in the 26S proteasome composed of a 20S core and two 19S regulatory subunits. Short oligopeptides are released from the proteasome and are degraded into tripeptides by tripeptidyl peptidase II followed by conversion to amino acids (AAs) by cellular tripeptidases. ATP, adenosine triphosphate; PPi, pyrophosphate.

In vivo studies on cancer patients suggested that TNF-α had no direct metabolic effect on muscle.[34] Thus, glutamine, alanine, phenylalanine, tyrosine, and total amino acid release into the perfusate did not increase during TNF-α treatment, suggesting that systemic metabolic changes were mediated through secondary, centrally produced factors. For some time, there were similar negative reports on the ability of TNF-α to induce direct protein catabolism in isolated muscle. However, more recent studies have shown TNF-α to directly induce protein degradation in murine myotubes through an increase in ubiquitin-dependent proteolysis.[35] In rats bearing the Yoshida AH-130 hepatoma, anti–TNF-α antibody inhibited the increased expression of ubiquitin and C8 proteasome subunit in skeletal muscle,[36] suggesting that TNF-α may be important in activating this proteolytic system during tumor growth.

The ubiquitin-proteasome proteolytic pathway has been considered to be the most important catabolic pathway responsible for intracellular protein degradation in muscle in cancer cachexia in both experimental animals[37,38] and patients with cancer.[39] Other proteolytic pathways, including lysosomal and calcium-activated pathways, contribute less than 15%–20% of total protein breakdown in muscles.[40] However, it has been suggested[41] that the calcium/calpain pathway releases myofilaments from the sarcomere for digestion by the proteasome and that this might be the rate-limiting step in the process. Also, lysosomal proteases, such as cathepsin B, may play a role in inducing muscle wasting during the early stages of lung cancer.[42]

Protein degradation by the ubiquitin system controls the intracellular concentration of many regulatory proteins. Proteins damaged by oxidation or mutation or that misfold or mislocalize are also good substrates for this system. Protein substrates for degradation are marked by the covalent attachment of a polyubiquitin chain, which is recognized by the 26S proteasome (Fig. 35.2). This is a barrel-shaped structure consisting of a 20S core and two 19S particles. A 19S particle mediates the binding and unfolding of a substrate protein, which requires adenosine triphosphate. At least six adenosine triphosphatases are associated with the 20S proteasome and their function is to provide a continuous supply of energy for protein degradation.[43] The 20S proteasome is composed of a stack of four rings: two outer α-rings and two inner β-rings in the order $\alpha\beta\beta\alpha$. The sites for proteolysis are on the inner surface of the β-rings. The proteasome releases short oligopeptides of mean lengths of 6–9 residues, which are further converted into tripeptides by the giant protease tripeptidyl peptidase II. The activity of this enzyme has been reported to be increased in muscle from septic rats,[44] but there have been no reports in cancer cachexia.

The main problem with invoking TNF-α as a mediator of cachexia in humans is that most studies have been unable to detect TNF-α[45] or have found that it did not correlate with weight loss.[46] This is in contrast with other conditions, such as chronic heart failure, in which a significant proportion of patients experience cardiac cachexia, a generalized wasting syndrome with poor prognosis and have increased serum levels of TNF-α.[47] There is also little evidence that TNF-α may act locally, because total LPL activity and messenger RNA for LPL did not differ in adipose tissue between cancer patients and control subjects.[45] In patients with invasive breast cancer, TNF-α correlated with the stage of disease, reflecting tumor size and metastasis.[48] However, in a single report of a study of 63 patients with pancreatic cancer using an enzyme immunoassay specific for TNF-α, investigators found serum levels to be detectable in 36.5% of patients, with higher levels being found in subjects with metastasis and body weight loss.[49] Serum levels of TNF-α inversely correlated with body weight and body mass index. It is not clear why these differences exist, but it would be interesting to determine TNF-α levels in weight-losing patients without metastasis.

IL-6

IL-6 production is a direct mediator of the APR during inflammation,[50] and it has been suggested that peripheral blood mononuclear cells from patients with cancer induce the hepatic APR primarily via an IL-6–dependent mechanism.[51] IL-6 has been implicated in the development of cachexia in mice bearing murine colon-26 adenocarcinoma.[52] Development of cachexia was associated with increasing serum levels of IL-6, whereas a monoclonal antibody to IL-6, but not to TNF-α, significantly suppressed progression of cachexia. However, serum levels of IL-6 were raised in mice into which two clones of this tumor were transplanted (clone 20 [cachexia inducing] and clone 5 [not cachexia inducing]), raising doubts about the role of IL-6 in the development of cachexia.[53] Levels of a tumor catabolic factor, proteolysis-inducing factor (PIF), showed a correlation with cachexia in these variants.[54] Thus, mice bearing the colon-26, clone 20 variant showed evidence for the presence of PIF in tumor, serum, and urine, whereas there was no evidence for the presence of PIF in tumor or body fluids of mice bearing the clone 5 tumors. This suggests that PIF and IL-6 may work together to induce cachexia in this model.[55] A similar conclusion was reached from colon-26 tumors transfected with the gene for IL-10, a cytokine synthesis inhibitory factor. Cachexia was suppressed, although IL-6 levels did not reach baseline, suggesting that an additional unknown factor may be responsible for the development of cachexia in this model.

There is some confusion about the ability of IL-6 to induce loss of muscle and adipose tissue, as observed in cachexia. Thus, atrophy of muscles was observed in IL-6 transgenic mice with increased mRNA levels for cathepsins (B and L) and ubiquitins (poly and mono).[56] However, when IL-6 was repeatedly administered to healthy mice over a 7-day period, there was no effect on food intake or body weight, although it did produce a hepatic APR.[57] Another member of the IL-6 superfamily, ciliary neurotrophic factor (CNTF), produced profound anorexia and lean tissue wasting, together with an APR at the same dose level. This finding suggests that IL-6 alone may not be able to induce tissue wasting and that the APR, although related, was not sufficient to produce cachexia. Both IL-6[58] and CNTF[57] were unable to induce myofibrillar protein degradation in an in vitro assay, suggesting that any effect that occurred was indirect. Llovera et al[59] showed that intravenous administration of TNF-α, IL-1, and IFN-γ caused an increased expression of both the 1.2- and the 2.4-kb ubiquitin mRNA transcripts in skeletal muscle, but that neither LIF nor IL-6 produced any change in ubiquitin gene expression. These results suggest that IL-6 may not be able to induce muscle protein degradation, even in vivo. Indeed, in a phase I study of IL-6 in which patients received between 1 and 10 μg/kg/day, weight loss was not a common side effect, despite a significant increase in acute-phase proteins.[60] Recent research suggests that CNTF appears not to act like a cytokine but instead activates hypothalamic leptin-like pathways in diet-induced obesity models unresponsive to leptin.[61] CNTF can suppress food intake without triggering hunger signals or associated stress responses that are usually associated with food deprivation.

Unlike the situation with TNF-α, significant increases in serum IL-6 have been found in weight-losing patients with non–small-cell lung cancer, when compared with patients with the same tumor but without weight loss.[62] In patients with colon cancer, serum IL-6 levels correlated with the APR.[63] It seems likely that IL-6 alone may be unable to induce the metabolic changes characteristic of cachexia, but it may act as a marker of the extent of the process and the APR.

IL-1

Administration of recombinant IL-1 in mice induces anorexia, weight loss, hypoalbuminemia, and acute-phase proteins.[64] The anorexigenic effect of IL-1 is greater than that of TNF-α, although they share similar effects on adipose tissue, such as suppression of LPL and enhancement of lipolysis. Intratumoral injection of IL-1 receptor antagonist into mice bearing colon-26 tumor was found to significantly reduce cachexia, without an effect on tumor burden.[65] However, tissue depletion and protein hypercatabolism in rats bearing the Yoshida AH-130 ascites hepatoma were unaffected by the administration of the IL-1 receptor antagonist, suggesting that IL-1 is not important in this model system for the development of cachexia.[66] Transfection of colon-26 cells with the gene for the IL-1 receptor antagonist also failed to abolish the capacity of the tumor to produce cachexia.[67] There was no correlation between serum IL-1 levels and cachexia or anorexia from a study of 61 patients with advanced and terminal cancer of several sites, including the pancreas.[46] These results raise doubts about a potential role of IL-1 in human cancer cachexia.

IL-2

IL-2 is another proinflammatory cytokine that may play a role in cancer cachexia. The serum concentration of soluble IL-2 receptor increased with the advance of cancer in patients with gastric and colorectal cancer and was highest in cachectic patients.[68] It was inversely correlated with serum concentrations of nutritional parameters, such as prealbumin and transferrin. In addition, the survival time of cachectic patients inversely correlated with soluble IL-2 receptor. These results suggest that soluble IL-2 receptor may be a marker of cachexia and the APR.

IFN-γ

Severe cachexia develops rapidly in nude mice inoculated with CHO cells constitutively producing mouse IFN-γ.[69] Passive immunization against IFN-γ before tumor cell inoculation prevented the cachexia, but IFN-γ by itself did not cause cachexia because both the release of IFN-γ and the presence of tumor cells were required. Administration of IFN-γ antibody to mice bearing the Lewis lung tumor reduced the depletion of body fat but had no effect on total body protein.[70] Like the other cytokines, IFN-γ inhibits LPL, although it is unlikely that a decrease in LPL alone could account for wasting of adipose tissue seen in cancer cachexia. Like TNF-α, IFN-γ caused an increased expression of the 1.2- and 2.4-kb transcripts of ubiquitin in skeletal muscle, whereas LIF and IL-6 produced no changes.[36] However, there have been no reports on the ability of IFN-γ to directly induce protein degradation in skeletal muscle. As with other cytokines, there is no correlation between serum IFN-γ levels and anorexia or cachexia in patients with advanced cancer.[46] Thus, there is no clear role for IFN-γ in tissue wasting in human cancer cachexia.

Leptin

Leptin is a cytokine secreted from adipocytes that is thought to represent the afferent signal in a feedback mechanism that regulates fat mass. Leptin modulates food intake and energy balance through its actions at specific receptors in the hypothalamus, and TNF-α, IL-6 and IL-1 increase ob gene expression and leptin secretion[71]; therefore, levels might be expected to be increased in cachexia if a local effect of these cytokines on adipose tissue were operative. However, in patients with pancreatic cancer, leptin concentrations, when corrected for body mass index, were lower than those reported for healthy subjects.[72] There was no association between increased leptin concentrations and weight loss or anorexia. In animal models of cachexia, serum leptin levels are proportional to body fat.[73] Thus, as fat levels decrease there is a corresponding decrease in leptin levels.

Tumor Catabolic Factors

The inability of cytokines to satisfy the criteria for the inducers of tissue wasting in cancer cachexia led to the search for tumor catabolic products that could be responsible for the degradation of adipose tissue and skeletal muscle.

Lipid-Mobilizing Factor

Patients with advanced cachexia can lose up to 85% of their total body fat,[4] and this appears to arise from an increase in lipid mobilization. Cancer patients have a high turnover of both glycerol and fatty acids, and the elevated mobilization of fatty acids is often evident before weight loss becomes established.[74] Fasting plasma glycerol concentrations are also much higher in weight-losing cancer patients than in weight-stable individuals.[75] There is also a twofold increase in the relative level of mRNA for hormone-sensitive lipase in adipose tissue of cancer patients compared with control subjects.[45] This results in an increase in serum triacylglycerol and free fatty acid levels. Increased mobilization of fatty acids has been observed, even in the presence of high plasma glucose concentrations,[76] and there is impaired suppression of lipid mobilization as well as continued oxidation of fatty acids on administration of glucose.[77] There is some evidence that the increase in lipid oxidation and energy expenditure may be mediated through a β-adrenergic receptor (β-AR) because the specific β-AR blocker atenolol and the nonspecific β-blocker propranolol significantly reduced REE, whole-body oxygen uptake, and

CO_2 production in weight-losing cancer patients.[78] In addition, patients with weight loss show increased plasma and urinary catecholamines, elevated heart rate, and increased fat oxidation.[75]

A LMF has been isolated from cachexia-inducing tumors of mice and men,[79] which may produce the observed effects on fat metabolism in cancer cachexia. LMF is a glycoprotein of an MW of 43 kDa, showing homology in amino acid sequence and immunoreactively with human plasma zinc α2-glycoprotein (ZAG). ZAG is a glycoprotein that was first isolated from human plasma,[80] and its name is derived from the ability to precipitate with zinc salts and its electrophoretic mobility in the region of the α_2-globulins. ZAG is closely related to antigens of the major histocompatibility complex in amino acid sequence and domain structure, although as a soluble protein, it lacks the amino acid sequence for transmembrane and cytoplasmic domains. Both LMF and ZAG have been shown to stimulate glycerol release from isolated murine epididymal adipocytes with a comparable dose-response profile.[81] Triglyceride hydrolysis occurs by stimulation of adenylate cyclase, and the resulting increase in cyclic adenosine monophosphate activates protein kinase A,[82] as in hormonal stimulation of lipolysis. Stimulation of adenylate cyclase by LMF involved both stimulatory (Gαs) and inhibitory (Gαi) guanine nucleotide-binding proteins.[82] LMF increased expression of Gαs and decreased expression of Gαi in 3T3L1 adipocytes in vitro.[83] Similar changes were seen in adipose tissue of cachectic mice bearing the MAC16 tumor, as well as in patients with cancer. This suggests that LMF may not only stimulate lipolysis directly but may also sensitize adipose tissue to other lipolytic stimuli.

Administration of LMF to obese mice caused weight loss through a specific reduction in carcass lipid, with no change in body water and a small, but nonsignificant, increase in lean body mass.[81] Weight loss was accompanied by decreased blood glucose levels due to increased glucose utilization by the brain, BAT, and skeletal muscle and increased overall lipid oxidation.[84] There was increased oxygen uptake by BAT, providing evidence for increased lipid utilization.[81] LMF induced an increase in mRNA levels for UCP1, 2, and 3 in BAT and an increase in UCP2 in both skeletal muscle and liver,[85] suggesting that it plays an important role in the utilization of excess lipid mobilized during fat catabolism. Thus, LMF not only induces direct lipid catabolism in adipose tissue but also stimulates consumption, with a net energy loss to the host.

Induction of lipolysis and stimulation of adenylate cyclase by LMF was attenuated by the specific β3-AR antagonist SR59230A.[86] LMF was found to bind to the human β3-AR to an extent similar to that of other β3-AR antagonists, although the affinity of binding was about 100-fold less. If LMF is involved in human cancer cachexia, this would explain why β-AR antagonists decreased oxidative metabolism of lipids and REE.[78] Like other β-AR antagonists, LMF stimulated protein synthesis and reduced degradation[87] and thus may play an important role in regulating loss of lean body mass in cancer cachexia.

Proteolysis-Inducing Factor

Wasting of skeletal muscle is associated with a decreased rate of protein synthesis[88] and an increased rate of degradation,[89] leading to elevated whole-body protein turnover,[90] which is apparent even in patients with small tumor burdens. The ubiquitin-proteasome proteolytic pathway appears to be mainly responsible for the increased protein breakdown.[39] Evidence for a circulatory factor capable of inducing muscle protein breakdown was provided from studies in mice bearing the cachexia-inducing MAC16 tumor[91] and from the sera of cancer patients with weight loss.[92]

PIF was purified from the MAC16 tumor and from the urine of patients with cancer cachexia with the use of an antibody cloned from splenocytes of mice with delayed cachexia after transplantation with the MAC16 tumor.[93] PIF was found to be a sulphated glycoprotein of an MW of 24kDa,[94] with extensive *N*- and *O*-glycosidic chains, which were shown to be responsible for both the immunoreactivity and biologic activity. The amino acid sequence of the peptide chain of PIF was found to be distinct from recognized cytokines[93] but has subsequently been shown to be 100% identical to an antimicrobial peptide, called dermicidin,[95] secreted by sweat glands and to Y-P30, a neuronal survival peptide,[96] although neither of these peptides are glycosylated. PIF was originally isolated from the urine of cachectic patients with pancreatic cancer but was also found in the urine of patients with carcinoma of the breast, ovary, lung, rectum, and liver if the weight loss exceeded 1 kg per month.[97] Patients with the same type of cancer but without weight loss showed no evidence of excretion of PIF, as did those with weight loss from causes other than malignancy. A correlation has been observed between PIF expression in gastrointestinal cancers, its detection in the urine, and weight loss.[98] PIF expression was located in the cytoplasm of tumor cells with the use of immunohistochemistry,[98] whereas a study in prostate cancer[99] in which in situ hybridization was used showed mRNA to be localized only in the epithetical cells of the tumor but not in stomal cells or in normal prostatic cells. There was a strong correlation between urinary PIF and development of cachexia in patients with prostatic cancer.[99] PIF was detected in the urine of 80% of patients with pancreatic cancer.[100] These patients had a significantly greater total weight loss and rate of weight loss than patients whose urine did not contain PIF. These results suggest a strong correlation between PIF production by human tumors and development of cancer cachexia.

Administration of PIF, isolated either from the MAC16 tumor[93] or from the urine of patients with pancreatic cancer,[97] to normal mice, produced marked weight loss (about 10%) over a 24-hour period. Body composition analysis showed specific loss of lean body mass,[101] with loss of skeletal muscle, but not visceral reserves,[37] as happens in cancer cachexia. Loss of gastrocnemius muscle resulted from an increase (by 50%) in protein degradation and a decrease (by 50%) in protein synthesis.[101] The effects of PIF were direct because inhibition of protein synthesis and stimulation of protein degradation occurred in murine myoblasts, as a surrogate model of skeletal muscle.[102] PIF produced increased mRNA and protein levels for E2 and proteasome subunits in skeletal muscle both in vitro and in vivo, confirming that it acts directly to stimulate the proteasome proteolytic pathway in muscle cells.[103] In hepatocytes, PIF activated the transcription factors NF-κB and STAT3, which resulted in the increased production of IL-8, IL-6, and C-reactive protein and in the decreased production of transferrin.[104] This suggests that PIF may play a crucial role in the inflammatory state associated with cancer cachexia. In addition, PIF has been shown to up-regulate expression of the cell surface adhesion molecules intracellular adhesion molecule-1 and vascular cell adhesion molecule in endothelial cells.[105] These can be up-regulated by proinflammatory cytokines, such as TNF-α, to mediate the interaction between cells.

PIF expression peaks during the embryonic period E8–E9 in the mouse,[104] which is a crucial stage in the patterning and eventual development of skeletal muscle. Because normal adult tissues do not express PIF, it seems likely that expression is normally switched off before birth, but that some tumor cells can reactivate expression, possibly through mutations that cause expression of a family of glycosidases, which convert the core peptide into a molecule that causes progressive degradation of skeletal muscle.

Treatment of Cachexia

Antagonists of PIF

Both loss of body weight in vivo[106] and protein degradation in vitro[102] induced by PIF are attenuated by treatment with the omega-3 polyunsaturated fatty acid eicosapentaenoic acid (EPA). In vitro studies suggest that EPA antagonizes the release of arachidonic acid from the membrane of muscle cells and the subsequent metabolism to eicosanoids.[102] One metabolite of arachidonic acid 15-hydroxyeicosatetraenoic acid was capable of inducing protein degradation, whereas the others were inactive in this respect. Studies in mice bearing the MAC16 tumor show that EPA effectively attenuates the development of cachexia in this model.[107] Preservation of skeletal muscle was attributed to a significant reduction in protein degradation without an effect on protein synthesis. EPA effectively attenuated the increased expression of key regulatory components of the ubiquitin-proteasome proteolytic pathway in skeletal muscle, possible by acting to prevent transcription.[108]

Administration of pure EPA orally to weight-losing patients with advanced pancreatic cancer effectively attenuated the weight loss, and this stabilization of weight persisted over the 12-week study period.[109] There was also stabilization of the APR. Similar weight stabilization was observed in patients who consumed a mixed triglyceride of EPA that provided about 2 g per day of EPA.[110] There was also stabilization of REE. Although nutritional supplementation alone has been shown to be ineffective in the treatment of cancer cachexia,[14] when patients with pancreatic cancer who experienced a weight loss of 2.9 kg/month consumed a nutritional supplement that provided 600 kcal, 32 g of protein, and 2 g of EPA, significant weight gain was seen at both 3 (median, 1 kg) and 7 weeks (median, 2 kg).[111] The weight gain was attributed solely to an increase in lean body mass. There was also a significant decrease in REE and a significant improvement in performance status and appetite. The production of IL-6 was significantly reduced, as was the proportion of patients excreting PIF in the urine, whereas there was an increase in serum insulin concentration and a decrease in the cortisol-to-insulin ratio.[112] These results suggest that EPA-containing nutritional supplements may be used to effectively reverse the process of cancer cachexia.

Antagonists of TNF-α

The synthetic progestins megestrol and medroxyprogesterone acetate are the major agents used in the treatment of cancer cachexia. Although the mechanism of action may be related to stimulation of appetite via neuropeptide Y in the ventromedial hypothalamus, they may act in part by down-regulating the synthesis and release of cytokines.[113] Thus, medroxyprogesterone acetate reduces levels of IL-1β, IL-6, and TNF-α produced in culture by phytohemagglutinin-stimulated peripheral blood mononuclear cells. A review of 15 randomized clinical trials of high-dose progestin therapy found a significant improvement in both appetite and body weight, although the effect on body weight was less than on appetite.[114] The duration of treatment lasted only 1–12 weeks, which probably overcame some of the side effects of therapy. Long-term treatment (>12 weeks) produced hypertension, edema, and thromboembolic events. This correlated with body composition measurements, which showed that with both megestrol[115] and medroxyprogesterone acetate,[116] the vast majority of the gained weight was due to adipose tissue and water (responsible for most of the weight gain), but there was no significant effect on fat-free mass. Thus, appetite stimulation produces the same effect on body composition as nutritional supplementation.[14]

Pentoxifylline has been reported to decrease TNF-α mRNA levels in patients with cancer, but a clinical trial in 35 patients with lung, gastrointestinal, and other tumors failed to demonstrate any beneficial effect on either anorexia or cachexia.[117]

Thalidomide is currently being evaluated for the treatment of cachexia because of its ability to reduce production of TNF-α by increasing the degradation rate of TNF-α mRNA, and it also blocks NF-κB-regulated genes through suppression of IκB kinase activity.[118] Adjunctive use of thalidomide in human immunodeficiency virus–infected patients receiving treatment for tuberculosis has been shown to promote weight gain.[119] A study of 10 patients with inoperable esophageal cancer administered thalidomide (200 mg daily for 2 weeks) found a gain in both body weight and lean body mass.[120] However, there was no change in food intake, as might be expected if it was working by suppression of TNF-α. Further studies are required to confirm the effectiveness of thalidomide and the mechanism of action.

Anticatabolic Agents

The anticatabolic actions of leucine and its metabolites, such as α-ketoisocaproate and β-hydroxy-β-methylbutyrate, on skeletal muscle result in decreased nitrogen and protein loss by inhibiting protein breakdown.[121] A recent clinical trial examined the effect of β-hydroxy-β-methylbutyrate, together with arginine and glutamine, on body weight and body composition in cachectic cancer patients.[122] There was an increase in bodyweight, which was attributed to an increase in lean body mass, suggesting that catabolism of intracellular proteins may be more important than decreases in protein synthesis in wasting of skeletal muscle in cancer cachexia.

Conclusion

Although cachexia is a complex, multifaceted syndrome, recent research has identified potential mediators of this condition and targets for therapy. Although anorexia frequently accompanies cachexia, it is becoming clear that the reduction of energy intake alone is not responsible for the wasting occurring in cachexia, and that anorexia and cachexia may be distinct and possibly unrelated phenomena. Loss of skeletal muscle is most damaging to the patient in both morbidity and mortality and appears to result from an increased protein breakdown, combined with a reduction in protein synthesis. Future studies will need to concentrate on the mechanisms by which this occurs, as well as the targets for existing therapies, which are successful in alleviating cachexia. Because cachexia results in a shorter-survival time for the patient with cancer, effective therapies would be expected to prolong life as well as improve quality of life. Although the best treatment for cachexia is eradication of the tumor, for many cancers, especially pancreatic cancer, this is not possible at the moment. However, effective treatment for cachexia should have the same benefits for the patient in terms of quality and quantity of life.

References

1. Parkin DM, Whelan SL, Ferlay J, et al. Cancer incidence in five continents. Lyon: IARC; 1997.
2. Oettle H, Arnold D, Hempel C, et al. The role of gemcitabine alone and in combination in the treatment of pancreatic cancer. *Anticancer Drugs.* 2000;11:771–786.
3. De Wys WD, Begg C, Lavin PT, et al. Prognostic effect of weight loss prior to chemotherapy in cancer patients. Am J Med 1980;69:491–497.
4. Fearon KCH. The mechanisms and treatment of weight loss in cancer. *Proc Nutr Soc.* 1992;51:251–265.
5. Bosneus I, Daneryd P, Svanberg E, et al. Dietary intake and resting energy expenditure in relation to weight loss in unselected cancer patients. *Int J Cancer.* 2001;93:380–383.
6. Okusaki T, Okada S, Ishii H, et al. Prognosis of advanced pancreatic cancer patients with reference to calorie intake. *Nutr Cancer.* 1998;32:55–58.
7. Wigmore SJ, Plester CE, Richardson RA, et al. Changes in nutritional status associated with unresectable pancreatic cancer. *Br J Cancer.* 1997;75:106–109.
8. Bistrain BR, Blackburn GL, Scrimshaw NS, et al. Cellular immunity in semistarved states in hospitalized adults. *Am J Clin Nutr.* 1975;28:1148–1155.
9. Jeejeebhoy KN. Muscle function and nutrition. *Gut.* 1986;27:25–39.
10. Moore FD. Energy and maintenance of body cell mass. *J Parent Ent Nutr.* 1980;4:228–259.
11. Andreyev HJN, Norman AR, Oates J, et al. Why do patients with weight loss have a worse outcome when undergoing chemotherapy for gastrointestinal malignancies? *Eur J Cancer.* 1998;4:503–509.
12. McDevitt TM, Tisdale MJ. Tumour associated hypoglycaemia in a murine cachexia model. *Br J Cancer.* 1992;66: 815–820.

13. Moley JF, Aamodt R, Rumble W, et al. Body cell mass in cancer bearing and anorexia patients. *JPEN*. 1987; 11:219–223.
14. Evans WK, Makuch R, Clarnon GH, et al. Limited impact of total parenteral nutrition on nutritional status during treatment for small cell lung cancer. *Cancer Res*. 1985; 45:3347–3353.
15. Downer S, Joel S, Albright A, et al. A double blind placebo controlled trial of medroxyprogesterone acetate (MPA) in cancer cachexia. *Br J Cancer.* 1993;67:1102–1105.
16. Maltoni M, Nanni O, Scarpi E, et al. High-dose progestins for the treatment of cancer anorexia-cachexia syndrome: a systematic review of randomised clinical trials. *Ann Oncol*. 2001;12:289–300.
17. Loprinzi CL, Schaid DJ, Dose AM, et al. Body composition changes in patients who gain weight while receiving megestrol acetate. *J Clin Oncol*. 1993;11:152–154.
18. Wadleigh R, Spaulding GM, Lumbersky B, et al. Dronabinol enhancement of appetite and cancer patients. *Proc Am Soc Oncol*. 1990;9:331.
19. Kardinal CG, Loprinzi CL, Schaid DJ, et al. A controlled trial of cyproheptadine in cancer patients with anorexia and/or cachexia. *Cancer.* 1990;65:2657–2661.
20. Fredrix EWHM, Soeters PB, Wouters EFM, et al. Energy balance in relation to cancer cachexia. *Clin Nutr.* 1990;9:319–324.
21. Falconer JS, Fearon KCH, Plester CE, et al. Cytokines, the acute-phase response and resting energy expenditure in cachectic patients with pancreatic cancer. *Ann Surg*. 1994;219:325–331.
22. Holroyde CP, Gabuzda TG, Putnam RC, et al. Altered glucose metabolism in metastatic carcinoma. *Cancer Res*. 1975;35:3710–3715.
23. Eden E, Edstrom S, Bennegard K, et al. Glucose flux in relation to energy expenditure in malnourished patients with and without cancer during periods of fasting and feeding. *Cancer Res*. 1984;45:1718–1724.
24. Collins P, Bing C, McColloch P, et al. Muscle UCP-3 mRNA levels are elevated in weight loss associated with gastrointestinal adenocarcinoma in humans. *Br J Cancer.* 2002;86:372–375.
25. Clapham JC, Arch JRS, Chapman H, et al. Mice overexpressing human uncoupling protein-3 in skeletal muscle are hyperphagic and lean. *Nature*. 2000;406:415–418.
26. Preston T, Slater C, McMillan DC, et al. Fibrinogen synthesis is elevated in fasting cancer patients with an acute phase response. *J Nutr.* 1998;128:1355–1360.
27. McMillan DC, Scott HR, Watson WS, et al. Longitudinal study of body cell mass depletion and the inflammatory response in cancer patients. *Nutr Cancer.* 1998;31:101–105.
28. Beutler B, Greenwald D, Hulmes JD, et al. Identity of tumour necrosis factor and the macrophage-secreted factor cachectin. *Nature*. 1985;316:552–554.
29. Grunfeld C, Wiking H, Neese R, et al. Persistence of the hypertriglyceridemic effect of tumor necrosis factor despite development of tachyphylaxis to its anorectic/cachectic effect in rats. *Cancer Res*. 1989;49:2554–2560.
30. Oliff A, Defo-Jones D, Boyer M, et al. Tumours secreting human TNF/cachectin induce cachexia in mice. *Cell*. 1987;50:555–563.
31. Zhang HH, Halbleib M, Ahmad F, et al. Tumour necrosis factor-α stimulates lipolysis in differentiated human adipocytes through activation of extracellular signal-related kinase and elevation of intracellular cyclic AMP. *Diabetes*. 2002;51:2929–2935.
32. Mahony SM, Tisdale MJ. Induction of weight loss and metabolic alterations by human recombinant tumour necrosis factor. *Br J Cancer.* 1988;58:345–349.
33. Tracey KJ, Morgello S, Kopin B, et al. Metabolic effects of cachectic/tumor necrosis factor are modified by site of production. *J Clin Invest*. 1990;86:2014–2024.
34. DeBlaauw I, Eggermont AMM, Deutz NEP, et al. TNF-α has no direct in vivo metabolic effect in human muscle. *Int J Cancer.* 1997;71:148–154.
35. Li YP, Schwartz RJ, Waddell ID, et al. Skeletal muscle myocytes undergo protein loss and reactive oxygen-mediated NF-κB activation in response to tumour necrosis factor α. *FASEB J*. 1998;12:871–880.
36. Llovera M, Carbo N, Garcin-Martinez C, et al. Anti-TNF treatment reverts increased muscle ubiquitin gene expression in tumor bearing rats. *Biochem Biophys Res Commun*. 1996;221:653–655.
37. Lorite MJ, Thompson MG, Drake JL, et al. Mechanism of muscle protein degradation induced by a cancer cachectic factor. *Br J Cancer.* 1998;78:850–856.
38. Temparis S, Asensi M, Taillandier D, et al. Increased ATP-ubiquitin-dependent proteolysis in skeletal muscle of tumor-bearing rats. *Cancer Res*. 1994;54:5568–5573.
39. Williams A, Sun X, Fischer JE, et al. The expression of genes in the ubiquitin-proteasome proteolytic pathway is increased in skeletal muscle from patients with cancer. *Surgery.* 199;126:744–750.
40. Lowell BB, Ruderman NB, Goodman MN. Evidence that lysosomes are not involved in the degradation of myofibrillar proteins in rat skeletal muscle. *Biochem J*. 1986; 234:237–240.
41. Hasslegren P-O, Fischer JE. Muscle cachexia: current concepts of intracellular mechanisms and molecular regulation. *Ann Surg*. 2001;233:9–17.
42. Jagoe RT, Redfern CPF, Roberts RG, et al. Skeletal muscle mRNA levels for cathepsin B, but not components of the ubiquitin-proteasome pathway are increased in patients with lung cancer referred for thoracotomy. *Clin Sci*. 2002; 102:353–361.
43. Tanaka K. Molecular biology of the proteasome. *Biochem Biophys Res Commun*. 1998;247:537–541.
44. Hasslegren P-O, Wray C, Mammen J. Molecular regulation of muscle cachexia: it may be more than the proteasome. *Biochem Biophys Res Commun*. 2002;290:1–10.
45. Thompson MP, Cooper ST, Parry BR, et al. Increased expression of the mRNA for the hormone-sensitive lipase in adipose tissue of cancer patients. *Biochem Biophys Acta*. 1993;1180:236–242.

46. Maltoni M, Fabbri L, Nanni O, et al. Serum levels of tumour necrosis factor and other cytokines do not correlate with weight loss and anorexia in cancer patients. *Support Care Cancer.* 1997;5:130–135.
47. Levine B, Kalman J, Mayer L, et al. Elevated circulating levels of tumor necrosis factor in severe chronic heart failure. *N Engl J Med.* 1990;323:236–241.
48. Sheen-Chen SM, Chen W-J, Eng H-L, et al. Serum concentration of tumour necrosis factor in patients with breast cancer. *Breast Cancer Res Treat.* 1997;43:211–215.
49. Karayiannakis AJ, Syrigos KN, Polychronidis A, et al. Serum levels of tumour necrosis factor-α and nutritional status in pancreatic cancer patients. *Anticancer Res.* 2001;21:1355–1358.
50. Oldenberg HS, Rogy MA, Lazarus DD, et al. Cachexia and the acute-phase protein response in inflammation are regulated by interleukin-6. *Eur J Immunol.* 1993;23:1889–1894.
51. O'Riordain MG, Falconer JS, Maingay J, et al. Peripheral blood cells from weight-losing cancer patients control the hepatic acute phase response by a primarily interleukin-6 dependent mechanism. *Int J Oncol.* 1999;15:823–827.
52. Strassman G, Fong M, Kenney JS, et al. Evidence for the involvement of interleukin-6 in experimental cancer cachexia. *J Clin Invest.* 89:1681–1684.
53. Soda K, Kawakami M, Kashii K, et al. Manifestations of cancer cachexia induced by colon 26 adenocarcinoma are not fully ascribable to interleukia-6. *Int Cancer.* 1995; 62:332–338.
54. Hussey HJ, Todorov PT, Field WN, et al. Effect of a fluorinated pyrimidine on cachexia and tumour growth in murine cachexia models: relationship with a proteolysis inducing factor. *Br J Cancer.* 2000;83:56–62.
55. Fujiki F, Mukaida N, Hirose K, et al. Prevention of adenocarcinoma colon 26-induced cachexia by interleukin 10 gene transfer. *Cancer Res.* 1997;57:94–99.
56. Tsujinaka T, Fujita J, Ebisui C, et al. Interleukin-6 receptor antibody inhibits muscle atrophy and modulates proteolytic systems in interleukin 6 transgenic mice. *J Clin Invest.* 1996;97:244–249.
57. Espat NJ, Auffenberg T, Rosenberg JJ, et al. Ciliary neurotrophic factor is catabolic and shares with IL-6 the capacity to induce an acute phase response. *Am J Physiol.* 1996;271:R185–R190.
58. Garcia-Martinez C, Lopez-Soriano FJ, Argiles JM. Interleukin-6 does not activate protein breakdown in rat skeletal muscle. *Cancer Lett.* 1994;76:1–4.
59. Llovera M, Carbo N, Lopez-Soriano J, et al. Different cytokines modulate ubiquitin gene expression in rat skeletal muscle. *Cancer Lett.* 1998;133:83–87.
60. Bouffet E, Philip T, Negrier C, et al. Phase I study of interleukin-6 in children with solid tumours in relapse. *Eur J Cancer.* 1997;33:1620–1626.
61. Lambert PD, Anderson KD, Sleeman MW, et al. Ciliary neurotrophic factor activates leptin-like pathways and reduces body fat, without cachexia or rebound weight gain, even in leptin-resistant obesity. *Proc Natl Acad Sci USA.* 2001;98:4652–4657.
62. Scott HR, McMillan DC, Crilly A, et al. The relationship between weight loss and interleukin 6 in non-small-cell lung cancer. *Br J Cancer.* 1996;73:1560–1562.
63. Fearon KC, McMillan DC, Preston T, et al. Elevated circulating interleukin-6 is associated with an acute phase response but reduced fixed hepatic protein synthesis in patients with cancer. *Ann Surg.* 1991;213:26–31.
64. Moldawer LL, Anderson C, Gelin J, et al. Regulation of food intake and hepatic protein synthesis by recombinant-derived cytokines. *Am J Physiol.* 1988;254:G450–G456.
65. Strassman G, Masui Y, Chizzonite R, et al. Mechanisms of experimental cancer cachexia: local involvement of IL-1 in colon-26 tumor. *J Immunol.* 1993;150:2341–2345.
66. Costelli P, Llovera M, Carbo N, et al. Interleukin-1 receptor antagonist (IL-1 ra) is unable to reverse cachexia in rats bearing an ascites hepatoma (Yoshida AH-130). *Cancer Lett.* 1995;95:33–38.
67. Yasumoto K, Mukaida N, Harada A, et al. Molecular analysis of the cytokine network involved in cachexia in colon 26 adenocarcinoma-bearing mice. *Cancer Res.* 1995;55: 921–927.
68. Shibata M, Takekawa M. Increased serum concentration of circulating soluble receptor for interleukin-2 and its effect as a prognostic indicator in cachectic patients with gastric and colorectal cancer. *Oncology.* 1997;56: 54–58.
69. Mathys P, Dijkmans R, Proost P, et al. Severe cachexia in mice inoculated with interferon-γ-producing tumour cells. *Int J Cancer.* 1991;49:77–82.
70. Mathys P, Heremans H, Opdenakker G, et al. Anti-interferon-γ antibody treatment, growth of Lewis lung tumours in mice and tumour-associated cachexia. *Eur J Cancer.* 1991;27:182–187.
71. Grunfeld C, Zhao C, Fuller J, et al. Endotoxin and cytokines induce expression of leptin, the ob gene product in hamsters. *J Clin Invest.* 1996;92:2152–2157.
72. Brown DR, Berkowitz DE, Breslow MJ. Weight loss is not associated with hyperleptinemia in humans with pancreatic cancer. *J Clin Endocrinol Metab.* 2001;86: 162–166.
73. Bing C, Brown M, King P, et al. Increased gene expression in brown fat uncoupling protein (UCP)1 and skeletal muscle UCP2 and UCP3 in MAC16-induced cancer cachexia. *Cancer Res.* 2000;60:2405–2410.
74. Shaw JH, Wolfe RR. Fatty acid and glycerol kinetics in septic patients and in patients with gastrointestinal cancer: the response to glucose infusion and parenteral feeding. *Ann Surg.* 1987;205:368–376.
75. Drott C, Persson H, Lundholm K. Cardiovascular and metabolic response to adrenaline infusion in weight-losing patients with and without cancer. *Clin Physiol.* 1989;9:427–439.
76. Waterhouse C, Kemperman JH. Carbohydrate metabolism in subjects with cancer. *Cancer Res.* 1971;31:1273–1278.
77. Edmonson JH. Fatty acid mobilization and glucose metabolism in patients with cancer. *Cancer.* 1966;19:277–280.

78. Hyltander A, Daneryd P, Sandstrom R, et al. Beta-adrenoceptor activity and resting energy metabolism in weight losing cancer patients. *Eur J Cancer.* 1990;36: 330–334.
79. Todorov PT, McDevitt TM, Meyer DJ, et al. Purification and characterization of a tumor lipid-mobilizing factor. *Cancer Res.* 1998;58:2353–2358.
80. Bürgi W, Schmid K. Preparation and properties of Zn-α2-glycoprotein of normal human plasma. *J Biol Chem.* 1961;236:1066–1074.
81. Hirai K, Hussey HJ, Barber MD, et al. Biological evaluation of a lipid-mobilizing factor isolated from the urine of cancer patients. *Cancer Res.* 1998;58:2359–2365.
82. Khan S, Tisdale MJ. Catabolism of adipose tissue by a tumour-produced lipid-mobilising factor. *Int J Cancer.* 1999;80:444–447.
83. Islam-Ali B, Khan S, Price SA, et al. Modulation of adipocyte G-protein expression in cancer cachexia by a lipid-mobilizing factor. *Br J Cancer.* 2001;85:758–763.
84. Russell ST, Tisdale MJ. Effect of a tumour-derived lipid-mobilising factor on glucose and lipid metabolism in vivo. *Br J Cancer.* 2002;87:580–584.
85. Bing C, Russell ST, Beckett EE, et al. Expression of uncoupling proteins-1, -2 and -3 mRNA is induced by an adenocarcinoma-derived lipid-mobilizing factor. *Br J Cancer.* 2002;86:612–618.
86. Russell ST, Hirai K, Tisdale MJ. Role of β3-adrenergic receptors in the action of a tumour lipid mobilizing factor. *Br J Cancer.* 2002;86:424–428.
87. Islam-Ali BS, Tisdale MJ. Effect of a tumour-produced lipid-mobilizing factor on protein synthesis and degradation. *Br J Cancer.* 2001;84:1648–1655.
88. Emery PW, Edwards RH, Rennie MJ, et al. Protein synthesis in muscle measured in vivo in cachectic patients with cancer. *Br Med J.* 1984;289:584–586.
89. Lundholm K, Bylund AC, Holm J, et al. Skeletal muscle metabolism in patients with malignant tumour. *Eur J Cancer.* 1976;12:465–473.
90. Fearon KC, Hansell DT, Preston T, et al. Influence of whole body turnover rate on resting energy expenditure in patients with cancer. *Cancer Res.* 1988;48:2590–2595.
91. Smith KL, Tisdale MJ. Mechanism of muscle degradation in cancer cachexia. *Br J Cancer.* 1993;68:314–318.
92. Belizario JE, Katz M, Chenker E, et al. Bioactivity of skeletal muscle proteolysis-inducing factors in the plasma proteins from cancer patients with weight loss. *Br J Cancer.* 1991;63:705–710.
93. Todorov P, Cariuk P, McDevitt T, et al. Characterization of a cancer cachectic factor. *Nature.* 1996;379:739–742.
94. Todorov PT, Deacon M, Tisdale MJ. Structural analysis of a tumor-produced sulphated glycoprotein capable of initiating muscle protein degradation. *J Biol Chem.* 1997;272: 12279–12288.
95. Schittek B, Hipfel R, Sauer B, et al. Dermicidin: a novel human antibiotic peptide secreted by sweat glands. *Nat Immunol.* 2001;2:1133–1137.
96. Cunningham TJ, Jing H, Akerblom I, et al. Identification of the human cDNA for new survival / evasion peptide (DSEP): studies in vitro and in vivo of overexpression by neural cells. *Exp Neurol.* 2002;177:32–39.
97. Cariuk P, Lorite MJ, Todorov PT, et al. Induction of cachexia in mice by a product isolated from the urine of cachectic cancer patients. *Br J Cancer.* 1997;76:606–613.
98. Cabal-Manzano R, Bhargava P, Torres-Duarte A, et al. Proteolysis-inducing factor is expressed in tumours of patients with gastrointestinal cancers and correlates with weight loss. *Br J Cancer.* 2001;84:1559–1601.
99. Wang Z, Corey E, Hass GM, et al. Expression of the human cachexia-associated protein (HCAP) in prostate cancer and in a prostate cancer animal model of cachexia. *Int J Cancer.* 2003;105:123–129.
100. Wigmore SJ, Todorov PT, Barber MD, et al. Characteristics of patients with pancreatic cancer expressing a novel cachectic factor. *Br J Surg.* 2000;87:53–58.
101. Lorite MJ, Cariuk P, Tisdale MJ. Induction of muscle protein degradation by a tumour factor. *Br J Cancer.* 1997;76:1035–1040.
102. Smith HJ, Lorite MJ, Tisdale MJ. Effect of a cancer cachectic factor on protein synthesis/degradation in murine C_2C_{12} myoblasts: modulation by eicosapentaenoic acid. *Cancer Res.* 1999;59:5507–5513.
103. Lorite MJ, Smith HJ, Arnold JA, et al. Activation of ATP-ubiquitin-dependent proteolysis in skeletal muscle in vivo and murine myoblasts in vitro by a proteolysis-inducing factor (PIF). *Br J Cancer.* 2001;85:297–302.
104. Watchorn TM, Waddell ID, Dowidar N, et al. Proteolysis-inducing factor regulates hepatic gene expression via the transcription factors NF-κB and STAT3. *FASEB J.* 2001; 15:562–564.
105. Watchorn TM, Waddell ID, Ross JA. Proteolysis-inducing factor differentially influences transcriptional regulation in endothelial subtypes. *Am J Physiol.* 2001;282: E763–E769.
106. Hussey HJ, Tisdale MJ. Effect of a cachectic factor on carbohydrate metabolism and attenuation by the eicosapentaenoic acid. *Br J Cancer.* 1999;80:1231–1235.
107. Beck SA, Smith KL, Tisdale MJ. Anticachectic and antitumor effect of eicosapentaenoic acid and its effect on protein turnover. *Cancer Res.* 1991;6089–6093.
108. Whitehouse AS, Smith HJ, Drake JL, et al. Mechanism of attenuation of skeletal muscle protein catabolism in cancer cachexia by eicosapentaenoic acid. *Cancer Res.* 2001;61:3604–3609.
109. Wigmore SJ, Barber MD, Ross JA, et al. Effect of oral eicosapentaenoic acid on weight loss in patients with pancreatic cancer. *Nutr Cancer.* 2000;36:177–184.
110. Wigmore SJ, Ross JA, Falconer JS, et al. The effect of polyunsaturated fatty acids on the progress of cachexia in patients with pancreatic cancer. *Nutrition.* 1996;12:S27–S30.
111. Barber MD, Ross JA, Voss AC, et al. The effect of an oral nutritional supplement enriched with fish oil on weight-

loss in patients with pancreatic cancer. *Br J Cancer.* 1999; 81:80–86.
112. Barber MD, Fearon KCH, Tisdale MJ, et al. Effect of fish oil-enriched nutritional supplement of metabolic mediators in patients with pancreatic cancer cachexia. *Nutr Cancer.* 2001;40:118–124.
113. Mantovani G, Maccio A, Esu S, et al. Medroxyprogesterone acetate reduces in vitro production of cytokines and serotonin involved in anorexia/cachexia and emesis by peripheral blood mononuclear cells of cancer patients. *Eur J Cancer.* 1997;33:602–607.
114. Maltoni M, Nanni O, Scarpi E, et al. High-dose progestins for the treatment of cancer anorexia-cachexia syndrome: a systematic review of randomised clinical trials. *Ann Oncol.* 2001;12:289–300.
115. Loprinzi CL, Schaid DJ, Dose AM, et al. Body composition changes in patients who gain weight while receiving megestrol acetate. *J Clin Oncol.* 1993;11:152–154.
116. Simons JP, Schols AMJ, Hoefnagels JM, et al. Effects of medroxyprogesterone acetate on food intake, body composition and resting energy expenditure in patients with advanced, nonhormone-sensitive cancer. *Cancer.* 1998;82: 553–560.
117. Goldberg RM, Loprinzi CL, Malliard JA. Pentoxifylline for treatment of cancer anorexia and cachexia? A randomized, double-blind, placebo-controlled trial. *J Clin Oncol.* 1995;13:2856–2859.
118. Keifer JA, Guttridge DC, Ashburner BP, et al. Inhibition of NK-κB activity by thalidomide through suppression of IκB kinase activity. *J Biol Chem.* 2001;276:22382–22387.
119. Reys-Teran G, Sierra-Madero JG, Martinez del Cerro V, et al. Effects of thalidomide on HIV-associated wasting syndrome: a randomized, double-blind, placebo controlled trial. *AIDS.* 1996;10:1501–1507.
120. Khan ZH, Simpson EJ, Cole AT, et al. Oesophageal cancer and cachexia: the effect of short-term treatment with thalidomide on weight loss and lean body mass. *Aliment Pharmacol Ther.* 2003;17:677–682.
121. Nissen S, Sharp R, Ray M, et al. Effect of leucine metabolite β-hydroxy-β-methylbutyrate on muscle metabolism during resistance-exercise training. *J Appl Physiol.* 1996;81:2095–2104.
122. May PE, Baker A, D'Olimpis JT, et al. Reversal of cancer-related wasting using oral supplementation with a combination of β-hydroxy-β-methylbutyrate, arginine and glutamine. *Am J Surg.* 2002;183:471–479.

CHAPTER

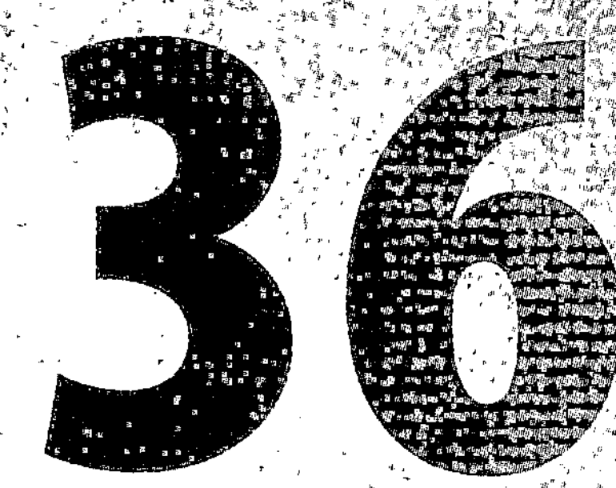

Target Discovery: Genomics/Proteomics

Christine A. Iacobuzio-Donahue, MD, PhD

The critical challenge in overcoming pancreatic cancer is to detect the disease early enough to allow for curative resection and to develop new approaches to treat established disease. Studies using global expression methodologies have provided a unique opportunity to better understand this lethal tumor and to meet these challenges. Specifically, expression profiling has advanced our understanding of pancreatic ductal adenocarcinoma in three important ways. First, more than 200 genes have been identified that are highly expressed in pancreatic duct adenocarcinomas but not in normal pancreatic ductal epithelium. Each of these highly expressed genes offers new opportunities for development of diagnostic tests or therapeutic targets. Second, many genes relating to the clinicopathologic features of infiltrating ductal adenocarcinomas have been identified, providing new insights into the biology of pancreatic cancer. Third, gene expression studies have revealed novel features related to the process of tissue invasion by pancreatic cancers. In this regard, new possibilities for drug delivery focused on tumor-stromal interactions have been identified. Each of these advances is discussed in more detail in the following sections.

Technical Aspects of Expression Profiling of Pancreatic Cancer

Before the knowledge gained from the use of expression profiling of pancreatic cancer can be discussed, a brief review of the relevant technical aspects related to expression profiling of pancreatic cancer is necessary. Four methods have revolutionized the ability to study pancreatic cancers and to have an impact on patient care. These methods include gene expression profiling technologies, such as serial analysis of gene expression (SAGE), complementary DNA (cDNA) microarrays, oligonucleotide arrays, or protein expression profiling methods such as proteomics.

Gene expression technologies, such as SAGE, cDNA microarrays or oligonucleotide arrays, can be used to determine the levels at which specific messenger RNAs (mRNAs) are expressed in samples of interest (Fig. 36.1). SAGE is a recently developed technique that allows one to obtain a quantitative and comprehensive profile of gene expression (see http://www.ncbi.nlm.nih.gov/SAGE/).[1] In SAGE, cellular mRNA transcripts are converted to

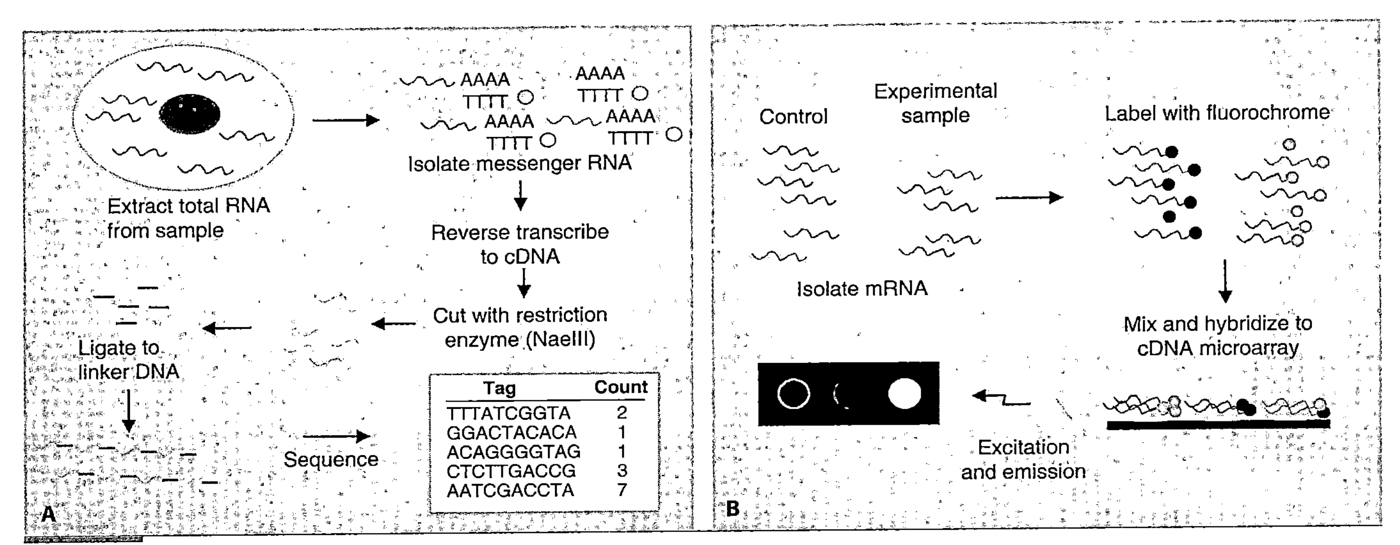

Figure 36.1
Diagrammatic representation of gene expression profiling. **(A)** Serial analysis of gene expression (SAGE). For this method, total RNA is extracted from the sample of interest (cell lines or tissues), and messenger RNA (mRNA) containing poly-A tails are isolated from this pool using poly-T oligonucleotides bound to beads. The isolated mRNA is digested with the NaeIII restriction enzyme to yield 9- to 10-bp tags, and these tags are ligated to a common repetitive DNA "linker." The resultant long fragments of DNA are then amplified and sequenced, with the abundance of each tag providing a quantitative measure of the number of transcripts from which the tag was derived in the original mRNA sample. **(B)** Complementary DNA (cDNA) microarrays. For this approach, both a control "reference" sample of mRNA (typically a pool of mRNAs from a variety of normal cell lines) and an experimental sample (cancer cell lines, normal or neoplastic tissues) are used. After extraction of total RNA and isolation of the mRNA as described in A, the control mRNA is labeled with Cy3-deoxyuridine triphosphate (dUTP), and the experimental samples are labeled with Cy5-dUTP. The two labeled samples are mixed in equal proportion and hybridized to the cDNA microarray chip where each spot contains multiple copies of cDNAs prepared from a single gene. The microarray chip is then scanned, and the relative fluorescence of each fluorochrome is determined to obtain a ratio of expression of the experimental sample to the reference sample.

cDNA and then cleaved at specific sites by restriction enzymes into small fragments of 10–14 bases, known as tags. These tags are linked together, amplified, and then sequenced. The abundance of each tag provides a quantitative measure of the number of transcripts from which the tag was derived in the total mRNA sample, thereby allowing expression levels for a particular tag to be compared between different samples. The ability to quantify gene expression is a major advantage of SAGE over other gene expression methodologies.

Alternative methods of gene expression analyses, such as cDNA microarrays and oligonucleotide arrays, have also shed light on the nature of pancreatic cancer. Unlike SAGE, cDNA microarray analyses involve the competitive hybridization of cDNAs derived from experimental and control samples to cDNA microarray chips, thus permitting the identification of relationships of global gene expression patterns among different sample types.[2] In contrast, oligonucleotide arrays allow cDNAs to be hybridized in a noncompetitive manner, with the intensity of signal reflecting in a linear fashion the amount of mRNA expression present in the original sample.[3] Finally, in proteomic methods, small amounts of protein are directly applied to biochips coated with specific chemical matrices (e.g., hydrophobic, cationic, anionic, normal phase) and analyzed by mass spectrometry to obtain a protein "fingerprint" of a sample.[4]

The Challenge of Studying Samples of Pancreatic Cancer

Although it has frequently been assumed that global expression profiling would be impossible in pancreatic tissues because of the high levels of RNases and other enzymes in the pancreas and because of the low neoplastic cellularity of most pancreatic cancers, in fact, these hurdles have been overcome by various approaches. Two sample types have proved useful for gene expression profiling in the pancreas. These include cultured cell lines (normal and malignant) and surgically resected pathological tissue specimens, both of which have inherent advantages and disadvantages for gene expression studies.

Pancreatic cell lines are very useful because they are pure populations of epithelial cells. One can therefore obtain an undiluted view of gene expression patterns. Additionally, neoplastic cell lines are particularly useful for evaluating the response of the neoplastic cells to various treatment strategies, delineating signaling cascades or cellular functions that may be altered by various experimental conditions. However, although cell lines are clearly useful, one must also appreciate their limitations. Cell lines are grown in artificial conditions that can result in the dysregulation of gene expression, particularly the down-regulation of gene expression related to the normal interactions of epithelial cells with their surrounding extracellular matrix components. Although this feature of cell lines may not affect some directed gene expression studies, one must nonetheless be aware of this limitation in interpreting gene expression data solely on the basis of the analysis of cell lines.

Because they represent the neoplasm in its "native" state, surgically resected tissue specimens are also essential for gene expression studies. However, two concerns exist regarding the use of surgically resected pancreatic tissue samples: (1) the predominance of non-neoplastic stromal cells within the tumor tissue specimens and (2) the extent of mRNA degradation in pancreatic tissues. Typically, resected pancreatic cancers are composed of a minor population of infiltrating neoplastic epithelial cells surrounded by a predominance of dense fibrous (or desmoplastic) non-neoplastic stroma (Fig. 36.2). This stroma contains proliferating fibroblasts; small, endothelial-lined vessels; inflammatory cells; and trapped residual atrophic parenchymal components of the organ invaded. A consistently low ratio of the infiltrating neoplastic epithelial cells to this abundant non-neoplastic desmoplastic response is unique to duct adenocarcinomas of the pancreas, in contrast to infiltrating carcinomas arising in other organ or tissue types. Microdissection or other methods of purification of the epithelial component have been used successfully to overcome this perceived obstacle.[5] Alternatively, some investigators have successfully used the approach of co-analyzing resected samples of chronic pancreatitis together with resected pancreatic cancers as a means to determine the genes that are solely overexpressed within the neoplastic tissues.[6]

The second common perception regarding the use of pancreatic tissues is that they contain a large amount of endogenous RNases, which can potentially interfere in the mRNA extraction methods preceding gene expression studies. RNases are a major secretory product of normal pancreatic acinar cells. However, there is commonly a significant loss of acinar cells within infiltrating pancreatic cancers that results from atrophy or destruction of the gland by the neoplasm, thus facilitating the study of mRNA expression patterns within these otherwise stromal rich tissues. Thus, with careful technique, adequate amounts of mRNA can be extracted from quickly frozen surgically resected samples.

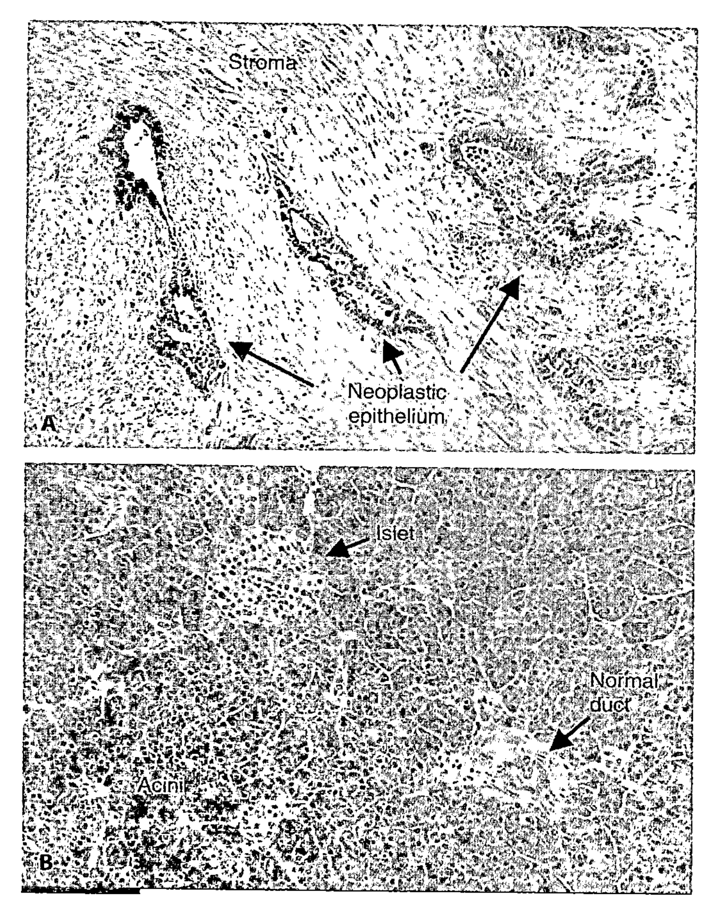

Figure 36.2
(A) Infiltrating pancreatic duct adenocarcinoma (×160). In this typical example of an infiltrating pancreatic duct adenocarcinoma, the non-neoplastic host stromal response (desmoplasia) accounts for most of the cellularity of the mass and is composed of proliferating fibroblasts, small vessels, and inflammatory cells. The neoplastic epithelium forms both glandular structures and individual cells, which infiltrate this stromal reaction. **(B)** Normal pancreas (×160). Normal pancreatic tissue is composed predominantly of acinar cells and islets (*upper left*), with a minority of the cellularity accounted for by the duct epithelial cells (*lower right*) from which almost all pancreatic cancers arise.

The availability and use of appropriate controls also pose a challenge in the study of pancreatic cancer. Normal pancreatic tissues contain a great predominance of acini and islet cells (Fig. 36.2), with duct epithelial cells, the presumed cell type of origin of pancreatic cancer, making up only a small proportion of bulk normal pancreas. Thus, expression profiling experiments that compare bulk normal pancreatic tissues with bulk resected pancreatic cancer tissues (composed predominantly of non-neoplastic stromal cells) largely reflect these differences in cell types and obscure any meaningful data. Microdissection of the duct epithelium may provide one method of enriching the normal samples,[5] whereas the use of non-neoplastic duct epithelial cells in culture is another alternative that we have used in several studies.[7]

Although each of these sample types alone can provide limited information about the gene expression patterns in pancreatic cancer, the analysis of these different sample types together can provide a comprehensive view of the gene expression patterns in pancreatic cancer and can account for both in vivo and in vitro expression specific patterns. Samples of normal pancreas can aid in identifying the contributions of trapped residual acinar and islet cells to the gene expression profiles detected in resected primary tumor tissues, whereas pancreatic cancer cell lines, when studied together with resected pancreatic cancer tissues, can be used to identify genes specifically expressed by the neoplastic epithelium. Likewise, genes expressed solely within resected pancreatic cancer tissues likely highlight genes whose expression relates to the non-neoplastic stromal elements but can also highlight genes expressed by the neoplastic epithelium due to tumor-stromal interactions.[8,9]

Expression Profiling of Pancreatic Cancer: Target Identification

Perhaps the most urgent need in the battle against pancreatic cancer is the identification of specific tumor markers for early diagnosis. Overexpressed genes that have been validated and now recognized as potentially important in pancreatic cancer include, but are not limited to: biglycan[10]; claudin 4[11,12]; coactosin-like 1[13]; fascin[14]; heat shock protein 47 (hsp47)[14]; hepatocarcinoma-intestine-pancreas/pancreatitis-associated-protein-1 (HIP/PAP-1)[15]; kunitz domain containing protein overexpressed in pancreatic cancer (Kop)[16]; mesothelin[17]; MUC4[18]; MUC5A/C, myoferlin[19,20]; prostate stem cell antigen (PSCA)[21]; syndecan-1[22]; S-100 proteins A4, A6 A10, A11, and P[7,19,23,24]; and transmembrane protease, serine 3 (TMPRSS3).[25] These potential tumor markers represent a variety of protein functions, including cell adhesion, cell motility, cytoskeletal assembly, proteolysis, and matrix remodeling. Some have now been validated as specific markers of pancreatic carcinoma and are discussed further in this chapter, whereas others are in the process of being confirmed (Table 36.1).

Mesothelin and PSCA were identified as highly expressed tags in SAGE libraries of pancreatic cancer cell lines, as compared with normal pancreatic duct epithelial cells.[17,21,26] Both mesothelin and PSCA encode glycosylphosphatidyl-inositol–anchored membrane-bound proteins, with a postulated role in cell adhesion.[27,28] Mesothelin immunolabeling can be seen in the vast majority (close to 100%) of pancreatic cancers, whereas PSCA immunolabeling is seen in 60% (Fig. 36.3). In contrast, the vast majority of normal ducts do not label for mesothelin. Pancreatic intraepithelial neoplasias (PanINs), the precursor lesions of pancreatic cancers, also are commonly negative for mesothelin protein, whereas PanINs show heterogeneous labeling for PSCA protein. The utility of applying mesothelin and PSCA immunolabeling to the diagnostic cytology of the pancreas has been shown. McCarthy et al[29] identified nine cytology specimens with features indicative, but not diagnostic, of pancreatic cancer, each with known follow-up. Six of these cases had an infiltrating pancreatic cancer on follow-up, with five of these six cases immunolabeling for either PSCA, mesothelin, or both. In contrast, none of three specimens that had a benign follow-up immunolabeled for PSCA or mesothelin protein.

Claudin 4 is a novel marker of pancreatic cancer also identified by SAGE, as well as by cDNA microarrays.[8] Claudin 4 is one of 15 members of the claudin gene family that play a role not only as a structural but also as a functional component of the tight junction barrier of normal epithelium.[30,31] Immunolabeling for claudin 4 has been found within virtually all primary (99%) or metastatic (100%) pancreatic cancer tissues analyzed (Fig. 36.3), as well as in most PanINs studied.[12] In all cases, immunolabeling was noted primarily in a membranous distribution. Claudin 4 protein is also detectable within normal breast, prostate, bladder, and gastrointestinal mucosa, although it is substantially less intense than that seen in pancreatic cancer tissues.

MUC4 and MUC5A/C are two of several apomucins that have been identified as highly expressed in pancreatic cancers by various gene expression methodologies. Apomucins are transmembrane glycoprotein complexes expressed by epithelial cells, with a putative role in epithelial protection.[32] Investigations of the expression of various apomucins have shown that MUC1, MUC4 and MUC5A, -5B, and -5C are differentially expressed in pancreatic adenocarcinoma as compared with normal pancreas, with MUC4 being detectable within 74% of pancreatic cancer tissues or cell lines, compared with 0% of normal pancreas or pancreatitis tissues.[18] These findings were confirmed in an immunohistochemical study by Swartz et al,[33] who showed MUC4 protein immunolabeling within 89% of pancreatic cancers and 85% of

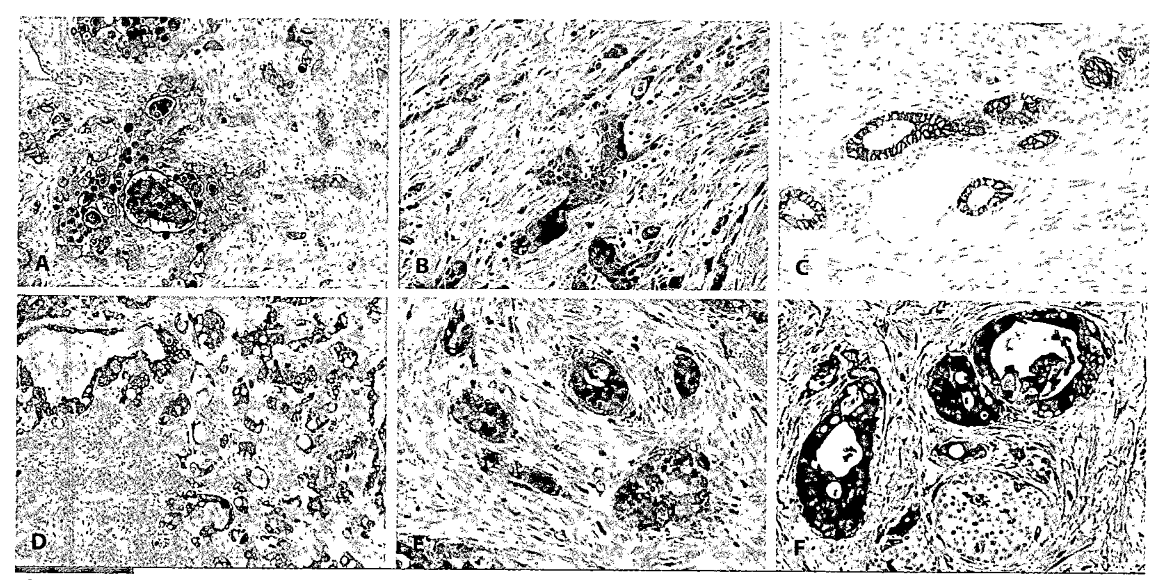

Figure 36.3
Immunohistochemical labeling of novel markers of pancreatic cancer identified by global gene expression analyses. **(A)** Mesothelin. Intense protein labeling is seen within the neoplastic epithelium in a membranous distribution. Luminal secretions also strongly label for mesothelin protein. **(B)** Prostate stem cell antigen (PSCA). Similar to mesothelin, the neoplastic epithelium labels for PSCA protein with membranous accentuation. Luminal secretions are also positive. **(C)** Claudin 4. Strong positive labeling of the neoplastic cells is seen, also in a membranous distribution. **(D)** MUC5A/C. The infiltrating carcinoma is strongly positive (seen in the top right), in contrast to the normal pancreas within the same section. **(E)** S-100A4. Neoplastic epithelium strongly labels for S-100A4 protein. Scattered positive labeling stromal cells are also seen, although not as strongly as the epithelium. **(F)** Fascin. Intensely positive cytoplasmic labeling is detected within the neoplastic epithelium. Scattered stromal cells are also positive, in contrast to the negative labeling normal islet present at bottom left.

high-grade PanINs (PanIN-3), compared with only 26% of low-grade PanIN lesions (PanIN-1 and -2). Similar findings have been reported for MUC5A/C, with 91% of pancreatic cancers showing strong positive membranous immunolabeling, in contrast to no cases of normal pancreatic duct epithelium labeling for MUC5A/C[26] (Fig. 36.3).

The S-100 proteins, fascin, hsp47, and HIP/PAP-1 have also been identified by global expression methodologies and also have potential as specific markers for pancreatic ductal adenocarcinomas. These genes encode for cytoplasmic proteins. S-100A4 is one of a family of sixteen S-100 calcium-binding proteins, all of which have an EF-hand domain that mediates their presumed role in tissue invasion and metastasis.[34] Immunohistochemical labeling for S-100A4 protein has been shown in 93% of invasive pancreatic ductal adenocarcinomas, compared with 4% of PanINs and 0% of normal pancreatic ducts[23] (Fig. 36.3). Fascin is also a promising novel marker of pancreatic cancer identified by oligonucleotide arrays. Fascin is an actin-bundling protein present in membrane ruffles, microspikes, and other motility-associated cell fibers.[35] Consistent with invasive cell behavior, fascin overexpression is associated with reduced cell-cell junction integrity and an increase of up to 17-fold in the motility of epithelial cells.[36] Among pancreatic duct adenocarcinomas, Maitra et al[14] found fascin immunolabeling in the neoplastic cells of 95% of cases studied, but not in 94% of the adjacent non-neoplastic pancreatic ducts. Fascin protein labeling was also found in a minority of PanINs, with 19% of PanINs showing some expression of fascin protein.[14]

Hsp47, another highly expressed protein in pancreatic cancers identified by oligonucleotide arrays, is thought to function in matrix remodeling and assembly. Also known as colligin, hsp47 is a collagen-specific chaperone that interacts transiently with procollagen during the process of folding, assembly, and transport from the endoplasmic reticulum in fibroblasts and myofibroblasts. Maitra et al[14] also showed that hsp47 protein immunolabeling was intense and virtually universal within ductal adenocarcinoma–associated stromal desmoplasia (100% of cases studied), although 65% of ductal adenocarcinomas also showed some labeling of hsp47 in the neoplastic epithelium. In contrast, labeling for hsp47 protein was absent in most (88%) of non-neoplastic pancreatic ducts.

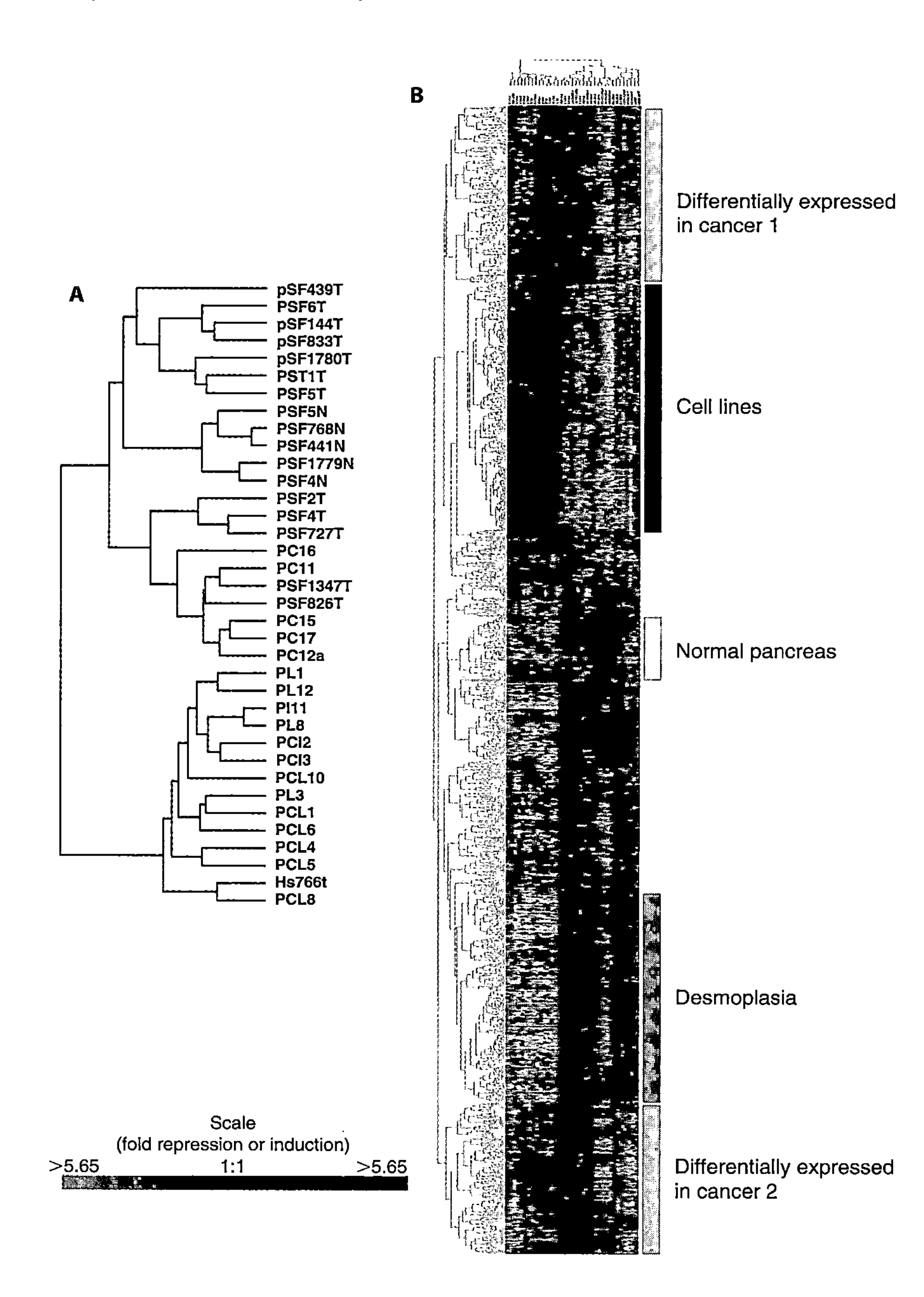

Figure 36.4
The gene expression profile of pancreatic cancer using complementary DNA (cDNA) microarrays. **(A)** Dendrogram representing the results of hierarchical cluster analysis of the gene expression patterns in 36 pancreatic samples, based on data for 1492 genes. Sample names highlighted in green are normal pancreatic tissue ($N = 5$), samples in red are pancreatic primary tumor tissue ($N = 17$), and samples listed in black are pancreatic cancer cell lines ($N = 14$). **(B)** Hierarchical cluster analysis of 1492 genes whose expression varied by at least two standard deviations from the mean in at least two samples. Five clusters of gene expression with similar patterns of variation in expression are highlighted, corresponding to acinar or islet gene expression in normal pancreas (white vertical bar), desmoplasia-associated gene expression (dark grey vertical bar), cell-line–specific expression (black vertical bar), and genes differentially expressed in pancreas cancers (light grey vertical bars). The ratio of the abundance of transcripts of each gene in a given sample to its median abundance across all cell lines or tissue samples is represented by the color of the corresponding cell in the TreeView-generated diagram. Green cells are those whose transcript levels were below the median; black, equal to the median; and red, greater than the median. Grey cells represent technically inadequate or missing data. Color saturation of each cell reflects the magnitude of the ratio relative to the mean for each gene. The complete dataset is freely available at http://genome-www.stanford.edu/pancreatic1. (From Iacobuzio-Donahue et al.[8]; with permission.)

In contrast to S-100 proteins, fascin, and hsp47, HIP/PAP-1 was identified with the use of proteomics technology analysis of pancreatic juice specimens. HIP/PAP-1 is a protein released from pancreatic acini during acute pancreatitis and is overexpressed in hepatocellular carcinoma.[37] Recently, quantification of HIP/PAP-1 in pancreatic juice and serum confirmed the significantly increased amounts of this protein in the samples from patients with pancreatic adenocarcinoma.[15] Moreover, Rosty et al[15] showed that patients with pancreatic juice HIP/PAP-1 at levels equal to or greater than 20 μg/mL were 21.9 times likelier to have pancreatic adenocarcinoma than were patients with levels less than 20 μg/mL.

New Insights Into the Biology of Pancreatic Ductal Adenocarcinoma

Gene expression profiling has also provided novel insight into the complex biology of pancreatic cancer (Fig. 36.4). Recent evidence provided through global gene expression profiling has revealed certain cellular processes as playing a more prominent role in pancreatic cancers than was previously recognized. For example, genes whose protein products are involved in cell membrane junctions and cell/matrix interactions have consistently been determined to be upregulated in pancreatic cancers by several investigators.[7,19,20,38-40] This observation could correspond to altered cellular attachments and cell surface architecture, resulting in aberrant cell-cell interactions that are a reproducible characteristic of cancer cells. Several ion-homeostasis–dependent proteins, especially those specific for the calcium ion, such as S-100A4, S-100A10, Trop-2, AIF-1, and ALG-2, are also overexpressed in pancreatic cancer.[7,19] The consistent expression of these genes in pancreatic cancers may indicate key homeostatic mechanisms necessary for cancer cell survival, and interference with these pathways may promote cancer cell death. Finally, several genes whose protein products may contribute to chemoradioresistance in pancreatic cancers have also been identified, such as ataxia-telangiectasia group D–associated protein (ATDC), topoisomerase II alpha (TOP2A), major vault protein, and transglutaminase II (TGM2).[7,19] ATDC protein is induced by ionizing radiation and suppresses the radiosensitivity of ataxia telangiectasia (A-T) fibroblast cell lines,[41] whereas expressed genes, such as topoisomerase II alpha[42] and transglutaminase II,[43] may relate to the chemotherapeutic resistance often observed for pancreatic cancers. Thus, global gene expression technologies can provide important insights into pancreatic carcinomas, many of which may affect how future chemotherapeutic or radiation therapies are designed and administered.

New Insights Into the Invasive Process within Pancreatic Cancers

Gene expression profiling of pancreatic cancer has also provided new insights into the process of tumor invasion. Gene expression studies of pancreatic cancer tissues have been used to identify expression patterns associated with the exuberant desmoplastic response.[19,39,44] Not surprisingly, a similar type cluster of genes has also been identified in infiltrating pancreas cancers with the use of SAGE by Ryu et al,[45] who termed these genes the *invasion-associated* genes of infiltrating pancreatic cancer. These genes are expressed in surgically resected pancreatic cancer tissues, but not in normal pancreas tissue or in cultured pancreatic cancer cell lines, thus reflecting the cellular components of the host stromal response that occur in the presence of infiltrating carcinoma.

Investigations into the cellular localization of these genes with the use of in situ hybridization have identified a specific architecture for the expression of these genes in invasive pancreatic carcinomas. Gene expression within invasive pancreatic cancers can be segregated into distinct and reproducible compartments: neoplastic epithelium, angioendothelium, juxtatumoral stroma (those stromal cells immediately adjacent to the invasive neoplastic epithelium),

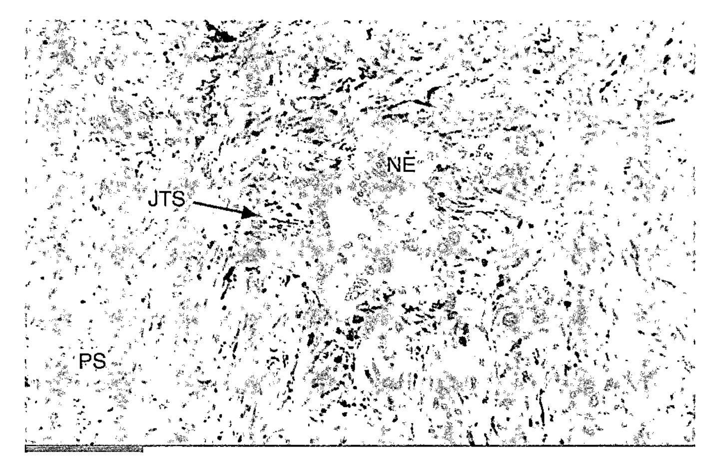

Figure 36.5
Juxtatumoral stromal expression in infiltrating pancreatic cancer. Shown is an example of in situ hybridization for ApoD expression. Strong positive labeling for ApoD-specific messenger RNA expression is seen in the stromal cells (JTS, juxtatumoral stroma) adjacent to the neoplastic epithelium (NE). In contrast, stromal cells not in contact with the neoplastic cells are negative (PS, panstromal).

and panstromal compartment (all stromal tissue within the host response) (Fig. 36.5). These findings indicate that a highly organized and structured process of tumor invasion exists in the pancreas. The finding of genes expressed by the neoplastic epithelium in invasive carcinomas, but not in cancer cell lines derived from invasive carcinomas, also highlights the importance of gene expression related to a neoplastic cell's interactions with its environment. Although these compartments of gene expression are distinct, potential lines of communication between different compartments may exist. To provide one example, α_2-macroglobulin is expressed by the juxtatumoral stroma, whereas the receptor for this gene product, α_2-macroglobulin receptor, is expressed by the neoplastic epithelium.[9] Thus, the host stromal response, and the juxtatumoral stroma in particular, may play an active role in the invasive process.[46] At the very least, studies using global gene expression have identified genes of the desmoplastic response that have potential for tumor-specific targeting of tumor-stromal interactions.

Potential Clinical Uses for Novel Targets Identified by Expression Profiling

The diversity in function of these highly expressed genes reflects the many cellular processes that are up-regulated in pancreatic cancer cells and establishes the utility of global expression platforms to identify novel tumor markers. Each of these proteins has immediate diagnostic utility for pancreatic carcinoma. For example, because mesothelin is only rarely expressed in normal pancreatic epithelium, mesothelin labeling can be used to support the diagnosis of infiltrating pancreatic ductal adenocarcinoma, particularly in small tissue samples or cytologic material. However, the presence of mesothelin immunolabeling in occasional PanINs or weak labeling of normal ducts indicates that mesothelin immunoreactivity by itself may not always be specific enough to render a diagnosis of infiltrating ductal adenocarcinoma. Therefore, whereas use of any one marker may have a limited sensitivity or specificity in detecting pancreatic cancer, the development of a panel of markers (e.g., mesothelin, S-100A4, fascin, and hsp47) may significantly increase the specificity of diagnosing pancreatic cancer without decreasing the sensitivity.[47]

Novel markers of pancreatic cancer also hold promise for the development of new screening tests for pancreatic cancer. For example, highly expressed membranous or secreted proteins, such as mesothelin and PSCA, may be shed into the blood or pancreatic secretions. If so, these proteins may serve as screening markers, not only for the identification of primary pancreatic cancers at an earlier stage but also for the identification of recurrent disease at an earlier phase when it may be more responsive to adjuvant therapies.

The development of tagged antibodies to one or more of these genes may also be useful for the diagnostic radiologic imaging of small primary pancreatic cancers or for novel therapeutic implications to combat pancreatic cancer. For example, in animal models, the use of tagged monoclonal antibodies to hsp47 has already been demonstrated as a feasible means for detection of solid tumors in vivo,[48] whereas others have shown feasibility in selectively targeting carcinomas expressing hsp47 with the use of peptides that are known to specifically bind to the hsp47 protein.[49] The same is true for therapeutic interventions. Immunotoxins targeted to PSCA or claudin 4 reduce tumor burden in xenografted tumors expressing these proteins.[11,50] Thus, the targeting of chemotherapeutic agents selectively to the neoplastic cells and stroma in pancreatic ductal adenocarcinoma can potentially increase efficacy while significantly reducing toxic side effects. Additionally, because cell- or antibody-based immunotherapies are safe and effective in patients with pancreatic cancer,[51,52] these proteins can form the basis for novel immunotherapies.

Future Directions

Our initial attempts to study pancreatic cancer with the use of global gene expression methodologies have revealed a wealth of information. Clearly, pancreatic ade-

Table 36.1 Examples of Novel Markers of Pancreatic Ductal Adenocarcinoma Identified by Gene Expression Profiling

Name	NORMAL CELLULAR FUNCTION	EXPRESSION IN PANCREATIC CANCER	POTENTIAL UTILITY
Claudin 4	Component of epithelial tight junctions	Overexpressed in neoplastic epithelium; membranous distribution	Molecular imaging immunotherapy
Fascin	Cytoskeletal protein, cellular motility	Overexpressed in neoplastic epithelium; cytoplasmic distribution	Diagnostic marker
HIP/PAP-1	Unknown	Normal acinar cells; released during acute/chronic pancreatitis	Screening marker in pancreatic juice
Hsp47	Collagen-specific chaperone	Desmoplastic stromal cells	Diagnostic marker/molecular imaging
Mesothelin	GPI-anchored protein, unknown adhesion	Overexpressed in neoplastic epithelium; membranous distribution	Diagnostic marker/immunotherapy/screening
MUC4	Apomucin, Epithelial Protection	Overexpressed in neoplastic epithelium; membranous distribution	Diagnostic marker/immunotherapy
PSCA	GPI-anchored protein, unknown adhesion	Overexpressed in neoplastic epithelium; membranous distribution	Diagnostic marker/immunotherapy/screening
S-100A4	S-100 calcium-binding protein	Overexpressed in neoplastic epithelium; cytoplasmic distribution	Diagnostic marker

nocarcinomas are complex tumors, as evidenced by the wide range of cellular functions represented by the genes determined to be differentially expressed by various investigators. However, these various methodologies have revealed similar findings regarding the genes or cellular processes that are most highly up-regulated in pancreatic cancers. These findings not only provide novel insight into the biology of pancreatic cancer but also identify numerous new targets for development into serologic markers or therapeutic regimens.

References

1. Velculescu VE, Zhang L, Vogelstein B, Kinzler KW. Serial analysis of gene expression. *Science*. 1995;270:484–487.
2. Shalon D, Smith SJ, Brown PO. A DNA microarray system for analyzing complex DNA samples using two-color fluorescent probe hybridization. *Genome Res*. 1996;6:639–645.
3. Wodicka L, Dong H, Mittmann M, et al. Genome-wide expression monitoring in Saccharomyces cerevisiae. *Nat Biotechnol*. 1997;15:1359–1367.
4. Issaq HJ, Veenstra TD, Conrads TP, Felschow D. The SELDI-TOF MS approach to proteomics: protein profiling and biomarker identification. *Biochem Biophys Res Commun*. 2002;292:587–592.
5. Crnogorac-Jurcevic T, Efthimiou E, Nielsen T, et al. Expression profiling of microdissected pancreatic adenocarcinomas. *Oncogene*. 2002;21:4587–4594.
6. Logsdon CD, Simeone DM, Binkley C, et al. Molecular profiling of pancreatic adenocarcinoma and chronic pancreatitis identifies multiple genes differentially regulated in pancreatic cancer. *Cancer Res*. 2003;63:2649–2657.
7. Ryu B, Jones J, Blades NJ, et al. Relationships and differentially expressed genes among pancreatic cancers examined by large-scale serial analysis of gene expression. *Cancer Res*. 2002;62:819–826.
8. Iacobuzio-Donahue CA, Maitra A, Olsen M, et al. Exploration of global gene expression patterns in pancreatic adenocarcinoma using cDNA microarrays. *Am J Pathol*. 2003;162:1151–1162.
9. Iacobuzio-Donahue CA, Ryu B, Hruban RH, Kern SE. Exploring the host desmoplastic response to pancreatic carcinoma: gene expression of stromal and neoplastic cells at the site of primary invasion. *Am J Pathol*. 2002;160:91–99.
10. Weber CK, Sommer G, Michl P, et al. Biglycan is overexpressed in pancreatic cancer and induces G1-arrest in pancreatic cancer cell lines. *Gastroenterology*. 2001;121:657–667.
11. Michl P, Buchholz M, Rolke M, et al. Claudin-4: a new target for pancreatic cancer treatment using Clostridium perfringens enterotoxin. *Gastroenterology*. 2001;121:678–684.
12. Nichols LS, Ashfaq R, Iacobuzio-Donahue CA. Claudin 4 protein expression in primary and metastatic pancreatic cancer: support for use as a therapeutic target. *Am J Clin Pathol*. 2004;121:226–230.
13. Nakatsura T, Senju S, Ito M, et al. Cellular and humoral immune responses to a human pancreatic cancer antigen, coactosin-like protein, originally defined by the SEREX method. *Eur J Immunol*. 2002;32:826–836.
14. Maitra A, Iacobuzio-Donahue C, Rahman A, et al. Immunohistochemical validation of a novel epithelial and a novel stromal marker of pancreatic ductal adenocarcinoma identified by global expression microarrays: sea urchin fascin homolog and heat shock protein 47. *Am J Clin Pathol*. 2002;118:52–59.
15. Rosty C, Christa L, Kuzdzal S, et al. Identification of hepatocarcinoma-intestine-pancreas/pancreatitis-associated protein I as a biomarker for pancreatic ductal adenocarcinoma by protein biochip technology. *Cancer Res*. 2002; 62:1868–1875.
16. Mueller-Pillasch F, Lacher U, Wallrapp C, et al. Cloning of a gene highly overexpressed in cancer coding for a novel KH-domain containing protein. *Oncogene*. 1997;14: 2729–2733.
17. Argani P, Iacobuzio-Donahue C, Ryu B, et al. Mesothelin is overexpressed in the vast majority of ductal adenocarcinomas of the pancreas: identification of a new pancreatic cancer marker by serial analysis of gene expression (SAGE). *Clin Cancer Res*. 2001;7:3862–3868.
18. Andrianifahanana M, Moniaux N, Schmied BM, et al. Mucin (MUC) gene expression in human pancreatic adenocarcinoma and chronic pancreatitis: a potential role of MUC4 as a tumor marker of diagnostic significance. *Clin Cancer Res*. 2001;7:4033–4040.
19. Iacobuzio-Donahue CA, Maitra A, Shen-Ong GL, et al. Discovery of novel tumor markers of pancreatic cancer using global gene expression technology. *Am J Pathol*. 2002;160: 1239–1249.
20. Han H, Bearss DJ, Browne LW, et al. Identification of differentially expressed genes in pancreatic cancer cells using cDNA microarray. *Cancer Res*. 2002;62:2890–2896.
21. Argani P, Rosty C, Reiter RE, et al. Discovery of new markers of cancer through serial analysis of gene expression: prostate stem cell antigen is overexpressed in pancreatic adenocarcinoma. *Cancer Res*. 2001;61:4320–4324.
22. Conejo JR, Kleeff J, Koliopanos A, et al. Syndecan-1 expression is up-regulated in pancreatic but not in other gastrointestinal cancers. *Int J Cancer*. 2000;88:12–20.
23. Rosty C, Ueki T, Argani P, et al. Overexpression of S100A4 in pancreatic ductal adenocarcinomas is associated with poor differentiation and DNA hypomethylation. *Am J Pathol*. 2002;160:45–50.
24. Crnogorac-Jurcevic T, Missiaglia E, Blaveri E, et al. Molecular alterations in pancreatic carcinoma: expression profiling shows that dysregulated expression of S100 genes is highly prevalent. *J Pathol*. 2003;201:63–74.
25. Wallrapp C, Hahnel S, Muller-Pillasch F, et al. A novel transmembrane serine protease (TMPRSS3) overexpressed in pancreatic cancer. *Cancer Res*. 2000;60:2602–2606.
26. Iacobuzio-Donahue CA, Ashfaq R, Maitra A, et al. Highly expressed genes in pancreatic ductal adenocarcinomas: a comprehensive characterization and comparison of the transcription profiles obtained from three major technologies. *Cancer Res*. 2003;63:8614–8622.
27. Chang K, Pastan I. Molecular cloning of mesothelin, a differentiation antigen present on mesothelium, mesotheliomas, and ovarian cancers. *Proc Natl Acad Sci USA*. 1996; 93:136–140.

28. Reiter RE, Gu Z, Watabe T, et al. Prostate stem cell antigen: a cell surface marker overexpressed in prostate cancer. *Proc Natl Acad Sci USA*. 1998;95:1735–1740.
29. McCarthy DM, Maitra A, Argani P, et al. Novel markers of pancreatic adenocarcinoma in fine-needle aspiration: mesothelin and prostate stem cell antigen labeling increases accuracy in cytologically borderline cases. *Appl Immunohistochem Mol Morphol*. 2003;11:238–243.
30. Colegio OR, Van Itallie C, Rahner C, Anderson JM. Claudin extracellular domains determine paracellular charge selectivity and resistance but not tight junction fibril architecture. *Am J Physiol Cell Physiol*. 2003;284:C1346–1354.
31. Van Itallie C, Rahner C, Anderson JM. Regulated expression of claudin-4 decreases paracellular conductance through a selective decrease in sodium permeability. *J Clin Invest*. 2001;107:1319–1327.
32. Carraway KL, Perez A, Idris N, et al. Muc4/sialomucin complex, the intramembrane ErbB2 ligand, in cancer and epithelia: to protect and to survive. *Prog Nucleic Acid Res Mol Biol*. 2002;71:149–185.
33. Swartz MJ, Batra SK, Varshney GC, et al. MUC4 expression increases progressively in pancreatic intraepithelial neoplasia. *Am J Clin Pathol*. 2002;117:791–796.
34. Schafer BW, Heizmann CW. The S100 family of EF-hand calcium-binding proteins: functions and pathology. *Trends Biochem Sci*. 1996;21:134–140.
35. Yamashiro S, Yamakita Y, Ono S, Matsumura F. Fascin, an actin-bundling protein, induces membrane protrusions and increases cell motility of epithelial cells. *Mol Biol Cell*. 1998;9:993–1006.
36. Grothey A, Hashizume R, Ji H, et al. C-erbB-2/ HER-2 upregulates fascin, an actin-bundling protein associated with cell motility, in human breast cancer cell lines. *Oncogene*. 2000;19:4864–4875.
37. Keim V, Iovanna JL, Rohr G, et al. Characterization of a rat pancreatic secretory protein associated with pancreatitis. *Gastroenterology*. 1991;100:775–782.
38. Gress TM, Wallrapp C, Frohme M, et al. Identification of genes with specific expression in pancreatic cancer by cDNA representational difference analysis. *Genes Chromosomes Cancer*. 1997;19:97–103.
39. Crnogorac-Jurcevic T, Efthimiou E, Capelli P, et al. Gene expression profiles of pancreatic cancer and stromal desmoplasia. *Oncogene*. 2001;20:7437–7446.
40. Gardner-Thorpe J, Ito H, Ashley SW, Whang EE. Differential display of expressed genes in pancreatic cancer cells. *Biochem Biophys Res Commun*. 2002;293:391–395.
41. Laderoute KR, Knapp AM, Green CJ, et al. Expression of the ATDC (ataxia telangiectasia group D-complementing) gene in A431 human squamous carcinoma cells. *Int J Cancer*. 1996;66:772–778.
42. Jarvinen TA, Tanner M, Rantanen V, et al. Amplification and deletion of topoisomerase II alpha associate with ErbB-2 amplification and affect sensitivity to topoisomerase II inhibitor doxorubicin in breast cancer. *Am J Pathol*. 2000;156:839–847.
43. Han JA, Park SC. Reduction of transglutaminase 2 expression is associated with an induction of drug sensitivity in the PC-14 human lung cancer cell line. *J Cancer Res Clin Oncol*. 1999;125:89–95.
44. Gress TM, Muller-Pillasch F, Lerch MM, et al. Expression and in-situ localization of genes coding for extracellular matrix proteins and extracellular matrix degrading proteases in pancreatic cancer. *Int J Cancer*. 1995;62:407–413.
45. Ryu B, Jones J, Hollingsworth MA, et al. Invasion-specific genes in malignancy: serial analysis of gene expression comparisons of primary and passaged cancers. *Cancer Res*. 2001;61:1833–1838.
46. Tlsty TD. Stromal cells can contribute oncogenic signals. *Semin Cancer Biol*. 2001;11:97–104.
47. Zhou W, Sokoll LJ, Bruzek DJ, et al. Identifying markers for pancreatic cancer by gene expression analysis. *Cancer Epidemiol Biomarkers Prev*. 1998;7:109–112.
48. Morino M, Yasuda T, Shirakami T, et al. HSP47 as a possible marker for malignancy of tumors in vivo. *In Vivo*. 1994;8:285–288.
49. Sauk JJ, Coletta RD, Norris K, Hebert C. Binding motifs of CBP2 a potential cell surface target for carcinoma cells. *J Cell Biochem*. 2000;78:251–263.
50. Saffran DC, Raitano AB, Hubert RS, et al. Anti-PSCA mAbs inhibit tumor growth and metastasis formation and prolong the survival of mice bearing human prostate cancer xenografts. *Proc Natl Acad Sci USA*. 2001;98:2658–2663.
51. Jaffee EM, Schutte M, Gossett J, et al. Development and characterization of a cytokine-secreting pancreatic adenocarcinoma vaccine from primary tumors for use in clinical trials. *Cancer J Sci Am*. 1998;4:194–203.
52. Jaffee EM, Hruban RH, Biedrzycki B, et al. Novel allogeneic granulocyte-macrophage colony-stimulating factor-secreting tumor vaccine for pancreatic cancer: a phase I trial of safety and immune activation. *J Clin Oncol*. 2001;19:145–156.

COMMENTARY

John V. Pearson, BS
Jeffrey M. Trent, PhD

In Chapter 36, Christine Iacobuzio-Donahue outlines the foundational contributions that genomic and proteomic approaches (including gene expression profiling) are beginning to make to the elucidation of the invasive process in pancreatic cancer. Furthermore and ultimately of most importance is the author's viewpoint that advances in this area will ultimately translate into a clinical setting. It is certainly believed that these technologies will lead to the identification of new diagnostic and therapeutic targets. This commentary provides additional information about the current state of our knowledge of genetic information derived from the completion of the final draft sequence of the human genome made available through the Human Genome Project.[1] The viewpoint to be addressed here is that our current understanding of the human genome is rudimentary at best and that our "annotation" is just the first step in an even more exciting phase, as techniques from the computational and systems theory disciplines are brought to bear on the genetic basis of disease.

Genomic techniques such as SAGE and cDNA and oligonucleotide microarrays can be used to examine gene expression patterns and transcript copy number, whereas proteomics approaches, including hybrid chromatography/mass spectroscopy techniques such as MALDI-TOF and SELDI-TOF, can provide information about the presence of gene products. The author takes time to differentiate whether cDNA or oligo-based approaches will provide more information and whether "competitive" hybridization (actually the relative ratio of information collected) will be of most value. Without devolving into discussion of how this technology is gravitating, regardless of platform provider, to oligo-based analysis, it is perhaps of most value to simply point out that first-generation tools exist for generating "lists" of genes that may be important in some biologic or clinical context and in this case in pancreatic cancer.

The author notes that, to date, these techniques have identified over 200 genes as being highly expressed in pancreatic duct adenocarcinomas when compared with expression in normal ductal epithelium. The appropriate follow-up question is this: What is the right technology to apply to validate these expression differences in an appropriate clinical context? Although some of these genes have been examined for their diagnostic significance, others have not been analyzed because of a lack of suitable validation tools (e.g., the easiest to consider would be the availability of antibodies that could be examined in large sample sets). For those targets with available antibodies, the identification of a minimal prognostic panel requires the evaluation and comparison of all targets on a large panel of pancreatic cancer samples with extensive clinical follow-up, now possible with the advent of tissue microarrays.[2] In addition, targets implicated by expression profiling could similarly be evaluated for their prognostic significance.

Although it is true that gene expression profiling can provide new insights into the biology of pancreatic cancer, it should be noted that fully characterizing even one gene implicated by SAGE or expression microarrays can be a significant undertaking. However, thanks to the development of many new tools that are publicly available, several approaches are now being routinely employed to help scientists prioritize which genes in their gene list are worthy of further investigation. The first of these involves annotation to add as much biologic detail as exists in the public databases via automated bioinformatic methods. Annotation databases can be loosely characterized according to the biologic entity they annotate. NCBI's LocusLink database[3] (now Entrez Gene) is a pan-species collection of information about genes and includes a rich variety of cross-links to other annotation databases. EBI's UniProt database[4] assembles information relating to gene products, and the Online Mendelian Inheritance in Man[5] database initially created by Dr. Victor McKusick at Johns Hopkins University and hosted at NCBI concentrates on genetic disorders. Other integrative initiatives include the Gene Ontology Consortium, which is defining a species-neutral system for classifying attributes of gene products.[6] The Gene Ontology system, when used by database curators to annotate their gene product collections, will provide a framework enabling researchers to start associating proteins across systems and species based on what the proteins do (biological process, molecular function) rather than what they are (sequence similarity, conserved domains, three-dimensional structure).

Once genes have been annotated, resources such as the Biomolecular Interaction Network Database,[7] the Kyoto Encyclopedia of Genes and Genomes,[8] and BioCarta's Proteomic Pathway Project can be used to investigate known regulatory relationships between the gene products. Unfortunately, although our knowledge of enzymatic and metabolic pathways is quite mature, our knowledge of cellular regulatory network functions is not, and many pathways in these pathway resources are incomplete. Consequently, a significant effort is being made to mine gene expression data for novel regulatory relationships.[9] Although today these efforts are largely in the domain of the basic research scientist, this information is being brought together in ways to provide benefit to the clinical community. Specifically, as work progresses matching gene expression signatures to treatment outcomes, provision of this information to practitioners who would use this is a focus of many groups.[10]

Other approaches used to analyze gene lists involve trying to identify the "master biologic switches," that is, those genes whose expression may not change appreciably but that have regulatory relationships with multiple genes on a gene list. Current strategies include transcription factor mapping and predictive methods. Predictive methods include efforts to find associations between genes by accessing the transcriptional levels of small predictor gene sets to predict the transcriptional state of a target gene.[11] The problem with these types of pathway mapping exercises is that use of any single gene has insufficient information content to predict, for example, outcome to a given experimental agent and certainly survival. Accordingly, we are moving forward to see the utility of gene sets, where a panel of genes (usually > 100) are combined to monitor and robustly predict something as complex as outcome or survival.

However, it must be recognized that the search for sets of genes that predict outcome comes with a huge cost. This "cost" is a mathematic one, specifically combinatorial studies, even ones that are based on relatively small gene panels and small predictor sets, require significant computing resources. As an example, if one merely examines a pool of 600 genes and tries to use the gene expression levels of all combinations of three genes to attempt to predict the expression level of a fourth gene requires evaluation of millions of pair-wise combinations. When one moves to all combinations of four genes that could predict a fifth gene, the number of calculations increases the problem space to billions of combinations! To put this seemingly esoteric discussion into the context of the reader of this commentary, it is increasingly clear that the study by any approach of any single gene is incapable of holding enough information to answer key clinical questions with certainty. It is therefore becoming important to look at combinations of genes to identify predictor gene sets that do have sufficient power. However, the computer requirements for employing the aforementioned combinatorial methods are daunting. For example, if one attempted to run on a typical desktop computer the aforementioned computational tools to identify a 3-gene predictive set from a pool of as few as 600, one would literally need to leave their computer running for years.[11] This illustrates that supercomputer resources are clearly required, and by using "computer clusters" where hundreds of computational nodes can be dedicated to the problem, the run time for these types of problems can be reduced from years to days or in some cases minutes. The point is that the merger of genetic tools with medicine is increasingly requiring the integration of computer science and a host of other systems approaches to maximize benefit to the scientist, physician, and ultimately the patient.

Moving beyond annotations, the emerging field of Systems Biology[12] suggests that one cannot understand a cell system simply by enumerating its components. Cellular systems are dynamic, and the topology, control, and communication systems must all be considered and integrated with information about the component genes and gene products in order to arrive at a model that is a reasonable approximation of the system. The point here again is not simply to note that the complex is becoming more complex but to suggest that in the postgenomic world gene expression information is only one tool in the toolkit and is most valuable when partnered with mathematic and computational techniques. Ultimately, it is integrative approaches coming from the intersection of multiple disciplines that will help translate genomic and proteomic information into treatments that provide beneficial clinical outcomes for patients with pancreatic cancer and other complex diseases.[13]

References

1. Lander ES, et al. Initial sequencing and analysis of the human genome. *Nature.* 2001;409:860–921.
2. Kallioniemi OP, Wagner U, Kononen J, Sauter G. Tissue microarray technology for high-throughput molecular profiling of cancer. *Hum Mol Genet.* 2001;10:657–662.
3. Pruitt KD, Katz KS, Sicotte H, Maglott DR. Introducing RefSeq and LocusLink: curated human genome resources at the NCBI. *Trends Genet.* 2000;16:44–47.
4. Apweiler R, Bairoch A, Wu CH, et al. UniProt: the Universal Protein knowledge base. *Nucleic Acids Res.* 2004;32 Database issue: D115–D119.
5. Hamosh A, Scott AF, Amberger J, Bocchini C, Valle D, McKusick VA. Online Mendelian Inheritance in Man (OMIM), a knowledgebase of human genes and genetic disorders. *Nucleic Acids Res.* 2002;30:52–55.
6. Harris MA, Clark J, Ireland A, et al. The Gene Ontology (GO) database and informatics resource. *Nucleic Acids Res.* 2004;32:Database issue:D258–D261.
7. Bader GD, Betel D, Hogue CD. BIND: the Biomolecular Interaction Network Database. *Nucleic Acids Res.* 2003;31:248–250.
8. Kanehisa M, Goto S, Kawashima S, Okuno Y, Hattori M. The KEGG resource for deciphering the genome. *Nucleic Acids Res.* 2004;32 Database issue:D277–D280.
9. Hashimoto RF, Kim S, Shmulevich I, Zhang W, Bittner ML, Dougherty ER. Growing genetic regulatory networks from seed genes. *Bioinformatics.* 2004;20:1241–1247.
10. Molidor R, Sturn A, Maurer M, Trajanoski Z. New trends in bioinformatics: from genome sequence to personalized medicine. *Exp Gerontol.* 2003;38:1031–1036.
11. Kim S, Dougherty ER, Chen Y. Multivariate measurement of gene expression relationships. *Genomics.* 2000;67:201–209.
12. Weston AD, Hood L. Systems biology, proteomics, and the future of health care: toward predictive, preventative, and personalized medicine. *J Proteome Res.* 2004;3:179–196.
13. Collins FS, Green ED, Guttmacher AE, et al. A vision for the future of genomics research. *Nature.* 2003;422:835–847.

CHAPTER 37

Gene Therapy and Virotherapy for Pancreatic Cancer

Masato Yamamoto, MD, PhD
David T. Curiel, MD, PhD

Concept of Cancer Gene Therapy for Pancreatic Cancer

Despite the number of efforts to improve the clinical outcome of pancreatic cancer patients, the prognosis of patients with unresectable carcinomas is still dismal.[1-4] New therapeutic modalities are urgently needed, and gene therapy represents one promising strategy. Initially, gene therapy encompassed the treatment of diseases caused by the impaired functionality of a specific gene by restoring that particular gene. However, as the development of gene delivery strategies progressed, the potential applications of gene therapy have expanded dramatically to include a large variety of schemes for the treatment of target diseases. Thus, gene therapy is better defined as "treatment of disease by introducing a gene with therapeutic effect or manipulating the disease-related gene." Additionally, a related field known as *virotherapy* is quickly emerging that exploits advanced virology along with viral vector design for gene therapy to eradicate cancer through the use of replicative viruses. As shown in Table 37.1, many of these methods have been attempted in the field of pancreatic cancer. In this chapter, we discuss the application of these new modalities to the treatment of pancreatic cancer.

Effectors Used for Pancreatic Cancer Gene Therapy

Various strategies have been investigated in the treatment of pancreatic cancer (Table 37.1). Although Table 37.1 includes only techniques reported in the context of pancreatic cancer, this covers most categories of cancer gene therapy. Cancer gene therapy is categorized into two distinct groups, depending on the target cell: (1) anti-tumor therapy based on direct cell killing and (2) anti-tumor therapy based on the manipulation of host cells. Some of the transgenes used for the first category are tumor selective, whereas others are not. For example, mutation compensation therapy with wild-type p53 expression is based on the concept that mutation of the proapoptotic *TP53* gene in cancer cells makes those cells selectively susceptible for wild-type p53–mediated apoptosis.[5] In this case, expression selectivity is not required, because the transgene does not harm normal cells. On the contrary, so-called suicide gene therapy with a transgene to

Table 37.1 Methods for Pancreatic Cancer Gene Therapy

Aim	Methods	Reported Transgene
Direct anti-tumor effect	Mutation compensation*	wt-p53,[14] p16(INK4a/CDKN2),[17]
	Suicide gene therapy*	thymidine kinase,[19,56,130-132] cytosine, deaminase,[133,134] UPRT,[135] nitroreductase,[136] CYP2B1[137]
	Blocking tumor growth cascade	
	Growth factor blockade	NK4 (HGF blockade)[20]
	Dominant-negative oncogene	DN-MEKK1,[21] DN-H-*ras*[22]
	Receptor with anti-tumor efficacy	SSTR-2[23,24]
	Apoptotic inducer†	TNF-α,[138] Bax,[139,140] p73,[141] E2F-1,[142,143] MDA-7,[140] fragile histidine triad (FHIT),[65] P21/WAF1,[144] Fas-estrogen receptor fusion protein[145]
	Antisense DNA and ribozymes	AS-CaSm,[146] AS-E-cadherin,[147] AS-PKC,[148]
	AS-AKT2,[149] rybozyme-K-*ras*[33]	
	Virotherapy*	Replicative HSV (hrR3, G207, NV1020),[66-68] herpesvirus saimiri,[150] E1b-deleted replicative adenovirus,[49,151] promoter-based CRAds,[63] E1a RNA stability-control CRFAds[74,75]
Indirect anti-tumor effect	Immunogene therapy through host cells	IL-2,[152-154] IL-4,[153,154] IL-13,[155] IL-12,[156] B7.1,[156] p202,[157] GM-CSF[9]
	Antivascularization therapy	Soluble Flk1,[51] soluble Flt-1[10]
	Metalloproteinase inhibitors	TIMP-1,[11,55] TIMP-2[55]

Abbreviations: HGF, hepatocyte growth factor; SSTR-2, somatostatin receptor type 2; TIMP, tissue inhibitor of metalloproteinase; wt, wild-type; UPRT, uracil phosphoribosyl transferase; TNF-α, tumor necrosis factor-α; MDA-7, melanoma differentiation-associated gene-7; HSV, herpes simplex virus; CRAd, conditionally replicative adenovirus; IL, interleukin; GM-CSF, granulocyte macrophage colony stimulating factor.

*Showing bystander effect.

†Some show bystander effect.

activate a prodrug requires selectivity of transgene expression because this method kills all the cells once the prodrug is converted to its active form, regardless of the nature of the cells.[6,7] The second category of cancer gene therapy achieves a therapeutic effect by manipulating host cells, including immunogene therapy to enhance the immune reaction of the host against neoplastic cells by activating immune cells or enhancing antigen presentation,[8,9] which is discussed by Drs. Laheru and Jaffee in Chapter 40 of this book. Other methods in this category involve modification of the blood supply to the tumor environment[10] and alteration of the surrounding stromal cell conditions.[11] This second group of strategies does not necessarily require selective gene expression.

Mutation Compensation

Mutation compensation methods take advantage of the fact that certain neoplasms lack the functionality of proapoptotic moieties such as p53, creating a situation in which transcomplementation of the defective gene induces apoptosis in a tumor-selective manner.[5] Because these effector genes do not harm normal cells carrying the normal gene, this method possesses intrinsic selectivity for cancer cells with a *TP53* mutation. Gene therapy with a *TP53*-expressing adenovirus vector was first applied for lung cancer[12] as well as pancreatic cancers.[13-16] Also, a *p16*-expressing adenovirus vector has also been applied for $p16^{INK4a/CDKN2}$ inactivated pancreatic cancer.[17]

Suicide Gene Therapy

Suicide gene therapy or virus-directed enzyme/prodrug therapy is an approach to the treatment of pancreatic cancer that uses combinations of nontoxic (or less toxic) prodrugs and enzymes such that a prodrug is converted into its active form, leading to a cytocidal effect[11] (Table 37.2). Usually, the selectivity of the system is controlled by the activity of the enzymes through targeted expression. To this end, α-fetoprotein promoter–based control has been

Table 37.2 Enzyme-Prodrug Combination for Suicide Gene Therapy

Enzyme	Origin	Prodrug
Thymidine kinase (TK)	HSV, VZV	Ganciclovir, acyclovir, penciclovir
Cytosine deaminase	*E. coli*, yeast	5-Fluorocytosine
UPRT	*E. coli*	5-Fluorouracil
Nitroreductase	*E. coli*	CB1954
CYP2B1	Rat	ifosfamide

Abbreviations: *E. coli*, *Escherichia coli*; HSV, herpes simplex virus; UPRT, uracil phosphoribosyl transferase; VZV, varicella-zoster virus.

applied in retroviral expression of thymidine kinase (TK) for hepatoma.[18] The first application in the field of pancreatic cancer was treatment with a retrovirus vector with carcinoembryonic antigen (CEA) promoter-driven TK expression.[19] Each system listed in Table 37.2 has its pros and cons. For example, in the TK-ganciclovir (GCV) system, the phosphorylated GCV can spread to adjacent cells via gap junction but does not leave the cells. In the cytosine deaminase and 5-fluorocytosine system, the activated form (5-fluorouracil) can diffuse to the surrounding area. Thus, the TK-GCV system should provide stricter localization, whereas the cytosine deaminase and 5-fluorocytosine system would achieve cytocidal effect in a larger area. These methods exhibit very dependable cytocidal effects in cells expressing the activating enzymes in vitro and in vivo. However, they require tight regulatory mechanisms to achieve tumor-selective expression of the enzymes because the fate of the cells is determined solely by the level of the converting enzyme, regardless of the nature of the cells. We discuss this "targeting" issue later in this chapter.

Blocking Tumor Growth Cascade

Strategies to block tumor growth signaling can be categorized into three subgroups. The first is receptor-level blocking of growth factors relevant to pancreatic cancer expansion (e.g., NK4: hepatocyte growth factor blocker[20]). This scheme does not require transgene expression in the neoplastic cells as long as the local concentration of the effector reaches an effective level. The second method is the use of dominant-negative (DN) oncogenes, which can block the relevant signal transduction in the cells (e.g., DN-MEKK1,[21] DN-H-Ras[22]). The third approach is the use of receptors with anti-tumor effect. In pancreatic cancers, the somatostatin receptor type 2 is known to show anti-tumor effect after tumor cell transduction.[23,24] The latter two systems require transgene expression in the target cancer cells for effect.

Inducers of Apoptosis

Various inducers of apoptosis have been applied to the treatment of pancreatic cancer. Although these genes can induce cancer cell death effectively, most of these molecules induce apoptotic cell death, regardless of the malignant potential of the cells. Thus, once again, tumor selectivity needs to be achieved via targeted gene introduction and/or its expression. Highly specific targeting needs to be achieved before these approaches can be realized clinically.[25] Another technical issue with the use of viral vectors for the delivery of these genes is that the expression of apoptotic inducers hampers the effective propagation of viral vectors in mammalian cells during production. This leads to limited or nonproductive replication of the vectors. To avoid this problem, host cells have been modified to be resistant to the expressed apoptotic inducer,[26] whereas strict switching has been incorporated into the vector system to suppress undesired transgene expression[27,28] during vector propagation.

Antisense Nucleotides and Ribozymes

Direct blocking of the function of a gene that is crucial for cancer growth with the use of nucleotides is a straightforward approach for the regulation of neoplasms. Because mutation of the *KRAS2* gene is frequently observed in patients with pancreatic cancer[29,30] and is critical for the malignant potential of these cancer cells,[31] this gene has been a good target of antisense/ribozyme strategies. Although several antisense oligonucleotides and ribozymes have exhibited antitumor effects,[32-34] the function of these agents requires high levels of in situ introduction of the nucleotides into each neoplastic cell. This is one of the key limiting factors of the clinical application of these methods to patients with cancer.

Virotherapy

Viral cytolysis is a widely known phenomenon in the field of virology. Thus, the use of various wild-type and modified viruses as cancer therapeutics is a rational approach. These viruses, which possess the ability to replicate within specific tissues, have been used in human clinical trials to achieve selective oncolysis of several types of neoplasms (Fig 37.1). Such viruses include adenoviruses,[35,36] mumps virus,[37] and West Nile virus.[38]

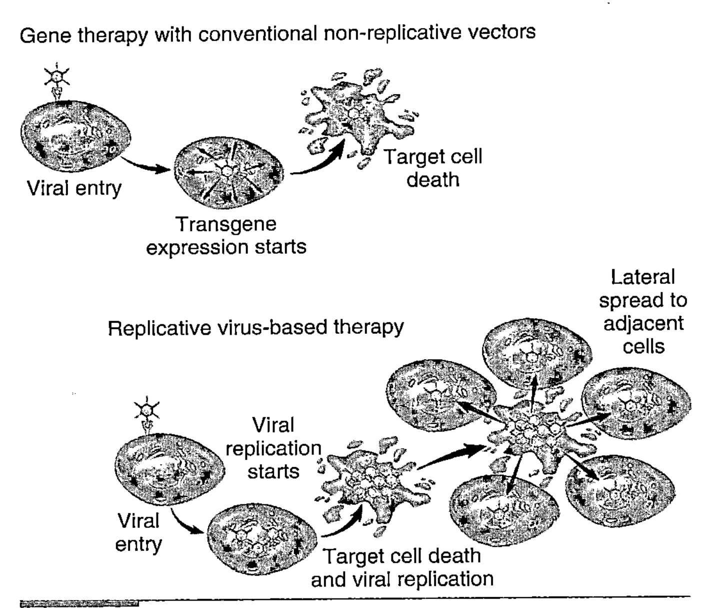

Figure 37.1
Replicative virus-based therapy. In conventional non-replicative vector–based gene therapy, the vector enters the target cell and expresses the effector gene to kill the tumor cells. In replicative virus–based therapy, the virus replicates in the initial infected target cell after entry and kills the cell by cytolysis through lytic infection. Subsequently, the released viruses infect surrounding target cells. The achievement of this lateral spread is a key for effective replicative virus–based therapy.

More recently, parvovirus H-1[39] and herpes simplex virus[40-44] (HSV) have been shown to achieve viral oncolysis of neoplastic cells. Because a major reason for the poor outcomes of cancer gene therapy clinical trials is insufficient transduction of the neoplasms, virotherapy offers a solution for this problem in that tumor-selective vector replication and lateral spread of the progeny would augment the therapeutic effect.[45-47] Initially, adenoviruses were one of the first wild-type viruses applied to cancer in the 1950s and 1960s.[35] Although these studies provided the background for virotherapy, the viruses used did not accomplish the expected therapeutic effect. Recently, advances in virology and the accumulated knowledge of vector modification have led to the development of advanced generation replicative viral agents. As shown in Table 37.3, these modalities achieve selective antitumor effect through scientifically designed mechanisms that control viral replication, and some are already at the stage of clinical evaluation. In the field of pancreatic cancer, conditionally replicative adenovirus ONYX-015 has been tested by direct injection into the carcinoma, but it did not show a clear therapeutic effect.[48,49]

Immunogene Therapy

The goal of immunogene therapy is to modulate the host immune system to fight against cancer cells. The strategy is discussed in detail by Drs. Laheru and Jaffee in Chapter 40.

Antivascularization Therapy

Carcinomas cannot develop to a detectable size without neovascularization, a process in which vascular endothelial growth factor plays a key role to recruit new vessels.[50] The blockade of vascular endothelial growth factor can therefore be used for antivascularization purposes. A soluble fragment of the vascular endothelial growth factor receptor (soluble Flk-1[51] and Flt-1[10]) has been used to treat pancreatic cancer.

Table 37.3 Replicative Viral Agents in Clinical Trials

Virus	Safety Feature	Reports in Pancreatic Cancer
Adenovirus	Mutation	Yes (ONYX-015)
	Promoter-based control of E1 and/or E4	Yes (RGD CRAd COX2F, dl331)
Herpesvirus	ICP-6 inactivation	Yes (hrR3)
	Deletion of UL-US joint region (including one γ34.5)	Yes (NV1020)
	ICP-6 inactivation and deletion of both γ34.5	Yes (G207)
	more than 20 other viruses	
Vaccinia virus	Vaccine strain	No
Epstein-Barr virus (EBV)	Requires immediate early proteins (BZLF1 or BRLF1)	No
Reovirus	Nonpathogenic, limited replication in Ras-activated cells	Yes (subtype 3)
Newcastle disease virus	Avian pathogen	No
Measles virus	Vaccine strain (Edmonston-B)	No

Metalloproteinase Inhibitors

Matrix metalloproteinase enzymes are involved in the proteolysis of the extracellular matrix, aiding neoplastic cell invasion and establishment of metastatic deposits.[52] In addition, matrix metalloproteinase enzyme expression is associated with neovascularization,[53] which is required to maintain the blood supply to the growing tumor. Tissue inhibitors of metalloproteinases are expressed in pancreatic cancers, and the balance of tissue inhibitor of metalloproteinase and matrix metalloproteinase enzyme expression is a key factor in pancreatic cancer development.[54] Based on this biology, the overexpression of tissue inhibitor of metalloproteinase has been successful in mouse models.[11,55]

The aforementioned modalities encompass the cancer gene therapy strategies proposed for pancreatic cancer. Most of these methods show promise for the future treatment of pancreatic cancer. Of note, some of these approaches are in preparation or are already in clinical trials.

Delivery Systems Used for Pancreatic Cancer Gene Therapy

Nonviral Gene Delivery

A big advantage of nonviral gene delivery is that this system only minimally invokes vector-derived immunogenicity. By contrast, viral vectors are widely known to induce various levels of immune reaction against viral components of the vectors. To date, the efficiency of nonviral gene delivery is lower than that of viral techniques. One possible reason is inefficient nuclear transport of the gene after endocytosis. Although several efforts have been made to improve nuclear localization, reports of in vivo efficacy of nonviral gene delivery systems in the field of pancreatic cancer are limited.[56] In several instances, this method was applied to the delivery of oligonucleotides (e.g., antisense oligonucleotide, ribozyme) and showed in vivo efficacy.[32,57,58] In these studies, the injection route was intraperitoneal. The enclosed environment of this administration site may have enhanced the delivery efficiency.

Nonreplicative Viral Vectors

A number of nonreplicative viral vectors have been used in gene therapy for pancreatic cancers. A retroviral vector was used for ex vivo gene transfer of pancreatic cancer cells for directed enzyme prodrug gene therapy using a CEA promoter-driven TK expression vector.[19] For in vivo transduction, inoculation of retroviral packaging cell lines for in situ vector production was used to compensate for the relatively low in vivo transduction efficiency after direct vector administration.[59] In this retroviral system, it was necessary to improve in vivo transduction efficiency to demonstrate clinical feasibility.

Adenoviral vectors have been used most frequently for pancreatic cancer gene therapy. Although the transduction efficiency of adenoviral vectors in pancreatic cancer is relatively high in comparison to other vectors, the efficiency of these vectors in pancreatic cancer is still much lower than those of other cancers because of the low levels of expression of the primary viral receptor (Coxsackie-adenovirus receptor [CAR]) by pancreatic cancer cells.[60] Of all viral vectors, adenoviral vectors are the most advanced in the context of vector modification because of their relatively simple infection process mediated by protein-protein interaction and the rich background information accumulated from the long history of adenovirus virology.[61] In the field of pancreatic cancer, antibody-based targeting (fibroblast growth factor [FGF] receptor[62]) and fiber modification-based infectivity enhancement (RGD in HI-loop[60,63]) have been reported.

Adeno-associated viral vectors have the advantage of long-term expression of transgenes.[64] This vector has been used for the expression of fragile histidine triad and showed promising in vivo effects.[65] Overall, each viral vector system has its advantages and limitations. Thus, selecting the optimal vector that best fits to the goal of the therapy is a key for success.

Virotherapy (Replicative Virus System)

The nature of pancreatic cancer defines some requirements for novel therapeutics. Because no gene delivery strategy can achieve transduction of 100% of the neoplastic cells, the therapeutic effectors need to be functional not only in the initially transduced cells but also in the surrounding cancer cells. Strategies with a so-called bystander effect or those that use an indirect anti-tumor effect via host cell modulation have the potential to achieve such widespread effects. Among them, virotherapy is one of the most promising approaches because the target cancer cells that are killed by the replicative agent become the producers of the next generation of viral progeny.[45] The extent of replicative virus spread would easily exceed the bystander effect accomplished through gap junction–mediated transportation or secretion of therapeutic effectors. In the field of pancreatic cancer, adenovirus,[48,49,63] HSV,[66-68] and reovirus[69] have been reported to be effective virotherapy agents in xenograft mouse models.

Adenovirus, dl1520 (ONYX-015), was the first oncolytic virus applied for pancreatic cancer.[48,49] Even though this

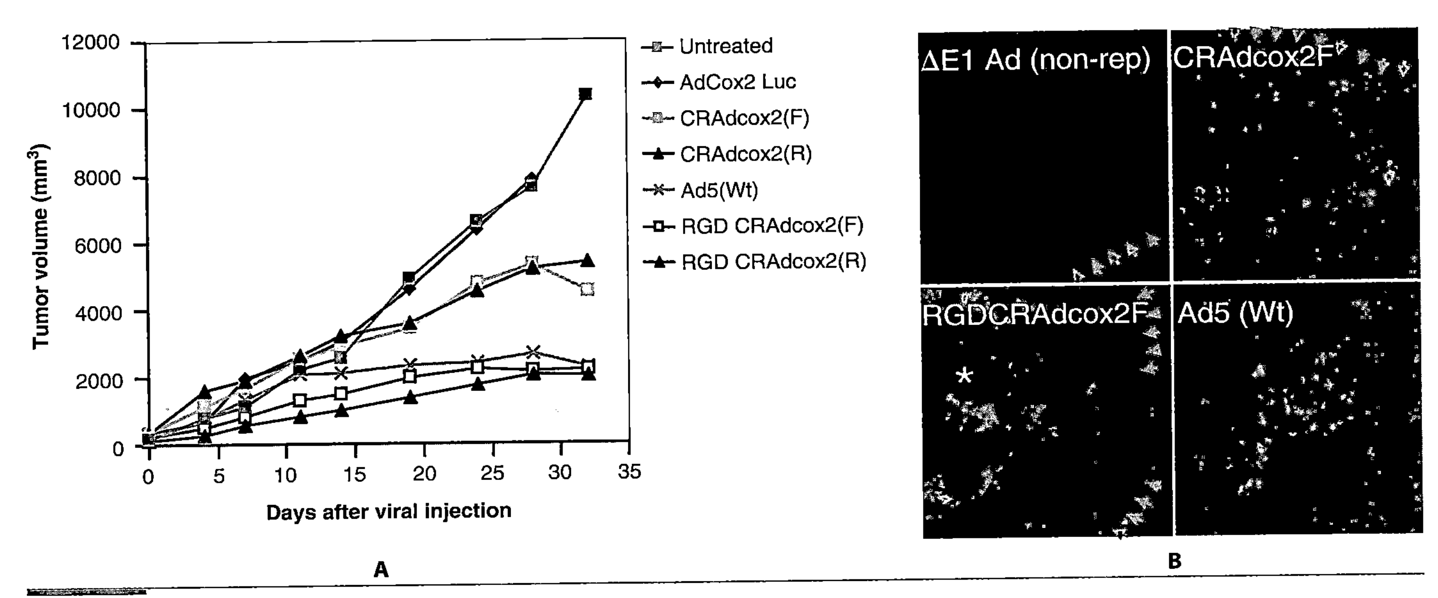

Figure 37.2
Functionality of infectivity-enhanced coxsackievirus (COX)-2 promoter-controlled conditionally replicative adenoviruses (CRAds). **(A)** Anti-tumor effect in subcutaneous xenograft model. In Hs766T human pancreatic cancer xenografts, 10^9 vp (viral particles) of the COX-2 CRAds with unmodified fiber (CRAdcox2F and CRAdcox2R) demonstrated some therapeutic effect, but it was not statistically significant from the control ($P > 0.05$, day 24). The RGD-modified COX-2 CRAds (RGD CRAdcox2F and RGD CRAdcox2R) showed a stronger anti-tumor effect, which was statistically significant when compared with the untreated group and the group that received nonreplicative control vectors ($P < 0.005$ at day 24, $P < 0.05$ at later points). **(B)** In vivo replication. After intratumoral injection of COX-2 CRAds adenoviral hexon protein was stained by immunostaining. Although there was no stained cell in the tumor with nonreplicative E1-deleted vector, tumors with CRAdcox2F, RGDCRAdcox2F, and Ad5(Wt) revealed cells expressing hexon. The outer edge of the tumor is shown with arrows. Necrosis in the center is shown with an asterisk.

virus showed promise in head and neck cancer clinical trials,[70] it did not show clear therapeutic benefit in pancreatic cancer (computed tomographically guided or intraoperative injection [phase I],[48] endoscopic ultrasonography–guided injection [phase I/II][49]). In an endoscopic ultrasonographic protocol, no viral replication was detected by in situ hybridization-based analysis of viral DNA. The expression of CAR in pancreatic cancer tends to be minimal (see detail in transduction efficacy section), and therefore, this deficiency would hamper secondary infection by progeny virus. The introduction of an RGD-4C motif in the HI-loop of the fiber knob region enhanced infectivity in pancreatic cancer by achieving CAR-independent infection through binding onto cell surface integrins.[60] This method was successfully applied with the use of a coxsackievirus (COX)-2 promoter–controlled conditionally replicative adenoviruses (CRAds) and was shown to dramatically enhance anti-tumor effect in a subcutaneous xenograft model of human pancreatic cancer (Fig. 37.2).[63] These findings serve as a proof-of-principle validation of infectivity-enhanced CRAds in this field.

Virotherapy using infectivity enhancements may lead to greater transduction of nonneoplastic tissues. Thus, a higher level of selectivity is needed for the safety of replicative vectors to avoid the problem of leaky replication in normal tissues.[45,46] Several methods have been proposed to increase the selectivity of CRAds. One technique is the optimization of tumor-specific promoter using promoter-controlled E1 expression–type CRAds. There are many promoters that are potentially applicable to the construction of pancreatic cancer CRAds. However, some of them are too weak to drive effective viral replication, and others become leaky when configured in an adenovirus vector (especially in CRAds). Among the best candidates, the COX-2 promoter shows a very high level of promoter activity comparable to that of the cytomegalovirus promoter, and the activity of the COX-2 promoter in normal liver is more than four orders lower than that of the cytomegalovirus promoter.[71] Because adenoviral vectors are associated with hepatotoxicity, low promoter activity in the liver is required to avoid this complication. COX-2 promoter–driven CRAds therefore show a nice therapeutic profile for the treatment of pancreatic cancer.[63]

A second strategy in the design of CRAd is to mutate the E1 region of the viral genome such that the defect can be compensated for only in a tumor cell environment. Based on this approach, a virus with an eight-amino-acid deletion in the CR2 (Δ24) and the one with additional 54-amino-acid deletion in CR1 region (CB016) have been proposed as selective oncolytic agents.[72,73]

A recent and novel approach is to control the stability of the E1 RNA. One such method uses the COX-2 3′-untranslated region to provide differential RNA stability, depending on the Ras activity of the target cell.[74] Another method relies on mutation of virus-associated RNAs that are necessary for inactivating protein kinase R to avoid an interferon response and promote viral replication. Virus-associated RNA mutant viruses cannot inactivate protein kinase R; therefore, viral replication occurs only in cells in which protein kinase R is inhibited through such mechanisms as Ras activation.[75] Because activating *KRAS2* mutations are one of the most frequently observed genetic alterations in pancreatic cancers, these strategies are suitable for pancreatic cancer CRAds.

To achieve greater selectivity and potency, CRAds have been designed based on critical virologic and oncologic features of adenovirus and pancreatic cancer. The combination of these strategies may achieve new-generation CRAds with better therapeutic profiles.

More than 20 HSV-based oncolytic viruses have been applied to the treatment of cancer. Among them, hrR3 (ICP-6 inactivation),[66] NV1020 (deletion of UL-US joint region, including one γ34.5),[67] and G207 (ICP-6 inactivation and deletion of both γ34.5)[67,68] have been tested for pancreatic cancer. Although one of the first-generation vectors, hrR3,[76] showed promise in mouse xenograft experiments,[42] this vector demonstrated residual neurotoxicity.[77] Another first-generation vector, NV1020, which was originally developed as a vaccine strain, has improved safety in rodents and primates[78] and was used as an oncolytic agent for non-central nervous system tumors.[79] A second-generation HSV vector, G207, contains multiple mutations to increase safety.[80] In *Aotus nancymai*, a New World owl monkey, inoculation of 10^9 plaque-forming units of G207 did not cause any adverse effects, even after intracerebral injection, whereas the parental F strain caused lethal encephalitis at a dose of 10^3 plaque-forming units.[81] The efficacy and safety data for replicative herpesvirus vectors are still accumulating. Although these studies have established feasibility and key fundamentals for the utility of replication-competent HSV vectors for the treatment of cancer, including those of pancreatic cancer origin, numerous significant hurdles need to be overcome for the full realization of this system.[47] The first obstacle is targeting. In contrast to adenovirus, in which transductional targeting has been relatively successful, targeting of HSV has been difficult because of complex mechanisms of infection. However, transcriptional targeting using tumor-specific promoters has already been successfully used in this system. The second hurdle that needs to be overcome is suboptimal spread of newly replicated virus as a result of the complex configuration of carcinomas, with physical barriers preventing viral spread. The third hurdle is neurovirulence. Even though second-generation vectors showed a nice safety profile in a very sensitive experimental owl monkey model, toxicity issues may still arise if less attenuated viruses need to be used to achieve stronger anti-tumor effects. In aggregate, despite several significant hurdles, replication-competent HSV vectors show promise for the treatment of solid tumors, including pancreatic cancer.

Reovirus is a double-stranded RNA virus commonly isolated from the respiratory and gastrointestinal tract of humans.[82] The most interesting molecular biologic feature of this virus is that it requires activated Ras for replication.[83] Based on this fact, pancreatic cancer is one of the best targets for this virus because *KRAS2*–activating mutations are frequently observed in pancreatic cancers. Indeed, this was the case when Etoh et al.[69] applied this virus in pancreatic cancer and showed anti-tumor effect and viral replication in the tumor.[69]

Theoretically, many viruses of human and other species origin have potential as a therapeutic agent for cancer. Because the power of replicative viral agents has been clearly validated, other viruses, including modified versions of existing viral agents, will perhaps be further applied in the same manner. Pancreatic cancer will continue to be a popular target of these new therapeutic modalities because of its dismal prognosis.

Problems of Current Pancreatic Cancer Gene Therapy and Efforts to Overcome Them

Transduction Efficiency

Cancer gene therapy clinical trials carried out to date have fallen short of their therapeutic expectations. These trials have demonstrated extremely limited tumor transduction frequencies and have suggested that this limitation may represent a fundamental barrier to realizing the full potential of cancer gene therapy.[84-87] Because the success of any gene therapy approach is fundamentally based on the ability to deliver the therapeutic gene to target cells with a requisite level of efficiency,[84,85,88,89] optimal tumor transduction is a key factor that must be addressed to realize gene therapy for pancreatic cancer. To date, viral vectors tend to have higher transduction efficiency than nonviral methods. There are two viral vectors that have been widely used for gene delivery to pancreatic cancer cells: (1) adenovirus-based system[90] and (2) HSV-based system.[47] Adenoviral vectors have been extensively used because of their high infectivity in a relatively wide range of tumor types.[91] However, the transduction of some types of cancer cells is poor because of low levels of expression of the primary adenovirus receptor, CAR.[91] Low CAR expression is typically the case for pancreatic cancers.[60] To overcome this problem, infection via Coxsackie-adenovirus receptor–independent mechanism is necessary. Interestingly, adenovirus has considerable versatility in the context of tropism modification based on capsid alteration. In particular, the fiber-knob region of adenovirus has several sites into which extrinsic peptide sequences for binding can be incorporated (e.g., HI-loop,[92] C-terminal[93]). The incorporation of an RGD motif that binds to integrins expressed on pancreatic cancer cells conferred high transduction efficiencies in CAR-negative cells through initial binding to integrins instead of to CAR.[94] Because infectivity of the progeny virus is one of the most important determining factors for the potency of replicative agents, infectivity enhancement should augment the potency of conditionally replicative adenoviruses. In fact, in the application of the aforementioned infectivity enhancement in CRAds, RGD-modified Δ24[95,96] and COX-2 CRAds[63] showed dramatically enhanced anti-tumor effects in vivo. Thus, infectivity enhancement is also a rational design for CRAds.

Although replication-competent HSV has been successfully applied to pancreatic cancers (see details in virotherapy section), suboptimal in vivo viral replication remains a barrier limiting the full potential of this system.[47] Infectivity enhancement based on transductional targeting for HSV is not easy because of its relatively complex infection mechanism. However, attempts to incorporate a syncytium-forming property might circumvent this problem[97]. The application of nonreplicative HSV vectors (amplicons) has been limited to vaccination purposes.[98] Should these agents be used for direct transduction of the cancer cells, improvement of transduction efficiency may be required.

Generally, for any vector types, higher transduction efficiency would reduce innate immune response to the vector because a much lower dose would be needed. So far, no incidence of severe adverse effects due to too high transduction has been reported in the context of cancer gene therapy. Because of the limitations outlined earlier, improvements in transduction will clearly be needed to realize the benefits of gene therapy in the field of pancreatic cancer. However, increased infectivity of the tumor may also augment transduction of normal cells; as a result, more selectivity may be required to maintain safety when these approaches are used. This balance between transduction efficiency and selectivity will be very important for the clinical utility of these new therapeutic modalities.

Selectivity

Because cancer gene therapy aims to selectively eliminate cancer cells, the effect of the treatment (usually cytocidal) needs to be limited to cancer cells to avoid adverse effects on normal cells. If the transgene itself is not toxic to normal cells, this selectivity requirement is of low priority. For example, adenoviral gene therapy with *p53* expression, which causes selective apoptotic cell death in *TP53* gene-mutated cancer cells while leaving surrounding normal cells intact, would not need further targeting for safety.[5] On the contrary, if the effector shows nonspecific cytocidal effect, some selectivity feature is necessary to avoid toxicity in normal organs. For example, in suicide gene therapy with HSV thymidine kinase as a transgene, virtually all cells expressing HSV thymidine kinase are killed after administration of GCV. Thus, tumor-specific expression of the effector is absolutely required to specifically kill cancer targets. In the case of adenoviral vectors, the vast majority of the vector injected or released into circulation localizes to the liver.[99] As a result, TK-expressing adenoviral vectors controlled with an ubiquitous promoter (e.g., cytomegalovirus immediate early promoter) showed lethal toxicity after administration of GCV.[71] This toxicity can be mitigated with the use of a selective promoter that is minimally active in the liver (e.g., COX-2 promoter).[71] These results clearly indicate the importance of selective expression of a toxic transgene for safety.

Selective expression can be achieved both transcriptionally and transductionally. Because the goal of targeting is to achieve maximal differential between cancer cells and background normal cells, the requirements for targeting are (1) high transgene expression at the requisite level for therapeutic effect and (2) minimal expression in nonneoplastic tissues below the level of toxicity. Transcriptional targeting uses selective promoters for the control of expression. For the adenovirus system, various tumor-specific promoters have been reported to achieve this goal in pancreatic cancer (e.g., CEA promoter,[19] MUC1 promoter,[100] COX-2 promoter[63,101]). However, when typical E1-deleted nonreplicative adenoviral vectors are used, the activity of enhancer/packaging signal region and cryptic transcription initiation sites can greatly affect the expression from promoters placed in the E1 region, leading to leaky expression of the transgene.[102,103] One way to enhance the fidelity of the promoter is to place an insulator between the viral sequence and the expression cassette.[103] Another approach is to move the enhancer/packaging signal to the right end of the viral genome,[104] which helps lower expression of the transgene from cryptic promoter sequences.[103]

Transductional targeting achieves selectivity at the level of gene delivery. This method is the most advanced for adenoviral vectors because this vector enters target cells via a well-defined mechanism on the basis of protein-protein interaction. There are two strategies in this targeting category. The first one is positively targeting the vector to the desired cells by incorporating a targeting motif in the vector capsid proteins,[105-107] using an antibody with targeting capability,[108] or substituting the fiber with that of another serotype fiber to achieve different tropism.[109-111] In the field of pancreatic cancer, FGF-2 conjugated with a Fab′2 fragment against the adenovirus knob region was successfully applied for in vitro adenoviral transduction of FGF-R–overexpressing pancreatic cancer cells.[62] The second transductional targeting approach is to improve the tumor/background ratio by reducing vector distribution to normal organ and/or by increasing tumor transduction. In order to reduce native hepatotropism, several vectors with capsid mutations have been reported.[112,113] Because the blood flow from the pancreas goes directly into the portal vein and then to the liver, untargeting the liver is an important issue when adenovirus is used for the treatment of pancreatic cancer. Dmitriev et al.[94] reported infectivity enhancement in CAR-negative cells by incorporating an RGD-4C motif into the adenoviral fiber[94] (described in the transduction efficiency section). Typically, pancreatic cancer cells express minimal CAR on their surface, in contrast to normal cells. The use of the aforementioned infectivity enhancement studies may improve the tumor/normal ratio to decrease toxicity.[60]

Monitoring Therapeutic Agents

To determine the functionality of the cancer gene therapy strategies, interval endpoint assays are needed to monitor treatment progress. These assays should be informative yet minimally invasive and would also be valuable for maintaining safety in clinical trials. For example, if the expression of TK could be monitored in normal organs, administration of the prodrugs could be halted if an undesired expression profile is observed. Such detection of transgene expression has been performed by immunoblotting or immunohistochemistry in biopsy specimens.[114] Although biopsy examination is informative, the invasiveness of this procedure is considerable, and the validity of the assay largely depends on the accessibility of the target organs to be tested. In the case of pancreatic cancer, biopsy evaluations would be difficult because of the limited accessibility of the organ.

Several efforts have been made to overcome this obstacle. One strategy is to use a secreted marker gene that could be detectable in the blood.[115] A soluble human carcinoembryonic antigen and β subunit of human chorionic gonadotropin has been successfully used to monitor tumor selective replication of an Edmonston-strain measles virus. However, monitoring secretory markers does not provide information on the cell types expressing the gene. Another strategy for monitoring therapy is imaging in which various established methods can be applied to the monitoring of transgene expression and/or viral replication. Radiologic imaging using radiolabeled substrates could be used to localize transgene expression with the use of radiolabeled prodrugs to image the localization of converting enzyme (e.g., 2′-fluoro-2′-deoxy-1 beta-D-aravinofuranosyl-5-iodouracil,[116,117] GCV[118,119] for TK) or radiolabeled ligand to image the localization of receptors (ligand peptides for somatostatin receptor-2[120] and dopamine receptor[121]). Labeling with a γ-ray emitter (e.g., ^{131}I, ^{99m}Tc) enables detection with γ-camera and single-photon emission computed tomography,[117] and labeling with a positron emitter (e.g., ^{18}F) enables detection with positron emission tomography.[121] Some radiolabeled ligand peptides have already been approved for clinical use in receptor imaging. In addition to radiologic imaging, optical imaging is also promising. Fluorescent proteins, like green fluorescent protein, have been used for in vitro imaging and were recently applied to in vivo imaging. Although this method does not require the administration of a tracer or substrate, it does require an excitation of a certain wavelength. Recently developed fluorescent proteins with red fluorescence (e.g., red fluorescent protein) could minimize nontarget tissue absorption.[122] Alternatively, luminescence-based optical imaging using luciferase genes can be applied for this purpose.[123,124] Although this latter method requires the administration of substrates, it has very high sensitivity relative to fluorescence imaging. In mice, luminescence imaging has been performed with minimal toxicity; however, its use and the application of fluorescence imaging have yet to be validated in humans. Both radiologic and optical imaging techniques may provide valid interval endpoints for clinical trials. The establishment of these methods will also be informative with regard to the in vivo properties of vectors in clinical settings. In aggregate, the wealth of the data from monitoring tools will not only help the planning of safer clinical trials but will also provide key information for future vector development.

In Vivo Experimental System

Mouse subcutaneous xenografts of human cancer cell lines have been most frequently used for in vivo evaluation of cancer gene therapy. In the case of replicative virus–based virotherapy, other animal systems are needed for the evaluation of toxicities because viruses have strict host requirements. For example, human adenoviruses do not replicate productively in mouse cells, confounding assessment of viral replication-based toxicity in mouse models. To address this complication, several models have been suggested. One model is the cotton rat, in which human adenovirus shows replication.[125-127] Although it is not clear how closely the viral replication in this system resembles that in humans, the fact that this is the only small animal system permissive for human adenovirus replication justifies the importance of this system. In addition to cotton rats, synergic models have been proposed to enhance understanding of the biology of replicative adenoviruses in their true host setting. One such system is the use of replicative canine adenovirus to treat spontaneous dog osteosarcoma. This unique model would provide valuable information on an oncolytic agent in its natural host. Such data would be translatable to humans because canine adenovirus is virologically very similar to human adenovirus.[128]

In the case of replicative HSV-based strategies, a strain of owl monkey *(Aotus nancymai)* provides a very useful model for analysis of toxicity.[81] This monkey is very sensitive to intracranial infection of HSV and experiences lethal encephalitis at a very lose dose.[81] This system has been successfully used for the preclinical safety evaluation of replicative HSV.

Overall, the development of experimental systems that more closely represent the clinical situation will increase the safety of cancer gene therapy modalities and will lead to a better understanding of the place of these strategies in clinical settings.

Conclusion

The fundamental genetic nature of pancreatic cancer and our improved understanding of which genes and pathways are targeted can be exploited through the development of new gene therapy modalities. The field of cancer gene therapy for pancreatic cancer is still too premature for its full potential to be realized. Although no method has proved to be clinically effective for cancers in general, many gene therapy modalities have been tested in the field of pancreatic cancer because of the strong need for novel therapeutics to improve this highly lethal form of cancer.

Since the initial recognized promise of gene therapy in the 1980s and the first gene therapy clinical trial for ADA deficiency in 1990, we have learned that there is no one ideal vector system appropriate for all diseases. A National Institutes of Health panel (co-chairs: Stuart H. Orkin, MD and Arno G. Motulsky, MD) published a report on the National Institutes of Health investment in gene therapy in 1995,[129] pointing out the lack of basic studies about vectors and disease pathophysiology. Since that time, the accumulation of basic data in the field of gene therapy has led to the development of new modalities with great promise. Although cancer gene therapy has not been established as a clinical option for patients, greater understanding of vector and effector design as well as pathophysiology will yield effective gene therapy agents for cancer. Perhaps in no other disease are novel therapeutics more needed than pancreatic cancer.

Acknowledgments

This manuscript is supported in part by National Institutes of Health grants R01 CA94084 (to D.T.C.), R01 DK63615 (to M.Y.), Department of Defense grant DAMD17-03-1-0104 (to M.Y.), P20CA101955 Project4 (to M.Y.), and an AVON Breast Cancer Research and Care Program grant (to M.Y.).

We appreciate Drs. Long P. Le, Pedro J. Ramirez, and Yaman Tekant for excellent advice and suggestions.

References

1. Jemal A, Tiwari RC, Murray T, Ghafoor A, Samuels A, Ward E, Feuer EJ, Thun MJ, American Cancer Society. Cancer Statistics, 2004. *CA Cancer J. Clin.* 2004;54:8–29.
2. Rosewicz S, Wiedenmann B. Pancreatic carcinoma. *Lancet.* 1997;349:485–489.
3. Gunzburg WH, Salmons B. Novel clinical strategies for the treatment of pancreatic carcinoma. *Trends Mol Med.* 2001;7:30–37.
4. Deininger MH, Schluesener HJ. Cyclooxygenases-1 and -2 are differentially localized to microglia and endothelium in rat EAE and glioma. *J Neuroimmunol.* 1999;95:202–208.
5. Roth JA, Swisher SG, Meyn RE. p53 tumor suppressor gene therapy for cancer. *Oncology (Huntingt).* 1999;13: 148–154.
6. Mullen CA. Metabolic suicide genes in gene therapy. *Pharmacol Ther.* 1994;63:199–207.
7. Fillat C, Carrio M, Cascante A, Sangro B. Suicide gene therapy mediated by the herpes simplex virus thymidine kinase gene/ganciclovir system: fifteen years of application. *Curr Gene Ther.* 2003;3:13–26.
8. Reilly RT, Machiels JP, Emens LA, Jaffee EM. Cytokine gene-modified cell-based cancer vaccines. *Methods Mol Med.* 2002;69:233–257.

9. Jaffee EM, Abrams R, Cameron J, et al. A phase I clinical trial of lethally irradiated allogeneic pancreatic tumor cells transfected with the GM-CSF gene for the treatment of pancreatic adenocarcinoma. *Hum Gene Ther.* 1998;9:1951–1971.
10. Hoshida T, Sunamura M, Duda DG, et al. Gene therapy for pancreatic cancer using an adenovirus vector encoding soluble flt-1 vascular endothelial growth factor receptor. *Pancreas.* 2002;25:111–121.
11. Bloomston M, Shafii A, Zervos EE, Rosemurgy AS. TIMP-1 overexpression in pancreatic cancer attenuates tumor growth, decreases implantation and metastasis, and inhibits angiogenesis. *J Surg Res.* 2002;102:39–44.
12. Zhang WW, Fang X, Mazur W, French BA, Georges RN, Roth JA. High-efficiency gene transfer and high-level expression of wild-type p53 in human lung cancer cells mediated by recombinant adenovirus. *Cancer Gene Ther.* 1994;1:5–13.
13. Cascallo M, Mercade E, Capella G, et al. Genetic background determines the response to adenovirus-mediated wild-type p53 expression in pancreatic tumor cells. *Cancer Gene Ther.* 1999;6:428–436.
14. Bouvet M, Bold RJ, Lee J, et al. Adenovirus-mediated wild-type p53 tumor suppressor gene therapy induces apoptosis and suppresses growth of human pancreatic cancer. *Ann Surg Oncol.* 1998;5:681–688.
15. Hwang RF, Gordon EM, Anderson WF, Parekh D. Gene therapy for primary and metastatic pancreatic cancer with intraperitoneal retroviral vector bearing the wild-type p53 gene. *Surgery.* 1998;124:143–150; discussion 150–151.
16. Kimura M, Tagawa M, Takenaga K, et al. Inability to induce the alteration of tumorigenicity and chemosensitivity of p53-null human pancreatic carcinoma cells after the transduction of wild-type p53 gene. *Anticancer Res.* 1997;17:879–883.
17. Calbo J, Marotta M, Cascallo M, et al. Adenovirus-mediated wt-p16 reintroduction induces cell cycle arrest or apoptosis in pancreatic cancer. *Cancer Gene Ther.* 2001;8:740–750.
18. Huber BE, Richards CA, Krenitsky TA. Retroviral-mediated gene therapy for the treatment of hepatocellular carcinoma: an innovative approach for cancer therapy. *Proc Natl Acad Sci USA.* 1991;88:8039–8043.
19. DiMaio JM, Clary BM, Via DF, Coveney E, Pappas TN, Lyerly HK. Directed enzyme pro-drug gene therapy for pancreatic cancer in vivo. *Surgery.* 1994;116:205–213.
20. Saimura M, Nagai E, Mizumoto K, et al. Intraperitoneal injection of adenovirus-mediated NK4 gene suppresses peritoneal dissemination of pancreatic cancer cell line AsPC-1 in nude mice. *Cancer Gene Ther.* 2002;9:799–806.
21. Hirano T, Shino Y, Saito T, et al. Dominant negative MEKK1 inhibits survival of pancreatic cancer cells. *Oncogene.* 2002;21:5923–5928.
22. Takeuchi M, Shichinohe T, Senmaru N, et al. The dominant negative H-ras mutant, N116Y, suppresses growth of metastatic human pancreatic cancer cells in the liver of nude mice. *Gene Ther.* 2000;7:518–526.
23. Rochaix P, Delesque N, Esteve JP, et al. Gene therapy for pancreatic carcinoma: local and distant antitumor effects after somatostatin receptor sst2 gene transfer. *Hum Gene Ther.* 1999;10:995–1008.
24. Benali N, Cordelier P, Calise D, et al. Inhibition of growth and metastatic progression of pancreatic carcinoma in hamster after somatostatin receptor subtype 2 (sst2) gene expression and administration of cytotoxic somatostatin analog AN-238. *Proc Natl Acad Sci USA.* 2000;97:9180–9185.
25. Tai YT, Strobel T, Kufe D, Cannistra SA. In vivo cytotoxicity of ovarian cancer cells through tumor-selective expression of the BAX gene. *Cancer Res.* 1999;59:2121–2126.
26. Lowe SL, Rubinchik S, Honda T, McDonnell TJ, Dong JY, Norris JS. Prostate-specific expression of Bax delivered by an adenoviral vector induces apoptosis in LNCaP prostate cancer cells. *Gene Ther.* 2001;8:1363–1371.
27. Arafat WO, Gomez-Navarro J, Xiang J, et al. An adenovirus encoding proapoptotic Bax induces apoptosis and enhances the radiation effect in human ovarian cancer. *Mol Ther.* 2000;1:545–554.
28. Kagawa S, Pearson SA, Ji L, et al. A binary adenoviral vector system for expressing high levels of the proapoptotic gene bax. *Gene Ther.* 2000;7:75–79.
29. Shibata D, Almoguera C, Forrester K, et al. Detection of c-K-ras mutations in fine needle aspirates from human pancreatic adenocarcinomas. *Cancer Res.* 1990;50:1279–1283.
30. Almoguera C, Shibata D, Forrester K, Martin J, Arnheim N, Perucho M. Most human carcinomas of the exocrine pancreas contain mutant c-K-ras genes. *Cell.* 1988;53:549–554.
31. Sirivatanauksorn V, Sirivatanauksorn Y, Lemoine NR. Molecular pattern of ductal pancreatic cancer. *Langenbecks Arch Surg.* 1998;383:105–115.
32. Aoki K, Yoshida T, Sugimura T, Terada M. Liposome-mediated in vivo gene transfer of antisense K-ras construct inhibits pancreatic tumor dissemination in the murine peritoneal cavity. *Cancer Res.* 1995;55:3810–3816.
33. Tsuchida T, Kijima H, Hori S, et al. Adenovirus-mediated anti-K-ras ribozyme induces apoptosis and growth suppression of human pancreatic carcinoma. *Cancer Gene Ther.* 2000;7:373–383.
34. Kijima H, Scanlon KJ. Ribozyme as an approach for growth suppression of human pancreatic cancer. *Mol Biotechnol.* 2000;14:59–72.
35. Smith RR, Heubner RJ, Rowe WP, Schatten WF, Homas LB. Studies on the use of viruses in the treatment of carcinoma of cervix. *Cancer.* 1956;9:1211–1218.
36. Bischoff JR, Kirn DH, Williams A, et al. An adenovirus mutant that replicates selectively in p53-deficient human tumor cells. *Science.* 1996;274:373–376.
37. Southam CM, Moore AE. Clinical studies of viruses as antineoplastic agents, with particular reference to Egypt 101 virus. *Cancer.* 1952;5:1025–1034.
38. Southam CM, Moore AE. Induced virus infection in man by Egypt isolated of West Nile virus. *J Trop Med Hyg.* 1954;3:19–50.
39. Telerman A, Tuynder M, Dupressoir T, et al. A model for tumor suppression using H-1 parvovirus. *Proc Natl Acad Sci USA.* 1993;90:8702–8706.

40. Martuza RL, Malick A, Markert JM, Ruffner KL, Coen DM. Experimental therapy of human glioma by means of a genetically engineered virus mutant. *Science*. 1991;252: 854–856.
41. Markert JM, Malick A, Coen DM, Martuza RL. Reduction and elimination of encephalitis in an experimental glioma therapy model with attenuated herpes simplex mutants that retain susceptibility to acyclovir. *Neurosurgery*. 1993;32:597–603.
42. Mineta T, Rabkin SD, Martuza RL. Treatment of malignant gliomas using ganciclovir-hypersensitive, ribonucleotide reductase-deficient herpes simplex viral mutant. *Cancer Res*. 1994;54:3963–3966.
43. Chambers R, Gillespie GY, Soroceanu L, et al. Comparison of genetically engineered herpes simplex viruses for the treatment of brain tumors in a SCID mouse model of human malignant glioma. *Proc Natl Acad Sci USA*. 1995;92:1411–1415.
44. Markert JM, Coen DM, Malick A, Mineta T, Martuza RL. Expanded spectrum of viral therapy in the treatment of nervous system tumors. *J Neurosurg*. 1992;77:590–594.
45. Alemany R, Balague C, Curiel DT. Replicative adenoviruses for cancer therapy. *Nat Biotechnol*. 2000;18:723–727.
46. Curiel DT. The development of conditionally replicative adenoviruses for cancer therapy. *Clin Cancer Res*. 2000;6:3395–3399.
47. Varghese S, Rabkin SD. Oncolytic herpes simplex virus vectors for cancer virotherapy. *Cancer Gene Ther*. 2002;9:967–978.
48. Mulvihill S, Warren R, Venook A, et al. Safety and feasibility of injection with an E1B-55 kDa gene-deleted, replication-selective adenovirus (ONYX-015) into primary carcinomas of the pancreas: a phase I trial. *Gene Ther*. 2001;8:308–315.
49. Hecht JR, Bedford R, Abbruzzese JL, et al. A phase I/II trial of intratumoral endoscopic ultrasound injection of ONYX-015 with intravenous gemcitabine in unresectable pancreatic carcinoma. *Clin Cancer Res*. 2003;9:555–561.
50. Ferrara N. VEGF and the quest for tumour angiogenesis factors. *Nat Rev Cancer*. 2002;2:795–803.
51. Tseng JF, Farnebo FA, Kisker O, et al. Adenovirus-mediated delivery of a soluble form of the VEGF receptor Flk1 delays the growth of murine and human pancreatic adenocarcinoma in mice. *Surgery*. 2002;132:857–865.
52. Stetler-Stevenson WG, Liotta LA, Kleiner DE, Jr. Extracellular matrix 6: role of matrix metalloproteinases in tumor invasion and metastasis. *FASEB J*. 1993;7:1434–1441.
53. Senger DR. Molecular framework for angiogenesis: a complex web of interactions between extravasated plasma proteins and endothelial cell proteins induced by angiogenic cytokines. *Am J Pathol*. 1996;149:1–7.
54. Bloomston M, Shafii A, Zervos EE, Rojiani A, Rosemurgy AS. MMP-2 and TIMP-1 are derived from, not in response to, pancreatic cancer. *J Surg Res*. 2002;102:35–38.
55. Rigg AS, Lemoine NR. Adenoviral delivery of TIMP1 or TIMP2 can modify the invasive behavior of pancreatic cancer and can have a significant antitumor effect in vivo. *Cancer Gene Ther*. 2001;8:869–878.
56. Aoki K, Yoshida T, Matsumoto N, et al. Gene therapy for peritoneal dissemination of pancreatic cancer by liposome-mediated transfer of herpes simplex virus thymidine kinase gene. *Hum Gene Ther*. 1997;8:1105–1113.
57. Aoki K, Furuhata S, Hatanaka K, et al. Polyethylenimine-mediated gene transfer into pancreatic tumor dissemination in the murine peritoneal cavity. *Gene Ther*. 2001; 8:508–514.
58. Aoki K, Yoshida T, Matsumoto N, Ide H, Sugimura T, Terada M. Suppression of Ki-ras p21 levels leading to growth inhibition of pancreatic cancer cell lines with Ki-ras mutation but not those without Ki-ras mutation. *Mol Carcinog*. 1997;20:251–258.
59. Carrio M, Romagosa A, Mercade E, et al. Enhanced pancreatic tumor regression by a combination of adenovirus and retrovirus-mediated delivery of the herpes simplex virus thymidine kinase gene. *Gene Ther*. 1999;6:547–553.
60. Wesseling JG, Bosma PJ, Krasnykh V, et al. Improved gene transfer efficiency to primary and established human pancreatic carcinoma target cells via epidermal growth factor receptor and integrin-targeted adenoviral vectors. *Gene Ther*. 2001;8:969–76.
61. Shenk T. Adenoviridae: the viruses and their replication. In: Fields B, Knipe D, Howley P, eds. *Virology*, Vol. 2, 3rd ed. Philadelphia: Lippincott-Raven; 1996: 2111–2148.
62. Kleeff J, Fukahi K, Lopez ME, et al. Targeting of suicide gene delivery in pancreatic cancer cells via FGF receptors. *Cancer Gene Ther*. 2002;9:522–532.
63. Yamamoto M, Davydova J, Wang M, et al. Infectivity enhanced, cyclooxygenase-2 promoter-based conditionally replicative adenovirus for pancreatic cancer. *Gastroenterology*. 2003;125:1203–1218.
64. Monahan PE, Samulski RJ. AAV vectors: is clinical success on the horizon? *Gene Ther*. 2000;7:24–30.
65. Dumon KR, Ishii H, Vecchione A, et al. Fragile histidine triad expression delays tumor development and induces apoptosis in human pancreatic cancer. *Cancer Res*. 2001; 61:4827–4836.
66. Kasuya H, Nishiyama Y, Nomoto S, Hosono J, Takeda S, Nakao A. Intraperitoneal delivery of hrR3 and ganciclovir prolongs survival in mice with disseminated pancreatic cancer. *J Surg Oncol*. 1999;72:136–141.
67. McAuliffe PF, Jarnagin WR, Johnson P, Delman KA, Federoff H, Fong Y. Effective treatment of pancreatic tumors with two multimutated herpes simplex oncolytic viruses. *J Gastrointest Surg*. 2000;4:580–588.
68. Lee JH, Federoff HJ, Schoeniger LO. G207, modified herpes simplex virus type 1, kills human pancreatic cancer cells in vitro. *J Gastrointest Surg*. 1999;3:127–131; discussion 132–133.
69. Etoh T, Himeno Y, Matsumoto T, et al. Oncolytic viral therapy for human pancreatic cancer cells by reovirus. *Clin Cancer Res*. 2003;9:1218–1223.
70. Khuri FR, Nemunaitis J, Ganly I, et al. A controlled trial of intratumoral ONYX-015, a selectively-replicating adenovirus, in combination with cisplatin and 5-fluorouracil

in patients with recurrent head and neck cancer. *Nat Med.* 2000;6:879–885.

71. Yamamoto M, Alemany R, Adachi Y, Grizzle WE, Curiel DT. Characterization of the cyclooxygenase-2 promoter in an adenoviral vector and its application for the mitigation of toxicity in suicide gene therapy of gastrointestinal cancers. *Mol Ther.* 2001;3:385–94.
72. Fueyo J, Gomez-Manzano C, Alemany R, Lee PS, McDonnell TJ, Mitlianga P, Shi YX, Levin VA, Yung WK, Kyritsis AP. A mutant oncolytic adenovirus targeting the Rb pathway produces anti- glioma effect in vivo. *Oncogene.* 2000;19:2–12.
73. Balague C, Noya F, Alemany R, Chow LT, Curiel DT. Human papillomavirus E6E7-mediated adenovirus cell killing: selectivity of mutant adenovirus replication in organotypic cultures of human keratinocytes. *J Virol.* 2001;75:7602–7611.
74. Ahmed A, Thompson J, Emiliusen L, et al. A conditionally replicating adenovirus targeted to tumor cells through activated RAS/P-MAPK-selective mRNA stabilization. *Nat Biotechnol.* 2003;21:771–777.
75. Cascallo M, Capella G, Mazo A, Alemany R. Ras-dependent oncolysis with an adenovirus VAI mutant. *Cancer Res.* 2003;63:5544–5550.
76. Goldstein DJ, Weller SK. Herpes simplex virus type 1-induced ribonucleotide reductase activity is dispensable for virus growth and DNA synthesis: isolation and characterization of an ICP6 lacZ insertion mutant. *J Virol.* 1988;62:196–205.
77. Yamada Y, Kimura H, Morishima T, Daikoku T, Maeno K, Nishiyama Y. The pathogenicity of ribonucleotide reductase-null mutants of herpes simplex virus type 1 in mice. *J Infect Dis.* 1991;164:1091–1097.
78. Meignier B, Longnecker R, Roizman B. In vivo behavior of genetically engineered herpes simplex viruses R7017 and R7020: construction and evaluation in rodents. *J Infect Dis.* 1988;158:602–614.
79. Meignier B, Martin B, Whitley RJ, Roizman B. In vivo behavior of genetically engineered herpes simplex viruses R7017 and R7020. II. Studies in immunocompetent and immunosuppressed owl monkeys *(Aotus trivirgatus)*. *J Infect Dis.* 1990;162:313–321.
80. Mineta T, Rabkin SD, Yazaki T, Hunter WD, Martuza RL. Attenuated multi-mutated herpes simplex virus-1 for the treatment of malignant gliomas. *Nat Med.* 1995;1:938–943.
81. Hunter WD, Martuza RL, Feigenbaum F, et al. Attenuated, replication-competent herpes simplex virus type 1 mutant G207: safety evaluation of intracerebral injection in nonhuman primates. *J Virol.* 1999;73:6319–26.
82. Nibert M, Schiff L, Fields B. Reoviruses and their replication. In: Fields B, Knipe D, Howley P, eds. *Virology,* Vol. 2. Philadelphia: Lippincott-Raven; 1996:1557–1596.
83. Coffey MC, Strong JE, Forsyth PA, Lee PW. Reovirus therapy of tumors with activated Ras pathway. *Science.* 1998;282:1332–1334.
84. Schmidt-Wolf G, Schmidt-Wolf IG. Human cancer and gene therapy. *Ann Hematol.* 1994;69:273–279.
85. Herrmann F. Cancer gene therapy: principles, problems, and perspectives. *J Mol Med.* 1995;73:157–163.
86. Seemayer TA, Cavenee WK. Molecular mechanisms of oncogenesis. *Lab Invest.* 1989;60:585–599.
87. Roth JA, Cristiano RJ. Gene therapy for cancer: what have we done and where are we going? *J Natl Cancer Inst.* 1997;89:21–39.
88. Culver KW, Blaese RM. Gene therapy for cancer. *Trends Genet.* 1994;10:174–178.
89. Freeman SM, Zwiebel JA. Gene therapy of cancer. *Cancer Invest.* 1993;11:676–688.
90. van Riel JM, Giaccone G, Pinedo HM. Pancreaticobiliary cancer: the future aspects of medical oncology. *Ann Oncol.* 1999;10[Suppl 4]:296–299.
91. Curiel DT. Strategies to adapt adenoviral vectors for targeted delivery. *Ann NY Acad Sci.* 1999;886:158–171.
92. Krasnykh V, Dmitriev I, Mikheeva G, Miller CR, Belousova N, Curiel DT. Characterization of an adenovirus vector containing a heterologous peptide epitope in the HI loop of the fiber knob. *J Virol.* 1998;72:1844–1852.
93. Wickham TJ, Tzeng E, Shears LL, 2nd, et al. Increased in vitro and in vivo gene transfer by adenovirus vectors containing chimeric fiber proteins. *J Virol.* 1997;71:8221–8229.
94. Dmitriev I, Krasnykh V, Miller CR, et al. An adenovirus vector with genetically modified fibers demonstrates expanded tropism via utilization of a coxsackievirus and adenovirus receptor-independent cell entry mechanism. *J Virol.* 1998;72:9706–9713.
95. Suzuki K, Alemany R, Yamamoto M, Curiel DT. The presence of the adenovirus E3 gene improves the oncolytic potency of conditionally replicative adenoviruses. *Clin Cancer Res.* 2002;8:3348–3359.
96. Suzuki K, Fueyo J, Krasnykh V, Reynolds PN, Curiel DT, Alemany R. A conditionally replicative adenovirus with enhanced infectivity shows improved oncolytic potency. *Clin Cancer Res.* 2001;7:120–126.
97. Fu X, Zhang X. Potent systemic antitumor activity from an oncolytic herpes simplex virus of syncytial phenotype. *Cancer Res.* 2002;62:2306–2312.
98. Delman KA, Zager JS, Bennett JJ, et al. Efficacy of multiagent herpes simplex virus amplicon-mediated immunotherapy as adjuvant treatment for experimental hepatic cancer. *Ann Surg.* 2002;236:337–342; discussion 342–343.
99. Brand K, Arnold W, Bartels T, et al. Liver-associated toxicity of the HSV-tk/GCV approach and adenoviral vectors. *Cancer Gene Ther.* 1997;4:9–16.
100. Batra SK, Kern HF, Worlock AJ, Metzgar RS, Hollingsworth MA. Transfection of the human Muc 1 mucin gene into a poorly differentiated human pancreatic tumor cell line, Panc1: integration, expression and ultrastructural changes. *J Cell Sci.* 1991;100(pt 4):841–849.
101. Wesseling JG, Yamamoto M, Adachi Y, et al. Midkine and cyclooxygenase-2 promoters are promising for adenoviral vector gene delivery of pancreatic carcinoma. *Cancer Gene Ther.* 2001;8:990–996.
102. Steinwaerder DS, Lieber A. Insulation from viral transcriptional regulatory elements improves inducible transgene expression from adenovirus vectors in vitro and in vivo. *Gene Ther.* 2000;7:556–567.

103. Yamamoto M, Davydova J, Takayama K, Alemany R, Curiel DT. Transcription initiation activity of adenovirus left-end sequence in adenovirus vectors with E1 deleted. *J Virol.* 2003;77:1633–1637.
104. Hearing P, Shenk T. The adenovirus type 5 E1A transcriptional control region contains a duplicated enhancer element. *Cell.* 1983;33:695–703.
105. Douglas JT, Miller CR, Kim M, et al. A system for the propagation of adenoviral vectors with genetically modified receptor specificities. *Nat Biotechnol.* 1999;17:470–475.
106. Dmitriev IP, Kashentseva EA, Curiel DT. Engineering of adenovirus vectors containing heterologous peptide sequences in the C terminus of capsid protein IX. *J Virol.* 2002;76:6893–6899.
107. Belousova N, Korokhov N, Krendelshchikova V, et al. Genetically targeted adenovirus vector directed to CD40-expressing cells. *J Virol.* 2003;77:11367–11377.
108. Curiel DT, Wagner E, Cotten M, et al. High-efficiency gene transfer mediated by adenovirus coupled to DNA-polylysine complexes. *Hum Gene Ther.* 1992;3:147–154.
109. Krasnykh VN, Mikheeva GV, Douglas JT, Curiel DT. Generation of recombinant adenovirus vectors with modified fibers for altering viral tropism. *J Virol.* 1996;70:6839–6846.
110. Shayakhmetov DM, Lieber A. Dependence of adenovirus infectivity on length of the fiber shaft domain. *J Virol.* 2000;74:10274–10286.
111. Havenga MJ, Lemckert AA, Ophorst OJ, et al. Exploiting the natural diversity in adenovirus tropism for therapy and prevention of disease. *J Virol.* 2002;76:4612–4620.
112. Einfeld DA, Schroeder R, Roelvink PW, et al. Reducing the native tropism of adenovirus vectors requires removal of both CAR and integrin interactions. *J Virol.* 2001;75: 11284–11291.
113. Smith TA, Idamakanti N, Rollence ML, et al. Adenovirus serotype 5 fiber shaft influences in vivo gene transfer in mice. *Hum Gene Ther.* 2003;14:777–787.
114. DeWeese TL, van der Poel H, Li S, et al. A phase I trial of CV706, a replication-competent, PSA selective oncolytic adenovirus, for the treatment of locally recurrent prostate cancer following radiation therapy. *Cancer Res.* 2001;61:7464–7472.
115. Peng KW, Facteau S, Wegman T, O'Kane D, Russell SJ. Non-invasive in vivo monitoring of trackable viruses expressing soluble marker peptides. *Nat Med.* 2002;8: 527–531.
116. Tovell DR, Yacyshyn HP, Misra HK, et al. Effect of acyclovir on the uptake of 131I-labelled 1-(2′fluoro-2′-deoxy-beta-D-arabinofuranosyl)-5-iodouracil in herpes infected cells. *J Med Virol.* 1987;22:183–188.
117. Zinn KR, Chaudhuri TR, Buchsbaum DJ, Mountz JM, Rogers BE. Simultaneous evaluation of dual gene transfer to adherent cells by gamma-ray imaging. *Nucl Med Biol.* 2001;28:135–144.
118. Tjuvajev JG, Avril N, Oku T, et al. Imaging herpes virus thymidine kinase gene transfer and expression by positron emission tomography. *Cancer Res.* 1998;58:4333–4341.
119. Gambhir SS, Barrio JR, Wu L, et al. Imaging of adenoviral-directed herpes simplex virus type 1 thymidine kinase reporter gene expression in mice with radiolabeled ganciclovir. *J Nucl Med.* 1998;39:2003–2011.
120. Zinn KR, Buchsbaum DJ, Chaudhuri TR, Mountz JM, Grizzle WE, Rogers BE. Noninvasive monitoring of gene transfer using a reporter receptor imaged with a high-affinity peptide radiolabeled with 99mTc or 188Re. *J Nucl Med.* 2000;41:887–895.
121. MacLaren DC, Gambhir SS, Satyamurthy N, et al. Repetitive, non-invasive imaging of the dopamine D2 receptor as a reporter gene in living animals. *Gene Ther.* 1999;6:785–791.
122. Knop M, Barr F, Riedel CG, Heckel T, Reichel C. Improved version of the red fluorescent protein (drFP583/DsRed/RFP). *Biotechniques.* 2002;33:592, 594, 596–598 passim.
123. Contag CH, Ross BD. It's not just about anatomy: in vivo bioluminescence imaging as an eyepiece into biology. *J Magn Reson Imaging.* 2002;16:378–387.
124. Rice BW, Cable MD, Nelson MB. In vivo imaging of light-emitting probes. *J Biomed Opt.* 2001;6:432–440.
125. Clyde WA, Jr. Experimental models for study of common respiratory viruses. *Environ Health Perspect.* 1980;35: 107–112.
126. Ginsberg HS, Prince GA. The molecular basis of adenovirus pathogenesis. *Infect Agents Dis.* 1994;3:1–8.
127. Prince GA, Porter DD, Jenson AB, Horswood RL, Chanock RM, Ginsberg HS. Pathogenesis of adenovirus type 5 pneumonia in cotton rats (*Sigmodon hispidus*). *J Virol.* 1993;67:101–111.
128. Morrison MD, Onions DE, Nicolson L. Complete DNA sequence of canine adenovirus type 1. *J Gen Virol.* 1997;78 (pt 4):873–878.
129. Orkin SH, Motulsky AG. *Report and Recommendation of the Panel to Assess the NIH Investment in Research on Gene Therapy.* Volume 1995 accessed from http://www.nih.gov/news/panelrep.html: NIH, 1995.
130. Rosenfeld ME, Vickers SM, Raben D, et al. Pancreatic carcinoma cell killing via adenoviral mediated delivery of the herpes simplex virus thymidine kinase gene. *Ann Surg.* 1997;225:609–618; discussion 618–620.
131. Block A, Chen SH, Kosai K, Finegold M, Woo SL. Adenoviral-mediated herpes simplex virus thymidine kinase gene transfer: regression of hepatic metastasis of pancreatic tumors. *Pancreas.* 1997;15:25–34.
132. Ohashi M, Kanai F, Tanaka T, et al. In vivo adenovirus-mediated prodrug gene therapy for carcinoembryonic antigen-producing pancreatic cancer. *Jpn J Cancer Res.* 1998;89:457–462.
133. Zhang SN, Yuan SZ, Zhu ZH, Wen ZF, Huang ZQ, Zeng ZY. Apoptosis induced by 5-flucytosine in human pancreatic cancer cells genetically modified to express cytosine deaminase. *Acta Pharmacol Sin.* 2000;21:655–659.
134. Evoy D, Hirschowitz EA, Naama HA, et al. In vivo adenoviral-mediated gene transfer in the treatment of pancreatic cancer. *J Surg Res.* 1997;69:226–231.
135. Oonuma M, Sunamura M, Motoi F, et al. Gene therapy for intraperitoneally disseminated pancreatic cancers by Escherichia coli uracil phosphoribosyltransferase (UPRT) gene mediated by restricted replication-competent adenoviral vectors. *Int J Cancer.* 2002;102:51–59.

136. McNeish IA, Green NK, Gilligan MG, et al. Virus directed enzyme prodrug therapy for ovarian and pancreatic cancer using retrovirally delivered E. coli nitroreductase and CB1954. *Gene Ther.* 1998;5:1061–1069.
137. Lohr M, Bago ZT, Bergmeister H, et al. Cell therapy using microencapsulated 293 cells transfected with a gene construct expressing CYP2B1, an ifosfamide converting enzyme, instilled intra-arterially in patients with advanced-stage pancreatic carcinoma: a phase I/II study. *J Mol Med.* 1999;77:393–398.
138. Sato T, Yamauchi N, Sasaki H, et al. An apoptosis-inducing gene therapy for pancreatic cancer with a combination of 55–kDa tumor necrosis factor (TNF) receptor gene transfection and mutein TNF administration. *Cancer Res.* 1998;58:1677–1683.
139. Pirocanac EC, Nassirpour R, Yang M, et al. Bax-induction gene therapy of pancreatic cancer. *J Surg Res.* 2002; 106:346–351.
140. Su Z, Lebedeva IV, Gopalkrishnan RV, et al. A combinatorial approach for selectively inducing programmed cell death in human pancreatic cancer cells. *Proc Natl Acad Sci USA.* 2001;98:10332–10337.
141. Rodicker F, Putzer BM. p73 is effective in p53-null pancreatic cancer cells resistant to wild-type TP53 gene replacement. *Cancer Res.* 2003;63:2737–2741.
142. Rodicker F, Stiewe T, Zimmermann S, Putzer BM. Therapeutic efficacy of E2F1 in pancreatic cancer correlates with TP73 induction. *Cancer Res.* 2001;61:7052–7055.
143. Elliott MJ, Farmer MR, Atienza C, Jr, et al. E2F-1 gene therapy induces apoptosis and increases chemosensitivity in human pancreatic carcinoma cells. *Tumour Biol.* 2002;23:76–86.
144. Joshi US, Dergham ST, Chen YQ, et al. Inhibition of pancreatic tumor cell growth in culture by p21WAF1 recombinant adenovirus. *Pancreas.* 1998;16:107–113.
145. Kawaguchi Y, Takebayashi H, Kakizuka A, Arii S, Kato M, Imamura M. Expression of Fas-estrogen receptor fusion protein induces cell death in pancreatic cancer cell lines. *Cancer Lett.* 1997;116:53–59.
146. Kelley JR, Fraser MM, Hubbard JM, Watson DK, Cole DJ. CaSm antisense gene therapy: a novel approach for the treatment of pancreatic cancer. *Anticancer Res.* 2003;23:2007–2013.
147. Takao S, Che X, Fukudome T, Natsugoe S, Ozawa M, Aikou T. Down-regulation of E-cadherin by antisense oligonucleotide enhances basement membrane invasion of pancreatic carcinoma cells. *Hum Cell.* 2000;13:15–21.
148. Denham DW, Franz MG, Denham W, et al. Directed antisense therapy confirms the role of protein kinase C-alpha in the tumorigenicity of pancreatic cancer. *Surgery.* 1998;124:218–223; discussion 223–224.
149. Cheng JQ, Ruggeri B, Klein WM, et al. Amplification of AKT2 in human pancreatic cells and inhibition of AKT2 expression and tumorigenicity by antisense RNA. *Proc Natl Acad Sci USA.* 1996;93:3636–3641.
150. Stevenson AJ, Giles MS, Hall KT, et al. Specific oncolytic activity of herpesvirus saimiri in pancreatic cancer cells. *Br J Cancer.* 2000;83:329–332.
151. Rothmann T, Hengstermann A, Whitaker NJ, Scheffner M, zur Hausen H. Replication of ONYX-015, a potential anticancer adenovirus, is independent of p53 status in tumor cells. *J Virol.* 1998;72:9470–9478.
152. Clary BM, Coveney EC, Blazer DG, 3rd, Philip R, Lyerly HK. Active immunotherapy of pancreatic cancer with tumor cells genetically engineered to secrete multiple cytokines. *Surgery.* 1996;120:174–181.
153. Kimura M, Tagawa M, Takenaga K, et al. Loss of tumorigenicity of human pancreatic carcinoma cells engineered to produce interleukin-2 or interleukin-4 in nude mice: a potentiality for cancer gene therapy. *Cancer Lett.* 1998;128:47–53.
154. Kimura M, Yoshida Y, Narita M, et al. Acquired immunity in nude mice induced by expression of the IL-2 or IL-4 gene in human pancreatic carcinoma cells and anti-tumor effect generated by in vivo gene transfer using retrovirus. *Int J Cancer.* 1999;82:549–555.
155. Kawakami K, Kawakami M, Husain SR, Puri RK. Potent antitumor activity of IL-13 cytotoxin in human pancreatic tumors engineered to express IL-13 receptor alpha2 chain in vivo. *Gene Ther.* 2003;10:1116–1128.
156. Putzer BM, Rodicker F, Hitt MM, Stiewe T, Esche H. Improved treatment of pancreatic cancer by IL-12 and B7.1 costimulation: antitumor efficacy and immunoregulation in a nonimmunogenic tumor model. *Mol Ther.* 2002; 5:405–412.
157. Wen Y, Yan DH, Wang B, et al. p202, an interferon-inducible protein, mediates multiple antitumor activities in human pancreatic cancer xenograft models. *Cancer Res.* 2001;61:7142–7147.

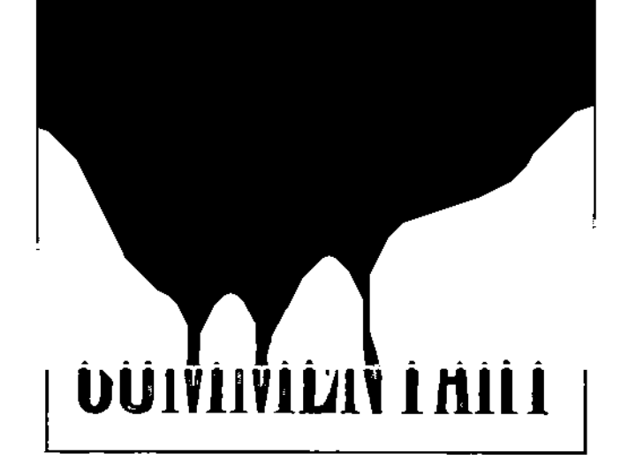

Bingliang Fang, PhD
Kelly K. Hunt, MD

Pancreatic cancer is the fourth leading cause of cancer-related deaths in the United States.[1,2] The median survival for patients with unresectable pancreatic cancer after diagnosis is 3–6 months, and the 5-year survival rate is less than 4% for all stages combined.[1] Clearly, new therapeutic approaches for the treatment of pancreatic cancer are needed. Chapter 37 provides comprehensive information on recent advances in gene therapy and virotherapy of pancreatic cancer.

Cancer is regarded as a genetic disease of somatic cells because multiple genetic alterations are required for development and maintenance of the malignant phenotype in cancer cells. Gene therapy or "nucleic acid-based medicine" aims to attack these genetic alterations directly. Like other conventional anticancer therapies (surgery, chemotherapy, radiotherapy), the ultimate goal of cancer gene therapy or virotherapy is to remove or destroy malignant cells. The specific cancer gene therapy or virotherapy strategies that might be employed in the treatment of pancreatic cancer, directly or indirectly, are well summarized in Chapter 37.

A large body of evidence now exists from various preclinical studies demonstrating that enforced overexpression or downregulation of various genetically encoded functions can lead to therapeutic benefits, suppressing tumor growth and prolonging survival of tumor-bearing animals. Moreover, these approaches can augment the response achieved with conventional therapeutics. Perhaps one of the best studied examples is the *TP53* tumor-suppressor gene. In many types of cancer, including pancreatic cancer, *TP53* gene therapy not only induces apoptosis in cancer cells but also dramatically augments the therapeutic effects of chemotherapy, radiotherapy, and antiangiogenesis therapy. This is because *TP53* function is required for effective antiangiogenic therapy[3] and for effective induction of apoptosis by ionizing radiation or various chemotherapeutic agents.[4] It is also conceivable that knocking down the expression of oncogenes, antiapoptosis genes, proangiogenesis genes, and chemoresistance or radioresistance-related genes by using antisense nucleotides, ribozymes, dominant-negative mutants, and small interfering RNAs[5,6] can directly trigger apoptosis, suppress angiogenesis, or dramatically reverse resistance to conventional therapies.

Virotherapy is based not on the premise of upregulating on downregulating a specific gene in cancer cells, but taking advantage of the fact that certain viruses will selectively replicate in tumor cells. The destructive effects of a replication-competent virus would be beneficial for cancer therapy as long as this destructive effect is specifically limited to tumor cells while sparing normal tissues. Thus, cancer virotherapy is exploring therapeutic applications of viruses that have substantial growth advantage in cancer cells over that of normal cells.

One unique difference between gene therapy/virotherapy and conventional chemotherapy is that the therapeutic components of gene therapy and virotherapy are large molecules or large particles that are usually only active after penetrating the nucleus. Therefore, the pharmacodynamics of gene therapy/virotherapy can be dramatically different from chemotherapy or protein-based therapy. On the other hand, once these molecules are inside of cells, local expression of therapeutic genes or replication of oncolytic viruses may provide a constitutive therapeutic effect at the cancer site without causing substantial systemic toxicity. Nevertheless, delivery of therapeutic genes or oncolytic virus to every tumor cell, especially in the case of metastatic disease, remains challenging. Thus, efficient delivery systems for cancer gene therapy are the hot topic in cancer gene therapy. This chapter briefly summarized the delivery systems for pancreatic cancer gene therapy, with a focus on oncolytic viruses or virotherapy.

The use of conditionally replicative virus for cancer therapy gained much attention after a report published in 1996 stated that an adenovirus with a mutation in the E1B region (designated dl1520 or ONYX-015) replicates specifically in *TP53*-mutated tumors.[7] Because *TP53* is the most frequently mutated gene in human cancers,[8] a virus that would specifically destroy *TP53*-null or -mutant cells would thus be regarded as a powerful anticancer agent. Although subsequent studies indicated that a lytic infection of cells with an E1B-mutated adenovirus did not depend on the cellular *TP53* status,[9,10] the notion that in situ amplification of replicative virus and the resulting burst of viral progeny from the lysed cancer cells could enhance the local spread and penetration of these vectors, thereby greatly increasing therapeutic efficacy, spurred the creation and testing of various other replicative viruses for cancer therapy.

As the authors of Chapter 37 have described, two techniques have been used to create oncolytic viruses. In the first, a tumor-specific promoter is used to control the expression of an essential gene for viral replication, such as adenoviral E1A. The promoters used in these studies included the COX-2 promoter,[11] the E2F promoter,[12] and the telomerase promoter.[13,14] The second approach uses viral mutants with defective functions that are required for viral replication in normal cells but that are dispensable for replication in cancer cells. For example, the E1A protein binds to the retinoblastoma protein pRb to trigger cell cycle progression into the S phase. An adenovirus (Ad-delta24) with a deletion of eight animo acids from the pRb-binding region of the E1A protein has been reported to replicate specifically in Rb-defective cells.[15]

The major problems in cancer gene therapy and virotherapy are similar to those of conventional anticancer therapies, although the approaches to solve these problems could be different. The first problem is resistance to treatment. In cultured cells, resistance to cancer gene therapy falls into one of two categories: resistance caused by insufficient expression of the therapeutic gene or resistance caused by reduced sensitivity to the therapeutic gene.[16] In the first case, the resistance might be caused by insufficient vector entry, low promoter activity, or increased degradation of the therapeutic gene product in the target cells. In the second case, the effects of the therapeutic gene are blocked even though the level of gene expression is high enough to destroy susceptible cells. Although the same can be true for in vivo or clinical situations, in vivo resistance to cancer gene therapy or virotherapy may be caused mainly by incomplete transduction or inefficient release of vector progeny in cancer cells. Chapter 37 discusses the role of the coxsackievirus-adenovirus receptor[17] in adenovirus infection and approaches to overcome the resistance to adenovirus-mediated transduction due to low coxsackievirus-adenovirus receptor expression, including modification of the adenoviral fiber knob with polylysine or arginine-glycine-aspartatic acid sequences to enhance transduction of refractory cells.[18-20]

The second problem is toxicity to normal cells at an effective dose of treatment to the cancer cells. In cancer therapy, the cytotoxic/oncolytic agents must be targeted directly to the cancer to minimize local or systemic toxicity reactions. As discussed in Chapter 37, strategies for targeted cancer gene therapy fall into two categories: using vectors that specifically transduce cancer cells (targeted transduction) and controlling transgene expression with tumor-specific promoters (targeted transcription). Targeted transduction can be achieved by reshaping preformed vector particles with bispecific conjugates or by modifying the genes encoding the surface proteins or viral vectors. However, finding candidate receptors present only in cancer cells could be challenging. For example, some of the potential tumor antigens, folate receptors, or growth factor receptors overexpressed in certain types of cancer cells are also present in a variety of normal cells. Even so, several groups have used phage display libraries and other techniques to identify peptides that can specifically bind to cancer cells or cancer vasculature.[21-24] Alternatively, the use of tissue- or tumor-specific promoters for selective transgene expression after nonselective gene delivery has been pursued in targeted cancer gene therapy. A number of promoters have been identified as being more active in cancer cells than their normal counterparts, including the telomerase promoter,[13,14] E2F promoter,[12] and COX-2 promoter,[11] as discussed previously here. More importantly, it has been shown that transgene expression from a weak, tumor-specific promoter can be dramatically augmented using a transcriptional factor, without loss of promoter specificity.[14,25] This augmentation happens because a small amount of a potent transcriptional factor, such as a GAL4/VP16[26] or a tetR/VP16 (tTA)[27] fusion protein, expressed from a tumor-specific promoter would be sufficient to activate target promoters upstream of a transgene and thereby increase transgene expression. These transcription-enhancing systems can be useful for targeted cancer gene therapy because high levels of therapeutic gene expression are key to the efficacy of cancer gene therapy.[28,29]

The authors also discussed the role of in vivo monitoring of vector distribution and transgene expression and relevant preclinical tumor models for better assessment of future clinical application. These are important issues in preclinical studies of cancer gene therapy and are critical for future development of gene therapy technology and for success of translating gene therapy to the clinics.

It is noteworthy that results of clinical trials of cancer gene therapy have shown that the effects of gene therapy, when used as a single agent, were often limited. One possible reason for this is that most of the reported clinical trials have been phase I or phase I/phase II trials that examined toxicity and dose escalation. Most of the patients entered in these trials had very advanced or metastatic disease or had failed to respond to chemotherapy, radiotherapy, or both. Nevertheless, a high rate of favorable clinical responses has been observed when cancer gene therapy was combined with conventional therapies, even in patients who failed to respond to conventional therapies.[30-33] As pointed out by the authors, gene therapy and virotherapy for pancreatic cancer are still too premature to realize their full potential. However, the investigation of these novel therapies may provide hope for patients with pancreatic cancer who are in great need of a fresh look at the treatment of this disease.

References

1. Jemal A, Tiwari RC, Murray T, Ghafoor A, Samuels A, Ward E, Feuer EJ, Thun MJ, American Cancer Society. Cancer Statistics, 2004. *CA Cancer J. Clin.* 2004;54:8–29
2. Shi X, Friess H, Kleeff J, Ozawa F, Buchler MW. Pancreatic cancer: factors regulating tumor development, maintenance and metastasis. *Pancreatology*. 2001;1:517–524.
3. Yu JL, Rak JW, Coomber BL, Hicklin DJ, Kerbel RS. Effect of p53 status on tumor response to antiangiogenic therapy. *Science*. 2002;295:1526–1528.
4. Lowe SW, Ruley HE, Jacks T, Housman DE. p53-dependent apoptosis modulates the cytotoxicity of anticancer agents. *Cell*. 1993;74:957–967.
5. Brummelkamp TR, Bernards R, Agami R. A system for stable expression of short interfering RNAs in mammalian cells. *Science*. 2002;296:550–553.
6. Elbashir SM, Harborth J, Lendeckel W, Yalcin A, Weber K, Tuschl T. Duplexes of 21-nucleotide RNAs mediate RNA interference in cultured mammalian cells. *Nature*. 2001;411:494–498.
7. Bischoff JR, Kirn DH, Williams A, et al. An adenovirus mutant that replicates selectively in p53-deficient human tumor cells. *Science*. 1996;274:373–376.
8. Hollstein M, Sidransky D, Vogelstein B, Harris CC. p53 mutations in human cancers. *Science*. 1991;253:49–53.

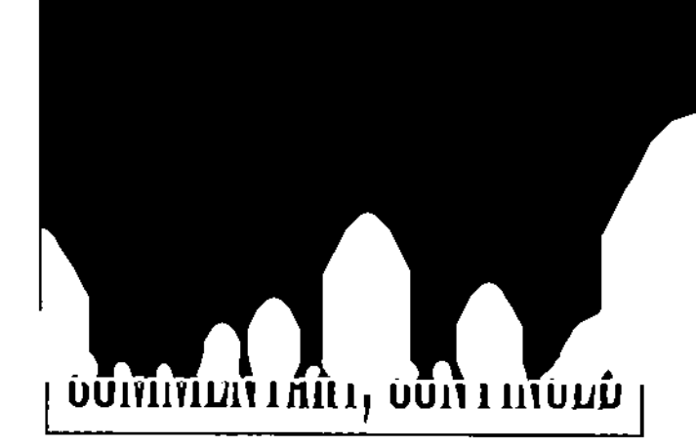

9. Hall AR, Dix BR, O'Carroll SJ, Braithwaite AW. p53-dependent cell death/apoptosis is required for a productive adenovirus infection. *Nat Med.* 1998;4:1068–1072.
10. Goodrum FD, Ornelles DA. p53 status does not determine outcome of E1B 55-kilodalton mutant adenovirus lytic infection. *J Virol.* 1998;72:9479–9490.
11. Yamamoto M, Alemany R, Adachi Y, Grizzle WE, Curiel DT. Characterization of the cyclooxygenase-2 promoter in an adenoviral vector and its application for the mitigation of toxicity in suicide gene therapy of gastrointestinal cancers. *Mol Ther.* 2001;3:385–394.
12. Parr MJ, Manome Y, Tanaka T, et al. Tumor-selective transgene expression in vivo mediated by an E2F-responsive adenoviral vector. *Nat Med.* 1997;3:1145–1149.
13. Gu J, Kagawa S, Takakura M, et al. Tumor-specific transgene expression from the human telomerase reverse transcriptase promoter enables targeting of the therapeutic effects of the *Bax* gene to cancers. *Cancer Res.* 2000;60:5359–5364.
14. Gu J, Fang B. Telomerase promoter-driven cancer gene therapy. *Cancer Biol Ther.* 2003;2:S64–S70.
15. Fueyo J, Alemany R, Gomez-Manzano C, et al. Preclinical characterization of the antiglioma activity of a tropism-enhanced adenovirus targeted to the retinoblastoma pathway. *J Natl Cancer Inst.* 2003;95:652–660.
16. Zhang L, Gu J, Lin T, Huang X, Roth JA, Fang B. Mechanisms involved in development of resistance to adenovirus-mediated proapoptotic gene therapy in DLD1 human colon cancer cell line. *Gene Ther.* 2002;9:1262–1270.
17. Bergelson JM, Cunningham JA, Droguett G, et al. Isolation of a common receptor for Coxsackie B viruses and adenoviruses 2 and 5. *Science.* 1997;275:1320–1323.
18. Wickham TJ, Roelvink PW, Brough DE, Kovesdi I. Adenovirus targeted to heparan-containing receptors increases its gene delivery efficiency to multiple cell types. *Nat Biotechnol.* 1996;14:1570–1573.
19. Wickham TJ, Tzeng E, Shears LL, II, et al. Increased in vitro and in vivo gene transfer by adenovirus vectors containing chimeric fiber proteins. *J Virol.* 1997;71:8221–8229.
20. Dmitriev I, Krasnykh V, Miller CR, et al. An adenovirus vector with genetically modified fibers demonstrates expanded tropism via utilization of a coxsackievirus and adenovirus receptor-independent cell entry mechanism. *J Virol.* 1998;72:9706–9713.
21. Arap W, Pasqualini R, Ruoslahti E. Cancer treatment by targeted drug delivery to tumor vasculature in a mouse model. *Science.* 1998;279:377–380.
22. Koivunen E, Arap W, Valtanen H, et al. Tumor targeting with a selective gelatinase inhibitor. *Nat Biotechnol.* 1999;17:768–774.
23. Nicklin SA, White SJ, Watkins SJ, Hawkins RE, Baker AH. Selective targeting of gene transfer to vascular endothelial cells by use of peptides isolated by phage display. *Circulation.* 2000;102:231–237.
24. Kolonin M, Pasqualini R, Arap W. Molecular addresses in blood vessels as targets for therapy. *Curr Opin Chem Biol.* 2001;5:308–313.
25. Koch P, Guo ZS, Kagawa S, Gu J, Roth JA, Fang B. Augmenting transgene expression from carcinoembryonic antigen (CEA) promoter via a GAL4 gene regulatory system. *Mol Ther.* 2001;3:278–283.
26. Sadowski I, Ma J, Triezenberg S, Ptashne M. GAL4-VP16 is an unusually potent transcriptional activator. *Nature.* 1988;335:563–564.
27. Gossen M, Bujard H. Tight control of gene expression in mammalian cells by tetracycline-responsive promoters. *Proc Natl Acad Sci USA.* 1992;89:5547–5551.
28. Lin T, Gu J, Zhang L, et al. Targeted expression of green fluorescent protein/Tumor necrosis factor-related apoptosis-inducing ligand fusion protein from human telomerase reverse transcriptase promoter elicits antitumor activity without toxic effect on primary human hepatocytes. *Cancer Res.* 2002;62:3620–3625.
29. Gerdes CA, Castro MG, Lowenstein PR. Strong promoters are the key to highly efficient, noninflammatory and noncytotoxic adenoviral-mediated transgene delivery into the brain in vivo. *Mol Ther.* 2000;2:330–338.
30. Roth JA, Grammer SF, Swisher SG, et al. Gene therapy approaches for the management of non-small cell lung cancer. *Semin Oncol.* 2001;28:50–56.
31. Swisher SG, Roth JA, Carbone DP. Genetic and immunologic therapies for lung cancer. *Semin Oncol.* 2002;29:95–101.
32. Kirn D. Clinical research results with dl1520 (ONYX-015), a replication-selective adenovirus for the treatment of cancer: what have we learned? *Gene Ther.* 2001;8:89–98.
33. Khuri FR, Nemunaitis J, Ganly I, et al. A controlled trial of intratumoral ONYX-015, a selectively-replicating adenovirus, in combination with cisplatin and 5-fluorouracil in patients with recurrent head and neck cancer. *Nat Med.* 2000;6:879–885.

CHAPTER

38

Antiangiogenic Therapy for Pancreatic Cancer

Chandrajit P. Raut, MD
Lee M. Ellis, MD

The Biology of Angiogenesis

Tumor angiogenesis is the establishment of a neovascular blood supply to the tumor derived from the existing blood vessels and augmented by circulating endothelial cells contributing to the growing vascular tree.[1-3] Angiogenesis is essential in the growth of malignant neoplasms.[4] A tumor mass larger than 0.25 mm in diameter exceeds the oxygen and nutrient diffusion limits of its vascular supply.[4-7] Therefore, additional growth requires tumors to develop a neovascular blood supply.[4-7] Angiogenesis also facilitates metastatic tumor cell dissemination because an increase in vascular density provides increased access of tumor cells to the circulation.[8] Once a distant metastatic deposit has been established, it must develop a neovascular supply for growth, similar to primary cancers.[6,9]

The Process of Angiogenesis

In homeostasis, the stimulatory signals provided by proangiogenic factors are counterbalanced by the inhibitory signals of antiangiogenic molecules (Table 38.1). The expression of angiogenic factors is induced by environmental stimuli, including hypoxia, acidosis, cytokines, growth factors, activated oncogenes, and loss of tumor-suppressor gene function.[5,10-15] The process of angiogenesis consists of multiple steps, including endothelial cell division, invasion, migration, differentiation/capillary tube formation, and maturation.[2] Various vascular effector molecules have been identified that cooperate to mediate specific steps in the angiogenic process, and efforts are under way to identify drugs that target these molecules to inhibit tumor angiogenesis.[2]

Angiogenesis in Pancreatic Adenocarcinoma

Although pancreatic adenocarcinoma may appear relatively hypovascular on imaging studies (compared with normal pancreas), pancreatic cancer relies on angiogenesis for growth and metastasis. Pancreatic cancer cells express proangiogenic factors, including vascular endothelial growth factor (VEGF), basic fibroblast growth factor (bFGF), interleukin-8, angiogenin, platelet-derived endothelial cell growth factor (PD-ECGF), platelet-derived growth factor, and tumor necrosis factor-α.[2,16,22] Similar to other tumors, expression of proangiogenic factors may correlate with a poor prognosis in pancreatic cancer.[17,18,22,23] The 1-year survival rates are significantly lower in patients with increased expression of

Table 38.1 Endogenous Pro- and Antiangiogenic Factors

Proangiogenic	Antiangiogenic
Angiogenin	Angiostatin
Fibroblast growth factors-1 and -2, [acidic and basic (aFGF, bFGF)]	Endostatin
Hepatocyte growth factor	Vasculostatin
Interleukin-8 (IL-8)	Interferons α, β, γ
Placenta growth factor	Platelet factor-4
Platelet-derived growth factor (PDGF)	Thrombospondins 1,2 (TSP-1,-2)
Platelet-derived endothelial cell growth factor (PD-ECGF)	Tissure inhibitors of metaolloproteinase 1,2,3
Tumor necrosis factor-α (TNF-α)	Tumstatin
Vascular endothelial growth factor (VEGF)	Others
Others	

proangiogenic factors.[22] Increased expression of VEGF and/or platelet-derived growth factor in pancreatic cancer specimens is associated with a higher-grade malignancy and a worse prognosis.[17,18] Tissue angiogenin expression is increased in human pancreatic cancers when compared with normal pancreatic tissue, and serum angiogenin levels are also significantly higher in patients with pancreatic cancer than in normal volunteers.[22]

Proangiogenic Factors as Targets for Therapy

Vascular Endothelial Growth Factor

VEGF is the prototypical proangiogenic molecule because it has been implicated in various steps throughout the process of angiogenesis. It was initially discovered because of its ability to increase vascular permeability and was first termed *vascular permeability factor*, or VPF.[24] The multifunctional VEGF family of molecules currently consists of six growth factors (VEGF-A, VEGF-B, VEGF-C, VEGF-D, VEGF-E, and placental growth factor). VEGF-A, which is more commonly referred to as VEGF, is a dimeric, disulfide-bonded, heparin-binding glycoprotein and is the best characterized of the VEGF family members.[25] Alternative splicing of the VEGF messenger RNA generates at least six different isoforms (121, 145, 165, 183, 189, and 206 amino acids in length) that have varying heparin affinities.[26] The different isoforms may have distinct functional properties in vivo that have not yet been fully elucidated in pancreatic cancer.[27]

VEGF family members bind with high affinity to three tyrosine kinase (TK) receptors that are typically expressed on endothelial cells: VEGF-R1 (Flt-1), VEGF-R2 (Flk-1/KDR), and VEGF-R3 (Flk-4).[28,29] Activation of VEGF-R2 by ligand binding leads to enhanced endothelial cell permeability and invasion and proliferation of endothelial cells; thus VEGF-R2 is a major target for antiangiogenic therapies.[28,30] VEGF may mediate blood flow through its effects on the vasodilator nitric oxide.[31] Moreover, VEGF may protect endothelial cells from apoptosis under stress conditions, such as nutrient deprivation and hypoxia,[32,33] thereby maintaining the integrity of the vascular system.[34] These effects are likely mediated through VEGF-R2 activation.

The role of VEGF-R1 in angiogenesis is less well defined. Transgenic mouse studies have demonstrated that mice that did not express VEGF-R1 died of vascular defects, whereas mice that lacked only the receptor TK domain of VEGF-R1 survived, suggesting that VEGF-R1 may act as a decoy receptor.[35] However, preclinical studies showed that antibodies directed against VEGF-R1 led to inhibition of the growth and, in some cases, regression of breast cancer xenografts in mice.[36] Interestingly, expression of VEGF-R1 was not restricted to the tumor-associated neovasculature but was also present on tumor epithelium.[36] Therefore, it was concluded that the anti–VEGF-R1 antibodies exerted not only antiangiogenic effects but also direct antitumoral effects. In contrast to VEGF-R1 and VEGF-R2, VEGF-R3 is expressed almost exclusively on lymphatic endothelial cells and is a major mediator of lymphangiogenesis.[28]

VEGF expression is tightly regulated by many factors. Hypoxia induces VEGF expression through an increase in the activity of hypoxia-inducible factor-Iα[37] that in turn increases VEGF transcription.[38] Other factors known to up-regulate VEGF expression in gastrointestinal malignancies include low pH, growth factors, intrinsic up-regulation of signal transduction pathways, and loss of tumor suppressor gene activity.[2,5,15,37,39,40]

Overexpression of VEGF correlates with high microvessel density in pancreatic cancer.[17,41] VEGF is overexpressed in pancreatic tumors[42] and correlates with local disease progression.[19,41] Fujimoto and colleagues[17] identified $VEGF_{121}$ and $VEGF_{165}$ as the predominant isoforms of VEGF expressed in pancreatic cancer. However, it is unknown whether other isoforms are expressed in pancreatic cancer and what their specific roles may be.[43] Although some studies suggest that VEGF overexpression is associated with a poor prognosis,[18] others have not found such a correlation, and thus the role of VEGF as a prognostic fac-

Table 38.2 Proangiogenic Factors Associated with Histopathologic and Clinicopathologic Features

Angiogenic Factor	↑ MVD	↑ Tumor Size	Poor Prognosis	↑ Metastases	References
VEGF	+*	+	+*	+	18,19,112-115
PD-ECGF	+		+	+	17,116
bFGF			+	+	22,117
TSP	+				60
Angiogenin			+		22

Abbreviations: bFGF, basic fibroblast growth factor; MVD, microvessel density; PD-ECGF, platelet-derived endothelial cell growth factor; TSP, thrombospondin; VEGF, vascular endothelial growth factor.

*Not supported by all studies.

tor remains controversial (Table 38.2).[17,19,37] Nevertheless, the role of VEGF as an important angiogenic factor in pancreatic cancer is best illustrated by studies that demonstrate decreased tumor growth with anti-VEGF therapies.[44,46]

Other Proangiogenic Factors

PD-ECGF is a 55-kDa polypeptide present in vivo as a 110-kDa homodimer.[47] It is also known as thymidine phosphorylase, an enzyme involved in pyrimidine nucleoside metabolism.[48] PD-ECGF induces endothelial cell chemotaxis through the degradation products of thymidine and indirectly stimulates angiogenesis.[49] PD-ECGF overexpression in pancreatic cancer in humans correlates with high microvessel density and poor prognosis (Table 38.2).[17]

Basic fibroblast growth factor (bFGF, FGF-2) belongs to a large family of at least 20 homologous polypeptide growth factors with an affinity for heparin and glycosaminoglycans.[50] bFGF promotes synthesis of proteinases[51]; stimulates endothelial cell migration and DNA synthesis[52]; induces the proliferation of tumor cells, stroma, and tumor-associated endothelial cells[53]; and promotes the formation of differentiated capillary tubes in vitro.[54] The biologic effects of bFGF are mediated by four structurally related receptor TKs: FGF-R1, -R2, -R3, and -R4.[55] Production of bFGF by pancreatic cancer cells may provide tumor cells a growth advantage through autocrine or paracrine means and may stimulate angiogenesis.[53] Overexpression of bFGF in pancreatic cancer is associated with a poor prognosis (Table 38.2).[23]

Thrombospondin (TSP) is a high-molecular-weight multifunctional glycoprotein that is secreted by fibroblasts, vascular smooth muscle cells, monocytes, and macrophages as well as neoplastic cells.[56] Of the five TSP subtypes (TSP-1, -2, -3, -4, and -5), TSP-1 and TSP-2 have been implicated in the inhibition of angiogenesis.[57] TSP-1 modulates endothelial cell adhesion, motility, and growth in a dose-dependent fashion.[58] At low concentrations, it inhibits angiogenesis, but at high concentrations, it stimulates neovascularization, thereby displaying both agonist and antagonist properties.[59] In contrast to studies in other tumor systems, pancreatic tumors with overexpression of TSP-1 have a higher microvessel density,[60] although this does not correlate with tumor grade or stage (Table 38.2).[57,60-65]

Angiogenin is a 14-kDa plasma protein with a high degree of homology with the ribonuclease A superfamily.[66] Angiogenin is a potent stimulator of angiogenesis and is up-regulated in human pancreatic cancer.[22] Increased cellular angiogenin messenger RNA levels and serum angiogenin levels correlate with significantly lower 1-year survival rates (Table 38.2).[22]

Antiangiogenic Strategies

Initially, antiangiogenic therapy was developed to inhibit blood vessel formation and, in turn, tumor growth. However, early clinical trials did not demonstrate any benefit from single-agent antiangiogenic therapy for almost all tumors, with the exception of renal cell carcinoma. Thus, the idea that antiangiogenic agents may be used for cytostatic or consolidation therapy requires further consideration. At present, it appears that antiangiogenic (more specifically, anti-VEGF) therapy enhances the efficacy of existing chemotherapeutic regimens.[67,68] We consider anti-VEGF therapy a modulator of drug delivery whereby effective antiangiogenic therapy may "normalize" the vasculature and improve the efficiency of blood flow.[69] This may seem counterintuitive because adequate blood supply is necessary for delivery of chemotherapeutic agents. As with any antineoplastic regimen, efficacy is best evaluated by overall survival rather than intermediate surrogate markers that may or may not have been validated.

Numerous strategies have been employed to develop and test antiangiogenic agents. At present, there are more than 40 antiangiogenic agents under development as well as hundreds of drugs/agents with antiangiogenic activity. The discussion below focuses on agents that have shown promise in preclinical and clinical studies in pancreatic cancer.

Antiangiogenic Therapy in Preclinical Models

Anti-VEGF Strategies

Because VEGF and its receptors are thought to play a key role in tumor angiogenesis, most of the antiangiogenic agents currently being tested target the VEGF ligand-receptor system. VEGF is an attractive target because its receptors are expressed almost exclusively on endothelial cells and are up-regulated on tumor endothelium compared with the surrounding normal endothelium.[70-72] Current antiangiogenic strategies targeting VEGF include neutralizing anti-VEGF antibodies,[73,74] anti-VEGF-R antibodies,[75] soluble hybrid VEGF receptors,[76] and VEGF-R TK inhibitors.[77] Although certain agents, such as inhibitors of cyclooxygenase-2 or the epidermal growth factor receptor, have been shown to indirectly inhibit angiogenesis through inhibition of VEGF expression in tumor cells,[78,79] this indirect antiangiogenic strategy is not discussed because of the fact that this approach is unlikely to be more effective at inhibiting angiogenesis than the direct approach described later.[79-81]

Preclinical studies with the VEGF-R TK inhibitor PTK 787/ZK222584 in orthotopic mouse models of pancreatic cancer demonstrated that blockade of VEGF-R signaling inhibited tumor growth and metastasis with minimal toxicity. Furthermore, this agent increased tumor cell and tumor-associated endothelial cell apoptosis.[82,83] The antineoplastic effect of this drug enhanced the activity of gemcitabine. In similar studies with an antibody specific to murine VEGF-R2 (DC101), combination therapy with gemcitabine inhibited tumor growth, reduced lymphatic metastases, increased tumor cell and tumor-associated endothelial cell apoptosis, and decreased tumor cell proliferation.[84]

In several preclinical models, anti-VEGF therapy increased therapeutic efficacy and delayed tumor growth when combined with radiation therapy.[85-87] Anti-VEGF therapy may increase the sensitivity of tumor endothelial cells to XRT because of inhibition of survival mechanisms. Alternately, "normalization" of blood flow as described by Jain and colleagues[69] may improve oxygen delivery and increase oxygen-free radical formation.

Endogenous Antiangiogenic Agents

Another class of antiangiogenic agents currently in various phases of preclinical and clinical trials includes the proteins or cleavage products of proteins produced endogenously in vivo. Many of these agents, such as angiostatin and endostatin, were discovered as products of primary tumors that could inhibit the growth and angiogenesis of distant metastases.[88,89] However, the exact mechanism of action for many of these agents has yet to be elucidated.

In a subcutaneous model of pancreatic cancer in mice, Kisker and colleagues[90] reported success in slowing tumor growth with low doses of endostatin and suppressing tumor growth altogether with high doses of this agent. In an orthotopic model of pancreatic cancer in mice, endostatin increased tumor-associated endothelial cell apoptosis and decreased interleukin-8 levels but did not have a significant impact on overall tumor size.[91]

Targeting Cyclooxygenase-2 in Tumor Endothelial Cells

The cyclooxygenase (COX) enzymes catalyze the rate-limiting step in the formation of prostaglandins and thromboxanes from arachidonic acid. The inducible isoform COX-2 is overexpressed in various solid tumors, including pancreatic cancer.[92-95] In vitro and in vivo studies have demonstrated that COX-2 inhibitors inhibit the production of proangiogenic factors VEGF and bFGF.[78,96-99] Perhaps more relevant is the fact that COX-2 inhibitors may directly affect the tumor neovasculature. In an orthotopic model of pancreatic cancer in mice, tumor-associated endothelial cells overexpressed COX-2, and treatment with COX-2 inhibitors significantly reduced microvessel density and increased both tumor cell and tumor-associated endothelial cell apoptosis.[100]

Overview of Clinical Trial Results

Anti-VEGF Therapy

Many strategies that target the VEGF ligand-receptor system are currently being studied in clinical trials (Table 38.3). Some of these agents, specifically the TK inhibitors, also demonstrate some (albeit less) activity against other TK receptors, such as EGF-R and platelet-derived growth factor receptor. Thus far, agents that target the

Table 38.3 Clinical Trials with Anti-VEGF Therapy in Pancreatic Cancer

Antiangiogenic Agent	Other Therapy	Pancreatic CA	Site
Phase I			
Bevacizumab	Capecitabine, XRT	Locally advanced	MDACC
Phase II			
Bevacizumab	Gemcitabine	Recur/stage III-IV	University of Chicago
Bevacizumab	Docetaxel	Recur/stage IV	FCCC
Phase III			
Bevacizumab	Gemcitabine	Recur/stage III-IV	Multicenter

Further details are available at *www.clinicaltrials.gov* and *www.cancer.gov*.

Abbreviations: FCCC, Fox Chase Cancer Center; MDACC, M. D. Anderson Cancer Center; VEGF, vascular endothelial growth factor; XRT, radiation therapy.

VEGF ligand-receptor system have shown relatively little toxicity in clinical trials compared with the toxicity of standard chemotherapy; however, adverse effects, such as hypertension, headaches, nausea, proteinuria, and thrombotic events, have been observed.[30,101] The long-term effects of antiangiogenic therapy are unknown.

At the 2003 meeting of the American Society of Clinical Oncology, Kindler and colleagues[68] reported the results from a National Cancer Institute-sponsored phase II multicenter trial in patients with unresectable pancreatic cancer (Table 38.4). Patients with confirmed unresectable pancreatic cancer who had not received prior chemotherapy for metastatic disease were included in the study. Patients received a combination of gemcitabine plus the recombinant humanized monoclonal anti-VEGF antibody bevacizumab (10 mg/kg intravenously every 2 weeks). Bevacizumab neutralizes all VEGF-A isoforms. The regimen was relatively well tolerated, with approximately a third of patients experiencing grade 3 or 4 leukopenia or neutropenia. However, there were no episodes of neutropenic fever. A few patients experienced variable nonhematologic toxicities, including fatigue, hyperglycemia, and slight elevation of liver function enzymes. Interestingly, hypertension was relatively rare, even though this is thought to be a "class effect" for this type of therapy. A partial response was identified in 27% of evaluable patients, greatly exceeding the 10% partial response rate in historic control subjects. In addition, 35% of patients exhibited stable disease, and only 23% of patients showed progression. Furthermore, at the time of reporting of the study, median survival had not yet been reached with a median follow-up of 6.2 months. The 6-month survival rate was 70%, and the estimated 1-year survival rate was 53%. The median time to progression was 6 months. This study demonstrates the promise of combining anti-VEGF therapy with standard chemotherapy. A randomized, double-blind, placebo-controlled, phase III trial is currently under way comparing gemcitabine plus placebo with gemcitabine plus bevacizumab (CALGB 80303).

Table 38.4 Comparison of Results from a Phase II Multicenter Clinical Trial of Bevacizumab and Gemcitabine Versus Historical Results from Gemcitabine Alone*

	Bevacizumab† + Gemcitabine (2003)	Gemcitabine‡ (2002)
Response rate	27%	5.6%
Median follow-up	6.2 months	—
Median survival	Not achieved	5.4 months
6-month survival	70%	<50%
1-year survival	53% (estimated)	<20%
Median time to progression	6 months	—

*Enrolled patients had unresectable pancreatic cancer with no prior therapy.
†Bevacizumab dose = 10 mg/kg intravenously every 2 weeks.
Phase II trial results were reported by Kindler et al.[68]
‡Gemcitabine results were obtained from the Eastern Cooperative Oncology Group Trial E2297 phase III study reported by Berlin et al.[117]

The improved response rates observed in this phase II clinical trial warrant further discussion. The response may be due in part to destruction of existing tumor vasculature, but this is likely a relatively minor mechanism of action. Anti-VEGF therapy may specifically eradicate the more inefficient, immature (pericyte-free) tumor microvasculature.[69] In turn, pericyte-covered vessels are left intact, resulting in redistribution of blood flow with an overall increase in tumor blood flow.[102,103] Furthermore, anti-VEGF therapy reduces tumor interstitial pressure.[86] Because high interstitial pressure impedes drug delivery, reduction of interstitial pressure should increase blood flow and delivery of therapeutic agents.[104] Thus, anti-VEGF therapy, by both eliminating inefficient tumor neovasculature and reducing tumor interstitial pressure, theoretically enables more efficient delivery of chemotherapy.[105-107]

Because preclinical models suggest that anti-VEGF therapy enhances the effectiveness of radiation therapy, combination therapy is currently under investigation. In a phase I clinical trial at the M.D. Anderson Cancer Center, Crane and colleagues[108] are combining bevacizumab with capecitabine and radiation therapy in patients with locally advanced pancreatic cancer. Preliminary results reported at the American Society of Clinical Oncology 2004 Gastrointestinal Cancers Symposium demonstrate that this novel combination is well tolerated. Of nine patients evaluable at a median follow-up of 6 months, one patient had a radiographic complete response, and the eight remaining patients had stable local disease; no patient experienced objective local tumor progression.

Endogenous Inhibitors of Angiogenesis

Angiostatin, endostatin, and thrombospondin analogues have all been studied in phase I clinical trials. There was a great deal of anticipation with regard to outcomes of the phase I endostatin trials. Although the drug could be safely administered, little activity was demonstrated in these trials.[109-111] As with other antiangiogenic agents, it is likely that endogenous inhibitors of angiogenesis will need to be combined with other therapeutic modalities in order to obtain any potential clinical benefit.

Conclusion

Currently, no other field in cancer research is undergoing such explosive growth as the field of angiogenesis. The results of this impressive body of research have led to the development of many novel potential antiangiogenic agents; more than 40 different agents are currently in clinical trials. Most of these agents have shown great promise in preclinical studies. The preclinical studies in pancreatic cancer described in this chapter have established that agents targeting proangiogenic factors are promising in xenograft models of human pancreatic cancer. By blocking the ligand-receptors with antibodies or inhibiting the receptors' TK function, investigators reported decreased pancreatic tumor growth, increased tumor cell and tumor-associated endothelial cell apoptosis, reduced microvessel density, fewer liver and lymphatic metastases, and improved survival of study animals. Moreover, minimal toxicity was associated with these treatments. Combination therapy with cytotoxic agents, such as gemcitabine, potentiated the therapeutic effects of the antiangiogenic agents, or vice versa. Phase II clinical trials with combination therapy of anti-VEGF therapy and chemotherapy are promising. Phase III trials are underway at the time of publication of this book and will yield important information about the impact of antiangiogenic therapy on current chemotherapeutic regimens. Any benefit observed with this type of therapy will likely be through the modulation and enhancement of other modalities, such as chemotherapy and radiation therapy. The ultimate clinical relevance of these agents will be determined when they are tested in humans in combination with other antineoplastic regimens.

References

1. Fidler IJ, et al. Critical determinants of neoplastic angiogenesis. *Cancer J.* 2000;6[Suppl 3]:S225–236.
2. Ellis LM, et al. Role of angiogenesis inhibitors in cancer treatment. *Oncology (Huntingt).* 2001;15[7 Suppl 8]:39–46.
3. Monestiroli S, et al. Kinetics and viability of circulating endothelial cells as surrogate angiogenesis marker in an animal model of human lymphoma. *Cancer Res.* 2001;61: 4341–4344.
4. Folkman J. Angiogenesis in cancer, vascular, rheumatoid and other disease. *Nat Med.* 1995;1:27–31.
5. Fidler IJ, Ellis LM. The implications of angiogenesis for the biology and therapy of cancer metastasis. *Cell.* 1994;79:185–188.
6. Folkman J. What is the evidence that tumors are angiogenesis dependent? *J Natl Cancer Inst.* 1990;82:4–6.
7. Liotta LA, Steeg PS, Stetler-Stevenson WG. Cancer metastasis and angiogenesis: an imbalance of positive and negative regulation. *Cell.* 1991;64:327–336.
8. Gannon G, et al. Overexpression of vascular endothelial growth factor-A165 enhances tumor angiogenesis but not metastasis during beta-cell carcinogenesis. *Cancer Res.* 2002;62:603–608.
9. Weidner N, et al. Tumor angiogenesis and metastasis: correlation in invasive breast carcinoma. *N Engl J Med.* 1991;324:1–8.
10. Maxwell PH, et al. Hypoxia-inducible factor-1 modulates gene expression in solid tumors and influences both angiogenesis and tumor growth. *Proc Natl Acad Sci USA.* 1997;94:8104–8109.
11. Rak J, et al. Mutant ras oncogenes upregulate VEGF/VPF expression: implications for induction and inhibition of tumor angiogenesis. *Cancer Res.* 1995;55:4575–4580.
12. Gerber HP, et al. Differential transcriptional regulation of the two vascular endothelial growth factor receptor genes: Flt-1, but not Flk-1/KDR, is up-regulated by hypoxia. *J Biol Chem.* 1997;272:23659–23667.

13. Dibbens JA, et al. Hypoxic regulation of vascular endothelial growth factor mRNA stability requires the cooperation of multiple RNA elements. *Mol Biol Cell.* 1999;10:907–919.
14. Bouck N, Stellmach V, Hsu SC. How tumors become angiogenic. *Adv Cancer Res.* 1996;69:135–174.
15. Akagi Y, et al. Regulation of vascular endothelial growth factor expression in human colon cancer by insulin-like growth factor-I. *Cancer Res.* 1998;58:4008–4014.
16. Bruns CJ, et al. In vivo selection and characterization of metastatic variants from human pancreatic adenocarcinoma by using orthotopic implantation in nude mice. *Neoplasia.* 1999;1:50–62.
17. Fujimoto K, et al. Expression of two angiogenic factors, vascular endothelial growth factor and platelet-derived endothelial cell growth factor in human pancreatic cancer, and its relationship to angiogenesis. *Eur J Cancer.* 1998;34:1439–1447.
18. Ikeda N, et al. Prognostic significance of angiogenesis in human pancreatic cancer. *Br J Cancer.* 1999;79:1553–1563.
19. Itakura J, et al. Enhanced expression of vascular endothelial growth factor in human pancreatic cancer correlates with local disease progression. *Clin Cancer Res.* 1997;3:1309–1316.
20. Kuniyasu H, et al. Relative expression of E-cadherin and type IV collagenase genes predicts disease outcome in patients with resectable pancreatic carcinoma. *Clin Cancer Res.* 1999;5:25–33.
21. Kuehn R, et al. Angiogenesis, angiogenic growth factors, and cell adhesion molecules are upregulated in chronic pancreatic diseases: angiogenesis in chronic pancreatitis and in pancreatic cancer. *Pancreas.* 1999;18:96–103.
22. Shimoyama S, et al. Increased angiogenin expression in pancreatic cancer is related to cancer aggressiveness. *Cancer Res.* 1996;56:2703–2706.
23. Yamanaka Y, et al. Overexpression of HER2/neu oncogene in human pancreatic carcinoma. *Hum Pathol.* 1993;24:1127–1134.
24. Dvorak HF, et al. Vascular permeability factor/vascular endothelial growth factor, microvascular hyperpermeability, and angiogenesis. *Am J Pathol.* 1995;146:1029–1039.
25. Senger DR, et al. Tumor cells secrete a vascular permeability factor that promotes accumulation of ascites fluid. *Science.* 1983;219:983–985.
26. Robinson CJ, Stringer SE. The splice variants of vascular endothelial growth factor (VEGF) and their receptors. *J Cell Sci.* 2001;114(pt 5):853–865.
27. Carmeliet P, et al. Impaired myocardial angiogenesis and ischemic cardiomyopathy in mice lacking the vascular endothelial growth factor isoforms VEGF164 and VEGF188. *Nat Med.* 1999;5:495–502.
28. Matsumoto T, Claesson-Welsh L. VEGF receptor signal transduction. *Sci STKE.* 2001;2001(112):RE21.
29. Neufeld G, et al. Vascular endothelial growth factor (VEGF) and its receptors. *FASEB J.* 1999;13:9–22.
30. Rosen LS. Clinical experience with angiogenesis signaling inhibitors: focus on vascular endothelial growth factor (VEGF) blockers. *Cancer Control.* 2002;9[2 suppl]:36–44.
31. Ku DD, et al. Vascular endothelial growth factor induces EDRF-dependent relaxation in coronary arteries. *Am J Physiol.* 1993;265(2 pt 2):H586–592.
32. Gerber HP, Dixit V, Ferrara N. Vascular endothelial growth factor induces expression of the antiapoptotic proteins Bcl-2 and A1 in vascular endothelial cells. *J Biol Chem.* 1998;273:13313–13316.
33. Gerber HP, et al. Vascular endothelial growth factor regulates endothelial cell survival through the phosphatidylinositol 3′-kinase/Akt signal transduction pathway: requirement for Flk-1/KDR activation. *J Biol Chem.* 1998;273:30336–30343.
34. Nor JE, et al. Vascular endothelial growth factor (VEGF)-mediated angiogenesis is associated with enhanced endothelial cell survival and induction of Bcl-2 expression. *Am J Pathol.* 1999;154:375–384.
35. Luttun A, et al. Revascularization of ischemic tissues by PlGF treatment, and inhibition of tumor angiogenesis, arthritis and atherosclerosis by anti-Flt1. *Nat Med.* 2002;8:831–840.
36. Wu Y, et al. A fully human monoclonal antibody against VEGFR-1 inhibits growth of human breast cancers [abstract 3005]. *Proc Am Assoc Cancer Res.* 2004;45.
37. Ellis LM, et al. Down-regulation of vascular endothelial growth factor in a human colon carcinoma cell line transfected with an antisense expression vector specific for c-src. *J Biol Chem.* 1998;273:1052–1057.
38. Kimura H, et al. Hypoxia response element of the human vascular endothelial growth factor gene mediates transcriptional regulation by nitric oxide: control of hypoxia-inducible factor-1 activity by nitric oxide. *Blood.* 2000;95:189–197.
39. Bouvet M, et al. Adenovirus-mediated wild-type p53 gene transfer down-regulates vascular endothelial growth factor expression and inhibits angiogenesis in human colon cancer. *Cancer Res.* 1998;58:2288–2292.
40. Mazure NM, et al. Induction of vascular endothelial growth factor by hypoxia is modulated by a phosphatidylinositol 3-kinase/Akt signaling pathway in Ha-ras-transformed cells through a hypoxia inducible factor-1 transcriptional element. *Blood.* 1997;90:3322–3331.
41. Ellis LM, et al. Vessel counts and vascular endothelial growth factor expression in pancreatic adenocarcinoma. *Eur J Cancer.* 1998;34:337–340.
42. Terris B, et al. Expression of vascular endothelial growth factor in digestive neuroendocrine tumours. *Histopathology.* 1998;32:133–138.
43. Tsuzuki Y, et al. Pancreas microenvironment promotes VEGF expression and tumor growth: novel window models for pancreatic tumor angiogenesis and microcirculation. *Lab Invest.* 2001;81:1439–1451.
44. Carmeliet P, Jain RK. Angiogenesis in cancer and other diseases. *Nature.* 2000;407:249–257.
45. Ferrara N. VEGF: an update on biological and therapeutic aspects. *Curr Opin Biotechnol.* 2000;11:617–624.
46. Kerbel RS. Tumor angiogenesis: past, present and the near future. *Carcinogenesis.* 2000;21:505–515.
47. Ishikawa F, et al. Identification of angiogenic activity and the cloning and expression of platelet-derived endothelial cell growth factor. *Nature.* 1989;338:557–562.

48. Furukawa T, et al. Angiogenic factor. *Nature*. 1992;356:668.
49. Haraguchi M, et al. Angiogenic activity of enzymes. *Nature*. 1994;368:198.
50. Burgess WH, Maciag T. The heparin-binding (fibroblast) growth factor family of proteins. *Annu Rev Biochem*. 1989;58:575–606.
51. Mignatti P, et al. In vitro angiogenesis on the human amniotic membrane: requirement for basic fibroblast growth factor-induced proteinases. *J Cell Biol*. 1989;108:671–682.
52. Moscatelli D, Presta M, Rifkin DB. Purification of a factor from human placenta that stimulates capillary endothelial cell protease production, DNA synthesis, and migration. *Proc Natl Acad Sci USA*. 1986;83:2091–2095.
53. Yamazaki K, et al. Expression of basic fibroblast growth factor (FGF-2)-associated with tumour proliferation in human pancreatic carcinoma. *Virchows Arch*. 1997;431:95–101.
54. Montesano R, et al. Basic fibroblast growth factor induces angiogenesis in vitro. *Proc Natl Acad Sci USA*. 1986;83:7297–7301.
55. Johnson DE, et al. The human fibroblast growth factor receptor genes: a common structural arrangement underlies the mechanisms for generating receptor forms that differ in their third immunoglobulin domain. *Mol Cell Biol*. 1991;11:4627–4634.
56. Zabrenetzky V, et al. Expression of the extracellular matrix molecule thrombospondin inversely correlates with malignant progression in melanoma, lung and breast carcinoma cell lines. *Int J Cancer*. 1994;59:191–195.
57. Tokunaga T, et al. Thrombospondin 2 expression is correlated with inhibition of angiogenesis and metastasis of colon cancer. *Br J Cancer*. 1999;79:354–359.
58. Taraboletti G, et al. Platelet thrombospondin modulates endothelial cell adhesion, motility, and growth: a potential angiogenesis regulatory factor. *J Cell Biol*. 1990;111:765–772.
59. Qian X, et al. Expression of thrombospondin-1 in human pancreatic adenocarcinomas: role in matrix metalloproteinase-9 production. *Pathol Oncol Res*. 2001;7:251–259.
60. Kasper HU, et al. Expression of thrombospondin-1 in pancreatic carcinoma: correlation with microvessel density. *Virchows Arch*. 2001;438:116–120.
61. Qian X, Tuszynski GP. Expression of thrombospondin-1 in cancer: a role in tumor progression. *Proc Soc Exp Biol Med*. 1996;212:199–207.
62. Tokunaga T, et al. Alterations in tumour suppressor gene p53 correlate with inhibition of thrombospondin-1 gene expression in colon cancer cells. *Virchows Arch*. 1998;433:415–418.
63. Gasparini G, et al. Thrombospondin-1 and -2 in node-negative breast cancer: correlation with angiogenic factors, p53, cathepsin D, hormone receptors and prognosis. *Oncology*. 2001;60:72–80.
64. Detmar M. The role of VEGF and thrombospondins in skin angiogenesis. *J Dermatol Sci*. 2000;24[Suppl 1]:S78–84.
65. Kazuno M, et al. Thrombospondin-2 (TSP2) expression is inversely correlated with vascularity in glioma. *Eur J Cancer*. 1999;35:502–506.
66. Strydom DJ, et al. Amino acid sequence of human tumor derived angiogenin. *Biochemistry*. 1985;24:5486–5494.
67. Hurwitz H, et al. Results of a phase III trial of bevacizumab in combination with bolus irinotecan, 5-fluourouracil, leucovorin as first-line therapy in subjects with metastatic CRC. *Proceedings of the American Society of Clinical Oncology*. 2003. Chicago, IL.
68. Kindler HL, et al. Bevacizumab plus gemcitabine in patients with advanced pancreatic cancer. i *Proceedings of the American Society of Clinical Oncology*. 2003. Chicago, IL.
69. Jain RK, Munn LL, Fukumura D. Dissecting tumour pathophysiology using intravital microscopy. *Nat Rev Cancer*. 2002;2:266–276.
70. Brown LF, et al. Increased expression of vascular permeability factor (vascular endothelial growth factor) and its receptors in kidney and bladder carcinomas. *Am J Pathol*. 1993;143:1255–1262.
71. Brown LF, et al. Expression of vascular permeability factor (vascular endothelial growth factor) and its receptors in adenocarcinomas of the gastrointestinal tract. *Cancer Res*. 1993;53:4727–4735.
72. Reinmuth N, et al. Induction of VEGF in perivascular cells defines a potential paracrine mechanism for endothelial cell survival. *FASEB J*. 2001;15:1239–1241.
73. Asano M, et al. Inhibition of tumor growth and metastasis by an immunoneutralizing monoclonal antibody to human vascular endothelial growth factor/vascular permeability factor121. *Cancer Res*. 1995;55:5296–5301.
74. Kim KJ, et al. Inhibition of vascular endothelial growth factor-induced angiogenesis suppresses tumour growth in vivo. *Nature*. 1993;362:841–844.
75. Witte L, et al. Monoclonal antibodies targeting the VEGF receptor-2 (Flk1/KDR) as an anti-angiogenic therapeutic strategy. *Cancer Metast Rev*. 1998;17:155–161.
76. Lin P, et al. Inhibition of tumor growth by targeting tumor endothelium using a soluble vascular endothelial growth factor receptor. *Cell Growth Differ*. 1998;9:49–58.
77. Shaheen RM, et al. Antiangiogenic therapy targeting the tyrosine kinase receptor for vascular endothelial growth factor receptor inhibits the growth of colon cancer liver metastasis and induces tumor and endothelial cell apoptosis. *Cancer Res*. 1999;59:5412–5416.
78. Chu J, et al. Potential involvement of the cyclooxygenase-2 pathway in the regulation of tumor-associated angiogenesis and growth in pancreatic cancer. *Mol Cancer Ther*. 2003;2:1–7.
79. Solorzano CC, et al. Optimization for the blockade of epidermal growth factor receptor signaling for therapy of human pancreatic carcinoma. *Clin Cancer Res*. 2001;7:2563–2572.
80. Bruns CJ, et al. Blockade of the epidermal growth factor receptor signaling by a novel tyrosine kinase inhibitor leads to apoptosis of endothelial cells and therapy of human pancreatic carcinoma. *Cancer Res*. 2000;60:2926–2935.
81. Bruns CJ, et al. Vascular endothelial growth factor is an in vivo survival factor for tumor endothelium in a murine model of colorectal carcinoma liver metastases. *Cancer*. 2000;89:488–499.

82. Baker CH, Solorzano CC, Fidler IJ. Angiogenesis and cancer metastasis: antiangiogenic therapy of human pancreatic adenocarcinoma. *Int J Clin Oncol.* 2001;6:59–65.
83. Solorzano CC, et al. Inhibition of growth and metastasis of human pancreatic cancer growing in nude mice by PTK 787/ZK222584, an inhibitor of the vascular endothelial growth factor receptor tyrosine kinases. *Cancer Biother Radiopharm.* 2001;16:359–370.
84. Bruns CJ, et al. Effect of the vascular endothelial growth factor receptor-2 antibody DC101 plus gemcitabine on growth, metastasis and angiogenesis of human pancreatic cancer growing orthotopically in nude mice. *Int J Cancer.* 2002;102:101–108.
85. Geng L, et al. Inhibition of vascular endothelial growth factor receptor signaling leads to reversal of tumor resistance to radiotherapy. *Cancer Res.* 2001;61:2413–2419.
86. Lee CG, et al. Anti-vascular endothelial growth factor treatment augments tumor radiation response under normoxic or hypoxic conditions. *Cancer Res.* 2000;60:5565–5570.
87. Jain RK. Tumor angiogenesis and accessibility: role of vascular endothelial growth factor. *Semin Oncol.* 2002;29[6 Suppl 16]:3–9.
88. O'Reilly MS, et al. Angiostatin: a novel angiogenesis inhibitor that mediates the suppression of metastases by a Lewis lung carcinoma. *Cell.* 1994;79:315–328.
89. O'Reilly MS, et al. Endostatin: an endogenous inhibitor of angiogenesis and tumor growth. *Cell.* 1997;88:277–285.
90. Kisker O, et al. Continuous administration of endostatin by intraperitoneally implanted osmotic pump improves the efficacy and potency of therapy in a mouse xenograft tumor model. *Cancer Res.* 2001;61:7669–7674.
91. Raut CP, et al. Direct effects of recombinant human endostatin on tumor cell IL-8 production are associated with increased endothelial cell apoptosis in an orthotopic model of human pancreatic cancer. *Cancer Biol Ther* 2004;3: 679–687.
92. Kokawa A, et al. Increased expression of cyclooxygenase-2 in human pancreatic neoplasms and potential for chemoprevention by cyclooxygenase inhibitors. *Cancer.* 2001;91:333–338.
93. Koshiba T, et al. Immunohistochemical analysis of cyclooxygenase-2 expression in pancreatic tumors. *Int J Pancreatol.* 1999;26:69–76.
94. Maitra A, et al. Cyclooxygenase 2 expression in pancreatic adenocarcinoma and pancreatic intraepithelial neoplasia: an immunohistochemical analysis with automated cellular imaging. *Am J Clin Pathol.* 2002;118: 194–201.
95. Molina MA, et al. Increased cyclooxygenase-2 expression in human pancreatic carcinomas and cell lines: growth inhibition by nonsteroidal anti-inflammatory drugs. *Cancer Res.* 1999;59:4356–4362.
96. Eibl G, et al. PGE(2) is generated by specific COX-2 activity and increases VEGF production in COX-2-expressing human pancreatic cancer cells. *Biochem Biophys Res Commun.* 2003;306:887–897.
97. Iniguez MA, et al. Cyclooxygenase-2: a therapeutic target in angiogenesis. *Trends Mol Med.* 2003;9:73–78.
98. Sawaoka H, et al. Cyclooxygenase inhibitors suppress angiogenesis and reduce tumor growth in vivo. *Lab Invest.* 1999;79:1469–1477.
99. Yoshida S, et al. COX-2/VEGF-dependent facilitation of tumor-associated angiogenesis and tumor growth in vivo. *Lab Invest.* 2003;83:1385–1394.
100. Raut CP, et al. Celecoxib inhibits angiogenesis by inducing endothelial cell apoptosis in human pancreatic tumor xerografts. *Cancer Biol Ther* 2004;3:•••–•••.
101. Yang JC, et al. A randomized trial of bevacizumab, an anti-vascular endothelial growth factor antibody, for metastatic renal cancer. *N Engl J Med.* 2003;349:427–434.
102. McCarty, Ellis, and Charnsangavej, unpublished observations
103. Benjamin LE, et al. Selective ablation of immature blood vessels in established human tumors follows vascular endothelial growth factor withdrawal. *J Clin Invest.* 1999;103:159–165.
104. Graff BA, et al. Intratumour heterogeneity in the uptake of macromolecular therapeutic agents in human melanoma xenografts. *Br J Cancer.* 2003;88:291–297.
105. Wildiers H, et al. Effect of antivascular endothelial growth factor treatment on the intratumoral uptake of CPT-11. *Br J Cancer.* 2003;88:1979–1986.
106. Salnikov AV, et al. Lowering of tumor interstitial fluid pressure specifically augments efficacy of chemotherapy. *FASEB J.* 2003;17:1756–1758.
107. Ma J, et al. Pharmacodynamic-mediated effects of the angiogenesis inhibitor SU5416 on the tumor disposition of temozolomide in subcutaneous and intracerebral glioma xenograft models. *J Pharmacol Exp Ther.* 2003;305:833–839.
108. Crane CH, et al. Preliminary results of a phase I study of rhuMab VEGF (bevacizumab) with concurrent radiotherapy (XRT) and capecitabine (CAP). ASCO Gastrointestinal Cancers Symposium. San Francisco, CA, 2004.
109. Eder JP Jr, et al. Phase I clinical trial of recombinant human endostatin administered as a short intravenous infusion repeated daily. *J Clin Oncol.* 2002;20:3772–3784.
110. Herbst RS, et al. Phase I study of recombinant human endostatin in patients with advanced solid tumors. *J Clin Oncol.* 2002;20:3792–3803.
111. Twombly R. First clinical trials of endostatin yield lukewarm results. *J Natl Cancer Inst.* 2002;94:1520–1521.
112. Ikeda N, et al. The association of K-ras gene mutation and vascular endothelial growth factor gene expression in pancreatic carcinoma. *Cancer.* 2001;92:488–499.
113. Niedergethmann M, et al. High expression of vascular endothelial growth factor predicts early recurrence and poor prognosis after curative resection for ductal adenocarcinoma of the pancreas. *Pancreas.* 2002;25:122–129.
114. Knoll MR, et al. Correlation of postoperative survival and angiogenic growth factors in pancreatic carcinoma. *Hepatogastroenterology.* 2001;48:1162–1165.
115. Seo Y, et al. High expression of vascular endothelial growth factor is associated with liver metastasis and a poor prognosis for patients with ductal pancreatic adenocarcinoma. *Cancer.* 2000;88:2239–2245.

116. Takao S, et al. Expression of thymidine phosphorylase is associated with a poor prognosis in patients with ductal adenocarcinoma of the pancreas. *Clin Cancer Res.* 1998;4:1619–1624.
117. Fujioka S, et al. Angiogenesis in pancreatic carcinoma: thymidine phosphorylase expression in stromal cells and intratumoral microvessel density as independent predictors of overall and relapse-free survival. *Cancer.* 2001;92:1788–1797.
118. Berlin JD, et al. Phase III study of gemcitabine in combination with fluorouracil versus gemcitabine alone in patients with advanced pancreatic carcinoma: Eastern Cooperative Oncology Group Trial E2297. *J Clin Oncol.* 2002;20:3270–3275.

39

Monoclonal Antibodies and Other Targeted Therapies for Pancreatic Cancer

Andrew H. Ko, MD
Margaret A. Tempero, MD

Although cytotoxic therapy remains the primary treatment modality for advanced pancreatic cancer, the current era of molecular therapeutics holds much promise for novel approaches to this disease in the future. We have already seen significant gains over the past decade in other cancer types with the approval of drugs that move beyond the realm of standard chemotherapy. For example, monoclonal antibodies represent a relatively new class of agents that now have proven efficacy in a variety of different tumors. Rituximab, an anti-CD20 chimeric antibody, plays an important role in the treatment of certain forms of non-Hodgkins' lymphoma, whereas Herceptin, an anti-HER-2/Neu antibody, is now commonly used for patients with metastatic breast cancer overexpressing this particular protein. The accompanying table lists currently approved antibodies and their indications for use (Table 39.1).

Another class of compounds generating a great deal of research and excitement is small molecule inhibitors. These are molecules specifically designed to target and disrupt a signaling pathway, enzyme, or cellular component implicated in the pathogenesis of a particular tumor type. Classic examples of small molecule inhibitors recently receiving Food and Drug Administration (FDA) approval include imatinib mesylate (Gleevec), an oral agent that inhibits the aberrant tyrosine kinase activity of the bcr-abl fusion protein in chronic myelogenous leukemia, and gefitinib (Iressa), which inhibits the tyrosine kinase activity of the epidermal growth factor receptor (EGFR) and has been approved for use in refractory non-small cell lung cancer. A number of additional agents, representing a broad range of mechanisms of action and directed against multiple different signaling pathways critical to tumor cell growth, are currently undergoing active preclinical and clinical testing as well for specific tumor types, including pancreatic cancer.

What impact will this revolution in molecular therapeutics have on the effectiveness of treatment for advanced pancreatic cancer in the future? There are certain obvious challenges specific to pancreatic cancer that represent major hurdles in terms of effective drug delivery and conduct of clinical trials of novel agents. For one, the dense desmoplastic reaction, which often engulfs the primary tumor in pancreatic cancer, may limit the accessibility of any systemic therapy to reach a significant portion of the tumor cells and effect its anti-tumor activity. Second, the lack of an ideal animal model that accurately recapitulates pancreatic tumor biology in human beings makes it difficult to translate exciting preclinical strategies into meaningful

Table 39.1 Monoclonal Antibodies Currently Approved for Use in Human Malignancies

Antibody	Target Antigen	Indication	Comments
Rituxan (rituximab)	CD20	B-cell non-Hodgkin's lymphoma	First mAb to receive FDA approval (1997)
Herceptin (trastuzumab)	HER-2/Neu	Breast cancer	
Mylotarg (gemtuzumab ozogamicin)	CD33	Acute myelogenous leukemia	Linked to antibiotic calicheamicin
Zevalin (ibritumomab Tiuxetan)	CD20	B-cell non-Hodgkin's lymphoma	Linked to Y-90 and In-111 isotopes
Erbitux (cetuximab)	EGFR	Colorectal cancer	
Avastin (bevacizumab)	VEGF	Colorectal cancer	Approved for use in combination with 5-FU–based cytotoxic regimen

patient-oriented results. Finally, many patients with advanced pancreatic cancer have significant constitutional symptoms, a poor performance status, and a rapidly deteriorating clinical course that at times precludes their ability to participate in clinical trials.

Despite these challenges, there is optimism that we will be able to make significant strides in the treatment of this almost uniformly fatal disease when it is detected in advanced stages. A number of clinical studies in advanced pancreatic cancer have been reported or are currently underway that are investigating these newer treatment strategies, some of which show a fair degree of promise or are at least provocative based on proof of principle. The purpose of this chapter is to highlight the available evidence regarding these novel therapies in pancreatic cancer. Discussion of these therapies will be divided into two main categories: antibodies and small molecule inhibitors.

EGFR: A "Prototype" Molecular Target

Many of the new agents discussed in this chapter target growth factor receptors or their ligands or a downstream signaling pathway of the receptor. This discussion provides rationale for developing antibodies or small molecules directed at these targets using EGFR as an example.

The EGFR (or ErbB-1) is a 170-kD protein that belongs to a family of other structurally related receptors, including HER-2/Neu (ErbB-2), HER-3 (ErbB-3), and HER-4 (ErbB-4), sometimes referred to as the type I growth receptor family. These receptors are part of a larger family of receptor tyrosine kinases (RTKs) that respond to extracellular signals and transduce these signals from the cell surface to the cytoplasm (Fig. 39.1). In its unbound state, EGFR exists as a monomer but after binding by a peptide ligand, such as EGF or transforming growth factor-α (TGF-α), undergoes dimerization (Fig. 39.2). This may involve either homodimerization or heterodimerization between EGFR and another member of the Erb-B receptor family. Dimerization leads to activation of the intracellular tyrosine kinase domain of the receptor, resulting in autophosphorylation and conformational change. Activation of the receptor then triggers a complex cascade of events[1-7], including activation of Ras and the Raf/Erk/MAP kinase pathways, which send signals to the nucleus of the cell and, ultimately, regulates gene expression of proteins critical to cell growth and cell cycle progression, such as cyclin D1. Furthermore, activated EGFR recruits and phosphorylates a number of other proteins, among them phosphatidylinositol-3-kinase, an enzyme that in turn activates the molecules protein kinase B/Akt, protein kinase C, and nuclear factor-κB (NF-κB), each of which is im-

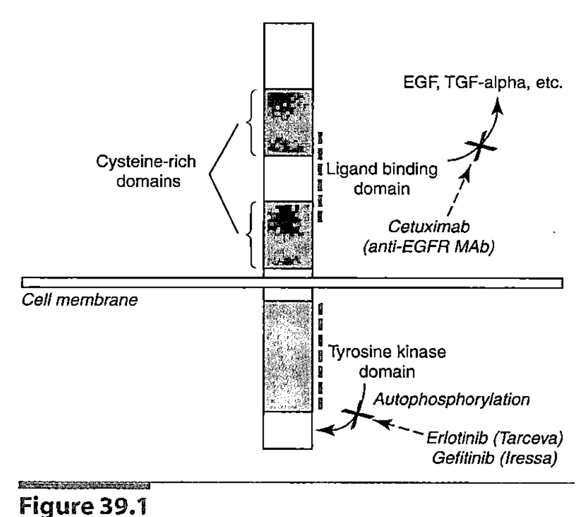

Figure 39.1
Structure of EGF receptor.

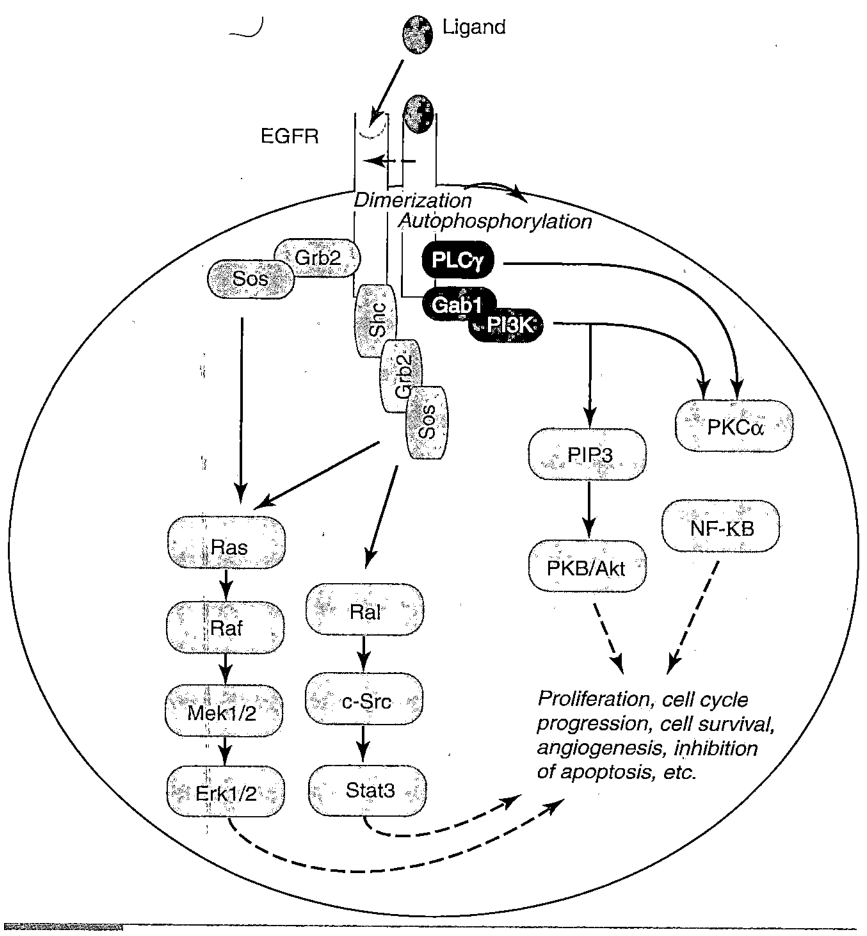

Figure 39.2
Schema of EGFR signaling.

portant in regulating cell growth and survival. EGF and TGF-α also induce vascular endothelial growth factor (VEGF),[8,9] thus suggesting a role of the EGFR pathway in mediating aspects of angiogenesis.

With this increasing understanding of how signaling through EGFR is intimately involved in controlling cellular proliferation and death, a great deal of attention has been turned to how this pathway may play a role not only in normal cells but also in malignant cells as well. There is, in fact, a large and growing body of evidence to suggest that this pathway may be critical in development and maintenance of the malignant phenotype in a variety of cancer subtypes and that increased EGFR expression is associated with poorer clinical outcomes.[10-15] In addition to overexpression of EGFR or its ligand(s), a mutant variant of the EGFR gene, referred to as EGFRvIII, has been discovered in several different human cancers. This mutation results in a deletion in the extracellular domain and constitutive activation of the tyrosine kinase domain, leading to cell proliferation independent of ligand binding.[16-18]

A great deal of evidence points to EGFR contributing to the development of pancreatic cancer. Murphy et al.[19] used an in vitro cell culture system to demonstrate that pancreatic cancer cells require a functional EGFR-mediated autocrine pathway for proliferation in serum-free conditions. Furthermore, a number of investigators have reported different rates of immunoreactivity for EGFR and its ligands in primary pancreatic cancer samples. Barton et al.[20] described a 95% immunoreactivity rate for TGF-α and a 12% rate for EGF in pancreatic tumor tissue. Yamanaka et al.[21] analyzed 87 human pancreatic carcinomas by immunohistochemical methods and found 43% showed overexpression for EGFR, 46% for EGF, and 54% for TGF-α. A recent study by Tobita et al.[22] of 77 cases of invasive ductal adenocarcinoma found 41.6% of the cases immunoreactive for EGFR, the majority of them showing a diffuse staining pattern.

The clinical implications of aberrant EGFR signaling in pancreatic cancer may be realized when considering that expression of these signaling components correlates with inferior patient outcomes. In the Yamanka et al. study, 38% of samples showed overexpression of both EGFR and either the TGF-α or EGF ligand; this coexpression pattern correlated with a more aggressive clinical course and worse patient outcomes.[21] Meanwhile, Tobita et al.[22] found that EGFR expression was associated with the presence of metastases, particularly liver based.

A number of agents have been specifically designed to inhibit EGFR-mediated signaling, including both monoclonal antibodies that compete for binding to EGFR, as well as small molecule inhibitors that directly disrupt the enzymatic activity of the RTK (reviewed in Mendelsohn and Baselga and Xiong and Abbruzzese).[7,23] These agents, particularly their study in the context of human pancreatic cancer, are discussed in greater detail in the subsequent sections.

One must sound a note of caution, however, that despite this seemingly solid rationale for pursuing anti-EGFR strategies in pancreatic cancer, levels of EGFR expression in tumors do not clearly correlate with response to anti-EGFR therapy either in vitro[24,25] or in vivo.[26-28] This lack of correlation has been shown in studies for both colorectal and head and neck carcinomas using an anti-EGFR antibody-based strategy and in a study for non-small cell lung cancer using a small molecule inhibitor.[26-28] Likely in a number of cancer types, critical downstream signals are activated via other receptors than EGFR,[7] and hence, a given tumor may not be as dependent on EGF and therefore less responsive to anti–EGFR-based therapy despite expressing high levels of EGFR. Conversely, increased levels of ligands, co-expression of EGFR mutants, and cross-talk with HER2 or other receptors may enhance EGFR-signaling output and potentially make a tumor responsive to EGFR inhibitors despite less than robust expression of the receptor.[29]

Antibodies

Introduction

Certainly one of the most critical determinants of success of monoclonal antibodies in the treatment of any malignancy is the selection of target antigen. Ideally, the antigen would be preferentially expressed by the tumor, with minimal to no expression in normal host cells. Other important features that may mediate the effectiveness of antibody therapy include genetic instability leading to aberrant antigens that escape binding by the therapeutic monoclonal antibody; the biologic function of the antigen (i.e., does it play a role in cellular growth, differentiation, and/or survival?), the density and stability of antigen expression on cell surfaces, and the degree of secretion of soluble antigen into the peripheral circulation, thus binding infused antibody and preventing the antibody from binding to the cell surface-based antigen.[30] In addition, antibodies are large molecules and do not always traffic easily through tumors with high interstitial pressure. Thus, there can be physical barriers preventing access of antibody to antigen.

Antibody-based treatment strategies have been further refined over time such that monoclonal murine antibodies, derived from the fusion of B lymphocytes from immunized mice with an immortal myeloma cell line (resulting in a hybridoma), have largely been supplanted by chimeric, humanized, or fully human mAbs produced by newer genetic engineering techniques. Antibodies composed mostly or entirely of human regions have the advantage over their murine counterparts with regard to (1) the potential of greater specificity for human tumor antigens and (2) a low frequency of the development of a host immune response (i.e., human antimouse antibody) negating the therapeutic effects of the antibody.

Antibodies can kill tumor cells via a variety of immune mechanisms: complement-mediated cytotoxicity, in which complement (specifically, C1q) is fixed to the Fc region of the antibody, resulting in activation of the complement cascade; antibody-dependent cell-mediated cytotoxicity (ADCC), in which any number of effector cells from the host immune system are recruited to lyse the target cell; and opsonization (phagocytosis), a function specifically carried out by neutrophils and mononuclear phagocytes.[30,31] Additionally, mAbs can interfere with tumor cell growth by preventing interaction between a cell signaling ligand and its receptor, leading to growth inhibition or apoptosis. This may take place either by antibody binding to one of the antigenic determinants of the ligand, sterically hindering ligand-receptor interaction (referred to as neutralization), or by antibody binding to the cell surface receptor, which can (1) act as a competitive inhibitor to the normal cell-signaling ligand and/or (2) result in internalization of the receptor–antibody complex and hence down-regulation of available cell surface receptors.[30,32] Finally, to take things even a step further, a number of additional approaches are under active development to effect potentially even greater therapeutic activity, moving beyond unconjugated antibody treatment into the realm of linkage of antibodies with drugs, toxins, or radiolabeled isotopes (Fig. 39.3).

Early Antibody Studies

Monoclonal antibody BW494 The first monoclonal antibody tested in pancreatic cancer, BW494, was developed by Bosslet et al.[33] in the 1980s. This murine immunoglobulin, IgG1 isotype, recognized a 200-kD glycoprotein antigen commonly present on pancreatic cancer cells and was demonstrated in in vitro studies to induce ADCC in pancreatic cancer cells in the presence of mononuclear cells.[33] Radiolabeling of this antibody with ^{131}Y or ^{111}I isotopes produced appropriate localization in tumor xenografts in nude mice, as well as in primary tumors and metastases in humans.[10,34] Furthermore, a single injection of ^{131}I-labeled antibody in nude mice suppressed tumor xenograft growth.[34] Based on these encouraging preclinical results, Buchler et al.[35-37] out of Germany conducted a series of clinical trials using BW494 in individuals with different stages of pancreatic cancer. A pilot study of 39 patients with advanced disease showed a partial remission in one patient and stable disease in an additional nine patients, with a median survival of 5 months. Eight of eight patients developed serum human antimouse antibody titers within 4 weeks after therapy had been initiated. Two phase II studies were subsequently conducted by this same group.[35] The

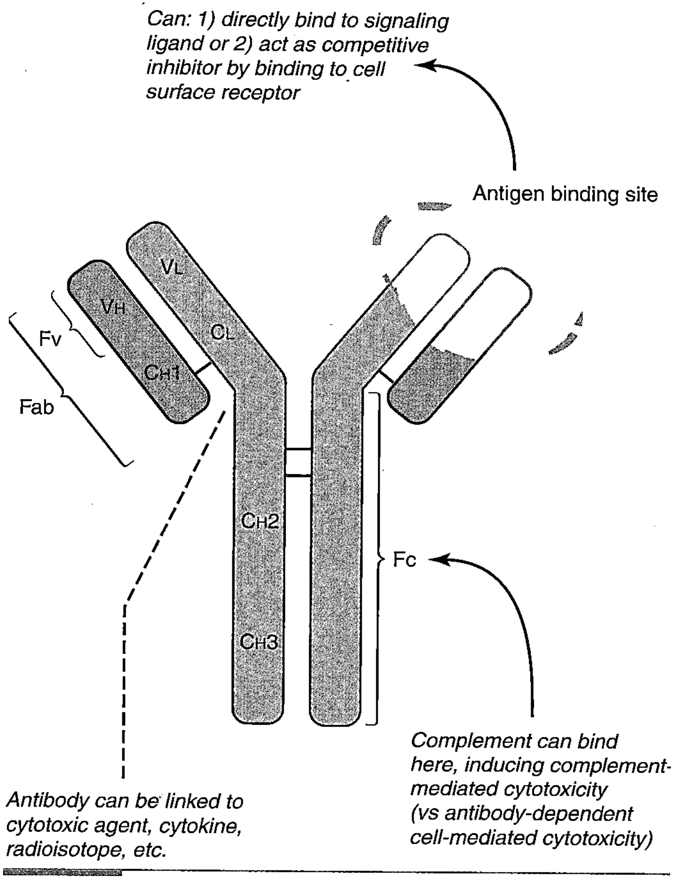

Figure 39.3
Antibody structure and mechanisms of anti-tumor activity.

first was a nonrandomized trial in 35 patients with locally advanced disease, in which no objective responses were seen, although 47% of patients showed stable disease for at least 3 months; the median survival was 6.5 months. In the second, 61 patients with resectable pancreatic cancer were randomized to receive either a series of postoperative infusions with BW494 antibody over a 10-day period or no further treatment. Kaplan-Meier estimates of survival showed no difference between the two groups (428 days for the treatment group and 386 for the control group).[38]

mAb 17-1A Murine mAb 17-1A was developed after immunization of mice with the colorectal cancer cell line SW1038.[39] This antibody, of immunoglobulin IgG_{2a} isotype, is directed against a 37-kD glycoprotein located on the cell surface of many adenocarcinomas, as well as on normal epithelial cells, including large and small bowel.[40-42] Furthermore, the 17-1A antigen has been demonstrated to be expressed in many pancreatic cancer cell lines.[43] The administration of mAb 17-1A to nude mice immediately after inoculation with human gastrointestinal cancer cells resulted in inhibition of explant growth, with increased numbers of macrophages found at the tumor site.[44] Given this provocative preclinical data, investigators in the mid-1980s began studying this antibody in the clinical setting for patients with advanced pancreatic cancer. An initial report by Sindelar et al.[45] suggested some anti-tumor activity in pancreatic cancer patients, with objective tumor regressions reported in 4 of 19 (21%) clinically evaluable patients when treated with either antibody alone or antibody absorbed onto autologous peripheral blood mononuclear cells (PBMCs). However, these responses did not correlate with the presence or absence of antiidiotype antibody formation. A subsequent study of 18 patients using mAb 17-1A admixed with autologous mononuclear cells failed to show any objective responses, although 3 of the 18 patients showed prolonged disease stabilization.[43]

A multicenter, phase II Eastern Cooperative Oncology Group study was performed in a group of 28 patients with advanced pancreatic cancer, using a more prolonged treatment course of mAb 17-1A than either of the previously mentioned studies to test the hypothesis that antigen saturation with repetitive and prolonged dosing might induce greater anti-tumor activity.[46] Patients were allowed to have received one prior chemotherapy regimen. Antibody therapy was given three times weekly for 8 consecutive weeks. Sixteen of the 28 patients were able to complete the full course of therapy; 6 were discontinued from treatment because of progressive disease, and 5 others were taken off the study because of hypersensitivity reactions, all occurring during the first 3 weeks of treatment. Of 22 patients evaluable for response, only 1 experienced a partial response. The mean progression-free survival was 50 days, and the mean overall survival was 82 days from the first infusion of antibody. Hence, the study investigators concluded that this treatment program was not effective in advanced pancreatic cancer.

Because of the potential of augmented ADCC by coadministration of γ-interferon with mAb 17-1A, several investigators have combined the two agents in clinical trial design. A phase II study was conducted by Tempero et al.[47] using recombinant γ-interferon (10^6 U/m^2 daily for 4 days) plus mAb 17-1A on days 2, 3, and 4. Of 25 evaluable patients, one objective response was observed (complete remission for 4 months in a patient with locally recurrent disease status post-Whipple resection and external beam radiation therapy (XRT), with stable disease lasting at least 2 months seen in an additional 9 patients. The median survival for the entire group was 5 months. Although correlative biologic studies demonstrated enhanced ADCC, as expected, in post-γ-interferon–treated patient PBMCs compared with pretreatment samples, this proof of principle did not translate into improved clinical benefit for this patient population.

Antibodies Against Growth Factor Receptors or Their Ligands

Cetuximab (Erbitux, IMC-C225) Cetuximab is a chimeric antibody (immunoglobulin G1 subclass) that competes with natural ligands (EGF, TGF-α) for binding to the EGF receptor. This antibody was engineered by fusing the variable region of M225 (a pure murine antibody) to the human constant region of IgG1. The result was a chimera that, compared with its murine counterpart, does not induce significant levels of neutralizing antibody and demonstrates greater affinity with EGFR. By preventing ligand-receptor binding, cetuximab inhibits activation of the tyrosine kinase enzymatic activity of EGFR, thus abrogating signal transduction pathways mediated by this receptor. A variety of preclinical studies have demonstrated that this antibody is effective at inhibiting the growth of a number of tumor xenografts in mouse models, including colon, skin, head and neck, lung, and pancreatic carcinomas.

A number of investigators have examined the activity of cetuximab on pancreatic cells in vitro and on pancreatic tumor xenografts in animal models.[48] Overholser et al.[48] found that treatment of the pancreatic cancer cell line BxPC-3 with 5 μg/cc of cetuximab could inhibit both EGF- and TGF-α–stimulated tyrosine phosphorylation of the EGF receptor. Furthermore, cetuximab inhibited DNA synthesis and colony formation in this cell line. The in vivo activity of cetuximab was also tested in nude mice with established BxPC-3 tumors. Cetuximab as a single agent showed promising cytostatic effects on the tumor xenografts, with a significant reduction in tumor volume at 10 weeks compared with the tumors in mice treated with vehicle alone. Additionally, the combination of cetuximab with 5-FU demonstrated enhanced antitumor activity compared with cetuximab alone, with actual tumor regressions (≥ 50% reduction in tumor volume) observed in 5 of 10 mice by 10 weeks. Histologic examination of cetuximab–treated tumors revealed significant necrosis, with decreased levels of tumor cell proliferation and increased tumor cell apoptosis.

Bruns et al.[49] confirmed the ability of cetuximab to inhibit EGFR autophosphorylation in the human pancreatic cancer cell line L3.6 pl. When these cells were established in the pancreas of nude mice, systemic therapy with either cetuximab alone or cetuximab in combination with gemcitabine led to a greater degree of tumor regression (median tumor volume reduction from 538 to 0.3 and 0 mm^3, respectively) than therapy with gemcitabine alone (median tumor volume 152 mm^3), including eradication of liver metastases.

Buchsbaum et al.[50] at the University of Alabama also demonstrated the potential benefit of adding cetuximab to other treatment modalities, including radiation, in a series of both in vitro and in vivo experiments. Two different pancreatic cancer cell lines, BxPC-3 and MiaPaCa-2, both expressing low levels of EGFR, were examined. As in the prior studies, cetuximab was shown to effectively inhibit EGF-induced tyrosine phosphorylation of the EGF receptor in both cell lines. However, although a 17% reduction in cell proliferation was noted in cetuximab–treated Bx-PC3 cells, no such reduction was observed in the similarly treated MiaPaCa-2 cell line. Treatment of both cell lines with various combinations of gemcitabine, 3 Gy of radiation, and cetuximab demonstrated that trimodality therapy produced rates of apoptosis and inhibition of cellular proliferation as high as, or higher than, any single- or dual-modality approach. However, when mice were implanted with either of these cell lines, only those harboring MiaPaCa-2 tumors demonstrated significant regression to cetuximab–based therapy, including 100% (eight of eight) complete responses to triple-modality therapy. None of the mice harboring BxPC-3 tumors, on the other hand, achieved similar dramatic complete regressions.

The explanation for these paradoxical findings remains uncertain, although they do reflect that much remains to be learned about how, if at all, cetuximab should be incorporated into therapy for pancreatic cancer. For example, the timing and schedule of administration of antibody relative to other modalities may be important considerations. For example, Huang et al.[51] showed that prolonged preincubation (6 weeks) with cetuximab led to a 42% down-regulation of EGFR expression in MiaPaCa-2 cells but no such down-regulation in BxPC-3 cells. This finding may at least partially be responsible for the increase in sensitivity of MiaPaCa-2 cells pretreated with cetuximab to subsequent gemcitabine and radiation treatment, whereas no such increase in sensitivity was seen in pretreated Bx-PC3 cells. Additionally, the possibility of parallel transactivating pathways that differ from one cell line to another may mediate sensitivity to cetuximab. There is evidence to suggest that the relative resistance of the Bx-PC3 cell line to combined-modality treatment may be due, at least in part, to transactivation of EGFR downstream signaling (i.e., Ras-MAP kinase) by other parallel pathways, such as fibroblast growth factor—rendering the inhibitory effects of cetuximab meaningless—a phenomenon that may not occur in other cell lines such as MiaPaCa-2.[51]

As described in the introductory section on EGFR signaling, activation of the signal transduction pathway leads to a complex cascade of events, and one of the pivotal questions regarding the use of cetuximab in pancreatic cancer is which downstream targets it may be affecting. Sclabas et al.[52] recently reported that blocking EGFR signaling in the human pancreatic cancer cell line MDA Panc-28 with cetuximab leads to a marked decrease in constitutive NF-κB binding activity, resulting in a decrease in the antiapoptotic gene bcl-xl. Thus, a primary mechanism by which this anti-EGFR antibody may be effecting its therapeutic activity is via targeting NF-κB pathway, which ultimately restores apoptosis in pancreatic cancer cells. Additionally, Bruns et al.[49] demonstrated in their orthotopic nude mouse model that cetuximab may also act via antiangiogenic mechanisms. These investigators showed that administration of cetuximab in these mice, either alone or in combination with gemcitabine, led to decreased production of both VEGF and interleukin-8, as well as decreased tumor microvessel density, compared with control mice or mice treated with gemcitabine alone.

The first clinical trial of cetuximab in pancreatic cancer was conducted by Abbruzzese et al.[53] at the M.D. Anderson Cancer Center. This was a phase II clinical trial testing the combination of gemcitabine and cetuximab in 41 patients, all of whom had advanced pancreatic cancer. Gemcitabine was administered weekly at 1,000 mg/m^2 per week, initially for 7 of 8 weeks and subsequently 3 of every 4 weeks if patients continued on study. Cetuximab was given at a loading dose of 400 mg/m^2, followed by weekly infusions of 250 mg/m^2. At the time of their presentation at the annual meeting of the American Society of Clinical Oncology in 2001, the investigators had observed an objective response in 5 of 41 patients after two courses of therapy (12%, all partial responses) and disease stabilization or minor responses in an additional 16 patients (39%). Median time to progression was 16 weeks. Mature survival data were not available at the time of the presentation. Dermatologic toxicity, fatigue, and fevers were the most common side effects seen, with acneiform rash and/or folliculitis occurring in greater than 50% of patients. Of interest, the investigators noted that 89% of patients screened for this study did test positive for EGFR expression.

At present, two cooperative group studies have been designed to study further the potential benefit that cetuximab may confer when given in combination with standard chemotherapy. A randomized phase II trial is being performed by the Eastern Cooperative Oncology Group, looking at the combination of docetaxel and irinotecan, with or without cetuximab, for patients with previously untreated advanced pancreatic cancer. Meanwhile, the Southwest Oncology Group has recently opened a phase III randomized study comparing gemcitabine plus cetuximab versus gemcitabine alone, also as first-line therapy for patients with advanced disease.

Trastuzumab (Herceptin) Trastuzumab, a recombinant humanized monoclonal antibody directed against the extracellular domain of the HER-2 (ErbB-2) receptor, has been approved for use in the treatment of HER-2/Neu-overexpressing metastatic breast cancer. Whether it may assume a role in the therapeutic armamentarium for pancreatic cancer remains to be seen. Specifically, the significance of the HER-2/Neu (c-erbB2) oncogene in pancreatic cancer has not yet been well established. A number of studies in the early- to mid-1990s examined c-erbB-2 expression in pancreatic cancer specimens, with rates of immunoreactivity ranging widely (7%–82%) depending on the specific antibody used.[54-60] Most recently, Novotny et al.[59] performed immunohistochemical analysis on 51 pancreatic adenocarcinomas and found that 10 samples (19.6%) showed overexpression of c-erbB-2. However, univariate analysis showed no correlation between overexpression of this oncogene with tumor size, grade, or stage at diagnosis; time from initial symptoms until diagnosis; or overall survival.

Similarly, Safran et al.[60] performed a retrospective analysis of 154 pancreatic cancer samples at Brown University for HER-2/Neu overexpression by immunohistochemistry. Staining was performed using the Dako HercepTest for p185^{HER2}. By definition, 2+ staining meant light to moderate staining encircling the cell membrane in greater than 10% of cells, whereas 3+ indicated moderate to intense staining encircling the cell membrane in greater than 10% of cells. This analysis found 23 cases with 2+ overexpression and an additional nine cases with 3+ overexpression, for a total of 32 of 154 samples (21%) that would be classified as having clear evidence of HER-2/Neu tumor overexpression.

Buchler et al.[61] from UCLA and Switzerland examined the effects of Trastuzumab on five different established pancreatic cancer cell lines (AsPC-1, Capan-1, HPAF-2, MiaPaCa-2, and PANC-1), each with different expression levels of HER-2 protein, as measured by both Western blotting and immunocytochemistry. Trastuzumab was added to cell monolayers at three different concentrations (1, 10, and 30 μg/ml) to determine effects on cell viability and growth. Inhibition of cell growth as measured by colorimetric assay was minimal after 24 hours in all cell lines but was more pronounced after 72 hours of antibody treatment. The greatest degree of growth suppression (approximately 15%) was observed in the MiaPaCa-2 cell line at the 30-μg/ml dose, correlating well with the high degree of HER-2 protein expression seen in this cell line. A dose-dependent effect of Trastuzumab was also seen, especially in the high-HER-2–expressing cell lines (MiaPaCa-2 and AsPC-1), in the soft agar assays examining the antibody's effects of anchorage-independent growth.

Two of these cell lines were then selected for orthotopic implantation into nude mice. After 7 weeks of tumor growth, Trastuzumab was given intraperitoneally 10 mg/kg three times a week. A statistically significant survival advantage was seen in the mice bearing xenograft tumors derived from the high-HER-2–expressing MiaPaCa-2 cell line treated with Trastuzumab compared with those treated with nonspecific IgG1 antibody. In contrast, the low-HER-2–expressing HPAF-2–bearing mice did not derive any noticeable survival advantage from treatment with Trastuzumab. In both mouse models, Trastuzumab treatment produced no significant difference in animal weight, ascites production, tumor volume, or number of metastatic lesions. No side effects were observed in the mice.

The first reported clinical study of Trastuzumab in patients with advanced pancreatic cancer was conducted by Safran et al.,[62] who performed a phase II study using gemcitabine in combination with Trastuzumab for patients with metastatic pancreatic cancer. Results were presented at the annual meeting of the American Society of Clinical Oncology in 2001. Patients were required to have documented tumor overexpression of HER-2/Neu (2+ or greater) by Dako immunohistochemistry and have measurable disease by radiographic criteria. The treatment strategy involved gemcitabine at a dose of 1,000 mg/m^2 weekly for 7 of 8 weeks and then 3 of every 4 weeks, with Trastuzumab given at a loading dose of 4 mg/kg during week 1 and 2 mg/kg weekly thereafter. Ten of the 21 patients (48%) had either radiographic or tumor marker evidence of response (decline in CA19-9 tumor marker by $>$ 50%). Median survival in this study was 7.5 months, with a 1-year survival rate of 24%. Marrow suppression and diarrhea were the main toxicities observed, although they were primarily less than or equal to grade 2; severe toxicities were far less common (16% rate of grade 3 or 4 neutropenia).

Bevacizumab (Arastin, rhuMAb VEGF) Although pancreatic cancer is not a grossly vascular tumor compared with some other tumor types, it does often contain foci of enhanced endothelial cell proliferation.[63] Moreover, several lines of data suggest that angiogenesis may be a critical aspect of pancreatic tumor development and growth: (1) Pancreatic cancer cell lines secrete VEGF-A, as well as express VEGFR-1 and VEGFR-2 and a variety of other proangiogenic factors.[64,65] (2) A positive correlation has been found between blood vessel density, tumor VEGF-A levels, and disease progression.[66-68] (3) Antiangiogenic therapies have proven effective in suppressing pancreatic tumor growth in mouse models, including TNP-470,[69] VEGF-A antisense molecule,[64] VEGF-A ribozyme,[70] and VEGFR-1– and VEGFR-2–containing adenoviral vectors.[71,72] These data are described in more detail elsewhere in this book.

At the 2003 annual meeting of the American Society of Clinical Oncology, Kindler et al.[73] presented results from their phase II study using a combination of gemcitabine and bevacizumab in the first-line treatment of advanced pancreatic cancer (gem 1,000 mg/m^2 days 1, 8, and 15 and bevacizumab 10 mg/kg days 1 and 15 of a 28-day cycle). Results have been encouraging, with the most recent update reporting a response rate of 21%, a time to disease progression of 5.8 months, and a 1-year survival rate of 37%[74] (compared with historical data using gemcitabine alone, or in combination with platinum agents: 1-year survival = 18%–36%). Treatment was overall very well tolerated. Because of these promising preliminary data, a larger multicenter study is currently in the planning stage through the Cancer and Leukemia Group B, with advanced pancreatic cancer patients randomized to receive either gemcitabine alone or gemcitabine in combination with bevacizumab.

Other Antibodies

The cancer-related cachexia so ubiquitous to pancreatic cancer patients is mediated in large part by the cytokine TNF-α. TNF-α is detectable in the serum in approximately one third of patients with advanced pancreatic cancer, and patients with detectable serum levels have a poorer nutritional status, reflected by significantly lower body weight and body mass index, lower hematocrit and hemoglobin values, and lower serum total protein and albumin levels compared with those with undetectable TNF-α levels.[75] Infliximab, a chimeric monoclonal IgG1 antibody directed against TNF-α (infliximab or Remicade), has been approved by the FDA for the treatment of rheumatoid arthritis and inflammatory bowel disease, but its role in improving cancer-related cachexia has yet to be firmly established. On this basis, an ongoing study is being conducted to determine the effects of this antibody on patients with pancreatic cancer-related cachexia.

A variety of other antibodies, directed against different tumor antigens of interest, have been or are currently being developed for study in pancreatic cancer. TAG-72, for instance, is a glycoprotein with high expression levels in pancreatic cancer,[76] and several radioimmunotherapy studies using an I-131–labeled antibody (originally termed B72.3 in its murine form, subsequently CC49 in its humanized version) against this antigen have been conducted in other solid tumor types, with disappointing results.[77-80] As a second example, chimeric monoclonal antibody directed against purified mucins of the human pancreatic cancer cell line SW1990,[81] termed c-Nd2, has been shown to be useful for radioimmunodetection when labeled with Indium-111 in patients with pancreatic cancer, with a diagnostic accuracy upward of 80%.[82] This antibody has also demonstrated ADCC both in vitro and in mouse models of pancreatic cancer,[83] suggesting its promise in the therapeutic realm, although no human clinical trials have been reported to date. Finally and most recently, selective, strong expression of the glycoprotein mesothelin was found in 16 of 18 primary human pancreatic cancer samples and appears to be a promising new target for directed therapy.[84] As a result, researchers have developed a recombinant immunotoxin, SS19(dsFv)PE38, consisting of the antimesothelin antibody (variable fragment) linked to a mutated Pseudomonas exotoxin.[85,86] The National Cancer Institute is now conducting a phase I study for patients with pancreatic and ovarian cancers, as well as mesotheliomas, using this immunotoxin.

Small Molecule Inhibitors

Introduction: Comparison to mAbs

As discussed previously, small molecule inhibitors are specifically designed to disrupt a particular signaling pathway, enzyme, or cellular component that plays some defined role in cell growth and tumorigenesis, taking advantage of molecular differences specific to tumor cells compared with normal cells. Although small molecule inhibitors may in some instances have the same primary target as monoclonal antibodies, such as disruption of signaling through EGFR, the activity profiles of these different classes of agents may be in fact quite dissimilar. Small molecule inhibitors, for instance, have the advantage of being more convenient for patients to receive (orally rather than intravenously) and are more rapidly distributed throughout the body than mAbs. On the other hand, small molecule inhibitors may be less specific for their target than mAbs and exhibit dose-limiting toxicities not generally seen with antibody therapy.[7] Most critically, tumors may be differentially responsive to one class of agents compared with another, even when they both are intended to disrupt the same signaling pathway. One novel strategy is to optimize the anti-tumor effects of these compounds by combining them. Preliminary in vitro data support this approach of combination treatment as a possible means to maximize antiproliferative activity.[87]

EGFR Inhibitors

PKI166 PKI166 (Novartis) is a selective oral tyrosine kinase inhibitor that inhibits the activity of both EGFR and the ErbB-2 receptor (HER-2/Neu).[88] This agent has been shown in a number of preclinical studies to have antitumor activity in pancreatic cancer cell lines and in xenografts implanted into nude mice, and it subsequently represented the first of this novel class of agents to be studied in the clinical arena as potential therapy for pancreatic cancer.[88-90] PKI166 appears to selectively inhibit EGFR tyrosine kinase by ATP-competitive inhibition, and proof of mechanism was established in a L3.6pl cell line, when incubation with PKI166 was shown to inhibit EGF-stimulated tyrosine phosphorylation of EGFR in a dose-dependent fashion.[88] PKI166 also enhanced the cytotoxicity mediated by gemcitabine in this same cell line.

Studies of PKI166 in murine tumor xenografts demonstrated promising activity, particularly in combination with gemcitabine.[88] Combined treatment of mice harboring L3.6pl pancreatic tumors with gemcitabine and PKI166 resulted in a decrease in pancreatic median tumor volume, a lower incidence of lymph node metastases, and a lower incidence of liver metastases compared with either agent alone. Median survival in mice treated with PKI166, either alone or in combination with gemcitabine, was greater than untreated mice or mice treated with gemcitabine alone. A dosing schedule of thrice-weekly oral administrations of PKI166 in combination with gemcitabine produced equivalent results as daily dosing, with less associated weight loss.[89]

Histologic and immunohistochemical analysis of the pancreata in PKI166-treated mice showed a significant reduction in tumor cell production of the proangiogenic molecules VEGF and interleukin-8, which in turn correlated with decreased microvessel density, increased apoptosis in tumor-associated endothelial cells, and decreased proliferating cell nuclear antigen (PCNA) staining.[90] Thus, part of the anti-tumor activity of this oral TK inhibitor appears to be via indirect antiangiogenic mechanisms.

Phase I and pharmacologic studies of PKI166 have now been performed in patients with advanced solid tumors. The maximum tolerated dose was either 750 mg orally once daily on a 2 week on/2 week off schedule[91] or

450 mg orally once daily with no treatment interruption.[92] The most common toxicities seen were skin rash, diarrhea, and elevated transaminases. In the U.S. trial, one partial response was seen in a patient with nonsmall lung cancer at the 450-mg/day dose level.[92] Two patients with advanced pancreatic cancer were included in this study at lower dose levels, neither of whom achieved partial response or disease stabilization.

Erlotinib (Tarceva, OSI-774) Erlotinib is another small molecule that inhibits the enzymatic activity of EGFR by binding to the ATP site of the tyrosine kinase region of the receptor.[93] Extensive preclinical studies have demonstrated the promise of this agent in many cancer subtypes, including pancreatic.[94] In vitro studies show that erlotinib inhibits the phosphorylation of the EGFR in a dose- and concentration-dependent manner, resulting in cell cycle arrest and induction of apoptosis, whereas tumor xenograft models confirm the potency of this agent, particularly when combined with conventional chemotherapy.[95]

Ng et al.[94] examined the effects of erlotinib alone and in combination with gemcitabine ± wortmannin (a PI-3Kinase inhibitor that promotes gemcitabine anti-tumor activity) in primary pancreatic xenografts implanted in severe combined immunodeficient (SCID) mice. Mice bearing tumors established from two pancreatic cancer patients (referred to as OCIP#2 and OCIP#7) were treated with various combinations of the previously mentioned three drugs. Their tumors were subsequently harvested and analyzed for phosphorylated and unphosphorylated EGFR, protein kinase B/Akt, and extracellular-regulated kinase (ERK1/2), the latter two molecules representing downstream targets of the EGFR signal transduction pathway. These investigators found that single-agent erlotinib significantly inhibited phosphorylation of EGFR in both tumor xenografts; however, phosphorylation of ERK was only decreased in one of two xenografts, and phosphorylation of protein kinase B (PKB) was decreased in neither. Hence, as the investigators note, it appears that the use of this inhibitor by itself cannot antagonize all of the potentially relevant pathways that mediate cell survival. However, intriguing possibilities lie in the combination of erlotinib with other antitumor agents: for example, erlotinib did increase the rate of apoptosis in both tumor xenografts when it was added to gemcitabine plus wortmannin, by approximately twofold.

Single-agent phase I studies and phase I studies in combination with chemotherapy have been performed that demonstrate the good safety profile of erlotinib, and they have shown that this agent can induce responses or prolonged periods of disease stabilization in a substantial number of patients with previously treated solid tumors. Hidalgo et al.[96] established 150 mg orally once daily, given in continuous uninterrupted fashion, as the recommended dose for disease-directed studies. Phase II and phase III studies have, at the time of this writing, either been completed or are ongoing in several tumor types.

A phase III trial was conducted by OSI Pharmaceuticals in collaboration with the National Cancer Institute of Canada Clinical Trials Group. This was an 800-patient randomized, controlled study assessing the use of erlotinib in combination with gemcitabine for untreated patients with advanced pancreatic cancer. An initial cohort was used to assess the safety of daily doses of erlotinib when combined with the approved dose and schedule of gemcitabine used in the treatment of pancreatic cancer. Results to date indicate the combination of 100 mg/day of erlotinib with gemcitabine 1,000 mg/m^2 weekly for 3 of 4 weeks, appears to be the appropriate dose for this patient population. Longer term follow-up of clinical efficacy has yet to be reported.

Other small molecule inhibitors of EGFR Gefitinib (Iressa, ZD1839) is another oral agent that, similar to Tarceva, blocks the tyrosine kinase activity of EGFR. Based on the results of a non-randomized phase II multicenter trial, this drug received FDA approval in 2003 as monotherapy treatment for patients with advanced non-small lung cancer in the third-line setting, after chemotherapy with both a platinum-based regimen and docetaxel. Large randomized studies adding gefitinib to chemotherapy in untreated patients with non-small lung cancer, however, failed to reveal any benefit. No studies have been published or reported to date examining gefitinib, either as monotherapy or in combination with other agents, in the treatment of pancreatic cancer.

Newer generations of anti-EGFR agents are also already in development, including those that irreversibly inhibit EGFR signaling and those that broadly inhibit all members of the erb-B receptor family. Phase I studies of these agents (CI-1033, EKB-569) have recently been completed.[97,98] Whether these compounds prove to have significantly better or different activity profiles compared with gefitinib or erlotinib, however, remains to be seen.

Other Oral Inhibitors

Exploiting the Ras-Raf-MAP kinase cascade Given that the overwhelming majority (90%) of pancreatic adenocarcinomas have activation of the K-ras oncogene,[99] targeting this protein and its effector molecules would appear to be a logical approach. The ras subfamily of GTP-binding proteins are membrane-bound molecules that transduce extracellular signals (including those of EGFR) and mediate a wide variety of cellular functions, including cell proliferation and survival (reviewed in Campbell et al.).[100] One of the posttranslational modifications necessary for localization of Ras to the plasma membrane is referred to as farnesylation because of the addition of a farnesyl group to the carboxy-terminal amino acids of the Ras protein. Inhibition of this step by drugs called farnesyl transferase inhibitors has been studied extensively in large randomized trials of pancreatic cancer, both as single agents and in combination with gemcitabine. However, efficacy appears to be limited.[101,102] The subject of farnesyl transferase inhibitors is covered in greater detail in other portions of this book.

One of the downstream targets of Ras is the family of mitogen-activated protein kinases (MAPKs), of which there are three main pathways: extracellular signal-regulated kinases (ERKs), c-Jun N-terminal kinases, and the p38 MAPKs.[103] The first of these, also termed the Raf/MEK/ERK pathway, has been an attractive target and is the furthest along in clinical development for possible therapeutic intervention. It is so called because membrane-bound Ras, in response to an extracellular signal, activates its primary mitogenic effector, the serine-threonine kinase Raf, with which it is bound. Activated Raf then phosphorylates another kinase called MAP kinase kinase (also referred to as MEK), which in turn activates ERK, also known as MAPK. This activated ERK protein can then translocate into the cell nucleus, where it has the ability to phosphorylate a number of transcription factors, leading to activation of gene expression and increased DNA synthesis and cell proliferation.

Although activation of the Raf-MEK-ERK signaling pathway represents one means by which cells undergo Ras-associated transformation, it is unclear the degree to which this represents the primary path mediating cell survival and proliferation in pancreatic cancer. Several studies have demonstrated that ERK1/2 plays an important role in controlling pancreatic cancer cell growth.[104-106] Others, on the other hand, have shown that despite oncogenic activation of K-ras and a corresponding increase in active Raf and MEK in pancreatic cancer cells, there was no corresponding increase in ERK1/2 activity.[107] Cross-talk between the ERK and P38 MAPK pathways may be one of the interactions required for pancreatic cancer proliferation.[108] Further evidence suggests that the c-Jun N-terminal kinase pathway may in fact be the more critical mediator of pancreatic cancer cell survival.[103]

Whether this suggests that the current generation of MAPK inhibitors are unlikely to show activity in pancreatic cancer remains uncertain. The three drugs at the forefront of clinical testing in solid tumors include ISIS 5132, a c-raf-1 antisense oligonucleotide; BAY 43-9006, an orally administered selective inhibitor of Raf-1; and CI-1040, an oral inhibitor of MEK. The first of these, ISIS 5132, is a phosphorothioate antisense oligodeoxynucleotide directed to the 3′ untranslated region of the c-raf-1 mRNA. Phase I clinical and pharmacokinetic studies using this compound in 31 patients with advanced solid tumors showed disease stabilization in 2 patients for greater than 7 months, with a corresponding decrease in c-raf-1 expression in PBMCs.[109,110] However, phase II studies using this antisense compound in hormone-refractory prostate, non-small cell lung, and colorectal cancer have produced disappointing results.[111-113]

Strumberg et al.[114] were the first to test the oral agent BAY 43-9006 in patients with advanced solid tumors, most of whom were heavily pretreated. Recently reported data from four separate phase I studies using a variety of dosing schedules showed that 38 of 115 patients receiving a dose of BAY 43-9006 of at least 200 mg orally twice a day achieved disease stabilization for more than 12 weeks, with 6 patients showing a minor or partial response.[115] Furthermore, proof of principle was established with evidence of inhibition of ERK1/2 in PBMCs at higher dose levels. Phase II studies using this agent are now ongoing.

CI-1040, meanwhile, has completed phase I testing in advanced solid tumors, with approximately 30% of patients demonstrating stable disease more than 12 weeks, and one patient with pancreatic cancer achieving a partial response lasting 6+ months.[116] Decreasing levels of phospho-MAPK in PBMCs were observed in a dose-dependent fashion.[117] Preliminary results of a phase II study using CI-1040 800 mg twice a day in patients with advanced non-small cell lung, breast, colon, and pancreatic cancers, however, failed to demonstrated significant anti-tumor activity.[118] Zero of 15 patients with previously untreated pancreatic cancer in this study had an objective response; one subject did show stable disease.

Proteasomal inhibitors Cellular proteins are tagged for degradation by undergoing a modification process called polyubiquitination. These ubiquitinated proteins enter a structure called the proteasome, which is present in high amounts in both the cytoplasm and nucleus of cells, where they subsequently undergo degradation through catalytic activities within the core of the proteasome. A number of proteasomal inhibitors are now being studied in malignant and inflammatory disorders based on the rationale that disruption of this ubiquitin–proteasomal pathway can alter cellular homeostatic mechanisms and ultimately result in cell death. Bortezomib (Velcade, PS-341) represents one such compound in this class of drugs, with high affinity, specificity, and selectivity for the catalytic activity of the proteasome. This agent has reversible activity and can prevent targeted proteolysis of a number of cellular proteins, including one called IκB, which binds to nuclear NF-κB and prevents NF-κB–mediated transcriptional activity. This drug has recently received approval in the treatment of refractory multiple myeloma based on phase II studies suggesting efficacy rates up to 35% in this patient population.

A number of preclinical studies suggest that this agent may have some applicability in the treatment of pancreatic cancer. PS-341 was found to induce apoptosis in several different pancreatic cancer cell lines in vitro and in tumor xenograft models and furthermore enhanced the cytotoxic effects of chemotherapy.[119-121] Different investigators have demonstrated that the potential effectiveness of PS-341 in pancreatic cancer may be mediated by decreased levels of the bcl-2 protein,[120] increased levels of the cyclin-dependent kinase inhibitor p21,[119] and reductions in tumor microvessel density and VEGF expression levels.[121] Based on these promising data, the North Central Cancer Treatment Group is currently conducting a randomized phase II study in chemotherapy-naïve patients with advanced pancreatic cancer looking at gemcitabine with or without bortezomib.

Future Possibilities: Looking Ahead

Although much of the focus of this chapter has been on agents that target the EGFR pathway because of the significant amount of clinical data already available on this subject, there are a number of other potential therapeutic targets that hold promise for success in the treatment of pancreatic cancer. For example, TGF-β signaling is known to be dysregulated in pancreatic tumorigenesis,[122] and exploitation of this pathway may prove to be fruitful in the rational design of new agents. Recently, Hedgehog, an important pathway regulating embryonic pancreatic development, has been identified as a key regulator in both the early and late stages of pancreatic cancer development;[123] this may represent yet another pathway amenable to targeted approaches when thinking about novel therapies specific for this disease in the future.

Although we are arriving at a greater understanding of the molecular basis of the development and maintenance of the pancreatic cancer phenotype, making the transition from identification of promising targets to the development of actual agents that can be used in the clinic and have a meaningful impact on patients remains a formidable challenge. We have learned important lessons from other targeted agents that have already been tested in clinical trials for pancreatic cancer patients, such as farnesyl transferase and matrix metalloproteinase inhibitors[101,102,124]—agents that appeared promising in preclinical testing and yet were met with disappointing results when tested in human subjects. Perhaps the greatest lesson lies in realizing the inherent problem of honing in on one target alone in a disease where multiple pathways are simultaneously involved in pathogenesis. In the future, combining two or more classes of compounds, including small molecule inhibitors, monoclonal antibodies, and standard chemotherapy—each targeting different aspects of pancreatic cancer development, growth, and spread—may lead to greater successes in the future for the treatment of this difficult disease.

References

1. Wells A. EGF receptor. *Int J Biochem Cell Biol.* 1999;31:637–643.
2. Ciardiello F, Tortora G. A novel approach in the treatment of cancer: targeting the epidermal growth factor receptor. *Clin Cancer Res.* 2001;7:2958–2970.
3. Yarden Y, Sliwkowski MX. Untangling the ErbB signalling network. *Nat Rev Mol Cell Biol.* 2001;2:127–137.
4. Olayioye MA, Neve RM, Lane HA, et al. The ErbB signaling network: receptor heterodimerization in development and cancer. *Embo J.* 2000;19:3159–3167.
5. Schlessinger J. Cell signaling by receptor tyrosine kinases. *Cell.* 2000;103:211–225.
6. Alroy I, Yarden Y. The ErbB signaling network in embryogenesis and oncogenesis: signal diversification through combinatorial ligand–receptor interactions. *FEBS Lett.* 1997;410:83–86.
7. Mendelsohn J, Baselga J. Status of epidermal growth factor receptor antagonists in the biology and treatment of cancer. *J Clin Oncol.* 2003;21:2787–2799.
8. Goldman CK, Kim J, Wong WL, et al. Epidermal growth factor stimulates vascular endothelial growth factor production by human malignant glioma cells: a model of glioblastoma multiforme pathophysiology. *Mol Biol Cell.* 1993;4:121–133.
9. Schreiber AB, Winkler ME, Derynck R. Transforming growth factor-alpha: a more potent angiogenic mediator than epidermal growth factor. *Science.* 1986;232:1250–1253.
10. Montz R, Klapdor R, Rothe B, et al. Immunoscintigraphy and radioimmunotherapy in patients with pancreatic carcinoma. *Nuklearmedizin.* 1986;25:239–244.
11. Aaronson SA. Growth factors and cancer. *Science.* 1991;254:1146–1153.
12. Grandis JR, Melhem MF, Gooding WE, et al. Levels of TGF-alpha and EGFR protein in head and neck squamous cell carcinoma and patient survival. *J Natl Cancer Inst.* 1998;90:824–832.

13. Porebska I, Harlozinska A, Bojarowski T. Expression of the tyrosine kinase activity growth factor receptors (EGFR, ERB B2, ERB B3) in colorectal adenocarcinomas and adenomas. *Tumour Biol.* 2000;21:105–115.
14. Woodburn JR. The epidermal growth factor receptor and its inhibition in cancer therapy. *Pharmacol Ther.* 1999;82: 241–250.
15. Salomon DS, Brandt R, Ciardiello F, et al. Epidermal growth factor-related peptides and their receptors in human malignancies. *Crit Rev Oncol Hematol.* 1995;19:183–232.
16. Nishikawa R, Ji XD, Harmon RC, et al. A mutant epidermal growth factor receptor common in human glioma confers enhanced tumorigenicity. *Proc Natl Acad Sci USA.* 1994;91:7727–7731.
17. Moscatello DK, Holgado-Madruga M, Godwin AK, et al. Frequent expression of a mutant epidermal growth factor receptor in multiple human tumors. *Cancer Res.* 1995; 55:5536–5539.
18. Moscatello DK, Holgado-Madruga M, Emlet DR, et al. Constitutive activation of phosphatidylinositol 3-kinase by a naturally occurring mutant epidermal growth factor receptor. *J Biol Chem.* 1998;273:200–206.
19. Murphy LO, Cluck MW, Lovas S, et al. Pancreatic cancer cells require an EGF receptor-mediated autocrine pathway for proliferation in serum-free conditions. *Br J Cancer.* 2001;84:926–935.
20. Barton CM, Hall PA, Hughes CM, et al. Transforming growth factor alpha and epidermal growth factor in human pancreatic cancer. *J Pathol.* 1991;163:111–116.
21. Yamanaka Y, Friess H, Kobrin MS, et al. Coexpression of epidermal growth factor receptor and ligands in human pancreatic cancer is associated with enhanced tumor aggressiveness. *Anticancer Res.* 1993;13:565–569.
22. Tobita K, Kijima H, Dowaki S, et al. Epidermal growth factor receptor expression in human pancreatic cancer: significance for liver metastasis. *Int J Mol Med.* 2003;11: 305–309.
23. Xiong HQ, Abbruzzese JL. Epidermal growth factor receptor-targeted therapy for pancreatic cancer. *Semin Oncol.* 2002;29:31–37.
24. Ciardiello F, Caputo R, Bianco R, et al. Antitumor effect and potentiation of cytotoxic drugs activity in human cancer cells by ZD-1839 (Iressa), an epidermal growth factor receptor-selective tyrosine kinase inhibitor. *Clin Cancer Res.* 2000;6:2053–2063.
25. Sirotnak FM, Zakowski MF, Miller VA, et al. Efficacy of cytotoxic agents against human tumor xenografts is markedly enhanced by coadministration of ZD1839 (Iressa), an inhibitor of EGFR tyrosine kinase. *Clin Cancer Res.* 2000;6:4885–4892.
26. Baselga J, Trigo J, Bourhis J, et al. Cetuximab (C225) plus cisplatin/carboplatin is active in patients with recurrent/metastatic squamous cell carcinoma of the head and neck progressing on a same dose and schedule platinum based agent. Orlando, FL: *Proceedings of the American Society of Clinical Oncology;* 2002;21:226a.
27. Saltz L, Rubin M, Hochster H, et al. Cetuximab (IMC-C225) plus irinotecan (CPT-11) is active in CPT-11-refractory colorectal cancer that expresses epidermal growth factor receptor. San Francisco: Proceedings of the American Society of Clinical Oncology; 2001;20:3a.
28. Perez-Soler R, Chachoua A, Huberman M, et al. A Phase II trial of the epidermal growth factor receptor (EGFR) tyrosine kinase inhibitor OSI-774, following platinum-based chemotherapy, in patients (pts) with advanced, EGFR-expressing, non-small cell lung cancer (NSCLC). San Francisco: Proceedings of the American Society of Clinical Oncology; 2001;20:310a.
29. Arteaga CL. Epidermal growth factor receptor dependence in human tumors: more than just expression? *Oncologist.* 2002;7(Suppl 4):31–39.
30. Maloney D. Monoclonal antibodies. In: Mendelsohn J, Howley P, Israel M, Liotta L, eds. *The Molecular Basis of Cancer* 2nd ed. Philadelphia: W.B. Saunders; 2001: 467–501.
31. Reff ME, Hariharan K, Braslawsky G. Future of monoclonal antibodies in the treatment of hematologic malignancies. *Cancer Control.* 2002;9:152–166.
32. Kim ES, Khuri FR, Herbst RS. Epidermal growth factor receptor biology (IMC-C225). *Curr Opin Oncol.* 2001;13: 506–513.
33. Bosslet K, Kern HF, Kanzy EJ, et al. A monoclonal antibody with binding and inhibiting activity towards human pancreatic carcinoma cells: I: immunohistological and immunochemical characterization of a murine monoclonal antibody selecting for well differentiated adenocarcinomas of the pancreas. *Cancer Immunol Immunother.* 1986;23:185–191.
34. Klapdor R, Lander S, Bahlo M, et al. Radioimmunotherapy of xenografts of human pancreatic carcinomas: intravenous and intratumoral application of 131I-labelled monoclonal antibodies. *Nuklearmedizin.* 1986;25:235–238.
35. Buchler M, Friess H, Malfertheiner P, et al. Studies of pancreatic cancer utilizing monoclonal antibodies. *Int J Pancreatol.* 1990;7:151–157.
36. Schulz G, Buchler M, Muhrer KH, et al. Immunotherapy of pancreatic cancer with monoclonal antibody BW 494. *Int J Cancer Suppl.* 1988;2:89–94.
37. Buchler M, Kubel R, Malfertheiner P, et al. Immunotherapy of advanced pancreatic carcinoma with the monoclonal antibody BW 494. *Dtsch Med Wochenschr.* 1988;113: 374–380.
38. Buchler M, Friess H, Schultheiss KH, et al. A randomized controlled trial of adjuvant immunotherapy (murine monoclonal antibody 494/32) in resectable pancreatic cancer. *Cancer.* 1991;68:1507–1512.
39. Koprowski H, Steplewski Z, Mitchell K, et al. Colorectal carcinoma antigens detected by hybridoma antibodies. *Somatic Cell Genet.* 1979;5:957–971.
40. Shen JW, Atkinson B, Koprowski H, et al. Binding of murine immunoglobulin to human tissues after immunotherapy with anticolorectal carcinoma monoclonal antibody. *Int J Cancer.* 1984;33:465–468.
41. Ernst CS, Sears HF, Herlyn M, et al. Detection of murine immunoglobulin in human tissues following therapeutic infusion of monoclonal antibody. *Hybridoma.* 1986;5 (Suppl 1):S79–S86.

42. Gottlinger HG, Funke I, Johnson JP, et al. The epithelial cell surface antigen 17-1A, a target for antibody-mediated tumor therapy: its biochemical nature, tissue distribution and recognition by different monoclonal antibodies. *Int J Cancer.* 1986;38:47–53.
43. Tempero MA, Haga Y, Sivinski C, et al. Immunotherapy with monoclonal antibody (Mab) in pancreatic adenocarcinoma. *Int J Pancreatol.* 1991;9:125–134.
44. Adams DO, Hall T, Steplewski Z, et al. Tumors undergoing rejection induced by monoclonal antibodies of the IgG2a isotype contain increased numbers of macrophages activated for a distinctive form of antibody-dependent cytolysis. *Proc Natl Acad Sci USA.* 1984;81:3506–3510.
45. Sindelar WF, Maher MM, Herlyn D, et al. Trial of therapy with monoclonal antibody 17-1A in pancreatic carcinoma: preliminary results. *Hybridoma.* 1986;5(Suppl 1):S125–132.
46. Weiner LM, Harvey E, Padavic-Shaller K, et al. Phase II multicenter evaluation of prolonged murine monoclonal antibody 17-1A therapy in pancreatic carcinoma. *J Immunother.* 1993;13:110–116.
47. Tempero MA, Sivinski C, Steplewski Z, et al. Phase II trial of interferon gamma and monoclonal antibody 17-1A in pancreatic cancer: biologic and clinical effects. *J Clin Oncol.* 1990;8:2019–2026.
48. Overholser JP, Prewett MC, Hooper AT, et al. Epidermal growth factor receptor blockade by antibody IMC-C225 inhibits growth of a human pancreatic carcinoma xenograft in nude mice. *Cancer.* 2000;89:74–82.
49. Bruns CJ, Harbison MT, Davis DW, et al. Epidermal growth factor receptor blockade with C225 plus gemcitabine results in regression of human pancreatic carcinoma growing orthotopically in nude mice by antiangiogenic mechanisms. *Clin Cancer Res.* 2000;6:1936–1948.
50. Buchsbaum DJ, Bonner JA, Grizzle WE, et al. Treatment of pancreatic cancer xenografts with Erbitux (IMC-C225) anti-EGFR antibody, gemcitabine, and radiation. *Int J Radiat Oncol Biol Phys.* 2002;54:1180–1193.
51. Huang ZQ, Buchsbaum DJ, Raisch KP, et al. Differential responses by pancreatic carcinoma cell lines to prolonged exposure to Erbitux (IMC-C225) anti-EGFR antibody. *J Surg Res.* 2003;111:274–283.
52. Sclabas GM, Fujioka S, Schmidt C, et al. Restoring apoptosis in pancreatic cancer cells by targeting the nuclear factor-kappaB signaling pathway with the anti-epidermal growth factor antibody IMC-C225. *J Gastrointest Surg.* 2003;7:37–43; discussion 43.
53. Abbruzzese J, Rosenberg A, Xiong Q, et al. Phase II study of anti-epidermal growth factor receptor (EGFR) antibody cetuximab (IMC-C225) in combination with gemcitabine in patients with advanced pancreatic cancer. San Francisco: Proceedings of the American Society of Clinical Oncology; 2001;20:130a.
54. Hall PA, Hughes CM, Staddon SL, et al. The c-erb B-2 proto-oncogene in human pancreatic cancer. *J Pathol.* 1990;161:195–200.
55. Satoh K, Sasano H, Shimosegawa T, et al. An immunohistochemical study of the c-erbB-2 oncogene product in intraductal mucin-hypersecreting neoplasms and in ductal cell carcinomas of the pancreas. *Cancer.* 1993;72:51–56.
56. Yamanaka Y, Friess H, Kobrin MS, et al. Overexpression of HER2/Neu oncogene in human pancreatic carcinoma. *Hum Pathol.* 1993;24:1127–1134.
57. Lei S, Appert HE, Nakata B, et al. Overexpression of HER2/Neu oncogene in pancreatic cancer correlates with shortened survival. *Int J Pancreatol.* 1995;17:15–21.
58. Day JD, Digiuseppe JA, Yeo C, et al. Immunohistochemical evaluation of HER-2/Neu expression in pancreatic adenocarcinoma and pancreatic intraepithelial neoplasms. *Hum Pathol.* 1996;27:119–124.
59. Novotny J, Petruzelka L, Vedralova J, et al. Prognostic significance of c-erbB-2 gene expression in pancreatic cancer patients. *Neoplasma.* 2001;48:188–191.
60. Safran H, Steinhoff M, Mangray S, et al. Overexpression of the HER-2/neu oncogene in pancreatic adenocarcinoma. *Am J Clin Oncol.* 2001;24:496–499.
61. Buchler P, Reber HA, Buchler MC, et al. Therapy for pancreatic cancer with a recombinant humanized anti-HER2 antibody (herceptin). *J Gastrointest Surg.* 2001;5:139–146.
62. Safran H, Ramanathan R, Schwartz J, et al. Herceptin and gemcitabine for metastatic pancreatic cancers that overexpress HER-2/neu. San Francisco: Proceedings of the American Society of Clinical Oncology; 2001;20:130a.
63. Korc M. Pathways for aberrant angiogenesis in pancreatic cancer. *Mol Cancer.* 2003;2:8.
64. Luo J, Guo P, Matsuda K, et al. Pancreatic cancer cell-derived vascular endothelial growth factor is biologically active in vitro and enhances tumorigenicity in vivo. *Int J Cancer.* 2001;92:361–369.
65. Itakura J, Ishiwata T, Shen B, et al. Concomitant overexpression of vascular endothelial growth factor and its receptors in pancreatic cancer. *Int J Cancer.* 2000;85:27–34.
66. Ikeda N, Adachi M, Taki T, et al. Prognostic significance of angiogenesis in human pancreatic cancer. *Br J Cancer.* 1999;79:1553–1563.
67. Itakura J, Ishiwata T, Friess H, et al. Enhanced expression of vascular endothelial growth factor in human pancreatic cancer correlates with local disease progression. *Clin Cancer Res.* 1997;3:1309–1316.
68. Seo Y, Baba H, Fukuda T, et al. High expression of vascular endothelial growth factor is associated with liver metastasis and a poor prognosis for patients with ductal pancreatic adenocarcinoma. *Cancer.* 2000;88:2239–2245.
69. Hotz HG, Reber HA, Hotz B, et al. Angiogenesis inhibitor TNP-470 reduces human pancreatic cancer growth. *J Gastrointest Surg.* 2001;5:131–138.
70. Tokunaga T, Abe Y, Tsuchida T, et al. Ribozyme mediated cleavage of cell-associated isoform of vascular endothelial growth factor inhibits liver metastasis of a pancreatic cancer cell line. *Int J Oncol.* 2002;21:1027–1032.
71. Hoshida T, Sunamura M, Duda DG, et al. Gene therapy for pancreatic cancer using an adenovirus vector encoding soluble flt-1 vascular endothelial growth factor receptor. *Pancreas.* 2002;25:111–121.
72. Ogawa T, Takayama K, Takakura N, et al. Anti-tumor angiogenesis therapy using soluble receptors: enhanced inhibition of tumor growth when soluble fibroblast growth factor receptor-1 is used with soluble vascular endothelial growth factor receptor. *Cancer Gene Ther.* 2002;9:633–640.

73. Kindler HL, Ansari R, Lester E, et al. Bevacizumab plus gemcitabine in patients with advanced pancreatic cancer. Chicago: Proceedings of the American Society of Clinical Oncology; 2003;22:259.
74. Kindler HL, Friberg G, Stadler WM, et al. Bevacizumab plus gemcitabine is an active combination in patients with advanced pancreatic cancer: interim results of an ongoing phase II trial from the University of Chicago Phase II Consortium. San Francisco: 2004 Gastrointestinal Cancers Symposium, 2004;x:84.
75. Karayiannakis AJ, Syrigos KN, Polychronidis A, et al. Serum levels of tumor necrosis factor-alpha and nutritional status in pancreatic cancer patients. *Anticancer Res.* 2001;21:1355–1358.
76. Tempero M, Takasaki H, Uchida E, et al. Co-expression of CA 19-9, DU-PAN-2, CA 125, and TAG-72 in pancreatic adenocarcinoma. *Am J Surg Pathol.* 1989;(13 Suppl 1):89–95.
77. Divgi CR, Scott AM, Gulec S, et al. Pilot radioimmunotherapy trial with 131I-labeled murine monoclonal antibody CC49 and deoxyspergualin in metastatic colon carcinoma. *Clin Cancer Res.* 1995;1:1503–1510.
78. Murray JL, Macey DJ, Kasi LP, et al. Phase II radioimmunotherapy trial with 131I-CC49 in colorectal cancer. *Cancer.* 1994;73:1057–1066.
79. Tempero M, Leichner P, Dalrymple G, et al. High-dose therapy with iodine-131-labeled monoclonal antibody CC49 in patients with gastrointestinal cancers: a phase I trial. *J Clin Oncol.* 1997;15:1518–1528.
80. Meredith RF, Bueschen AJ, Khazaeli MB, et al. Treatment of metastatic prostate carcinoma with radiolabeled antibody CC49. *J Nucl Med.* 1994;35:1017–1022.
81. Hirayama K, Chung YS, Sawada T, et al. Characterization and biodistribution of a mouse/human chimeric antibody directed against pancreatic cancer mucin. *Cancer.* 1995; 75:1545–1553.
82. Sawada T, Nishihara T, Yamamoto A, et al. Preoperative clinical radioimmunodetection of pancreatic cancer by 111 In-labeled chimeric monoclonal antibody Nd2. *Jpn J Cancer Res.* 1999;90:1179–1186.
83. Nishihara T, Sawada T, Yamamoto A, et al. Antibody-dependent cytotoxicity mediated by chimeric monoclonal antibody Nd2 and experimental immunotherapy for pancreatic cancer. *Jpn J Cancer Res.* 2000;91:817–824.
84. Hassan R, Laszik Z, Lerner MR, et al. Mesothelin, a cell surface glycoprotein, as a target for tumor specific therapy of pancreatic cancer. Chicago: Proceedings of the American Society of Clinical Oncology; 2003;22:283.
85. Chowdhury PS, Chang K, Pastan I. Isolation of anti-mesothelin antibodies from a phage display library. *Mol Immunol.* 1997;34:9–20.
86. Chowdhury PS, Pastan I. Improving antibody affinity by mimicking somatic hypermutation in vitro. *Nat Biotechnol.* 1999;17:568–572.
87. Bos M, Mendelsohn J, Kim YM, et al. PD153035, a tyrosine kinase inhibitor, prevents epidermal growth factor receptor activation and inhibits growth of cancer cells in a receptor number-dependent manner. *Clin Cancer Res.* 1997;3:2099–2106.
88. Bruns CJ, Solorzano CC, Harbison MT, et al. Blockade of the epidermal growth factor receptor signaling by a novel tyrosine kinase inhibitor leads to apoptosis of endothelial cells and therapy of human pancreatic carcinoma. *Cancer Res.* 2000;60:2926–2935.
89. Solorzano CC, Baker CH, Tsan R, et al. Optimization for the blockade of epidermal growth factor receptor signaling for therapy of human pancreatic carcinoma. *Clin Cancer Res.* 2001;7:2563–2572.
90. Baker CH, Solorzano CC, Fidler IJ. Blockade of vascular endothelial growth factor receptor and epidermal growth factor receptor signaling for therapy of metastatic human pancreatic cancer. *Cancer Res.* 2002;62:1996–2003.
91. Hoekstra R, Dumez H, van Oosterom A, et al. A phase I and pharmacological study of PKI166, an epidermal growth factor receptor tyrosine kinase inhibitor, administered orally in a two weeks on, two weeks off scheme to patients with advanced cancer. Orlando, FL: Proceedings of the American Society of Clinical Oncology; 2002;21:86a.
92. Murren J, Papadimitrakopoulou V, Sizer K, et al. A phase I, dose-escalating study to evaluate the biological activity and pharmacokinetics of PKI166, a novel tyrosine kinase inhibitor, in patients with advanced cancers. Orlando, FL: Proceedings of the American Society of Clinical Oncology; 2002;21:95a.
93. Kim TE, Murren JR. Erlotinib OSI/Roche/Genentech. *Curr Opin Investig Drugs.* 2002;3:1385–1395.
94. Ng SS, Tsao MS, Nicklee T, et al. Effects of the epidermal growth factor receptor inhibitor OSI-774, Tarceva, on downstream signaling pathways and apoptosis in human pancreatic adenocarcinoma. *Mol Cancer Ther.* 2002;1: 777–783.
95. Grunwald V, Hidalgo M. Development of the epidermal growth factor receptor inhibitor OSI-774. *Semin Oncol.* 2003;30:23–31.
96. Hidalgo M, Siu LL, Nemunaitis J, et al. Phase I and pharmacologic study of OSI-774, an epidermal growth factor receptor tyrosine kinase inhibitor, in patients with advanced solid malignancies. *J Clin Oncol.* 2001;19: 3267–3279.
97. Rinehart J, Wilding G, Willson JK, et al. A phase I clinical and pharmacokinetic/food study of oral CI-1033, a pan-erb B tyrosine kinase inhibitor, in patients with advanced solid tumors. Chicago: Proceedings of the American Society of Clinical Oncology; 2003;22:205.
98. Hidalgo M, Erlichman C, Rowinsky E, et al. Phase I trial of EKB-569, an irreversible inhibitor of the epidermal growth factor receptor, in patients with advanced solid tumors. Orlando, FL: Proceedings of the American Society of Clinical Oncology; 2002;21:17a.
99. Almoguera C, Shibata D, Forrester K, et al. Most human carcinomas of the exocrine pancreas contain mutant c-K-ras genes. *Cell.* 1988;53:549–554.
100. Campbell SL, Khosravi-Far R, Rossman KL, et al. Increasing complexity of Ras signaling. *Oncogene.* 1998;17:1395–1413.
101. Bramhall SR, Rosemurgy A, Brown PD, et al. Marimastat as first-line therapy for patients with unresectable pancreatic cancer: a randomized trial. *J Clin Oncol.* 2001;19:3447–3455.

102. Bramhall SR, Schulz J, Nemunaitis J, et al. A double-blind placebo-controlled, randomised study comparing gemcitabine and marimastat with gemcitabine and placebo as first line therapy in patients with advanced pancreatic cancer. *Br J Cancer.* 2002;87:161–167.
103. Hirano T, Shino Y, Saito T, et al. Dominant negative MEKK1 inhibits survival of pancreatic cancer cells. *Oncogene.* 2002;21:5923–5928.
104. Ehlers RA, Zhang Y, Hellmich MR, et al. Neurotensin-mediated activation of MAPK pathways and AP-1 binding in the human pancreatic cancer cell line, MIA PaCa-2. *Biochem Biophys Res Commun.* 2000;269:704–708.
105. Douziech N, Calvo E, Laine J, et al. Activation of MAP kinases in growth responsive pancreatic cancer cells. *Cell Signal.* 1999;11:591–602.
106. Douziech N, Lajas A, Coulombe Z, et al. Growth effects of regulatory peptides and intracellular signaling routes in human pancreatic cancer cell lines. *Endocrine.* 1998;9:171–183.
107. Yip-Schneider MT, Lin A, Barnard D, et al. Lack of elevated MAP kinase (Erk) activity in pancreatic carcinomas despite oncogenic K-ras expression. *Int J Oncol.* 1999;15:271–279.
108. Ding XZ, Adrian TE. MEK/ERK-mediated proliferation is negatively regulated by P38 map kinase in the human pancreatic cancer cell line, PANC-1. *Biochem Biophys Res Commun.* 2001;282:447–453.
109. O'Dwyer PJ, Stevenson JP, Gallagher M, et al. c-raf-1 depletion and tumor responses in patients treated with the c-raf-1 antisense oligodeoxynucleotide ISIS 5132 (CGP 69846A). *Clin Cancer Res.* 1999;5:3977–3982.
110. Stevenson JP, Yao KS, Gallagher M, et al. Phase I clinical/pharmacokinetic and pharmacodynamic trial of the c-raf-1 antisense oligonucleotide ISIS 5132 (CGP 69846A). *J Clin Oncol.* 1999;17:2227–2236.
111. Tolcher AW, Reyno L, Venner PM, et al. A randomized phase II and pharmacokinetic study of the antisense oligonucleotides ISIS 3521 and ISIS 5132 in patients with hormone-refractory prostate cancer. *Clin Cancer Res.* 2002;8:2530–2535.
112. Cripps MC, Figueredo AT, Oza AM, et al. Phase II randomized study of ISIS 3521 and ISIS 5132 in patients with locally advanced or metastatic colorectal cancer: a National Cancer Institute of Canada clinical trials group study. *Clin Cancer Res.* 2002;8:2188–2192.
113. Coudert B, Anthoney A, Fiedler W, et al. Phase II trial with ISIS 5132 in patients with small-cell (SCLC) and non-small cell (NSCLC) lung cancer: a European Organization for Research and Treatment of Cancer (EORTC) Early Clinical Studies Group report. *Eur J Cancer.* 2001;37: 2194–2198.
114. Strumberg D, Schuehly U, Moeller JG, et al. Phase I clinical, pharmacokinetic and pharmacodynamic study of the Raf kinase inhibitor BAY 43-9006 in patients with locally advanced or metastatic cancer. San Francisco: Proceedings of the American Society of Clinical Oncology; 2001;20:83a.
115. Strumberg D, Awada A, Piccart M, et al. Final report of the phase I clinical program of the novel raf kinase inhibitor BAY 43-9006 in patients with refractory solid tumors. San Francisco: Proceedings of the American Society of Clinical Oncology; 2001;22:203.
116. LoRusso P, Adjei A, Meyer M, et al. A phase I clinical and pharmacokinetic evaluation of the oral MEK inhibitor, CI-1040, administered for 21 consecutive days, repeated every 4 weeks in patients with advanced cancer. Orlando, FL: Proceedings of the American Society of Clinical Oncology; 2002;21:81a.
117. Mitchell D, Reid J, Parchment R, et al. Pharmacokinetics and pharmacodynamics of the oral MEK inhibitor, CI-1040, following multiple dose administration to patients with advanced cancer. Orlando, FL: Proceedings of the American Society of Clinical Oncology; 2002.
118. Waterhouse D, Rinehwart J, Adjei A, et al. A phase 2 study of an oral MEK inhibitor, CI-1040, in patients with advanced nonsmall-cell lung, breast, colon, or pancreatic cancer. Chicago: Proceedings of the American Society of Clinical Oncology; 2003;22:204.
119. Shah SA, Potter MW, McDade TP, et al. 26S proteasome inhibition induces apoptosis and limits growth of human pancreatic cancer. *J Cell Biochem.* 2001;82:110–122.
120. Bold RJ, Virudachalam S, McConkey DJ. Chemosensitization of pancreatic cancer by inhibition of the 26S proteasome. *J Surg Res.* 2001;100:11–17.
121. Nawrocki ST, Bruns CJ, Harbison MT, et al. Effects of the proteasome inhibitor PS-341 on apoptosis and angiogenesis in orthotopic human pancreatic tumor xenografts. *Mol Cancer Ther.* 2002;1:1243–1253.
122. Friess H, Berberat P, Schilling M, et al. Pancreatic cancer: the potential clinical relevance of alterations in growth factors and their receptors. *J Mol Med.* 1996;74:35–42.
123. Thayer SP, Di Magliano MP, Heiser PW, et al. Hedgehog is an early and late mediator of pancreatic cancer tumorigenesis. *Nature.* 2003;425:851–856.
124. Cohen SJ, Ho L, Ranganathan S, et al. Phase II and pharmacodynamic study of the farnesyltransferase inhibitor R115777 as initial therapy in patients with metastatic pancreatic adenocarcinoma. *J Clin Oncol.* 2003;21:1301–1306.

CHAPTER 40

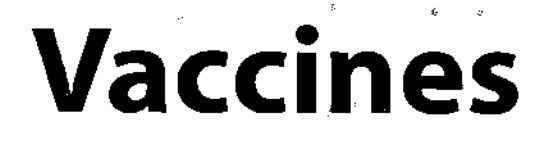

Vaccines

Daniel A. Laheru, MD
Elizabeth M. Jaffee, MD

Vaccines have the potential to provide non–cross-resistant mechanisms of anti-tumor activity that can be integrated with surgery, radiation therapy, and chemotherapy. A major advantage of immune-based therapies is their ability to specifically target the transformed tumor cell relative to the normal cell of origin. Less severe nonspecific toxicities are therefore expected than occur with other cancer treatment modalities. It has been more than 100 years since the first reported attempts to activate a patient's immune system to eradicate cancer. Although numerous subsequent vaccine studies demonstrated clinically significant treatment effects, active immunotherapy has not yet become an established cancer treatment modality. However, numerous advances have allowed the design of more specific cancer vaccine approaches: sequencing of the human genome, gene microarray technology, and a greater understanding into the mechanisms of T-cell regulation. These advances have resulted in improved systemic anti-tumor immune responses in animal models. Many of these vaccine approaches have been developed for clinical testing. They range from whole tumor cell to antigen-targeted recombinant viral vaccines that enhance tumor-specific antibody and cellular responses. A few pancreatic cancer–associated antigens have been identified as candidate targets of both antibody and cellular responses, particularly T-cell responses. Currently, vaccine approaches either target a small group of candidate antigens expressed by the tumor or rely on whole tumor cells as the source of immunogens. However, with the recent sequencing of the human genome and the development of rapid methods for identifying genes that are differentially expressed by tumor cells, many more candidate immune targets are expected to be identified. These antigens may serve as immunogens for pancreatic cancer treatment as well as prevention. Finally, recent insights into overcoming immune tolerance to cancer has led to the development of integrated vaccine and immune modulating therapies that are undergoing initial testing in the clinics. This chapter reviews the important features of an effective anti-tumor immune response, discusses the results of some of the more promising strategies that are currently in clinical development, and speculates on what can be expected in the near future.

Features of the Immune System that Are Required for Effective Immunity Against Cancer

The immune system comprises a number of cell types which, when activated, are extremely efficient at recognizing and killing their target (Fig. 40.1). In particular,

B cells and T cells each possess vast arrays of clonally distributed antigen receptors that enable them to recognize foreign antigens and to discriminate self from non-self. In fact, it has been estimated that both T and B cells can express more than a million different antigen-specific receptors through recombination of the genes encoding for their receptor at the time of maturation in the thymus and bone marrow, respectively. Therefore, the immune system has an unlimited capability to recognize antigenic differences between normal and malignant cells, whether they are in the form of the product of a new genetic alteration, a reactivated embryonic gene, or an overexpressed gene. Other cell types that are likely involved in immune recognition of cancer include professional antigen-presenting cells (APCs), particularly dendritic cells, macrophages, and natural killer cells. This complex network of cellular interactions is depicted in Fig. 40.1.

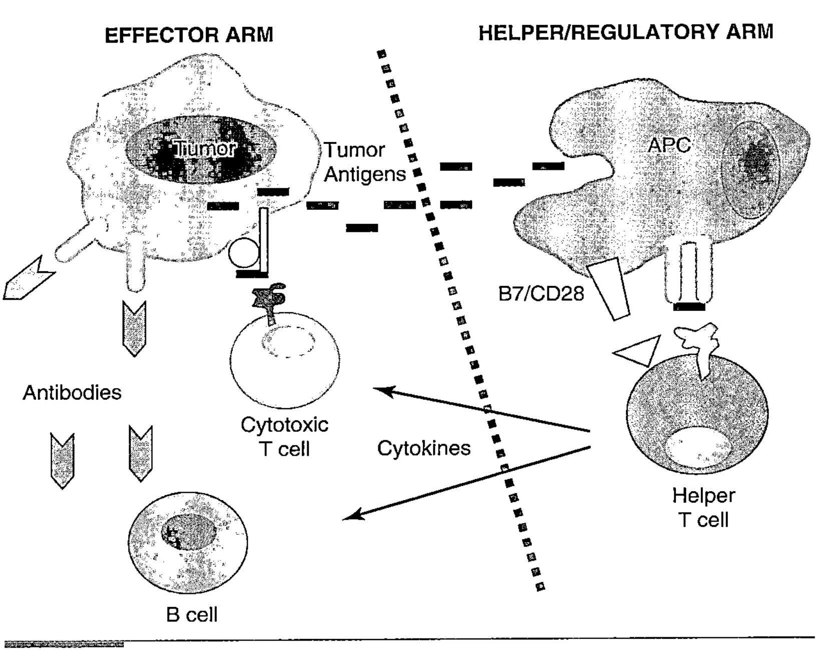

Figure 40.1
Two components of an effective anti-tumor immune response. Effective vaccines must initially prime the helper/regulatory arm of the immune response (composed of professional antigen-presenting cells [APCs] and CD4+ T cells) before the effector arm (B cells and CD8+ T cells) can be activated.

The B-cell receptor is a surface immunoglobulin with the ability to bind antigens that are intact soluble molecules or whole proteins expressed on a cell surface. Therefore, special antigen processing is not required for B-cell receptor or soluble antibody binding to its antigen. In contrast, the T-cell receptor (TCR) recognizes fragments of the antigenic protein bound to human leukocyte antigen (HLA) class I and II molecules on another cell. This peptide-HLA complex is formed as a result of fragmentation of proteins within specialized cellular compartments and subsequent association with a binding site on the HLA molecule (Fig. 40.2).

Two forms of T-cell antigen processing exist.[1-5] Professional APCs (macrophages, B cells, and dendritic cells) have the ability to capture extracellular proteins that are released by the tumor through secretion, shedding, or tumor lysis. These proteins are subsequently internalized via endocytosis and are processed through the exogenous pathway. These proteins are taken up into low-pH vesicles (the lysosomal compartment), where they undergo fragmentation. Peptide fragments (10–25 amino acids in length) then bind to the HLA class II protein before expression of the complex on the cell surface. This complex is recognized exclusively by CD4+ helper T cells in the context of engagement of a second co-stimulatory or regulatory molecule and its ligand, including the B7 and tumor necrosis factor family of immune regulatory molecules (Fig. 40.3).[6-8] In the presence of both types of signals, activated CD4+ T cells can amplify the CD8+ T-cell response (also referred to as cytotoxic T lymphocytes [CTLs] because they have the ability to lyse tumor). In addition, memory CD4+ T cells are generated and play the key role in the maintenance of protective immunity.

In contrast, pancreatic tumor cells cannot process and present antigen through the exogenous pathway, because they usually do not derive from professional APCs. However, all cells, including tumor cells, have the ability to process and present antigens that derive from cellular proteins through the endogenous pathway.[1,4,8,9] Any protein within a tumor cell can gain access to the cytosol and undergo enzymatic degradation into 8–10 amino acid fragments by proteasomes. The peptide fragments are subsequently transported into the endoplasmic reticulum via the transporter of antigen processing (TAP), where they bind to HLA class I molecules and are transported to the cell surface for recognition by CD8+ T cells. CD8+ T cells exclusively recognize antigen in this way. In general, CD4+ T cells provide helper or regulatory function, whereas CD8+ T cells carry out direct tumor lysis (Fig. 40.1). A few candidate pancreatic antigens recognized by B and T cells have already been identified and fall into several categories, including reactivated embryonic genes (carcinoembryonic anti-

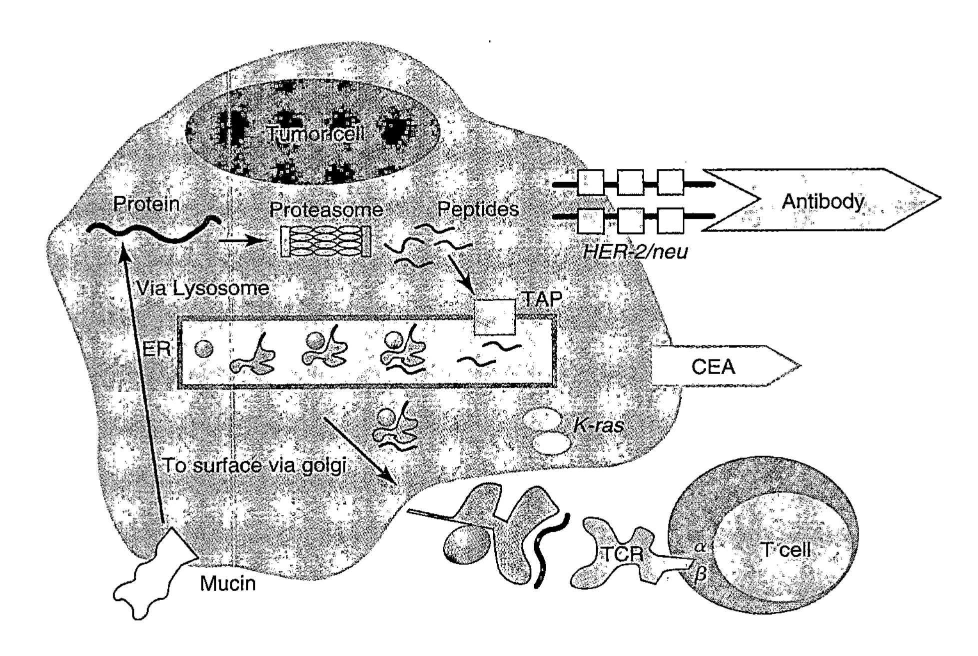

Figure 40.2
Vaccines have specificity and unlimited recognition capacity. Any protein within a tumor cell (nuclear, cytoplasmic, or cell surface) can gain access to the cytosol and be processed and presented on human leukocyte antigen (HLA) I molecules to T cells. Surface molecules can also be recognized by secreted antibodies.

gen), mutated oncogenes/suppressor genes (*KRAS2* and *TP53*), altered mucins (MUC1), and overexpressed tissue-specific genes (*Her2/neu*). We have recently identified a new candidate T-cell target, mesothelin, which is overexpressed by most pancreatic cancers.[10]

Tumors Use Multiple Mechanisms to Evade Immune Recognition

Despite these unique features of the immune system that make it possible to recognize self from non-self, it has long been recognized that human cancers are, in general, poorly immunogenic. For cancers to proliferate, tumor cells must develop local and systemic mechanisms that allow them to escape immune recognition.[11] Local mechanisms include loss of tumor antigen expression, down-regulation of HLA class I expression (the surface molecules that present tumor antigens to T cells), secretion of factors that inhibit immune function (e.g., tumor growth factor beta [TGF-β], and changes in tumor vasculature that impede immune access. Systemic mechanisms include lack of co-stimulatory factors (usually provided by professional APCs) available for facilitating immune priming and induction of regulatory factors that suppress tumor-specific immune cell activation, augmentation, and survival. Dissection of the complex mechanisms involved in immune tolerance to tumors is ongoing in preclinical models and in patients.[12-16] For immune-based therapies to be successful at treating pancreatic cancer,

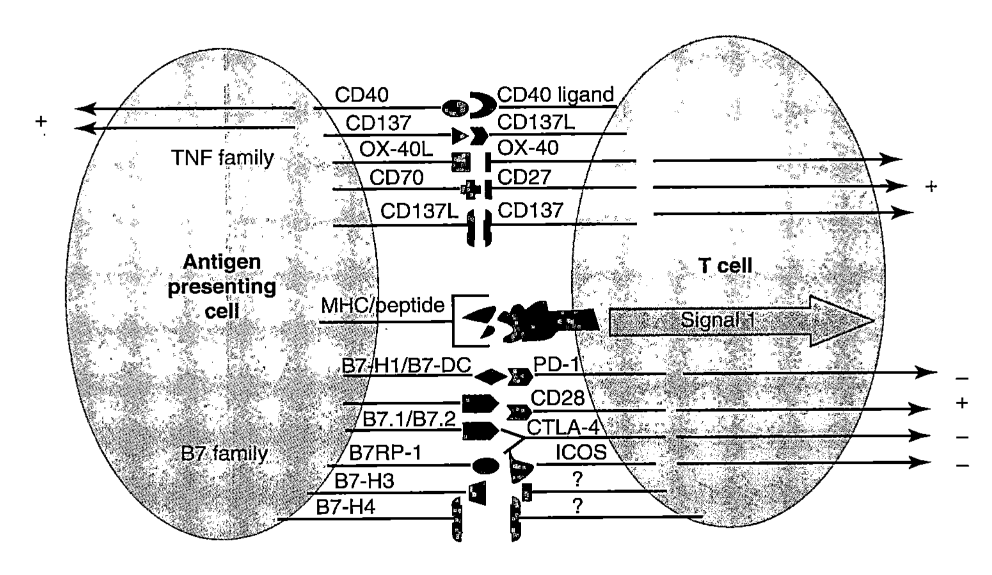

Figure 40.3
T-cell activation requires modulation of the B7 and tumor necrosis factor (TNF) family of immune regulatory molecules. A growing number of co-stimulatory and down-regulatory molecules and their ligands have been identified on T cells and professional antigen-presenting cells (APCs). Agonist and antagonist antibodies can be used to modulate these molecules to produce more effective T-cell activation and longevity.

Table 40.1 Observed Mechanisms of Immune Evasion

Local Mechanisms	Systemic Mechanisms
Lack of co-stimulation 1. B7 and TNF family of molecules 2. Adhesion molecules: ICAM	Alterations in TCR signaling 1. Down-modulation of TCR-ζ chain 2. Down-modulation of NFκ-B
Down-regulation and/or genetic loss 1. HLA class I molecules 2. β2-microglobulin 3. TAP transporter molecules	Cancer cachexia due to secretion of immunosuppressive cytokines 1. TGF-β 2. IL-10 3. IL-1 4. IL-6
Dysregulation of death signals	Loss of co-stimulation 1. B7 and TNF family of molecules 2. Adhesion molecules: ICAM
Tumor secretion of suppressive cytokines 1. TGF-β1 and TGF-β2 2. IL-10	Induction of T-regulatory cells

Abbreviations: TNF, tumor necrosis factor; HLA, human leukocyte antigen; ICAM, intracellular adhesion molecule; TAP, transporter of antigen processing; TCR, T-cell receptor; TGF, tumor growth factor; IL, interleukin.

they must incorporate strategies that can bypass these mechanisms of immune evasion. Recognized features of these local and systemic mechanisms by which tumors evade immune recognition are described in the following sections and are listed in Table 40.1.

Local Processes

It is clear that the tumor and its microenvironment play a critical role in immune evasion. In the local tumor environment, loss of appropriate signaling may occur by down-regulation of HLA class I molecules through processes such as loss of expression of HLA class I alleles and β2-microglobulin and down-regulation of TAP, which transports antigenic peptides to the site in the cell, where they bind to newly synthesized HLA molecules for presentation to T cells.[11] Such alterations within the tumor cell are not uncommon because tumors have unstable genomes. The instability of the genome is also responsible for the frequently described loss of tumor antigen expression. In addition to the loss of appropriate antigen recognition molecules on the tumor cell, alterations can occur at the level of the TCR on the T cell's surface. The TCR is noncovalently associated with an array of largely intracytoplasmic subunits that form the CD3 complex and are responsible for converting TCR-antigen/major histocompatibility complex/co-stimulatory signal recognition to downstream signal transduction pathways, such as upregulation of interleukin (IL)-2, that ultimately lead to T-cell activation and amplification.[17-20] Expression of the TCR-ζ chain, which is the large intracytoplasmic homodimer associated with the CD3 complex, is selectively reduced in patients with pancreatic adenocarcinoma and other solid tumors.[21,22] Although the precise mechanism is unknown, TCR-ζ down-regulation is thought to occur through caspase-3–mediated apoptosis.[23,24] The loss of expression has been demonstrated not only in peripheral blood but also in the T cells infiltrating delayed-type hypersensitivity (DTH) sites of autologous tumor after vaccination with antigen.[16,21] Functionally, the loss of TCR-ζ chain expression is manifested by decreases in the production of both interferon gamma and IL-4, two cytokines associated with immune activation. However, increases in TCR-ζ expression with parallel increases in both interferon gamma and IL-4 can occur in response to tumor-targeted vaccination.[21]

Although the TCR-antigen/HLA/co-stimulatory molecule interaction is critical for effective activation of CTL against tumor antigen, effective CTL activation is not sufficient for tumor response, because tumor cells have evolved other local mechanisms of immune escape. For example, most pancreatic adenocarcinoma tumor cell lines are resistant to Fas-mediated apoptosis, presumably through overexpression of protein tyrosine phosphatase FAP-1.[22] In addition, pancreatic adenocarcinoma cell lines kill activated CTLs by the mechanism of Fas ligand–induced apoptosis.[25-28] Additional local mechanisms of immune escape occur, including tumor cell secretion of immunosuppressive cytokines, such as TGF-β1, TGF-β2, and IL-10, which can further limit host defenses by interfering with the production of inflammatory cytokines and/or the recruitment of APCs to the tumor microenvironment.[29-32]

Systemic Processes

Efficient immune priming against tumor cells is dependent on TCR recognition of specific peptide fragments derived from the tumor cell in the context of the appropriate HLA class I molecule and co-stimulatory molecules. The context in which the antigen is presented to the T cell appears to determine whether the T cell subsequently becomes activated. In the absence of the appropriate co-stimulatory signals, engagement of the TCR can lead to ignorance, anergy, or even apoptotic T-cell death.[33-35] The list of molecules involved in the immune regulation of T cell responses is expanding rapidly (Fig. 40.3).

Even in the presence of appropriate co-stimulatory signals, systemic mechanisms are in place to actively regulate all types of antigen-specific immune responses, including tumor-specific immune responses. In fact, some chemotherapeutic agents (cyclophosphamide and some of the alkylating agents) can enhance immune-based therapies when given in sequence with them.[36-38] It was not until recently that studies have been able to provide a mechanism for this observation. It is now clear that tumors induce a regulatory T-cell response (previously called suppressor T cells) that secrete cytokines, including IL-10, that turn off activated T cells and may induce T-cell apoptosis. The induction of these regulatory cells appears to be tumor antigen specific, although these T cells function in an antigen-unrestricted manner.[39] The induction of these regulatory T cells is likely a natural mechanism by which the host immune system provides checks and balances to control all types of immune responses. This response is one of many natural mechanisms of regulation that need to be temporarily overcome to effectively induce systemic immune responses to pancreatic cancer (Fig. 40.4).

It has been extremely difficult to identify other systemic causes of immune escape because the processes involved are invariably multifactorial. However, the syndrome of cancer cachexia (see Chapter 35) is thought to play a significant role in systemic immune suppression associated with pancreatic adenocarcinoma. Most patients with pancreatic cancer have the characteristics of this syndrome, including weight loss through depletion of adipose tissue and skeletal muscle mass, as well as the development of secondary states of immune deficiency, as manifested by suppressed DTH responses to common antigens.[40,41] Cytokines that have been implicated in the production of cachexia are known immunosuppressive cytokines, including IL-1, IL-6, IL-10, and TGF-β, whereas others are thought to be proinflammatory, such as tumor necrosis factor-α and interferon gamma.[42] Therefore, the precise interplay between these known inhibitory and proinflammatory cytokines and the mechanisms by which these effects lead to immune suppression remain unknown.

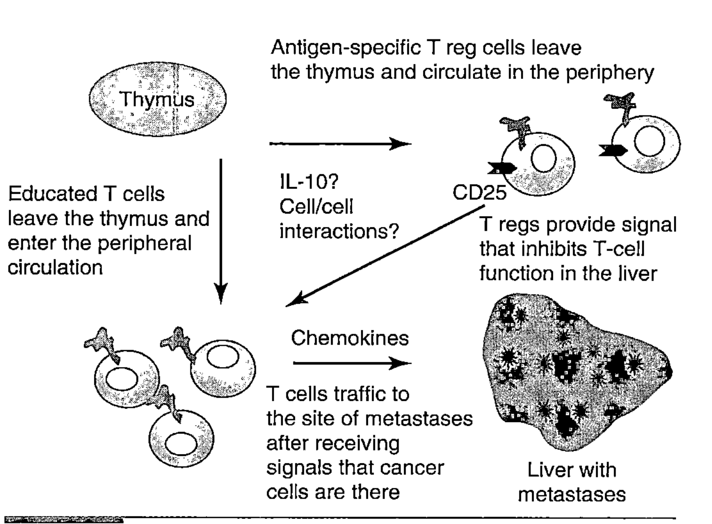

Figure 40.4
T regulatory cells are a recognized mechanism of immune tolerance that must be bypassed to achieve effective immunization. T-regulatory cells are typically CD4+CD25+ T cells that are selected in the thymus and released into the peripheral circulation, where they naturally prevent unchecked T-cell responses. They also prevent effective immunization against cancer antigens. Agents are available to selectively deplete these T cells before immunization.

Vaccines in Practice

The goal of cancer vaccine therapy is to recruit and activate tumor-specific T cells that have the ability to directly lyse a tumor cell or, in some cases, activate B cells that secrete antibodies that assist in lysing the tumor cell. Vaccines have at least four advantages over other cancer modalities. First, tumor-specific T cells act via a mechanism that is distinct from chemotherapy or radiation therapy and represent a non–cross-resistant treatment with an entirely different spectrum of toxicities. Second, the immune system is capable of recognizing a broad diversity of potential antigens while orchestrating selective as well as specific cytotoxic responses. This feature may be essential in recognizing and eliminating a heterogenous tumor population while avoiding normal tissue toxicity. Third, vaccine approaches can also generate antigen-specific memory T-cell responses that are capable of being reactivated if tumor cells expressing the same antigen profile recur. Fourth, the induction of cellular immune responses has the added benefit of allowing natural access to the microenvironment of the tumor.

Preclinical animal models assessing vaccine potency have been able to eliminate small burdens of established tumors, a situation that corresponds to the state of minimal residual disease commonly found after resection of human tumors.[33] Translation of these vaccine approaches into therapies for patients with pancreatic cancers are in early phases of clinical development.[43-45] Examples of the different vaccine approaches that are currently undergoing clinical testing are discussed in the following sections.

Peptide- and Protein-Based Vaccines

Although significant progress has been made in our understanding of the biology of pancreatic cancer at the genetic level, specific pancreatic tumor antigens that can serve as rejection targets have not yet been identified. However, point mutations in various oncogenes (*KRAS2*) or tumor-suppressor genes (*TP53*, *p16*, *DPC4*, *BRCA2*, *Her2/neu*) have been associated with different histologically defined precursor lesions (see Chapter 3)[46-48] and are being studied as candidate immune targets. Mutated *KRAS2* is one example of an attractive immune target because it is mutated in >90% of pancreatic adenocarcinomas.[49-52] The *ras p21* proto-oncogenes, including *KRAS2*, *N-ras*, and *H-ras*, encode proteins that are important for regulating cellular events, including growth and differentiation. Point mutations at codons 12, 13, and 61 have been identified in many cancers, including pancreatic adenocarcinoma.[46,51-52] These mutations encode distinct proteins that are potential immunogens. The major advantage of a protein- or peptide-based vaccine is the ability to deliver high doses of the potential immunogen safely and at a relatively modest cost. However, vaccine approaches that employ peptides and proteins have several limitations. First, the vaccine approaches that will be most successful at optimally priming with the peptide and/or protein have not yet been determined. Second, proteins that are identified as a candidate-immunogen based on the criteria that they are overexpressed in pancreatic adenocarcinoma may turn out not to be the most relevant target of the immune response. Third, the most successful vaccine approaches will likely require targeting multiple tumor antigens because antigen loss variants are one mechanism by which cancers escape immune recognition.[11]

Mutated *KRAS2*–based vaccines have been the most extensively studied peptide/protein–based vaccine approach in patients with pancreatic adenocarcinoma. In preclinical models, vaccination with mutant *KRAS2* peptides induces both major histocompatibility complex class I– and II–restricted T-cell responses. *KRAS2*–specific T-cell responses have also been elicited in patients treated with vaccines that consist of *KRAS2* peptides that contain a point mutation at codon 12.[52-53] In one study, 12 patients with advanced disease whose tumors expressed *KRAS2* mutations at codon 12 were treated with subcutaneous injections of a 13-amino-acid peptide vaccine at various doses (100–1500 μg) once a week for 4 weeks. The vaccine resulted in local skin reactions but was otherwise safe. Postvaccination $CD4^+$ and/or HLA-A2–restricted $CD8^+$ CTL responses were identified in 3/8 evaluable patients.[54] In the second study, an additional 19 patients with metastatic disease whose tumors also expressed *KRAS2* mutations at codon 12 were co-administered the 13-amino-acid peptide vaccine subcutaneously once a week for 4 weeks with either recombinant granulocyte macrophage colony stimulating factor (GM-CSF) or IL-2. The vaccine was well tolerated when administered with either cytokine. Stable disease was noted in 3/9 patients who received peptide + IL-2 and in 2/10 patients who received peptide + GM-CSF.[55] In the final study, patients with either resected (10 patients) or advanced pancreatic adenocarcinoma (38 patients) were intradermally administered a 17-amino-acid peptide containing either the specific *KRAS2* codon 12 mutation (resected disease) or a mixture of four *KRAS2* peptides containing the four most common mutations (advanced disease). Human GM-CSF (40 μg) was administered intradermally 15 minutes before peptide vaccination. Patients were vaccinated weekly for 4 weeks and were given booster injections at weeks 6 and 10. Peptide vaccination was well tolerated in all 48 patients. Of the 48 vaccinated patients, 43 were evaluable for induction of immune response. A positive DTH (measured as >5-mm induration 48 hours after vaccination) was observed in 21/43 patients. In addition, the peptide vaccine elicited a positive mutated *KRAS2*–specific proliferative T-cell response in the peripheral blood of 17/43 evaluable patients. The mean survival of patients after resection was 25.6 months. In the group with advanced disease, stable disease was present in 11/34 evaluable patients. An immune response (defined as either a positive DTH or a proliferative T-cell response) was observed in 20 of the 34 treated patients, including all 11 patients demonstrating stable disease. The median survival in the group who demonstrated an immune response was 148 days, versus 61 days in the group that did not demonstrate an immune response ($P = 0.0002$).[56] This and other vaccines under clinical development are listed in Table 40.2.

Heat shock proteins (HSPs) are ubiquitous and highly conserved cellular proteins that are up-regulated during cell stress. They are thought to bind to cellular proteins that become damaged when a cell experiences stress, thereby facilitating the protein's refolding to an active conformation. In the nonstressed environment, HSPs are thought to have multiple functions, including helping newly synthesized polypeptides fold, assisting in protein transport, and associating with peptides generated during protein degradation. They are also thought to stimulate macrophage and dendritic cell activation and assist in representation of peptides. Preclinical studies have shown that HSPs isolated from tumor cells can serve as potent vaccines by taking advantage of their role as a peptide transporter and as a stimulator of APCs.[57,58] This approach has recently been tested in patients with resected pancreatic adenocarcinoma from whom HSPs could be obtained and purified. Eligible patients were administered 5 mg of protein (HSP-96) subcutaneously weekly for 4 weeks. The vaccine was well tolerated. In addition, an increase in postvaccination $CD8^+$ T cells specific for autologous tumor was measured by Enzyme-Linked-Immunospot (ELISPOT) in one patient.[59] A follow-up clinical trial using this approach is currently under investigation (Table 40.2).

Table 40.2 Comparison of Results of Pancreatic Cancer Vaccine Clinical Trials

Approach	Stage	Results	Reference
MUC1 (105 amino acids, 5 repetitions)	NS	Phase I: 24 patients received 100μg of peptide with BCG given every 3 weeks for 3 total injections. 1 patient with stable disease.	Goydos et al, *J Surg Res.* 1996;63:298–304.
Recombinant vaccinia-CEA (rV-CEA) and avipox-CEA in a prime boost approach	IV	Phase I: 18 patients (1 patient with pancreatic carcinoma). Patients received either 1 dose of rV-CEA followed by 3 weekly doses of avipox-CEA or 3 weekly doses of avipox-CEA followed by 1 dose of rV-CEA. CEA-specific T-cell responses were seen in 6/6 HLA-A2$^+$ patients receiving the rV-CEA followed by the avipox-CEA vaccine.	Marshall et al, *J Clin Oncol.* 2000;18 :3964–3973.
Canarypox virus/CEA/B7.1	IV	Phase I: 18 patients with advanced adenocarcinoma including pancreatic adenocarcinoma, received intramuscular injections of 4.5×10^6 up to 4.5×10^8 PFUs every 4 weeks for 3 months. Stable disease was associated with increased T-cell responses in 3 patients. All doses were well tolerated.	Horig et al, *Ca Immunol Immunother.* 2000;49: 504–514.
MUC1 mixed with SB-AS2 adjuvant	I, II, III	Phase I: patients received MUC1 vaccine admixed with SB-AS2 adjuvant. Induced an HLA-A2–restricted T-cell response in 1 patient.	Ramanathan et al, *Proc ASCO.* 2000;19:1791.
KRAS2 peptide (17 amino acid) administered with GM-CSF	I, II, III, IV	Phase II: 10 patients with resected disease and 38 patients with advanced disease, DTH response to peptide or T-cell proliferation associated with stable disease in 11/43 evaluable patients. Mean survival of resected patients was 25.6 months.	Gjertsen et al, *Int J Cancer.* 2001;92:441–450.
GM-CSF whole tumor cell	I, II, III	Phase I: 14 patients received 10^7, 5×10^7, 10^8, or 5×10^8 vaccine cells sequenced with adjuvant chemotherapy. DTH responses to autologous tumor correlated with vaccine dose and disease-free survival in 3/14 patients.	Jaffee et al, *J Clin Oncol.* 2001;19:145–156.
Heat shock protein vaccine	I, II, III	Pilot study: patients with resected disease received 5 mg of HSP-96 subcutaneously, weekly for 4 weeks. Well tolerated. Postvaccination CD8$^+$ T-cell response in 1 patient.	*Antigenics Biodrugs.* 2002;16:72–74.
G17DT, an immunoconjugate, amino terminal of gastrin-17 conjugated to diphtheria toxoid	IV I, II, III	Phase II: 30 patients, given 3 doses of 100 or 250 μg of G17DT on weeks 0, 2, and 6. 20 patients produced an antibody response with a significant survival difference (217 vs 121 days, $P = 0.0023$) for antibody responders. These responses were seen with 250-μg dose.	Brett et al, *J Clin Oncol.* 2002;20:4225-4231.

Abbreviations: NS, not specified; BCG, bacille Calmette-Guérin; CEA, carcinoembryonic antigen; DC, dendritic cell; DTH, delayed-type hypersensitivity; HSP, heat shock protein; mRNA, messenger RNA; PFU, plaque-forming unit; MUC1, mucin-1; GM-CSF, granulocyte macrophage colony stimulating factor; DTH, delayed-type hypersensitivity; EGF-R, epidermal growth factor receptor; Ca, cancer.

Continued

Table 40.2 Comparison of Results of Pancreatic Cancer Vaccine Clinical Trials—*Continued*

Approach	Stage	Results	Reference
CEA pulsed autologous DC	I, II, III	Pilot study, 3 patients received autologous, monocyte-derived DCs loaded with mRNA encoding CEA monthly for 6 months. Injection site reactions were observed without other toxicity.	Morse et al, *Int J Gastrointest Cancer.* 2002;32:1–6.
GM-CSF whole tumor cell	IV IV	Phase II: 60-patient study	Jaffee et al, In progress
GM-CSF whole tumor cell		Phase II: 20-patient study	Jaffee et al, In progress
Mesothelin-specific immunotoxin		Phase I: patients with mesothelioma, ovarian Ca, and pancreatic Ca	In progress

Glycoproteins as Antigens

Mucin-1 (MUC1) is a glycosylated transmembrane protein that is uniquely characterized by an extracellular domain that consists of a variable number of tandem repeats of 20 amino acids rich in proline, serine, and threonine residues. Although normally present lining ductal epithelial surfaces, including the gastrointestinal tract, MUC1 is overexpressed on the cell surface of many cancers, including pancreatic adenocarcinoma.[60,61] There is also evidence to suggest that MUC1 protein expression is associated with an increased risk of metastasis and poor prognosis.[62] Data from animal and phase I clinical studies have demonstrated that HLA-unrestricted T cells isolated from patients with MUC1-expressing tumors can recognize these exposed epitopes and can induce MUC1-specific DTH responses.[63] More recently, immunization with MUC1 peptide has been shown to induce an HLA-A2–restricted T-cell response[64] (Table 40.2).

Carcinoembryonic antigen (CEA) is another glycoprotein that is overexpressed in pancreatic cancers. Although it is known to be a member of the immunoglobulin supergene family, the exact function of CEA is unclear.[65,66] A CEA-vaccine approach has been tested in 18 patients with CEA-expressing advanced tumors, including one patient with pancreatic adenocarcinoma.[67] A recombinant vaccinia virus containing the CEA gene (*rV-CEA*) was generated because the vaccinia virus is capable of infecting APCs and could therefore potentially present CEA to both $CD4^+$ and $CD8^+$ T cells. In addition, a second recombinant anti-CEA vaccine, avipox-CEA (ALVAC) was generated. The avipox virus is similar to the vaccinia virus but is not capable of infecting mammalian cells and would therefore pose a decreased risk for a systemic infection. Furthermore, because patients have not had prior exposure to avipox viruses (in contrast to vaccinia viruses, which were used to eradicate smallpox), prior viral vector immunity capable of eliminating the vaccine before it has time to induce anti-tumor immunity would be less likely. Patients were assigned to one of two cohorts. The first cohort received one subcutaneous vaccination of *rV-CEA* followed by three vaccinations of ALVAC at 4-week intervals. The second cohort received vaccinations 4 weeks apart in the reverse sequence. In addition, 9/18 patients who had no evidence of disease progression after the first series of vaccinations went on to receive two additional vaccinations with ALVAC + 100 μg of GM-CSF followed by ALVAC + GM-CSF + IL-2. The vaccine in both sequences was well tolerated, with only mild skin reactions noted. No objective responses were observed in either sequence. However, CEA-specific T-cell responses measured by ELISPOT occurred in 6/6 HLA-$A2^+$ patients receiving the *rV-CEA* vaccine followed by the ALVAC. In contrast, CEA-specific T-cell responses occurred in only 2/5 patients who received the ALVAC vaccine before the *rV-CEA* vaccine. Subsequent vaccinations when co-administered with GM-CSF continued to demonstrate an increase in CEA-specific T-cell responses. A second CEA vaccine study using this same approach combined with GM-CSF is ongoing (Table 40.2).

Whole Tumor Cell Vaccines

The major limitation of defined antigen-based vaccines is the lack of identified pancreatic tumor antigens that are the known targets of the immune response. Until a panel of pancreatic tumor-specific antigens are discovered, the whole tumor cell represents the best source of immunogens.

A whole tumor cell vaccine approach involves the use of autologous or allogeneic tumor cells to stimulate an immune response. However, studies aimed at dissecting anti-tumor immune responses have confirmed that most tumors are not naturally immunogenic.[68] Evidence from preclinical models suggests that the failure of the immune system to reject spontaneously arising tumors is unrelated to the absence of sufficiently immunogenic tumor antigens. Instead, the problem is derived from the immune system's inability to appropriately respond to these antigens.[33] The importance of the local release of stimulatory cytokines to provide an immunologic boost and attract other immune cells has been extensively examined. These findings have led to the concept that a tumor cell can become more immunogenic if it is engineered to secrete immune-activating cytokines.

Tumor cells genetically modified to secrete immune-activating cytokines have been extensively studied for their ability to induce systemic anti-tumor immune responses.[69] Preclinical studies have shown that these vaccines can induce immune responses potent enough to cure mice of pre-established tumor.[33] In one comparison study of 10 cytokines, GM-CSF was the most potent, generating systemic immunity that was dependent on both $CD4^+$ and $CD8^+$ T cells.[70] GM-CSF is involved in the recruitment and differentiation of bone marrow–derived dendritic cells, and dendritic cells are known to be the most efficient APCs at activating T cells.[70,71] In addition, GM-CSF is produced by activated $CD4^+$ T helper cells, further supporting the concept that this cytokine may function by priming immune effector cells.[69,71,72] Studies aimed at optimizing this cytokine-secreting tumor vaccine approach confirmed that GM-CSF secretion must be at the site of relevant tumor antigen. Simple injection of soluble GM-CSF along with the appropriate tumor cells does not provide sustained local levels required to provide a sufficient immunologic boost.[73] This information suggested that the mere presence of GM-CSF was not sufficient. Rather, the sustained release and the duration of GM-CSF secretion appeared to be critical for priming the immune response. Furthermore, high levels must be sustained for several days. In the preclinical data, it appeared that a minimum of 35 ng/10^6 cells/24 hours is necessary to generate effective anti-tumor immunity.[33]

A GM-CSF–secreting tumor vaccine was first tested in patients with renal cell carcinoma. Lethally irradiated autologous renal cell carcinoma cells transduced with the GM-CSF gene were prepared and tested in a phase I trial of patients with metastatic renal cell carcinoma. Although the maximally tolerated dose as well as the dose of maximal bioactivity could not be determined because of technical difficulty of expanding each patient's tumor cells beyond 4×10^7 cells, a dose of 4×10^7 cells resulted in postvaccination DTH responses against autologous tumor cells that were similar to those measured in mouse studies testing this vaccine approach. Other immune parameters, including histologic evaluation of the vaccine biopsy and DTH sites, revealed similar immune infiltrates when compared with preclinical models. The vaccine was well tolerated at all vaccine doses tested. The most common side effects were local induration and erythema at the vaccine site.[74] A similar spectrum of toxicities were subsequently observed in autologous prostate and melanoma studies and in allogeneic pancreatic and prostate vaccine studies.[75,76]

Although the use of autologous tumor cells may preserve unique antigens expressed by each patient's cancer, the development of an autologous vaccine requires that extensive processing, in vitro expansion, and regulatory testing be performed for each individual patient vaccine. In the case of metastatic disease, the development of autologous tumor vaccine would also require the ability to obtain adequate tissue. These limitations preclude the use of autologous cellular vaccines for most cancers, including pancreatic adenocarcinoma. Recent data support the immunologic rationale for using allogeneic cells as the source of immunogen. First, studies evaluating human melanoma antigens have demonstrated that most antigens identified so far are shared among at least 50% of other patient melanomas, regardless of whether they have the same HLA type. In addition, there are data to support the hypothesis that the professional APCs that present immunogen to specific T cells in the context of HLA are host derived. Therefore, the vaccine cells do not need to be HLA compatible with the host's immune system as long as they can release cellular proteins (the tumor antigens) for uptake by the professional APCs (macrophages and dendritic cells) that are attracted to the vaccine site by GM-CSF. Tumor antigens are taken up by the APC's exogenous processing pathway. However, these antigens also gain access to the cytosol for processing onto HLA class I through the recently defined cross-priming mechanism.[33,69] Taken together, the data suggest that relevant tumor antigens can be delivered by an allogeneic tumor and still sufficiently mount an effective $CD4^+$ and $CD8^+$ T-cell response against a tumor.

The results of a phase I study using irradiated allogeneic pancreatic tumor cell lines transfected with GM-CSF as adjuvant treatment administered in sequence with adjuvant chemoradiation in patients with resected adenocarcinoma of the pancreas was recently reported.[77] Fourteen patients with stage 2 or 3 disease received an initial vaccination 8 weeks after pancreaticoduodenectomy. This was a dose escalation study in which three patients each received 1×10^7, 5×10^7, and 1×10^8 cells.

An additional five patients received 5×10^8 vaccine cells. Study patients were jointly enrolled in an adjuvant chemoradiation protocol for 6 months. After the completion of adjuvant chemoradiation, patients were reassessed, and those who were still in remission were treated with three additional vaccinations given 1 month apart at the same dose that they received for the first vaccination. This was the first GM-CSF–secreting vaccine study to escalate the vaccine dose to 5×10^8 GM-CSF–secreting cells. However, toxicities remained mostly limited to grade I/II local reactions at the vaccine site. In addition, there were self-limited systemic rashes, including one documented case of Grover's syndrome.[78] Systemic GM-CSF levels were evaluated as an indirect measure of the longevity of vaccine cells at the immunizing site. This pancreatic vaccine study is the first GM-CSF vaccine clinical trial to measure low but detectable serum GM-CSF levels in patients. As was observed in preclinical studies,[33,70] GM-CSF levels peaked at 48 hours after vaccination. In addition, serum GM-CSF levels could be detected for up to 96 hours after vaccination. These data, together with data from preclinical models, would suggest that detectable serum GM-CSF levels may serve as a biomarker of immune response. The vaccine sites were also evaluated as a measure of the local immune reaction to the vaccine. Eleven of 14 patients demonstrated a local inflammatory response similar to that observed in preclinical models[33,70] and autologous GM-CSF vaccine clinical trials.[74-76] Postvaccination DTH responses to autologous tumor cells have been used in previously reported vaccine studies as a surrogate to identify and characterize specific immune responses associated with vaccination.[79] In the pancreatic cancer vaccine trial, postvaccination DTH responses to autologous tumor cells were observed in one of three patients receiving 1×10^8 vaccine cells and in two of four patients receiving 5×10^8 vaccine cells. These data support previous findings that this vaccine approach is safe and can induce tumor-directed immune responses. Follow-up studies are ongoing to determine whether these promising effects on immune activation will translate into a true clinical benefit for patients with pancreatic cancer (Table 40.2).

A Look to the Future

More Rapid Methods for Identifying Pancreatic Tumor Antigens

There are significant challenges that must be overcome if immune-based therapies are to play an important role in the treatment of advanced cancer. First, immune-based strategies must be able to circumvent the genetic alterations within a tumor cell that result in their ability to evade immunologic recognition and eradication. Typically, genetic alterations result in the loss of antigen expression or the ability to adequately present antigen to T cells. One possible solution to this problem is to design polyvalent vaccines that target immunity against several tumor-rejection antigens. However, there are currently only a few candidate antigens expressed by pancreatic cancer that may serve as relevant immune targets. Three methods are routinely used for identifying potential new targets (Table 40.3). The first method uses serum to screen phage display libraries prepared from tumor cells to iden-

Table 40.3 Methods Currently Employed to Identify New Tumor Antigens

Method	Advantages	Disadvantages
cDNA library screening 1. Requires T cells 2. Requires tumor cells	Unbiased T cells pick antigen	1. Requires expertise in generating T-cell lines/clones 2. Requires expertise in generating tumor cell lines 3. Tedious, requiring large amounts of time
SEREX phage display library screening 1. Requires immunized serum 2. Requires tumor cells	Unbiased B cells pick antigen	1. Requires B cells and tumor cells 2. May not easily lead to relevant T-cell antigens 3. Tedious, requiring large amounts of time
Functional genomic screening 1. Requires immunized lymphocytes 2. Requires known overexpressed proteins	Rapid identification of cancer associated gene products that are recognized by T cells	1. No method for prioritizing screening of overexpressed antigens 2. Can be a fishing expedition

Abbreviations: cDNA, complementary DNA; SEREX, serological analysis of recombinant cDNA expression.

tify candidate antibody targets.[80] Proteins identified by this method can subsequently be screened for recognition by tumor-specific T cells. The second method employs tumor-specific T cells to screen complementary DNA libraries prepared from tumor cells to directly identify candidate antigens.[80] These methods have successfully identified a panel of melanoma-associated antigens as well as a number of nonmelanoma tumor antigens.[80] However, these techniques are tedious and slow and require significant manpower with both T-cell and molecular cloning expertise. An "indirect" antigen discovery method has also been successfully used to identify numerous candidate-tumor antigens that are recognized by T cells. However, this approach has also been slow because it depends on the existence of identified tumor-associated proteins. Until recently, the number of known pancreatic tumor–associated proteins have been few in number and include mostly mutated oncogene or tumor-suppressor proteins that would not be expected to serve as shared tumor antigens. With the recent sequencing of the human genome[81,82] and the availability of rapid gene profiling techniques, such as Serial Analysis of Gene Expression (SAGE),[83,84] it is now possible to more effectively identify pancreatic tumor proteins that can be characterized by "indirect" antigen discovery methods (see Chapter 36). As an example, we have used immunized lymphocytes from patients enrolled in a phase I study of an allogeneic GM-CSF–secreting tumor vaccine[77] to screen differentially expressed pancreatic proteins and have identified mesothelin as a new candidate-immune target expressed by pancreatic cancers.[87]

Combinatorial Vaccine Approaches Hold Promise for Overcoming Mechanisms of Immune Tolerance

It is unlikely that vaccines alone will be able to overcome mechanisms that functionally inactivate tumor-specific T cells, a recognized problem that limits the application of immunotherapy for the treatment of most patients with advanced cancer. Consequently, it might be possible to enhance the effects of vaccine-based approaches by combining cytoreductive and/or immune-modulating doses of chemotherapy with the tumor cell cytotoxic specificity of vaccines. Both combinations have been shown to overcome peripheral tolerance to tumor antigens in preclinical models.[36-38] In one preclinical mammary tumor model, immune-modulating doses of either paclitaxel, cyclophosphamide, or doxorubicin administered in sequence with a GM-CSF–transfected *Her2/Neu* vaccine enhanced the anti-tumor immune response to levels that were potent enough to overcome tolerance and result in the cure of tumor-bearing mice.[37] In another study, the combination of a Herceptin-like antibody to rat *Her2/Neu* administered in sequence with a GM-CSF–transfected *Her2/Neu* vaccine demonstrated a synergistic enhancement capable of curing larger *Her2/Neu*–expressing metastases.[85] In yet other studies, the administration of antagonistic antibodies that target co-stimulatory T-cell molecules or antagonistic antibodies that target down-regulatory T-cell molecules enhances the potency of vaccines when given to tumor-bearing, tolerized mice.[86] This data, together with earlier studies, provide the rationale to integrate tumor vaccines into current treatment modalities. Many of these approaches are now being tested in clinical trials in patients with a range of cancers, including pancreatic cancer (Table 40.2).

Conclusion

Immunotherapy is an attractive therapeutic approach in the management of pancreatic adenocarcinoma because it represents a non–cross-resistant therapy while adding minimal additional toxicities. However, both the inherent instability of the tumor genome and tumor tolerance mechanisms are significant practical obstacles that must be overcome if immune-based approaches for pancreatic cancer can achieve their promise. Recent advances in both tumor immunology and vaccine design have already resulted in promising preliminary data from phase I studies, and many additional trials are already in progress. Ultimately, the success of immune-based therapies against pancreatic cancer will depend on the development of multiple strategies that can be applied in synergy with immunotherapy. Although a substantial amount of work remains, the possibility of designing an effective vaccine approach for pancreatic adenocarcinoma has become a goal to achieve.

References

1. Germain RN. Immunology: The ins and outs of antigen processing and presentation. *Nature.* 1986;322:687–689.
2. Steinman RM. The dendritic cell system and its role in immunogenicity. *Annu Rev Immunol.* 1991;9:271–296.
3. Pieters J. MHC class II restricted antigen processing and presentation. *Adv Immunol.* 2000;75:159–208.
4. Solheim JC. Class I MHC molecules: assembly and antigen presentation. *Immunol Rev.* 1999;172:11–19.
5. Hammerling GJ, Vogt AB, Kropshofer H. Antigen processing and presentation—towards the millennium. *Immunol Rev.* 1999;172:5–9.
6. Chen L, Ashe S, Brady WA, et al. Costimulation of antitumor immunity by the B7 counterreceptor for the T lymphocyte molecules CD28 and CTLA-4. *Cell.* 1992;71:1093–1102.

7. Schwartz RH. Costimulation of T lymphocytes: the role of CD28, CTLA-4, and B7/BB1 in interleukin-2 production and immunotherapy. *Cell.* 1992;71:1065–1068.
8. Lechler R, Aichinger G, Lightstone L. The endogenous pathway of MHC class II antigen presentation. *Immunol Rev.* 1996;151:51–79.
9. Ostrand-Rosenberg S. Tumor immunotherapy: the tumor cell as an antigen presenting cell. *Curr Opin Immunol.* 1994;6:722–727.
10. Argani P, Iacobuzio-Donahue C, Ryu B, et al. Mesothelin is overexpressed in the vast majority of ductal adenocarcinomas of the pancreas: identification of a new pancreatic cancer marker by SAGE. *Clin Cancer Res.* 2001;7:3862–3868.
11. Marincola FM, Jaffee EM, Hicklin DJ, et al. Escape of human solid tumors from T-cell recognition: molecular mechanisms and functional significance. *Adv Immunol.* 2000;74:181–273.
12. Radoja S, Frey AB. Cancer induced defective cytotoxic T lymphocyte effector function: another mechanism how antigenic tumors escape immune-mediated killing. *Mol Med.* 2000;6:465–479.
13. Restifo NP, Esquivel F, Kawakami Y, et al. Identification of human cancers deficient in antigen processing. *J Exp Med.* 1993;177:265–272.
14. Correa MR, Ochoa AC, Ghosh P, et al. Sequential development of structural and functional alterations in T cells from tumor bearing mice. *J Immunol.* 1997;158:5292–5296.
15. Levitsky HI. Augmentation of host immune responses to cancer: overcoming the barrier of tumor antigen-specific T-cell tolerance. *Cancer J Sci Am.* 2000;6[supp3]:S281–S290.
16. von Bernstorff W, Voss M, Freichel S, et al. Systemic and local immunosuppression in pancreatic cancer patients. *Clin Cancer Res.* 2001;7[suppl]:925s–932s.
17. Klausner RD, Samelson LE. T cell antigen receptor activation pathways: the tyrosine kinase connection. *Cell.* 1991;64:875–878.
18. Irving BA, Weiss A. The cytoplasmic domain of the T cell receptor ζ chain is sufficient to couple to receptor associated signal transduction pathways. *Cell.* 1991;64:891–901.
19. Samelson LE, Patel MD, Weissman AM, et al. Antigen activation of murine T cells induces tyrosine phosphorylation of a polypeptide associated with the T cell antigen receptor. *Cell.* 1986;46:1083–1090.
20. Siegel JN, Klausner RD, Rapp UR, et al. T cell receptor engagement stimulates c-raf associated kinase activity via a protein kinase C dependent pathway. *J Biol Chem.* 1990;265:18472–18480.
21. Schmielau J, Nalesnik MA, Finn OJ. Suppressed T-cell receptor ζ chain expression and cytokine production in pancreatic cancer patients. *Clin Cancer Res.* 2001;7:933s–939s.
22. Ungefroren H, Voss M, Bernstorff WV, et al. Immunological escape mechanisms in pancreatic carcinoma. *Ann NY Acad Sci.* 1999;880:243–251.
23. Takahashi A, Kono K, Amemiya H, et al. Elevated caspase-3 activity in peripheral blood T cells coexists with increased degree of T cell apoptosis and down regulation of TCR zeta molecules in patients with gastric cancer. *Clin Cancer Res.* 2001;7:74–80.
24. Gastman BR, Johnson DE, Whiteside TL, et al. Caspase mediated degradation of T cell receptor zeta chain. *Cancer Res.* 1999;59:1422–1427.
25. Kornmann M, Ishiwata T, Kleef J, et al. Fas and Fas-ligand expression in human pancreatic cancer. *Ann Surg.* 2000;231:368–379.
26. Elnemr A, Ohta T, Yachie A, et al. Human pancreatic cancer cells express nonfunctional Fas receptors and counterattack lymphocytes by expressing Fas ligand; a potential mechanism for immune escape. *Int J Oncol.* 2001;18:33–39.
27. Von Bernstorff W, Spanjaard RA, Chan AK, et al. Pancreatic cancer cells can evade immune surveillance via nonfunctional Fas (APO-1/CD95) receptors and aberrant expression of Fas ligand. *Surgery.* 1999;125:73–84.
28. Ungefroren H, Voss M, Jansen M, et al. Human pancreatic adenocarcinomas express Fas and Fas ligand yet are resistant to Fas mediated apoptosis. *Cancer Res.* 1998;58:1741–1749.
29. Restifo NP, Kawakami Y, Marincola F, et al. Molecular mechanisms used by tumors to escape immune recognition: immunogenetherapy and the cell biology of major histocompatibility complex class I. *J Immunol.* 1993;14:182–190.
30. Ganss R, Hanahan D. Tumor microenvironment can restrict the effectiveness of activated antitumor lymphocytes. *Cancer Res.* 1998;58:4673–4681.
31. Blobe GC, Schiemann WP, Lodish HF. Role of transforming growth factor beta in human disease. *N Engl J Med.* 2000;342:1350–1358.
32. Bellone G, Turletti A, Artusio E, et al. Tumor associated transforming growth factor beta and interleukin 10 contribute to a systemic Th2 immune phenotype in pancreatic carcinoma patients. *Am J Pathol.* 1999;155:537–547.
33. Greten TF, Jaffee EM. Cancer vaccines. *J Clin Oncol.* 1999;17:1047–1060.
34. Matzinger P. Tolerance, danger, and the extended family. *Annu Rev Immunol.* 1994;12:991–1045.
35. Jenkins MK, Schwartz RH. Antigen presentation by chemically modified splenocytes induces antigen-specific T cell unresponsiveness in vitro and in vivo. *J Exp Med.* 1987;165:302–319.
36. Berd D, Maguire HC, Mastrangelo MJ. Induction of cell-mediated immunity to autologous melanoma cells and regression of metastases after treatment with a melanoma cell vaccine preceded by cyclophosphamide. *Cancer Res.* 1986;46:2572–2577.
37. Machiels JP, Reilly RT, Emens L, et al. Cyclophosphamide, doxorubicin, and paclitaxel enhance the anti-tumor immune response of GM-CSF secreting whole cell vaccines in tolerized mice. *Cancer Res.* 2001;61:3689–3697.
38. Proietti E, Greco G, Garrone B, et al. Importance of cyclophosphamide-induced bystander effect on T cells for a successful tumor eradication in response to adoptive immunotherapy in mice. *J Clin Invest.* 1998;101:429–441.
39. Wolf AM, Wolf D, Steurer M, et al. Increase of regulatory T cells in the peripheral blood of cancer patients. *Clin Cancer Res.* 2003;9:606–612.
40. Wigmore SJ, Todorov PT, Barber MD, et al. Characteristics of pancreatic cancer expressing a novel cancer cachectic factor. *Br J Surg.* 2000;87:53–58.

41. Tisdale MJ. Biology of cachexia. *J Natl Cancer Inst.* 1997; 89:1763–1773.
42. Fearon KC, Barber MD, Falconer JS, et al. Pancreatic cancer as a model: inflammatory mediators, acute phase response and cancer cachexia. *World J Surg.* 1999;23:584–588.
43. DiMagno E, Reber HA, Tempero MA. AGA technical review on the epidemiology, diagnosis, and treatment of pancreatic ductal adenocarcinoma. *Gastroenterology.* 1999;117: 1463–1484.
44. Tempero M. Biologic therapy of gastrointestinal cancer. *Cancer Treat Res.* 1998;98:227–237.
45. Laheru DA, Jaffee EM. Potential role of tumor vaccines in GI malignancies. *Oncology (Huntingt).* 2000;14:245–256.
46. Hruban RH, Goggins M, Parsons J, et al. Progression model for pancreatic cancer. *Clin Cancer Res.* 2000;6:2969–2972.
47. Abbruzzese JL. Molecular diagnosis of pancreatic and biliary cancer: ready for broad implementation? *Cancer J.* 2000;6:282–284.
48. Saforafas GH, Tsiotou AG, Tsiotos GG. Molecular biology of pancreatic cancer; oncogenes, tumor suppressor genes, growth factors, and their receptors from a clinical perspective. *Cancer Treat Rev.* 2000;26:29–52.
49. Bos JL. Ras oncogenes in human cancer: a review. *Cancer Res.* 1989:49:4682–4689.
50. Flanders TY, Foulkes WD. Pancreatic adenocarcinoma: epidemiology and genetics. *J Med Genet.* 1996:33:889–898.
51. Hruban RH, Van Mansfeld AD, Offerhaus GJ, et al. K-ras oncogene activation in adenocarcinoma of the pancreas. *Am J Pathol.* 1993;143:545–554.
52. Gjertsen MK, Bakka A, Breivik J, et al. Vaccination with mutant ras peptides and induction of T-cell responsiveness in pancreatic carcinoma patients carrying the corresponding ras mutation. *Lancet.* 1995;346:1399–1400.
53. Bergmann-Leitner ES, Kantor JA, Shupert WL, et al. Identification of a human CD8+ T lymphocyte neo-epitope created by a ras codon 12 mutation which is restricted by the HLA-A2 allele. *Cell Immunol.* 1998;187:103–116.
54. Khleif SN, Abrams S, Allegra C, et al. The generation of CD4+ and CD8+ T cell responses from patients vaccinated with mutant ras peptides corresponding to the patient's own ras mutation. *Proc ASCO.* 1997;19:1566.
55. Wojtowicz ME, Hamilton MJ, Bernstein S, et al. Clinical trial of mutant ras peptide vaccination along with IL-2 or GM-CSF. *Proc ASCO.* 2000;19:1818.
56. Gjertsen MK, Buanes T, Rosseland AR, et al. Intradermal ras peptide vaccination with granulocyte-macrophage colony stimulating factor as adjuvant: clinical and immunological responses in patients with pancreatic adenocarcinoma. *Int J Cancer.* 2001;92:441–450.
57. Wang XY, Kaneko Y, Repasky E, Subjeck JR. Heat shock proteins and cancer immunotherapy. *Immunol Invest.* 2000;29:131–137.
58. Janetzki S, Blachere NE, Srivastava PK. Generation of tumor specific cytotoxic T lymphocytes and memory T cells by immunization with tumor derived heat shock protein gp96. *J Immunother.* 1998;21:269–276.
59. Lewis JJ, Janetzki S, Livingston PO, et al. Pilot trial of vaccination with autologous tumor derived gp96 heat shock protein-peptide complex (HSPPC-96) in patients with resected pancreatic adenocarcinoma. *Proc ASCO.* 1999;18:1687.
60. Finn OJ, Jerome KR, Henderson RA, et al. MUC-1 epithelial tumor mucin-based immunity and vaccines. *Immunol Rev.* 1995;145:61–89.
61. Apostopopoulos V, McKenzie IF. Cellular mucins: targets for immunotherapy. *Crit Rev Immunol.* 1994;14:293–309.
62. Mukherjee P, Ginardi AR, Madsen CS, et al. Mice with spontaneous pancreatic cancer naturally develop MUC-1 specific CTLs that eradicate tumors when adoptively transferred. *J Immunol.* 2000;165:3451–3460.
63. Brossart P, Heinrich K, Stuhler G. Identification of HLA-A2 restricted T cell epitopes derived from the MUC-1 tumor antigen for broadly applicable vaccine therapies. *Blood.* 1999;12:4309–4317.
64. Ramanathan RK, Lee K, Mckolanis J, et al. Phase I study of a MUC-1 synthetic vaccine admixed with SB-AS2 adjuvant in resected and locally advanced pancreatic cancer. *Proc ASCO.* 2000;19:1791.
65. Compton C, Fenoglio-Preiser CM, Pettigrew N, Fielding LP. American Joint Committee on Cancer Prognostic Factors Consensus Conference: Colorectal working group. *Cancer.* 2000;88:1739–1757.
66. Hammarstrom S. The carcinoembryonic antigen (CEA) family: structures, suggested functions and expression in normal and malignant tissues. *Semin Cancer Biol.* 1999;9(2):67–81.
67. Marshall JL, Hoyer RJ, Toomey MA, et al. Phase I study in advanced cancer patients of a diversified prime and boost vaccination protocol using recombinant vaccinia virus and recombinant nonreplicating Avipox virus to elicit anticarcinoembryonic antigen immune responses. *J Clin Oncol.* 2000;18:3964–3973.
68. Restifo NP. Cancer vaccines: basic principles. In: Rosenberg SA, ed. *The Principles and Practice of the Biologic Therapy of Cancer.* 3rd ed. Philadelphia: Lippincott Williams & Wilkens; 2000:571–584.
69. Pardoll DM, Jaffee EM. Cancer vaccines: clinical applications. In: Rosenberg SA, ed. *The Principles and Practice of the Biologic Therapy of Cancer.* 3rd ed. Philadelphia: Lippincott Williams & Wilkens; 2000:647–662.
70. Dranoff G, Jaffee EM, Golumbek P, et al. Vaccination with irradiated tumor cells engineered to secrete murine GM-CSF stimulates potent, specific and long lasting anti-tumor immunity. *Proc Natl Acad Sci USA.* 1993;90:3539–3543.
71. Huang AY, Golumbek PT, Ahmadzadeh M, et al. Role of bone marrow derived cells in presenting MHC class I restricted tumor antigens. *Science.* 1994;264:961–965.
72. Nakazaki Y, Tani K, Lin ZT, et al. Vaccine effect of granulocyte-macrophage colony stimulating factor or CD80 gene transduced murine hematopoietic tumor cells and their cooperative enhancement of anti-tumor immunity. *Gene Ther.* 1998;5:1355–1362.
73. Golumbek PT, Azhari R, Jaffee EM, et al. Controlled release biodegradable cytokine depots: a new approach to cancer vaccine design. *Cancer Res.* 1993;53:1–4.
74. Simons JW, Jaffee EM, Weber C, et al. Bioactivity of human GM-CSF gene transduced autologous renal vaccines. *Cancer Res.* 1997;57:1537–1546.

75. Simons JW, Mikhak B, Chang JF, et al. Induction of immunity to prostate cancer antigens: results of a clinical trial of vaccination with irradiated autologous prostate tumor cells engineered to secrete granulocyte-macrophage colony stimulating factor using ex vivo gene transfer. *Cancer Res.* 1999;59:5160–5168.
76. Soiffer R, Lynch T, Mihm M, et al. Vaccination with irradiated autologous melanoma cells engineered to secrete human granulocyte-macrophage colony-stimulating factor generates potent antitumor immunity in patients with metastatic melanoma. *Proc Natl Acad Sci USA.* 1998;95:13141–13146.
77. Jaffee EM, Hruban R, Biedzycki B, et al. A novel allogeneic GM-CSF secreting tumor vaccine for pancreatic cancer: a phase I trial of safety and immune activation. *J Clin Oncol.* 2001;19:145–156.
78. Davis MP, Dinneen AB, Landa N, et al. Grover's disease: clinicopathologic review of 72 cases. *Mayo Clin Proc.* 1999;74:229–234.
79. Snozl M, Marincola FM. Cancer vaccines: basic principles. In: Rosenberg SA, ed. *The Principles and Practice of the Biologic Therapy of Cancer.* 3rd ed. Philadelphia: Lippincott Williams & Wilkens; 2000:617–631.
80. Boon T, Van Den Eynde BJ. Cancer vaccines; cancer antigens. In: Rosenberg SA, ed. *The Principles and Practice of the Biologic Therapy of Cancer.* 3rd ed. Philadelphia: Lippincott Williams & Wilkens; 2000:493–504.
81. Lander ES, Linton LM, Birren B, et al. Initial sequencing and analysis of the human genome. *Nature.* 2001;409: 860–921.
82. Venter JC, Adams MD, Myers EW, et al. The sequence of the human genome. *Science.* 2001;291:1304–1351.
83. Velculescu VE, Zhang L, Vogelstein B, et al. Serial analysis of gene expression. *Science.* 1995;270:484–487.
84. Zhang L, Zhou W, Velculescu VE, et al. Genome expression profiles in normal and cancer cells. *Science.* 1997; 276:1268–1272.
85. Wolpoe ME, Lutz ER, Ercolini AM, et al. HER-2/neu-specific monoclonal antibodies collaborate with Her-2/neu-targeted GM-CSF secreting whole tumor cell vaccination to augment CD8+ T cell effector function and tumor-free survival in Her-2/neu transgenic mice. *J Immunol.* 2003;171:2161–2169.
86. Pardoll DM. Spinning molecular immunology into successful immunotherapy. *Nat Rev Immunol.* 2002;2:227–238.
87. Thomas AM, Santarsiero LM, Lutz E, et al. Mesothelin-specific $CD8^+$ T cells responses provide evidence of invivo Cross-priming by antigen-presenting cells in vaccinated pancreatic cancer patients. *J Exp Med.* 2004;200:297–306.

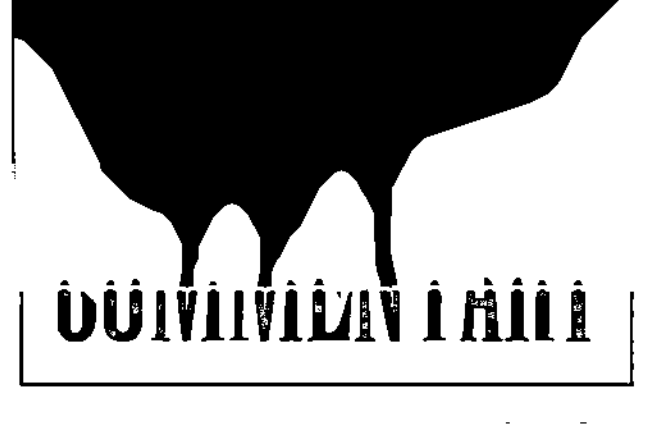

Jonathan J. Lewis, MD, PhD

A decade ago, it seemed rational that our rapidly increasing knowledge of the molecular identities of tumor antigens and a deeper understanding of basic immunology would point the way to an effective therapeutic cancer vaccine.[1] Significant progress has been made, and objective responses after immune based treatments are observed in a small number of patients. Despite this progress, we do not yet have a cancer vaccine in any type of cancer that can reliably and consistently induce tumor destruction or improve patient survival.[2]

There is now incontrovertible evidence that precursor frequencies of tumor-specific T cells can be increased after immunization using several different antigens, including antigens that are nonmutated "self" tissue differentiation antigens, as well as various unique antigens.[3-7] The presence of increased anti-tumor T-cell precursors after vaccination has been convincingly demonstrated in both mice and humans, using tetramer or ELISPOT analysis, real-time reverse transcription-polymerase chain reaction, among other techniques. The correlation of causality in terms of this increase in frequency with clinical response has been difficult.

Part of this difficulty reflects the pitfalls of early stage human clinical trials. Because of human heterogeneity, clinical trials are less efficient than laboratory studies. Because of this inefficiency, animal models may be useful in the correlation of immune and tumor response and the optimization of vaccine schedule, mode of delivery, and adjuvants and cofactor molecules. Unfortunately, there are no good, consistent models in which large, established, nonimmunogenic tumors could be induced to regress using a cancer vaccine given alone. Most successful cancer vaccine models in mice are based on the prevention of challenge or based on the treatment of tiny tumor burdens. In human studies, in the absence of a clinical response rate that is significantly above the background variability that is observed in any diverse patient cohort, it is often difficult to interpret data accurately. We are not yet sure of the correct or most efficient outcome measurement when assessing vaccination effects in early-stage human studies.[2]

In the very well-written Chapter 40 by Dr. Laheru and Dr. Jaffee, an excellent summary of current approaches to vaccination in pancreatic cancer is presented. This reflects a large experience in the development of pancreatic cancer vaccines.[8-12] They summarize the current and completed clinical trials and the multitude of various approaches. It is important to note that for phase 1 or phase 2 clinical trials, interpretations of data are often confounded by variables inherent in any early, nonrandomized clinical trial. Thus, in the absence of a clinical response rate that is significantly above the background variability that is observed in any diverse patient cohort, it is often difficult to interpret data accurately. There is fundamental artificiality when reducing any diverse set of clinical data to a single outcome. We are not yet sure of the correct or most efficient outcome measurement when assessing vaccination effects in early stage human studies.[2]

There are sufficient data to support the notion that therapeutic cancer vaccines can induce antitumor immune responses in humans with cancer including pancreatic cancer. How best to translate this increase in immune responsiveness to consistently and reproducibly induce objective cancer regression or increased survival remains unclear at this time. Despite monumental advances in our understanding of molecular and cellular immunology, we have thus far been unable to translate this into a proven and measurable clinical benefit. Vaccines and immunotherapy in pancreatic cancer will need to overcome the inherent instability of the tumor genome as well as tumor tolerance mechanisms. I concur fully with the authors that the ultimate success of immune-based therapies against pancreatic cancer will depend on the development of multiple strategies that can be applied in synergy with immunotherapy.

References

1. Lewis JJ, Houghton AN. Definition of tumor antigens suitable for vaccine construction. *Semin Cancer Biol.* 1995;6:321–327.
2. Restifo NP, Lewis JJ. Therapeutic cancer vaccines. In: DeVita VT, Rosenberg SA, Hellman S, eds. *Cancer: Principles and Practice of Oncology.* Baltimore: Lippincott; 2004:45–57.
3. Coulie PG, Karanikas V, Lurquin C, et al. Cytolytic T-cell responses of cancer patients vaccinated with a MAGE antigen. *Immunol Rev.* 2002;188:33–42.
4. Lewis JJ, Janetzki S, Schaed S, et al. Evaluation of CD8(+) T-cell frequencies by the Elispot assay in healthy individuals and in patients with metastatic melanoma immunized with tyrosinase peptide. *Int J Cancer.* 2000;87:391–398.
5. Rosenberg SA, Yang JC, Schwartzentruber DJ, et al. Immunologic and therapeutic evaluation of a synthetic peptide vaccine for the treatment of patients with metastatic melanoma. *Nat Med.* 1998;4:321–327.
6. Belli F, Testori A, Rivoltini L, et al. Vaccination of metastatic melanoma patients with autologous tumor-derived heat shock protein gp96-peptide complexes: clinical and immunologic findings. *J Clin Oncol.* 2002;20:4169–4180.
7. Lewis JJ, Janetzki S, Livingston PO, et al. Pilot trial of vaccination with autologous tumor-derived gp96 heat shock protein-peptide complex (HSPPC-96) in patients with resected pancreatic adenocarcinoma. *Proc Am Soc Clin Oncol.* 1999;17:1687.
8. Jaffee EM, Abrams R, Cameron J, et al. A phase I clinical trial of lethally irradiated allogeneic pancreatic tumor cells transfected with the GM-CSF gene for the treatment of pancreatic adenocarcinoma. *Hum Gene Ther.* 1998;9:1951–1971.

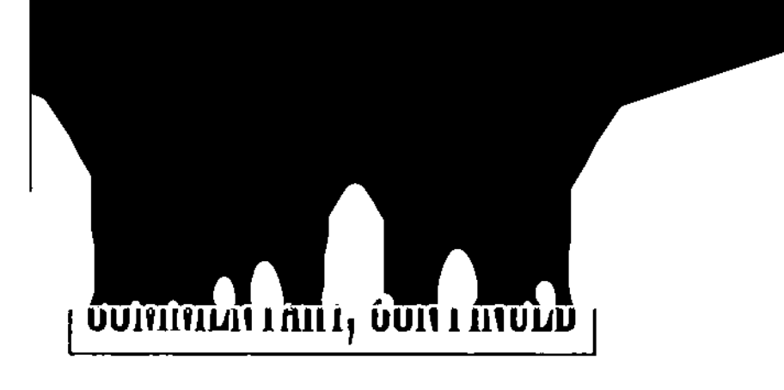

9. Jaffee EM, Hruban RH, Biedrzycki B, et al. Novel allogeneic granulocyte-macrophage colony-stimulating factor-secreting tumor vaccine for pancreatic cancer: a phase I trial of safety and immune activation. *J Clin Oncol.* 2001;19:145–156.
10. Jaffee EM, Hruban RH, Canto M, Kern SE. Focus on pancreas cancer. *Cancer Cell.* 2002;2:25–28.
11. Laheru D, Biedrzycki B, Jaffee EM. Immunologic approaches to the management of pancreatic cancer. *Cancer J.* 2001;7:324–337.
12. Yeo TP, Hruban RH, Leach SD, et al. Pancreatic cancer. *Curr Probl Cancer.* 2002;26:176–275.

3

Endocrine Pancreas

CHAPTER 41

Tumors of the Endocrine System

David S. Klimstra, MD

The endocrine neoplasms of the pancreas represent an important subset of pancreatic neoplasms, both because of the distinctive endocrine paraneoplastic syndromes that may be present and because these neoplasms are often less aggressive and more amenable to curative surgical therapy than are carcinomas of the exocrine pancreas. From a pathological standpoint, pancreatic endocrine neoplasms (PENs) represent a diagnostic challenge because of the wide range of histologic patterns that exist. Variability in clinical behavior has frustrated attempts to sharply define benign and malignant categories of PENs, and attention has recently been directed toward defining prognostic factors and understanding the genetic alterations underlying these neoplasms.

The Normal Endocrine Pancreas

In the normal pancreas, the endocrine cells are largely found within the islets of Langerhans, although approximately 10% of pancreatic endocrine cells are extrainsular, usually distributed within the ducts.[1] During development, all of the pancreatic endocrine cells originate from the embryonic ducts and are therefore of endodermal origin.[2] The histologic appearance and cellular composition of the islets differ between the regions of the pancreas derived from the dorsal and ventral embryologic pancreatic primordial (Fig. 41.1). Most (90%) islets consist of roughly spherical collections of cells derived from the embryonic dorsal pancreas. These compact islets are abundant in the body and tail but are also found in the head of the gland and contain predominantly α and β cells, with minor populations of pancreatic polypeptide (PP) and δ cells.[3] In the portion of the head of the pancreas derived from the embryonic ventral pancreas (essentially, the uncinate process), the islets have a trabecular configuration and are rather ill-defined, with interposition between cords of acinar cells. These diffuse islets also contain many β cells but are predominantly (70%) composed of PP cells, with few δ and α cells.[3]

General Features and Classification

PENs account for roughly 2%–4% of clinically detected pancreatic neoplasms. Because endocrine microadenomas are relatively common incidental findings, the prevalence of PENs at autopsy (between 1% and 10% of autopsies[1,4]) is significantly higher than the clinical prevalence. Males and females are equally affected. PENs may arise at any age,[5] but most occur between the ages of 30 and 60 years;

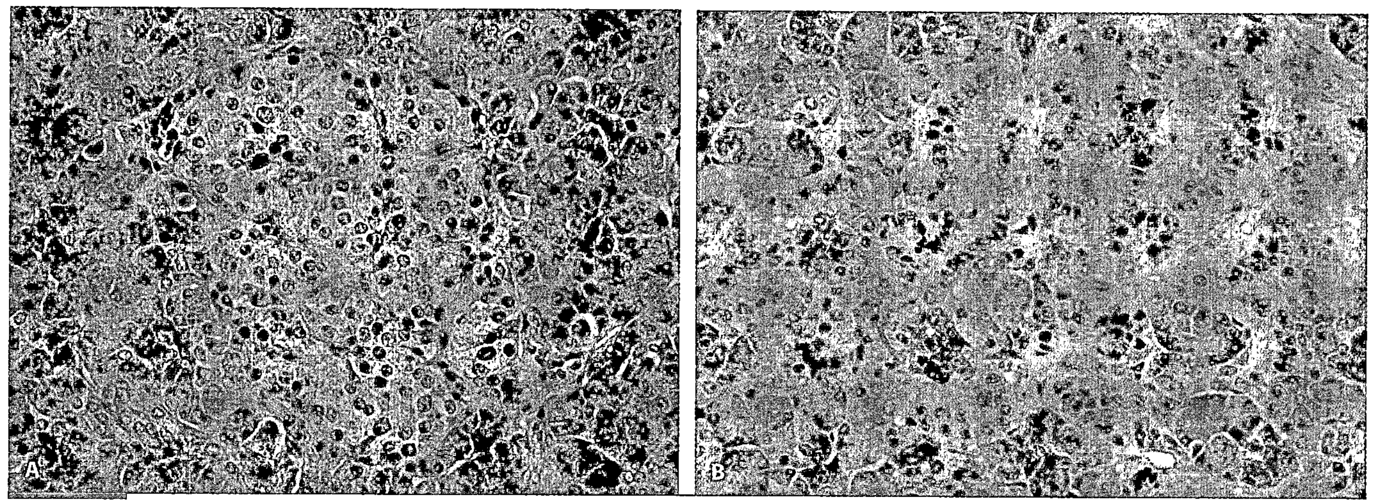

Figure 41.1
Normal pancreatic islets. Compact islets (**A**) are roughly spherical, consisting of closely packed lobules of endocrine cells separated by capillaries. Diffuse islets (**B**) are less well circumscribed and have a trabecular arrangement, with interposed acini between the endocrine cells.

those arising in patients with multiple endocrine neoplasia 1 (MEN1) syndrome occur at a younger age.

Several different classification systems can be applied to endocrine neoplasms of the pancreas (Table 41.1). Most are in the well-differentiated category, in the sense that they retain the organoid architecture typical of endocrine organs and have a relatively low proliferative rate. PENs measuring less than 0.5 cm are designated as endocrine microadenomas. Microadenomas are the only PENs that can be regarded as completely benign. Most of the remainder of well-differentiated PENs are low- to intermediate-grade malignancies, and despite numerous studies on prognostic factors, no specific classification system has achieved widespread acceptance. Finally, a small group of primary pancreatic neoplasms qualify as high-grade endocrine carcinomas because of their diffuse architecture, high proliferative rate, and abundant necrosis.

The well-differentiated PENs are also subclassified on the basis of the presence and type of associated clinical syndrome caused by inappropriate hormone secretion by the tumor. PENs are designated as insulinoma, glucagonoma, gastrinoma, and so on if the patient exhibits characteristic clinical findings in the presence of elevated serum levels of the responsible peptide or bioamine. These "functional" PENs are listed in Table 41.2. PENs without a clinical syndrome are termed "nonfunctional," although most of these also exhibit some evidence of hormone production if serum peptide levels are measured or immunohistochemistry is employed to detect them.[6] A nonfunctional PEN that is documented to produce a specific hormone may be designated on the basis of the corresponding cell type (e.g., "α-cell neoplasm", "β-cell neoplasm"), but they should not be labeled as functional tumors in the absence of the appropriate clinical syndrome.[1] The presence or absence of an associated clinical syndrome has prognostic significance; there-

Table 41.1 Classification of Pancreatic Endocrine Neoplasms

Classification
Endocrine microadenoma
Well-differentiated pancreatic endocrine neoplasm
Functional pancreatic endocrine neoplasm
Insulinoma
Glucagonoma
Somatostatinoma
VIPoma
Gastrinoma
Carcinoid tumor
Other ectopic and mixed hormone producing neoplasms
Nonfunctional pancreatic endocrine neoplasm (not otherwise specified)
PPoma
Poorly differentiated endocrine carcinoma
Small cell carcinoma
Large cell endocrine carcinoma
Mixed endocrine carcinomas
Mixed ductal-endocrine carcinoma
Mixed acinar-endocrine carcinoma
Mixed acinar-endocrine-ductal carcinoma

Abbreviations: VIPoma, vasoactive intestinal polypeptide-secreting tumor; PPoma, pancreatic polypeptide-secreting tumor.

Table 41.2 Functional Pancreatic Endocrine Neoplasms

	Cell Type	Syndrome	Clinical Findings
Insulinoma	β cell	Insulinoma syndrome	Hypoglycemia
Glucagonoma	α cell	Glucagonoma syndrome	Skin rash, stomatitis, diabetes, weight loss
Somatostatinoma	δ cell	Somatostinoma syndrome	Diabetes, cholelithiasis
VIPoma	Unknown	Verner-Morrison syndrome	Watery diarrhea, hypokalemia, achlorhydria
Gastrinoma	G cell	Zollinger-Ellison syndrome	Peptic ulcers

Abbreviations: VIPoma, vasoactive intestinal polypeptide-secreting tumor.

fore, the relevant clinical distinction is between "syndromic" and "nonsyndromic" PENs. However, the functional and nonfunctional terminology is entrenched in the lexicon. Rare PENs have been described that exhibit expression of PP by immunohistochemistry, associated with increases in serum PP levels.[7,8] Although these neoplasms have been designated "PPomas," no known clinical syndrome is associated with PP hypersecretion, so PPomas are categorized as nonfunctional PENs. Many PENs producing somatostatin, calcitonin, and neurotensin also fall into the nonfunctional group.

Based on surgical studies, approximately one third of all PENs are nonfunctional[1,9-11]; in patients with MEN1 with multiple PENs, a greater proportion of the individual tumors are nonfunctional,[12] but most patients with MEN1 have at least one PEN that is functional.[1,13,14] Insulinomas are the most common functional tumors (45%), followed by gastrinomas (20%), glucagonomas (13%), vasoactive intestinal polypeptide-secreting tumors (VIPomas) (10%), and somatostatinomas (5%). PENs producing other unusual syndromes (e.g., Cushing's syndrome, carcinoid syndrome, acromegaly) occur but are rare.[15-17]

PENs may be associated with a number of genetic syndromes, most importantly MEN1 and von Hippel-Lindau (VHL) syndromes.[18,19] In these cases, the genetic abnormality underlying the syndrome plays a role in the development of the PENs, which often are multiple.[20,21] The pathological features of these PENs are generally similar to those occurring sporadically, although the PENs in patients with VHL syndrome may have clear-cell features and may be associated with a serous cystic neoplasm.[22]

Pathological Features

The gross appearance of PENs is generally that of a circumscribed, solid mass composed of tan, uniform, fleshy parenchyma (Fig. 41.2). Larger PENs are multinodular,

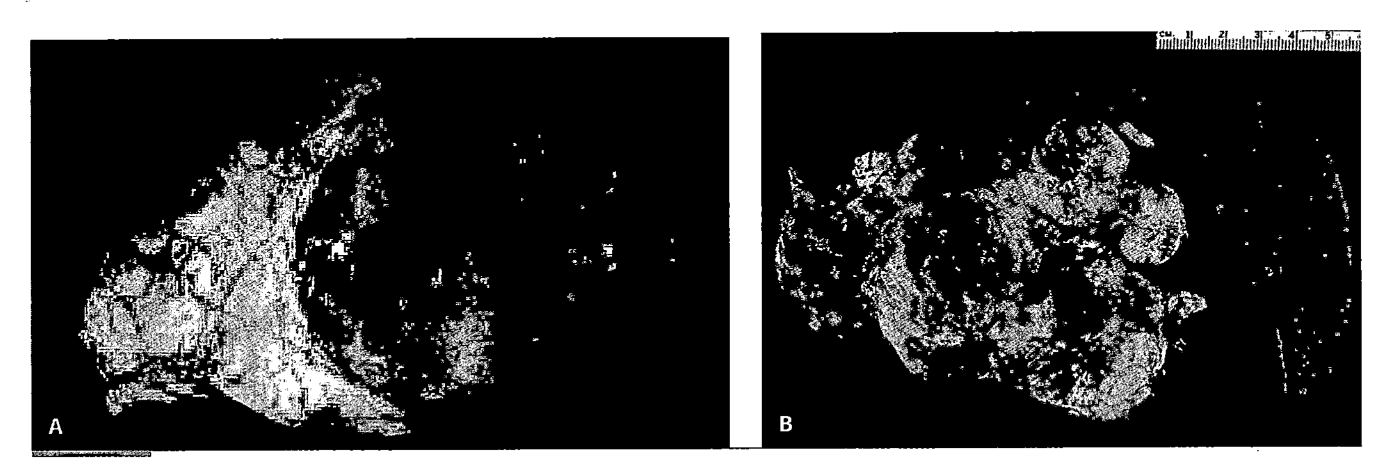

Figure 41.2
Gross appearance of pancreatic endocrine neoplasms. Some examples are relatively small and circumscribed **(A)**, consisting of a uniform tan neoplasm sharply demarcated from the surrounding pancreas. Larger examples **(B)** exhibit a more multinodular pattern. In this case, there is extensive hemorrhage and cystic degeneration, with gross invasion of the spleen.

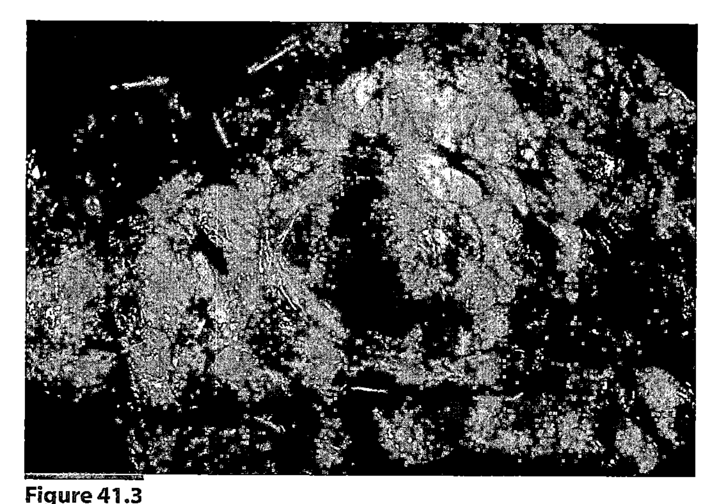

Figure 41.3
Cystic pancreatic endocrine neoplasm. A central unilocular cyst is separated from a fibrous capsule by a thin rim of tan tumor parenchyma.

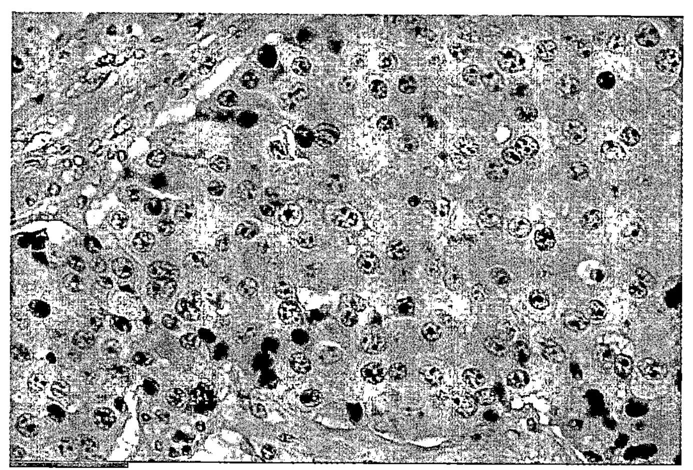

Figure 41.5
Cytologic features of pancreatic endocrine neoplasms. The nuclei are round to oval and relatively uniform, and the chromatin is coarsely granular. The cytoplasm is moderate in amount and amphophilic.

with fibrous septa dividing the neoplasm. Some examples have more abundant fibrous stroma, imparting a firm consistency. Cystic change is a less common phenomenon,[23] usually in the form of a single central locule lined by a thin rim of neoplastic cells (Fig. 41.3).

Most PENs have an expansile growth pattern, and small neoplasms may be completely surrounded by a fibrous capsule. It is common to find invasive growth, however, including extension into the adjacent tissues, such as the residual pancreatic parenchyma, the peripancreatic soft tissues, vessels, or adjacent organs (e.g., the spleen).

PENs are histologically characteristic at both the architectural and cytologic levels. Many different architectural arrangements have been recognized, all collectively referred to as "organoid" patterns. Cells are arranged in regular nests, ribbons, or trabecula, and it is common for more than one pattern to be found in different regions of a single neoplasm (Fig. 41.4). The trabecular pattern is particularly characteristic, and when thin, complex trabecula are interwoven, the term *gyriform* is applied to the architecture. The cytology of PENs is often similar to that of other well-differentiated endocrine neoplasms, such as carcinoid tumors. The nuclei are usually round to oval and uniform (Fig. 41.5), although scattered enlarged nuclei are not uncommon. The chromatin is coarsely granular and clumped, imparting the classic "salt and pepper" appearance characteristic of well-differentiated endocrine neoplasms in general. Nucleoli may be inconspicuous, although many PENs have easily identifiable or even prominent nucleoli.

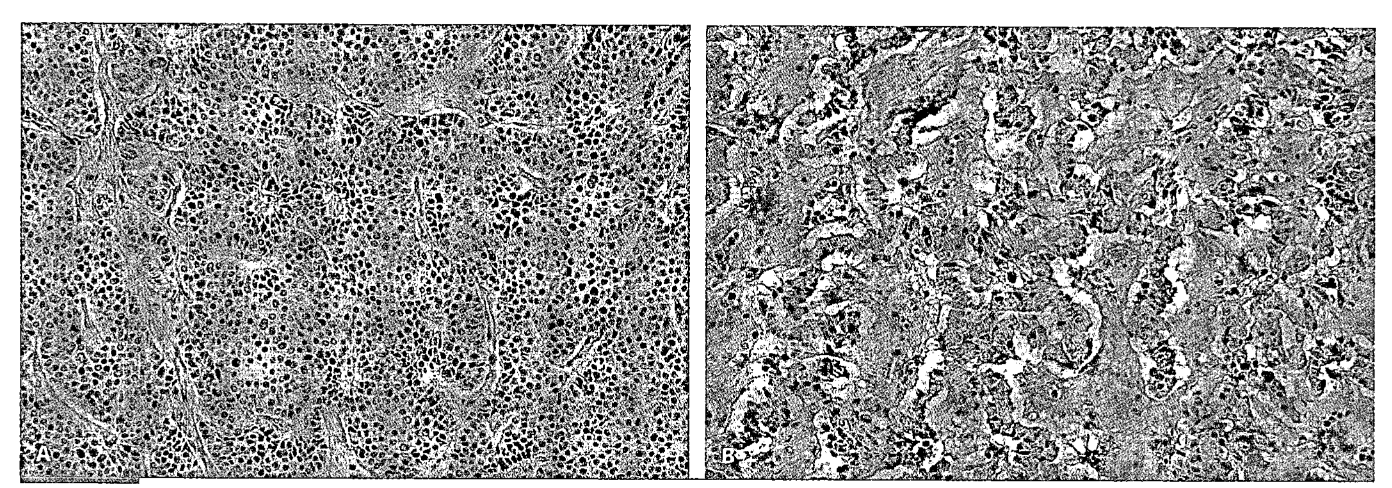

Figure 41.4
Architectural patterns of pancreatic endocrine neoplasms. Many examples demonstrate a nesting pattern **(A)**, with thin fibrovascular septa separating relatively uniform neoplastic cells. In the gyriform pattern **(B)**, thin interanastamosing trabecula of endocrine cells are found.

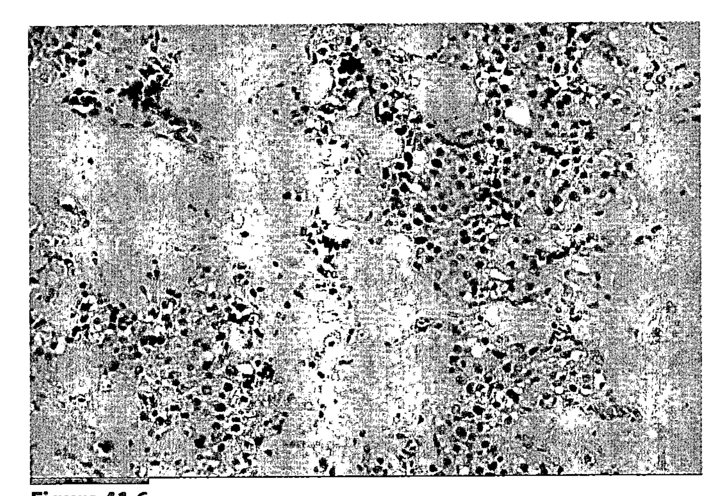

Figure 41.6
Some pancreatic endocrine neoplasms demonstrate abundant hyalinized stroma between the nests of neoplastic endocrine cells.

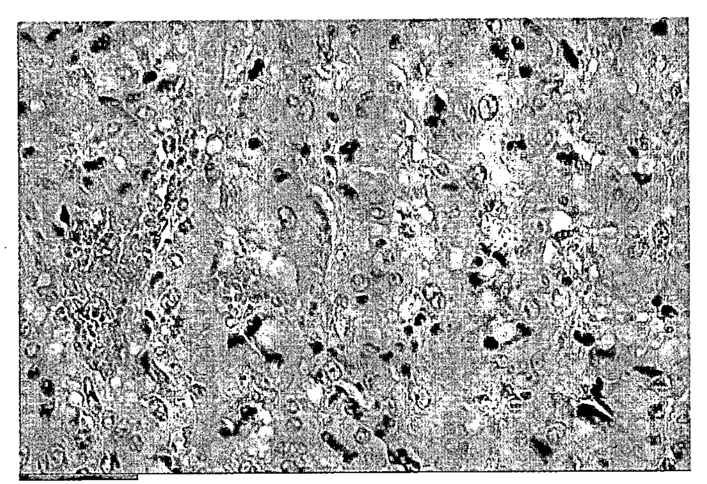

Figure 41.8
Pleomorphic pancreatic endocrine neoplasm. The nuclei are enlarged and atypical, but there is also abundant cytoplasm, and the mitotic rate is not increased.

The aforementioned architectural and cytologic features are key to recognizing PENs, but there are many variations in histology that may cause diagnostic dilemmas. The range of patterns one may encounter in PENs exceeds that of nearly all other endocrine neoplasms. The stroma varies considerably in amount. Some PENs have nearly no collagen within the neoplasm (Fig. 41.4A); there is only a thin (but abundant) fibrovascular stroma separating the cellular nests. Other examples contain abundant, hyalinized, or amyloid-like stroma that results in the appearance of sparse, thin epithelial cords compressed by broad bands of collagen (Fig. 41.6). Calcifications may be found, including psammoma bodies.[24] The quantity and the appearance of the cytoplasm also vary. A moderate amount of amphophilic-to-basophilic cytoplasm is typical, but PENs with oncocytic cytoplasm[25-27] or clear-cell change have been described (Fig. 41.7). The latter type is reportedly more common in patients with VHL syndrome.[22] Some PENs have scant cytoplasm and the resulting high nucleus-to-cytoplasm ratio that may cause confusion with small-cell carcinomas or primitive neuroectodermal tumors. The nuclear morphology may also vary; PENs with marked nuclear pleomorphism have been reported,[28] and these cases are commonly confused with ductal carcinomas or other high-grade neoplasms (Fig. 41.8). In these instances, the nuclear atypia is not generally accompanied by an increased proliferative rate and does not appear to have adverse prognostic significance.

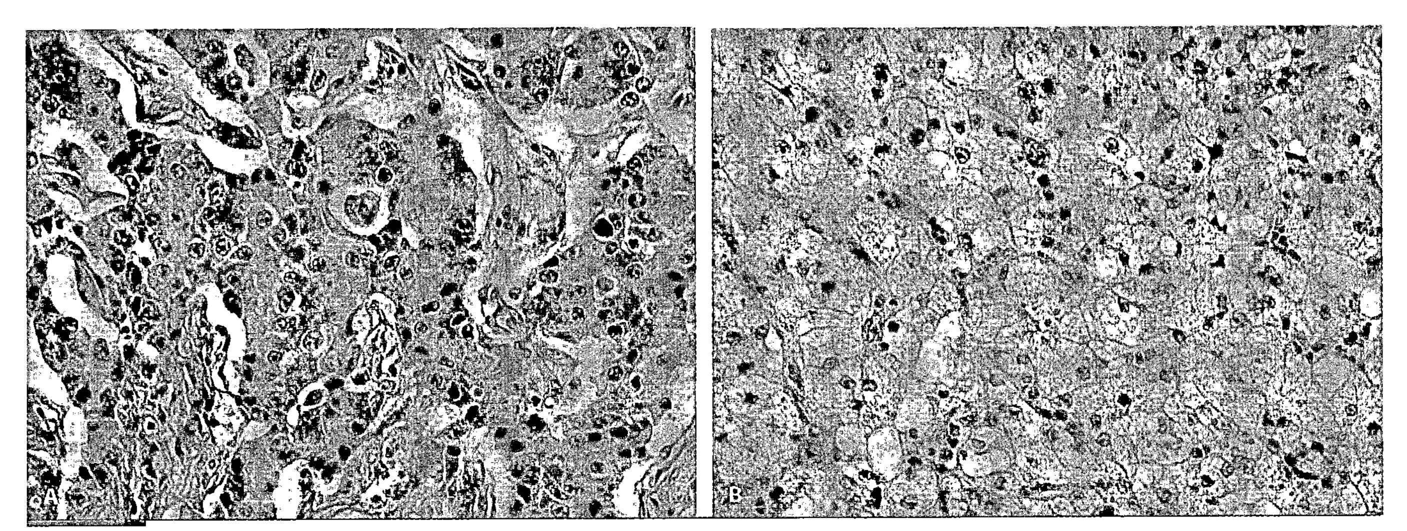

Figure 41.7
Less common patterns of pancreatic endocrine neoplasms (PENs). Oncocytic PENs **(A)** have abundant, granular eosinophilic cytoplasm due to numerous mitochondria. Clear-cell PENs **(B)** have foamy-to-clear cytoplasm due to accumulation of numerous small vesicles.

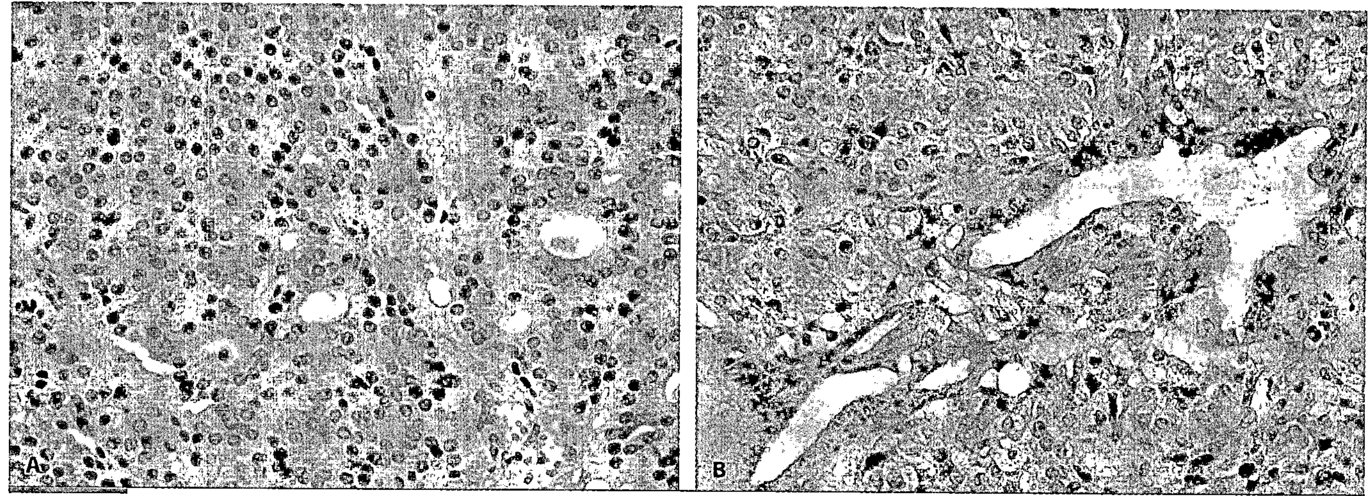

Figure 41.9
Glands in pancreatic endocrine neoplasms (PENs). In some cases, the neoplastic endocrine cells form lumina (A), where each gland is formed of cells similar to those in the solid regions of the neoplasm. In other PENs (B), nonneoplastic ductules are entrapped within the tumor. There is very close juxtaposition between the neoplastic endocrine cells and the nonneoplastic glandular epithelium.

Mitotic rate is an important measure of aggressiveness in PENs. Well-differentiated PENs are defined to have less than 10 mitotic figures per 10 high-power microscopic fields (hpf); neoplasms with 10 or more mitoses per 10 hpf are considered high-grade endocrine carcinomas (pg. 586). In many PENs, mitotic figures are nearly undetectable, a search of 30 to 50 hpf (or more) being required to find even a single mitotic figure. Some PENs have a higher proliferative rate, and the finding of 2 or more mitoses per 50 hpf places a PEN in a worse prognostic category.[29] Necrosis is also variably present; most commonly it is accompanied by an increase in proliferative rate and signifies a more aggressive PEN.

Glands may also be found in PENs and may take several forms. In some cases, the neoplastic endocrine cells form lumina (Fig. 41.9A). Although these gland-forming PENs may be mistaken for adenocarcinomas, the cells lining the lumina retain endocrine differentiation and are cytologically similar to the more abundant solid areas that are typically present. In other cases, nonneoplastic ductules are entrapped within PENs.[30,31] The neoplastic endocrine cells are often closely juxtaposed to the ductules, but they are cytologically distinct (Fig. 41.9B). Finally, true mixed ductal-endocrine carcinomas occur (see "Mixed" Endocrine Neoplasms).

Immunohistochemistry and Electron Microscopy

Once the diagnosis of PENs is suspected on the basis of the histologic features, several methods can be used to confirm the diagnosis. Classical silver staining techniques to demonstrate neurosecretory granules have largely been replaced by immunohistochemistry. Expression of general endocrine markers, including chromogranin, synaptophysin, and neural cell adhesion molecule (CD56), is detectable in essentially all PENs.[32] Synaptophysin expression is commonly more diffuse, and some PENs may demonstrate only focal staining for chromogranin (Fig. 41.10). Expression of peptides, such as insulin, glucagon, PP, somatostatin, gastrin, or vasoactive intestinal polypeptide, is common, and most functional PENs can be shown to produce the appropriate peptide by immunohistochemistry.[6] In addition, minor cell populations producing a variety of other peptides are commonly detectable.[33-35] Nonfunctional PENs also contain various peptide cell types, usually (but not inevitably) making up less than 25% of the total cell population. Other "ectopic" peptides are often produced as well, and exhaustive immunohistochemical labeling for species, such as is achieved with adrenocorticotropic hormone, bombesin, calcitonin, neurotensin, and so on, identifies additional secretory products.

Many PENs also immunolabel for glycoproteins, such as carcinoembryonic antigen and CA19.9,[29,36,37] especially those with gland formation. Focal acinar differentiation may also be present in scattered cells that label for trypsin or chymotrypsin.[37,38] A subset of PENs expresses CD99, as do normal islet cells. Labeling of PENs with the proliferation marker MIB1 demonstrates a relatively low proliferative rate, in keeping with their low mitotic rate. Generally, 1%–5% of the nuclei are labeled, but some examples demonstrate labeling of up to 10% of cells.[1]

Although many elegant studies documented the utility of electron microscopy for the diagnosis of PENs, this

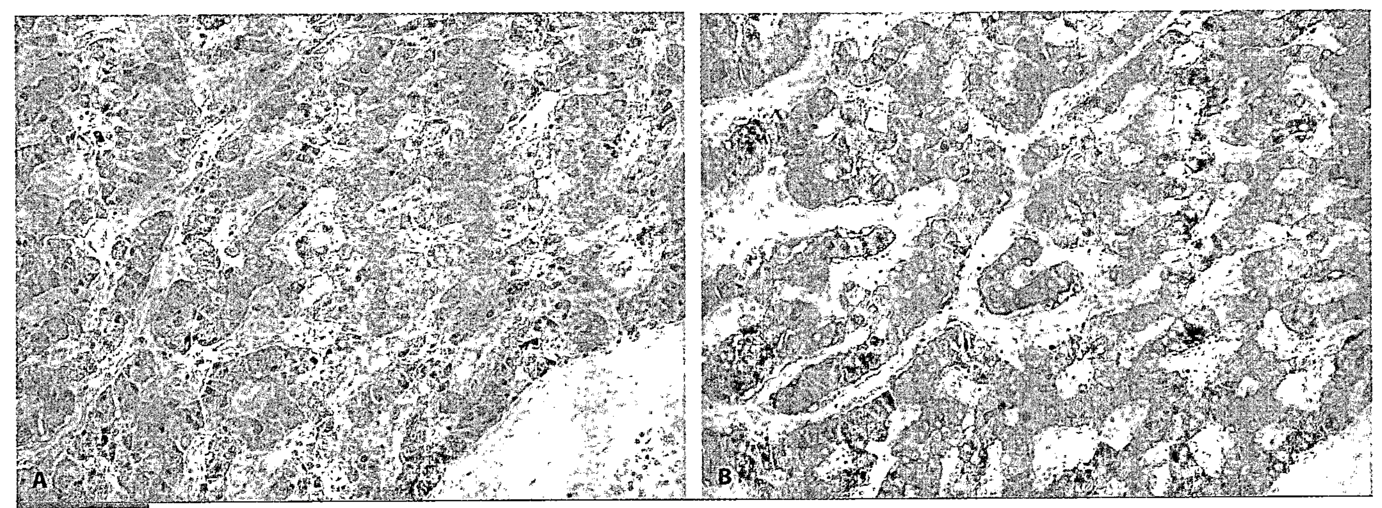

Figure 41.10
Immunohistochemical staining of pancreatic endocrine neoplasms (PENs). Most label with both chromogranin (A) and synaptophysin (B). In some PENs, the synaptophysin staining is more intense and diffuse.

technique has largely been supplanted by immunohistochemistry. If ultrastructural examination is performed, PENs contain relatively abundant 100- to 350-nm dense core neurosecretory granules.[39,40] Most have a nonspecific morphology, with dense core content separated by a halo from the limiting membrane. Secretory granules morphologically characteristic of α or β cells are sometimes found in the corresponding functional PENs.[35,41]

Functional Pancreatic Endocrine Neoplasms

From a purely morphologic standpoint, there are no specific microscopic findings that distinguish the different types of functional PENs.[42-44] Insulinomas are usually small; many cases measure less than 2 cm, presumably because insulinomas are exquisitely symptomatic and are detected at an early stage. Certain histologic features were classically described to be characteristic of specific functional PENs, such as stromal amyloid in insulinomas or gland formation in gastrinomas, but none are sufficiently specific to allow distinction from other types of PENs. Somatostatinomas occurring in the periampullary duodenum (glandular duodenal carcinoids) do have a distinctive appearance, including well-formed glands, eosinophilic cytoplasm, and numerous psammoma bodies,[45] but pancreatic somatostatinomas do not share these features.

Cytologic Findings

Fine-needle aspiration is a sensitive technique for the preoperative diagnosis of PENs.[46-49] Aspirates of PENs produce relatively cellular smears with a clean background. The cells are arranged in clusters and individually. Nuclei are round to oval and uniform, and the characteristic endocrine chromatin pattern is often present. The nuclei are eccentrically located, producing a plasmacytoid configuration to the cells (Fig. 41.11). Endocrine differentiation may be documented by immunohistochemical labeling for chromogranin or synaptophysin to confirm the diagnosis.[50]

Molecular Genetic Features

Recent cytogenetic and molecular studies have identified many chromosomal alterations in PENs. Interestingly, activation of oncogenes does not appear to play a major role in the development of these tumors. Com-

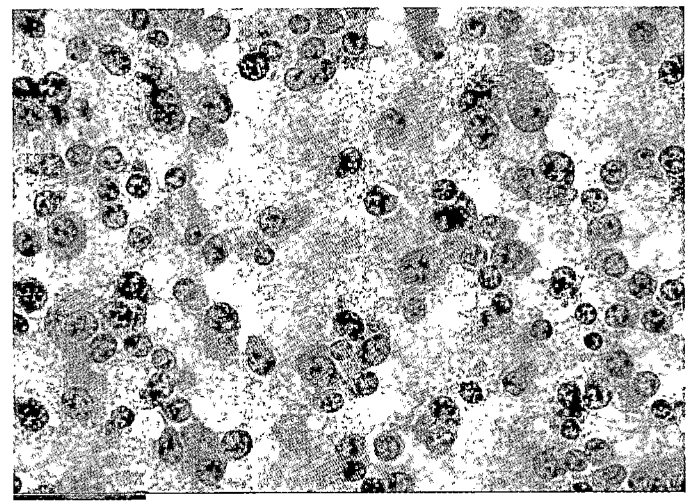

Figure 41.11
Fine-needle aspirate smear of pancreatic endocrine neoplasm. The cells are arranged individually and in loose clusters. Many exhibit a plasmacytoid appearance, with eccentrically located nuclei. The chromatin pattern is coarsely granular, characteristic of well-differentiated endocrine neoplasms.

parative genomic hybridization studies demonstrate that chromosomal losses are more common than gains.[51-53] In PENs arising in patients with MEN1 or VHL syndromes, the genetic defect responsible for the syndrome is involved in the pathogenesis of the pancreatic neoplasms.[20,21,54] PENs arising in MEN1 patients show a germline mutation in the *menin* gene on chromosome 11q13 coupled with a somatic (acquired) loss of the normal copy of this gene. Studies on sporadic PENs have also detected relatively common losses at 11q13 or elsewhere on the short arm of chromosome 11 (70%), but specific *menin* gene mutations are present in only approximately 20% of the neoplasms, suggesting involvement of another tumor-suppressor gene.[55-62] Interestingly, insulinomas have a much lower frequency of mutations in the *menin* gene than most other functional PENs and nonfunctional PENs. The VHL gene is usually normal in sporadic PENs.[63]

The chromosomal alterations that have been described in sporadic PENs are relatively consistent and include gains at 4p, 4q, 5q, 7p, 7q, 9q, 12q, 14q, 17p, 17q, and 20q and losses at 1p, 3p, 6q, 9p, 10p, 10q, 11q, 18q, 22q, Y, and X.[51-53,64,65] Some of these losses are associated with more aggressive clinical behavior. The specific genes involved at most of these loci have yet to be determined.

Many of the genes targeted in the development of ductal adenocarcinomas of the pancreas have been examined in PENs, and most of these are not targeted in PENs.[57,66-68] In particular, *KRAS2*, *TP53*, *p16*, and *SMAD4* are not mutated in most PENs, although the *p16* gene is inactivated via hypermethylation of the promoter in 40% of cases.[69-71] *HER2/neu* amplification is also not commonly detected.[72] It appears that promotor methylation, rather than mutation, may be a relatively common mechanism of tumor-suppressor gene inactivation in PENs.[69]

Other studies have examined gene expression in PENs to determine which genes are significantly over- or underexpressed relative to normal islet cells. Overexpressed genes include putative oncogenes, growth factors, and cell adhesion and migration molecules, whereas the cell cycle regulator *p21*, the cell surface glycoprotein MIC2 (CD99), and putative metastasis-suppressor genes are among those underexpressed.[73] Data from these studies may shed light on pathways important in tumorigenesis in PENs, and some of these species may prove to be prognostically relevant.

Some of the genetic alterations in PENs are more commonly detected in larger or more advanced-stage neoplasms, suggesting that there is continuing genetic progression in PENs that parallels clinical progression. Fewer gains and losses of genetic material occur in smaller PENs (<2 cm), although losses at 1p and 11q and gains at 9q are already present.[53] In fact, some data suggest that smaller PENs may represent poly- or oligoclonal proliferations from which more aggressive monoclonal neoplasms may arise.[74]

Natural History and Prognostic Considerations

The natural history of PENs is highly variable. Small neoplasms without adverse prognostic features are readily curable by surgical resection. Many insulinomas fall into this category because they generally measure less than 2 cm when detected. Most other functional and all nonfunctional PENs are usually larger at diagnosis, and the outcome is much less favorable.[75] Approximately 50%–80% of these neoplasms recur or metastasize,[1,10,76-79] and up to 30% of patients already have metastatic disease at first presentation. Functional PENs with mixed or "ectopic" syndromes are reportedly more aggressive.[15,16] The 5-year survival after surgical resection for nonfunctioning PENs is 65%, but the 10-year survival is only 45%.[29]

Metastases usually occur first in regional lymph nodes and liver,[80] with more distant metastases developing late in the course of the disease. Despite the high rate of metastasis, relatively long survival is typical. Because the disease progresses slowly, many patients live for several years or even longer than a decade after the appearance of metastases. Unfortunately, metastatic PENs are relatively resistant to chemotherapy, and cure is unlikely after metastases develop.

One of the most controversial aspects of PENs is the predicting of their clinical behavior. For many years, attempts were made to separate PENs into benign and malignant categories; recently, a borderline malignant potential category was proposed as well.[1] Because some PENs that demonstrate malignant behavior have deceptively bland histologic features, it was believed that few pathological parameters accurately stratify PENs, and only the finding of locally invasive growth, large-vessel invasion, or distant metastases could be considered absolute criteria of malignancy. Even with these criteria, however, some "malignant" PENs do not recur after resection and some "benign" PENs lacking these features ultimately prove lethal. Subsequently, it was recognized that PENs treated by surgical resection have had the natural history of the neoplasm interrupted, and that a completely resected PEN that does not recur may not have been biologically benign, because malignant neoplasms can be cured by early surgical intervention.

Current studies have focused on defining prognostic parameters to predict which resected PENs are most likely to recur or metastasize, essentially treating all clinically relevant PENs as malignant neoplasms.[29] The exception is the endocrine microadenoma, which can be accepted as benign. Of course, most microadenomas are incidental findings without clinical symptoms. Features of prognostic significance in PENs include tumor size, mitotic rate, presence of necrosis, extrapancreatic invasion, and vascular invasion, in addition to the presence of nodal or distant metastases.[1,29,81] Peptide production detected in the serum or by immunohistochemistry is not a prognostic factor for nonfunctional PENs.[29] Nuclear pleomorphism is also not a useful predictor[28]; however, some studies have demonstrated a correlation between overall nuclear grade and prognosis.[29] Other factors reportedly predictive of more aggressive behavior include loss of progesterone receptor expression,[82,83] aneuploidy,[84,85] increased Ki67 or proliferating cell nuclear antigen labeling index,[86] loss of heterozygosity of chromosome 17p13,[12] loss of heterozygosity of chromosome 22q,[65] increased fractional allelic loss,[64] up-regulated CD44 isoform expression,[87,88] and immunohistochemical expression of cytokeratin 19.[89] Other allelic losses associated with malignant behavior include loss of chromosomes 1p,[90] 3p,[51,66,91] 6q,[51,92] and X.[93] Aberrant methylation of tumor-suppressor gene promoters is also more commonly detected in advanced-stage PENs,[69] as is up-regulation of vascular endothelial growth factor C.[94] Loss of *p27* expression[95] and methylation of the promotor of the DNA mismatch repair gene *hMLH1*[96] appear to be markers of indolent behavior.

Although no uniform grading system has been used for PENs (other than the distinction from high-grade endocrine carcinomas), a proposal has been made to use the mitotic rate and presence of necrosis to separate low-grade PENs from an intermediate-grade category.[29] Under that proposal, cases demonstrating two or more mitoses per 50 hpf or the presence of necrosis are considered intermediate grade, whereas those lacking these features are considered low grade. Alternatively, PENs have been separated into benign, borderline, and low-grade malignant categories on the basis of a combination of tumor size, mitotic rate, vascular invasion, gross local invasion, and metastases.[1,97]

Differential Diagnosis

The pathological differential diagnosis for PENs includes acinar cell carcinoma, pancreatoblastoma, solid-pseudopapillary tumor, and ductal adenocarcinoma. Features helpful for separating these entities are presented in Table 41.3. The first three share with PENs a solid, hypercellular appearance and a nesting growth pattern.

Table 41.3 Differential Diagnosis of Pancreatic Endocrine Neoplasms

	Histologic Findings	Immunohistochemical Findings
Pancreatic endocrine neoplasm	Organoid architecture, hyalinized stroma, coarsely clumped chromatin, few mitosis	Chromogranin (+) Synaptophysin (+)
Acinar cell carcinoma	Solid and acinar patterns, granular eosinophilic cytoplasm, prominent nucleoli, plentiful mitoses	Trypsin (+) Chymotrypsin (+) Chromogranin (F) Synaptophysin (F)
Pancreatoblastoma	Solid and acinar patterns, squamoid corpuscles, cellular stroma	Trypsin (+) Chymotrypsin (+) Chromogranin (F) Synaptophysin (F)
Solid-pseudopapillary tumor	Solid and pseudopapillary patterns, nuclear grooves, hyaline cytoplasmic globules, foamy histiocytes	Vimentin (+) α_1-Antitrypsin (+) Chromogranin (−) Trypsin (−)
Ductal adenocarcinoma	Simple glands, intracellular mucin, desmoplastic stroma, marked nuclear atypia	Chromogranin (F)

Abbreviations: +, positive; −, negative; F, focally positive.

Acinar cell carcinoma and pancreatoblastoma exhibit acinar differentiation and demonstrate well-formed acinar structures and granular, eosinophilic cytoplasm.[98-100] Pancreatoblastomas also have distinctive squamoid corpuscles and a hypercellular stromal component. Both acinar cell carcinoma and pancreatoblastoma consistently produce pancreatic exocrine enzymes and can be distinguished from PENs by immunohistochemical labeling for trypsin and chymotrypsin, which are usually diffusely expressed. However, both acinar cell carcinoma and pancreatoblastoma may also contain a minor component of endocrine cells, so focal labeling for chromogranin and synaptophysin may be found. Solid-pseudopapillary tumors and PENs have many histologic similarities but can be distinguished by the presence of pseudopapillae, nuclear grooves, aggregates of foamy tumor cells and histocytes, and collections of large hyaline globules.[101] On immunohistochemistry, solid-pseudopapillary tumors do express CD56 and often also synaptophysin, but they are never positive for chromogranin. The hyaline globules of solid-pseudopapillary tumors stain for α_1-antitrypsin, and there is consistent positivity for CD10 and nuclear accumulation of β-catenin. Solid-pseudopapillary tumors express vimentin but are negative or only focally positive for keratin. Pancreatic ductal adenocarcinomas are generally not difficult to distinguish from PENs, with the exception of PENs that exhibit gland formation. Even in such PENs, the glands are found within larger nests of cells, in contrast to the individual infiltrating glands of ductal adenocarcinomas, and intracellular mucin is not present. Ductal adenocarcinomas usually also have a higher mitotic rate and more significant nuclear pleomorphism.

Endocrine microadenomas may be confused with enlarged non-neoplastic islets.[102] Immunohistochemical staining for islet peptides is helpful. Non-neoplastic islets retain the normal proportions and distribution of peptide cell types, whereas microadenomas generally have a predominance of one cell type (commonly α or PP cells).

"Mixed" Endocrine Neoplasms

Minor endocrine elements are relatively common in predominantly exocrine pancreatic neoplasms. Thus, it should not be surprising that rare neoplasms exist in which both endocrine and exocrine components are significantly represented. These "mixed" neoplasms have been arbitrarily defined to contain more than 25% of each component, and endocrine, acinar, and ductal lines of differentiation may all be represented (Fig. 41.12). Reported mixed neoplasms that contain an endocrine component include mixed ductal-endocrine carcinoma, mixed acinar-endocrine carcinoma, and mixed acinar-endocrine-ductal carcinoma.[103-109] In most reported examples, the exocrine elements predominate. The different cell types are usually intimately intermixed, and immunohistochemical labeling is often necessary to detect the various lines of differentiation. Ductal differentiation in the form of lumen formation or expression of glycoproteins such as CA19.9 is common in conventional PENs[50] and

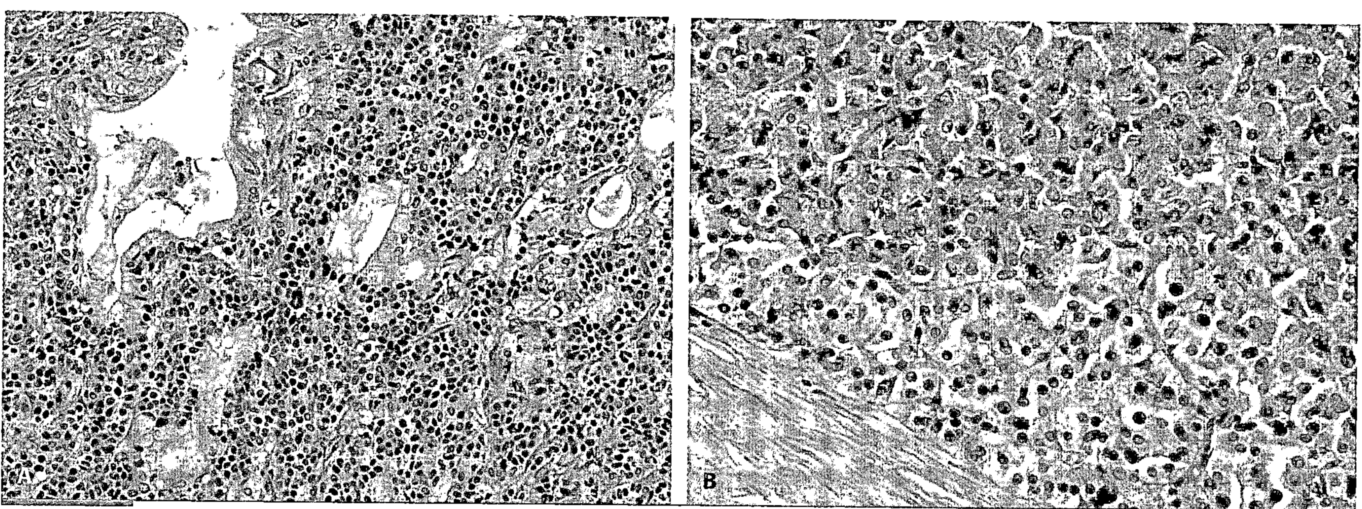

Figure 41.12
Mixed endocrine carcinomas. In mixed ductal-endocrine carcinomas **(A)**, there are solid nests of endocrine cells mixed with neoplastic ductal structures that contain mucin and markedly atypical nuclei. A mixed acinar-endocrine carcinoma **(B)**, contains well-differentiated endocrine cells with round, centrally located nuclei and pale cytoplasm (*bottom*) as well as acinar elements that have basally located nuclei with prominent nucleoli and granular, eosinophilic cytoplasm (*top*).

does not constitute sufficient evidence for a diagnosis of mixed ductal-endocrine carcinoma. Rather, a separate distinct gland-forming component with intracellular mucin production should be found combined with the endocrine elements. Most reported mixed pancreatic neoplasms have demonstrated aggressive clinical behavior, paralleling that of the more aggressive exocrine component.

High-Grade Endocrine Carcinoma

High-grade endocrine carcinomas are extremely rare in the pancreas. These neoplasms are related to small-cell carcinomas,[110-112] and metastasis from sites such as the lung have to be excluded before an example can be accepted as primary in the pancreas. Most patients are older adults, similar to the distribution of ductal adenocarcinomas. The neoplasms are often large and metastatic at diagnosis, so resected examples are few. Histologically, high-grade endocrine carcinomas may be composed of either small or large cells (Fig. 41.13). The neoplastic cells grow in diffuse sheets and have a markedly infiltrative growth pattern. There is often little nesting or other architectural patterns. The principle feature that separates this group from well-differentiated PENs is the proliferative rate. More than 10 mitoses per 10 hpf should be found, and often the rate is 50 or more. In addition, there is abundant necrosis. A diagnosis of small-cell carcinoma may be rendered for a high-grade endocrine carcinoma when cells with minimal cytoplasm and fusiform nuclei with a granular chromatin pattern and inconspicuous nucleoli predominate. In other high-grade endocrine carcinomas, the cells are larger, with moderate amounts of cytoplasm, the nuclei are round, and nucleoli are prominent. These large-cell endocrine carcinomas must be distinguished from poorly differentiated carcinomas lacking endocrine differentiation, so immunohistochemical labeling for chromogranin or synaptophysin must be performed for the diagnosis to be confirmed. High-grade endocrine carcinomas of the pancreas are highly aggressive neoplasms, with a natural history equal to or more virulent than that of ductal adenocarcinomas.

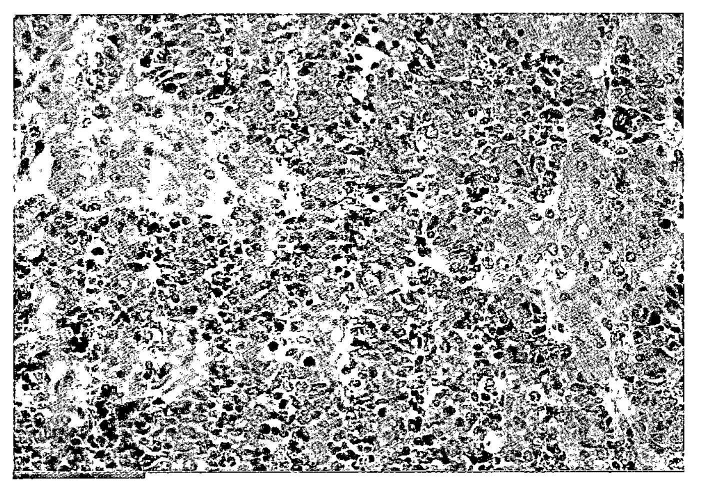

Figure 41.13
Small-cell carcinoma of the pancreas. This high-grade endocrine carcinoma is composed of sheets of small cells with fusiform nuclei and minimal cytoplasm. The mitotic rate is very high, consistent with the high-grade nature of this neoplasm.

References

1. Solcia E, Capella C, Klöppel G. *Tumors of the Pancreas*. 3rd series. Washington, DC: Armed Forces Institute of Pathology; 1997.
2. Conklin JL. Cytogenesis of the human fetal pancreas. *Am J Anat*. 1962;111:181–189.
3. Klimstra DS. Pancreas. In: Sternberg SS, ed. *Histology for Pathologists*. 2nd ed. Philadelphia: Lippincott-Raven; 1997: 613–647.
4. Kimura W, Kuroda A, Morioka Y. Clinical pathology of endocrine tumors of the pancreas: analysis of autopsy cases. *Dig Dis Sci*. 1991;36:933–942.
5. Shorter NA, Glick RD, Klimstra DS, et al. Malignant pancreatic tumors in childhood and adolescence: the Memorial Sloan-Kettering experience, 1967 to present. *J Pediatr Surg*. 2002;37:887–892.
6. Mukai K, Grotting JC, Greider MH, Rosai J. Retrospective study of 77 pancreatic endocrine tumors using the immunoperoxidase method. *Am J Surg Pathol*. 1982;6:387–399.
7. Larsson LI, Schwartz T, Lundqvist G, et al. Occurrence of human pancreatic polypeptide in pancreatic endocrine tumors: possible implication in the watery diarrhea syndrome. *Am J Pathol*. 1976;85:675–684.
8. Tomita T, Kimmel JR, Friesen SR, et al. Pancreatic polypeptide in islet cell tumors: morphologic and functional correlations. *Cancer*. 1985;56:1649–1657.
9. Broughan TA, Leslie JD, Soto JM, Hermann RE. Pancreatic islet cell tumours. *Surgery*. 1986;99:671–678.
10. Kent RB, van Heerden JA, Weiland LH. Nonfunctioning islet cell tumors. *Ann Surg*. 1981;193:185–190.
11. Klöppel G, Heitz PU. Pancreatic endocrine tumors. *Pathol Res Pract*. 1988;183:155–168.
12. Gumbs AA, Moore PS, Falconi M, et al. Review of the clinical, histological, and molecular aspects of pancreatic endocrine neoplasms. *J Surg Oncol*. 2002;81:45–53.
13. Klöppel G, Willemer S, Stamm B, et al. Pancreatic lesions and hormonal profile of pancreatic tumors in multiple endocrine neoplasia type I: an immunocytochemical study of nine patients. *Cancer*. 1986;57:1824–1832.
14. Le Bodic MF, Heymann MF, Lecomte M, et al. Immunohistochemical study of 100 pancreatic tumors in 28 patients with multiple endocrine neoplasia, type I. *Am J Surg Pathol*. 1996;20:1378–1384.
15. Clark ES, Carney JA. Pancreatic islet cell tumor associated with Cushing's syndrome. *Am J Surg Pathol*. 1984;8:917–924.
16. Doppman JL, Nieman LK, Cutler GB, et al. Adrenocorticotropic hormone–secreting islet cell tumors: are they always malignant? *Radiology*. 1994;190:59–64.

17. Gordon DL, Lo MC, Schwartz MA. Carcinoid of the pancreas. *Am J Med.* 1971;51:412–415.
18. Hammel PR, Vilgrain V, Terris B, et al. Pancreatic involvement in von Hippel-Lindau disease. *Gastroenterology.* 2000;119:1087–1095.
19. Hull MT, Warfel KA, Muller J, Higgins JT. Familial islet cell tumors in von Hippel-Lindau's disease. *Cancer.* 1979;44:1523–1526.
20. Chandrasekharappa SC, Guru SC, Manickam P, et al. Positional cloning of the gene for multiple endocrine neoplasia-type 1. *Science.* 1997;276:404–407.
21. Latif F, Tory K, Gnarra J, et al. Identification of the von Hippel-Lindau disease tumor suppressor gene. *Science.* 1993;260:1317–1320.
22. Hoang MP, Hruban RH, Albores-Saavedra J. Clear cell endocrine pancreatic tumor mimicking renal cell carcinoma: a distinctive neoplasm of von Hippel-Lindau disease. *Am J Surg Pathol.* 2001;25:602–609.
23. Ligneau B, Lombard-Bohas C, Partensky C, et al. Cystic endocrine tumors of the pancreas: clinical, radiologic, and histopathologic features in 13 cases. *Am J Surg Pathol.* 2001;25:752–760.
24. Greider MH, DeSchryver-Kecskemeti K, Kraus FT. Psammoma bodies in endocrine tumors of the gastroenteropancreatic axis: a rather common occurrence. *Semin Diagn Pathol.* 1984;1:19–29.
25. Carstens PH, Cressman FK, Jr. Malignant oncocytic carcinoid of the pancreas. *Ultrastruct Pathol.* 1989;13:69–75.
26. Gotchall J, Traweek ST, Stenzel P. Benign oncocytic endocrine tumor of the pancreas in a patient with polyarteritis nodosa. *Hum Pathol.* 1987;18:967–969.
27. Pachioni D, Papotti M, Macri L, et al. Pancreatic oncocytic endocrine tumors: cytologic features of two cases. *Acta Cytol.* 1996;40:742–746.
28. Zee S, Hochwald S, Conlon K, et al. Pleomorphic pancreatic endocrine neoplasms (PENs): a variant commonly confused with adenocarcinoma. *Mod Pathol.* 2001;14:1212A.
29. Hochwald SN, Zee S, Conlon KC, et al. Prognostic factors in pancreatic endocrine neoplasms: an analysis of 136 cases with a proposal for low-grade and intermediate-grade groups. *J Clin Oncol.* 2002;20:2633–2642.
30. Deshpande V, Selig MK, Nielsen GP, et al. Ductulo-insular pancreatic endocrine neoplasms: clinicopathologic analysis of a unique subtype of pancreatic endocrine neoplasms. *Am J Surg Pathol.* 2003;27:461–468.
31. van Eeden S, de Leng WWJ, Offerhaus GJA, et al. Ductulo-insular tumors of the pancreas: endocrine tumors with entrapped non-neoplastic ductules. *Am J Surg Pathol.* 2004; 28:813–820.
32. Lloyd RV, Mervak T, Schmidt K, et al. Immunohistochemical detection of chromogranin and neuron-specific enolase in pancreatic endocrine neoplasms. *Am J Surg Pathol.* 1984;8:607–614.
33. Heitz PU, Kasper M, Polak JM, Kloppel G. Pancreatic endocrine tumors: immunocytochemical analysis of 125 tumors. *Hum Pathol.* 1982;13:263–271.
34. Larsson LI, Grimelius L, Hakanson R, et al. Mixed endocrine pancreatic tumors producing several peptide hormones. *Am J Pathol.* 1975;79:271–284.
35. Liu TH, Tseng HC, Zhu Y, et al. Insulinoma: an immunocytochemical and morphologic analysis of 95 cases. *Cancer.* 1985;56:1420–1429.
36. Arihiro K, Inai K. Malignant islet cell tumor of the pancreas with multiple hormone production and expression of CEA and CA19-9. *Acta Pathol Jpn.* 1991;41:150–157.
37. Kamisawa T, Tu Y, Egawa N, et al. Ductal and acinar differentiation in pancreatic endocrine tumors. *Dig Dis Sci.* 2002;47:2254–2261.
38. Yantiss RK, Chang HK, Farraye FA, et al. Prevalence and prognostic significance of acinar cell differentiation in pancreatic endocrine tumors. *Am J Surg Pathol.* 2002;26:893–901.
39. Erlandson RA. *Diagnostic Transmission Electron Microscopy of Tumors.* New York: Raven Press; 1994.
40. Fitzpatrick B, Ordonez NG, Mackay B. Islet cell tumor. *Ultrastr Pathol.* 1991;15:579–584.
41. Greider MH, Elliott DW. Electron microscopy of human pancreatic tumors of islet cell origin. *Am J Pathol.* 1964;44:663–678.
42. Bordi C, Ravazzola M, Baetens D, et al. A study of glucagonomas by light and electron microscopy and immunofluorescence. *Diabetes.* 1979;28:925–936.
43. Capella C, Polak JM, Buffa R, et al. Morphologic patterns and diagnostic criteria of VIP-producing endocrine tumors: a histologic, histochemical, ultrastructural, and biochemical study of 32 cases. *Cancer.* 1983;52:1860–1874.
44. Donow C, Pipeleers-Marichal M, Schroder S, et al. Surgical pathology of gastrinoma: site, size, multicentricity, association with multiple endocrine neoplasia type 1, and malignancy. *Cancer.* 1991;68:1329–1334.
45. Griffiths DF, Jasani B, Newman GR, et al. Glandular duodenal carcinoid: a somatostatin rich tumor with endocrine associations. *J Clin Pathol.* 1984;37:164–169.
46. al-Kaisi N, Weaver MG, Abdul-Karim FW, Siegler E. Fine needle aspiration cytology of neuroendocrine tumors of the pancreas: a cytologic, immunocytochemical and electron microscopic study. *Acta Cytol.* 1992;36:655–660.
47. Bell DA. Cytologic features of islet-cell tumors. *Acta Cytol.* 1987;31:485–492.
48. Collins BT, Cramer HM. Fine-needle aspiration cytology of islet cell tumors. *Diagn Cytopathol.* 1996;15:37–45.
49. Sneige N, Ordonez NG, Veanattukalathil S, Samaan NA. Fine-needle aspiration cytology in pancreatic endocrine tumors. *Diagn Cytopathol.* 1987;3:35–40.
50. Labate AM, Klimstra DL, Zakowski MF. Comparative cytologic features of pancreatic acinar cell carcinoma and islet cell tumor. *Diagn Cytopathol.* 1997;16:112–116.
51. Speel EJ, Richter J, Moch H, et al. Genetic differences in endocrine pancreatic tumor subtypes detected by comparative genomic hybridization. *Am J Pathol.* 1999;155:1787–1794.
52. Stumpf E, Aalto Y, Hoog A, et al. Chromosomal alterations in human pancreatic endocrine tumors. *Genes Chromosomes Cancer.* 2000;29:83–87.
53. Zhao J, Moch H, Scheidweiler AF, et al. Genomic imbalances in the progression of endocrine pancreatic tumors. *Genes Chromosomes Cancer.* 2001;32:364–372.
54. Lubensky IA, Pack S, Ault D, et al. Multiple neuroendocrine tumors of the pancreas in von Hippel-Lindau disease patients: histopathological and molecular genetic analysis. *Am J Pathol.* 1998;153:223–231.

55. Asteria C, Anagni M, Fugazzola L, et al. MEN1 gene mutations are a rare event in patients with sporadic neuroendocrine tumors. *Eur J Intern Med.* 2002;13:319–323.
56. Cupisti K, Hoppner W, Dotzenrath C, et al. Lack of MEN1 gene mutations in 27 sporadic insulinomas. *Eur J Clin Invest.* 2000;30:325–329.
57. Gortz B, Roth J, Krahenmann A, et al. Mutations and allelic deletions of the MEN1 gene are associated with a subset of sporadic endocrine pancreatic and neuroendocrine tumors and not restricted to foregut neoplasms. *Am J Pathol.* 1999;154:429–436.
58. Hessman O, Lindberg D, Einarsson A, et al. Genetic alterations on 3p, 11q13, and 18q in nonfamilial and MEN 1-associated pancreatic endocrine tumors. *Genes Chromosomes Cancer.* 1999;26:258–264.
59. Komminoth P. Review: multiple endocrine neoplasia type 1, sporadic neuroendocrine tumors, and MENIN. *Diagn Mol Pathol.* 1999;8:107–112.
60. Shan L, Nakamura Y, Nakamura M, et al. Somatic mutations of multiple endocrine neoplasia type 1 gene in the sporadic endocrine tumors. *Lab Invest.* 1998;78:471–475.
61. Wang EH, Ebrahimi SA, Wu AY, et al. Mutation of the MENIN gene in sporadic pancreatic endocrine tumors. *Cancer Res.* 1998;58:4417–4420.
62. Zhuang Z, Vortmeyer AO, Pack S, et al. Somatic mutations of the MEN1 tumor suppressor gene in sporadic gastrinomas and insulinomas. *Cancer Res.* 1997;57:4682–4686.
63. Moore PS, Missiaglia E, Antonello D, et al. Role of disease-causing genes in sporadic pancreatic endocrine tumors: MEN1 and VHL. *Genes Chromosomes Cancer.* 2001;32:177–181.
64. Rigaud G, Missiaglia E, Moore PS, et al. High resolution allelotype of nonfunctional pancreatic endocrine tumors: identification of two molecular subgroups with clinical implications. *Cancer Res.* 2001;61:285–292.
65. Wild A, Langer P, Celik I, et al. Chromosome 22q in pancreatic endocrine tumors: identification of a homozygous deletion and potential prognostic associations of allelic deletions. *Eur J Endocrinol.* 2002;147:507–513.
66. Chung DC, Smith AP, Louis DN, et al. A novel pancreatic endocrine tumor suppressor gene locus on chromosome 3p with clinical prognostic implications. *J Clin Invest.* 1997;100:404–410.
67. Moore PS, Orlandini S, Zamboni G, et al. Pancreatic tumours: molecular pathways implicated in ductal cancer are involved in ampullary but not in exocrine nonductal or endocrine tumorigenesis. *Br J Cancer.* 2001;84:253–262.
68. Pellegata NS, Sessa F, Renault B, et al. K-ras and p53 gene mutations in pancreatic cancer: ductal and nonductal tumors progress through different genetic lesions. *Cancer Res.* 1994;54:1556–1560.
69. House MG, Herman JG, Guo MZ, et al. Aberrant hypermethylation of tumor suppressor genes in pancreatic endocrine neoplasms. *Ann Surg.* 2003;238:423–431.
70. Muscarella P, Melvin WS, Fisher WE, et al. Genetic alterations in gastrinomas and nonfunctioning pancreatic neuroendocrine tumors: an analysis of p16/MST1 tumor suppressor gene inactivation. *Cancer Res.* 1998;58:237–240.
71. Serrano J, Goebel SU, Peghini PL, et al. Alterations in the p16INK4a/CDKN2A tumor suppressor gene in gastrinomas. *J Clin Endocrinol Metab.* 2000;85:4146–4156.
72. Goebel SU, Iwamoto M, Raffeld M, et al. Her-2/neu expression and gene amplification in gastrinomas: correlations with tumor biology, growth, and aggressiveness. *Cancer Res.* 2002;62:3702–3710.
73. Maitra A, Hansel DE, Argani P, et al. Global expression analysis of well-differentiated pancreatic endocrine neoplasms using oligonucleotide microarrays. *Clin Cancer Res.* 2003;9:5988–5995.
74. Perren A, Roth J, Muletta-Feurer S, et al. Clonal analysis of sporadic pancreatic endocrine tumours. *J Pathol.* 1998; 186:363–371.
75. Brentjens R, Saltz L. Islet cell tumors of the pancreas: the medical oncologist's perspective. *Surg Clin North Am.* 2001;81:527–542.
76. Dial PF, Braasch JW, Rossi RL, et al. Management of nonfunctioning islet cell tumors of the pancreas. *Surg Clin North Am.* 1985;65:291–299.
77. Eckhauser FE, Cheung PS, Vinik AI, et al. Nonfunctioning malignant neuroendocrine tumors of the pancreas. *Surgery.* 1986;100:978–988.
78. Liu TH, Zhu Y, Cui QC, et al. Nonfunctioning pancreatic endocrine tumors: an immunohistochemical and electron microscopic analysis of 26 cases. *Pathol Res Pract.* 1992; 188:191–198.
79. Venkatesh S, Ordonez NG, Ajani J, et al. Islet cell carcinoma of the pancreas: a study of 98 patients. *Cancer.* 1990;65:354–357.
80. Eriksson B, Oberg K, Skogseid B. Neuroendocrine pancreatic tumors: clinical findings in a prospective study of 84 patients. *Acta Oncol.* 1989;28:373–377.
81. La Rosa S, Sessa F, Capella C, et al. Prognostic criteria in nonfunctioning pancreatic endocrine tumours. *Virchows Arch.* 1996;429:323–333.
82. Pelosi G, Bresaola E, Bogina G, et al. Endocrine tumors of the pancreas: Ki-67 immunoreactivity on paraffin sections is an independent predictor for malignancy: a comparative study with proliferating-cell nuclear antigen and progesterone receptor protein immunostaining, mitotic index, and other clinicopathologic variables. *Hum Pathol.* 1996;27:1124–1134.
83. Viale G, Doglioni C, Gambacorta M, et al. Progesterone receptor immunoreactivity in pancreatic endocrine tumors: an immunocytochemical study of 156 neuroendocrine tumors of the pancreas, gastrointestinal and respiratory tracts, and skin. *Cancer.* 1992;70:2268–2277.
84. Bottger T, Seidl C, Seifert JK, et al. Value of quantitative DNA analysis in endocrine tumors of the pancreas. *Oncology.* 1997;54:318–323.
85. Kenny BD, Sloan JM, Hamilton PW, et al. The role of morphometry in predicting prognosis in pancreatic islet cell tumors. *Cancer.* 1989;64:460–465.
86. Clarke MR, Baker EE, Weyant RJ, et al. Proliferative activity in pancreatic endocrine tumors: association with function, metastases, and survival. *Endocr Pathol.* 1997;8:181–187.
87. Imam H, Eriksson B, Oberg K. Expression of CD44 variant isoforms and association to the benign form of endocrine pancreatic tumours. *Ann Oncol.* 2000;11:295–300.
88. Komminoth P, Seelentag WK, Saremaslani P, et al. CD44 isoform expression in the diffuse neuroendocrine system. II. Benign and malignant tumors. *Histochem Cell Biol.* 1996;106:551–562.

89. Deshpande V, Muzikansky A, Ferandez del Castillo C. Cytokeratin 19 is a powerful predictor of survival in pancreatic endocrine tumors. *Mod Pathol.* 2003;16:272A.
90. Ebrahimi SA, Wang EH, Wu A, et al. Deletion of chromosome 1 predicts prognosis in pancreatic endocrine tumors. *Cancer Res.* 1999;59:311–315.
91. Barghorn A, Komminoth P, Bachmann D, et al. Deletion at 3p25.3-p23 is frequently encountered in endocrine pancreatic tumours and is associated with metastatic progression. *J Pathol.* 2001;194:451–458.
92. Barghorn A, Speel EJ, Farspour B, et al. Putative tumor suppressor loci at 6q22 and 6q23-q24 are involved in the malignant progression of sporadic endocrine pancreatic tumors. *Am J Pathol.* 2001;158:1903–1911.
93. Missiaglia E, Moore PS, Williamson J, et al. Sex chromosome anomalies in pancreatic endocrine tumors. *Int J Cancer.* 2002;98:532–538.
94. Hansel DE, Rahman A, Hermans J, et al. Liver metastases arising from well-differentiated pancreatic endocrine neoplasms demonstrate increased VEGF-C expression. *Mod Pathol.* 2003;16:652–659.
95. Rahman A, Maitra A, Ashfaq R, et al. Loss of p27 nuclear expression in a prognostically favorable subset of well-differentiated pancreatic endocrine neoplasms. *Am J Clin Pathol.* 2003;120:685–690.
96. House MG, Herman JG, Guo MZ, et al. Prognostic value of hMLH1 hypermethylation and microsatellite instability in pancreatic endocrine neoplasms. *Surgery.* 2003;134:902–908.
97. Solcia E, Rindi G, Paolotti D, et al. Clinicopathological profile as a basis for classification of the endocrine tumours of the gastroenteropancreatic tract. *Ann Oncol.* 1999;10[suppl 2]:S9–15.
98. Klimstra DS, Heffess CS, Oertel JE, Rosai J. Acinar cell carcinoma of the pancreas: a clinicopathologic study of 28 cases. *Am J Surg Pathol.* 1992;16:815–837.
99. Klimstra DS, Wenig BM, Adair CF, Heffess CS. Pancreatoblastoma: a clinicopathologic study and review of the literature. *Am J Surg Pathol.* 1995;19:1371–1389.
100. Ordonez NG. Pancreatic acinar cell carcinoma. *Adv Anat Pathol.* 2001;8:144–159.
101. Klimstra DS, Wenig BM, Heffess CS. Solid-pseudopapillary tumor of the pancreas: a typically cystic carcinoma of low malignant potential. *Semin Diagn Pathol.* 2000;17:66–80.
102. Bartow SA, Mukai K, Rosai J. Pseudoneoplastic proliferation of endocrine cells in pancreatic fibrosis. *Cancer.* 1981;47:2627–2633.
103. Kashiwabara K, Nakajima T, Shinkai H, et al. A case of malignant duct-islet cell tumor of the pancreas: immunohistochemical and cytofluorometric study. *Acta Pathol Jpn.* 1991;41:636–641.
104. Klimstra DS, Rosai J, Heffess CS. Mixed acinar-endocrine carcinomas of the pancreas. *Am J Surg Pathol.* 1994;18:765–778.
105. Kloppel G. Mixed exocrine-endocrine tumors of the pancreas. *Semin Diagn Pathol.* 2000;17:104–108.
106. Ohike N, Jurgensen A, Pipeleers-Marichal M, Kloppel G. Mixed ductal-endocrine carcinomas of the pancreas and ductal adenocarcinomas with scattered endocrine cells: characterization of the endocrine cells. *Virchows Arch.* 2003;442:258–265.
107. Okada Y, Mori H, Tsutsumi A. Duct-acinar-islet cell tumor of the pancreas. *Pathol Int.* 1995;45:669–676.
108. Reid JD, Song-Lim Y, Petrelli M, Jaffe R. Ductuloinsular tumors of the pancreas. *Cancer.* 1982;49:908–915.
109. Schron DS, Mendelsohn G. Pancreatic carcinoma with duct, endocrine, and acinar differentiation: a histologic, immunocytochemical, and ultrastructural study. *Cancer.* 1984;54:1766–1770.
110. Chetty R, Clark SP, Pitson GA. Primary small cell carcinoma of the pancreas. *Pathology.* 1993;25:240–242.
111. O'Connor TP, Wade TP, Sunwoo YC, et al. Small cell undifferentiated carcinoma of the pancreas: report of a patient with tumor marker studies. *Cancer.* 1992;70:1514–1519.
112. Reyes CV, Wang T. Undifferentiated small cell carcinoma of the pancreas: a report of five cases. *Cancer.* 1981;47:2500–2502.

COMMENTARY

Susanne van Eeden, MD
G. Johan A. Offerhaus, MD, PhD

"Unfortunately I have to open my communication with the confession that I am in no way in a position to present the complete results of a successful research, but at the most to contribute some sporadic observations, which give an idea that the construction of the examined object is much more complicated than heretofore suspected."

This citation comes from the thesis by Paul Langerhans, published in 1869, in which he first describes the pancreatic endocrine cell clusters that were later to be named after him, without being aware of their functional significance.[1]

It is now clear that the pancreas is an organ that consists of an exocrine part, containing acini and ductal structures, and an endocrine component, composed of cells organized in the islets described by Langerhans. Since his time, significant progress has been made at both the morphologic and molecular level in understanding embryonic pancreatic development, the physiologic role of the pancreatic islet cells, and the related pathologic conditions.

As described in the chapter on pancreatic endocrine neoplasms (PENs) by Klimstra, the pancreatic endocrine cells arise from progenitor cells in the primitive ducts of the pancreatic primordia. One of the transcription factors essential in the formation of these ducts and also for the functioning of mature beta cells is the pancreatic duodenal homeobox 1 protein (Pdx1), which belongs to the homeodomain family of proteins. Other transcription factors of the homeodomain family and basic helix-loop-helix family subsequently involved in the endocrine differentiation of ductal progenitor cells are hepatocyte nuclear factor 6, neurogenin 3, NeuroD1/BETA2, Pax4, Nkx2.2, Nkx6.1, Pax6, and Isl1.[2] Although most endocrine cells separate from the ducts and migrate into the exocrine pancreas, forming the islets of Langerhans, some of them remain at their site of origin, and also some cells with stem cell capacities are thought to remain in the mature pancreas.[3]

This understanding of the embryologic development of the endocrine pancreas is important with respect to the pathogenesis of PENs because it is now believed that PENs originate from a common precursor cell that proliferates and differentiates toward an endocrine phenotype. If this is the case, the transcription factors involved in normal embryonic pancreatic development might prove to be important in tumorigenesis as well, and it is therefore conceivable that these transcription factors will play a role in diagnosis and prognostication in the near future. A recently described transgenic mouse model, in which PENs developed after infection with a c-*myc* oncogene-bearing retrovirus under the control of the pancreas-specific elastase promoter, supports this notion. The expression of Pdx1 and the endocrine-specific transcription factors Nkx2.2, Pax6, and Isl1 has been observed in these neoplasms.[4]

Although our understanding of the biology of PENs has grown, it remains surprisingly difficult to predict the clinical behavior of a PEN. Assessment of associated clinical findings, tumor size, gross local invasion, metastasis, and vascular invasion allows PENs to be subdivided into either functioning or nonfunctioning neoplasms of benign behavior, uncertain behavior, low-grade malignancy, and high-grade malignancy in the *Revised Classification of Neuroendocrine Tumours of the Lung, Pancreas and Gut* by Capella et al.[5] Although the prognostic value of these parameters is disputed, validation of the Capella classification in a group of 82 sporadic PENs shows a statistically significant difference in survival between the neoplasms of different grades.[6] Based on the classification by Capella et al., the World Health Organization (WHO) separates PENs into either functioning or nonfunctioning neoplasms of benign behavior, tumors of uncertain behavior, well-differentiated carcinomas, and poorly differentiated carcinomas/small-cell carcinomas,[7] but with different cut-off points for tumor size, with the addition of mitotic activity and proliferation rate (measured by Ki67 labeling). This latter system also does not separate insulinomas from the other PENs. The new WHO classification does not contain significant changes from the old classification, but the terms *macroadenoma* and *borderline tumor* are replaced in order to emphasize the ambiguous clinical behavior rather than implying a certain inherent tumor biology.

As Klimstra indicates, PENs can be classified in more than one way, but because the parameters mentioned earlier seem to be of at least some value and in order to obtain consistent classification and comparable research results, it deserves consideration to consequently follow the WHO guidelines in classifying PENs until more accurate prognostic parameters have been established.

Because PENs are well-vascularized neoplasms and angiogenesis is an important feature of tumorigenesis, the prognostic value of tumor microvessel density and the expression of the angiogenic factors of the vascular endothelial growth factor family and their receptors have been investigated recently. Although one study shows that low microvessel density is an unfavorable prognostic factor, and although, as mentioned by Klimstra, a role for vascular endothelial growth factor-C in tumor progression has been suggested, the results of different studies are not consistent and do not provide parameters that can be used in clinical practice.[8-10]

One group of PENs of which the aggressive behavior is easily predictable microscopically on the basis of cell type, high proliferative activity, and presence of necrosis is the poorly differentiated/small-cell carcinomas. However, as Klimstra indicates, these neoplasms are rare, and before a diagnosis of a poorly differentiated PEN is made, a metastasis from a primary tumor elsewhere, especially a bronchial carcinoma, has to be excluded. In these cases, the clinical data and imaging techniques are important. Additionally, a staining for thyroid transcription factor 1 might be of use, but it should be interpreted with caution. This protein is expressed in the nucleus of normal thyroidal and pulmonary epithelial cells and in a large number of the (adeno)carcinomas derived from these tissues. Positivity for thyroid transcription factor 1 has been reported in 90% of the small-cell carcinomas of the lung, but also in small-cell carcinomas from other sites, such as the prostate and urinary bladder.[11] Therefore, both positive and negative labeling results have to be correlated with the other available data before a final diagnosis is made.

Another important differential diagnosis on the other side of the spectrum mentioned by Klimstra is the one of endocrine microadenomas versus enlarged nonneoplastic islets. Enlarged nonneoplastic islets can be seen in islet cell hyperplasia, which is a poorly defined and rare condition that should not be confused with the much more frequently observed aggregation of islets in chronic pancreatitis, caused by atrophy of the exocrine pancreas. Islet cell hyperplasia is defined as an increase in islet mass due to increased islet size and/or islet number.[12] If the islets cells contain enlarged pleomorphic nuclei, if ductuloinsular complexes consisting of endocrine cell nests budding off ducts are observed, and if the patient presents with persistent hyperinsulinemic hypoglycemia, indicative of beta-cell dysfunction, the term *nesidioblastosis* is frequently used. Islet cell hyperplasia predominantly occurs in newborns but has also been described in adults. In newborns, it can be associated with maternal diabetes, erythroblastosis fetalis, hereditary tyrosinemia, or Beckwith-Wiedemann syndrome, but in these conditions, the histologic features of nesidioblastosis are usually not very prominent.[12,13] Nesidioblastosis can be focal or diffuse. Especially the focal form, also referred to as *focal adenomatous hyperplasia*, has features reminiscent of an endocrine microadenoma. But in contrast to the conventional microadenoma, in which only one cell type is found, the focal variant of nesidioblastosis contains a mixture of different cell types. In some sporadic cases of neonatal focal nesidioblastosis, somatic loss of the maternal allele of the imprinted chromosome region 11p15 has been described, which encodes numerous candidate genes.[14] In a part of these cases, the paternal allele of the high-affinity sulfonylurea receptor (*SUR1*) gene, involved in insulin secretion by beta cells and also on chromosome 11p15, shows a germline mutation.[15] The fact that not only germline mutations, but also somatic genetic alterations have been found, suggests that these lesions might be clonal and maybe should be regarded as a functioning variant of a microadenoma. Although generally the age of the patients (newborns vs adults) and the clinical presentation (hypoglycemia vs asymptomatic coincidental finding) differ, it might turn out that both lesions are more similar than previously thought from a pathogenic point of view.

Extensive discussion of diffuse nesidioblastosis, which is usually not in the differential diagnosis of a PEN, is beyond the scope of this commentary. However, the combination of islet cell hyperplasia and the presence of multiple pancreatic endocrine microadenomas should be mentioned here as a typical feature of multiple endocrine neoplasia type 1 syndrome, because as described by Klimstra, most of these patients experience clinically relevant PENs in the course of their disease.

In his chapter, Klimstra emphasizes that the difference between functioning and nonfunctioning PENs is based on the presence or absence of a clinical syndrome with increased serum peptide levels and that immunohistochemical evidence of hormone production does not automatically mean that a PEN is clinically functioning. In addition, negative stains do not rule out the diagnosis of a functioning PEN; hormones can be released from the neoplastic cells so quickly that immunohistochemical stains are negative. It is also possible that the neoplasm produces a slightly modified hormone that cannot be recognized by the antibodies used for immunohistochemistry.

The differential diagnosis of PENs discussed by Klimstra is important not only in histology but also in interpreting fine-needle aspirates. PENs can be confused with acinic cell carcinoma, solid-pseudopapillary (Hamoudi) neoplasm, and pancreatoblastoma. Cytologic features suggestive of acinic cell carcinoma are prominent nucleoli and granular cytoplasm.[16] A solid-pseudopapillary neoplasm is characterized by papillary clusters with fibrovascular stalks. The neoplastic cells contain abundant metachromatic material, nuclear grooves, and foamy macrophages, and necrosis is often present.[16] In a pancreatoblastoma, multiple cell types can be observed in the same neoplasm: small cells with dark nuclei and scanty cytoplasm and larger epithelial cells, occasionally in an acinar arrangement, with abundant granular-to-vacuolated cytoplasm and more prominent nucleoli.[16] In addition to the cytologic features, the patient characteristics (pancreatoblastoma in children, solid-pseudopapillary neoplasm in young females) and imaging techniques can be helpful in making the correct diagnosis.

All in all, it is obvious that our knowledge on the endocrine pancreas and its diseases has increased immensely since the days of Paul Langerhans. However, the words cited from his thesis are still true concerning PENs: we are not yet in a position to present the complete results of a successful research, but we can contribute some observations. Perhaps in the future, the pathogenesis of PENs will be unraveled, their biologic behavior will be fully understood, and the construction of the examined object seem not as complicated as heretofore suspected.

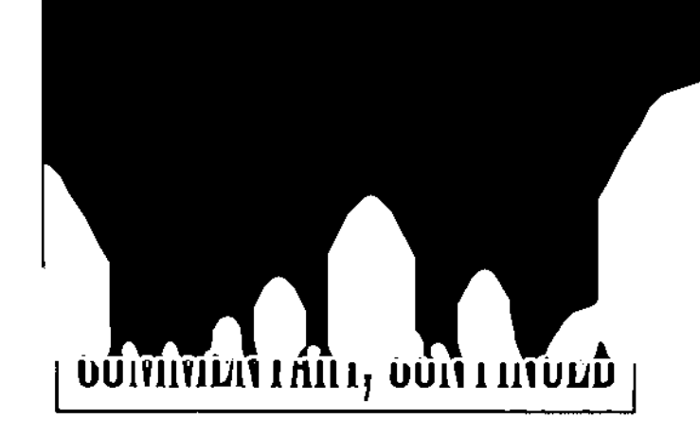

References

1. Howard JM, Hess W. The endocrine pancreas. In: Howard JM, Hess W, eds. *History of the Pancreas. Mysteries of a Hidden Organ*. New York: Kluwer Academic/Plenum Publishers; 2002:99–164.
2. Schwitzgebel VM. Programming of the pancreas. *Mol Cell Endocrinol*. 2001;185:99–108.
3. Holland AM, Góñez JL, Harrison LC. Progenitor cells in the adult pancreas. *Diabetes Metab Res Rev*. 2004;20:13–27.
4. Lewis BC, Klimstra DS, Varmus HE. The c-myc and PyMT oncogenes induce different tumor types in a somatic mouse model for pancreatic cancer. *Genes Dev*. 2003;17:3127–3138.
5. Capella C, Heitz PU, Höfler H, Solcia E, Klöppel G. Revised classification of neuroendocrine tumours of the lung, pancreas and gut. *Virchows Arch*. 1995;425:547–560.
6. Heymann MF, Joubert M, Nemeth J, et al. Prognostic and immunohistochemical validation of the Capella classification of pancreatic neuroendocrine tumours: an analysis of 82 sporadic cases. *Histopathology*. 2000;36:421–432.
7. Klöppel G, Heitz PU, Capella C, Solcia E. Endocrine tumours of the pancreas. In: Solcia E, Klöppel G, Sobin LH, in collaboration with 9 pathologists from 4 countries. *Histological Typing of Endocrine Tumours*. 2nd ed. Heidelberg: Springer-Verlag; 2000:56–60.
8. Marion-Audibert AM, Barel C, Gouysse G, et al. Low microvessel density is an unfavorable histoprognostic factor in pancreatic endocrine tumors. *Gastroenterology*. 2003;125:1094–1104.
9. Hansel DE, Rahman A, Hermans J, et al. Liver metastases arising from well-differentiated pancreatic endocrine neoplasms demonstrate increased VEGF-C expression. *Mod Pathol*. 2003;16:652–659.
10. La Rosa S, Uccella S, Finzi G, Albarello L, Sessa F, Capella C. Localization of vascular endothelial growth factor and its receptors in digestive endocrine tumors: correlation with microvessel density and clinicopathological features. *Hum Pathol*. 2003;34:18–27.
11. http://immunoquery.com
12. Lubensky I. Endocrine pancreas. In: LiVolsi V, Asa SL, eds. *Endocrine Pathology*. Philadelphia: Churchill Livingstone; 2002:205–235.
13. Lloyd RV, Douglas BR, Young WF. Diffuse neuroendocrine system. In: West-King D, ed. *Endocrine Diseases, Atlas of Nontumor Pathology*. Washington, DC: American Registry of Pathology, Armed Forces Institute of Pathology; 2001:259–308.
14. de Lonlay P, Fournet JC, Rahier J, et al. Somatic deletion of the imprinted 11p15 region in sporadic persistent hyperinsulinemic hypoglycemia of infancy is specific of focal adenomatous hyperplasia and endorses partial pancreatectomy. *J Clin Invest*. 1997;100:802–807.
15. Verkarre V, Fournet JC, de Lonlay P, et al. Paternal mutation of the sulfonylurea receptor (SUR1) gene and maternal loss of 11p15 imprinted genes lead to persistent hyperinsulinism in focal adenomatous hyperplasia. *J Clin Invest*. 1998;102:1286–1291.
16. Greenberg ML. Pancreas. In: Gray W, ed. *Diagnostic Cytopathology*. New York: Churchill Livingstone; 1995:415–434.

CHAPTER

Sporadic Gastrinoma

Chandu Vemuri, MD
Gerard M. Doherty, MD

Definition of Disease

Sporadic gastrinomas are functional neuroendocrine tumors that develop outside of familial genetic syndromes and secrete the gastrointestinal hormone gastrin. These tumors can cause the clinical features of Zollinger-Ellison syndrome, due to hypergastrinemia that causes elevated gastric acid output. The clinical result can be a severe ulcer diathesis.

Gastrinoma and the Zollinger-Ellison syndrome is a classic example of a functional pancreatic endocrine tumor. The management is complex because of the need to evaluate and treat both the functional hormonal syndrome and the potential malignancy. When these patients are diagnosed and treated, it is critical that the definitions and diagnostic criteria be kept clearly in mind. The diagnosis of Zollinger-Ellison syndrome (gastrinoma) requires the demonstration of simultaneous elevations of serum gastrin and gastric acid output. Other common causes of hypergastrinemia (e.g., atrophic gastritis) are frequently mistaken for gastrinoma but do not meet these simple diagnostic definitions.

History of Discovery of Gastrinoma

The description of gastrinoma and the Zollinger-Ellison Syndrome is relatively recent, having occurred within the past 50 years. In 1955, Zollinger and Ellison described the original two cases of gastrinoma.[1] In 1960, Gregory and colleagues[2] identified gastrin within the pancreatic tumors of a patient with Zollinger-Ellison syndrome.

The early treatment of Zollinger-Ellison syndrome was focused on managing the severe ulcer diathesis. At that time, the only truly effective way to manage the ulcers was total gastrectomy. This removed the parietal cell mass of the stomach and eliminated acid output by eliminating the end organ for gastrin effect. Major breakthroughs in the treatment of patients with gastrinoma occurred in the late 1970s and throughout the 1980s, with the development of H_2-receptor antagonists. These medications block the production of acid in patients with gastrinoma, allowing the nonoperative management of patients' hyperacidity. In turn, this changed the operative strategy from one of controlling acid output to one of controlling potential malignancy. Once the efficacy of these medications had been clearly demonstrated by the mid-1980s, it was no longer necessary to operate to decrease the acid output in these patients. Patients could all have their ulcer disease and diarrhea suppressed with H_2-receptor antagonists. The subsequent development of proton pump inhibitors, which are more potent inhibitors of acid output, has made this nonoperative management of acid output more clear. These medications can be taken less frequently and in smaller doses than was often necessary with the H_2-receptor antagonists.

Subsequent significant developments in the management of gastrinoma have included the introduction of somatostatin receptor scintigraphy, which has added to the generally improved options for imaging pancreatic endocrine tumors. In addition, larger operative series defined the role of surgery in controlling the metastatic disease from gastrinoma, in addition to demonstrating that many of the primary tumors are in the wall of the duodenum rather than the pancreas. The current focus of study and area for improvement is in the management of disseminated disease.

Pathology

Pathophysiology

The pathophysiology of Zollinger-Ellison syndrome and gastrinoma is dictated by the effects of gastrin and its hypersecretion. All of the symptoms that develop early in Zollinger-Ellison syndrome are secondary to the elevated gastric acid hypersecretion stimulated by gastrin. Late in the course of disease, patients can experience the effects of distant metastases, including liver failure and bone fractures. However, the main symptom complex is dominated by gastric acid hypersecretion, which can cause peptic ulcer disease, severe gastroesophageal reflux disease, and significant diarrhea. All of these effects are resolved when the gastric acid hypersecretion is controlled.

The direct effect of the gastrin is to stimulate the gastric mucosa, including the parietal cell mass. The parietal cell hyperplasia causes a marked increase in the secretory capacity of the stomach. The basal acid output of the stomach is increased because of the increased mass, and the maximum acid output is also substantially increased because of the increased number of parietal cells. This increased gastric acid output causes substantial symptoms of gastroesophageal reflux in many patients. In addition, the increased acid load delivered to the duodenum and jejunum causes ulcers in these areas. It also overwhelms the capability of the pancreas and small bowel to neutralize the gastric acid, leading to significant diarrhea. Control of either the hypergastrinemia by tumor resection or suppression of acid output with proton pump inhibitors completely resolves the ulcer disease, symptoms of gastroesophageal reflux, and diarrhea.

Chronic elevations of gastrin also stimulate the enterochromaffin-like cells. These cells in the lining of the stomach can develop into gastric carcinoid tumors. This is less frequent in the sporadic setting than it is in the setting of gastrinoma in patients with multiple endocrine neoplasia type 1.

Gross Pathology

Primary gastrinoma tumors can occur throughout the head, body, and tail of the pancreas as well as in the submucosa of the duodenum. In addition to these typical sites, rarely, primary gastrinomas can occur in the wall of the stomach, jejunum, or gallbladder. Tumors have also been described primarily occurring in the liver, kidney, mesentery, ovary, heart, and omentum.[3-9] In older series, there are often large numbers of patients who have either no tumor identified or a tumor identified only in lymph nodes. Once the frequency of duodenal wall primary tumors was more widely appreciated in the mid-1980s, most endocrine surgeons added longitudinal duodenotomy, with careful palpation of the lining of the duodenum, to the abdominal exploration. This has greatly decreased the number of tumors not found at operation for gastrinoma.

Overall, approximately 40% of all tumors are located in the duodenum, and a very similar number of tumors are located in the pancreas.[10] The tumors in the pancreas tend to be larger and are more frequently associated with liver metastasis. However, even primary duodenal tumors less than 5 mm in diameter can be associated with both lymph node and liver metastasis. Overall, at least two thirds of gastrinomas are clearly malignant, with the presence of metastatic disease in lymph nodes and/or the liver. For the remaining third, the definition of malignancy is somewhat difficult because the histologic criteria for distinction between benign and malignant gastrinoma are not clear.

Histology

Gastrinomas, like other neuroendocrine tumors of the gastrointestinal tract, are typically fairly bland-appearing, well-differentiated tumors (Fig. 42.1). The tumors generally contain little necrosis and are made up of monotonous cuboidal cells with few mitoses, and fine granular, eosinophilic cytoplasm. The growth patterns can display trabecular, gyriform, or glandular morphology; however, these morphologic differences do not predict clinical behavior.

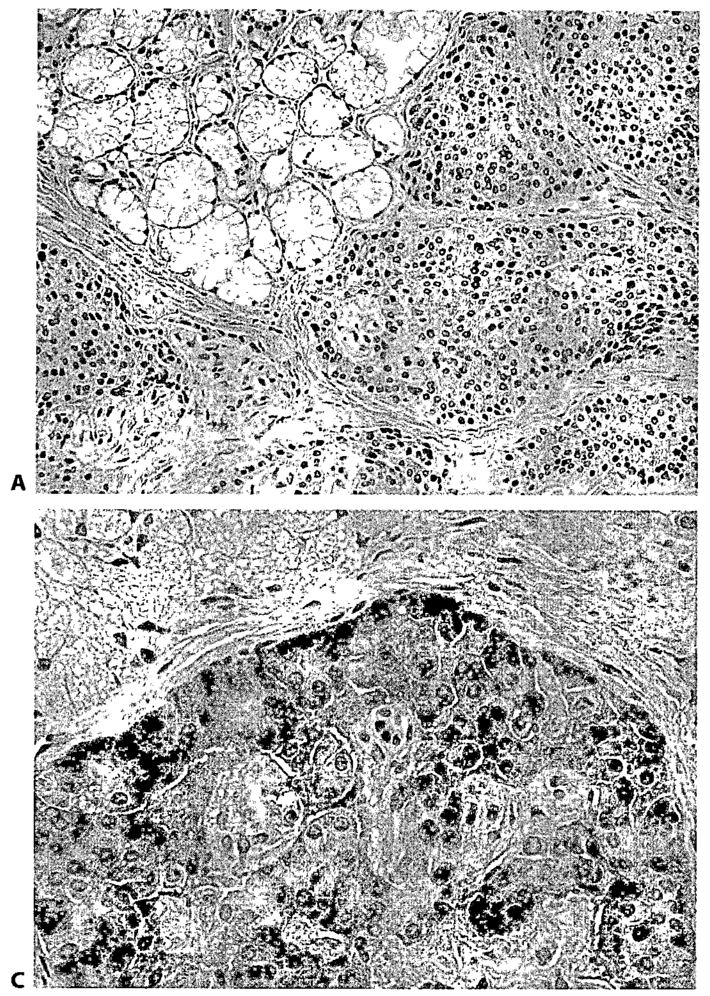

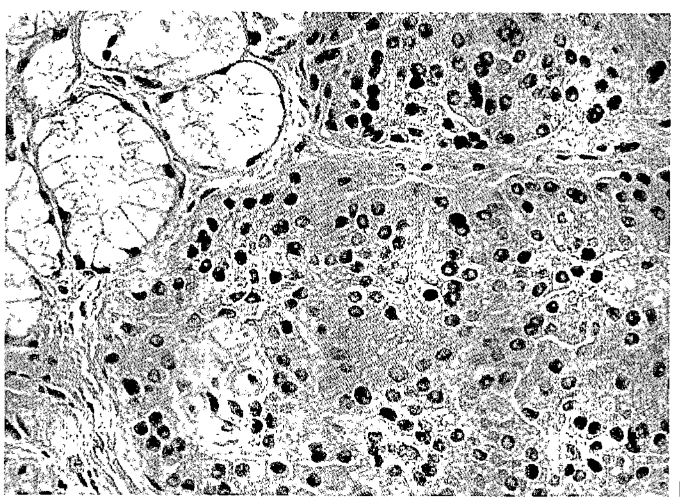

Figure 42.1
Histology of gastrinoma. **(A)** Monotonous cuboidal cell appearance of gastrinoma (original magnification 200 ×). **(B)** Higher-power view of gastrinoma (original magnification 400×). **(C)** Gastrin immunohistochemistry demonstrating strong cytoplasmic staining. (Photomicrographs courtesy of Thomas Giordano, MD, Department of Pathology, University of Michigan.)

Immunohistochemically, most gastrinomas stain positively for gastrin. Many gastrinomas also contain chromogranin A, in addition to one or more of the less frequently expressed hormones, including pancreatic polypeptide, somatostatin, insulin, and neuron-specific enolase.[11] Conversely, however, not all tumors that express gastrin immunohistochemically should be clinically designated as gastrinomas. Gastrin is expressed in many neuroendocrine tumors that do not cause the Zollinger-Ellison syndrome.[11] In general, there is substantial overlap in the immunohistochemical hormonal expression of various neuroendocrine tumors. The dominant hormonal syndrome is typically used to designate the tumor (e.g., gastrinoma, insulinoma, somatostatinoma).

Occasionally, gastrinomas, like other gastrointestinal tract neuroendocrine tumors, can appear quite aggressive. The tumors are poorly differentiated histologically. This pattern can be associated with aggressive growth, metastasis, and poor prognosis. These tumors do not tend to respond significantly to systemic therapy.

Epidemiology

Gastrinomas typically appear in the third through sixth decades of life. Among the functional pancreatic endocrine tumors, insulinoma is more common than gastrinoma. However, gastrinomas are far more frequently malignant than insulinomas. Gastrinoma is thus the most common functional malignant pancreatic endocrine tumor.

Between 15% and 25% of people with gastrinoma are from multiple endocrine neoplasia type I families. The management of gastrinoma in these cases requires a different set of considerations than the management of sporadic gastrinoma. Patients with multiple endocrine neoplasia type 1 generally have multiple small tumors and typically cannot be cured by operation. This chapter deals specifically with gastrinomas in the sporadic setting.

Clinical Presentation

Patients with Zollinger-Ellison syndrome present with symptoms of elevated acid output (Table 42.1).[12-15] Late in the disease, patients may experience symptoms of right upper quadrant pain from liver replacement or bone pain; however, early in the disease, the symptoms are almost entirely due to the gastric acid hypersecretion. Patients have often had symptoms for many years before the diagnosis of gastrinoma. This is due both to the rarity of Zollinger-Ellison syndrome and to the commonplace occurrence of unrelated peptic ulcer disease or gastroesophageal reflux disease.[16] In one recent series, the mean duration of symptoms before diagnosis was 6.4 years.[17]

The common symptoms of gastric acid hypersecretion include abdominal pain, reflux symptoms, and diarrhea. All of these symptoms are treatable by suppressing the acid output. The diarrhea occurs because of the increased acid load from the stomach into the small bowel.

Occasionally, patients present with complications of gastrinoma, such as bleeding and perforated peptic ulcer disease, or with esophageal strictures from severe gastroesophageal reflux disease. The recent widespread availability of very potent acid suppression medication has decreased the incidence of these complications. Many people are empirically given these medications, which effectively decrease gastric acid hypersecretion, before the development of severe complications.

Diagnosis

Differential Diagnosis

The differential diagnosis of the Zollinger-Ellison syndrome includes all of the more common causes of upper abdominal pain and ulcer disease. The most frequent of these is idiopathic peptic ulcer disease, which may be related to *Helicobacter pylori* infection (Table 42.2).

The clinical situations that should lead one to suspect Zollinger-Ellison syndrome and to test for it include evidence of unusual or complicated peptic ulcer disease. Such issues could include perforation or bleeding of the ulcer itself, the presence of severe diarrhea, the absence of *H. pylori* infection, or the failure of the ulcer to heal after adequate *H. pylori* treatment and acid-suppression therapy. Also, the presence of a pancreatic tumor or hypercalcemia or nephrolithiasis should suggest gastrinoma in the setting of multiple endocrine neoplasia type 1. Recurrence of a previously treated ulcer should also prompt evaluation for gastrinoma.

Other findings that should prompt evaluation for gastrinoma include the documentation of hypergastrinemia or hypercalcemia in a patient with abdominal symptoms. In addition, patients with gastric carcinoid tumors should be evaluated for evidence of gastrinoma if gastric acid secretion is present (most carcinoids associated with achlorhydria).

Table 42.1 Clinical Presentation of Patients with Zollinger-Ellison Syndrome

Patients and Symptoms	Ellison and Wilson,[14] 1964 ($N = 260$) No. (%)	Mignon et al.,[13] 1986 ($N = 144$) No. (%)	Mignon and Cadiot,[12] 1998 ($N = 127$) No. (%)	Roy et al.,[15] 2000 ($N = 203$) No. (%)
% with MEN	54 (21%)	34 (24%)	0 (0%)	0 (0%)
Pain	241 (93%)	37 (26%)	ND	159 (78%)
Diarrhea	18 (7%)	21 (15%)	67 (53.4%)	146 (72%)
Heartburn	ND	ND	ND	85 (42%)
Nausea	ND	ND	ND	57 (28%)
Vomiting	ND	ND	ND	52 (26%)
Weight loss	ND	ND	ND	37 (18%)
Bleeding	ND	ND	ND	55 (27%)
Pain + bleeding	ND	ND	ND	44 (22%)
Pain + diarrhea	78 (30%)	70 (49%)	ND	113 (56%)
Peptic ulcer			114 (90%)	

Abbreviations: MEN, multiple endocrine neoplasia; ND, Not determined.

Table 42.2 Differential Diagnosis of Gastrinoma and Signs/Symptoms that Suggest Gastrinoma

Differential Diagnosis	Signs/Symptoms Suggestive of Gastrinoma
Idiopathic peptic ulcer disease	Diarrhea
	Negative *Helicobacter pylori*
	Chronic diarrhea during fasting
	Weight loss
	Long history of persistent symptoms
Idiopathic GERD	Complications (e.g., perforation)
	Refractory to treatment
	Positive family history of PUD or GERD
	Prominent gastric folds
	Multiple peptic ulcers
	Ulcers in uncommon locations
	Esophageal stricture
	Gastric outlet obstruction

Abbreviations: GERD, gastroesophageal reflux disease; PUD, peptic ulcer disease.

Screening Tests

For patients who fall into the categories in which gastrinoma might be suspected, the initial study that should be performed is a fasting serum gastrin level. The serum gastrin level is nearly always increased in patients with gastrinoma. However, most patients with an elevated serum gastrin level do not have gastrinoma. Hypergastrinemia is most frequently a physiologic response to low gastric acid output, as can commonly occur with pernicious anemia. This situation can also be drug induced from the use of proton pump inhibitors or H_2 antagonists. Other causes of an elevated gastrin level can include chronic renal failure or prior gastric surgery.

The most concerning situation that can cause elevated fasting serum gastrin level in a patient with prior gastric surgery is the retained gastric antrum syndrome. This occurs in patients who have had a partial gastrectomy with Billroth 2 reconstruction, in which a portion of the antrum has been left attached to the duodenum. When that occurs, the antrum attached to the duodenum is disconnected from the proximal stomach and therefore is not exposed to gastric acid. This leads to chronic hypergastrinemia and chronic hypertrophy of the gastrin-producing G-cells in the distal stomach. This also causes very high gastric acid output if any of the parietal cell mass has been preserved in the proximal stomach. These patients can have severe ulcer disease and may require surgical correction; however, they do not have gastrinoma.

Other causes of chronic hypergastrinemia associated with elevated gastric acid output include gastric outlet obstruction and short-bowel syndrome, as well as gastrinoma.

Confirmatory Tests

Once suspected by the clinical situation and the presence of hypergastrinemia, the diagnosis of gastrinoma must be confirmed by measurement of simultaneous fasting serum gastrin levels and gastric acid output. An elevation in fasting serum gastrin with increased acid output is diagnostic of gastrinoma in most patients, particularly if the possibility of retained gastric antrum syndrome is excluded. If the gastric pH is less than 2.5 and the serum gastrin level is greater than 1000 pg/mL, then the diagnosis of Zollinger-Ellison syndrome is clear. However, if the serum gastrin level is increased only to between 100 and 1000 pg/mL and the fasting gastric pH is less than 2.5, then there are some other possible diagnoses in the differential such as of *H. pylori*–related peptic ulcer disease. In this situation, a secretin stimulation test is a useful provocative examination to document an abnormal response of gastrin to intravenous secretin. After the infusion of secretin, if the serum gastrin increases by 200 pg/mL or more, then gastrinoma is confirmed. The secretin test is rarely associated with false-positive results, but it can have a false-negative result (approximately 10%). If the diagnosis of gastrinoma is strongly suspected and the secretin test result is equivocal, then the diagnosis may be confirmed using a calcium infusion test.[18] For this test, a 3-hour infusion of 5 mg/kg of calcium (as calcium gluconate) is administered. An increase in the serum gastrin level by more than 395 pg/mL confirms the diagnosis of gastrinoma. The diagnosis of gastrinoma should be made biochemically before anatomic localization studies are performed. This avoids the situation in which a series of nondiagnostic x-ray studies are performed in a patient whose label of gastrinoma is unfounded.

Localization Tests

Once the diagnosis of gastrinoma has been confirmed biochemically the next immediate step in management is medical control of acid output, which should precede further evaluation and localization of the tumor. After gastric acid hypersecretion is controlled, localization of the tumor should be attempted. The accurate localization of the sites of tumor is important for determination of prognosis and planning of definitive surgical therapy.

There are a wide variety of useful tests, including conventional noninvasive imaging methods, such as

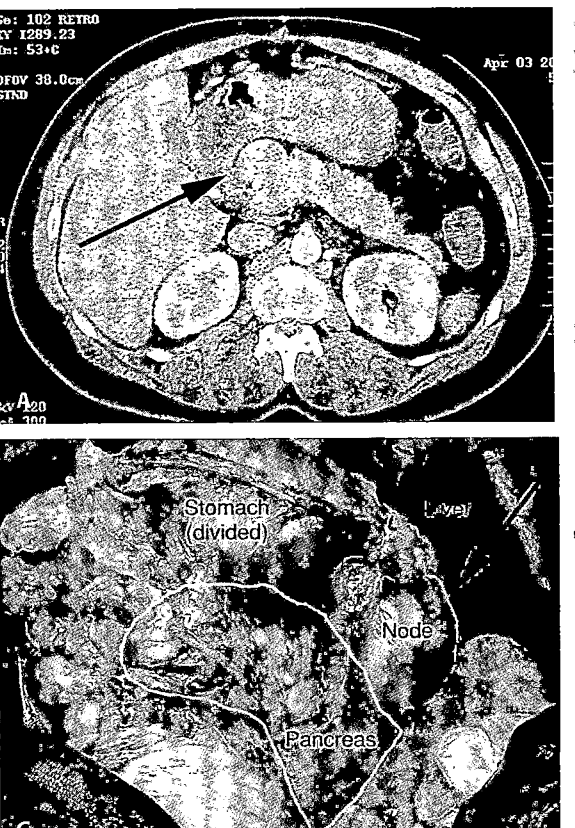

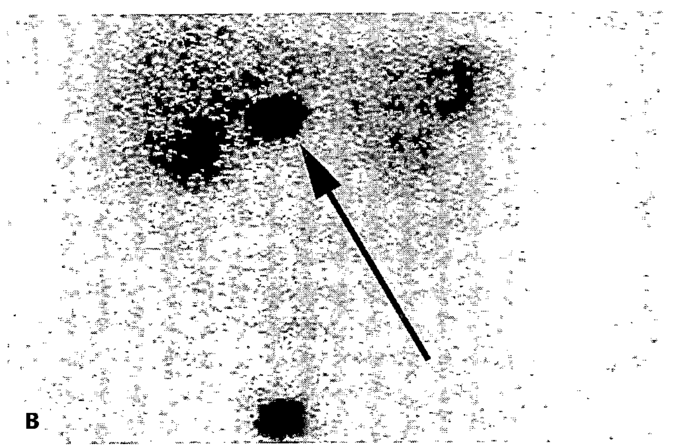

Figure 42.2
Imaging and gross findings in a patient with gastrinoma. **(A)** Computed tomographic scan of the abdomen reveals a mass near the head of the pancreas (*arrow*). **(B)** Somatostatin receptor scintigraphy (SRS) shows an intense focus of uptake in the right upper quadrant (*arrow*). **(C)** Abdominal exploration shows a large lymph node containing metastatic gastrinoma, adjacent to the duodenum, which contained a small primary tumor.

computed tomographic scanning, ultrasound, and magnetic resonance imaging. In addition, invasive testing with angiography or selected venous sampling is possible.[19] Finally, functional testing using either somatostatin receptor scintigraphy or fluorodeoxyglucose positron emission tomography can potentially localize disease (Fig. 42.2).

A straightforward start for the localization of these tumors is to perform computed tomography of the abdomen and pelvis and somatostatin receptor scintigraphy. These tests are complementary and can define anatomic abnormalities as well as demonstrate their function. In order to evaluate specific findings on either computed tomography scan or somatostatin receptor scintigraphy, magnetic resonance imaging of the liver may be helpful. Occasionally, endoscopic ultrasonography is also helpful for defining lesions in the pancreas or peripancreatic lymph nodes.[20] However, endoscopic ultrasound is not very useful for identifying abnormalities in the duodenum.

Invasive localization tests, such as angiography with or without the intra-arterial injection of secretin and measurement of gastrin in hepatic veins, or direct portal venous sampling, can identify specific regions where the gastrinomas reside.[21] These studies have the advantage of not relying on the tumor size for their sensitivity. However, the clinical impact of intra-arterial secretin stimulation or portal venous sampling localization is not clear. One could recommend use of such studies if all other imaging studies are negative and duodenal gastrinomas are suspected. However, an alternative to this approach is operative exploration with the assumption that the tumors must be there. Intraoperative localization tests are discussed in the surgical treatment section.

Treatment

Acid-Suppression Therapy

One of the most critical steps in the treatment of patients with Zollinger-Ellison syndrome is the adequate suppression of gastric acid output. As the cause of the symptoms, signs, and complications of the syndrome, the gastric acid output is an essential functional issue. With current medical options, it is possible to control the gastric acid output in every patient with gastrinoma. The current medications of choice are the proton pump inhibitors, such as omeprazole, lansoprazole, and pantoprazole. The prior generation of medications (H_2-receptor antagonists), such as cimetidine, ranitidine, and famotidine, all work as well but require larger and more frequent doses. For this reason, the proton pump inhibitors are substantially more clinically effective.

The goal of medical therapy for gastric acid output is to suppress the hypersecretion to below 10 mEq/hr for the hour before the next dose of drug. Proper management of gastric acid secretion thus requires gastric acid output determination at the initiation of therapy and then at least annually during treatment. One effective approach is to use omeprazole (60 mg total daily dose) and to document suppression of acid output within 1 hour of the next subsequent dose. If the acid secretion remains above 10 mEq/hr, then the dose should be increased to 80 mg/day (40 mg orally twice a day). In a recent National Institutes of Health study, all patients with gastrinoma had initial control of their gastric acid output on omeprazole, at 60 mg orally twice a day or less.[22]

Patients may require increases in their dose of antisecretory medication over time. Although long-term tachyphylaxis does not appear to occur with proton pump inhibitors, patients may require increased medication due to tumor progression. Conversely, many patients can have reduction in their dose over time; this occurs because omeprazole is labile in gastric acid. Once the gastric acid hypersecretion has been controlled, the omeprazole is effective in smaller doses. Thus, nearly all patients with uncomplicated Zollinger-Ellison syndrome have acid output controlled on omeprazole, 20 mg twice daily, as a long-term dose.

Long-term acid suppression with omeprazole or other proton pump inhibitors decreases the absorption of protein-bound vitamin B12 and iron. Prospective studies have demonstrated that the vitamin B12 levels in particular decrease over time. Iron stores have not been shown to decrease clinically. For this reason, patients receiving long-term acid-suppression therapy with proton pump inhibitors over a period of years should have serum vitamin B12 level determinations at least annually and the vitamins should be replenished if necessary.

In the acute situation, when oral acid-suppression therapy is not an option, such as in preparation for abdominal operation, parenteral therapy is necessary. An intravenous infusion of H_2-receptor antagonists is completely effective if the dosing is appropriate. An effective regimen includes an initial bolus dose of ranitidine of 150 mg, followed by a continuous intravenous infusion of 1 mg/kg of body weight per hour. Gastric acid secretion should be determined after 4 hours. If the gastric ph is less than 2.5 or the gastric acid output is greater than 10 mEq/hr, then the ranitidine infusion dose should be increased by 0.5–1.0 mg/kg/hr until these goals are reached.

Even after an apparently successful and complete resection of gastrinoma and in patients with Zollinger-Ellison syndrome, gastric acid hypersecretion may persist. This is presumably secondary to hypertrophy of the parietal cell mass over a period of years before treatment. In the perioperative recovery period and afterward, gastric acid suppression must be continued to prevent complications from acid oversecretion. The same acid output criteria can be used to titrate the dose of proton pump inhibitor in this situation.

Surgical Therapy

The only potentially curative option for patients with gastrinoma is complete surgical resection. The rationale for surgical resection in this group is clear.[23,24] If the condition is untreated, the natural history of gastrinoma is one of indolent but gradual progression, with the development of liver metastasis and death in at least a proportion of the patients. In a study from the National Institutes of Health, 23% (six of 26) of patients with gastrinoma who did not have liver metastases at diagnosis and who did not have resection went on to develop liver metastases over an average of 8.7 (1.5–19) years.[24] Two of these six patients died of metastatic disease. In contrast, only three of 98 patients who underwent operative resection of their gastrinoma developed liver metastases. This was a statistically significant difference. Although this was not a randomized study, the implication is very compelling.

The operative approach for patients with gastrinoma is dictated by the extent of disease.[25] In general, the principle is to perform a low-morbidity, complete resection of the disease with preservation of the maximum amount of normal pancreas. In practice, this leads to distal pancreatectomy and peripancreatic lymph node dissection for tumors in the distal body or tail of the pancreas (very rare location). For amenable tumors in the head of the pancreas, a local enucleation of the tumor is generally carried out. For tumors in the duodenum, a full-thickness duodenal local resection is generally effective.[10] The overwhelming majority of sporadic gastrinomas are located in the pancreatic head, uncinate process, or duodenum (within the gastrinoma triangle). For all patients, a peripancreatic and adjacent lymphadenectomy should be included. For most patients with limited disease, a pancreaticoduodenectomy is avoided. This procedure can involve significant morbidity and is typically not justified given the indolent nature and lack of local aggressiveness of gastrinoma. However in selected situations, pancreaticoduodenectomy may be the best option.[26]

For all patients who have gastrinoma in and around the head of the pancreas and particularly for those in whom a primary tumor is not readily identified, a duodenotomy with palpation of the wall of the duodenum between thumb and forefinger is helpful to find duodenal wall submucosal gastrinomas. These tumors can be quite small (3–10 mm), even when associated with much larger deposits of tumor in adjacent lymph nodes.

The most life-threatening aspect of gastrinoma is the development of distant metastasis. Usually, the initial site of metastasis beyond lymph nodes is the liver. Patients with resectable liver metastasis may benefit from an aggressive operative approach. However, many patients have diffuse liver metastasis that are not amenable to surgical resection. In this situation, medical management is preferable.

Many patients with distant metastases develop bone metastases as well. These lesions can be quite indolent but may become symptomatic. Systemic therapy to try to arrest the growth of the tumor can be helpful for some patients. For people who become symptomatic from skeletal lesions, radiation therapy can be helpful. All patients with metastatic disease must have active management of their gastric acid hypersecretion in order to avoid complications of the Zollinger-Ellison syndrome.

The outcome of aggressive therapy for gastrinoma results in approximately 25% of patients becoming long-term disease-free survivors. This appears to have a beneficial effect in decreasing the number of people who develop liver metastases. In addition, an evaluation of those patients with primary duodenal gastrinomas demonstrated that in 63 patients managed at the National Institute of Health, the 10-year disease specific survival was 100% and the disease-free survival was 60%. The prognosis was better for patients who did not have lymph node metastasis at operation. These data indicate that exploration and resection for patients who have disease that is amenable to removal is followed by a generally excellent prognosis.[10]

Systemic Tumor Therapy

The options for systemic therapy for patients with malignant gastrinomas include cytotoxic chemotherapy and somatostatin analogues. A variety of systemic chemotherapeutic agents have been used. The most frequently used first-line regimen is streptozotocin and 5-fluorouracil. This regimen yields approximately 50% objective responses that include symptomatic improvement and/or biochemical reduction in gastrin levels. Significant tumor regression occurs in one quarter to one third of patients. The toxicity of streptozotocin includes nausea and vomiting in nearly all patients. Long-term use of streptozotocin requires monitoring of renal function because renal toxicity can be significant. A second-line therapeutic option is etoposide and cisplatin, which is effective in small-cell lung cancer but has not been very effective in pancreatic endocrine tumors (unless dedifferentiated). The effect of either regimen on survival has not been established.

Somatostatin analogues are used to try to take advantage of the expression of type 2 somatostatin receptors on most gastrinomas. Somatostatin analogues can suppress gastrin released from tumors; however, this is not as clinically useful because the acid output can be suppressed by proton pump inhibitors. Recent information from the National Institutes of Health implies that octreotide is also an effective anti-tumor agent for patients with progressive malignant disease.[27] In 53% of their 15 patients, octreotide had an anti-growth effect. There was a very low incidence of serious side effects. Seven of the eight patients in whom octreotide was deemed useful had tumor stabilization, and one of the eight had a decrease in tumor size. The mean duration of this effect was greater than 2 years.

The timing of initiation of systemic therapy for patients with gastrinoma is not established. Many clinicians initiate therapy only when progression of disease has been demonstrated. Given the low toxicity of somatostatin analogues, it is reasonable and appropriate to begin therapy at the time of the diagnosis of unresectable distant disease.[27]

Conclusion

Gastrinoma is a disease characterized by both a functional syndrome that must be appropriately managed to avoid life-threatening complications, and an indolent, but potentially life-threatening, malignant tumor. Appreciation and careful management of each of these aspects will lead to prolonged survival for most patients with this disease.

References

1. Zollinger RM, Ellison EH. Primary peptic ulceration of the jejunum associated with islet cell tumors of the pancreas. *Ann Surg*. 1955;142:709–728.
2. Gregory RA, Tracy HJ, French JM, Sircus W. Extraction of a gastrin-like substance from a pancreatic tumor in a case of Zollinger-Ellison syndrome. *Lancet*. 1960;1:1045–1048.
3. Herrmann ME, Ciesla MC, Chejfec G, DeJong SA, Yong SL. Primary nodal gastrinomas. *Arch Pathol Lab Med*. 2000; 124:832–835.
4. Norton JA, Doherty GM, Fraker DL, et al. Surgical treatment of localized gastrinoma within the liver: a prospective study. *Surgery*. 1998;124:1145–1152.
5. Somogyi L, Mishra G. Diagnosis and staging of islet cell tumors of the pancreas. *Curr Gastroenterol Rep*. 2000;2:159–164.
6. Perrier ND, Batts KP, Thompson GB, et al. An immunohistochemical survey for neuroendocrine cells in regional pancreatic lymph nodes: a plausible explanation for primary nodal gastrinomas. *Surgery*. 1995;118:957–965.
7. Ellison EC. Forty year appraisal of gastrinoma: back to the future. *Ann Surg*. 1995;222:511–521.
8. Arnold WS, Fraker DL, Alexander HR, Weber HC, Norton JA, Jensen RT. Apparent lymph node primary gastrinoma. *Surgery*. 1994;116:1123–1129.
9. Goletti O, Chiarugi M, Buccianti P, et al. Resection of liver gastrinoma leading to persistent eugastrinemia: case report. *Eur J Surg*. 1992;158:55–57.
10. Zogakis TG, Gibril F, Libutti SK, et al. Management and outcome of patients with sporadic gastrinoma arising in the duodenum. *Ann Surg*. 2003;238:42–48.
11. Gurevich L, Kazantseva I, Isakov VA, et al. The analysis of immunophenotype of gastrin-producing tumors of the pancreas and gastrointestinal tract. *Cancer*. 2003;98:1967–1976.
12. Mignon M, Cadiot G. Diagnostic and therapeutic criteria in patients with Zollinger-Ellison syndrome and multiple endocrine neoplasia type 1. *J Intern Med*. 1998;243:489–494.
13. Mignon M, Ruszniewski R, Haffar S, Rigaud D, Rene E, Bonfils S. Current approach to the management of tumoral process in patients with gastrinoma. *World J Surg*. 1986;10:702–709.
14. Ellison EH, Wilson SD. The Zollinger-Ellison syndrome: reappraisal and evaluation of 260 registered cases. *Ann Surg*. 1964;160:512–530.
15. Roy PK, Venzon DJ, Shojamanesh H, et al. Zollinger-Ellison syndrome: clinical presentation in 261 patients. *Medicine*. 2000;79:379–411.
16. Ellison EC, Sparks J. Zollinger-Ellison syndrome in the era of effective acid suppression: are we unknowingly growing tumors? *Am J Surg*. 2003;186:245–248.
17. Jensen JC, Gardner JD. Zollinger-Ellison syndrome: clinical presentation, pathology, diagnosis and treatment. In: Dannenberg A, Zakim D, eds. *Peptic Ulcer and Other Related Diseases*. Armonk, NY: Academic Research Associates, 1991:117–212.
18. Wada M, Komoto I, Doi R, Imamura M. Intravenous calcium injection test is a novel complementary procedure in differential diagnosis for gastrinoma. *World J Surg*. 2002; 26:1291–1296.
19. Turner JJ, Wren AM, Jackson JE, Thakker RV, Meeran K. Localization of gastrinomas by selective intra-arterial calcium injection. *Clin Endocrinol*. 2002;57:821–825.
20. Zimmer T, Scherubl H, Faiss S, Stolzel U, Riecken EO, Wiedenmann B. Endoscopic ultrasonography of neuroendocrine tumours. *Digestion*. 2000;62:45–50.
21. Cohen MS, Picus D, Lairmore TC, Strasberg SM, Doherty GM, Norton JA. Prospective study of provocative angiograms to localize functional islet cell tumors of the pancreas. *Surgery*. 1997;122:1091–1100.
22. Metz DC, Pisegna JR, Fishbeyn VA, Benya RV, Jensen RT. Control of gastric acid hypersecretion in the management of patients with Zollinger-Ellison syndrome. *World J Surg*. 1993;17:468–480.
23. Macfarlane MP, Fraker DL, Alexander HR, Norton JA, Jensen RT. A prospective study of surgical resection of duodenal and pancreatic gastrinomas in MEN-1. *Surgery*. 1995;118:973–9.
24. Fraker DL, Norton JA, Alexander HR, Venzon DJ, Jensen RT. Surgery in Zollinger-Ellison syndrome alters the natural history of gastrinoma. *Ann Surg*. 1994;220:320–330.
25. Kato M, Imamura M, Hosotani R, et al. Curative resection of microgastrinomas based on the intraoperative secretin test. *World J Surg*. 2000;24:1425–1430.
26. Norton JA, Kivlen M, Li M, Schneider D, Chuter T, Jensen RT. Morbidity and mortality of aggressive resection in patients with advanced neuroendocrine tumors. *Arch Surg*. 2003;138:859–866.
27. Shojamanesh H, Gibril F, Louie A, et al. Prospective study of the antitumor efficacy of long-term octreotide treatment in patients with progressive metastatic gastrinoma. *Cancer*. 2002;94:331–343.

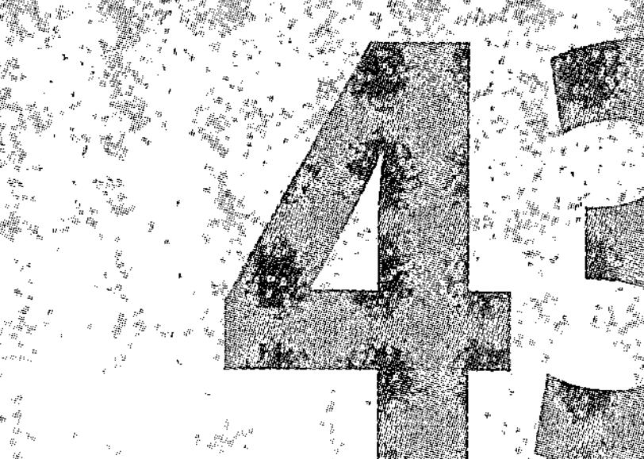

CHAPTER 43

Sporadic Insulinoma

Michael J. Demeure, MD

Insulinomas, although rare, are the most common neuroendocrine tumor of the pancreas. The incidence is approximately four cases per million person-years. The median age at diagnosis is 47 years, with a range of 8 to 82 years. There is a slight female predominance in that 59% of the cases occur in women.[1] The majority of these tumors are solitary, benign, and readily curable with surgical removal. Up to 16% are malignant, and in 4%–10% of the cases, insulinomas occur as part of the Multiple Endocrine Neoplasia type 1 (MEN-1) syndrome.[2,3] These MEN-1–associated insulinomas require a different surgical approach than do sporadic ones.[4] Perhaps because of their rarity, the presence of an insulinoma may not be considered in the diagnosis of a patient with atypical symptoms. A thorough understanding of the clinical presentation as well as diagnostic and imaging options is necessary for the proper care of patients with these interesting tumors.

History

The discovery of insulin was reported by Banting and Best in 1922.[5] In this report, they described a series of experiments on dogs with diabetes in which they were able to lower serum blood sugar with a series of injections of extracts from duct-ligated pancreas. At the time he began his studies, Banting was an orthopedic surgeon in London, Ontario, who took time away from his clinical activities. Charles Best was a fourth-year medical student who joined Banting to work in the lab of Dr. J. J. R. Macleod at the University of Toronto. Banting sold his car to pay for the dogs used in his experiments.[6] Banting and Best first developed a model for diabetes by removing the pancreas of dogs. The difficulties in isolating insulin from pancreatic extracts stemmed from the presence of digestive enzymes degrading the insulin that was present. This was overcome by using pancreas from fetal calves before 4 months of gestation.[7] Ultimately, their work led to a report later the same year in the *Canadian Medical Journal* on the initial treatment of three cases of patients with diabetes mellitus with pancreatic extracts.[8]

Progress in the understanding of the pathologic effects of excess insulin came rapidly as evidenced in an article by Seale Harris in 1924.[9] It was known that hyperthyroidism could precede hypothyroidism in some cases. Similarly, Seale reasoned that dysfunction, other than hypoinsulinism, of the islets of Langerhans resulting in hyperinsulism was possible. He noted the symptoms of excess insulin in diabetic patients and observed similar symptoms in nondiabetic patients. Similar reports followed from Jonas[10] and John.[11]

In 1926, Shields Warren described a series of 20 patients in whom islet cell tumors were observed at autopsy.[12] Wilder et al.[13] at the Mayo Clinic had been involved in the early clinical work on insulin and had reported a patient who had severe spontaneous bouts of hypoglycemia. This 40-year-old patient, who was himself a physician, had been suffering from progressively worsening "sudden attacks of faintness and weakness" for 18 months. He found he could control his symptoms by eating between meals or consuming sweet drinks. His attacks worsened to the point of collapse, and resuscitation became possible only with intravenous injections of dextrose solutions. As no medical treatment could offer control of the disease, William J. Mayo operated on this man and found liver metastases originating from an islet cell cancer arising in the tail of the pancreas. In 1929, Howland et al.[14] reported the first patient with an insulinoma diagnosed during life who was cured by surgical extirpation. This patient was a 52-year-old woman who had formerly practiced law. She had a 6-year history of symptoms, including exhaustion, convulsions, and coma associated with vomiting and sweats. Initially, a light meal at the early onset of symptoms was sufficient to ward off an attack, but later this did not suffice. An islet cell tumor of the pancreas producing hyperinsulinism was diagnosed, and so Roscoe R. Graham performed an operative exploration. The result was the enucleation of a 2-cm mass from the body of the pancreas and the first curative resection of a benign insulinoma.

Clinical Presentation and Biochemical Evaluation

Accounts of the clinical presentations of the patients described previously here nicely detail many of the symptoms and signs of hypoglycemia. A classic report by Whipple and Franz[15] in 1935 detailed the history of discovery leading to the appreciation of the disease state associated with hyperinsulinism and insulin producing islet cell tumors. They reviewed the cases reported to date and added six cases of their own on which they operated to the series. Their description of the symptoms associated with insulinoma is now referred to as Whipple's triad:

1. The patient exhibits signs and symptoms of hypoglycemia during fasting.
2. At the time of symptoms, serum glucose is ≤45 mg/dl.
3. The symptoms are relieved by oral or intravenous administration of glucose.

The symptoms and signs commonly associated with hypoglycemia include neuroglycopenic symptoms such as confusion, blurred vision, weakness, or headache and autonomic symptoms, including anxiety, sweating, hunger, and palpitations. A delay in the diagnosis is not uncommon, as these patients are often diagnosed with psychiatric or neurologic disorders. In one series, patients with insulinomas had symptoms for approximately 3 years before diagnosis.[16] It may be to the chagrin of a treating physician that the observation of hypoglycemia leading to a diagnosis of insulinoma is first observed by a nurse or paramedic who routinely checks a fingerstick blood glucose level as part of protocol treatment of a poorly responsive patient.

The essential diagnostic test for a suspected insulinoma is a supervised 72-hour fast, during which patients are observed for signs and symptoms of hypoglycemia. Approximately 70% of patients with insulinomas will develop hypoglycemic symptoms within 24 hours, and up to 98% will do so within 72 hours. Every 6 hours, simultaneous blood draws for blood glucose, insulin, and C-peptide levels should be drawn. If the blood glucose drops below 60 mg/dl, blood draws should be done more frequently, and the test should be concluded if the patient develops symptoms and a blood glucose level below 40 mg/dl. An inappropriately high insulin level in the face of hypoglycemia, that is, an insulin to glucose ratio greater than 0.3, secures the diagnosis of an insulinoma. Levels of C-peptide and proinsulin should also be elevated in these patients. If they are not, one should look for insulin antibodies, the detection of which should alert the clinician to the use of exogenous insulin. Patients should also undergo a sulfonylurea screen to exclude the surreptitious use of oral hypoglycemic agents.

In equivocal cases, stimulatory tests with secretagogues such as tolbutamide, leucine, glucagon, or calcium have been suggested. These tests have proven to be neither sensitive nor specific.[17,18] The C-peptide suppression test may be more reliable. This test is predicated on the observation that insulin and C-peptide secretion by an insulinoma is autonomous and not suppressed by low serum glucose levels. Plasma C-peptide levels are measured at 15-minute intervals after the injection of 0.1-mU/kg body weight bovine or porcine insulin. A fall in C-peptide levels suggests normal suppression of secretion, thus excluding an insulinoma, whereas persistently inappropriately elevated C-peptide levels are indicative of an insulinoma.[19]

Pathology

Insulinomas arise from the β-islet cells of the pancreas that are components of a diffuse neuroendocrine cell system derived from specialized ectoderm.[20] Pancreatic islet cell

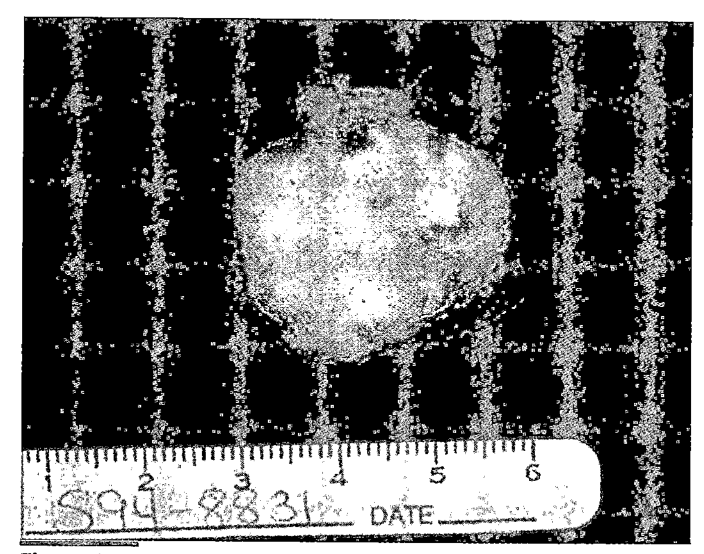

Figure 43.1
Gross appearance of a benign insulinoma removed by enucleation.

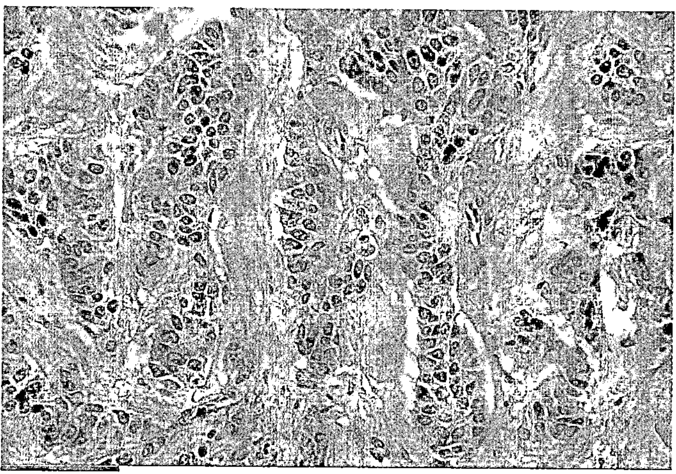

Figure 43.2
Microscopic appearance of a benign insulin producing islet cell tumor.

tumors may produce more than one peptide, but they are classified according to the clinical syndrome that predominates or the hormone that is demonstrated in most abundance in the serum.[21] The majority of insulinomas are solitary, well-demarcated tumors measuring 1–2 cm in diameter (Fig. 43.1). They are of a firm consistency and grossly similar to other tumors of neuroendocrine origin such as parathyroid adenomas and pheochromocytoma. Rarely, some islet cell tumors, including insulinomas, may present as cystic pancreatic neoplasms.[22,23] By microscopy, insulinomas form solid nests with areas exhibiting a trabecular pattern but often also have glandular or gland-like elements (Fig. 43.2).[24] Electron microscopy demonstrates the endocrine nature of these tumors with many electron-dense secretory granules in the cytoplasm.[25]

Anatomy and Localization

Imaging studies should be performed after diagnosis is confirmed by biochemical investigations. Before an operation for insulinoma, most, if not all, endocrine surgeons would agree that one should exclude metastatic disease to the liver by either computerized tomography (CT) or magnetic resonance imaging (MRI). The reasons for selecting one modality over another are varied but include institutional expertise and the ease of obtaining one study compared with the other. This author prefers MRI because the properties of neuroendocrine tumors allow for enhancement with T2 weighting or with gadolinium contrast. Beyond this area of general agreement, the optimum and most cost-effective preoperative localization algorithm for a sporadic insulinoma remain an area of debate. Some authors have written that beyond excluding metastases no preoperative imaging is required and that surgeons should employ careful bimanual palpation of the pancreas with intraoperative high-resolution ultrasonography. This approach should allow identification of at least 90% of insulinomas.[26] Virtually all insulinomas are to be found in the pancreas. Those who argue for more extensive imaging before operation cite the financial and emotional costs of a failed exploration.

CT has the advantages of being widely available, relatively inexpensive, and noninvasive. Unfortunately, the sensitivity for identifying an insulinoma is as low as 11%–17%,[27,28] but in one series it was a respectable 73%.[29] Imaging technology continues to improve with faster spiral CT providing dynamic imaging and thin slices, and thus, sensitivity may improve. In one recent series from the Mayo Clinic, 19 of 30 (63%) insulinomas were identified using multiphasic CT, including arterial, pancreatic, and portal venous phases.[30] Most tumors were hyperenhancing on at least one phase, usually an early phase. Retrospective analysis of the images in the 11 patients, in whom no insulinoma was prospectively identified, showed the tumor in six. MRI may be better than CT. Theoni et al.[31] reported identification of 85% of 20 functional small islet cell tumors, including 18 insulinomas using MRI with a 1.5-T magnet. Images were best seen with T2-weighted fast spin echo or spoiled gradient-echo; however, in some cases, gadolinium enhancement improved identification of the tumor. In another series of 26 patients with insulinomas, MRI with a 0.5-T magnet was 92% sensitive.[32] If the MRI or CT localizes the insulinoma, this author will proceed to operation at this point but if the localizing studies are negative, then additional imaging tests are used.

Endoscopic ultrasound (EUS) has been touted by many, but results are largely dependent on the operator. The sensitivity is generally reported to be in the 70%–95% range; however, sensitivity is likely to be less for tumors in the region of the pancreatic tail.[33] The addition of EUS in the evaluation of patients in whom CT or MRI has not identified the primary tumor has been shown to be cost-effective if one then can forego more expensive tests such as venous sampling or angiography.[34] This group of investigators from the University of Michigan argues that for patients with a sporadic insulinoma, EUS should be the initial diagnostic test. A CT or MRI to exclude metastatic disease should only be done for tumors larger than 3 cm by EUS because smaller tumors are rarely malignant. In a recent series from France, using the combination of thin-cut, dual-phase helical CT and EUS, insulinomas were correctly identified in all 32 patients seen from 1987 to 2000.[35] This latter regimen seems a cost-effective and efficient preoperative imaging protocol.

Nuclear medicine imaging or somatostatin receptor scintigraphy (SRS) of insulinomas with ^{111}In-pentectreotide relies on the finding that most insulinomas have somatostatin receptor subtypes 2 and 5 and, in one series, SRS had a sensitivity of 60%.[36] SRS for the localization of insulinomas is not usually favored because of a relatively low sensitivity and the availability of other modalities.[37,38] The sensitivity of SRS is improved when tomographic images (SPECT or Single Photon Emission Computed Tomography) are obtained in addition to planar images, and thus, SPECT should be routinely done when SRS is employed.[39]

The sensitivity of more invasive imaging techniques such as angiography (36%–55%) and transhepatic portal venous sampling (55%–100%) are not appreciably better than the less invasive techniques discussed.[40,41] In 1987, Imamura et al.[42] reported on a technique to identify gastrinomas by selective injection of the arteries supplying the duodenum and pancreas with secretin. Blood was sampled from the hepatic veins, and a rise in gastrin levels was seen after injection into the artery supplying the region of the gastrinoma. Doppman et al.[43] adapted this test to locate an insulinoma in four patients using calcium as the secretagogue. Calcium infusion causes a rise in insulin and C-peptide levels within 30 to 60 seconds.[40,44] The group from the National Institutes of Health later reported their experience with selective arterial calcium stimulation in 31 patients with insulinomas and reported a sensitivity of 94%.[45]

Conduct of the Operation

Before proceeding with an operation, it is essential to have a secure biochemical diagnosis of endogenous hypoglycemia due to an insulin-producing tumor. Iatrogenic, factitious, or drug-induced causes of hypoglycemia should be excluded. Accordingly then, if one follows these tenets, inappropriate laparotomies for an incorrect diagnosis should be rare events.[46] One should have available the capacity for rapid intraoperative glucose monitoring and ideally, the rapid assay for insulin that is now available.[47] A rise in serum glucose after removal of a pancreatic tumor is indicative of a curative operation and gratifying to the surgical team. Intraoperative ultrasound with a high frequency (10–12 mHz) probe is an important adjunct to the exploration. If the surgeon is not very familiar with interpretation of ultrasound finding, he should have a radiologist available to come to the operating room. If one chooses not to do preoperative localizing tests, as Grant et al.[48] stated, one is placing "consummate faith in the combined techniques of surgical exploration and intraoperative ultrasonography."

The abdomen is entered via either a midline incision or a bilateral subcostal incision. Mechanical retractors facilitate exposure. A careful and thorough exploration with particular attention to the liver as well as portal and peripancreatic lymph nodes is conducted to assess for possible metastases. Even if preoperative studies have identified the location of the insulinoma, the entire pancreas should still be explored because 13%–24% of patients have multiple insulinomas.[49,50]

For tumors of the head of the pancreas, an extensive Kocher maneuver is done by incising the lateral peritoneal attachments of the duodenum. In this manner, one can fully mobilize the pancreatic head to allow careful palpation and ultrasound evaluation of the head and uncinate process. At this time, one should also inspect the periaortic lymph nodes behind the head of the pancreas. One must then decide whether the tumor may be safely enucleated or whether a pancreaticoduodenectomy is needed.

For tumors of the body or tail of the pancreas, the lesser sac is entered through the gastrocolic omentum. The stomach is retracted in an upward direction, and the anterior surface of the pancreas identified. The peritoneum along the superior and inferior aspects of the body and tail of the pancreas is incised. The pancreas can then be palpated between the thumb and forefinger or between the fingers of two hands. Often, an insulinoma can be seen on the anterior surface of the pancreas. They typically appear as a reddish tan to brown nodule. A tumor that is not visible may be felt as a firm area within the pancreatic parenchyma. Intraoperative ultrasound is a useful adjunct not only to identify the tumor but also to establish its location in relationship to the pancreatic duct and splenic vessels. In some cases, resection is safer than enucleation. For multiple lesions in the body and tail, a distal pancreatectomy is advisable. As most insulinomas are benign, a spleen-preserving distal pancreatectomy is generally preferred to an en bloc resection of the tail of the pancreas and spleen.

For enucleation, one must have good exposure and control of the pancreas. The lesion is approached with a fine hemostat, electrocautery, and small hemostatic clips. The site of the tumor resection should be carefully inspected for evidence of the leakage of clear watery fluid indicative of pancreatic juice. Administration of 1 mg of secretin stimulates increased production of pancreatic juice and may facilitate identification of an injury to the pancreatic duct. If identified, pancreatic resection should be considered. Alternatively, one can anastomose the defect in the pancreas to a Roux limb of jejunum. If no leak is present the defect in the resection bed may be gently closed or plugged with omentum. Some have advocated the use of tissue sealants, but there is no proof that pancreatic fistula rates are reduced. Similarly, the perioperative use of somatostatin analogues such as octreotide or vapreotide does not appear to reduce the rate of pancreatic fistula formation after pancreatic resection,[51] and thus, it does not seem likely that it would be of benefit in preventing a pancreatic leak after enucleation. This author places closed-suction drains near the tumor resection site.

Because they are generally small and benign, insulinomas are perhaps the pancreatic tumors best suited for resection by a laparoscopic approach. In 1996, Gagner et al.[52] reported a series of 12 patients with islet cell tumors of the pancreas, most of them insulinomas, who underwent attempts at either laparoscopic distal pancreatectomy or enucleation of their tumors. One could question the success of this early experience as four patients were converted to open procedures, and in two patients, the insulinoma was not found. The threshold was, however, crossed, and several reports have followed demonstrating that laparoscopic surgery for insulinomas is possible and offers the advantages of minimally invasive surgery to this group of patients.[53,54] The list of laparoscopic procedures reported now includes distal pancreatectomy with preservation of the spleen.[55] Limitations remain and include a relatively high fistula rate and the technical demands of the procedure with associated prolonged operative times. A hand-assist approach may be ideal in some cases because one may need to palpate the pancreas for a small insulinoma, and the patient will derive the benefits of a small incision. Presently, the laparoscopic approach is not indicated for insulinomas in the setting of MEN-1 or for malignant or large tumors. The report by Fernandez-Cruz et al.[53] contains an excellent description of the laparoscopic conduct of the operation, and the reader is referred to it for details of the procedure.

In the event that pancreatic exploration is unsuccessful in locating an insulinoma, a distal pancreatectomy should be done only if one has established that the location of the insulinoma is in the pancreatic tail, by means of an invasive test such as selective venous sampling with arterial stimulation. Despite recommendations by some authors in the past,[56] a "blind" distal pancreatectomy should not be done. Such authors recommended up to a 90% distal pancreatectomy because they said an occult insulinoma is found in 46%–90% of cases.[2,57] This approach is no longer recommended. It is just as likely, or perhaps more so, that the missed insulinoma is in the pancreatic head or uncinate as it is in the tail. If the tail is resected and the insulinoma is not removed, one may be left with the prospect of needing to remove the remaining pancreas with a pancreaticoduodenectomy. In such a situation it is better to close the patient's abdomen, control the hypoglycemic symptoms with medications, and embark on a search for the missing insulinoma or establish whether the patient has a rare case of adult nesidioblastosis.

Glucose levels should be closely monitored during the operation. Intravenous infusion with dextrose solution is used to maintain the serum glucose level in an acceptable range. One typically sees a rise in the serum glucose level within 20 minutes after successful removal of an insulinoma; however, this response may be delayed.[58] One should be cautious, however, because false positives and negatives do occur.[59] Generally, the serum glucose levels will rise to the 200- to 300-mg/dl range for several days to 3 weeks after successful surgery, and then gradually, blood sugar levels will return to normal.[60] Recently, Carniero et al.[47] reported on the use of a rapid chemiluminescent assay for insulin. Assay results were available within 8 minutes, making this assay a useful intraoperative adjunct. In this report, eight consecutive patients underwent pancreatic resection for insulinomas. In the perioperative period, the patients were infused with 10% dextrose at a rate sufficient to maintain their blood sugar levels near 150 mg/dl. Blood levels of insulin were determined at the start of surgery, during dissection of the pancreatic tumor, and after removal of the insulinoma. Using the intraoperative insulin assay, these authors recommend that the criteria for a successful curative resection be as follows: (1) the return of insulin levels to normal (10–86 pmol/L) 15 minutes after tumor removal and (2) an insulin to glucose ratio of less than 0.4. These authors do warn that diazoxide may interfere with performance of this assay in these patients. An advantage of this particular system (Future Diagnostics, Wijchen, Netherlands) is that the insulin assay can be done with the same equipment that is used for the intraoperative parathyroid hormone assay. Otherwise, the purchase of such equipment for use in a rare number of cases would be difficult to justify from a financial perspective alone. These authors also suggest that one do a fine-needle aspirate of any suspicious nodule and eject the contents into 1 ml of saline. One should see a high insulin level in the saline if the tumor biopsied is an insulinoma. The optimum criteria for prediction of a postoperative cure, remain to be established. Proye et al.[61] suggested that one should see normal peripheral and portal vein blood insulin levels 20 minutes after resection.

Adult Nesidioblastosis

Organic hyperinsulinism caused by hypertrophy of the β-islet cells is a well-known phenomenon in neonates but a rare event in adults.[62,63] The Mayo Clinic group has reported on a series of 10 patients with what they term noninsulinoma pancreatogenous hypoglycemia.[64] These patients all had biochemical evidence suggestive of an insulinoma, yet no tumor was found. Preoperative selective arterial calcium stimulation guided surgeons to a distal pancreatectomy. Pathologic examination of the operative specimens demonstrated islet cell hypertrophy or nesidioblastosis. Eight of the 10 patients had improvement in their hypoglycemia. It would seem that intraoperative insulin and glucose monitoring would be particularly useful in this patient population to guide the extent of pancreatic resection.

Malignant Insulinomas

Approximately 10% of insulinomas are malignant. The behavior of malignant insulinomas tends to be fairly indolent, although progressive. One 60-year study from the Mayo Clinic found a 10-year survival rate of 29%.[1] A malignant insulinoma (Fig. 43.3) should be suspected if the primary tumor is larger than 3 cm. In all cases, one should carefully evaluate the liver and peripancreatic lymph nodes for evidence of metastatic disease. Suspicious nodes should be sampled for histopathology. For lesions in the body and tail, an en bloc distal pancreatectomy and splenectomy with nodal dissection should be done. For malignant insulinomas of the pancreatic head or uncinate, a Whipple procedure is recommended. Even if a cure is not possible, an aggressive surgical approach to debulk tumor and resect liver metastases is warranted to ameliorate hypoglycemic symptoms. Although there are no prospective randomized series, single-institution retrospective series suggest that complete surgical resection can improve survival. McEntee et al.[65] reviewed their experience with 17 patients who underwent complete resection of neuroendocrine metastases to the liver. Of these, 11 (65%) were alive and free of disease at a mean follow-up interval of 19 months.

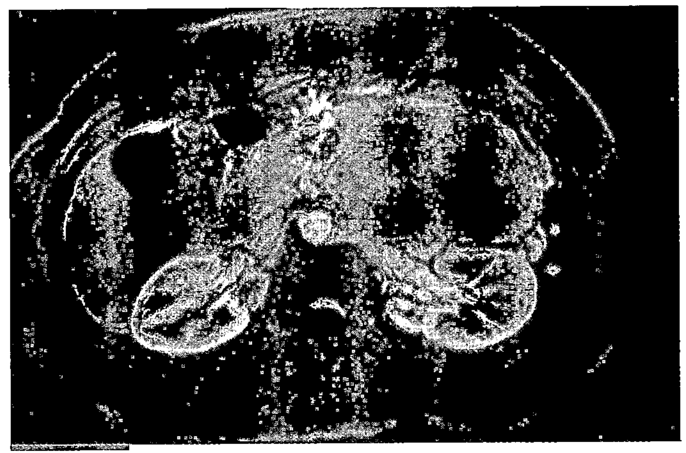

Figure 43.3
Large malignant insulin producing islet cell cancer of the pancreatic body and tail.

Although there is increasing anecdotal experience with hepatic artery embolization (HAE) or chemoembolization, there are few series that demonstrate efficacy of these techniques. In order to treat unresectable, liver dominant or exclusive disease, interventional radiologists can introduce catheters selectively into the hepatic arteries. The premise for this treatment modality is that the metastases derive their blood supply predominantly from the arterial rather than the portal system. Embolization deprives the tumors of nutrient blood flow, whereas the hepatic parenchyma can survive on portal flow. Embolization after the instillation of chemotherapy is thought to enhance the activity of the cytotoxic drugs because the lack of arterial flow slows washout of the drugs from the liver, hopefully enhancing the antitumor effect. Chamberlain et al.[66] from Memorial Sloan-Kettering studied the efficacy of surgery, HAE, and medical therapy in 85 patients with hepatic neuroendocrine metastasis from 1992 to 1998. There were 59 (69%) nonfunctional islet cell tumors included in this study. Patients were offered

HAE if they were not candidates for surgical resection and their pain or hormonal symptoms were refractory to pharmacologic treatment. A small number of patients (n = 7) were embolized to attempt to control aggressive tumor growth. Embolization was conducted using polyvinyl alcohol particles to embolize the lobe of the liver that had the greatest tumor burden. There were 59 separate embolization sessions in 33 patients. Symptoms were palliated in 94% of the patients undergoing HAE. The procedure-related mortality of both surgical resection and HAE was 6%. Yao et al.[67] from Northwestern University recently reported their series of 36 patients with liver metastases from neuroendocrine tumors. Twenty of these patients underwent chemoembolization with cisplatin, doxorubicin, and mitomycin C combined with viscous collagen agent or ethiodol and polyvinyl alcohol particles. Seven of these patients had clinical or radiographic effects of tumor response that were sustained for more than 1 year, although all patients eventually developed progressive disease.

Liver transplantation for metastatic islet-cell tumors remains controversial. Proponents argue that for multifocal, unresectable liver disease, in the absence of distant metastases outside the liver, transplantation provides relief of symptoms in both functioning and nonfunctioning neoplasms. Several small studies have shown limited efficacy and even increased length of survival compared with historic controls for patients undergoing liver transplantation. The largest series was from the multicenter French experience and included 31 patients, the reported 5-year actuarial survival was 36% with 5 patients surviving longer than 5 years.[68] This is noteworthy because patients in this study were selected after failing other treatments. Only 16% of the study patients had not undergone any prior medical or surgical treatment. Enthusiasm, however, should be tempered by the high operative mortality of 19%. Patients with carcinoid tumors faired much better than the rest of the group (40% actuarial survival at 5 years compared with 0%), including those with metastatic islet cell carcinoma.

Medical Control of Hypoglycemia

The standard agent for the medical management of problematic hypoglycemia in patients with insulinomas is diazoxide. It is used for patients before surgery, after failed surgery, or for those whose tumors are not resectable. Diazoxide is a nondiuretic benzothiazine derivative introduced during the 1950s as an antihypertensive agent.[69] It was soon appreciated that hyperglycemia was a side-effect of the medication,[70] and it later became recognized that diazoxide was effective in controlling hypoglycemia in patients harboring insulinomas.[71] The initial starting dose is 5 mg/kg, given in divided doses three times per day, and is titrated for biochemical control. Treatment with diazoxide controls symptoms well in 78%–97% of patients.[69,72] The principal side effects are usually mild and not problematic. These include hirsutism, hypotension, rash, nausea, and weight gain caused by sodium and fluid retention.[72] Administration of diazoxide should be discontinued the evening before surgery so as not to interfere with intraoperative monitoring of glucose levels.[69]

Octreotide acetate (Sandostatin) is a synthetic cyclic octapeptide that is analogous to and exerts similar pharmacologic actions as the natural gut hormone somatostatin. Somatostatin is a 14 amino acid peptide that binds to five different somatostatin receptor subtypes in humans. Like somatostatin, octreotide is a potent inhibitor of insulin, growth hormone, glucagon, gastrin, vasoactive intestinal peptide, secretin, motilin, pancreatic polypeptide, and serotonin; it decreases splanchnic blood flow. Octreotide is typically used as an adjunct to therapy in functional islet cell tumors to decrease the release of the biologically active peptide hormones responsible for the patient's symptoms and to decrease the hormone's effects on target organs. Currently, the Food and Drug Administration has approved the use of octreotide for the treatment of acromegaly, symptoms related to carcinoid syndrome, or profuse watery diarrhea associated with vasoactive intestinal peptidomas. It is not normally used in patients with insulinomas, but monthly injections of long-acting octreotide may be beneficial for patients whose hypoglycemia is difficult to control. Preclinical data suggest that octreotide may inhibit tumor growth by decreasing the effects of mediators of cell proliferation such as insulin-like growth factors, epidermal growth factors, and transforming growth factor-α. This may be the basis for tumor regression on octreotide therapy seen in anecdotal reports. Some have suggested that octreotide in high doses (500–1,000 mg three times daily) could have cytoreductive activity. A multicenter study in Italy conducted on 58 patients with islet cell tumors showed ultrasound confirmed stabilization of disease in 47% of patients at 6 months and 22% of patients at 1 year.[73] The 3% rate of tumor regression seen in this study was disappointing. No studies have shown an increase in survival due to treatment with octreotide. The usual starting dose is 100–150 mcg injected subcutaneously three times daily, but higher doses are often required. Octreotide has also recently become available in a long-acting injectable depot suspension (Sandostatin LAR). Long-acting octreotide maintains all of the pharmacologic effects as the immediate-release form of the drug. It is administered by intramuscular injection every 4 weeks at a dose of 20–30 mg. Although more expensive, benefits of the long-acting form of the drug include improved patient comfort by avoiding thrice daily injections and a potential cost savings that might be realized by avoiding home nurse visits or hospitalization.

In 1992, Moertel et al.[74] published their classic study on the use of chemotherapy for metastatic islet cell tumors. In this multicenter trial, patients who had unresectable or metastatic islet cell carcinoma were randomly assigned to receive one of three chemotherapy regimens. These included streptozocin plus fluorouracil, streptozocin plus doxorubicin, or chlorozotocin alone. This study included 105 patients that were not categorized by their specific islet cell neoplasm subtype. The response was determined by both changes in tumor size as documented by CT scan and/or by reduction serum hormone level. The streptozocin-doxorubicin combination had the highest response rates, with 69% of patients showing documented tumor response. Median survival was also highest for the streptozocin-doxorubicin group (2.2 years) compared with the streptozocin-fluorouracil (1.4 years) and streptozocin only groups (1.5 years). The degree to which this study can be extrapolated to insulin producing neoplasms is unclear, but there does appear to be benefit in using this chemotherapeutic regimen in the management of nonoperable disease. A limitation of this study is the lack of a matched, control group that did not receive chemotherapy.

References

1. Service FJ, McMahon MM, O'Brien PC, et al. Functioning insulinoma-incidence, recurrence and long-term survival of patients: a 60-year study. *Mayo Clin Proc.* 1991;66: 711–719.
2. Stephanini P, Carboni M, Patrassi N, Basoli A. Beta-islet tumors of the pancreas: results of a study of 1067 cases. *Surgery.* 1974;75:597–609.
3. Burns AR, Dackiw APB. Insulinoma. *Curr Treat Options Oncol.* 2003;4:309–317.
4. Demeure MJ, Klonoff DC, Karam JH, Duh Q-Y, Clark OH. Insulinomas associated with multiple endocrine neoplasia type 1: the need for a different surgical approach. *Surgery.* 1991;110:998–1005.
5. Banting FG, Best C. Internal secretion of pancreas. *J Lab Clin Med.* 1922;7:251–266.
6. Freisen SR. *Classic descriptions of neuroendocrine syndromes of the pancreas and gut.* Austin, TX: RG Landes; 1993:58–91.
7. Bliss M. Banting's, Best's, and Collip's accounts of the discovery of insulin. *Bull Hist Med.* 1982;56:554–568.
8. Banting FG, Best CH, Collip JB, Campbell W, Fletcher AA. Pancreatic extracts in the treatment of diabetes mellitus. *Canad Med A J.* 1922;12:141.
9. Harris S. Hyperinsulinism and dysinsulinism. *JAMA.* 1924;83:729–733.
10. Jonas L. Hypoglycemia. *Med Clin North Am.* 1924;8:949–958.
11. John HJ. Hyperinsulinism. *Surg Gynecol Obstet.* 1927;44: 190–193.
12. Warren S. Adenomas of islands of Langerhans. *Am J Pathol.* 1926;2:335–340.
13. Wilder RM, Allan FN, Power MH, Robertson HE. Carcinoma of the islets of the pancreas: hyperinsulinism and hypoglycemia. *JAMA.* 1927;89:348–355.
14. Howland G, Campbell WR, Maltby EJ, Robinson WL. Dysinsulinism: convulsions and coma due to islet cell tumor of the pancreas, with operation and cure. *JAMA.* 1929;93: 674–679.
15. Whipple AO, Franz VK. Adenoma of islet cells with hyperinsulinism. *Am Surg.* 1935;101:1299–1355.
16. Grant CS. Insulinoma. *Surg Oncol Clin North Am.* 1998;7: 819–844.
17. Service FJ, Dale AJD, Elveback IR, et al. Insulinoma: clinical and diagnostic features of 60 consecutive cases. *Mayo Clin Proc.* 1976;51:417–429.
18. Arnold R, Frank M, Bülchman G. Insulinoma and persistent neonatal hyperinsulinemic hypoglycemia (nesidioblastosis). In: Beger HG, Warshaw AL, Bücher MW, et al., eds. *The Pancreas.* Oxford, UK: Blackwell Science; 1998: 1187–1202.
19. Turner RC, Keding I. Plasma proinsulin, C-peptide and insulin in diagnostic suppression test for insulinomas. *Diabetologia.* 1977;13:571–577.
20. Pearce AGE. Peptides in brain and intestine. *Nature.* 1976;262:92–94.
21. Heitz PU, Kasper M, Polak JM, Klöppel G. Pathology of the endocrine pancreas. *J Histochem Cytochem.* 1979;27: 1401–1402.
22. Pareja-Megía MJ, Ríos-Martin JJ, García-Escudero A, Gonzáles-Cámpora R. Papillary and cystic insulinoma of the pancreas. *Histopathology.* 2002;40:488–489.
23. Grogan JR, Saeian K, Taylor AJ, Quiroz F, Demeure MJ, Komorowski RA. Making sense of mucin-producing pancreatic tumors. *AJR Am J Roentgenol.* 2001;176:921–929.
24. Heitz PU, Klöppel G. Pancreatic endocrine tumors. *Path Res Pract.* 1988;183:155–168.
25. Greider MH, Elliott DW. Electron microscopy of human pancreatic tumors of islet cell origin. *Am J Pathol.* 1964;44:663–678.
26. Boukhman MP, Karam JM, Shaver J, Siperstein AE, DeLorimier AA, Clark OH. Localization of insulinomas. *Arch Surg.* 1999;134;818–823.
27. Gianello P, Gigot JF, Berthet F, et al. Pre- and intraoperative localization of insulinomas: report of twenty-two observations. *World J Surg.* 1988;12:389–397.
28. Doherty GM, Doppman JL, Shawker TH, et al. Results of a prospective strategy to diagnose, localize and resect insulinomas. *Surgery.* 1991;110:989–997.
29. Bottger TC, Weber W, Beyer J, Junginger T. Value of tumor localization in patients with insulinoma. *World J Surg.* 1990;14:107–114.

30. Felder JL, Fletcher JG, Reading CC, et al. Preoperative detection of pancreatic insulinomas on multiphasic helical CT. *AJR Am J Roentgenol.* 2003;181:775–780.
31. Theoni RF, Mueller-Lisse UG, Chan R, Do NK, Shyn PB. Detection of small, functional islet cell tumors in the pancreas: selection of MR imaging sequences for optimal sensitivity. *Radiology.* 2000;214:483–490.
32. Catalano C, Pavone P, Laghi A, et al. Localization of pancreatic insulinomas with MR imaging at 0.5 T. *Acta Radiol.* 1999;40:644–648.
33. Grant CS. Surgical aspects of hyperinsulinemic hypoglycemia. *Endocrinol Clin North Am.* 1999;28:533–554.
34. Bansal R, Tierney W, Carpenter S, Thompson N, Scheiman JM. Cost effectiveness of EUS for preoperative localization of pancreatic endocrine tumors. *Gastrointest Endosc.* 1999;49:19–25.
35. Gouya H, Vignaux O, Augui J. CT, endoscopic sonography, and a combined protocol for preoperative evaluation of pancreatic insulinomas. *AJR Am J Roentgenol.* 2003;181:987–992.
36. Bertherat F, Tenenbaum K, Perlemoine C, et al. Somatostatin receptors 2 and 5 are the major somatostatin receptors in insulinomas: an *in vivo* and *in vitro* study. *J Clin Endocrinol Metab.* 2003;88:5353–5360.
37. Lamberts SW, Kenning EP, Reubi JC. The role of somatostatin and its analogues in the diagnosis and treatment of tumors. *Endocr Rev.* 1991;12:450–482.
38. Perry RR, Vinik AI. Diagnosis and management of functioning islet cell tumors. *J Clin Endocrinol Metab.* 1195;80: 2273–2278.
39. Schillaci O, Massa R, Scopinaro F. 111In-pentecreotide scintigraphy in the detection of insulinomas: importance of SPECT imaging. *J Nucl Med.* 2000;41:459–462.
40. Won JGS, Tseng H-S, Yan A-H, et al. Intra-arterial calcium stimulation test for detection of insulinomas: detection rate, responses to pancreatic peptides, and its relationship to differentiation of tumor cells. *Metabolism.* 2003;52:1320–1329.
41. Hiramoto JS, Feldstein VA, LaBerge JM, Norton JA. Intraoperative ultrasound and preoperative localization detects all occult insulinomas. *Arch Surg.* 2001;136: 1020–1025.
42. Imamura M, Takahashi K, Adashi H, et al. Usefulness of selective arterial secretin injection test for localization of gastrinomas in the Zollinger-Ellison syndrome. *Ann Surg.* 1987;205:230–239.
43. Doppman JL, Miller JL, Chang R, et al. Insulinoma: localization with selective intraarterial injection of calcium. *Radiology.* 1991;178:237–241.
44. Prentki M, Matschinsky FM. Ca2+, camp, and phospholipids-derived messengers in coupling mechanisms of insulin secretion. *Physiol Rev.* 1987;67:1185–1248.
45. Brown CK, Bartlett DL, Doppman JL, et al. Intraarterial calcium stimulation and intraoperative ultrasonography in the localization and resection of insulinomas. *Surgery.* 1997;122:1189–1194.
46. Rothmund M, Angelini L, Brunt M, et al. Surgery for benign insulinoma: an international review. *World J Surg.* 1990;14:393–399.
47. Carniero DM, Levi JU, Irvin GL III. Rapid insulin assay for intraoperative confirmation of complete resection of insulinomas. *Surgery.* 2002;132:937–943.
48. Grant CS, vanHeerden JA, Charboneau JW, et al. Insulinoma: the value of intraoperative ultrasonography. *Arch Surg.* 1988;123:843–847.
49. Fajans SS, Vinik AI. Insulin-producing islet cell tumors. *Endocrinol Metab Clin North Am.* 1989;18:45–74.
50. Stefanini P, Carboni M, Patrassi N, Basoli A. Beta-islet cell tumors of the pancreas: results of a study on 1067 cases. *Surgery.* 1974;75:597–609.
51. Sarr MG, Pancreatic Surgery Group. The potent somatostatin analogue vapreotide does not decrease pancreas-specific complications after elective pancreatectomy: a prospective, multicenter, double-blinded, randomized, placebo-controlled trial. *JACS.* 2003;196:556–565.
52. Gagner M, Pomp A, Herrera MF. Early experience with laparoscopic resections of islet cell tumors. *Surgery.* 1996;120:1051–1054.
53. Fernandez-Cruz L, Sáenz A, Astudillo E, et al. Outcome of laparoscopic pancreatic surgery: endocrine and nonendocrine tumors. *World J Surg.* 2002;26:1057–1065.
54. Berends FJ, Cuesta MA, Kazemier G, et al. Laparoscopic detection and resection of insulinomas. *Surgery.* 2000;128:386–391.
55. Park AE, Heniford BT. Therapeutic laparoscopy of the pancreas. *Ann Surg.* 2002;236:149–158.
56. Kaplan EL, Lee C-H. Recent advances in the diagnosis and treatment of insulinomas. *Surg Clin North Am.* 1979;59: 119–129.
57. Edis AJ, McIlrath DC, van Heerden JA, Fulton RE, Sheedy PF, Service FJ, Dale AJ. Insulinoma: current diagnosis and surgical management. *Curr Prob Surg.* 1976;13(10):1-45.
58. Thompson GB. Insulinoma. In: Prinz RA, Staren ED, eds. *Endocrine Surgery.* Georgetown, TX: Landes Bioscience; 2000:222–228.
59. Harrison TS, Child CG III, Fry WJ, et al. Current surgical management of functioning islet-cell tumors of the pancreas. *Ann Surg.* 1973;178:485–495.
60. Kaplan EL, Lee C-H. Recent advancements in the diagnosis and treatment of insulinomas. *Surg Clin North Am.* 1979;59:119–129.
61. Proye CA, Pattou F, Carnaille B, Lefebvre J, Decoulx M, d'Herbomez M. Intraoperative insulin measurement during surgical management of insulinomas. *World J Surg.* 1998;22:1218–1224.
62. Stefanini P, Carboni M, Patrassi N, Basoli A. Hypoglycemia and insular hyperplasia. *Ann Surg.* 1974;180:130–135.
63. Harrison TS, Fajans SS, Floyd JC, Jr, et al. Prevalence of diffuse pancreatic beta islet cell disease with hyperinsulinism: problems in recognition and management. *World J Surg.* 1984;8:583–589.
64. Thompson GB, Service FJ, Andrews JC, et al. Noninsulinoma pancreatogenous hypoglycemia syndrome: an update in 10 surgically treated patients. *Surgery.* 2000;128:937–945.
65. McEntee GP, Nagorney DM, Kvols LK, Moertel CG, Grant CS. Cytoreductive hepatic surgery for neuroendocrine tumors. *Surgery.* 1990;108:1091–1096.

66. Chamberlain R, Canes D, Brown KT, et al. Hepatic neuroendocrine metastases: does intervention alter outcomes? *J Am Coll Surg.* 2000;190:432–445.
67. Yao KA, Talamonti MS, Nemcek A, et al. Indications and results of liver resection and hepatic chemoembolization for metastatic gastrointestinal neuroendocrine tumors. *Surgery.* 2001;120:677–685.
68. Le Treut Y, Delpero J, Dousset B, et al. Results of liver transplantation in the treatment of metastatic neuroendocrine tumors: a 31-case French multicentric report. *Ann Surg.* 1997;225:355–364.
69. Goode PN, Farndon JR, Anderson J, Johnston IDA, Morte JA. Diazoxide in the management of patients with insulinoma. *World J Surg.* 1986;10:586–592.
70. Finnerty FA. Discussion. In: Moyer JH, ed. *Hypertension: The First Hahnemann Symposium on Hypertensive Disease.* Philadelphia: WB Saunders; 1959:653.
71. Le Quesne LP, Nabarro JDN, Kurtz A, Zweig S. The management of insulinoma tumours of the pancreas. *Br J Surg.* 1979;66:373–378.
72. Gill GV, Rauf O, MacFarland IA. Diazoxide treatment for insulinoma: a national UK survey. *Postgrad Med J.* 1997;73:640–641.
73. Di Bartolomeo M, Bajetta E, Buzzoni R, Mariani L, Carnaghi C, Somma L, Zilembo N. Clinical efficacy of ocretotide in the treatment of metastatic neuroendocrine tumors: A study by the Italian Trials in Medical Oncology Group. *Cancer.* 1996;77(2):402-8.
74. Moertel CG, Lefkopoulo M, Lipsitz S, Hahn RG, Klaasen D. Streptozocin-doxorubicin, streptozocin-fluorouracil or chlorozotocin in the treatment of advanced islet-cell carcinoma. *N Engl J Med.* 1992;326(8):519–523.

CHAPTER 44

Rare Functioning Tumors: VIPoma, Glucagonoma, Somatostatinoma

Geoffrey B. Thompson, MD

In a 27-year period at the Mayo Clinic, 322 patients were treated for islet cell tumors. Ninety-three percent of these tumors were made up of insulinomas, gastrinomas, or seemingly nonfunctioning islet cell tumors. The remaining 7% were composed of a wide range of rare functioning tumors, including those that secrete adrenocorticotropic hormone, corticotropin-releasing factor, parathyroid hormone–like substances, serotonin, calcitonin, growth hormone or growth hormone–releasing factor, and cholecystokinin. The most common of these rare functioning tumors today are those that secrete vasoactive intestinal peptide (VIP), glucagon, and somatostatin.[1] A discussion of these last three tumors and their associated syndromes is the basis for this chapter (Tables 44.1 and 44.2).

VIPoma

Fewer than 300 reported cases of VIP-secreting islet cell tumors have been reported in the medical literature.[2] The syndrome associated with VIP excess has been called the Verner-Morrison syndrome, WDHA syndrome (watery diarrhea, hypokalemia, achlorhydria), WDHH syndrome (watery diarrhea, hypokalemia, hypochlorhydria), and pancreatic cholera.[1,3]

In 1958, Verner and Morrison described two patients with severe, watery diarrhea, both of whom died of dehydration and renal failure despite vigorous intravenous fluid resuscitation.[3,4] It was not until 1970 that VIP was isolated from bovine intestine.[5]

It is now known that VIP is a neuropeptide that is distributed widely throughout the central nervous system.[6] VIP can also be found in peptidergic neurons adjacent to blood vessels within the splanchnic nervous system that include the small intestine, large bowel, and pancreatic exocrine ducts.[3]

VIP exerts its effects by interacting with a specific adenylate cyclase–coupled receptor. Seventy-five percent of VIPomas arise within the pancreas; 20% are neurogenic in origin (ganglioneuroblastomas, ganglioneuromas, and neuroblastomas), and 5% are extrapancreatic and nonneurogenic (duodenum, jejunum).[2,7]

VIP has several physiologic functions that include augmentation of peristalsis, stimulation of pancreatic fluid and bicarbonate secretion, inhibition of solute absorption, and stimulation of intestinal water and ion secretion.[8] VIP directly inhibits gastric acid secretion, thus causing hypochlorhydria.[9] VIP also has a direct vasodilator effect that can lead to flushing.[10] Questions remain as to whether other substances contribute to the syndrome;

Table 44.1 Evaluation

Tumor	Site of Origin	Clinical Syndrome	Diagnosis	Localization
VIPoma	75% pancreatic (75% in the body/tail) 20% neurogenic 5% in the duodenum, jejunum	Watery diarrhea, hypokalemia, achlorhydria, hypercalcemia, hypophosphatemia, nephrolithiasis, glucose intolerance	Plasma VIP levels >1000 pg/mL	CT, SRS, IOUS, Ca^{2+} stimulation testing
Glucagonoma	100% pancreatic (90% in the body/tail)	80% glucose intolerance, 67% NME, 85% NNA, deep venous thrombosis, stomatitis, glossitis, cheilosis, vulvovaginitis	Plasma glucagon levels >1000 pg/mL	CT, SRS, IOUS
Somatostatinoma	50%–65% in the pancreatic head 35%–50% in the duodenum,[a] ampulla,[a] small bowel	Glucose intolerance Steatorrhea, gallstones, hypochlorhydria	Increased plasma somatostatin levels	CT, SRS, EUS, IOUS

[a]More common in patients with neurofibromatosis.
Abbreviations: NME, necrolytic migratory erythema; NNA, normochromic, normocytic anemia; CT, computed tomography; SRS, somatostatin-receptor scintigraphy; IOUS, intraoperative ultrasonography; EUS, endoscopic ultrasonography; VIP, vasoactive intestinal polypeptide; VIPoma, vasoactive intestinal polypeptide-secreting tumor.

these substances include histidine isoleucine and prostaglandin E, both potent secretagogues found to be increased in some patients with VIPomas.[11,12]

The VIPoma syndrome typically occurs in middle-aged adults; 10% occur in children younger than 10 years. Seventy-five percent of the pancreatic tumors arise within the body and tail. At least 50% of these are malignant, with more than half being metastatic to lymph nodes or liver by the time of diagnosis.[1,8] Ninety percent of the neurogenic tumors are benign, and 4% of the patients belong to a multiple endocrine neoplasia type 1 kindred.[1] The tumors are generally solitary, ranging in size from 2 to 6 cm. Islet cell hyperplasia and nesidioblastosis have been described in association with the VIPoma syndrome.[8]

The pathophysiologic effects of increased VIP levels and perhaps other peptides give rise to the VIPoma syndrome. The predominant symptom is that of a profuse, secretory diarrhea, typically producing 3 L or more of tea-colored stool per day.[13] Volumes of less than 700 mL/24 hours rule out a VIPoma syndrome.[14] Plasma VIP levels are typically two- to ten-fold above the upper limit of normal range (200 pg/mL). Most patients exhibit VIP levels

Table 44.2 Management

Tumor	Percent Malignant	Treatment	Palliation
VIPoma	50% 50% metastatic at diagnosis	Distal pancreatectomy ± splenic preservation Whipple procedure Enucleation Gradient-guided pancreatic resection	Liver resection, RFA, sandostatin, LAR, HAE, chemotherapy, immunotherapy, TPN, indomethacin, steroids
Glucagonoma	80% 50% metastatic at diagnosis	Distal pancreatectomy/splenectomy, regional lymphadenectomy	Liver resection, radiofrequency ablation, sandostatin, HAE, chemotherapy, immunotherapy, TPN
Somatostatinoma	Most	Whipple procedure	Liver resection, RFA, HAE, chemotherapy

Abbreviations: RFA, radiofrequency ablation; HAE, hepatic artery embolization; TPN, total parenteral nutrition; VIPoma, vasoactive intestinal polypeptide-secreting tumor; LAR, long-acting release.

greater than 1000 pg/mL.[14] Secretion may be episodic, so multiple blood samples may be required.

If the cause of diarrhea is uncertain, stool cultures should be obtained and a fasting state instituted to rule out infectious or osmotic causes (e.g., lactose intolerance). In contrast to the VIPoma syndrome, the Zollinger-Ellison syndrome is characterized by acid hypersecretion, an ulcer diathesis, and diarrhea that can be abated with nasogastric suction. The somatostatinoma syndrome is characterized by steatorrhea, and the malignant carcinoid syndrome is associated with elevated 24-hour urinary 5-hydroxyindole acetic acid levels.[8]

Once the diagnosis is established, treatment and localization should begin promptly. Failure to intervene can result in serious dehydration, electrolyte imbalance, and metabolic acidosis. If the condition is left untreated, death can result from cardiac arrhythmia and acute renal failure. Other consequences include glucose intolerance, hypophosphatemia, hypercalcemia, and nephrolithiasis.[1] Because most of these tumors are large and intrapancreatic, computed tomography (CT) remains the most cost-effective imaging modality for localization.[1,3] Somatostatin-receptor scintigraphy (SRS)[15-17] is a useful adjunct to CT if it can be obtained quickly,[18,19] because the mainstay of preoperative stabilization is treatment with somatostatin analogue along with intravenous fluid and electrolyte therapy.[10] Once somatostatin has been given, SRS becomes less reliable because of receptor binding. If somatostatin analogue has already been administered, positron-emission tomography scanning[20,21] or magnetic resonance imaging[22,23] can then be used for staging. Other adjuncts for control of diarrhea include intravenous steroids and indomethacin, the latter because of its inhibitory action on prostaglandin E synthesis.[1] Sandostatin is very effective at decreasing circulating VIP levels, decreasing stool volume, and reversing many of the metabolic and electrolyte abnormalities.[18,19]

Once the patient has been stabilized, surgical resection may be undertaken. Because most VIPomas are large, malignant, and located in the pancreatic body and tail, distal pancreatectomy, splenectomy, and regional lymphadenectomy should be performed.[1,3] Enucleation, splenic-preserving distal pancreatectomy,[24] and laparoscopic approaches[25] should be considered only for small tumors (<2 cm). Larger tumors confined to the pancreatic head or uncinate require pancreatoduodenectomy. Intraoperative ultrasonography should be used routinely to rule out multiple tumors and liver metastases, as well as to guide surgical enucleation.[26]

In individuals with profound secretory diarrhea, increased plasma VIP levels, and negative results on conventional imaging (CT, SRS), other modalities should be used, including endoscopic ultrasonography,[27] extended upper endoscopy, positron-emission tomography,[21] and metaiodobenzylguanidine scanning. If all else fails, one can consider the use of selective arterial calcium stimulation[28,29] with hepatic vein sampling for VIP. There are, however, no published data on the reliability of this test for VIP-secreting tumors or VIP-associated nesidioblastosis. In the past, blind distal pancreatectomies have been considered after extrapancreatic and neurogenic tumors have been ruled out, because the vast majority of such neoplasms are found in the pancreatic body and tail. The use of the calcium stimulation test may allow for a more accurate gradient-guided resection in these rare situations.

Patients with limited hepatic disease should not be denied surgical intervention.[30-34] Resection of the primary tumor helps control hormonal sequelae[35] and prevents potential complications from locally advanced disease, such as duodenal obstruction or gastrointestinal bleeding from direct invasion of the stomach, duodenum, or colon, or from gastric varices secondary to splenic vein occlusion. Liver resections, metastasectomies, and radiofrequency ablation can all be used for hepatic tumor debulking.[35-37] Patients with diffuse liver metastases that are unresponsive to conventional treatment modalities may be candidates for orthotopic liver transplantation when all extrahepatic disease has been controlled.[38] The gallbladder should be removed in all patients who have metastatic disease and/or large primary tumors to facilitate the future use of somatostatin analogue[39] and hepatic artery embolization,[40] to prevent their potential complications (gallstones, ischemic cholecystitis) should their use become necessary in the future. Further discussion of advanced islet cell carcinoma can be found in Chapter 51.

Glucagonomas

Glucagonomas rank below insulinomas and gastrinomas in terms of frequency (1 case per 20–200 million population).[41] A patient with a malignant islet cell tumor with signs and symptoms of what we would now call the *glucagonoma syndrome* was first reported on by Becker et al in 1942.[42] In 1966, McGavran et al[43] described a similar patient with a glucagon-secreting α-cell tumor. However, it was left to Mallinson et al,[44] in 1974, to clearly elucidate the syndrome in a published series of nine patients.

Glucagon, a peptide hormone produced by the pancreatic α cells, is an important counter-regulatory hormone involved in glucose metabolism.[3] Glucagon is stored and released in response to hypoglycemia or stress. It is

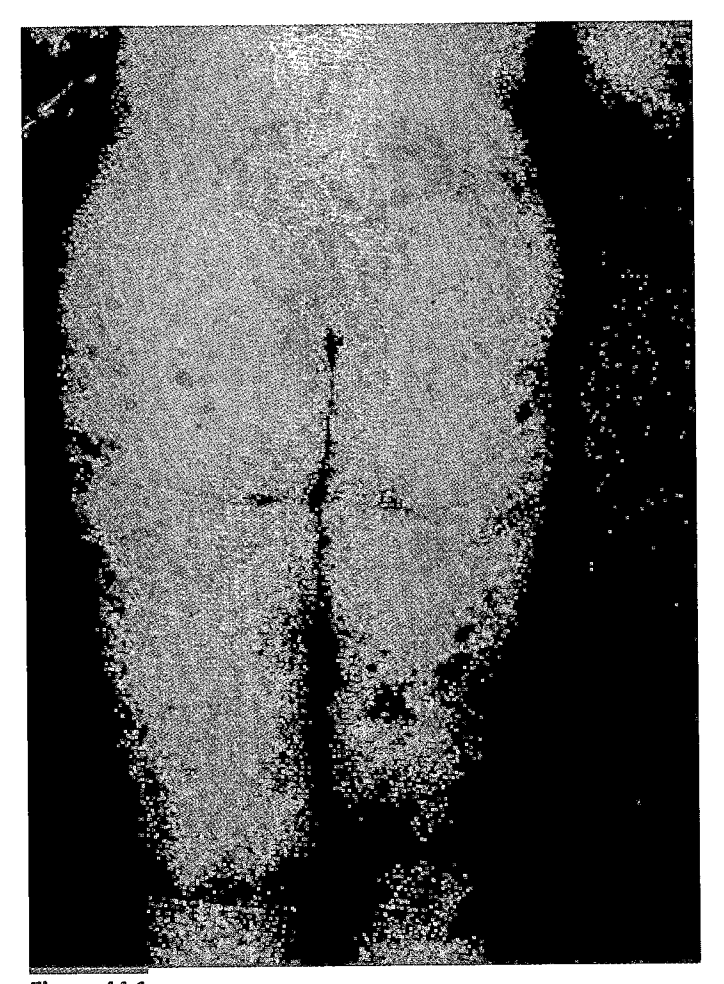

Figure 44.1
Necrolytic migratory erythema (NME) in a middle-aged woman with the glucagonoma syndrome.

a potent stimulator of gluconeogenesis, glycogenolysis, and ketogenesis. It also inhibits glycolysis and lipogenesis.[1] It is the exaggeration of these effects that leads to the biochemical and clinical features of the glucagonoma syndrome (diabetes and skin rash).[3]

More than 80% of patients with a glucagonoma display some degree of glucose intolerance. It is usually not severe and often goes undiagnosed for many years until the effects of metastatic disease become apparent or the patient experiences the necrotizing skin rash characteristic of the glucagonoma syndrome (Fig. 44.1).[45] This necrolytic migratory erythema occurs in approximately two thirds of patients with the glucagonoma syndrome.[46-48] The association of this rash and the clinical finding of glucose intolerance strongly suggest the presence of a glucagonoma. The rash begins most frequently in the intertriginous areas and in the skin around the mouth, vagina, and anus. It eventually involves the trunk, thighs, extremities, and face. The rash begins as erythematous patches that spread annularly or serpiginously to become confluent. The erythematous plaques become raised and develop central bullae that slough, leaving necrotic centers and serous crusts. Healing takes place within 2–3 weeks, leaving behind hyperpigmented sites. The process is chronic, recurrent, and migratory.[1] The rash is attributed to the hypoaminoacidemia that results from the profound catabolic effects of glucagon. Interestingly, parenteral administration of amino acids has been shown to ameliorate the dermatitis. Zinc and essential fatty deficiencies have also been postulated to contribute to the necrolytic migratory erythema.[46-48]

A normochromic, normocytic anemia occurs in about 85% of patients with the glucagonoma syndrome[49] and may be related to glucagon's ability to depress erythropoiesis.[50]

Stomatitis, glossitis, and chronic vulvovaginitis also occur in this syndrome.[49] Weight loss can be quite severe and may be explained by excessive lipolysis and gluconeogenesis. Both muscle and visceral protein stores are significantly diminished.[50]

Deep venous thrombosis and thromboembolism are quite common in patients with the glucagonoma syndrome. The exact etiology of this is not clear, but fatal pulmonary embolism is a common cause of death.[51] Long-term anticoagulant therapy is often required to prevent such lethal events. Preoperative preparation may require placement of a vena caval filter.

Diarrhea occurs in a small number of patients with the glucagonoma syndrome.[8] Glucagonomas, like many functional endocrine tumors, produce and secrete other peptides, some of which may enhance intestinal motility.[52]

Because most of the clinical findings in patients with the glucagonoma syndrome are nonspecific, it is not until the cutaneous manifestations appear that the diagnosis is considered. This delay is probably responsible for the high rate of metastatic spread and the attainment of large tumor size before clinical detection. Although a skin biopsy may be diagnostic, it is the finding of hyperglucagonemia that is confirmatory. Normal glucagon levels range from 25 to 250 pg/mL.[44] Glucagon levels can be increased in patients with renal failure, cirrhosis, hepatic failure, or severe stress, but levels rarely exceed 500 pg/mL. In patients with the glucagonoma syndrome, the level is often greater than 1000 pg/mL.

More than 80% of glucagonomas are malignant and large (3–35 cm), and more than half of the patients with glucagonomas have metastatic disease (regional lymph nodes and/or liver) at the time of diagnosis. Multiple tumors are distinctly unusual, and rarely are these tumors associated with the multiple endocrine neoplasia type 1 syndrome. Ninety percent of glucagonomas can be easily found in the body and tail of the pancreas, consistent with the known α-cell distribution within the normal

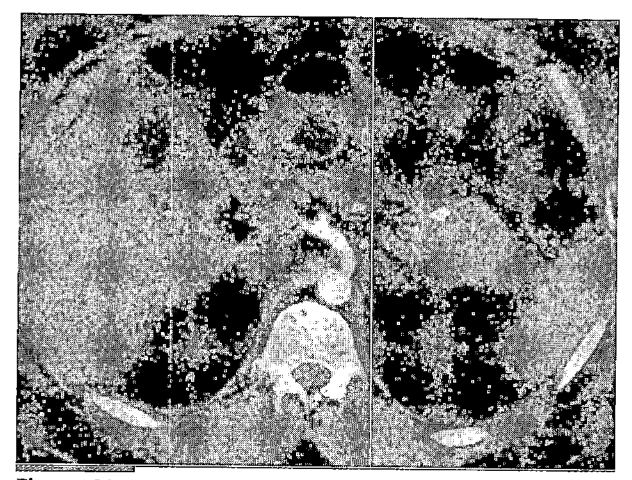

Figure 44.2
Computed tomographic scan of large glucagonoma in the tail of the pancreas.

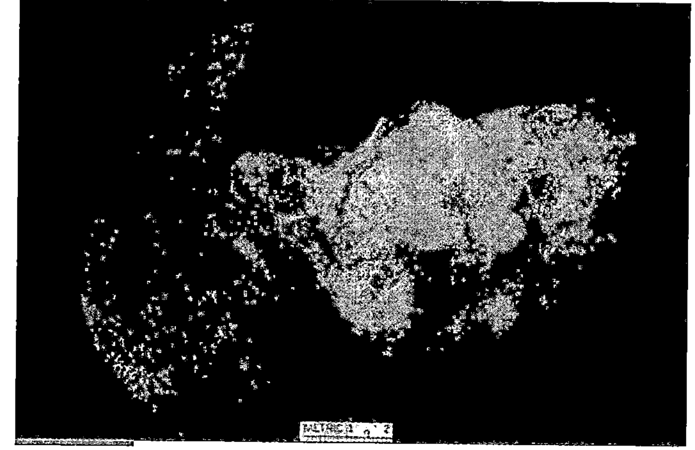

Figure 44.4
Resected glucagonoma (distal pancreatectomy/splenectomy specimen).

pancreas. Glucagonomas have no histologic features distinct from other islet cell neoplasms. As with all islet cell tumors, local invasion, metastatic disease, and, to a lesser extent, size (>2 cm) determine malignancy. Immunostaining tends to be positive for glucagon, but other peptides may stain as well. Gastrin production has been associated with some glucagonomas, and metastases are capable of altering their hormonal profile.[53]

Localization with CT (Fig. 44.2) and staging with SRS (Fig. 44.3) are generally all that are needed given the large size and somatostatin-rich receptor status of the tumors.[15-17] The preoperative use of parenteral hyperalimentation, somatostatin analogue, and anticoagulants/filters will greatly improve the existing catabolic state and lessen the risk of fatal perioperative embolic complications.[1]

Surgical resection or debulking is the mainstay of therapy and may be curative when the tumor is identified in its earliest stage. The surgical management is essentially identical to that described for VIPomas. With a preponderance of malignant tumors in the body and tail (≥90%), distal pancreatectomy and splenectomy (Fig. 44.4) with regional lymphadenectomy are the surgical procedures of choice.

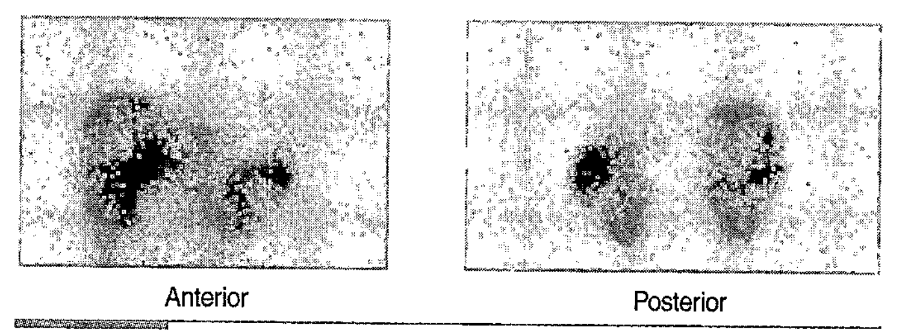

Figure 44.3
Somatostatin-receptor scintigraphy (SRS) demonstrating multiple hepatic metastases.

Resolution of the necrotizing skin rash is rapid after complete tumor removal (Fig. 44.5). Patients with limited hepatic disease are treated in a fashion similar to that described for the VIPoma syndrome. Patients with advanced disease are discussed in greater detail in Chapter 48.

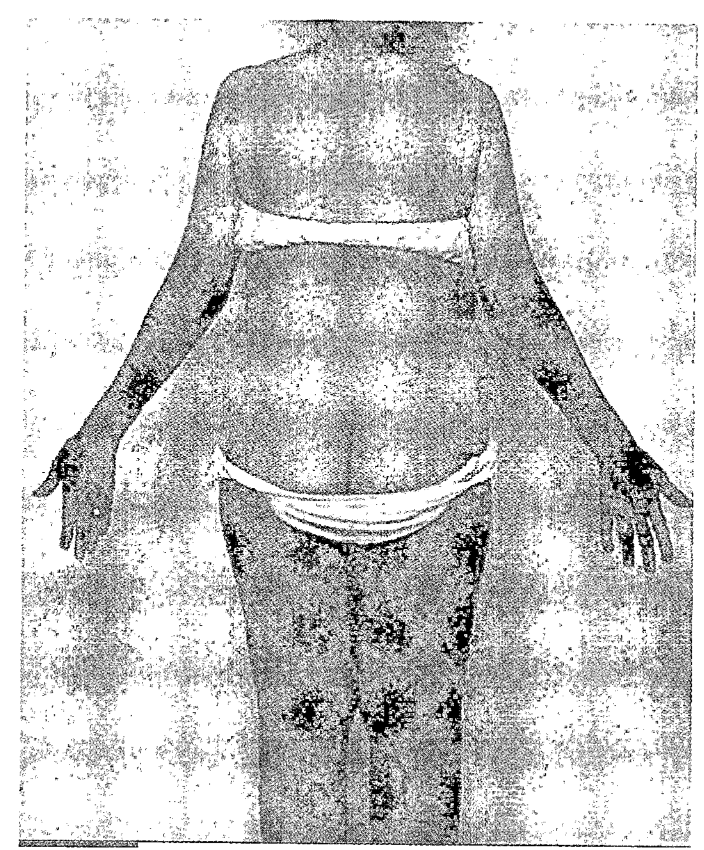

Figure 44.5
Resolution of necrolytic migratory erythema 3 months after surgical resection of a glucagonoma and normalization of glucagon levels.

In a retrospective, multicenter series of 233 patients with the glucagonoma syndrome, the 10-year survival rate was 51.6% in those presenting with metastatic disease, versus 64.3% in those without metastatic disease ($P < 0.001$).[54] In a series from the Mayo Clinic (21 patients), all had metastatic disease at presentation. Nine of twenty-one (43%) had tumor-related deaths at a mean of 4.9 years after diagnosis.[55]

Somatostatinomas

Ganda et al[56] and Larsson et al[57] first reported the somatostatinoma syndrome in 1977. The syndrome is characterized by steatorrhea, diabetes mellitus, hypochlorhydria, and cholelithiasis. It is rare that all four manifestations are present in a given patient. Somatostatin, a cyclic polypeptide, was first identified in 1968 in the hypothalamus[3]; its principal function was shown to be inhibition of growth hormone secretion. Since that time, somatostatin has also been localized to the pancreatic D cell, stomach, duodenum, and small intestine. It is a universal inhibitor of peptide release. The mean age of onset is 51 years, and the sex distribution is equal.[8] The tumors tend to be large and solitary. Two thirds of these tumors occur in the pancreas; two thirds of those tumors are found in the pancreatic head. Other primary sites include the duodenum, the ampulla of Vater, and the small bowel. Most of these tumors are malignant. They may rarely be associated with other familial endocrinopathies, such as neurofibromatosis and multiple endocrine neoplasia type 1.[58]

Duodenal somatostatinomas are more frequent in von Recklinghausen's disease[58,59]; therefore, pheochromocytomas must be ruled out before surgery.[3] There is also a weak association between celiac disease and duodenal somatostatinomas.[60]

Somatostatin has significant inhibitory effects (direct and indirect) on various gastroenteropancreatic peptides and appears to play a pivotal role in the maintenance of nutrient homeostasis.[8] All of the clinical findings in the somatostatinoma syndrome can be explained on the basis of inhibition of peptide secretion secondary to somatostatin excess. Diabetes mellitus is secondary to suppression of insulin secretion, hypochlorhydria is secondary to suppression of gastrin and gastric acid secretion, and steatorrhea is secondary to decreased pancreatic exocrine secretion and impaired fat absorption. Gallstones are common and are likely due to suppression of cholecystokinin secretion and perhaps to inhibition of biliary motility by somatostatin.[61] The constellation of symptoms, along with the increased circulating somatostatin levels, confirm the diagnosis.[62-64] Fifteen percent to 30% demonstrate multisecretory activities, including calcitonin production.[65] Calcium may be used to provoke somatostatin release in these patients.[66] Pancreatic tumors tend to be larger and more often present with the syndrome. Duodenal tumors tend to be smaller and can present with bleeding, ampullary obstruction, or jaundice. Both are metastatic in more than half of cases. Duodenal tumors often display characteristic psammoma bodies under light microscopy.[64] Because of the large size of these tumors, CT and SRS are very sensitive localizing modalities. Endoscopic fine-needle aspiration has been used successfully to identify small periampullary tumors.[67] The surgical management is similar to that described for glucagonomas and VIPomas. However, with the predominance of somatostatinomas in the head of the pancreas and the duodenum, a Whipple procedure is often necessary. Resecting a large primary or debulking hepatic metastases may effectively palliate symptoms for prolonged periods. Treatment of advanced disease can be found in Chapter 48.

In a literature review, House et al[63] found that even in the presence of synchronous metastases, 5-year overall survival approached 40%. Predictors of an unfavorable prognosis include size >3 cm, poor cytologic differentiation, nodal metastases, and incomplete surgical resection. In another large international review (173 patients), by Soga and Yakuwa,[68] the overall 5-year survival rate was 75%; the survival rate was 60% in patients with metastases and 100% in those without metastatic disease.

References

1. van Heerden JA, Thompson GB. Islet cell tumours of the pancreas. In: Trede M, Carter DC, eds. *Surgery of the Pancreas*. Edinburgh: Churchill Livingstone; 1993;545–561.
2. Soga J, Yakuwa Y. VIPoma/diarrheogenic syndrome: a statistical evaluation of 241 reported cases. *J Exp Clin Cancer Res*. 1998;17:389–400.
3. Doherty GM. VIPoma, glucagonoma, and other rare islet cell tumors. In: Doherty GM, Skogseid B, eds. *Surgical Endocrinology*. Philadelphia: Lippincott Williams & Wilkins; 2001;375–379.
4. Verner JV, Morrison AB. Islet cell tumor and a syndrome of refractory watery diarrhea and hypokalemia. *Am J Med*. 1958;25:374–380.
5. Said SI, Mutt V. Polypeptide with broad biological activity: isolation from small intestine. *Science*. 1970;169:1217–1218.
6. Roczen RL, Andersen KD. Gastrointestinal hormones in disease. *Probl Gen Surg*. 1994;11:21–52.
7. Cellier C, Yaghi C, Cuillerier E, et al. Metastatic jejunal VIPoma: beneficial effect of combination therapy with interferon-alpha and 5-fluorouracil. *Am J Gastroenterol*. 2000;95:289–293.
8. Mozell E, Stenzel P, Wolterine EA, et al. Functional endocrine tumors of the pancreas: clinical presentation, diagnosis and treatment. *Curr Probl Surg*. 1990;27:309–386.

9. Holm-Bentzen M, Schulta A, Fahrenkrug J, et al. Effect of VIP on gastric acid secretion in man. *Hepatogastroenterology*. 1980;27[suppl]:S126.
10. O'Dorisio TM, Mekhjian HS, Gaginella TS. Medical therapy of VIPomas. *Endocrinol Metab Clin North Am*. 1989; 18:545–556.
11. Anaganostides AA, Christofides ND, Tatemoto K, et al. Peptide histidine isoleucine: a secretagogue in human jejunum. *Gut*. 1984;25:381–385.
12. Jaffe BM, Condon S. Prostaglandins E and F in endocrine diarrheagenic syndromes. *Ann Surg*. 1976;184:516–524.
13. Krejs G. VIPoma syndrome. *Am J Med*. 1987;82:37–48.
14. Bloom SR, Long RG, Bryant MG, et al. Clinical, biochemical and pathological studies in 62 VIPomas. *Gastroenterology*. 1980;78:1143.
15. Briganti V, Matteini M, Ferri P, et al. Octreoscan SPET evaluation in the diagnosis of pancreas neuroendocrine tumors. *Cancer Biother Radiopharm*. 2001;16:515–524.
16. Thomason JW, Martin RS, Fincher ME. Somatostatin receptor scintigraphy: the definitive technique for characterizing vasoactive intestinal peptide-secreting tumors. *Clin Nucl Med*. 2000;25:661–664.
17. Krausz Y, Bar-Ziv J, de Jong RB, et al. Somatostatin-receptor scintigraphy in the management of gastroenteropancreatic tumors. *Am J Gastroenterol*. 1998;93:66–70.
18. Arnold R, Wied M, Behr TH. Somatostatin analogues in the treatment of endocrine tumors of the gastrointestinal tract. *Expert Opin Pharmacother*. 2002;3:643–656.
19. Tomassetti P, Migliori M, Corinaldesi R, Gullo L. Treatment of gastroenteropancreatic neuroendocrine tumours with octreotide LAR. *Aliment Pharmacol Ther*. 2000;14:557–560.
20. Nishiguchi S, Shiomi S, Ishizu H, et al. A case of glucagonoma with high uptake on F-18 fluorodeoxyglucose positron emission tomography. *Ann Nucl Med*. 2001;15:259–262.
21. Schillaci O, Corleto VD, Annibale B, et al. Single photon emission computed tomography procedure improves accuracy of somatostatin receptor scintigraphy in gastro-entero pancreatic tumours. *Ital J Gastroenterol Hepatol*. 1999;2:S186–S189.
22. Semelka RC, Custodio CM, Cem Balci N, Woosley JT. Neuroendocrine tumors of the pancreas: spectrum of appearances on MRI. *J Magn Reson Imaging*. 2000;11:141–148.
23. Mortele KJ, Oei A, Bauters W, et al. Dynamic gadolinium-enhanced MR imaging of pancreatic VIPoma in a patient with Verner-Morrison syndrome. *Eur Radiol*. 2001;11:1952–1955.
24. Kimura W, Inoue T, Futakawa N, et al. Spleen-preserving distal pancreatectomy with conservation of the splenic artery and vein. *Surgery*. 1996;120:885–890.
25. Fernandez-Cruz L, Saenz A, Astudillo E, et al. Outcome of laparoscopic pancreatic surgery: endocrine and neuroendocrine tumors. *World J Surg*. 2002;26:1057–1065.
26. Norton JA, Cromack DT, Shawker TH, et al. Intraoperative ultrasound localization of islet cell tumors: a prospective comparison to palpation. *Ann Surg*. 1988;207:160–168.
27. Anderson MA, Carpenter S, Thompson NW, et al. Endoscopic ultrasound is highly accurate and directs management in patients with neuroendocrine tumors of the pancreas. *Am J Gastroenterol*. 2000;95:2271–2277.
28. Imamura M, Minematsu S, Suzuki T, et al. Usefulness of selective arterial secretin injection test for localization of gastrinoma in the Zollinger-Ellison syndrome. *Ann Surg*. 1987;205:230–239.
29. Rosato FE, Bonn J, Shapiro M, et al. Selective arterial stimulation of secretin in localization of gastrinomas. *Surg Gynecol Obstet*. 1999;171:196–200.
30. Azimuddin K, Chamberlain RS. The surgical management of pancreatic neuroendocrine tumors. *Surg Clin North Am*. 2001;81:511–525.
31. Phan GQ, Yeo CJ, Hruban RH, et al. Surgical experience with pancreatic and peripancreatic neuroendocrine tumors: review of 125 patients. *J Gastrointest Surg*. 1998;2:472–482.
32. Hellman P, Andersson M, Rastad J, et al. Surgical strategy for large or malignant endocrine pancreatic tumors. *World J Surg*. 2000;24:1353–1360.
33. Lo CY, van Heerden JA, Thompson GB, et al. Islet cell carcinoma of the pancreas. *World J Surg*. 1996;20:878–883.
34. Brentjens R, Saltz L. Islet cell tumors of the pancreas: the medical oncologist's perspective. *Surg Clin North Am*. 2001;81:527–542.
35. Nagorney DM, Bloom SR, Polak JM, et al. Resolution of recurrent Verner-Morrison syndrome by resection of metastatic VIPoma. *Surgery*. 1983;93:348–353.
36. Sarmiento JM, Que FG, Grant CS, et al. Concurrent resections of pancreatic islet cell cancers with synchronous hepatic metastases: outcomes of an aggressive approach. *Surgery*. 2002;132:976–982.
37. Hellman P, Ladjevardi S, Skogseid B, et al. Radiofrequency tissue ablation using cooled tip for liver metastases of endocrine tumors. *World J Surg*. 2002;26:1052–1056.
38. Hengst K, Nashan B, Avenhaus W, et al. Metastatic pancreatic VIPoma: deteriorating clinical course and successful treatment by liver transplantation. *Z Gastroenterol*. 1998;36:239–245.
39. Buscombe JR, Caplin ME, Hilson AJ. Long-term efficacy of high-activity 111in-pentetreotide therapy in patients with disseminated neuroendocrine tumors. *J Nucl Med*. 2003;44:1–6.
40. Case CC, Wirfel K, Vassilopoulou-Sellin R. Vasoactive intestinal polypeptide-secreting tumor (VIPoma) with liver metastases: dramatic and durable symptomatic benefit from hepatic artery embolization, a case report. *Med Oncol*. 2002;19:181–187.
41. Nightingale KJ, Davies MG, Kingsnorth AN. Glucagonoma syndrome: survival 24 years following diagnosis. *Dig Surg*. 1999;16:68–71.
42. Becker SW, Kahn D, Rothman S. Cutaneous manifestations of internal malignant tumors. *Arch Dermatol Syph*. 1942;45: 1069–1080.
43. McGavran MH, Unger RH, Recant L, et al. A glucagon-secreting alpha-cell carcinoma of the pancreas. *N Engl J Med*. 1966;274:1408–1413.
44. Mallinson CN, Bloom SR, Warin AP, et al. A glucagonoma syndrome. *Lancet*. 1974;2:1–5.
45. Alkemade JA, van Tongeren JH, van Haelst UJ, et al. Delayed diagnosis of glucagonoma syndrome. *Clin Exp Dermatol*. 1999;24:455–457.
46. Barazzoni R, Zanetti M, Tiengo A, Tessari P. Protein metabolism in glucagonoma. *Diabetologia*. 1999;42:326–329.

47. Chao SC, Lee JY. Brittle nails and dyspareunia as first clues to recurrences of malignant glucagonoma. *Br J Dermatol.* 2002;146:1071–1074.
48. Chastain MA. The glucagonoma syndrome: a review of its features and discussion of new perspectives. *Am J Med Sci.* 2001;321:306–320.
49. Leichter SB. Clinical and metabolic aspects of glucagonoma. *Medicine.* 1980;59:100–113.
50. Naets JP, Gans M. Inhibitory effect of glucagon on erythropoiesis. *Blood.* 1980;55:997–1002.
51. Bloom SR, Polak JM. Glucagonoma syndrome. *Am J Med.* 1987;82:25–36.
52. Polak JM, Adrian TE, Bryant MG, et al. Pancreatic polypeptide in insulinomas, gastrinomas, VIPomas and glucagonomas. *Lancet.* 1976;1:328–330.
53. Balian A, Fromont C, Naveau S, et al. A particularly aggressive combined glucagonoma and gastrinoma syndrome. *Eur J Gastroenterol Hepatol.* 1999;11:1417–1419.
54. Soga J, Yakuwa Y. Glucagonomas/diabetico-dermatogenic syndrome (DDS): a statistical evaluation of 407 reported cases. *J Hepatobiliary Pancreat Surg.* 1998;5:312–319.
55. Wermers RA, Fatourechi V, Wynne AG, et al. The glucagonoma syndrome: clinical and pathologic features in 21 patients. *Medicine.* 1996;75:53–63.
56. Ganda OP, Weir GC, Soeldner JS, et al. "Somatostatinoma": a somatostatin-containing tumor of the endocrine pancreas. *N Engl J Med.* 1977;296:963–967.
57. Larsson L-I, Hirsch MA, Holst JJ, et al. Pancreatic somatostatinoma: clinical features and physiologic implications. *Lancet.* 1977;1:666–668.
58. Usui M, Matsuda S, Suzuki H, et al. Somatostatinoma of the papilla of Vater with multiple gastrointestinal stromal tumors in a patient with von Recklinghausen's disease. *J Gastroenterol.* 2002;37:947–953.
59. Chetty R, Essa A. Heterotopic pancreas: periampullary somatostatinoma and type I neurofibromatosis: a pathogenetic proposal. *Pathology.* 1999;31:95–97.
60. Frick EJ Jr, Kralstein JR, Scarlato M, et al. Somatostatinoma of the ampulla of Vater in celiac sprue. *J Gastrointest Surg.* 2000;4:388–391.
61. Maselli MA, Piepoli AL, Pezzolla F, et al. Effect of somatostatin on human gallbladder motility: an in vitro study. *Neurogastroenterol Motil.* 1999;11:47–53.
62. Tanaka S, Yamasaki S, Matsushita H, et al. Duodenal somatostatinoma: a case report and review of 31 cases with special reference to the relationship between tumor size and metastasis. *Pathol Int.* 2000;50:146–152.
63. House MG, Yeo CJ, Schulick RD. Periampullary pancreatic somatostatinoma. *Ann Surg Oncol.* 2002;9:869–874.
64. Green BT, Rockey DC. Duodenal somatostatinoma presenting with complete somatostatinoma syndrome. *J Clin Gastroenterol.* 2001;33:415–417.
65. Sugimoto F, Sekiya T, Saito M, et al. Calcitonin-producing pancreatic somatostatinoma: report of a case. *Surg Today.* 1998;28:1279–1282.
66. Vezzadini C, Poggioli R, Casoni I, et al. Use of calcium provocative test in the diagnosis of gastroenteropancreatic endocrine tumors. *Panminerva Med.* 1996;38:255–258.
67. Guo M, Lemos LB, Bigler S, et al. Duodenal somatostatinoma of the ampulla of Vater diagnosed by endoscopic fine needle aspiration biopsy: a case report. *Acta Cytol.* 2001;45:622–626.
68. Soga J, Yakuwa Y. Somatostatinoma/inhibitory syndrome: a statistical evaluation of 173 reported cases as compared to other pancreatic endocrinomas. *J Exp Clin Cancer Res.* 1999;18:13–22.

CHAPTER 45

Pancreatic Endocrine Neoplasms in Multiple Endocrine Neoplasia Type 1

Maria A. Kouvaraki, MD, PhD
Suzanne E. Shapiro, MS
Jeffrey E. Lee, MD
Douglas B. Evans, MD

Multiple endocrine neoplasia type 1 (MEN1) is a hereditary disease that is transmitted in an autosomal dominant pattern with more than 95% penetrance of at least one clinical manifestation by the age of 40 years.[1-5] Its prevalence is estimated to be between 2 and 20 per 100,000 individuals.[3] Wermer first described MEN1 in 1954 as "adenomatosis of endocrine glands" affecting several members of a family in two consecutive generations. Wermer was the first to propose a genetic basis for the disease; more specifically, he suggested that the disease was transmitted by a single autosomal dominant gene with a high degree of penetration.[6-8]

Initial linkage and loss of heterozygosity studies localized the *MEN1* gene to chromosome 11q13,[9,10] and in 1997, this gene was identified and cloned.[11] It has been suggested that the protein product of the *MEN1* gene, menin, functions as a tumor suppressor.[11-13] Affected individuals inherit a mutated *MEN1* allele, and inactivation of the remaining *MEN1* allele through a spontaneous somatic mutation results in tumor development in specific tissues.

Patients with MEN1 develop various combinations of functioning (i.e., hypersecretion of one or more hormones) and nonfunctioning tumors within the parathyroid glands (90%–97%), pancreatic islet cells and duodenum (30%–80%), and the anterior pituitary gland (20%–65%).[2,3,14,15] A wide spectrum of tumors including adrenal tumors (5%–41%), foregut carcinoid tumors (2%–8%), lipoma (0.9%), thyroid neoplasms (8%–27%), malignant melanoma (0.5%), and testicular teratoma (0.5%) is also seen in MEN1 patients.[5,15] Endocrine tumors associated with MEN1 usually become clinically evident in late adolescence or young adulthood. The most common clinical manifestations include functional effects of hormone hypersecretion such as hypercalcemia (hyperparathyroidism), ulcer diathesis (hypergastrinemia), or hypoglycemia (insulinoma). Hyperparathyroidism is usually the first clinical manifestation of the syndrome, typically appearing between the ages of 20 and 25 years, but sometimes as late as the fifth decade of life, and may occur in up to 97% of affected individuals.[5] In addition, hyperparathyroidism is present in most asymptomatic gene carriers and is often synchronously diagnosed in MEN1 patients who present with other clinical manifestations of the disease. Pancreatic islet cell neoplasms are the second most common manifestation of MEN1, and these tumors, when functioning, may secrete various hormones including gastrin, insulin, glucagon, and pancreatic polypeptide (PP). Among the functioning tumors, gastrinomas are the most common and account for up to 60% of functioning pancreatic tumors in MEN1.[15] Insulinomas are the next most frequent functioning pancreatic tumor, accounting for 10%–33% of all MEN1-associated hormonally active pancreatic tumors.[4,15,16] Insulinomas are more common in younger patients (< 40 years), whereas gastrinomas and somatostatinomas typically occur in older patients (> 40 years).[5]

Complications from hypercalcemia and peptic ulcer disease rarely cause death in patients with MEN1 syndrome, as was the case before the development of proton pump inhibitors. Progressive metastatic neuroendocrine (islet cell) carcinoma now represents the greatest health risk to patients with MEN1 and is currently the major cause of disease-specific mortality in these patients.[17] Up to 50% of MEN1 patients with malignant pancreatic neoplasms will develop liver metastasis. The surgical management of pancreatic neuroendocrine tumors in patients with MEN1 remains controversial because MEN1-associated pancreatic tumors have unique characteristics when compared with pancreatic tumors of sporadic etiology. First, MEN1-associated pancreatic tumors are almost always multifocal, and second, they are usually distributed throughout the pancreatic parenchyma,[18] with or without a hormonal excess syndrome. Unlike the situation with medullary thyroid cancer in MEN2 (where total thyroidectomy is performed as a prophylactic procedure), total pancreatectomy would result in insulin dependence and pancreatic exocrine insufficiency, both of which may result in significant patient morbidity. Therefore, the timing and proper extent of pancreatic resection remain controversial.

Also in contrast to multiple endocrine neoplasia type 2 (MEN2), the relationship between genotype and phenotype in MEN1 is still unclear.[3,19,20] Therefore, genotype cannot be used to guide the timing and extent of pancreatic resection. Currently patient demographics and clinical features of MEN1 such as patient age, sites of tumor involvement, and tempo of disease progression vary extensively among patients with MEN1 and even among members within the same family (with the same genetic mutation). This chapter reviews the available data necessary to develop an appropriate surgical strategy for patients with MEN1-associated pancreatic neoplasms.

The Genetics of MEN1

Molecular Genetics of MEN1

The *MEN1* gene, identified by positional cloning, maps to chromosomal region 11q13.[11] The *MEN1* gene contains 10 exons, the first of which is not translated.[11] Consistent with Knudson's two-hit hypothesis, patients with MEN1 receive the first "hit" through an inherited germline mutation, and tumor formation is caused by the second "hit," in which the remaining MEN1 allele is lost through somatic mutation. This suggests that MEN1 functions as a tumor suppressor gene.[9,10]

The *MEN1* gene encodes a 610-amino acid nuclear protein called menin.[11] Menin interacts with several transcription factors, including *junD*,[13] Smad3,[21] nuclear factor-κB,[22] and Pem,[23] suggesting that menin plays a role in the regulation of cell proliferation and apoptosis. Menin directly binds to the activated protein-1 (AP-1) transcription factor *junD* and thus inhibits *junD*-dependent transcription. Mutant menin is likely to be an inactive truncated protein not capable of binding junD, resulting in uncontrolled *junD*-dependent transcription.[12,13] The AP-1 transcription factor group of proteins consists of Jun members (*c-Jun*, which is the cellular counterpart of the *v-Jun* oncogene, *JunB*, and *JunD*) and Fos members (c-Fos, FosB, Fra1, and Fra2). None of the other AP-1 proteins has been found to interact with menin.[13] Recently, menin has been shown to also have a role in DNA repair through its interaction with the 32-kDa subunit of replication protein A (RPA2)[24] and the protein FANCD2, which is defective in patients with Fanconi anemia.[22] In addition, studies using animal models indicated that although MEN1-null mice die in utero,[25,26] conditional homozygous inactivation of the *MEN1* gene in the pituitary gland and endocrine pancreas bypasses embryonic lethality and produces β-cell hyperplasia in less than 4 months as well as insulinomas and prolactinomas after 9 months.[27]

More than 350 germline mutations have been reported in this gene, which are distributed throughout exons 2 through 10 as well as in splice sites within the noncoding introns.[28] The most frequent mutations involve codons 83, 84, 209–211, and 514–516.[11,29-33] Interestingly, somatic mutations of the *MEN1* gene have been reported as the most frequent mutations in several sporadic endocrine tumors in patients without MEN1, including parathyroid adenomas (21%), gastrinomas (33%), insulinomas (17%), and bronchial carcinoids (36%).[34-36]

Whereas a strong correlation between genotype and phenotype characterizes MEN2 syndrome, most published observations have failed to report such a correlation in MEN1.[37] Different mutations of the *MEN1* gene have been identified in different families with the same clinical manifestations of the syndrome.[38-40] Conversely, the same mutation of the *MEN1* gene has been found in different kindreds with different spectra of clinical features.[41] However, recently Bartsch et al.[19] suggested a possible genotype-phenotype association in MEN1 patients with pancreatic endocrine tumors (PETs).[19] This study reported that patients who carried nonsense or frameshift mutations (resulting in a truncated protein) of the C- or N-terminal regions (exons 2, 9, or 10) of the *MEN1* gene had a higher incidence of malignant tumors (55% vs 10%) and a shorter disease-free survival compared with patients with missense mutations in the same regions or with all other mutations outside those regions. However, this study included a small number of patients, and no statistical analysis was performed. A recent study published from our institution showed that all patients with frameshift mutations had a PET. Furthermore, glucagonomas appeared to be associated with frameshift mutations in exon 2. An association was also suggested between pituitary tumors and frameshift mutations in exon 2, whereas bronchial and thymic carcinoids were more frequently associated with mutations in exon 10. However, our data did not demonstrate a significant association between the specific type or location of *MEN1* mutation and the development of metastatic disease in patients with PETs. The small number of patients with lymph node and distant organ metastases in our study limited the power of our analysis. Other studies suggesting a possible *MEN1* genotype-phenotype association showed that patients with MEN1 and triple-organ involvement (i.e., parathyroid, pancreas, and pituitary) or aggressive phenotypes with malignancies share truncating mutations.[42,43] In addition, a mild variant of MEN1 called "familial isolated hyperparathyroidism" has been associated with missense mutations occurring mainly between exons 3 and 7.[44-46]

Genetic Testing and Counseling Issues

Genetic testing for MEN1 is currently available for clinical use. Entire sequencing of the nine coding exons (exons 2 through 9) is estimated to identify mutations in approximately 75%–90% of patients with MEN1 depending on the techniques and experiences of individual laboratories. Therefore, a significant proportion of families with clinical MEN1 (involvement of two or more principle endocrine glands: parathyroid, pituitary, and pancreas) will not have an identifiable *MEN1* mutation; these families are considered noninformative with respect to genetic testing. At-risk relatives from noninformative families can obtain screening only through clinical means according to the guidelines outlined later in this chapter.

Although consensus guidelines for MEN1 genetic testing are still being developed, compelling reasons to consider genetic testing include but are not limited to (1) confirmation of a clinical diagnosis or atypical presentation, (2) identification of at-risk relatives through presymptomatic screening, and (3) cessation of clinical screening in relatives who test negative for a mutation previously identified within the kindred.[1] The genetic testing process should be carefully supervised under the direction of a genetic counselor who is qualified to discuss testing options and alternatives as well as the potential benefits, risks, and limitations of genetic testing. For example, some individuals may experience adverse psychologic emotions from learning their inherited cancer risk. These emotions may include denial, anger, sorrow, and survivor's guilt. Additional potential risks of genetic testing include the revelation of unanticipated information (e.g., nonpaternity) and the threat of discrimination when attempting to secure employment or insurance. After genetic counseling, patients should be well informed to provide written informed consent.

Presymptomatic genetic testing can identify carrier status as many as 20 years before disease is clinically manifested.[47] Because of the lack of consensus on prophylactic intervention and the inability to predict the clinical pattern of future disease, the importance of presymptomatic screening remains controversial.[48] We currently recommend that at-risk relatives consider presymptomatic genetic analysis at an age when MEN1 manifestations typically first appear (i.e., late adolescence or early adulthood) or when the patient develops the maturity to participate in the informed consent process.[49] In lieu of genetic testing, at-risk relatives should be clinically screened for associated individual neoplasms.

The Natural History of Pancreatic Tumors in MEN1

Pancreatic neuroendocrine carcinoma in MEN1 is often an indolent disease, making assessment of its natural history difficult. Almost all patients with *MEN1* syndrome will develop islet cell hyperplasia or a discrete pancreatic neoplasm during their lifetime.[50] Approximately 50% of MEN1-associated pancreatic neoplasms are functional and produce clinical symptoms because of the hypersecretion of one or more pancreatic hormones such as gastrin and/or insulin (Table 45.1). Nonfunctioning pancreatic neuroendocrine tumors are defined as those without clinical evidence of peptide hypersecretion and occur in the remaining 50% of MEN1 patients.[4] However, most clinically nonfunctioning pancreatic tumors are associated with some degree of elevation of one or more pancreatic hormones such as PP.[43] Patients with nonfunctioning tumors usually come to medical attention because of symptoms related to local tumor growth.[16]

Immunohistochemical studies have been used to better characterize the cell of origin and the functional

Table 45.1 Frequency of Different Pancreatic Endocrine Tumors in Surgically Treated Patients with MEN1

		Number of Patients (%)				
Authors	Total†	Insulinoma	Gastrinoma	Vipoma	Glucagonoma	Nonfunctioning or PPoma
Kloppel et al.[51]	9	2/9 (22)	2/9 (22)	1/9 (11)	0/9	4/9 (44)*
Sheppard et al.[86]	9	2/9 (22)	7/9 (78)	1/9 (11)	0/9	0/9
Samaan et al.[104]	11	2/11 (18)	4/11 (36)	0/11	2/11 (18)	3/11 (27)
Tisell and Ahlman[103]	5	3/5 (60)	0/5	0/5	1/5 (20)	NA
Pipeleers-Marichal et al.[53]	7	1/7 (14)	6/7 (86)	0/7	0/7	0/7
Grama et al.[89]	27	7/27 (26)	14/27 (52)	0/27	0/27	7/27 (26)
Thompson et al.[91]	48	7/48 (15)	38/48 (79)	0/48	0/48	3/48 (6)
Lowney et al.[64]	43	10/48 (21)	12/48 (25)	2/48 (4)	0/48	24/48 (50)
Bartsch et al.[19]	16	4/21 (19)	9/21 (43)	1/21 (5)	0/21	5/21 (24)
Lairmore et al.[93]	21	3/21 (14)	2/21 (10)	1/21 (5)	0/21	15/21 (71)
Total	196	41 (21)	94 (46)	6 (3)	3 (1)	61 (31)

Abbreviation: NA, not available.
* Only the largest tumor is reported.
† Some patients had more than one type of pancreatic endocrine tumor.

status of various endocrine tumors of the pancreas in MEN1 patients. The clinical syndrome caused by hormone hypersecretion is not necessarily associated with immunohistochemical expression of only one hormone. Pancreatic neoplasms in MEN1 patients frequently express insulin (insulinomas), glucagon (glucagonomas), and PP (PPomas).[51] Gastrin-producing tumors (gastrinomas) are often small and not amenable to immunohistochemical staining. Somatostatin-producing tumors (somatostatinomas) are rare, and immunohistochemical staining for vasoactive intestinal polypeptide (VIP) and neurotensin is rarely positive.[51]

Gastrinoma is the most common functioning islet cell tumor associated with MEN1.[14,15,52,53] MEN1-associated gastrinomas often occur within the gastrinoma triangle (pancreatic head and the first and second portions of the duodenum), and in contrast to sporadic gastrinomas, they can also occur in the body and tail of the pancreas and more distal duodenum.[51,53-57] In fact, sporadic and MEN1-associated gastrinomas are more commonly located in the duodenum than the pancreas.[56,58] Most of the duodenal tumors are small (often only 2 to 3 mm in diameter or less), multicentric, and located within the submucosal layer of the duodenum.[53,56,58] Duodenal gastrinomas frequently coexist with other functioning and nonfunctioning neuroendocrine tumors located throughout the pancreas. Despite their small size, these tumors metastasize frequently (minimum of 40%) to the peripancreatic and periduodenal lymph nodes; however, liver metastases are much less common.[15,53,59] Interestingly, liver metastases from sporadic gastrinomas located in the duodenum (in contrast to the pancreas) are rare; however, less is known about the natural history of MEN1-associated pancreatic and duodenal tumors partly because of the mutifocality of these tumors.[16,53,56,58,60]

In patients with sporadic gastrinomas, liver metastases may be more frequent in patients whose primary tumors are of increased size (> 3 cm).[60-62] It is not known whether such data can be applied to patients with MEN1-associated gastrinomas; few studies (involving small numbers of patients) have attempted to correlate the size of the primary tumor with the incidence of synchronous or metachronous liver metastasis.[60,61,63] Furthermore, one would assume that studies that correlate the size of the primary tumor with the presence of synchronous liver metastases overestimate the size of the primary tumor as there is no way to determine how long the metastases were present. For example, Weber et al.[60] reported that the size of the primary tumor did correlate with the presence of synchronous liver metastases; however, only two of the patients (with synchronous liver metastases) had MEN1, and the size of their primary tumor was not provided. In addition, only 3 of 34 patients with MEN1-associated gastrinomas developed metachronous liver metastases.[60] Cadiot et al.[61] analyzed the primary tumor size in eight patients with MEN1-associated gastrinomas who developed metachronous liver metastases; primary tumor size was 3 cm or larger in four patients, less than 3 cm in three patients, and unknown in the remaining patient.[61] The authors did not report how many patients had surgical excision of the primary tumor before the development of metachronous liver metastases. Finally, Mignon et al.[63] reported seven MEN1 patients with metachronous liver metastases. This study documented that two of seven patients had primary tumors larger than 3 cm in size, but the sizes of the primary tumors in the remaining five patients were unknown. In contrast, the report by Lowney et al.[64] does not support a correlation between the size of the primary tumor and the risk of metastasis. This study reported only a single patient with metachronous liver metastasis, and the primary tumor size in this patient was not reported. These investigators considered lymph node metastases as evidence of distant disease. This is not incorrect; however, the metastatic potential of neuroendocrine neoplasms is usually based on the presence or absence of distant organ (liver, lung, and bone) metastases because lymph node metastases are common and do not accurately predict the development of distant organ disease as is the case in other more common solid tumors. Clearly, the number of patients with MEN1-related gastrinomas (or other neuroendocrine pancreatic tumors) is too small and their follow-up too brief to assess accurately a possible relationship between tumor size and malignant potential, especially with respect to the development of distant metastases to liver, lung, or bone.

As mentioned, lymph node metastases do not appear to be a consistent marker of distant organ metastasis as occurs in other solid tumors, nor do they predict early mortality in patients with MEN1.[60,65] Obviously, lymph node metastases can be detected only if lymph nodes are removed by the surgeon and histologically examined by the pathologist. Furthermore, studies have probably underestimated the frequency of lymph node metastases because of the absence of uniform criteria for histologic sectioning of lymph nodes.[66-68] Despite probable underreporting, lymph node metastases are common in patients with MEN1-related PETs, occurring in 39%–55% of patients, and are thought to be even more common in patients with duodenal gastrinomas.[56,58,64,69] The uncertain biologic significance of lymph node metastases combined with inconsistencies in lymph node assessment justify the use of liver metastases (or other distant metastases) as the proper endpoint for studies examining the malignant potential of neuroendocrine tumors in patients with MEN1. Furthermore, the definition of a malignant PET should probably include only those patients with distant organ metastases. However, currently it is best to assume that all PETs, regardless of the presence or absence of hormone production or the immunohistochemical profile, have the biologic ability to metastasize to distant organs. Ongoing research into the molecular profiling of PETs may alter this conclusion in the future.

Some investigators have suggested that liver metastases from gastrinomas tend to have a less aggressive natural history in MEN1 patients compared with patients with sporadic gastrinomas.[61,63,70] For example, Mignon et al.[63] reported 2 of 17 patients (12%) with MEN1-related gastrinomas died of liver metastasis compared with 20 of 56 deaths (36%) in patients with sporadic gastrinomas. The percentage of patients with liver metastases was similar between the two groups. However, this study did not report the duration of follow-up for either group, making it impossible to exclude lead-time bias. Weber et al.[60] reported that a significantly higher percentage of patients with sporadic gastrinomas had liver metastases at the time of diagnosis (22% compared with 6% of MEN1 patients), but the development of metachronous liver metastases did not differ significantly between patients with MEN1-associated and sporadic gastrinomas (9% and 5%, respectively). Thus, the superior survival suggested for patients with MEN1-associated gastrinomas is probably due to the lower frequency of (synchronous) metastatic disease at presentation, a function of lead-time bias due to screening of at-risk patients. However, Gibril et al.[71] suggested that there is a subset of MEN1 patients with gastrinomas in which tumors exhibit aggressive growth. The patients with aggressive tumors appeared to have higher serum gastrin levels, liver or bone metastases, increased frequency of gastric carcinoids, pancreatic gastrinomas larger than 3 cm in size, and a shorter duration from the onset of symptoms of gastrin hypersecretion to the development of liver metastasis.[71] In summary, the results of these studies suggest that the natural history of PETs (nonfunctioning and gastrin-producing) in patients with MEN1 remains poorly defined and unpredictable. There is not a clinically relevant association between primary tumor size or location and the incidence of distant metastatic disease in patients with MEN1.

Insulinomas are the second most frequent functioning pancreatic tumor, occurring in approximately 10%–20% of patients with MEN1.[4,5,72,73] Insulinomas arise from the β-cells of the pancreas and are often multifocal throughout the pancreas. In contrast to gastrinomas, insulinomas are not found in the duodenum and are rarely malignant (9%–20%).[74,75] However, within specific kindreds, insulin- and proinsulin-producing tumors can be highly malignant.[76] When distant metastases occur, they are typically present in the liver. In approximately 10% of MEN1-associated tumors, insulinoma may coexist with gastrinoma.[77]

Glucagonomas arise from α-cells of the pancreatic islets and occur in fewer than 3% of MEN1 patients.[5,78] Notably, glucagonoma hypersecretion in a patient with MEN1 does not always produce a clinical syndrome. The asymptomatic nature of glucagonomas, especially when tumor size is small (< 3 cm), complicates the diagnosis. As such, small glucagonomas are usually diagnosed as clinically occult tumors found during routine screening of MEN1 patients with abdominal imaging. Glucagonomas are located most frequently within the pancreatic tail and body; however, unlike insulinomas, these tumors tend to be large, and the majority are malignant (50%–80%).[63,78,79]

VIPomas arise from VIP secreting δ-cells of the pancreas and are rare in patients with MEN1.[80] These tumors are almost exclusively located within the body and tail of the pancreas (90%)[72] and are associated with significant malignant potential (66%).[63] Somatostatinomas also arise from δ-cells but are exceedingly rare in patients with MEN1. Somatostatinomas may metastasize to the liver; however, the exact incidence of liver metastases is unknown because of the rarity of these neoplasms.[63]

PPomas are commonly considered within the group of nonfunctioning PETs. Hypersecretion of PP does not lead to a recognized clinical syndrome.[51] PPomas are located most frequently in the pancreatic head but can be found anywhere within the pancreas.[81,82] These tumors arise from F cells (or PP cells or D_2 cells). PPomas may metastasize to the liver, and it has been suggested that large tumor size is a predictor of metastasis.[82] By definition, nonfunctioning PETs are not associated with an elevated level of peptide hormone. MEN1-related nonfunctioning PETs are almost exclusively malignant (80%–100%) and are associated with both lymph node and liver metastasis.[83,84]

Surgical Management of Pancreatic Tumors in MEN1

1. **Gastrinoma:** MEN1 patients with clinical evidence of hyperparathyroidism and gastrinoma have been reported to show a reduction in fasting gastrin levels and basal acid output after parathyroidectomy. Parathyroidectomy is accepted as the initial surgical procedure for these patients.[2,85] In contrast, the role of surgery in the management of MEN1 patients with Zollinger-Ellison syndrome (ZES) is not clear. Gastrin levels rarely return to normal after surgery, and control of acid hypersecretion without surgery is now possible with the introduction of Na^+-K^+-ATPase inhibitors (e.g., omeprazole). However, correction of hypercalcemia or medical control of increased acid production because of hypergastrinemia obviously does not address the malignant potential of gastrin-producing neoplasms in the pancreas or duodenum.[63,86,87] Thus, the long-term survival of MEN1 patients with gastrinoma is dependent on the biologic behavior of the tumor and the effectiveness of surgical therapy.

   Skogseid et al.[76,88,89] and Thompson[16,90-92] advocated early surgical intervention for all MEN1 patients with gastrinomas.[16,76,88-92] They consider a distal pancreatectomy with enucleation (after ultrasound localization) of any tumor within the pancreatic head in all patients with biochemical or radiographic evidence of a gastrinoma.[16,90-92] Duodenotomy is considered essential for all MEN1 patients with elevated basal or stimulated gastrin levels, as small duodenal gastrinomas are frequently present (87%) and cannot be found without opening the duodenum.[91] They also perform a peripancreatic and portal lymph node dissection to include those lymph nodes in the porta hepatis and along the common hepatic artery proximally to the celiac axis.[16,90-92] Bartsch et al.[19] and Lairmore et al.[93] also advocate surgery for all MEN1 patients with hypergastrinemia. According to these authors, pancreaticoduodenectomy is the procedure of choice for MEN1-related gastrinomas[19] and for very large PETs within the head and uncinate process of the pancreas, especially when regional lymph nodes metastases are present.[93]

   Norton et al.[94] and Jensen[95] have advocated a much less aggressive approach for the management for MEN1-associated gastrinomas.[94-96] They suggest surgical resection of tumors 2.5 cm in size or larger.[50,59,97,98] Before 1994, these authors reserved operation for gastrinomas larger than 3 cm.[62] The rationale for this strategy is that major pancreatic operations are associated with significant morbidity and possible mortality, and therefore, pancreatic resection should not be performed unless there is a clinically significant risk for the development of distant metastases.[60,98] These authors recommended enucleation for gastrinomas located within the head of the pancreas and segmental pancreatic resection or enucleation for tumors located within the body or the tail.[50,59] Mignon et al.[63,77] suggested that surgery is not curative for MEN1 patients with hypergastrinemia. Although pancreatic tumors larger than 3 cm may be associated with synchronous or metachronous liver metastases, these authors do not feel that surgery is likely to prevent the development of liver metastasis.[77] For tumors localized within the duodenum, Mignon suggested duodenal transillumination and exploration with enucleation of any tumor. The report from the Group d'Etude des neoplasies Endocriniennes Multiples de type 1 in France agreed with this strategy.[99]

Published reports on the surgical management of MEN1-related gastrinoma appear in Table 45.2. Distal pancreatectomy with or without enucleation of tumors in the head or the uncinate process of the pancreas was performed in 130 patients (52%), enucleation or nonanatomic resection of tumor in 25 (10%), pancreaticoduodenectomy in 14 (6%), and total pancreatectomy in 3 (1%). Duodenotomy was performed in 87 (35%) of 251 patients with gastrinoma. The criteria for cure of gastrinoma included a normal serum gastrin level (fasting, lower than 100 pg/ml; nonfasting, lower than 200 pg/ml), a negative secretin test, and no evidence of tumor on imaging studies. The reported biochemical cure rates were generally low yet ranged from 0%–87% in various studies. However, a normal basal gastrin level (nonstimulated) was achieved in a much higher percentage of patients (67%–91%). The 10-year overall survival for patients with MEN1-associated gastrinomas ranged from 71%–100%, demonstrating the rather indolent progression of disease seen in most patients. Indolent tumor growth, long survival duration, and a rare disease make for a natural history that is difficult to document accurately. In the absence of accurate natural history data, one cannot expect to achieve consensus on treatment recommendations.

2. **Insulinoma**: There is general consensus that patients with insulinoma syndrome should be managed with surgery. Mignon et al.[63,77] suggested that in MEN1-associated insulinoma, removal of the functionally dominant islet cell areas is essential, but near total or total pancreatectomy should be avoided.[63,77] Bartsch et al.[19] and Lairmore et al.[93] also suggested that all MEN1 patients with hyperinsulinism should be treated with surgery.[19] A combination of enucleation and/or distal pancreatectomy can be used in patients with insulinoma. Table 45.3 summarizes the surgical approaches used to treat insulinomas in MEN1 patients in 12 reported series. Sixty-nine patients underwent surgery for MEN1-associated insulinoma syndrome. Distal pancreatectomy was performed in 32 (46%), enucleation in 13 (19%), total pancreatectomy in 3 (4%), and pancreaticoduodenectomy in 2 (3%), one of which had a large insulinoma within the pancreatic head.[93] With a follow-up period ranging from several months to 18 years, cure (defined as normal levels of glucose and insulin and no evidence of tumor on imaging studies) was achieved in 57%–100% of patients. Persistent or recurrent hypoglycemia was reported only in patients who had simple enucleation in the absence of distal pancreatectomy. The 10-year overall survival for patients with MEN1-associated insulinomas approaches 100% in most published series. Lairmore et al.[93] and Bartsch et al.[19] have reported an overall survival of 67% (two of three) and 83% (five of six), respectively.[19,93] Neither of the two deaths in these series were related to progressive insulinoma or complications of hypoglycemia.[19] Given the difficulty of extrapolating treatment recommendations from such small numbers of patients, it appears that a logical surgical approach is similar to the operation for gastrinoma: distal subtotal pancreatectomy and enucleation of ultrasound-visible disease in the pancreatic head and uncinate process.
3. **Nonfunctioning PETs**: Nonfunctioning tumors of the pancreas, including PPomas, represent as many as 71% of surgically treated pancreatic tumors in the published MEN1 population (Table 45.4). In Table 45.4, 39 patients with nonfunctioning pancreatic tumors underwent surgery; eight of these patients underwent a distal pancreatectomy with enucleation of other tumors in the pancreatic head or uncinate process. With a follow-up period ranging from 5 to 19 years, four patients experienced disease recurrence, one with liver metastasis and one with lung metastasis (Table 45.4). Several surgical strategies have been proposed for the management of clinically nonfunctioning neuroendocrine pancreatic tumors in MEN1 patients. The most aggressive approach is advocated by Skogseid et al.,[76,88,89] who suggest that pancreatic imaging is ineffective for the early detection of MEN1-associated pancreatic tumors. They obtain biochemical markers annually from the age of 15 years, and surgery is recommended if peptide levels increase, even in the absence of radiographic evidence of a pancreatic neoplasm. All patients with elevations in at least two pancreatic peptides were found at surgery to have a grossly visible pancreatic or duodenal tumor, with an average size of 1.3 cm.[88,100] According to this protocol, the appropriate surgical approach includes intraoperative ultrasonography, duodenotomy (if ZES is diagnosed), subtotal distal pancreatectomy, and enucleation of any tumor within the pancreatic head or uncinate process.

Table 45.2 Surgical Management of MEN1-Associated Gastrinoma (Zollinger-Ellison Syndrome)

	Number of Patients									Follow-Up
Authors	MEN1 and ZES	Surgery	PD or TP	Duodenotomy	DP ± Enucleation	Enucleation or NAR	Biochemical Cure (%)	m-LM (%)	DOD (%)	
Kloppel et al.[51]	NA	2	1 (PD)	NA	0	1	2/2 (100%)*	NA	NA	NA
van Heerden et al.[169]	25	10	1 (PD)†	NA	4	5	0/10	NA	0/10	Mean: 79.75 m
Sheppard et al.[86]	22	7	0	2	6	1	0/7	NA	NA	Range: 3–84 m
Samaan et al.[104]	6	4	1 (TP)	2	2	1‡	1/4 (25%)	1/4 (25%)	0/4	NA
Thompson et al.[170]	NA	6	0	6	6	0	1/6 (17%) 5/6 (83%)*	0/6	0/6	Mean: 7 y (5–144 m)
Pipeleers-Marichal et al.[53]	NA	7	2 (PD)‖	2	4	1‡	4/7 (57%)*	NA	NA	NA
Grama et al.[89]	19	14	NA	5	NA	NA	0/14	2/19 (11%)	4/19 (21%)	Range: 7–14 y
Thompson[69]	11	11	0	11	10¶	1‡	3/11 (27%) 10/11 (91%)*	0/11	0/11	Range: 3 m–14 y
Cherner and Sawyers[171]	1	1	0	0	1	0	0/1	0/1	0/1	16 m
Thompson et al.[172]	NA	3	0	3	3	0	0/3	0/3	0/3	NA
Melvin et al.[173]	19	17	NA	NA	NA	NA	1/17 (6%)	NA	4/19 (21%)	Mean: 14 y (1–39 y)
Mignon et al.[63]	36	33	3 (PD)	9	21	9	1/33 (3%)	7/33 (21%)	2/33 (6%)	Median: 95 m (17–278 m)
Thompson[91]	43	38	NA	38	38	0	33% 67%*	1/38 (3%)	0/38	Up to 19 y
Cadiot et al.[61]	NA	48	5 (PD) 1 (TP)	NA	32	4	NA	8/48 (17%)	3/48 (6%)	Median: 102 m (12–366 m)
Lowney et al.[64]	NA	12	NA	NA	NA	NA	NA	0/12	0/12	NA
Norton et al.[59]	NA	28	NA	NA	NA	NA	0/28	NA	NA	Median: 5 ±7 y
Bartsch et al.[19]	21	8	3 (PD)§	7	3	2	87%	0/8	NA	Median: 53 m (1–198 m)
Lairmore et al.[93]	NA	2	0	2	NA	1	NA	0/2	0/2	Range: 1.5–6.8 y
Total	203	251	17	87	130	25	Range: 0%–100%	0%–25%	0%–21%	Range: 3 m–21 y

Abbreviations: DOD, dead of disease; DP, distal pancreatectomy; m, months; m-LM, metachronous liver metastases; NA, not available; NAR, nonanatomic resection; PD, pancreaticoduodenectomy; y, years; ZES, Zollinger-Ellison syndrome.

* Eugastrinemic.

† Reoperation after recurrence (prior simple enucleation of duodenal tumor).

‡ Excision of the tumor from duodenum.

‖ One patient has both PD and distal pancreatectomy.

¶ Three patients had reoperation after recurrence (prior simple enucleation of duodenal tumor).

§ Two patients had reoperations after recurrence.

Table 45.3 Surgical Management of MEN1-Associated Insulinoma

	Number of Patients							Follow-Up
Authors	Surgery	PD or TP	DP	Enucleation or NAR	Cure	m-LM	DOD	
Kloppel et al.[51]	2	0	0	2	2/2 (100%)	0/2	0/2	NA
Tisell et al.[102,103]	3	2 (TP)	1	0	2/3 (67%)	NA	0/3	Range: 3.5–9+ y
Sheppard et al.[86]	2	0	1	1	100%	NA	0/2	Range: 3–84 m
Samaan et al.[104]	2	0	2	0	100%	0/2	0/2	Range: 18 m–7 y
Demeure et al.[74]	6	0	5	1*	5/6 (84%)†	NA	0/6	Up to 15 y
Grama et al.[89]	7	0	NA	NA	4/7 (57%)	1/7 (14%)	0/7	Range: 7–14 y
O'Riordain et al.[174]	18	1 (TP)	12	5	16/18 (89%)	0/18	4/18 (22%)	Median: 10.3 y (1.7–18.8 y)
Lo et al.[75]	3	0	2	1‡	2/3 (67%)†	0/3	0/3	Mean: 26 m (6–57 m)
Thompson[91]	7	0	7	0	100%	0/7	0/7	Up to 18 y
Lowney et al.[64]	10	NA	NA	NA	NA	1/10 (10%)	1/10 (10%)	NA
Bartsch et al.[19]	6‖	1¶	2	3	100%	0/6	0/6	Median: 41 m (1–181 m)
Lairmore et al.[93]	3	1	NA	NA	NA	NA	1/3 (33%)§	Range: 1.5 y–6.8 y
Total	69	5	32	13	Range: 57%–100%	0%–14%	0%–33%	Range: 3 m–21 y

Abbreviations: DOD, dead of disease; DP, distal pancreatectomy; m, months; m-LM, metachronous liver metastases; NA, not available; NAR, nonanatomic resection; PD, pancreaticoduodenectomy; TP, total pancreatectomy; y, years.

* Reoperation: total pancreatectomy: no recurrence.

† 100% cure after reoperation.

‡ Reoperation: distal pancreatectomy: no recurrence.

‖ Two patients had gastrinoma and insulinoma.

¶ The patient underwent PD because of concomitant gastrinoma.

§ One perioperation death.

Table 45.4 Surgical Management of MEN1-Associated Nonfunctioning and Other Rare PETs

Authors	Number of Patients								Follow-Up
	Surgery	PD or TP	Duodenotomy	DP	Enucleation or NAR	Biochemical Cure (%)	m-LM	DOD	
Kloppel et al.[51]	4 (NPET)*	0	NA	4	0	0/4	NA	1/4 (25%)	NA
	1 (VIP)	1(PD)	NA	0	0	NA	NA	NA	NA
Tisell et al.[102,103]	1 (SOM/GLU)	1	0	0	0	0/1	0/1	1/1 (100%)	NA
Sheppard et al.[86]	1 (VIP)	0	0	1	0	100%	NA	NA	17 m
Samaan et al.[104]	2 (GLU)	0	0	2	0	1/2 (50%)	0/2	1/2 (50%)	NA
Grama et al.[89]	7	NA	NA	NA	NA	NA	1/7 (14%)	4/7 (57%)	Range: 7–14 y
Thompson[91]	3 (NPET)	0	3	3	0	NA	0/3	0/3	Up to 19 y
Lowney et al.[64]	19 (NPET)*	NA	NA	NA	NA	16/19† (84%)	0/19	0/19	NA
	2 (VIP)	NA	NA	NA	NA	NA	0/2	0/2	Up to 21 y
Bartsch et al.[19]	3 (NPT)	0	0	3	0	3/3 (100%)‡	0/3	0/3	Median: 78 m (1–198 m)
	1 (VIP)	0	0	1	0	0/1	1/1 (100%)	0/1	Median: 78 m (1–198 m)
Lairmore et al.[93]	15 (NPET)*	NA	NA	NA	NA	NA	NA	NA	Range: 1.5–6.8 y
	1 (VIP)	NA	NA	NA	NA	NA	NA	NA	Range: 1.5–6.8 y
Total	60	2‖	3‖	14‖	0‖	21‖	2‖	7‖	Range: 17 m–21 y

Abbreviations: DP, distal pancreatectomy; DOD, dead of disease; GLU, glucagonoma; m, months; m-LM, metachronous liver metastases; NA, not available; NAR, nonanatomic resection; NPET, nonfunctioning pancreatic endocrine tumors; PD, pancreaticoduodenectomy; SOM, somatostatinoma; TP, total pancreatectomy; VIP, VIPoma; y, years.

* PPomas included with nonfunctioning tumors

† Two of 19 patients recurred.

‡ Imaging studies were positive in two patients.

‖ Insufficient information to total.

Thompson[16,90,91] advocates surgery in all MEN1 patients with a nonfunctioning PET greater than 1 cm found on endoscopic ultrasound (EUS). This operation, now commonly referred to as the "Thompson procedure," includes distal pancreatectomy (at the level of the superior mesenteric vein), enucleation of any identified lesions in the pancreatic head or uncinate process, and regional lymphadenectomy.[16,90,91] In the absence of gastrin hypersecretion, duodenal exploration is not performed.

Fraker and Norton[96] suggested surgical resection for nonfunctioning PETs that are 2 to 3 cm or larger.[50,59,94-98] The rationale for this strategy is based on their experience in patients with sporadic gastrinomas in which primary tumor size appeared to correlate with metastatic potential.[60,98] Mignon and Cadiot[77] also suggested surgery for nonfunctioning PETs larger than 3 cm.[77]

Bartsch et al.[19] suggested that patients with nonfunctioning PETs should undergo surgery if tumor size is larger than 1 cm.[19] Pancreaticoduodenectomy may be necessary for very large tumors that are located within the head and uncinate process of the pancreas in close proximity to the pancreatic duct or tumors with synchronous metastatic disease in regional lymph nodes.[19]

Brandi et al.[1] published a consensus statement on the management of MEN1 patients and confirmed that surgery should be considered the main treatment for insulinoma. For MEN1-related gastrinoma, this group was less enthusiastic about surgery because of the finding that few patients have a normal serum level of gastrin after operation. Their consensus statement reflects the difficulty in developing treatment recommendations, especially with regard to major abdominal surgery, when there are limited data on which to base recommendations. It is reasonable to conclude that patients with MEN1-related PETs should be managed at a center experienced with the global management of this disease and specifically the operative management of complex pancreatic malignancies. Both an in-depth knowledge of the disease and the technical aspects of pancreatic surgery are necessary components for a favorable outcome.

The 2003 National Comprehensive Cancer Network also provided treatment guidelines for patients with MEN1-related neuroendocrine tumors. This publication suggests that patients with radiographically occult presumed sporadic gastrinomas (no primary tumor has been found by preoperative imaging studies) may be observed or referred for surgery. Surgery for all forms of functioning and nonfunctioning tumors should include distal pancreatectomy, duodenotomy, enucleation of any palpable or ultrasound-visible tumors in the pancreatic head, and regional lymphadenectomy (Thompson procedure).[101] Tumors in the pancreatic head that cannot be enucleated would obviously require pancreaticoduodenectomy.[101]

Total pancreatectomy to cure nonfunctioning PETs in MEN1 patients is rarely recommended because of the resulting endocrine and exocrine insufficiency. Some authors suggest that total pancreatectomy is warranted in patients with multifocal tumors in the setting of a strong family history of metastatic PET.[102-104] Hopefully, future studies will elucidate a genotype-phenotype correlation in MEN1 syndrome and thus define the subset of MEN1 patients who need to be treated with total pancreatectomy. At M.D. Anderson Cancer Center, we currently operate on all MEN1 patients with evidence of PETs on computed tomography (CT) imaging. We concur that the Thompson procedure is the most appropriate operation for these patients. In rare cases with large tumors within the head of the pancreas that are not amenable to enucleation, pancreatoduodenectomy is an appropriate alternative. Table 45.5 summarizes the extent of metastatic disease as well as MEN1-related deaths in patients with PETs from 22 published series.

4. **VIPoma, Glucagonoma:** Clinical studies have suggested that VIPomas and glucagonomas represent a relatively small percentage of MEN1-associated pancreatic tumors (Table 45.1). Two of the three surgically treated patients with glucagonomas (Table 45.4) underwent distal pancreatectomy with enucleation of synchronous tumors within the head or the uncinate process of the pancreas. Tisell and Ahlman[103] reported a patient with metastatic disease due to glucagonoma who underwent debulking surgery; this patient died 4 years after surgery. Of the five operated patients with VIPomas, only two underwent distal pancreatectomy with a cure in both. The limited number of surgically treated patients with VIPoma reported in the literature precludes any definite conclusions unique to the prognosis of these specific tumors.

Authors' Recommendations for the Surgical Management of MEN1-Associated PETs

Tables 45.2–45.5 illustrate the small number of surgically treated patients with MEN1-associated PETs from which we are asked to develop treatment recommendations.

Table 45.5 Development of Metastatic Disease in Patients with MEN1 and PETs

	Number of Patients					
Authors	**MEN1/PETs**	**MEN1/Surgery**	**LNM**	**s-LM**	**m-LM**	**Deaths**
Tisell et al.[102,103]	8*	5	NA	1	NA	1/8
Samaan et al.[104]	14	11	NA	3	1	NA
Sheppard et al.[86]	24	9	3	NA	NA	NA
Thompson[69]	16	11	3	0	NA	1/11
Grama et al.[89]	33	27	NA	7	4	NA
Cherner and Sawyers[171]	1	1	NA	1	NA	0/1
Mignon et al.[63]	45	36	NA	7	7	8/45
Melvin et al.[173]	19	17	3	NA	6	48% at 20 y
Pipeleers-Marichal et al.[56]	18	18	7	1	NA	At least 2 patients died†
Weber et al.[60]	34	18	NA	2	3	NA
Skogseid et al.[88]	24	20	NA	6	NA	NA
Skogseid et al.[100]	NA	25	NA	3	NA	NA
Mutch et al.[97]	20	14	1	1	NA	NA
Burgess et al.[87]	NA	NA	NA	NA	9	NA
Thompson[91]	NA	48	NA	1	1	1/48 at 10 y
Jensen[95]	44	28	NA	2	6	NA
Norton et al.[59]	NA	28	NA	NA	4	4/28
Lowney et al.[64]	48	43	11	2	1	2/48
Cadiot et al.[61]	77	48	5	NA	8	NA
Bartsch et al.[19]	21	16	NA	NA	1	2/21‡
Lairmore et al.[93]	NA	21	NA	2	NA	1/21
Gibril et al.[71]	57	41	24	3	9	1/57
Total	503	485	57‖	42‖	60‖	23‖

Abbreviations: LM, liver metastasis; LNM, lymph node metastasis; m-LM, metachronous liver metastasis; NA, not available; s-LM, synchronous liver metastasis; y, years.

* Two patients were treated in other hospitals

† This information is taken from previously published data on the same series of patients.[53]

‡ One patient died from metastatic thymoma.

‖ Insufficient information to total.

From an endocrine perspective, patients with ZES (gastrinoma) and insulinoma syndrome should receive surgical treatment. Although the results with surgery for ZES in patients with MEN1 have been suboptimal with respect to rendering patients eugastrinemic, advances in surgical technique, the routine use of intraoperative ultrasound, and the appreciation that the duodenum harbors small tumors in the majority of patients provide an optimistic outlook for surgery performed by experienced pancreatic surgeons. Even if postoperative stimulated gastrin levels remain abnormal, control of gastric acid production may be improved by a reduction in tumor burden. In addition, PETs may be a unique neoplasm in oncology and one in which overall tumor burden may be related to metastatic potential. Although this concept is foreign to the management of other solid tumors, patients with sporadic and familial PETs may receive a survival advantage by maintaining a tumor volume as low as possible, even if all gross or microscopic disease cannot be removed. For this reason, the management of such patients is very much an art as well as a science.

With regard to patients with tumors other than gastrinomas or insulinomas, oncologic concerns become even more compelling. In such patients, it seems most appropriate to operate when disease is confirmed on imaging studies (contrast-enhanced multidetector CT). The operation described by Thompson appears to be the most logical approach, thereby removing all visible tumor while decreasing the overall islet cell mass (and therefore the volume of at-risk pancreas; Fig. 45.1). This clearly represents a compromise procedure by leaving islet cell mass

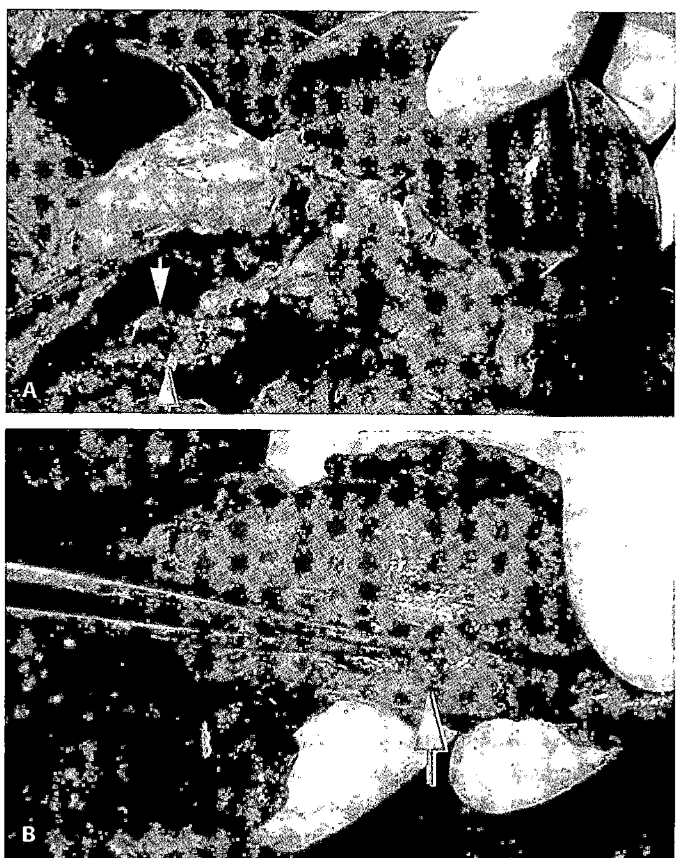

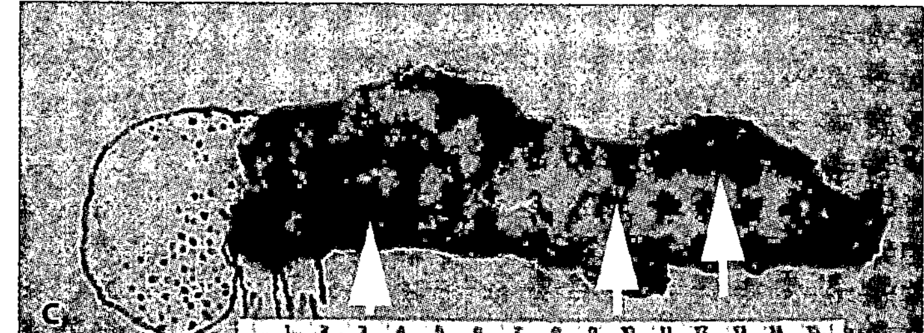

Figure 45.1
Intraoperative photographs of selected aspects of the operative procedure for islet cell neoplasms in the setting of MEN1 as described by Thompson consisting of distal subtotal pancreatectomy, enucleation of islet cell neoplasms in the pancreatic head, and peripancreatic and portal lymphadenectomy (due to the high frequency of regional lymph node metastases especially in patients without distant organ metastases). **(A)** The distal pancreas has been separated from the splenic vessels (*the yellow arrow marks the splenic artery, and the blue arrow marks the splenic vein*) by dividing the many small tributaries from the pancreatic body and tail to these vessels. The pancreatic body is elevated with a right-angle clamp to illustrate how the entire body of the pancreas can be separated from the splenic artery and vein. The spleen is preserved whenever possible, and the authors prefer to preserve the splenic artery and vein rather than to attempt splenic preservation on just the short gastric vessels. **(B)** One can see a close-up photograph of a small tumor (*blue arrow*) extending to the surface of the pancreas. **(C)** The resected body and tail of the pancreas appears with multiple islet cell neoplasms of different sizes marked with yellow arrows.

in the pancreatic head and therefore increasing the risk of metachronous neoplasms while preventing the complications of insulin-dependent diabetes associated with total pancreatectomy. The goal of this operation is to delay the need for total pancreatectomy (assuming patients may develop metachronous neoplasms in the remaining pancreas and therefore require completion total pancreatectomy) and thereby avoid the long-term complications of type 1 diabetes especially in young patients. Very long-term follow-up will be necessary to further elucidate the wisdom of this approach.

Treatment of Metastatic Disease

Medical treatment of patients with advanced neuroendocrine carcinoma of the pancreas attempts to control symptoms of hormonal excess and prevent tumor growth and metastasis.[105] In patients with gastrinoma, acid hypersecretion is now effectively controlled with H^+/K^+-ATPase inhibitors (omeprazole) in almost every patient. In contrast, medical management of insulinoma is rarely effective and indicated only in patients with a high surgical risk or those who have previously failed surgical treatment.[106] Diazoxide or somatostatin analogues may be used for this purpose. For VIPomas or metastatic carcinoid tumors, regimens such as corticosteroids, indomethacin, metoclopramide, and lithium carbonate have been successful for symptomatic patients.[52,81] Octreotide may also control watery diarrhea in most patients with VIPomas.

Controlled trials of chemotherapy and radiation treatment modalities have not been performed in MEN1 patients with malignant PETs because of the small number of patients available for study. Therefore, empiric treatment based on our larger experience with sporadic disease is usually the basis for therapy. A multimodality approach with somatostatin analogue, systemic triple chemotherapy consisting of Adriamycin, 5-fluorouracil (5-FU), streptozocin, and biotherapy with interferon-α is commonly applied. In addition, hepatic artery embolization has been proposed by several investigators.[52,107-110]

Octreotide is a human somatostatin analogue that inhibits the secretion of different peptide hormones from neuroendocrine tumors, which express somatostatin receptors. These receptors mediate the antiproliferative and antisecretory action of somatostatin. Octreotide analogues are effective in controlling hormone-related symptoms in patients with gastrinoma, but their efficacy with respect to tumor response (tumor size) remains controversial.[110-112] Burgess et al.[113] reported rapid symptomatic improvement and biochemical response in MEN1 patients with gastrinomas; gastrin levels decreased by at least 25% of the pretreatment level.[113] These investigators also reported that the size of hepatic metastases in patients with metastatic disease was reduced by up to 15% after treatment with octreotide.[113] Other investigators also found objective biochemical or tumor response to octreotide.[114,115] Octreotide has been used as palliative therapy for metastatic insulinoma, but it is not generally recommended, as insulinomas usually do not possess somatostatin receptors and thus octreotide only rarely improves hypoglycemic symptoms.[52,106,116] Octreotide has a well-established role in the systemic management of unresectable or metastatic VIPomas and hormonally active metastatic carcinoid tumors.[113]

Systemic chemotherapy has been evaluated in sporadic PETs, with variable rates of tumor response, and these data are used as a basis for the treatment of MEN1 patients with metastatic neuroendocrine carcinoma. The most commonly used chemotherapeutic agents include streptozocin, 5-FU, doxorubicin, chlorozotocin, and dacarbazine. Streptozocin-based combination chemotherapy (usually with 5-FU and doxorubicin) has a response rate of up to 63% in patients with sporadic disease.[117,118] Recent data from our institution suggest that the response rate is probably closer to 35%–40%.[119] Grama et al.[89] reported a biochemical response of 25% in MEN1 patients treated with this regimen.[89] Response to streptozocin-based combination chemotherapy may be associated with the histologic type of PET. It has been suggested that malignant insulinoma and VIPoma have superior response to streptozocin and 5-FU than do gastrinomas and nonfunctioning PETs.[107] Interferon-α alone or in combination with somatostatin has been used in the treatment of patients with sporadic metastatic PETs and has therefore been proposed for patients with MEN1-associated malignant PETs.[120] For gastrinomas, the administration of human leukocyte interferon may be beneficial.[105]

Selective hepatic artery embolization of metastatic tumor can control hormonal symptoms and reduce tumor burden. The metastatic lesions in the liver are typically hypervascular with a blood supply derived from the hepatic artery.[107,120,121] However, there are currently no specific guidelines concerning the optimal timing of embolization. It is not clear whether liver embolization should be attempted early in the course of the disease or after response or failure of systemic therapy. The indolent and often variable nature of disease progression in patients with metastatic PETs makes for a very heterogeneous population that is difficult to study. It is very hard to determine the impact of various treatment interventions versus the frequently witnessed variations in tumor progression; for example, one cannot often differentiate the impact of therapy from stable disease unrelated to treatment response. Patient management is therefore often based on the judgment of an experienced clinician combined with a knowledge of the overall tumor burden and tempo of disease progression. Finally, the role of radiotherapy is predominantly in the palliative management of metastases to bone, skin, or brain.[43]

Emerging Data on the Importance of Carcinoid Tumors

Carcinoids occur in 2%–8% of MEN1 patients.[5,15] They are usually foregut in origin, located mainly in the thymus, bronchus, or stomach. Most carcinoid tumors are malignant and therefore represent the second leading cause of MEN1-related death after malignant PETs.[98,122]

MEN1-related thymic carcinoids are rare (0%–6%), aggressive, and occur more often in men.[40,123,124] Thymic carcinoids are usually diagnosed after age 45, and the diagnosis is usually delayed because patients are generally asymptomatic.[38,125] When symptoms do occur, they are due to tumor compression and include dysarthria, dyspnea, cough, and chest and neck discomfort.[40,125] Most thymic carcinoids in MEN1 patients are malignant (up to 50% have hepatic metastases at the time of diagnosis) and frequently are the cause of disease-specific mortality.[15,38] Prophylactic transcervical thymectomy during neck exploration for parathyroidectomy is recommended in MEN1 patients to both remove a supernumerary ectopic parathyroid and reduce the volume of thymic tissue and thereby possibly prevent the development of a thymic carcinoid tumor.[4] The treatment of choice for an established thymic carcinoid tumor is surgical excision, which may prevent local disease progression and facilitate the use of adjuvant therapy.[38,125] Adjuvant therapy includes radiotherapy, chemotherapy, and interferon-α.[38,125] Brandi et al.[1] recommended CT imaging every 3 years to screen at-risk MEN1 patients for thymic carcinoids; however, in kindreds with a history of thymic carcinoids, more frequent screening with chest CT or magnetic resonance imaging (MRI) may be reasonable.[1,15,40]

MEN1-associated bronchial carcinoids are also rare neoplasms occurring in only 8% of MEN1 patients, and in contrast to thymic carcinoids, bronchial tumors are more prevalent in women.[5,15] Bronchial carcinoids may rarely secrete adrenocorticotropic hormone (ACTH) or growth hormone releasing hormone (GHRH). Although rare, these neoplasms may also produce atypical carcinoid syndrome or foregut carcinoid syndrome as a result of histamine secretion by the tumor cells. Foregut carcinoid tumors rarely secrete serotonin because of a lack of the enzyme aromatic amino acid decarboxylase. Dominant symptoms include flushing and headache. Flushing with foregut tumors tends to be prolonged, purple in color, and distributed predominantly in the face and neck.[126] Bronchospasm, cutaneous edema, and hypotension may also be present. In contrast, with midgut carcinoids cutaneous flushing is usually short in duration and pink-red in color. Other symptoms of midgut carcinoids include watery diarrhea caused by bowel hypermotility, abdominal pain, perspiration, hypotension, and cardiac valvular fibrosis resulting in right-sided heart failure. The symptoms may be paroxysmal and may vary in intensity over time. Carcinoid symptoms can be precipitated by a particular "trigger" agent such as alcohol, cheese, coffee, chocolate, red wine, or exercise. Like sporadic bronchial carcinoids, 66% of MEN1-associated bronchial carcinoid tumors are centrally located in the pulmonary lobes, and the remaining tumors may be peripheral. Pulmonary carcinoids in MEN1 patients are usually classified as low-grade typical or intermediate-grade atypical carcinoid. Metastases to regional lymph nodes or to the liver have only rarely been reported.[127] High-grade large-cell and small-cell neuroendocrine carcinoma have not been described in MEN1 patients. Bronchial carcinoid tumors seen on imaging studies may be confused with bronchogenic carcinomas of the lung. Surgical excision is the preferred treatment, and radiation therapy is used for patients with regional lymph node metastases.

Type II gastric carcinoids arise from histamine-secreting enterochromaffin-like cells (ECL cells) in up to 30% of MEN1 patients with ZES.[15] Type I gastric carcinoids are due to secondary hypergastrinemia in the setting of achlorhydria, chronic atrophic gastritis, and pernicious anemia, and type III gastric carcinoids are sporadic in origin and not associated with hypergastrinemia. Type III gastric carcinoids are thought to have a much greater malignant potential than types I and II, which rarely metastasize to distant sites. Hypergastrinemia in MEN1-associated ZES results in marked ECL cell proliferation, which eventually may lead to carcinoid tumor formation.[95,128-134] These tumors are multifocal in up to 92% of patients and are usually very small (80% are less than 2 cm).[135] They are distributed throughout the fundus or corpus of the stomach and are accompanied by diffuse argyrophilic cell hyperplasia of ECL cells or dysplasia in the entire oxyntic mucosa, which is not atrophic.[136,137] Gastric carcinoids in MEN1 patients usually occur in association with gastrin-producing duodenal tumors.[53] These neoplasms demonstrate a relatively low malignant potential and metastasize to lymph nodes in up to one third of patients and rarely to the liver.[135,138] The natural history of gastric carcinoids in MEN1 patients is not well studied because they are so uncommon. Recently, it has been found that gastric carcinoid tumors express vesicular monoamine transporter type 2, which is used as a histologic marker to distinguish carcinoids and their metastases from PETs.[15]

Upper endoscopy with biopsy will accurately assess the size, number, and extent of carcinoid tumors in the stomach. Submucosal lesions are not amenable to direct inspection, and thus, an EUS may be valuable in the diagnosis of these tumors especially when deep biopsy specimens are obtained.[138] Somatostatin receptor scintigraphy has a sensitivity of 75% and specificity of 95% in localizing gastric carcinoid tumors.[139] Abdominal CT scan, MRI, and somatostatin receptor scintigraphy may all be useful in detecting distant metastases. Although the precise malignant potential is unknown, distant metastases from type II gastric carcinoid tumors are very rare. Therefore, when possible, type II gastric carcinoids should be removed endoscopically, especially if such lesions are small and relatively few in number.[138,140] Patients should be followed by endoscopy at 6- to 12-month intervals.[138,141] The role for surgery (gastrectomy) in type II gastric carcinoids is unclear due to the limited clinical experience with this tumor in MEN1.[142,143] Long-acting somatostatin analogues administered for at least 6 months may facilitate regression of early-stage tumors.[142,144-146]

Clinical Screening in MEN1

Screening in the Affected Patient with MEN1

1. **Pancreatic screening:** Recent studies, including unpublished data from our institution, demonstrate that malignant neuroendocrine carcinoma rather than peptic ulcer disease is the main cause of death in MEN1 patients.[17,98,122,127,147] This lends support to a more traditional oncologic approach to this disease—namely, routine clinical, biochemical, and radiographic assessment, and surgical resection of disease that is apparent on high-quality imaging studies. Biochemical screening of at-risk patients may include serum levels of glucagon, gastrin, PP, and chromogranin

A (CgA). CgA is a glycoprotein released into the bloodstream from neuroendocrine cells and is considered a sensitive immunohistochemical marker to identify the neuroendocrine origin of tumor cells.[148-150] Plasma CgA is elevated in 60%–100% of patients with either functioning and nonfunctioning PETs; the sensitivities and specificities of the CgA measurements reported in various studies range between 70%–100%.[150-152] The sensitivity of CgA is reported to be superior to other serum tumor markers such as neuron specific enolase and the α-subunit of glycoprotein hormones.[149,150,153] The degree of elevation in CgA appears to correlate with tumor volume in patients with neuroendocrine tumors.[149,151] Granberg et al.[151] reported that all MEN1 patients with radiographically imaged tumors and 60% of those with CT-occult biochemically functional pancreatic neoplasms had elevated serum levels of CgA.[151] Approximately 44% of MEN1 patients without radiographic or biochemical evidence of a pancreatic neoplasm may also have an elevated CgA. This may represent a false-positive result, but most likely it is due to CgA secretion from an otherwise undetectable pancreatic tumor or less likely, from other MEN1-associated neoplasms.[151] Goebel et al.[150] demonstrated that changes in the serum levels of CgA over time are related to tumor volume.[150] However, no data exist to determine the efficacy of this marker as a screening tool. The level of CgA cannot differentiate between specific types of endocrine tumors. CgA may be normal when tumor volume is low, and serum CgA levels drawn on different days may vary considerably.[149,151] Repeat measurements are necessary when using CgA for treatment monitoring. Despite its poor utility in tumor screening, CgA is a useful marker in the postoperative monitoring of patients who had elevated levels before tumor removal. Although CgA is considered the best tumor marker currently available for use in patients with PETs, it is probably an overused test of limited clinical utility.[149,150,153]

Gastrinomas produce gastrin, and therefore, this peptide may be used as a tumor marker to aid diagnosis and response to treatment. Burgess et al.[87] suggested that plasma gastrin levels correlate with the extent of tumor burden.[87] The level of serum gastrin may indicate malignant disease; serum levels of gastrin greater than 1000 to 1500 pg/ml have been suggested to correlate with liver metastasis.[53,76,88,154] However, other investigators have not reproduced the association between gastrin levels and tumor volume.[150] Skogseid and Doherty reported that all patients with malignant pancreatic tumors had elevations of at least four peptide hormones.[155]

Elevated levels of PP have also been reported to be a marker of islet cell neoplasms in MEN1 patients.[156] Serum PP levels increase with age in normal individuals and also may be elevated in various diseases such as diabetes mellitus, chronic renal insufficiency, and peptic ulcer disease.[156-158] PP levels should be considered abnormally high only if they are three times the age-matched normal basal level.[156,159] Fasting serum levels of PP show a sensitivity of 88%–95% and a specificity of 95%–100% to determine the presence of a neuroendocrine pancreatic tumor in MEN1 patients.[97,156] Elevations in PP levels that are more than 4.5 times the basal level after meal stimulation suggest the presence of some degree of islet cell hyperplasia.[97,156] There is no consensus on the clinical significance and an elevated PP level in the absence of a neoplasm on imaging studies.

Currently no specific guidelines exist for the frequency of abdominal imaging in patients with MEN1 (Table 45.6). Thompson et al.[16,90,91,160-162] suggested that pancreatic screening for all patients with MEN1, even asymptomatic patients, should include annual or semiannual biochemical testing and an initial EUS, which should be repeated every 3 years if no tumor is found or after 1 year if a small PET ($\leq$ 1 cm in size) is identified. If a tumor is seen on EUS and is larger then 1 cm, then it should be removed surgically; EUS should then be repeated every 2 years to monitor the residual pancreas.[161] In addition, this protocol includes a CT of the abdomen and an octreoscan to exclude metastatic disease.[16,91,161] The rationale behind this aggressive screening protocol is to detect pancreatic neoplasms early and excise them before metastasis occurs.[90] Other investigators advocate EUS every 2 years in all MEN1 patients.[90,98,160] We currently do not perform EUS for PET screening in MEN1 patients unless the tumor is seen on CT or MRI. In patients at high risk for the development of islet cell tumors (by family history), we currently recommend CT imaging every 1 to 2 years beginning at age 20 or earlier if islet cell carcinoma has been diagnosed at an earlier age within the patient's family. The frequency of CT imaging is also based on the aggressiveness of the tumor in the individual kindred. Other investigators believe that imaging studies should be repeated every 3 to 4 years.[99,163,164] MRI, selective angiography, or somatostatin receptor scintigraphy (octreoscan) have all been proposed as screening studies with similar

Table 45.6. Recommendations for MEN1 Diagnostic Screening

		Age of	Biochemical	Imaging		
Authors	Institution	Onset	Screening	Frequency	Screening	Frequency
Skogseid et al.[76,88,100,175]	Uppsala, Sweden	15 y	ins, PP, gastrin, c-p, chromogranin A, glucagon, Glc, proinsulin	Annually	NA	Every 3–5 y
Demeure et al.[74]	University of California	NA	Fasting ins, ins/Glc ratio, Fasting test for 24–72 h, provocating tests	NA	NA	NA
Mignon et al.[63,77]	Bichat–Claude Bernard Hospital, France/GENEM	NA	Ca, u-Ca, P, PTH, prolactin, fasting Glc, c-p, K, free cortisol, urinary-free cortisol	Patients with ZES/ 6 months	Sella turcica CT or MRI, EUS, abdominal CT, octreoscan	In ZES/6–12 m
Mutch et al.[97]	Washington University School of Medicine, St. Louis, MO	15 y	PP, fasting Glc	Annually	CT. If CT(+), then octreoscan, MRI	Abnormal biochemical tests or signs and symptoms
Chanson et al.[99]	GENEM	NA	ins, gastrin, PP, Ca, u-Ca, P, PTH, prolactin, fasting Glc, c-p, K, dexamethasone test, FSH, LH, glu, GH, secretin test	Annually	abd-CT, abd-US, EUS in ZES, octreoscan, MRI/CT brain	Every 3–5 y
Lowney et al.[64]	Washington University School of Medicine St. Louis, MO	NA	Biochemical hormone screening or directed biochemical tests	NA	Somatostatin receptor scintigraphy	Patients who exhibit symptoms or who had abnormal biochemical screening
Thakker[105]	Nuffield Department of Medicine, University of Oxford, UK	Early childhood	Ca, prolactin, gastrin, other gastrointestinal hormones	Annually	Abdominal imaging	Every 5–10 y
Thompson et al.[91,161,162]	The University of Michigan hospitals	NA	Serum gastrin levels and, if elevated, a secretin stimulation test	Every 6m-1 y	EUS in all MEN1 patients. If EUS (+), a CT for liver metastasis	Every 1–3 y

Continued

Table 45.6 Recommendations for MEN1 Diagnostic Screening—*Continued*

Authors	Institution	Age of Onset	Biochemical Screening	Imaging Frequency	Screening	Frequency
Norton et al.[59]	National Institutes of Health	NA	Fasting serum gastrin levels	NA	Somatostatin receptor scintigraphy	NA
Bartsch et al.[19]	Philipps-University Marburg, Germany	NA	Fasting and stimulating hormone tests	Annually	CT, somatostatin receptor scintigraphy	Annually
Karges et al.[164]	University of Ulm, Germany	10–12 y	Ca, PTH, prolactin, gastrin	Annually	Abdominal US MRI anterior pituitary, EUS or CT or MRI	Every 3–4 y*
Lairmore et al.[93]	Washington.University School of Medicine St. Louis, MO	NA	Biochemical screening	Annually	Selective radiographic °localizing studies	Patients with elevated tumor markers, onset of signs or symptoms

Abbreviations: NA, not available; ZES, Zollinger-Ellison syndrome; US, ultrasound; CT, computer tomography; h, hours; m, months; y, years; Ca, calcium; u-Ca, urinary calcium; glu, glucagon; P, Phosphorous; K, Potassium; c-p, c-peptide; GH, growth hormone; FSH, follicle stimulating hormone; LH, Luteinizing hormone; abd, abdominal; EUS, endoscopic ultrasound; MRI, magnetic resonance imaging; PP, pancreatic polypeptide; ins, insulin; PTH, parathyroid hormone.
*When indicated annually.

sensitivities.[16,19,59,64,100,165] CT and MRI are noninvasive and clearly the tests of choice for pancreatic imaging in at-risk MEN1 patients.

2. **Screening of other endocrine glands:** Continued tumor surveillance for MEN1-related neoplasms is recommended for all MEN1 patients. It is reasonable for asymptomatic MEN1 patients (confirmed to be affected through genetic testing) to undergo a complete physical examination and biochemical (serum levels of prolactin, total and ionized calcium, phosphorus, intact parathyroid hormone, PP, CgA, and gastrin) and imaging studies (CT of chest and abdomen) at an interval appropriate for the patient's age and kindred-associated risk. Patients who have been surgically treated for an MEN1-associated PET should undergo postoperative abdominal CT imaging approximately 3 months after resection to create a baseline for further follow-up imaging. Long-term surveillance of these patients, according to National Comprehensive Cancer Network guidelines, should include physical examination and assessment of biochemical tumor markers every 6 months for the first 3 years and annually after year 4.[101] At M.D. Anderson Cancer Center, we advocate abdominal and chest CT scans every 12–24 months based on risk factor assessment to include the patient's personal and family history.

Screening in the Healthy Relative at Risk for MEN1

The frequency of diagnostic evaluations and the exact tests that should be performed in relatives at risk for MEN1 (based on the presence of an established family history without genetic confirmation in the proband or the patient in question) are not clearly defined. Diagnostic screening of kindred members with *MEN1* syndrome leads to earlier tumor detection by approximately two decades.[100,166] The aim of screening (both patients who are known to be affected and those relatives at risk for MEN1) is to detect abnormalities at a presymptomatic stage and thus to reduce morbidity and mortality resulting from MEN1-related malignancies.[122] We advocate yearly biochemical screening, including serum levels of prolactin, total and ionized calcium, intact parathyroid hormone, fasting glucose, gastrin, PP, and CgA. Other investigators propose similar biochemical screening.[19,59,63,89-91,93,155,163,164,167,168] In addition to biochemical screening, we recommend radiographic screening for PETs and carcinoid tumors to include contrast-enhanced CT scanning of the abdomen and chest. The use and frequency of CT imaging in patients of unknown MEN1 status within an affected kindred are controversial, and clear recommendations are not available.

References

1. Brandi ML, Gagel RF, Angeli A, et al. Guidelines for diagnosis and therapy of MEN type 1 and type 2. *J Clin Endocrinol Metab.* 2001;86:5658–5671.
2. Brandi ML, Marx SJ, Aurbach GD, Fitzpatrick LA. Familial multiple endocrine neoplasia type I: a new look at pathophysiology. *Endocr Rev.* 1987;8:391–405.
3. Ki Wong F, Burgess J, Nordenskjold M, Larsson C, Tean Teh B. Multiple endocrine neoplasia type 1. *Semin Cancer Biol.* 2000;10:299–312.
4. Burgess JR, Greenaway TM, Shepherd JJ. Expression of the MEN-1 gene in a large kindred with multiple endocrine neoplasia type 1. *J Intern Med.* 1998;243:465–470.
5. Trump D, Farren B, Wooding C, et al. Clinical studies of multiple endocrine neoplasia type 1 (MEN1). *Q J Med.* 1996;89:653–669. Erratum in *Q J Med.* 1996;89:957–958.
6. Danowski TS, Mateer FM, Longabaugh EE. Endocrine adenomatosis (polyendocrine disease). Familial occurrences. *Acta Med Scand.* 1962;172:559–566.
7. Wermer P. Genetic aspects of adenomatosis of endocrine glands. *Am J Med.* 1954;16:363–371.
8. Johnson GJ, Summerskill WH, Anderson VE, Keating FR Jr. Clinical and genetic investigation of a large kindred with multiple endocrine adenomatosis. *N Engl J Med.* 1967;277:1379–1385.
9. Nakamura Y, Larsson C, Julier C, et al. Localization of the genetic defect in multiple endocrine neoplasia type 1 within a small region of chromosome 11. *Am J Hum Genet.* 1989;44:751–755.
10. Larsson C, Skogseid B, Oberg K, Nakamura Y, Nordenskjold M. Multiple endocrine neoplasia type 1 gene maps to chromosome 11 and is lost in insulinoma. *Nature.* 1988;332:85–87.
11. Chandrasekharappa SC, Guru SC, Manickam P, et al. Positional cloning of the gene for multiple endocrine neoplasia-type 1. *Science.* 1997;276:404–407.
12. Guru SC, Goldsmith PK, Burns AL, et al. Menin, the product of the MEN1 gene, is a nuclear protein. *Proc Natl Acad Sci USA.* 1998;95:1630–1634.
13. Agarwal SK, Guru SC, Heppner C, et al. Menin interacts with the AP1 transcription factor JunD and represses JunD-activated transcription. *Cell.* 1999;96:143–152.
14. Marx S, Spiegel AM, Skarulis MC, Doppman JL, Collins FS, Liotta LA. Multiple endocrine neoplasia type 1: clinical and genetic topics. *Ann Intern Med.* 1998;129:484–494.
15. Gibril F, Schumann M, Pace A, Jensen RT. Multiple endocrine neoplasia type 1 and Zollinger-Ellison syndrome: a prospective study of 107 cases and comparison with 1009 cases from the literature. *Medicine (Baltimore).* 2004;83:43–83.
16. Thompson NW. Multiple endocrine neoplasia type I: surgical therapy. *Cancer Treat Res.* 1997;89:407–419.
17. Carty SE, Helm AK, Amico JA, et al. The variable penetrance and spectrum of manifestations of multiple endocrine

neoplasia type 1. *Surgery*. 1998;124:1106–1113; discussion 1113–1114.
18. Thompson NW, Lloyd RV, Nishiyama RH, et al. MEN I pancreas: a histological and immunohistochemical study. *World J Surg*. 1984;8:561–574.
19. Bartsch DK, Langer P, Wild A, et al. Pancreaticoduodenal endocrine tumors in multiple endocrine neoplasia type 1: surgery or surveillance? *Surgery*. 2000;128: 958–965.
20. Kouvaraki MA, Lee JE, Shapiro SE, et al. Genotype-phenotype analysis in multiple endocrine neoplasia type 1. *Arch Surg*. 2002;137:641–647.
21. Kaji H, Canaff L, Lebrun JJ, Goltzman D, Hendy GN. Inactivation of menin, a Smad3-interacting protein, blocks transforming growth factor type beta signaling. *Proc Natl Acad Sci USA*. 2001;98:3837–3842.
22. Heppner C, Bilimoria KY, Agarwal SK, et al. The tumor suppressor protein menin interacts with NF-kappaB proteins and inhibits NF-kappaB-mediated transactivation. *Oncogene*. 2001;20:4917–4925.
23. Lemmens IH, Forsberg L, Pannett AA, et al. Menin interacts directly with the homeobox-containing protein Pem. *Biochem Biophys Res Commun*. 2001;286:426–431.
24. Sukhodolets KE, Hickman AB, Agarwal SK, et al. The 32-kilodalton subunit of replication protein A interacts with menin, the product of the MEN1 tumor suppressor gene. *Mol Cell Biol*. 2003;23:493–509.
25. Bertolino P, Radovanovic I, Casse H, Aguzzi A, Wang ZQ, Zhang CX. Genetic ablation of the tumor suppressor menin causes lethality at mid-gestation with defects in multiple organs. *Mech Dev*. 2003;120:549–560.
26. Crabtree JS, Scacheri PC, Ward JM, et al. A mouse model of multiple endocrine neoplasia, type 1, develops multiple endocrine tumors. *Proc Natl Acad Sci USA*. 2001;98: 1118–1123.
27. Biondi CA, Gartside MG, Waring P, et al. Conditional inactivation of the MEN1 gene leads to pancreatic and pituitary tumorigenesis but does not affect normal development of these tissues. *Mol Cell Biol*. 2004;24:3125–3131.
28. UMD-MEN1 Mutation Database (vol. 2004). GENEM, 2002.
29. Agarwal SK, Kester MB, Debelenko LV, et al. Germline mutations of the MEN1 gene in familial multiple endocrine neoplasia type 1 and related states. *Hum Mol Genet*. 1997;6:1169–1175.
30. Giraud S, Zhang CX, Serova-Sinilnikova O, et al. Germline mutation analysis in patients with multiple endocrine neoplasia type 1 and related disorders. *Am J Hum Genet*. 1998;63:455–467.
31. Teh BT, Kytola S, Farnebo F, et al. Mutation analysis of the MEN1 gene in multiple endocrine neoplasia type 1, familial acromegaly and familial isolated hyperparathyroidism. *J Clin Endocrinol Metab*. 1998;83:2621–2626.
32. Poncin J, Abs R, Velkeniers B, et al. Mutation analysis of the MEN1 gene in Belgian patients with multiple endocrine neoplasia type 1 and related diseases. *Hum Mutat*. 1999;13:54–60.
33. Sakurai A, Shirahama S, Fujimori M, et al. Novel MEN1 gene mutations in familial multiple endocrine neoplasia type 1. *J Hum Genet*. 1998;43:199–201.
34. Debelenko LV, Brambilla E, Agarwal SK, et al. Identification of MEN1 gene mutations in sporadic carcinoid tumors of the lung. *Hum Mol Genet*. 1997;6:2285–2290.
35. Heppner C, Kester MB, Agarwal SK, et al. Somatic mutation of the MEN1 gene in parathyroid tumours. *Nat Genet*. 1997;16:375–378.
36. Zhuang Z, Vortmeyer AO, Pack S, et al. Somatic mutations of the MEN1 tumor suppressor gene in sporadic gastrinomas and insulinomas. *Cancer Res*. 1997;57:4682–4686.
37. Wautot V, Vercherat C, Lespinasse J, et al. Germline mutation profile of MEN1 in multiple endocrine neoplasia type 1: search for correlation between phenotype and the functional domains of the MEN1 protein. *Hum Mutat*. 2002;20:35–47.
38. Teh BT, Zedenius J, Kytola S, et al. Thymic carcinoids in multiple endocrine neoplasia type 1. *Ann Surg*. 1998;228:99–105.
39. Petty EM, Green JS, Marx SJ, Taggart RT, Farid N, Bale AE. Mapping the gene for hereditary hyperparathyroidism and prolactinoma (MEN1Burin) to chromosome 11q: evidence for a founder effect in patients from Newfoundland. *Am J Hum Genet*. 1994;54:1060–1066.
40. Teh BT, McArdle J, Chan SP, et al. Clinicopathologic studies of thymic carcinoids in multiple endocrine neoplasia type 1. *Medicine (Baltimore)*. 1997;76:21–29.
41. Bassett JH, Forbes SA, Pannett AA, et al. Characterization of mutations in patients with multiple endocrine neoplasia type 1. *Am J Hum Genet*. 1998;62:232–244.
42. Calender A. Genetic testing in multiple endocrine neoplasia and related syndromes. *Forum (Genova)*. 1998;8:146–159.
43. Skogseid B, Doherty GM. *Surgical Endocrinology*. Philadelphia: Lippincott Williams and Wilkins; 2001.
44. Teh BT, Esapa CT, Houlston R, et al. A family with isolated hyperparathyroidism segregating a missense MEN1 mutation and showing loss of the wild-type alleles in the parathyroid tumors letter. *Am J Hum Genet*. 1998;63:1544–1549.
45. Fujimori M, Shirahama S, Sakurai A, et al. Novel V184E MEN1 germline mutation in a Japanese kindred with familial hyperparathyroidism. *Am J Med Genet*. 1998;80: 221–222.
46. Kassem M, Kruse TA, Wong FK, Larsson C, Teh BT. Familial isolated hyperparathyroidism as a variant of multiple endocrine neoplasia type 1 in a large Danish pedigree. *J Clin Endocrinol Metab*. 2000;85:165–167.
47. Gagel R, Marx S. Multiple endocrine neoplasia. In: Larsen P, Kronenberg H, Melmed S, et al., eds. *Williams Textbook of Endocrinology*. 10th ed. Philadelphia: W.B. Saunders; 2003:1717–1762.
48. Glascock MJ, Carty SE. Multiple endocrine neoplasia type 1: fresh perspective on clinical features and penetrance. *Surg Oncol*. 2002;11:143–150.
49. Shapiro SE, Cote GC, Lee JE, Gagel RF, Evans DB. The role of genetics in the surgical management of familial endocrinopathy syndromes. *J Am Coll Surg*. 2003;197:818–831.
50. Norton JA, Alexander HR, Fraker DL, Venzon DJ, Gibril F, Jensen RT. Comparison of surgical results in patients

with advanced and limited disease with multiple endocrine neoplasia type 1 and Zollinger-Ellison syndrome. *Ann Surg.* 2001;234:495–505; discussion 505–506.
51. Kloppel G, Willemer S, Stamm B, Hacki WH, Heitz PU. Pancreatic lesions and hormonal profile of pancreatic tumors in multiple endocrine neoplasia type I: an immunocytochemical study of nine patients. *Cancer.* 1986; 57:1824–1832.
52. Pannett AA, Thakker RV. Multiple endocrine neoplasia type 1. *Endocr Relat Cancer.* 1999;6:449–473.
53. Pipeleers-Marichal M, Somers G, Willems G, et al. Gastrinomas in the duodenums of patients with multiple endocrine neoplasia type 1 and the Zollinger-Ellison syndrome. *N Engl J Med.* 1990;322:723–727.
54. Stabile BE, Morrow DJ, Passaro E. The gastrinoma triangle: operative implications. *Am J Surg.* 1984;147:25–31.
55. Norton JA. Neuroendocrine tumors of the pancreas and duodenum. *Curr Probl Surg.* 1994;31:77–156.
56. Pipeleers-Marichal M, Donow C, Heitz PU, Kloppel G. Pathologic aspects of gastrinomas in patients with Zollinger-Ellison syndrome with and without multiple endocrine neoplasia type I. *World J Surg.* 1993;17:481–488.
57. Bhagavan BS, Slavin RE, Goldberg J, Rao RN. Ectopic gastrinoma and Zollinger-Ellison syndrome. *Hum Pathol.* 1986;17:584–592.
58. Donow C, Pipeleers-Marichal M, Schroder S, Stamm B, Heitz PU, Kloppel G. Surgical pathology of gastrinoma: site, size, multicentricity, association with multiple endocrine neoplasia type 1, and malignancy. *Cancer.* 1991;68:1329–1334.
59. Norton JA, Fraker DL, Alexander HR, et al. Surgery to cure the Zollinger-Ellison syndrome. *N Engl J Med.* 1999;341: 635–644.
60. Weber HC, Venzon DJ, Lin JT, et al. Determinants of metastatic rate and survival in patients with Zollinger-Ellison syndrome: a prospective long-term study. *Gastroenterology.* 1995;108:1637–1649.
61. Cadiot G, Vuagnat A, Doukhan I, et al. Prognostic factors in patients with Zollinger-Ellison syndrome and multiple endocrine neoplasia type 1: Groupe d'Etude des Neoplasies Endocriniennes Multiples (GENEM and groupe de Recherche et d'Etude du Syndrome de Zollinger-Ellison (GRESZE). *Gastroenterology.* 1999;116:286–293.
62. Fraker DL, Norton JA, Alexander HR, Venzon DJ, Jensen RT. Surgery in Zollinger-Ellison syndrome alters the natural history of gastrinoma. *Ann Surg.* 1994;220:320–328; discussion 328–330.
63. Mignon M, Ruszniewski P, Podevin P, et al. Current approach to the management of gastrinoma and insulinoma in adults with multiple endocrine neoplasia type I. *World J Surg.* 1993;17:489–497.
64. Lowney JK, Frisella MM, Lairmore TC, Doherty GM. Pancreatic islet cell tumor metastasis in multiple endocrine neoplasia type 1: correlation with primary tumor size. *Surgery.* 1998;124:1043–1048; discussion 1048–1049.
65. Delcore R, Cheung LY, Friesen SR. Outcome of lymph node involvement in patients with the Zollinger-Ellison syndrome. *Ann Surg.* 1988;208:291–298.
66. Cox CE. Clinical relevance of serial sectioning of sentinel nodes and the detection of micrometastatic nodal disease in breast cancer. *Ann Surg Oncol.* 1998;5:297–298.
67. Jannink I, Fan M, Nagy S, Rayudu G, Dowlatshahi K. Serial sectioning of sentinel nodes in patients with breast cancer: a pilot study. *Ann Surg Oncol.* 1998;5:310–314.
68. Mies C, Schlesselman JJ. Detection of "occult" lymph node metastasis in breast cancer: should pathologists go the extra mile? *Adv Anat Pathol.* 2000;7:149–152.
69. Thompson NW. Surgical treatment of the endocrine pancreas and Zollinger-Ellison syndrome in the MEN 1 syndrome. *Henry Ford Hosp Med J.* 1992;40:195–198.
70. Malagelada JR, Edis AJ, Adson MA, van Heerden JA, Go VL. Medical and surgical options in the management of patients with gastrinoma. *Gastroenterology.* 1983;84:1524–1532.
71. Gibril F, Venzon DJ, Ojeaburu JV, Bashir S, Jensen RT. Prospective study of the natural history of gastrinoma in patients with MEN1: definition of an aggressive and a nonaggressive form. *J Clin Endocrinol Metab.* 2001;86:5282–5293.
72. Delcore R, Friesen SR. Gastrointestinal neuroendocrine tumors. *J Am Coll Surg.* 1994;178:187–211.
73. Rasbach DA, van Heerden JA, Telander RL, Grant CS, Carney JA. Surgical management of hyperinsulinism in the multiple endocrine neoplasia, type 1 syndrome. *Arch Surg.* 1985;120:584–589.
74. Demeure MJ, Klonoff DC, Karam JH, Duh QY, Clark OH. Insulinomas associated with multiple endocrine neoplasia type I: the need for a different surgical approach. *Surgery.* 1991;110:998–1004; discussion 1004–1005.
75. Lo CY, Lam KY, Fan ST. Surgical strategy for insulinomas in multiple endocrine neoplasia type I. *Am J Surg.* 1998;175: 305–307.
76. Skogseid B, Eriksson B, Lundqvist G, et al. Multiple endocrine neoplasia type 1: a 10-year prospective screening study in four kindreds. *J Clin Endocrinol Metab.* 1991;73:281–287.
77. Mignon M, Cadiot G. Diagnostic and therapeutic criteria in patients with Zollinger-Ellison syndrome and multiple endocrine neoplasia type 1. *J Intern Med.* 1998;243: 489–494.
78. Thakker RV. Multiple endocrine neoplasia type 1. *Endocrinol Metab Clin North Am.* 2000;29:541–567.
79. Boden G. Glucagonomas and insulinomas. *Gastroenterol Clin North Am.* 1989;18:831–845.
80. Smith SL, Branton SA, Avino AJ, et al. Vasoactive intestinal polypeptide secreting islet cell tumors: a 15-year experience and review of the literature. *Surgery.* 1998;124: 1050–1055.
81. Friesen SR. Tumors of the endocrine pancreas. *N Engl J Med.* 1982;306:580–590.
82. Orci L, Malaisse-Lagae F, Baetens D, Perrelet A. Pancreatic-polypeptide-rich regions in human pancreas. *Lancet.* 1978;2:1200–1201.
83. Kent RB III, van Heerden JA, Weiland LH. Nonfunctioning islet cell tumors. *Ann Surg.* 1981;193:185–190.
84. Dial PF, Braasch JW, Rossi RL, Lee AK, Jin GL. Management of nonfunctioning islet cell tumors of the pancreas. *Surg Clin North Am.* 1985;65:291–299.

85. Norton JA, Cornelius MJ, Doppman JL, Maton PN, Gardner JD, Jensen RT. Effect of parathyroidectomy in patients with hyperparathyroidism, Zollinger-Ellison syndrome, and multiple endocrine neoplasia type I: a prospective study. *Surgery.* 1987;102:958–966.
86. Sheppard BC, Norton JA, Doppman JL, Maton PN, Gardner JD, Jensen RT. Management of islet cell tumors in patients with multiple endocrine neoplasia: a prospective study. *Surgery.* 1989;106:1108–1117; discussion 1117–1118.
87. Burgess JR, David R, Parameswaran V, Greenaway TM, Shepherd JJ. The outcome of subtotal parathyroidectomy for the treatment of hyperparathyroidism in multiple endocrine neoplasia type 1. *Arch Surg.* 1998;133:126–129.
88. Skogseid B, Oberg K, Eriksson B, et al. Surgery for asymptomatic pancreatic lesion in multiple endocrine neoplasia type I. *World J Surg.* 1996;20:872–876; discussion 877.
89. Grama D, Skogseid B, Wilander E, et al. Pancreatic tumors in multiple endocrine neoplasia type 1: clinical presentation and surgical treatment. *World J Surg.* 1992;16:611–618; discussion 618–619.
90. Thompson NW. Current concepts in the surgical management of multiple endocrine neoplasia type 1 pancreatic-duodenal disease: results in the treatment of 40 patients with Zollinger-Ellison syndrome, hypoglycaemia or both. *J Intern Med.* 1998;243:495–500.
91. Thompson NW. Management of pancreatic endocrine tumors in patients with multiple endocrine neoplasia type 1. *Surg Oncol Clin North Am.* 1998;7:881–891.
92. Gauger PG, Thompson NW. Early surgical intervention and strategy in patients with multiple endocrine neoplasia type 1. *Best Pract Res Clin Endocrinol Metab.* 2001;15:213–223.
93. Lairmore TC, Chen VY, DeBenedetti MK, Gillanders WE, Norton JA, Doherty GM. Duodenopancreatic resections in patients with multiple endocrine neoplasia type 1. *Ann Surg.* 2000;231:909–918.
94. Norton JA, Doppman JL, Jensen RT. Curative resection in Zollinger-Ellison syndrome: results of a 10-year prospective study. *Ann Surg.* 1992;215:8–18.
95. Jensen RT. Management of the Zollinger-Ellison syndrome in patients with multiple endocrine neoplasia type 1. *J Intern Med.* 1998;243:477–488.
96. Fraker DL, Norton JA. The role of surgery in the management of islet cell tumors. *Gastroenterol Clin North Am.* 1989;18:805–830.
97. Mutch MG, Frisella MM, DeBenedetti MK, et al. Pancreatic polypeptide is a useful plasma marker for radiographically evident pancreatic islet cell tumors in patients with multiple endocrine neoplasia type 1. *Surgery.* 1997;122:1012–1019; discussion 1019–1020.
98. Doherty GM, Olson JA, Frisella MM, Lairmore TC, Wells SA, Jr, Norton JA. Lethality of multiple endocrine neoplasia type I. *World J Surg.* 1998;22:581–586; discussion 586–587.
99. Chanson P, Cadiot G, Murat A. Management of patients and subjects at risk for multiple endocrine neoplasia type 1: MEN 1: GENEM 1: Groupe d'Etude des Neoplasies Endocriniennes Multiples de type 1. *Horm Res.* 1997;47:211–220.
100. Skogseid B, Oberg K, Akerstrom G, et al. Limited tumor involvement found at multiple endocrine neoplasia type I pancreatic exploration: can it be predicted by preoperative tumor localization? *World J Surg.* 1998;22:673–677; discussion 667–678.
101. Clark OH, Ajani J, Benson AB III, et al. (2003, 01/14/04). NCCN Oncology Practice Guidelines v.1.2003 (Version 1.2003). National Comprehensive Cancer Network, Inc. Available: http://www.nccn.org/physician_gls/f_guidelines.html [2004, 02-3-2004].
102. Tisell LE, Ahlman H, Jansson S, Grimelius L. Total pancreatectomy in the MEN-1 syndrome. *Br J Surg.* 1988; 75:154–157.
103. Tisell LE, Ahlman H. Treatment of the pancreatic disease of multiple endocrine neoplasia type 1 (MEN 1). *Acta Oncol.* 1989;28:415–417.
104. Samaan NA, Ouais S, Ordonez NG, Choksi UA, Sellin RV, Hickey RC. Multiple endocrine syndrome type I: clinical, laboratory findings, and management in five families. *Cancer.* 1989;64:741–752.
105. Thakker RV. Multiple endocrine neoplasia: syndromes of the twentieth century. *J Clin Endocrinol Metab.* 1998;83: 2617–2620.
106. Veldhuis JD, Norton JA, Wells SA, Jr, Vinik AI, Perry RR. Surgical versus medical management of multiple endocrine neoplasia (MEN) type I. *J Clin Endocrinol Metab.* 1997; 82:357–364.
107. Eriksson BK. Systemic therapy for neuroendocrine tumors of the pancreas. In: Skogseid B, Doherty GM, eds. *Surgical Endocrinology.* Philadelphia: Lippincott Williams and Wilkins; 2001;1.
108. Eriksson BK, Larsson EG, Skogseid BM, Lofberg AM, Lorelius LE, Oberg KE. Liver embolizations of patients with malignant neuroendocrine gastrointestinal tumors. *Cancer.* 1998;83:2293–2301.
109. Pisegna JR, Slimak GG, Doppman JL, et al. An evaluation of human recombinant alpha interferon in patients with metastatic gastrinoma. *Gastroenterology.* 1993;105:1179–1183.
110. Arnold R, Trautmann ME, Creutzfeldt W, et al. Somatostatin analogue octreotide and inhibition of tumour growth in metastatic endocrine gastroenteropancreatic tumours. *Gut.* 1996;38:430–438.
111. Maton PN. The use of the long-acting somatostatin analogue, octreotide acetate, in patients with islet cell tumors. *Gastroenterol Clin North Am.* 1989;18:897–922.
112. Kvols LK, Buck M, Moertel CG, et al. Treatment of metastatic islet cell carcinoma with a somatostatin analogue (SMS 201-995). *Ann Intern Med.* 1987;107:162–168.
113. Burgess JR, Greenaway TM, Parameswaran V, Shepherd JJ. Octreotide improves biochemical, radiologic, and symptomatic indices of gastroenteropancreatic neoplasia in patients with multiple endocrine neoplasia type 1 (MEN-1): implications for an integrated model of MEN-1 tumorigenesis. *Cancer.* 1999;86:2154–2159.
114. Mozell EJ, Cramer AJ, O'Dorisio TM, Woltering EA. Long-term efficacy of octreotide in the treatment of Zollinger-Ellison syndrome. *Arch Surg.* 1992;127:1019–1024; discussion 1024–1026.

115. Shojamanesh H, Gibril F, Louie A, et al. Prospective study of the antitumor efficacy of long-term octreotide treatment in patients with progressive metastatic gastrinoma. *Cancer.* 2002;94:331–343.
116. Krenning EP, Kwekkeboom DJ, Oei HY, et al. Somatostatin-receptor scintigraphy in gastroenteropancreatic tumors: an overview of European results. *Ann N Y Acad Sci.* 1994;733:416–424.
117. Moertel CG, Lefkopoulo M, Lipsitz S, Hahn RG, Klaassen D. Streptozocin-doxorubicin, streptozocin-fluorouracil or chlorozotocin in the treatment of advanced islet-cell carcinoma. *N Engl J Med.* 1992;326:519–523.
118. Rivera E, Ajani JA. Doxorubicin, streptozocin, and 5-fluorouracil chemotherapy for patients with metastatic islet-cell carcinoma. *Am J Clin Oncol.* 1998;21:36–38.
119. Kouvaraki MA, Ajani JA, Hoff P, et al. Fluorouracil, Doxorubicin, and Streptozocin in the treatment of patients with locally advanced and metastatic pancreatic endocrine carcinomas. *J Clin Oncol.* 2004;22:in press.
120. Eriksson B, Oberg K. An update of the medical treatment of malignant endocrine pancreatic tumors. *Acta Oncol.* 1993;32:203–208.
121. Ackerman NB, Lien WM, Silverman NA. The blood supply of experimental liver metastases: 3: the effects of acute ligation of the hepatic artery or portal vein. *Surgery.* 1972;71:636–641.
122. Geerdink EA, Van der Luijt RB, Lips CJ. Do patients with multiple endocrine neoplasia syndrome type 1 benefit from periodical screening? *Eur J Endocrinol.* 2003;149: 577–582.
123. Duh QY, Hybarger CP, Geist R, et al. Carcinoids associated with multiple endocrine neoplasia syndromes. *Am J Surg.* 1987;154:142–148.
124. Manes JL, Taylor HB. Thymic carcinoid in familial multiple endocrine adenomatosis. *Arch Pathol.* 1973;95:252–255.
125. Gibril F, Chen YJ, Schrump DS, et al. Prospective study of thymic carcinoids in patients with multiple endocrine neoplasia type 1. *J Clin Endocrinol Metab.* 2003;88: 1066–1081.
126. Caplin ME, Buscombe JR, Hilson AJ, Jones AL, Watkinson AF, Burroughs AK. Carcinoid tumour. *Lancet.* 1998;352: 799–805.
127. Wilkinson S, Teh BT, Davey KR, McArdle JP, Young M, Shepherd JJ. Cause of death in multiple endocrine neoplasia type 1. *Arch Surg.* 1993;128:683–690.
128. Bordi C, D'Adda T, Azzoni C, Pilato FP, Caruana P. Hypergastrinemia and gastric enterochromaffin-like cells. *Am J Surg Pathol.* 1995;19(Suppl 1):S8–S19.
129. Lehy T, Cadiot G, Mignon M, Ruszniewski P, Bonfils S. Influence of multiple endocrine neoplasia type 1 on gastric endocrine cells in patients with the Zollinger-Ellison syndrome. *Gut.* 1992;33:1275–1279.
130. Peghini PL, Annibale B, Azzoni C, et al. Effect of chronic hypergastrinemia on human enterochromaffin-like cells: insights from patients with sporadic gastrinomas. *Gastroenterology.* 2002;123:68–85.
131. Tang LH, Modlin IM, Lawton GP, Kidd M, Chinery R. The role of transforming growth factor alpha in the enterochromaffin-like cell tumor autonomy in an African rodent mastomys. *Gastroenterology.* 1996;111:1212–1223.
132. Tang LH, Luque EA, Efstathiou JA, et al. Gastrin receptor expression and function during rapid transformation of the enterochromaffin-like cells in an African rodent. *Regul Pept.* 1997;72:9–18.
133. Hakanson R, Sundler F. Trophic effects of gastrin. *Scand J Gastroenterol Suppl.* 1991;180:130–136.
134. Hakanson R, Sundler F. Histamine-producing cells in the stomach and their role in the regulation of acid secretion. *Scand J Gastroenterol Suppl.* 1991;180:88–94.
135. Rindi G, Bordi C, Rappel S, La Rosa S, Stolte M, Solcia E. Gastric carcinoids and neuroendocrine carcinomas: pathogenesis, pathology, and behavior. *World J Surg.* 1996;20: 168–172.
136. Rindi G, Luinetti O, Cornaggia M, Capella C, Solcia E. Three subtypes of gastric argyrophil carcinoid and the gastric neuroendocrine carcinoma: a clinicopathologic study. *Gastroenterology.* 1993;104:994–1006.
137. Solcia E, Capella C, Fiocca R, Rindi G, Rosai J. Gastric argyrophil carcinoidosis in patients with Zollinger-Ellison syndrome due to type 1 multiple endocrine neoplasia: a newly recognized association. *Am J Surg Pathol.* 1990; 14:503–513.
138. Modlin IM. Gastric carcinoid tumors. In: Skogseid DA, ed. *Surgical Endocrinology.* Philadelphia: Lippincott Williams and Wilkins; 2000;1:441–446.
139. Gibril F, Reynolds JC, Lubensky IA, et al. Ability of somatostatin receptor scintigraphy to identify patients with gastric carcinoids: a prospective study. *J Nucl Med.* 2000;41:1646–1656.
140. Borch K, Renvall H, Kullman E, Wilander E. Gastric carcinoid associated with the syndrome of hypergastrinemic atrophic gastritis: a prospective analysis of 11 cases. *Am J Surg Pathol.* 1987;11:435–444.
141. Gilligan CJ, Lawton GP, Tang LH, West AB, Modlin IM. Gastric carcinoid tumors: the biology and therapy of an enigmatic and controversial lesion. *Am J Gastroenterol.* 1995;90:338–352.
142. Tomassetti P, Salomone T, Migliori M, Campana D, Corinaldesi R. Optimal treatment of Zollinger-Ellison syndrome and related conditions in elderly patients. *Drugs Aging.* 2003;20:1019–1034.
143. Bordi C, Corleto VD, Azzoni C, et al. The antral mucosa as a new site for endocrine tumors in multiple endocrine neoplasia type 1 and Zollinger-Ellison syndromes. *J Clin Endocrinol Metab.* 2001;86:2236–2242.
144. Tomassetti P, Migliori M, Caletti GC, Fusaroli P, Corinaldesi R, Gullo L. Treatment of type II gastric carcinoid tumors with somatostatin analogues. *N Engl J Med.* 2000;343:551–554.
145. Ruszniewski P, Laucournet H, Elouaer-Blanc L, Mignon M, Bonfils S. Long-acting somatostatin (SMS 201-995) in the management of Zollinger-Ellison syndrome: evidence for sustained efficacy. *Pancreas.* 1988;3:145–152.
146. Ferraro G, Annibale B, Marignani M, et al. Effectiveness of octreotide in controlling fasting hypergastrinemia and related enterochromaffin-like cell growth. *J Clin Endocrinol Metab.* 1996;81:677–683.

147. Dean PG, van Heerden JA, Farley DR, et al. Are patients with multiple endocrine neoplasia type I prone to premature death? *World J Surg.* 2000;24:1437–1441.
148. Deftos LJ. Chromogranin A: its role in endocrine function and as an endocrine and neuroendocrine tumor marker. *Endocr Rev.* 1991;12:181–187.
149. Nobels FR, Kwekkeboom DJ, Coopmans W, et al. Chromogranin A as serum marker for neuroendocrine neoplasia: comparison with neuron-specific enolase and the alpha-subunit of glycoprotein hormones. *J Clin Endocrinol Metab.* 1997;82:2622–2628.
150. Goebel SU, Serrano J, Yu F, Gibril F, Venzon DJ, Jensen RT. Prospective study of the value of serum chromogranin A or serum gastrin levels in the assessment of the presence, extent, or growth of gastrinomas. *Cancer.* 1999;85:1470–1483.
151. Granberg D, Stridsberg M, Seensalu R, et al. Plasma chromogranin A in patients with multiple endocrine neoplasia type 1. *J Clin Endocrinol Metab.* 1999;84:2712–2717.
152. Bernini GP, Moretti A, Ferdeghini M, et al. A new human chromogranin 'A' immunoradiometric assay for the diagnosis of neuroendocrine tumours. *Br J Cancer.* 2001;84: 636–642.
153. Peracchi M, Conte D, Gebbia C, et al. Plasma chromogranin A in patients with sporadic gastro-entero-pancreatic neuroendocrine tumors or multiple endocrine neoplasia type 1. *Eur J Endocrinol.* 2003;148:39–43.
154. Stabile BE, Braunstein GD, Passaro E, Jr. Serum gastrin and human chorionic gonadotropin in the Zollinger-Ellison syndrome. *Arch Surg.* 1980;115:1090–1095.
155. Skogseid B, Doherty GM. Multiple endocrine neoplasia type 1: clinical and genetic features. *Ital J Gastroenterol Hepatol.* 1999;31(Suppl 2):S131–S134.
156. Friesen SR, Tomita T, Kimmel JR. Pancreatic polypeptide update: its roles in detection of the trait for multiple endocrine adenopathy syndrome, type I and pancreatic polypeptide-secreting tumors. *Surgery.* 1983;94:1028–1037.
157. Floyd JC Jr, Fajans SS, Pek S, Chance RE. A newly recognized pancreatic polypeptide; plasma levels in health and disease. *Recent Prog Horm Res.* 1976;33:519–570.
158. Berger D, Crowther RC, Floyd JC, Jr, Pek S, Fajans SS. Effect of age on fasting plasma levels of pancreatic hormones in man. *J Clin Endocrinol Metab.* 1978;47:1183–1189.
159. Strodel WE, Vinik AI, Eckhauser FE, Thompson NW. Hyperparathyroidism and gastroenteropancreatic hormone levels. *Surgery.* 1985;98:1101–1106.
160. Thompson NW, Czako PF, Fritts LL, et al. Role of endoscopic ultrasonography in the localization of insulinomas and gastrinomas. *Surgery.* 1994;116:1131–1138.
161. Gauger PG, Scheiman JM, Wamsteker EJ, Richards ML, Doherty GM, Thompson NW. Role of endoscopic ultrasonography in screening and treatment of pancreatic endocrine tumours in asymptomatic patients with multiple endocrine neoplasia type 1. *Br J Surg.* 2003;90: 748–754.
162. Doherty GM, Thompson NW. Multiple endocrine neoplasia type 1: duodenopancreatic tumours. *J Intern Med.* 2003;253:590–598.
163. Hai N, Kosugi S. Gene diagnosis and clinical management of multiple endocrine neoplasia type 1 (MEN1). *Biomed Pharmacother.* 2000;54(Suppl 1):47s–51s.
164. Karges W, Schaaf L, Dralle H, Boehm BO. Concepts for screening and diagnostic follow-up in multiple endocrine neoplasia type 1 (MEN1). *Exp Clin Endocrinol Diabetes.* 2000;108:334–340.
165. Meko JB, Doherty GM, Siegel BA, Norton JA. Evaluation of somatostatin-receptor scintigraphy for detecting neuroendocrine tumors. *Surgery.* 1996;120:975–983; discussion 983–984.
166. Lips CJ, Koppeschaar HP, Berends MJ, Jansen-Schillhorn van Veen JM, Struyvenberg A, Van Vroonhoven TJ. The importance of screening for the MEN 1 syndrome: diagnostic results and clinical management. *Henry Ford Hosp Med J.* 1992;40:171–172.
167. Skogseid B, Oberg K. Prospective screening in multiple endocrine neoplasia type 1. *Henry Ford Hosp Med J.* 1992; 40:167–170.
168. Skogseid B, Rastad J, Oberg K. Multiple endocrine neoplasia type 1: clinical features and screening. *Endocrinol Metab Clin North Am.* 1994;23:1–18.
169. van Heerden JA, Smith SL, Miller LJ. Management of the Zollinger-Ellison syndrome in patients with multiple endocrine neoplasia type I. *Surgery.* 1986;100:971–977.
170. Thompson NW, Bondeson AG, Bondeson L, Vinik A. The surgical treatment of gastrinoma in MEN I syndrome patients. *Surgery.* 1989;106:1081–1085; discussion 1085–1086.
171. Cherner JA, Sawyers JL. Benefit of resection of metastatic gastrinoma in multiple endocrine neoplasia type I. *Gastroenterology.* 1992;102:1049–1053.
172. Thompson NW, Pasieka J, Fukuuchi A. Duodenal gastrinomas, duodenotomy, and duodenal exploration in the surgical management of Zollinger-Ellison syndrome. *World J Surg.* 1993;17:455–462.
173. Melvin WS, Johnson JA, Sparks J, Innes JT, Ellison EC. Long-term prognosis of Zollinger-Ellison syndrome in multiple endocrine neoplasia. *Surgery.* 1993;114:1183–1188.
174. O'Riordain DS, O'Brien T, van Heerden JA, Service FJ, Grant CS. Surgical management of insulinoma associated with multiple endocrine neoplasia type I. *World J Surg.* 1994;18:488–493; discussion 493–494.
175. Skogseid B, Oberg K. Experience with multiple endocrine neoplasia type 1 screening. *J Intern Med.* 1995;238:255–261.

CHAPTER

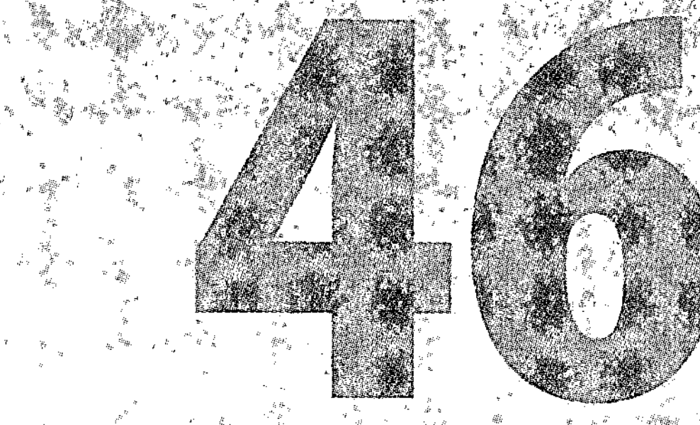

The von Hippel–Lindau Syndrome

Eric Jonasch, MD

The von Hippel–Lindau (VHL) syndrome is a pleiotropic syndrome that most commonly produces retinal, cerebellar, spinal, adrenal, renal, and pancreatic lesions. The incidence has been estimated to be between 1in 35,000 and 1 in 40,000.[1,2] With the discovery of the *VHL* gene in 1993,[3] the advent of genetic testing for VHL, and improved imaging techniques, early detection and management of the lesions associated with VHL are now possible. These advances have resulted in improved survival and quality of life for many individuals and families living with this disease. Nonetheless, many challenges still face both the patient and the treating physician.

A summary of the lesions attributed to VHL and their location can be found in Table 46.1. In terms of morbidity, the most serious lesions are the hemangioblastomas and retinal angiomata, with loss of vision and loss of neurologic function still possible, despite the most up-to-date treatments. From a mortality standpoint, renal cell carcinomas and pancreatic neuroendocrine tumors (NETs) are true cancers and can result in dissemination and death.

At least three distinct phenotypes have been defined for VHL. Table 46.2 outlines the classification developed by the National Cancer Institute.[4] The major difference is the absence of pheochromocytomas in the type 1 category. Type 1 VHL is usually associated with large deletions of the *VHL* gene, whereas type 2 syndromes are associated with nonsense, missense, and frameshift mutations.[1]

Eighty percent of VHL cases have a familial origin, and the remaining 20% are likely de novo mutations.[5] In 1964, before the era of genetic testing, Melmon and Rosen[6] proposed a set of clinical diagnostic criteria for VHL.[7] If a family history of retinal or central nervous system hemangioblastoma was present, only one hemangioblastoma or visceral lesion (renal tumors, pancreatic cysts or tumors, pheochromocytoma, papillary cystadenomas of the epididymis) was necessary for a diagnosis of VHL disease to be made. If no family history was present, two or more hemangioblastomas or one hemangioblastoma and a visceral manifestation were required for diagnosis. Although still very useful, this classification is now complementary to genetic testing, which should be performed if possible in patients with suspected VHL.

History

The first description of pancreatic involvement in VHL was published in 1884, when Pye-Smith[8] reported on a case of a patient with cystic disease of the cerebellum in combination with cysts of the pancreas.

Table 46.1 Frequency of Lesions and Age at Onset of von Hippel-Lindau Disease Lesions

Mean (range) Age	Frequency of Onset (years)	Patients (%)
Central nervous system		
Retinal hemangioblastomas	25 (1–67)	25–60
Endolymphatic sac tumors	22 (12–50)	10
Craniospinal hemangioblastomas		
Cerebellum	33 (9–78)	44–72
Brainstem	32 (12–46)	10–25
Spinal cord	33 (12–66)	13–50
Lumbosacral nerve roots	Unknown	<1
Supratentorial	Unknown	<1
Visceral		
Renal cell carcinoma or cysts	39 (16–67)	25–60
Pheochromocytomas	30 (5–58)	10–20
Pancreatic tumor or cyst	36 (5–70)	35–70
Epididymal cystadenoma	Unknown	25–60
Broad-ligament cystadenoma	Unknown (16–46)	Unknown

See references

Table 46.2 Genotype-Phenotype Classification in Families with von Hippel-Lindau Disease*

	Clinical Characteristics
Type 1	Retinal hemangioblastomas CNS hemangioblastomas Renal cell carcinoma Pancreatic neoplasms and cysts
Type 2A	Pheochromocytomas Retinal hemangioblastomas CNS hemangioblastomas
Type 2B	Pheochromocytomas Retinal hemangioblastomas CNS hemangioblastomas Renal cell carcinoma Pancreatic neoplasms and cysts
Type 2C	Pheochromocytomas only

*Endolymphatic sac tumors and cystadenomas of the epididymis and broad ligament have been assigned specific von Hippel–Lindau types.
Abbreviation: CNS, central nervous system.

The German ophthalmologist Eugen von Hippel, who published the first full description of the retinal vascular abnormality in 1904,[9] based his initial work on the observations of two patients: Otto Mayer and Otto Mobius.[6] On Mr. Mayer's demise in 1921, an autopsy was performed that revealed, among other things, pancreatic cysts.[10] One year later, Berblinger[11] published postmortem findings on another case of angiomatosis retinae with a brain tumor and pancreatic cysts.[6] The pathologist Arvid Lindau published a paper in 1926 describing 40 cases with cystic cerebellar tumors and associated these cases with the presence of cysts of the kidneys, pancreas, and epididymis.[9] Sixteen of the cases described by Lindau were drawn from his own practice, and of these, eight had pancreatic cysts.[6]

Cystadenomas, also referred to as microcystic adenomas, were initially reported in 1931 by Knodel[12] and in 1934 by Hughes[13]. Pancreatic hemangioblastomas were reported in 1947 by Bockhoven and Levatin[14] and in 1959 by Bird and Mendelow.[15]

In 1965, Melmon and Rosen[6] published an article in which they coined the term "von Hippel–Lindau" to describe the constellation of central nervous system and visceral lesions documented in the familial syndrome.[7] In their publication, they described the presence of pancreatic cysts and cystadenomas but did not describe the presence of pancreatic NETs in this patient population.[6] In 1968, Legre et al.[16] published an article describing a patient with clinical VHL who had an insulinoma in the head of the pancreas. Numerous case reports describing NETs in patients with VHL were published afterward.[17-23] In 1988, Jennings and Gaines[24] formally proposed that NETs be included as part of the VHL syndrome.

Very few cases of pancreatic adenocarcinoma and pancreatic renal cell carcinoma metastases in VHL patients have been published.[25,26] It is not clear whether the incidence of primary pancreatic adenocarcinoma is any higher in patients with VHL than in the general population, and genetically, these patients do not possess the *VHL* mutation.[25]

Incidence

Pancreatic manifestations of VHL occur between 0 to greater than 90% of the time within cohorts of patients with VHL (Table 46.3), with a fairly wide variation among families. Pancreatic lesions can be the only abdominal manifestation in a subset of patients[27] and can precede any other manifestation.

Cysts, serous cystadenomas, and NETs are clearly associated with VHL. Rare cases of adenocarcinoma and metastases from renal cell carcinoma have also been seen in this population.

Table 46.3 Pancreatic Manifestations of von Hippel–Lindau Syndrome

Manifestation Type	Frequency	Treatment
Cysts	0%–93%	Observation/cyst aspiration if symptomatic
Serous cystadenoma	Uncommon	Observation
Neuroendocrine tumor	5%–17%	Resection
Renal cell carcinoma metastasis	Extremely rare	Consider resection
Hemangioblastoma	Rare	Observation: resection if growth or symptoms occur
Adenocarcinoma	Rare: unclear association	Resection

Cysts and serous cystadenomas are the most common pancreatic lesions in VHL. These are found in anywhere from 0% to nearly 100% of patients with VHL (Table 46.4), depending on the cohort being analyzed.[27,28] Although they are not malignant themselves, they can grow to a substantial size and compress adjacent normal pancreatic parenchyma. This can result in endocrine and exocrine insufficiency, closure of bile ducts,[29] and compression of adjacent small intestine.[6,7,30]

NETs are somewhat less common but potentially lethal manifestations of VHL, occurring in 5%–17% of patients with VHL,[29-31,34] and may occur in the presence or absence of pancreatic cystic disease.[7,23,31-33] NETs are characteristically solid and are generally smaller than cysts and cystadenomas. NETs are frequently nonfunctional,[7,30,34] although a few case reports exist in the literature describing hormonal secretion by pancreatic NETs.[20,23]

In a recent report, Libutti et al.[30] screened a series of 256 patients with VHL for pancreatic lesions. A total of 30 solid masses were found in 30 (12%) of the patient population. Of the 18 patients with pathological material available, 17 had NETs.[30] These tumors possess the ability to metastasize, in particular when they reach sizes in excess of 3 cm. Of the 30 patients described, four had confirmed metastatic disease. There is an association between neuroendocrine pancreatic tumors and pheochromocytomas, another common manifestation in patients with VHL, which leads to interesting questions on the nature of the VHL mutation necessary to generate the specific phenotypic manifestations of the disease.[22,24,30,34]

Pancreatic metastases from renal cell carcinoma are an extremely rare manifestation in patients with VHL, with only one case report in the literature.[26] In cases of

Table 46.4 Cohorts of Patients with von Hippel–Lindau Syndrome

Reference	Patients	Pancreas Involvement	Cysts	Cystadenomas	NET
Hammel et al.[51]	158	122	112 (70.9)	15 (9.5)	15 (9.5)
Hough et al.[27]	52	29	21	2	6
Neumann et al.[28]	66	11	8	2	1
Lamiell et al.[38]	43	16	13	Not available	5
Green et al.[52]	38	2	2	Not available	0
Horton et al.[18]	29*	23	21	Not available	2
Cheng et al.[29]	11	10	7	2	1

Abbreviation: NET, neuroendocrine tumor.
*Cases evaluated at autopsy.

pancreatic metastases in the context of sporadic renal cell carcinomas, the prognosis appears to be better than with metastases to other organ sites, and surgery can play an important role in the management of this situation.[35-37]

Lamiell et al.[38] reported on two cases of pancreatic adenocarcinomas in their cohort of patients with VHL, and a few other case reports exist in the literature.[39]

Pathology and Genetics

Little is known about what drives the generation of specific lesion subtypes in VHL. The pancreas replicates the neuroendocrine and cystic lesions seen in other organs but fails to demonstrate the hemangioblastomas so commonly occurring in the central nervous system. The following section outlines the histologic information available on the major pancreatic lesions in patients with VHL, followed by the available genetic information. As more detailed analyses are published, improved genotype-phenotype correlations may become possible, ultimately leading to a precise understanding of the pathogenesis of these lesions.

Histology

Cysts Cysts are composed of epithelium-lined collections of serous fluid and range in size from a few millimeters to more than 10 cm.[7] They are found throughout the pancreas and are often multiple.[32]

Serous cystadenomas Serous cystadenomas, also referred to as *microcystic adenomas*, are grapelike clusters of multiple microscopic and macroscopic (2 mm–2 cm in diameter) cysts separated by thickened walls of stroma.[7,27] They are often arranged in a stellate pattern with a central nidus, which may be calcified or scarlike.[7,28,40] The cysts are lined with cubic epithelial cells, which are rich in glycogen but are not mucus secreting.[32] An analysis by Mohr et al.[41] demonstrated occasional entrapped islets of Langerhans within the fibrous stroma. Light microscopy revealed a predominant population of bland, cuboidal, and flattened serous epithelial cells with clear and/or amphophilic cytoplasm. A secondary population of numerous endothelial cells forming capillaries and closely intermixed with epithelial cells was consistently seen on hematoxylin and eosin stains in all benign cysts, microscopic serous cystadenomas, and macroscopic serous cystadenomas. Nuclear atypia, mitoses, and necrosis were absent in all lesions. The cells were strongly positive for cytokeratins AE1/AE3 and MAK 6 and rich in intracytoplasmic glycogen on periodic acid–Schiff and periodic acid–Schiff after diastase digestion. Immunohistochemistry revealed a third cell type in all lesions: a smooth muscle cell, which was strongly positive for vimentin and smooth muscle actin.

Neuroendocrine tumors Lubensky et al. provided a detailed histologic and genetic analysis of NETs in pancreatic lesions from patients with VHL.[25] Morphologically, the tumors were characterized by solid, trabecular and/or glandular architecture and prominent stromal collagen bands. Sixty percent of tumors revealed at least focally clear-cell cytology. All tumors were positive for panendocrine immunohistochemical markers (chromogranin A or synaptophysin); 35% of tumors demonstrated focal positivity for pancreatic polypeptide, somatostatin, insulin and/or glucagons. In addition, a lack of immunostaining for pancreatic and gastrointestinal hormones was observed in 65% of tumors. Dense core neurosecretory granules were evident by electron microscopic evaluation, and the clear cells demonstrated abundant intracytoplasmic lipid.

Genetic Correlation

In VHL patients, 15%–20% of patients have large germline deletions, 27% have missense mutations, 27% have nonsense or frameshift mutations, and the remainder have no deletion or mutation detected. Presence of pheochromocytoma is usually associated with a nonsense, missense, or frameshift mutation.

Pancreatic cystic lesions and NETs have been shown to possess the *VHL* gene mutation. In the publication by Mohr et al.,[41] DNA samples from 27 microdissected benign cysts and serous cystadenomas from three patients with known germline mutations were found to have loss of heterozygosity at the *VHL* locus in 24 of 27 cases.[41] In the analysis of NETs from Lubensky et al.,[25] six cases of NET and one case of adenocarcinoma were subjected to genetic analysis. All NET cases showed allelic loss of the second copy of the *VHL* gene, and in the one case in which both NET and adenocarcinoma were present, the adenocarcinoma was negative for loss of heterozygosity at the *VHL* locus, whereas the NET was positive. This finding casts further doubt on the likelihood that pancreatic adenocarcinoma arises as a direct consequence of VHL in this patient population.

VHL mutations are not involved in the generation of sporadic or multiple endocrine neoplasia–associated NETs. Hessman et al.[42] demonstrated that 3p mutations along with 11q13 and 18q mutations were common in both sporadic and multiple endocrine neoplasia–associated pancreatic NETs, and the 3p mutations were associated with a more aggressive phenotype. On closer analysis of the 3p locus, Chung et al.[43] determined that patients with sporadic pancreatic NETs lacked a *VHL* mutation, although an allelic loss occurred at 3p25, centromeric to the VHL locus, in 33% of 43 patients studied.

The association between pancreatic manifestations of VHL and specific genetic mutations was evaluated by Hes et al.[44] The presence of pancreatic cysts was associated with deletions within the *VHL* gene. In these 35 patients, there were no cases of pheochromocytoma, supporting the finding that type I phenotypes are associated with gene deletions. Pheochromocytomas and NETs are commonly found in the same patients.[24,30,34] For example, in a study by Marcos et al.,[45] 10 patients of 25 (40%) with NETs were also diagnosed with pheochromocytomas. Nonetheless, cases of both pancreatic cysts and pheochromocytoma occurring within the same patient exist, underscoring the complexity of the genotype-phenotype relationship.

Clinical Management

Signs, Symptoms, and Physical Examination

Cysts and cystadenomas Most patients with VHL are asymptomatic from cysts and cystadenomas. However, because of the mass effect of enlarging cystic lesions, patients may experience abdominal pain, early satiety, obstructive jaundice,[40] intestinal obstruction, pancreatitis,[29,46,47] or symptoms of exocrine or endocrine pancreatic insufficiency.[6,7,27,48] In rare instances, a mass may be palpable on physical examination.[6,49]

NETs Primary NETs are usually clinically silent as well, unless locally advanced disease or dissemination occurs. Generally, NETs do not secrete bioactive substances, although case reports of endocrinopathies caused by pancreatic NETs exist. Vasoactive intestinal polypeptide, calcitonin,[23] insulin, glucagon, gastrin, and somatostatin[20] have been reported.

Imaging Manifestations

In 1964, Melmon and Rosen[6] recommended regular roentgenographic evaluation of the kidneys with angiography in patients with the diagnosis of VHL to screen for clinically silent renal cell carcinomas. However, not until the advent of high-quality computed tomography (CT) and ultrasound imaging did it became practical to evaluate the pancreas.

For cystic lesions, the available imaging techniques have been reported to have comparable diagnostic value.[7,9,31] Neumann et al.[28] advocated for the use of ultrasound for the screening of pancreatic lesions because of its lower cost and potential morbidity (dye load, radiation) when compared with CT scans. On CT, cyst walls enhance poorly, if at all. Calcifications are common throughout the pancreas.[7] Serous cystadenomas are suggested by a focal enlargement of the pancreas composed of small cysts, radially aligned with a central calcified scar.[7]

Because of their smaller size and makeup, NETs are harder to detect on ultrasound. On CT, they generally produce intense enhancement and may contain calcification.[7] As the tumor enlarges, areas of necrosis may appear. Because of their potential for metastatic spread when they are larger than 3 cm, it is important that these lesions are detected early. Marcos et al.[45] reported on the radiographic characteristics of 29 pathologically defined NETs from 25 patients with VHL. Eighteen of the tumors were less than 3 cm and enhanced homogeneously on CT. Of the remaining 11 larger tumors, an increased incidence of heterogeneous enhancement was observed, and necrosis was present in three lesions. Two of the 11 also manifested hepatic metastases.

The most recent National Cancer Institute screening guidelines[4] recommend a combination of ultrasound, CT, and magnetic resonance imaging. Table 46.5 summarizes these recommendations.

Diagnostic Procedures

For most patients with cystic disease, no further diagnostic procedures are necessary, because of the absence of malignant potential for these lesions. For all solid

Table 46.5 Recommended Intervals for Screening in At-Risk Individuals

Test	Start Age (frequency)
Ophthalmoscopy	Infancy (yearly)
Plasma or 24-hr urinary catecholamines and metanephrines	2 years of age (yearly and when blood pressure is raised)
MRI of craniospinal axis[a]	11 years of age (yearly)
CT and MRI of internal auditory canals[a]	Onset of symptoms (hearing loss, tinnitus, vertigo, or unexplained difficulties of balance)
Ultrasound of abdomen	8 years of age (yearly; MRI as clinically indicated)
CT of abdomen[a]	18 years of age or earlier if clinically indicated (yearly)
Audiologic function tests	When clinically indicated

[a]Imaging that are generally recommended before and after contrast infusion.
Abbreviations: CT, computed tomography; MRI, magnetic resonance imaging.

lesions, a tissue diagnosis should be obtained either in a diagnostic or a therapeutic maneuver. If a biopsy fails to provide diagnostic material, repeat biopsy or laparotomy may be necessary, because of the possible dissemination of these lesions.

Serum and urine tests potentially provide data aiding in the detection of NETs, but because of the low incidence of functional tumors, they are neither sensitive nor specific enough for routine use.

Management

Cysts In the report by Melmon and Rosen[6] in 1964, the authors stated that "the cystic lesions of the pancreas and kidney should be left alone." Although this may be sound advice for most cases, some patients experience substantial and serious morbidity from the compressive effects of the cysts. Choyke et al.[7] described the percutaneous drainage of cysts and the instillation of hypertonic saline to prevent reaccumulation. In addition, stent placement may sometimes be necessary,[38,40,46,50] as may be the replacement of pancreatic enzymes in cases of exocrine pancreatic insufficiency.

Neuroendocrine tumors Because of the high probability of malignant disease, all solid pancreatic lesions need to monitored very closely and generally require surgical resection if they are larger than 3 cm. If the lesions are smaller than 1 cm, biopsy is a reasonable first step. Lesions smaller than 1 cm can be monitored with imaging every 6–12 months initially, and every 12 months thereafter once growth kinetics have been established. For lesions between 1 and 3 cm, a case-by-case assessment is advised.[31]

Once NETs metastasize, there are no satisfactory treatments. Various chemotherapies have been tried with little success. Local ablative techniques, including radiofrequency ablation, may be tried but do not ultimately provide curative therapy.

Conclusion

Despite defining the causative genetic lesion, VHL remains a puzzle and a challenge for both patients and physicians. The multiple pancreatic manifestations are an example of the complex changes that occur with this mutation.

Fortunately, as we are armed with a better understanding of the natural history of the various lesions, the advent of genetic testing, and good imaging technology, the morbidity and mortality of the pancreatic manifestations of VHL have decreased. Early detection of NETs and appropriate surgical intervention can effectively prevent dissemination and death. Nevertheless, no preventive systemic therapies are available, nor do effective therapies exist to deal with metastatic NETs once they develop. In addition, the histologically benign cystic pancreatic manifestations of VHL themselves can decrease quality of life.

The combination of an improved molecular understanding of VHL coupled with the expanding availability of targeted molecules may change the treatment of VHL in the next few years and improve both the quality and the quantity of life enjoyed by individuals with this disease.

References

1. Neumann HP, Wiestler OD. Clustering of features of von Hippel-Lindau syndrome: evidence for a complex genetic locus. *Lancet*. 1991;337:1052–1054.
2. Maher ER, Iselius L, Yates JR, Littler M, Benjamin C, Harris R, et al. von Hippel-Lindau disease: a genetic study. *J Med Genet*. 1991;28:443–447.
3. Latif F, Tory K, Gnarra J, et al. Identification of the von Hippel-Lindau disease tumor suppressor gene. *Science*. 1993;260:1317–1320.
4. Lonser RR, Glenn GM, Walther M, et al. von Hippel-Lindau disease. *Lancet*. 2003;361:2059–2067.
5. Sgambati MT, Stolle C, Choyke PL, et al. Mosaicism in von Hippel-Lindau disease: lessons from kindreds with germline mutations identified in offspring with mosaic parents. *Am J Hum Genet*. 2000;66:84–91.
6. Melmon KL, Rosen SW. Lindau's Disease. Review of the literature and study of a large kindred. *Am J Med*. 1964;36:595–617.
7. Choyke PL, Glenn GM, Walther MM, Patronas NJ, Linehan WM, Zbar B. von Hippel-Lindau disease: genetic, clinical, and imaging features. *Radiology*. 1995;194:629–642.
8. Pye-Smith PH. Cyst of the cerebellum with numerous small cysts in the pancreas and the kidneys. *Trans R Pathol Soc*. 1884;36:17–21.
9. Hes FJ, Feldberg MA. von Hippel-Lindau disease: strategies in early detection (renal-, adrenal-, pancreatic masses). *Eur Radiol*. 1999;9:598–610.
10. Brandt R. Zur Frage der Angiomatosis retinae. *Arch Ophthal*. 1921;106:127.
11. Berblinger W. Zur auffassung von der sogenannten v. Hippelschen Krankheit der Netzhaut (Capillaeres Haemangiom im verlaengerten Mark). *Arch Ophthal*. 1922;110:395.
12. Knodel G. Zur Kenntnisder v. Hippelschen Erkrankung (Angiomatosis retinae). *Virchows Arch Pathol Anat*. 1931;281:886.
13. Hughes RF. A case of Lindau's disease. *CMAJ*. 1934;31:537.
14. Bockhoven S, Levatin P. Treatment of Lindau's disease: report of a case. *Arch Ophthalmol*. 1947;38:461.
15. Bird AV, Mendelow H. Lindau's disease in a South African family: a report on 3 further cases. *Br J Surg*. 1959;47:173.
16. Legre PJ, Giuen CI, Clement JP, Pietri H. Maladie de von Hippel-Lindau, cancer de la tete du pancreas adenome Langerhansien hypoglyemient. *Presse Med*. 1968;40:1911–1914.

17. Hardwig P, Robertson DM. von Hippel-Lindau disease: a familial, often lethal, multi-system phakomatosis. *Ophthalmology*. 1984;91:263–270.
18. Horton WA, Wong V, Eldridge R. von Hippel-Lindau disease: clinical and pathological manifestations in nine families with 50 affected members. *Arch Intern Med*. 1976;136:769–777.
19. Andersson A, Bergdahl L. Insulomas and multiple endocrine neoplasia. *Acta Chir Scand*. 1976;142:297–300.
20. Probst A, Lotz M, Heitz P. von Hippel-Lindau's disease, syringomyelia and multiple endocrine tumors: a complex neuroendocrinopathy. *Virchows Arch A Pathol Anat Histol*. 1978;378:265–272.
21. Hull MT, Warfel KA, Muller J, Higgins JT. Familial islet cell tumors in Von Hippel-Lindau's disease. *Cancer*. 1979;44:1523–1526.
22. Mulshine JL, Tubbs R, Sheeler LR, Gifford RW, Jr. Clinical significance of the association of the von Hippel-Lindau disease with pheochromocytoma and pancreatic apudoma. *Am J Med Sci*. 1984;288:212–216.
23. Cornish D, Pont A, Minor D, Coombs JL, Bennington J. Metastatic islet cell tumor in von Hippel-Lindau disease. *Am J Med*. 1984;77:147–150.
24. Jennings CM, Gaines PA. The abdominal manifestation of von Hippel-Lindau disease and a radiological screening protocol for an affected family. *Clin Radiol*. 1988;39:363–367.
25. Lubensky IA, Pack S, Ault D, et al. Multiple neuroendocrine tumors of the pancreas in von Hippel-Lindau disease patients: histopathological and molecular genetic analysis. *Am J Pathol*. 1998;153:223–231.
26. Chambers TP, Fishman EK, Hruban RH. Pancreatic metastases from renal cell carcinoma in von Hippel-Lindau disease. *Clin Imaging*. 1997;21:40–42.
27. Hough DM, Stephens DH, Johnson CD, Binkovitz LA. Pancreatic lesions in von Hippel-Lindau disease: prevalence, clinical significance, and CT findings. *AJR Am J Roentgenol*. 1994;162:1091–1094.
28. Neumann HP, Dinkel E, Brambs H, et al. Pancreatic lesions in the von Hippel-Lindau syndrome. *Gastroenterology*. 1991;101:465–471.
29. Cheng TY, Su CH, Shyr YM, Lui WY. Management of pancreatic lesions in von Hippel-Lindau disease. *World J Surg*. 1997;21:307–312.
30. Libutti SK, Choyke PL, Bartlett DL, et al. Pancreatic neuroendocrine tumors associated with von Hippel-Lindau disease: diagnostic and management recommendations. *Surgery*. 1998;124:1153–1159.
31. Hes FJ, van der Luijt RB, Lips CJ. Clinical management of von Hippel-Lindau (VHL) disease. *Neth J Med*. 2001;59:225–234.
32. Girelli R, Bassi C, Falconi M, et al. Pancreatic cystic manifestations in von Hippel-Lindau disease. *Int J Pancreatol*. 1997;22:101–109.
33. Choyke PL, Filling-Katz MR, Shawker TH, et al. von Hippel-Lindau disease: radiologic screening for visceral manifestations. *Radiology*. 1990;174(pt 1):815–820.
34. Binkovitz LA, Johnson CD, Stephens DH. Islet cell tumors in von Hippel-Lindau disease: increased prevalence and relationship to the multiple endocrine neoplasias. *AJR Am J Roentgenol*. 1990;155:501–505.
35. Law CH, Wei AC, Hanna SS, et al. Pancreatic resection for metastatic renal cell carcinoma: presentation, treatment, and outcome. *Ann Surg Oncol*. 2003;10:922–926.
36. Sohn TA, Yeo CJ, Cameron JL, Nakeeb A, Lillemoe KD. Renal cell carcinoma metastatic to the pancreas: results of surgical management. *J Gastrointest Surg*. 2001;5:346–351.
37. Faure JP, Tuech JJ, Richer JP, Pessaux P, Arnaud JP, Carretier M. Pancreatic metastasis of renal cell carcinoma: presentation, treatment and survival. *J Urol*. 2001;165:20–22.
38. Lamiell JM, Salazar FG, Hsia YE. von Hippel-Lindau disease affecting 43 members of a single kindred. *Medicine (Baltimore)*. 1989;68:1–29.
39. Fill WL, Lamiell JM, Polk NO. The radiographic manifestations of von Hippel-Lindau disease. *Radiology*. 1979;133:289–295.
40. Beerman MH, Fromkes JJ, Carey LC, Thomas FB. Pancreatic cystadenoma in von Hippel-Lindau disease: an unusual cause of pancreatic and common bile duct obstruction. *J Clin Gastroenterol*. 1982;4:537–540.
41. Mohr VH, Vortmeyer AO, Zhuang Z, et al. Histopathology and molecular genetics of multiple cysts and microcystic (serous) adenomas of the pancreas in von Hippel-Lindau patients. *Am J Pathol*. 2000;157:1615–1621.
42. Hessman O, Lindberg D, Einarsson A, et al. Genetic alterations on 3p, 11q13, and 18q in nonfamilial and MEN 1-associated pancreatic endocrine tumors. *Genes Chromosomes Cancer*. 1999;26:258–264.
43. Chung DC, Smith AP, Louis DN, Graeme-Cook F, Warshaw AL, Arnold A. A novel pancreatic endocrine tumor suppressor gene locus on chromosome 3p with clinical prognostic implications. *J Clin Invest*. 1997;100:404–410.
44. Hes F, Zewald R, Peeters T, et al. Genotype-phenotype correlations in families with deletions in the von Hippel-Lindau (VHL) gene. *Hum Genet*. 2000;106:425–431.
45. Marcos HB, Libutti SK, Alexander HR, et al. Neuroendocrine tumors of the pancreas in von Hippel-Lindau disease: spectrum of appearances at CT and MR imaging with histopathologic comparison. *Radiology*. 2002;225:751–758.
46. Jackaman FR. Polycystic pancreas: Lindau's disease. *J R Coll Surg Edinb*. 1984;29:121–122.
47. Tenner S, Roston A, Lichtenstein D, Sica G, Carr-Locke D, Banks PA. von Hippel-Lindau disease complicated by acute pancreatitis and Evan's syndrome. *Int J Pancreatol*. 1995;18:271–275.
48. Thompson RK, Peters JI, Sirinek KR, Levine BA. von Hippel-Lindau syndrome presenting as pancreatic endocrine insufficiency: a case report. *Surgery*. 1989;105:598–604.
49. Davison C, Brock S, Dyke CG. Retinal and central nervous hemangioblastomas with visceral changes (von Hippel-Lindau's disease). *Bull Neurol Inst N York*. 1936;5:72.
50. Deboever G, Dewulf P, Maertens J. Common bile duct obstruction due to pancreatic involvement in the von Hippel-Lindau syndrome. *Am J Gastroenterol*. 1992;87:1866–1868.
51. Hammel PR, Vilgrain V, Terris B, et al. Pancreatic involvement in von Hippel-Lindau disease: the Groupe Francophone d'Etude de la Maladie de von Hippel-Lindau. *Gastroenterology*. 2000;119:1087–1095.
52. Green JS, Bowmer MI, Johnson GJ. von Hippel-Lindau disease in a Newfoundland kindred. *CMAJ*. 1986;134:133–138, 146.

CHAPTER 47

Nonfunctioning Pancreatic Endocrine Tumors

Carmen C. Solorzano, MD
Jeffrey E. Lee, MD

Pancreatic endocrine tumors (PETs) (also called neuroendocrine or islet cell tumors) are uncommon neoplasms. The incidence of clinically significant PET is 3.6 to 4 per million population per year; nonfunctioning PET is reported to account for 15%–53% of all PETs.[1-3] Histologically, nonfunctioning PETs, like functioning PETs, are classified as amine precursor uptake and decarboxylation neoplasms (APUDomas) and share cytochemical features with melanoma, pheochromocytoma, carcinoid tumors, and medullary thyroid carcinoma.[4] PETs, like other APUDomas, have the capacity to synthesize and secrete polypeptide products that can have specific endocrine hormone activity.

PETs are considered functional if they are associated with a clinical syndrome caused by APUD hormone release or nonfunctioning if not associated with clinical symptoms. Pancreatic polypeptide (PP)–producing tumors (PPomas) are included in the latter category, as the hormone generally causes no specific symptoms. The majority of nonfunctioning PETs are malignant, as defined by their potential for uncontrolled local growth and distant metastases.[4,5]

Etiology and Molecular Biology

No environmental, behavioral, or epidemiologic risk factors for development of nonfunctioning PET have been identified. PETs, including nonfunctioning PETs, are associated with multiple endocrine neoplasia type 1 (MEN1) and von Hippel-Lindau (VHL). MEN1 is an autosomal dominant inherited disorder characterized by the near-universal development of hyperparathyroidism, along with frequent pituitary adenomas and PETs.[6] PETs can be identified in 30%–80% of patients with MEN1. Gastrinomas and nonfunctioning PETs or PPomas are the most common PETs in patients with MEN1. The development of metastatic disease in patients with MEN1 and PET is uncommon before the age of 30 years; however, metastasis from PET is a frequent cause of mortality in this patient population.[7,8]

The MEN1 syndrome is caused by mutations in the *MEN1* gene, located on chromosome 11.[9] This 9-kb gene consists of 10 exons and encodes a 610-amino acid protein called menin.[10] Menin is a unique gene product with no homology to known proteins. It has no localization or signal peptide, and its mechanism of tumor suppression is unknown. Menin is a nuclear protein that interacts with multiple transcription factors, including JunD, nuclear factor-κB, Smad3, Pem, Nm23H1, glial fibrillary acidic protein, and vimentin.[11-13] Binding to JunD suppresses activated protein-1 activity and suppresses Ras-mediated tumor formation[10-14]; it has been postulated that these mechanisms are related to its role as a tumor-suppressor gene. To date, over 300 unique *MEN1* mutations have been identified in 49%–87% of MEN1 kindreds screened.[15-17] *MEN1* mutations are generally inactivating and usually lead to a truncated protein. Categories of mutations identified include frameshift, nonsense, splice, and missense mutations, as well as deletions. Mutations may involve intron as well as exon sequences. The mutations identified have been distributed throughout the gene; rare "warm spots" have been identified.[18] In contrast to the experience with *RET* mutations in MEN2 patients, to date, no genotype–phenotype correlation has been identified for MEN1 patients with *MEN1* mutations, including for MEN1 patients with PETs.[19-24]

Several investigators have sought to identify evidence for a role for the *MEN1* gene in patients with both MEN1-associated and sporadic PETs. In one investigation, a loss of heterozygosity (LOH) was identified at the *MEN1* locus within the pancreatic tumor specimens of 23 of 27 patients (85%) with MEN1.[24] In another investigation, among 31 patients with sporadic PETs (functioning and nonfunctioning), mutations in MEN1 were identified in 12 patients (39%), LOH in 12 patients (39%), and both in 7 patients (23%).[25] These investigations taken together suggest that *MEN1* is responsible for the development of PETs in patients with MEN1 and that this same gene may also play a role in the development of some, although not all, sporadic PETs.

VHL is an autosomal dominant inherited disorder characterized by the development of retinal and central nervous system hemangiomas, renal cell carcinomas, pheochromocytomas, and PETs.[26] PETs develop in 15%–20% of patients with VHL.[27,28] Full penetrance of VHL occurs by the age of 65 years; however, there is great variability in the clinical manifestations of the disease. The VHL syndrome is due to mutations in the *VHL* gene, located on chromosome 3 (3p25). Genetic testing is 95% sensitive in identifying mutations. The VHL gene has 3 exons, 712 nucleotides, and codes for a 213 amino acid protein. The protein binds to elongin B and elongin C transcription factors. Occasional *VHL* mosaicism may occur.[29] Pancreatic cystic neoplasms (separately from PETs) have been shown to demonstrate LOH at the *VHL* locus.[30] To date, PETs in patients with VHL have not been examined for LOH. Although a genotype-phenotype association for pheochromocytoma in VHL has been identified,[31] no such association has yet been described for PETs in patients with VHL. Interestingly, LOH of chromosome 3p as well as deletion of chromosome 3 has been described in sporadic PETs, and LOH of chromosome 3p and deletion of chromosome 3 have been linked to the development of metastatic disease in patients with sporadic PETs.[24,32,33] These data suggest that the *VHL* gene (as well as perhaps other 3p genes) is involved in the development and progression of PETs. Other genetic loci altered in sporadic PETs identified by genome-wide allelotyping include 3q, 11p, 16p, and 22q. Other markers investigated have included *cyclin-D1*, $p16^{INK4}$, *Smad4/DPC*, *HER-2/neu*, and *p53*. No link between these markers and prognosis of PETs has been identified.

Histology and Diagnosis

Differences in tumor biology, prognosis, and treatment strategies emphasize the importance of differentiating pancreatic endocrine from pancreatic exocrine tumors. Although the histologic features of PET are often characteristic, immunohistochemistry can be helpful in confirming the presence of a PET.[4] General neuroendocrine immunohistochemical markers that may be useful include synaptophysin, chromogranin A (CgA), and neuron-specific enolase (NSE). Nonfunctioning PETs may lose CgA staining, whereas synaptophysin and NSE staining are usually preserved. Specific pancreatic neuroendocrine immunohistochemical markers that can be commonly identified in nonfunctioning PETs include PP and glucagon. As with functioning PETs, however, the intensity of immunohistochemical staining for these peptides does not directly correspond to serum levels of the hormone or to the severity of any clinical symptoms. In equivocal cases, electron microscopy of PETs can be helpful in identifying characteristic ultrastructural electron-dense secretory granules.

The histology of a nonfunctioning PET is not a reliable predictor of its biologic behavior. The presence of nodal or distant metastases is obviously confirmatory of malignancy. However, size and standard histologic features such as nuclear pleomorphism, mitotic activity, or the presence of local or vascular invasion are less reliable criteria. Therefore, because patients with nonfunctioning PETs as a group are at risk for the development of metastatic disease, these tumors are generally considered malignant or potentially malignant.[4,5]

Serum Markers

A number of serum markers have been evaluated for their clinical utility in the diagnosis and management of patients with nonfunctioning PET. Nonfunctioning PETs can secrete a variety of peptide hormones, proteins, and glycoproteins, including PP,[34-38] CgA,[39,40] NSE,[41] and the β or β subunits of human chorionic gonadotropin.[39,42]

Up to 75% of nonfunctioning PETs are associated with increased serum levels of PP.[33,43,44] Nonfunctioning PETs without elevated PP and PETs with elevated PP (PPomas) do not appear to differ in presentation or biologic behavior.[45] PP has been investigated as a marker for patients with MEN1[46,47] and as a marker for metastatic disease in patients with known PETs.[35] Unfortunately, measurements of PP have proven to be of limited value in these patients. PP levels are poorly correlated with tumor burden, often do not normalize after surgical resection, have wide intrapatient variability, and are often falsely elevated, even in patients without pancreatic tumors. For these reasons, treatment decisions are not based on the plasma level of PP. Elevated plasma levels of PP do not establish the diagnosis of a PPoma even in the presence of a pancreatic mass. PP levels can be elevated in patients with functioning PETs as well as in patients with nonpancreatic carcinoid tumors. Importantly, elevated plasma levels of PP can occur after a meal in normal individuals, as well as in patients with chronic inflammatory disorders, acute diarrhea, chronic renal failure, diabetes, pancreatitis, alcohol abuse, a bowel resection, and advanced age.[48,49,50]

CgA has been suggested as the best general neuroendocrine serum marker available for the evaluation and management of patients with nonfunctioning PET.[40] In a study that evaluated levels of CgA, NSE, and the α subunit of glycoprotein hormones in a series of 211 patients with a variety of neuroendocrine tumors, elevated serum CgA levels were seen in 9 of 13 patients (69%) with nonfunctioning PETs. Among all 211 patients, CgA levels were correlated with tumor burden. However, the specificity of CgA is not equal to that of the hormonal secretory products of other neuroendocrine tumors (parathyroid hormone in patients with hyperparathyroidism, calcitonin in patients with medullary thyroid cancer).[48] Therefore, CgA levels are not generally clinically helpful in monitoring patients with nonfunctioning PETs for disease recurrence or response to therapy.

Clinical Presentation, Initial Evaluation, and Patient Selection

Nonfunctioning PETs typically present in the fourth or fifth decade of life.[51,52] The most common clinical presentation of patients with nonfunctioning PET is local symptoms from the primary pancreatic tumor or from liver metastases. Nonfunctioning PETs are usually solitary tumors except in patients with MEN1 in whom they are characteristically multiple. Nonfunctioning PETs have a predilection for the pancreatic head (approximately 60%).[53-56]

The proper diagnostic and treatment strategies for patients with presumed malignant neoplasms of the periampullary region remain a source of controversy and confusion. Unlike functioning neuroendocrine tumors of the pancreas and duodenum, nonfunctioning PETs and PPomas do not manifest a specific clinical syndrome. Patients may present similar to patients with pancreatic adenocarcinoma: with fatigue, weight loss, nausea, and/or abdominal discomfort.[1,2,57] In addition, patients with pancreatic head tumors may present with jaundice.[1,2] Patients with nonfunctioning PET associated with MEN1 may present with asymptomatic masses identified on screening evaluation. Likewise, patients with sporadic PET may present with incidentally identified pancreatic masses identified on abdominal imaging studies performed for unrelated reasons.[1] Nonfunctioning PET should be considered in the differential diagnosis of such patients, particularly in the setting of a characteristic appearance on radiographic imaging studies. On contrast-enhanced computed tomography (CT), a PET usually appears hypervascular or hyperdense (Fig. 47.1A) when imaged with intravenous contrast enhancement.[58,59] PETs may contain calcifications (Fig. 47.1B). PETs may also mimic other pancreatic tumor processes; they may be hypodense compared with adjacent pancreatic parenchyma, similar to pancreatic adenocarcinomas, and they may contain cystic components (Fig. 47.1C). In part because of the lack of specific associated hormonal symptoms, the majority of patients with nonfunctioning PET do not present until they have locally advanced, unresectable, or metastatic disease.

At our institution, we continue to use objective CT criteria to define potentially resectable pancreatic tumors (of exocrine or endocrine origin).[58,60-62] Determination of resectability of the primary tumor is based on the relationship of the mass to the superior mesenteric artery (SMA) and superior mesenteric vein (SMV). A tumor that encases the celiac axis or the superior mesenteric artery is considered unresectable. Some investigators have suggested that palliative pancreatic resection (debulking) in patients with unresectable neuroendocrine tumors may provide relief from hormonal or local tumor-related symptoms and improve the efficacy of chemotherapy by decreasing overall tumor burden.[51,63,64] However, most of these reports included patients with functioning tumors and syndromes of hormone excess. No available data exist to support debulking procedures in patients with unresectable nonfunctioning islet cell carcinomas. Incomplete resection (debulking) for nonfunctioning islet cell carcinoma of the pancreas is not performed at our institution

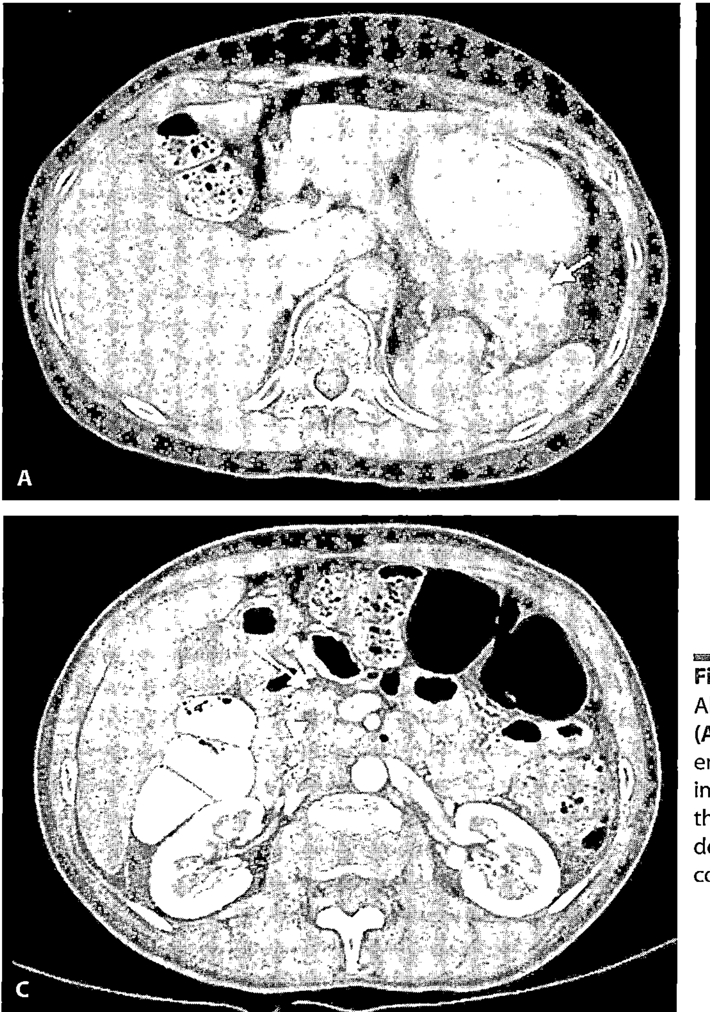

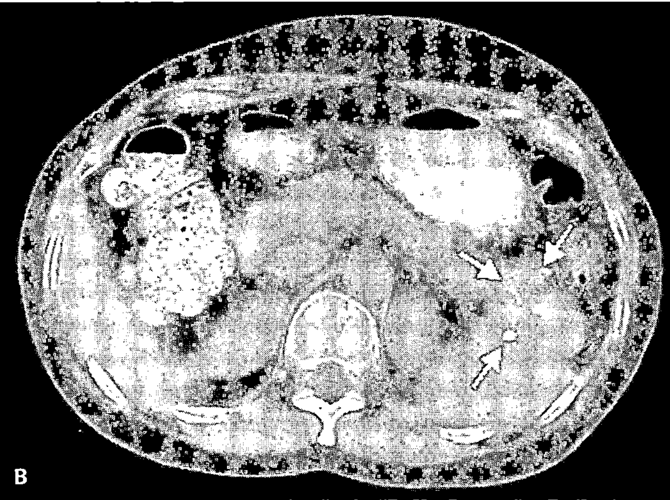

Figure 47.1
Abdominal CT imaging studies of patients with nonfunctioning PETs. **(A)** intravenous contrast-enhanced imaging study demonstrating an enhancing mass in the tail of the pancreas (*arrow*). **(B)** Nonenhanced image of the patient shown in **(A)** demonstrating calcifications within the tumor (*arrows*). **(C)** Intravenous contrast-enhanced imaging study demonstrating a hypodense mass (*arrow*) within the pancreatic head containing a cystic component (*arrowhead*).

because of the favorable survival duration of patients with locally advanced disease not treated surgically and the potential morbidity of palliative pancreatic resection.[53,65-67]

Tumors to the right of the SMA and SMV, originating in the pancreatic head or uncinate process, may cause obstruction of the intrapancreatic portion of the common bile duct, gastric outlet obstruction, and/or pain because of invasion of the retroperitoneal mesenteric plexus. Unlike adenocarcinomas in this region, nonfunctioning PETs occasionally grow to an enormous size (Fig. 47.2), with minimal symptoms. Patients may have little in the way of discomfort and may not develop jaundice despite the considerable size of these tumors (Fig. 47.3). Neuroendocrine pancreatic tumors arising to the left of the SMA and SMV can present an even greater diagnostic challenge. Patients may complain of vague, poorly localized upper abdominal pain, or dyspepsia. In contrast to patients with adenocarcinoma of the body or tail of the pancreas, they may not have significant weight loss, cachexia, back pain, or other signs of advanced disease. Neoplasms of the stomach (gastrointestinal stromal tumors), colon (locally advanced adenocarcinoma), adrenal gland (adrenocortical carcinoma, pheochromocytoma), and kidney (renal cell carcinoma) can be confused with PETs, especially if clinical evidence of peptide production is subtle or absent. A standard radiographic evaluation and biochemical screening can help prevent unexpected findings at laparotomy (Fig. 47.4).

In patients with presumed sporadic nonfunctioning PET, surgical resection is the preferred treatment if technically possible. After surgical resection, one does not usually consider additional treatment in the absence of radiographically demonstrable metastatic disease, even if the plasma level of PP or CgA remains elevated. Furthermore, treatment of established metastatic disease is generally based on the observed rate of tumor progression and the degree of tumor burden, rather than on PP or CgA levels.

Our experience with reoperative pancreaticoduodenectomy underscores the importance of an accurate preoperative diagnosis.[68] Four patients from this series had nonfunctioning PET and serve to illustrate this concept. At initial surgical exploration at an outside institution, the first of the four patients was felt to have a locally advanced, unresectable tumor of the pancreatic head. Intraoperative biopsies were interpreted as adenocarcinoma, and she was treated with radiation therapy and systemic chemotherapy. After referral to our institution, the diagnosis was revised to islet cell carcinoma (nonfunctioning PET) after review of the intraoperative biopsy material. The other three patients in our series underwent prereferral exploration for planned pancreaticoduodenectomy in the absence of preoperative tissue confirmation of malignancy. Intraoperative frozen section biopsies were inconclusive, and the surgeons involved were not prepared to proceed with resection in the absence of a positive

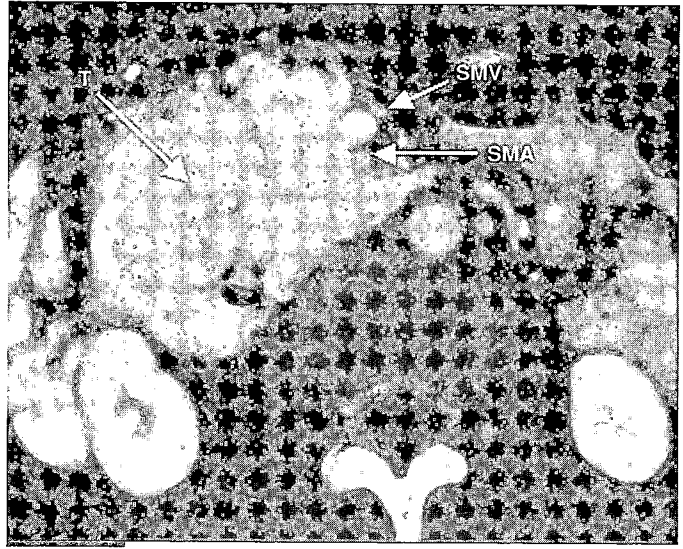

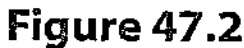

Figure 47.2
Abdominal CT imaging study of a patient with a large nonfunctioning PET. The tumor (T) involved the SMV; the SMA was marginally free. The patient was not jaundiced, and there was no preoperative evidence for metastatic disease. The patient underwent a complete resection of his tumor; extirpation required resection of a segment of the SMV, with reconstruction using autologous internal jugular vein. Final histopathology revealed a pancreatic neuroendocrine carcinoma, absent nodal metastases, and focal tumor invasion of the SMV. The patient remains free of disease 10 years after his surgery.

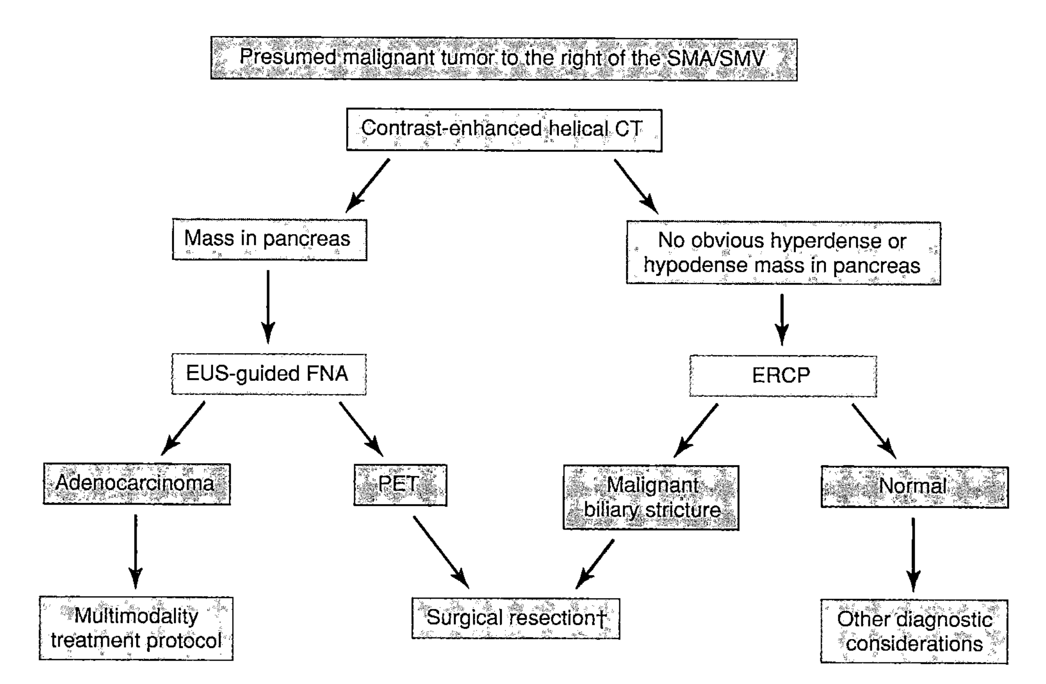

Figure 47.3
Strategy for evaluation of a patient with a tumor presenting to the right of the SMA/SMV. EUS = endoscopic ultrasound; FNA = fine-needle aspiration biopsy; ERCP = endoscopic retrograde pancreatography. SMA = superior mesenteric artery; SMV = superior mesenteric vein; PET = pancreatic endocrine tumors.

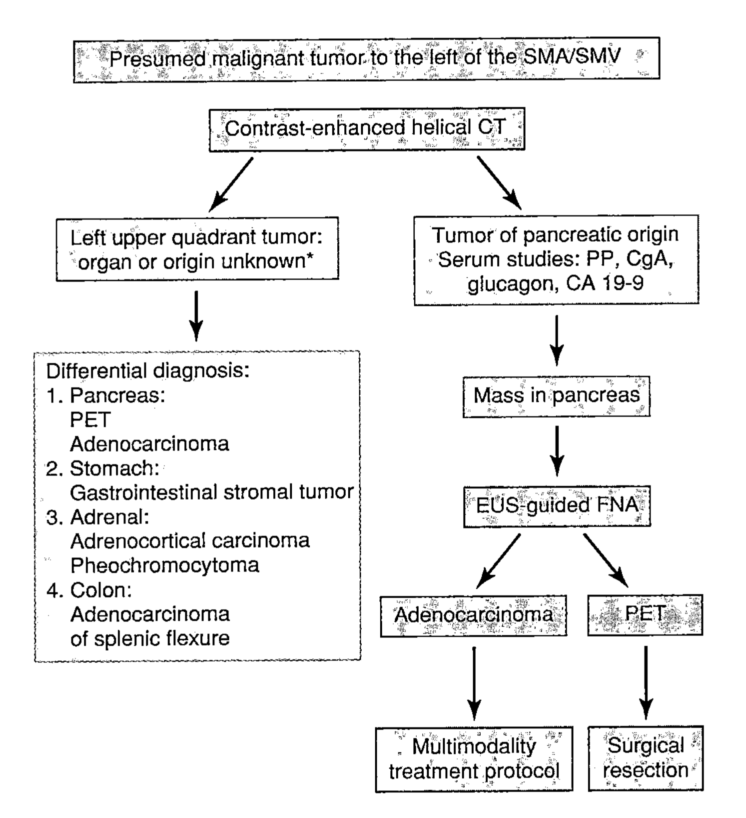

Figure 47.4
Strategy for evaluation of a patient with a tumor presenting to the left of the SMA/SMV.

biopsy. The diagnosis of PET was confirmed on permanent section histology in only one of these three patients before reoperative pancreaticoduodenectomy. These four patients serve to illustrate both the inaccuracy of intraoperative assessment of resectability (best determined by high-quality preoperative cross-sectional imaging studies), and the common mistake of assuming that biopsy confirmation of malignancy can always be achieved at the time of laparotomy (best determined, if at all, by preoperative fine-needle aspiration biopsy).[58] Accurate preoperative imaging will improve the likelihood that patients who undergo operation will have resectable tumors, avoid unnecessary operations in patients with locally advanced disease, and minimize the need for intraoperative biopsy. Many surgeons will not proceed with pancreaticoduodenectomy in the absence of tissue confirmation of cancer. Although we do not share this view, we acknowledge its relevance in the general surgical community. For those surgeons who require biopsy proof of malignancy before proceeding with pancreaticoduodenectomy, the biopsy should be performed under endoscopic ultrasound guidance. Reports of endoscopic ultrasound-guided FNA of the pancreas have demonstrated its accuracy and safety.[69-71]

In patients with MEN1, tumors may arise anywhere within the pancreas.[52,72] Increased levels of PP indicate the presence of hyperplastic, neoplastic, or malignant cells.[46] The standard goal of operation in patients with MEN1 is to palliate symptoms of hormonal excess (insulin, gastrin). Only recently have surgeons considered the oncologic aspects of pancreatic neoplasia in this disease.[73] In patients with MEN1 who have a pancreatic neoplasm (functioning or nonfunctioning) with no evidence of metastatic disease at diagnosis, the only way to potentially prevent the development of liver metastases (if not already microscopically present) would be to perform a total pancreaticoduodenectomy. Traditional wisdom has argued that this treatment, with its long-term metabolic side effects, is excessive for the majority of patients, who will not develop metastatic disease. Ideally, one would then like to remove identifiable tumor while leaving enough pancreas to preserve endogenous glycemic control. One would like to be able to monitor patients with a simple test that can identify recurrent neoplasm before the development of metastatic disease. Although increased basal and meal-stimulated PP levels may arguably identify patients with MEN1 and pancreatic neoplasia,[46] the serum level of PP cannot be used to assess a patient's risk of developing metastatic disease.[35-43]

One of our recent patients illustrated the continued need for such a tool. A 30-year-old male of known MEN1 kindred sought a second opinion on the appropriateness of complete pancreaticoduodenectomy. He had undergone a distal pancreatectomy at the age of 24 years for insulin- and glucagon-producing tumors of the body and tail of the pancreas. His father and uncle had both died of hepatic metastases from PETs. The serum PP level was increased, at 422 pg/ml, up from 331 pg/ml the year previously. The glucagon level was mildly increased at 280 pg/ml, and the gastrin and vasoactive intestinal polypeptide levels were within normal ranges. CT demonstrated a small area of low density with a rim of hypervascular enhancement in the pancreatic head, but there was no evidence of extrapancreatic disease. The increased PP level and the abnormality on the CT argued for the presence of persistent tumor in the pancreatic head. However, a normal basal PP level and a normal CT would not exclude the possibility of metachronous additional PETs in the setting of MEN1, in which diffuse multifocal disease is the rule. Knowledge of the natural history of pancreatic neoplasia in MEN1 (diffuse, multifocal) is of much greater value than the presence or absence of an increased PP level. One could certainly support total pancreaticoduodenectomy in a patient as described here with MEN1 and a strong family history of malignant tumors (as defined by the documentation of metastasis to distant organs). Unfortunately, there is no way to exclude the possibility of microscopic hepatic metastases already being present at the time of proposed radical pancreatic surgery. The potential long-term complications of total pancreaticoduodenectomy—insulin-dependent diabetes, exocrine pancreatic insufficiency, and a gastrointestinal dysfunction—make treatment decisions difficult in the MEN1 patient with a strong family history of malignant PET. Unfortunately, serial monitoring of the serum level of PP, as one would monitor the carcinoembryonic antigen level in a patient with colorectal carcinoma, is of little clinical utility.

Because of the characteristic multiplicity of the PETs in patients with MEN1 as well as low rates of clinical cure, some investigators have discouraged early surgery in patients with PET in the setting of MEN1.[74] In the 1999 National Cancer Institute (NCI) series reporting surgical treatment of patients with the Zollinger-Ellison syndrome, 28 patients had MEN1. All patients with MEN1 who underwent operation had relatively large tumors (3 cm or greater) by the time they had their surgery. No patient with MEN1 was free of disease at 10 years.

In contrast to the NCI approach, other investigators have recommended a more aggressive approach, including consideration for treatment of patients with only biochemical evidence for disease.[57,73] Size is an imperfect predictor of malignant behavior; metastatic disease may be present in patients with MEN1 even when the primary tumors are small,[75] and the NCI results are discouraging with regard to long-term disease-free survival. Therefore, Thompson[75a] has recommended that patients with pancreatic tumors of any size identified on preoperative imaging evaluation (CT and endoscopic ultrasound) be considered for operation. Selected patients with MEN1 and biochemical evidence for gastrinoma without imaging evidence for disease may also be considered for operation after regionalization of their tumors via hepatic vein sampling for gastrin. A standardized operative approach is taken in these patients, with full mobilization of the pancreas, intraoperative ultrasound, resection of pancreatic body and tail tumors via a distal subtotal pancreatectomy, enucleation of tumors in the pancreatic head, a portal, peripancreatic and periduodenal lymph node dissection, and a duodenotomy with palpation of the duodenal wall and resection of any identified tumors in patients with hypergastrinemia. In contrast to the NCI experience, an aggressive surgical approach in 11 patients with gastrinoma in the setting of MEN1 resulted in normal serum gastrin levels in 10 of 11 patients after follow-up ranging from 3 months to 14 years.[73] Although the oncologic benefit of resection in such patients is unproven, an aggressive approach such as described previously here is reasonable in selected patients, particularly those with hypergastrinemia who are from MEN1 kindreds in which there is a history of malignant PET with hepatic metastasis, as well as any good-risk MEN1 patient with pancreatic tumors identified on imaging studies.

Operative Management

The goals of operative resection of nonfunctioning PETs are to improve local disease control and to increase quality and length of patient survival. These goals must be tempered by the potential operative morbidity and the long-term complications of insulin dependence and gastrointestinal dysfunction. Data from our institution have demonstrated that resection of a primary tumor in the presence of metastatic disease does not prolong patient survival.[53,65]

Survival data for 163 patients treated at M.D. Anderson Cancer Center for nonfunctioning PET were analyzed based on disease extent and treatment of the primary tumor.[65] The overall median survival duration and the 5-year survival rate from the time of diagnosis were 3.2 years and 43%, respectively. Patients found to have metastatic disease at the time of diagnosis had a median survival of 2.2 years compared with 7.1 years for patients with localized, nonmetastatic disease ($P <$ 0.0001). Although nonfunctioning PETs are believed to have an indolent growth pattern in comparison to ductal adenocarcinoma of the pancreas, it is important to note that the majority of patients in this series died of metastatic PET. Furthermore, only 42 of the 163 patients (26%) were able to receive a potentially curative resection of their primary tumor. As expected, a survival advantage was demonstrated for patients who underwent complete resection of the primary tumor in the absence of metastatic disease. However, only 20 of the 42 patients (48%) who underwent resection of the primary tumor were alive and without evidence of recurrent disease at last follow-up. Therefore, it is inappropriate based on these data to assume that complete resection of the primary tumor in the absence of metastatic disease corresponds to a long-term cure.

Of the 20 patients in our series who had locally advanced primary tumors in the absence of metastatic disease,

12 (60%) died of disease. Ten of these 12 patients had tumors in the head of the pancreas. Before death, these 10 patients had a median of two hospital admissions each for complications related to their primary tumor process or attempts to treat that tumor process: biliary obstruction, gastric outlet obstruction, gastrointestinal hemorrhage, or treatment-related toxicity. These data demonstrate that primary tumors to the right of the superior mesenteric vessels are associated with significant patient morbidity and are best managed by pancreaticoduodenectomy, occasionally requiring in-continuity vascular or adjacent organ resection for adequate local–regional control (Fig. 47.5).

The median survival in our series for patients presenting with metastatic disease ranged from 1.8 to 3 years. Although the survival duration of patients with metastatic nonfunctioning PET is clearly superior to that of patients with metastatic adenocarcinoma of the pancreas, the majority of patients with metastatic nonfunctioning PET will die of disease within 2 years of diagnosis. Therefore, both regional and systemic therapies along with investigational protocol-based treatments should be considered at the time of diagnosis in these patients. The difference in survival duration between patients in our series with metastatic disease who either did or did not undergo resection of their primary tumor did not achieve statistical significance despite the inherent selection bias in favor of those who underwent resection of the primary tumor (i.e., those who underwent resection of the primary tumor were those most likely to have less extensive extrapancreatic disease and a better performance status).

Unlike tumors in the pancreatic head, pancreatic body and tail tumors rarely cause symptoms and therefore are often metastatic at diagnosis. Patients with liver metastases from primary tumors in the pancreatic body and tail achieved no benefit from distal pancreatectomy in the absence of significant symptoms related to the primary tumor. Therefore, in the absence of a symptomatic primary tumor, there is little role for pancreatectomy in treating nonfunctioning PETs of the body or tail in the presence of unresectable extrapancreatic metastatic disease. This concept may change as strategies for the management of hepatic metastases become more successful.[76-80] There may, however, be a place for pancreaticoduodenectomy in selected good-risk patients with nonfunctioning PET of the pancreatic head who have low-volume extrapancreatic metastatic disease. Tumors of the pancreatic head, in contrast to tumors of the distal pancreas, may erode into the duodenum, resulting in gastrointestinal hemorrhage, or may cause biliary or gastric outlet obstruction; such complications may be better managed with resection of the primary tumor rather than palliative bypass procedures.

Finally, despite anecdotal reports of successful combined resection of the primary tumor and distant metastases,[63,64,81] such an aggressive surgical approach was possible in only 4 of 101 patients who presented with metastases in our series. The extrapancreatic metastatic disease was not amenable to surgical resection (in the opinion of the treating physicians at our institution) in the other 97 patients who had metastatic disease at the time of initial diagnosis.

The previously mentioned data emphasize the importance of making patient treatment decisions based on a sound knowledge of the natural history and patterns of failure for nonfunctioning PET. Figure 47.5 outlines our treatment schema for the patient with a sporadic nonfunctioning PET. In the presence of hepatic metastases, we would consider resection of the primary tumor in only patients with a good performance status and low-volume metastatic disease. The classic scenario is a young patient who presents with biliary obstruction caused by an islet

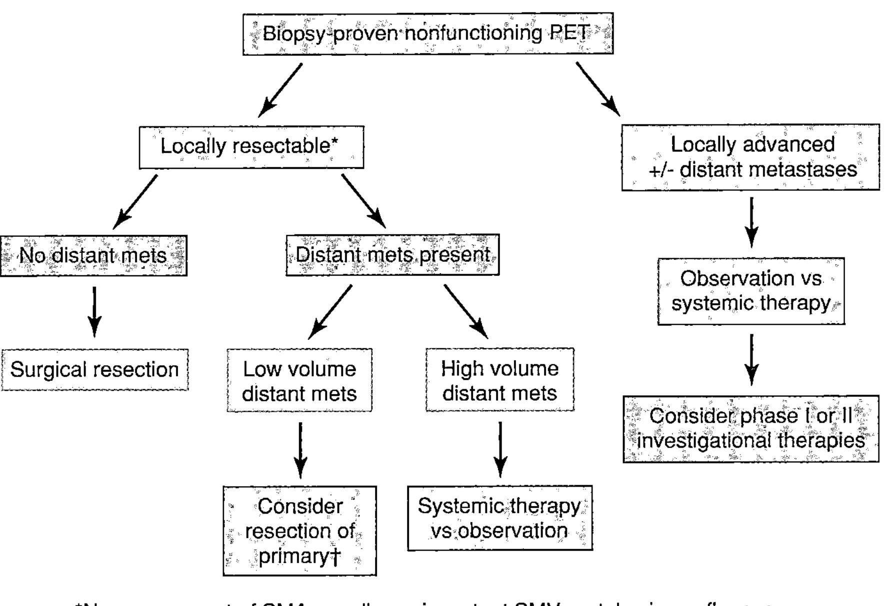

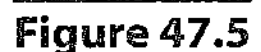

Figure 47.5
Strategy for treatment of a patient presenting with a biopsy-proven nonfunctioning PET.

cell carcinoma of the pancreatic head; at the time of laparotomy, multiple 1-cm nodules are seen in the liver, and biopsy confirms metastatic disease. Our data suggest that this patient has a high probability of incurring major morbidity because of uncontrolled growth of the primary tumor before death from metastatic disease and, therefore, would benefit from resection of the primary tumor. In contrast, distal pancreatic tumors would not be resected in the presence of metastatic disease unless they are causing symptoms or resection would influence treatment (e.g., patients who may be candidates for hepatic transplantation if the primary tumor were controlled).

Extended Surgical Resection

Occasionally, nonfunctioning PET will require an extended operation to achieve a complete resection. Our criteria for pancreatic resection include the absence of arterial encasement as well as a patent superior mesenteric-portal venous (SM-PV) confluence. Similar to our philosophy in the local–regional management of pancreatic adenocarcinoma,[68,82] we do not perform debulking operations for nonfunctioning PET. However, the variable tumor biology of islet cell tumors results in a subset of patients who have large primary tumors yet who do not have demonstrable distant metastatic disease. The technical limitations to successful resection in these patients are either arterial encasement (SMA, hepatic artery [HA], or celiac axis) or venous encasement or occlusion (SM-PV confluence). Data from our institution have demonstrated the safety of segmental resection of the SM-PV confluence when necessary to allow complete resection.[60,63] Unlike other authors, we prefer to preserve the splenic vein–portal vein confluence when possible in order to minimize the risk of gastric hemorrhage from the development of sinistral portal hypertension. Preserving the confluence, however, limits the mobility of the divided SMV and prevents direct reanastomosis between the SMV and portal vein in many patients. Our preferred conduit for interposition grafting in this situation is the internal jugular vein.[62] We do not advocate resection of the SMA because of the historically high morbidity and mortality associated with this procedure; therefore, at this time, encasement of the SMA remains a contraindication to surgical resection of nonfunctioning PET.

Locally advanced tumors of the cephalad portion of the head and neck of the pancreas may encase the celiac axis or HA without involving the SMA. We have a small experience with resection and reconstruction of both the HA and the SM-PV confluence with saphenous vein and jugular vein, respectively. If the left gastric artery is not involved, the stomach can be preserved. Typically, large tumors of the neck and body of the pancreas involve the HA and the left gastric and splenic arteries near their origin, and tumor extirpation requires upper abdominal exenteration, with removal of the stomach and spleen, in addition to total pancreaticoduodenectomy. Our experience with this procedure in two patients suggests that nutritional management is the major long-term complication; both patients have failed to return to their preoperative weights. The combination of total pancreaticoduodenectomy plus total gastrectomy leads to long-term gastrointestinal dysfunction, especially when combined with an extensive retroperitoneal dissection, with removal of the celiac and mesenteric neural plexus.[83-85] For these reasons, such resections should be reserved for highly selected patients and should only be performed when complete tumor extirpation appears possible based on preoperative imaging studies.

Because the median survival is 5 years in patients with unresected nonmetastatic nonfunctioning PET, it becomes difficult to recommend operation as the complexity, and therefore, potential morbidity of the surgical procedure increases. Patients and physicians are less accepting of the up-front risks of operative therapy as survival time without operation increases and the potential operative morbidity increases. With further advances in operative technique and nutritional support, the extent of surgical resection advisable in patients with nonmetastatic islet cell carcinoma may increase. At this time, we are highly selective in our use of extended pancreaticoduodenectomy when total gastrectomy and/or HA revascularization may be necessary.

Treatment of Locally Advanced Disease

The appropriate management of patients with locally advanced, surgically unresectable neuroendocrine carcinoma of the pancreas in the absence of extrapancreatic metastatic disease remains a difficult therapeutic dilemma. At present, we prefer to treat biliary or gastric outlet obstruction in these patients with surgical bypass rather than endoscopic or transhepatic stenting because of their relatively long median survival and the potential morbidity of nonsurgical methods of long-term palliation. For oncologic treatment, cytotoxic chemotherapy is considered when there is radiographic evidence of disease progression or the development of symptoms. Octreotide or interferon-α[76,86,87] can result in disease stabilization; however, these therapies rarely result in a radiographically definable treatment response. In general, we have not used local–regional chemoradiation for locally advanced PET. In the absence of pain of visceral origin, external-beam radiation therapy probably has minimal palliative benefit. Furthermore, many patients have such extensive local–regional disease that the radiation therapy fields required would be so large as to result in significant gastrointestinal toxicity. The experience with radiation therapy for locally advanced pancreatic neuroendocrine carcinoma is anecdotal.[88]

Treatment of Metastatic Disease

The management of patients with metastatic islet cell carcinoma of the pancreas is difficult to define accurately in a simple algorithmic approach. Despite anecdotal reports of successful combined resection of the primary tumor and distant metastases,[63,64,81] such an aggressive surgical approach was only possible in 4 of 101 patients presenting with metastases in our series. The extrapancreatic metastatic disease was not amenable to surgical resection (in the opinion of the treating physicians at this institution) in the other 97 patients in our series who had metastatic disease at the time of initial diagnosis. In 16 of these 97 patients (17%), the primary tumor was resected despite the presence of unresectable extrapancreatic metastatic disease. This clearly would not have been the approach taken if the diagnosis were exocrine pancreatic cancer. The modest improvement in survival in these 16 patients (median survival, 3 years) compared with the 81 patients with metastatic disease who did not undergo surgery (median survival, 1.8 years) did not achieve statistical significance and is most likely due to selection bias.

Based on our data, we can develop general therapeutic guidelines for patients with metastatic pancreatic neuroendocrine carcinoma. In the absence of a symptomatic primary tumor, pancreatic resection in the presence of unresectable extrapancreatic metastatic disease is probably not indicated. There may, however, be a place for pancreaticoduodenectomy in selected good-risk patients with neuroendocrine carcinoma of the pancreatic head who have low-volume extrapancreatic metastatic disease. Tumors of the pancreatic head, in contrast to tumors of the distal pancreas, may erode into the duodenum, resulting in gastrointestinal hemorrhage, or may cause biliary or gastric outlet obstruction; such complications may be better managed with resection of the primary tumor rather than palliative bypass procedures. The rationale for aggressive management of the primary tumor despite the presence of extrapancreatic disease may be more compelling as treatments for metastatic disease become more effective. Treatments involving systemic chemotherapy, radiopharmaceuticals, HA embolization, radiofrequency ablation (RFA), cryotherapy, and liver transplantation[89-92] remain areas of active investigation that may ultimately significantly change stage-specific treatment recommendations.

Streptozocin remains the single most active systemic agent for treating patients with metastatic islet cell carcinoma, including metastatic nonfunctioning PET. Combination therapy of streptozocin with 5-fluorouracil (5-FU) is associated with improved response rates and survival duration.[93] Doxorubicin is also an effective agent in combination with 5-FU. Currently, the combination of streptozocin with doxorubicin may be the first-line combination of choice based on the results of a prospective randomized trial that demonstrated superiority in response rates and duration of response for this combination compared to streptozocin plus 5-FU or chlorozotocin alone.[94] We would consider chemotherapy in patients with unresectable local–regional PET who either develop radiographic evidence of disease progression or who have symptoms (e.g., pain) related to their primary tumor process. Patients with distant metastases from PET with radiographic evidence for disease progression or significant symptomatology are also candidates for either standard combination systemic therapies, as outlined previously here or for protocol-based treatments.

Liver-directed resectional and ablative therapies may be considered in patients whose disease is confined to the liver, especially if symptomatic or if their tumors demonstrate radiographic evidence of disease progression. Multiple retrospective reports have documented the safety of hepatic resection,[63,64,81,95-97] cryosurgical ablation or RFA,[77,98,99] in the treatment of selected patients with PET metastatic to the liver. Although the oncologic benefit of an aggressive approach in patients with metastatic nonfunctional PET remains unproven, in selected patients with relatively low-volume and indolent disease confined to the liver, these approaches seem reasonable.

HA embolization or chemoembolization[100-103] may be considered in patients with hepatic metastases from nonfunctioning PET. Although insufficient comparative data exist to make firm recommendations, we would favor HA embolization in patients (1) not considered candidates for surgical resection or RFA because of the extent of liver involvement, (2) whose performance status makes them poor candidates for an open operation, (3) who develop recurrence limited to the liver following resection or RFA, and (4) with relatively indolent liver-only disease in the presence of extrapancreatic disease. Isolation perfusion of the liver for hepatic metastases from PET, as performed at the NCI, remains an investigational procedure.[104]

Liver transplantation may be justified in selected highly symptomatic patients with metastatic neuroendocrine carcinoma confined to the liver.[79,80,85] In the United States, however, limitations on the availability of livers for transplant and the good performance status of most patients with metastatic PET results in a situation in which these patients are too low on transplant priority lists to be considered active candidates until their cancer has progressed to the point that they are effectively excluded.

Conclusion

Whereas patients with nonfunctioning PET or PPoma have a relatively prolonged survival duration compared with patients with adenocarcinoma of the pancreas, the majority of patients who do not undergo a potentially curative resection die of disease less than 5 years after diagnosis. The decision to proceed with operative resection of the primary pancreatic tumor should be based on its location in the pancreas, the extent of resection required (with its inherent early and late morbidity), and the presence or absence of metastatic disease. Systemic therapy and regional therapies, along with investigational protocol-based treatments, should be considered at the time of diagnosis for patients with a good performance status who have locally advanced primary tumors or metastatic disease.

References

1. Kent RB, van Heerden JA, Weiland LH. Nonfunctioning islet cell tumors. *Ann Surg.* 1981;193:185–190.
2. Lo CY, van Heerden JA, Thompson GB, et al. Islet cell carcinoma of the pancreas. *World J Surg.* 1996;20:878–883.
3. Alexander HR, Jensen RT. Pancreatic endocrine tumors. In: DeVita VT Jr, Hellman S, Rosenberg SA, eds. *Cancer Principles and Practice of Oncology* (6th ed). Philadelphia: Lippincott; 2001:1788–1813.
4. Kloppel G, Schroder S, Heitz PU. Histopathology and immunopathology of pancreatic endocrine tumors. In: Mignon M, Jensen RT, eds. *Endocrine Tumors of the Pancreas: Recent Advances in Research and Management.* Basel, Switzerland: S. Karger; 1995:120.
5. Eriksson B, Oberg K. PPomas and nonfunctioning endocrine pancreatic tumors: clinical presentation, diagnosis, and advances in management. In: Mignon M, Jensen RT, eds. *Endocrine Tumors of the Pancreas: Recent Advances in Research and Management.* Basel, Switzerland: S. Karger; 1995:208.
6. Skogseid B, Eriksson B, Lundqvist G, et al. Multiple endocrine neoplasia type 1: a 10–year prospective screening study in four kindreds. *J Clin Endocrinol Metab.* 1991;73:281.
7. Doherty GM, Olson JA, Frisella MM, et al. Lethality of multiple endocrine neoplasia type I. *World J Surg.* 1998;22:581–586; discussion 586–587.
8. Dean PG, van Heerden JA, Farley DR, et al. Are patients with multiple endocrine neoplasia type I prone to premature death? *World J Surg.* 2000;24:1437–1441.
9. Chandrasekharappa SC, Guru SC, Manickam P, et al. Positional cloning of the gene for multiple endocrine neoplasia-type 1. *Science.* 1997;276:404–407.
10. Marx SJ, Agarwal SK, Heppner C, et al. The gene for multiple endocrine neoplasia type 1: recent findings. *Bone.* 1999;25:119–122.
11. Poisson A, Zablewska B, Gaudray P. Menin interacting proteins as clues toward the understanding of multiple endocrine neoplasia type 1. *Cancer Lett.* 2003;189:1–10.
12. Gobl AE, Berg M, Lopez-Egido JR, et al. Menin represses JunD-activated transcription by a histone deacetylase-dependent mechanism. *Biochim Biophys Acta.* 1999;1447: 51–56.
13. Agarwal SK, Guru SC, Heppner C, et al. Menin interacts with the AP1 transcription factor JunD and represses JunD-activated transcription. *Cell.* 1999;96:143–152.
14. Yumita W, Ikeo Y, Yamauchi K, et al. Suppression of insulin-induced AP-1 transactivation by menin accompanies inhibition of c-Fos induction. *Int J Cancer.* 2003;103:738–744.
15. Bassett JH, Forbes SA, Pannett AA, et al. Characterization of mutations in patients with multiple endocrine neoplasia type 1. *Am J Hum Genet.* 1998;62:232–244.
16. Mutch MG, Dilley WG, Sanjurjo F, et al. Germline mutations in the multiple endocrine neoplasia type 1 gene: evidence for frequent splicing defects. *Hum Mutat.* 1999;13: 175–185.
17. Bartsch D, Kopp I, Bergenfelz A, et al. MEN1 gene mutations in 12 MEN1 families and their associated tumors. *Eur J Endocrinol.* 1998;139:416–420.
18. Teh BT, Kytola S, Farnebo F, et al. Mutation analysis of the MEN1 gene in multiple endocrine neoplasia type 1, familial acromegaly and familial isolated hyperparathyroidism. *J Clin Endocrinol Metab.* 1998;83: 2621–2626.
19. Wataru Y, Ikeo Y, Yamauchi K, et al. Suppression of insulin-induced AP-1 transactivation by menin accompanies inhibition of c-Fos induction. *Int J Cancer.* 2003;103:738–744.
20. Giraud S, Zhang CX, Serova-Sinilnikova O, et al. Germline mutation analysis in patients with multiple endocrine neoplasia type 1 and related disorders. *Am J Hum Genet.* 1998;63:455–467.
21. Kouvaraki MA, Lee JE, Shapiro SE, et al. Genotype-phenotype analysis in multiple endocrine neoplasia type 1. *Arch Surg.* 2002;137:641–647.
22. Poncin J, Abs R, Velkeniers B, et al. Mutation analysis of the MEN1 gene in Belgian patients with multiple endocrine neoplasia type 1 and related diseases. *Hum Mutat.* 1999; 13:54–60.
23. Wautot V, Vercherat C, Lespinasse J, et al. Germline mutation profile of MEN1 in multiple endocrine neoplasia type 1: search for correlation between phenotype and the functional domains of the MEN1 protein. *Hum Mutat.* 2002;20:35–47.

24. Hessman O, Lindberg D, Einarsson A, et al. Genetic alterations on 3p, 11q13, and 18q in nonfamilial and MEN 1-associated pancreatic endocrine tumors. *Genes Chromosomes Cancer.* 1999;26:258–264.
25. Wang EH, Ebrahimi SA, Wu AY, et al. Mutation of the menin gene in sporadic pancreatic endocrine tumors. *Cancer Res.* 1998;58:4417–4420.
26. Friedrich CA. Von Hippel-Lindau syndrome: a pleomorphic condition. *Cancer.* 1999;86(11 Suppl):2478–2482.
27. Hammel PR, Vilgrain V, Terris B, et al. Pancreatic involvement in von Hippel-Lindau disease: the Groupe Francophone d'Etude de la Maladie de von Hippel-Lindau. *Gastroenterology.* 2000;119:1087–1095.
28. Libutti SK, Choyke PL, Bartlett DL, et al. Pancreatic neuroendocrine tumors associated with von Hippel-Lindau disease: diagnostic and management recommendations. *Surgery.* 1998;124:1153–1159.
29. Sgambati MT, Stolle C, Choyke PL, et al. Mosaicism in von Hippel-Lindau disease: lessons from kindreds with germline mutations identified in offspring with mosaic parents. *Am J Hum Genet.* 2000;66:84–91.
30. Mohr VH, Vortmeyer AO, Zhuang Z, et al. Histopathology and molecular genetics of multiple cysts and microcystic (serous) adenomas of the pancreas in von Hippel-Lindau patients. *Am J Pathol.* 2000;157:1615–1621.
31. Hes F, Zewald R, Peeters T, et al. Genotype-phenotype correlations in families with deletions in the von Hippel-Lindau (VHL) gene. *Hum Genet.* 2000;106:425–431.
32. Guo SS, Arora C, Shimoide AT, Sawicki MP. Frequent deletion of chromosome 3 in malignant sporadic pancreatic endocrine tumors. *Mol Cell Endocrinol.* 2002;190:109–114.
33. Hessman O, Skogseid B, Westin G, Akerstrom G. Multiple allelic deletions and intratumoral genetic heterogeneity in MEN1 pancreatic tumors. *J Clin Endocrinol Metab.* 2001;86:1355–1361.
34. Strodel WE, Vinik AI, Lloyd RV, et al. Pancreatic polypeptide-producing tumors. Silent lesions of the pancreas? *Arch Surg.* 1984;119:508–514.
35. Langstein HN, Norton JA, Chiang V, et al. The utility of circulating levels of human pancreatic polypeptide as a marker for islet cell tumors. *Surgery.* 1990;108:1109–1115.
36. Choksi UA, Sellin RV, Hickey RC, Samaan NA. An unusual skin rash associated with a pancreatic polypeptide-producing tumor of the pancreas. *Ann Intern Med.* 1988;108:64–65.
37. Mutch MG, Frisella MM, DeBenedetti MK, et al. Pancreatic polypeptide is a useful plasma marker for radiographically evident pancreatic islet cell tumors in patients with multiple endocrine neoplasia type 1. *Surgery.* 1997;122:1012–1019; discussion 1019–1020.
38. Adrian TE, Uttenthal LO, Williams SJ, Bloom SR. Secretion of pancreatic polypeptide in patients with pancreatic endocrine tumors. *N Engl J Med.* 1986;315:287–291.
39. Stridsberg M, Oberg K, Li Q, et al. Measurements of chromogranin A, chromogranin B (secretogranin I), chromogranin C (secretogranin II) and pancreastatin in plasma and urine from patients with carcinoid tumours and endocrine pancreatic tumours. *J Endocrinol.* 1995;144:49–59.
40. Nobels FR, Kwekkeboom DJ, Coopmans W, et al. Chromogranin A as serum marker for neuroendocrine neoplasia: comparison with neuron-specific enolase and the alpha-subunit of glycoprotein hormones. *J Clin Endocrinol Metab.* 1997;82:2622–2628.
41. Granberg D, Stridsberg M, Seensalu R, et al. Plasma chromogranin A in patients with multiple endocrine neoplasia type 1. *J Clin Endocrinol Metab.* 1999;84:2712–2717.
42. Prinz RA, Marangos PJ. Serum neuron-specific enolase: a serum marker for nonfunctioning pancreatic islet cell carcinoma. *Am J Surg.* 1983;145:77–81.
43. Eriksson B. Tumor markers for pancreatic endocrine tumors, including chromogranins HCG-alpha and HCG-beta. In: Mignon M, Jensen RT, eds. *Endocrine Tumors of the Pancreas: Recent Advances in Research and Management.* Basel, Switzerland: S. Karger; 1995:121.
44. Chiang HC, O'Dorisio TM, Huang SC, et al. Multiple hormone elevations in Zollinger-Ellison syndrome: prospective study of clinical significance and of the development of a second symptomatic pancreatic endocrine tumor syndrome. *Gastroenterology.* 1990;99:1565–1575.
45. Pilato FP, D'Adda T, Banchini E, Bordi C. Nonrandom expression of polypeptide hormones in pancreatic endocrine tumors: an immunohistochemical study in a case of multiple islet cell neoplasia. *Cancer.* 1988;61:1815–1820.
46. Jensen RT, Norton JA. Management of metastatic pancreatic endocrine tumors. In: Feldman M, Scharschmidt BF, Sleisenger MH, eds. *Gastrointestinal and Liver Disease.* Philadelphia: WB Saunders; 1998:871.
47. Friesen SR, Tomita T, Kimmel JR. Pancreatic polypeptide update: its roles in detection of the trait for multiple endocrine adenopathy syndrome, type I and pancreatic polypeptide-secreting tumors. *Surgery.* 1983;94:1028–1037.
48. Skogseid B, Eriksson B, Lundqvist G, et al. Multiple endocrine neoplasia type 1: a 10-year prospective screening study in four kindreds. *J Clin Endocrinol Metab.* 1991; 73:281–287.
49. Vinik AI, Moattari AR. Treatment of endocrine tumors of the pancreas. *Endocrinol Metab Clin North Am.* 1989;18: 483–518.
50. Peracchi M, Tagliabue R, Quatrini M, Reschini E. Plasma pancreatic polypeptide response to secretin. *Eur J Endocrinol.* 1999;141:47–49.
51. Thompson GB, van Heerden JA, Grant CS, et al. Islet cell carcinomas of the pancreas: a twenty-year experience. *Surgery.* 1988;104:1011–1017.
52. Friesen SR. Tumors of the endocrine pancreas. *N Engl J Med.* 1982;306:580–590.
53. Evans DB, Skibber JM, Lee JE, et al. Nonfunctioning islet cell carcinoma of the pancreas. *Surgery.* 1993;114:1175–1181.
54. Cheslyn-Curtis S, Sitaram V, Williamson RC. Management of non-functioning neuroendocrine tumours of the pancreas. *Br J Surg.* 1993;80:625–627.
55. Madura JA, Cummings OW, Wiebke EA, et al. Nonfunctioning islet cell tumors of the pancreas: a difficult diagnosis but one worth the effort. *Am Surg.* 1997;63:573–577.
56. Thompson NW, Eckhauser FE. Malignant islet-cell tumors of the pancreas. *World J Surg.* 1984;8:940–951.
57. Grama D, Skogseid B, Wilander E, et al. Pancreatic tumors in multiple endocrine neoplasia type 1: clinical presentation and surgical treatment. *World J Surg.* 1992;16:611–618.

58. Fuhrman GM, Charnsangavej C, Abbruzzese JL, et al. Thin-section contrast-enhanced computed tomography accurately predicts the resectability of malignant pancreatic neoplasms. *Am J Surg.* 1994;167:104–111.
59. Van Hoe L, Gryspeerdt S, Marchal G, et al. Helical CT for the preoperative localization of islet cell tumors of the pancreas: value of arterial and parenchymal phase images. *AJR Am J Roentgenol.* 1995;165:1437–1439.
60. Fuhrman GM, Leach SD, Staley CA, et al. Rationale for en bloc vein resection in the treatment of pancreatic adenocarcinoma adherent to the superior mesenteric–portal vein confluence: Pancreatic Tumor Study Group. *Ann Surg.* 1996;223:154–162.
61. Bold RJ, Charnsangavej C, Cleary KR, et al. Major vascular resection as part of pancreaticoduodenectomy for cancer: radiologic, intraoperative, and pathologic analysis. *J Gastrointest Surg.* 1999;3:233–243.
62. Cusack JC Jr, Fuhrman GM, Lee JE, Evans DB. Managing unsuspected tumor invasion of the superior mesenteric-portal venous confluence during pancreaticoduodenectomy. *Am J Surg.* 1994;168:352–354.
63. Carty SE, Jensen RT, Norton JA. Prospective study of aggressive resection of metastatic pancreatic endocrine tumors. *Surgery.* 1992;112:1024–1031.
64. McEntee GP, Nagorney DM, Kvols LK, et al. Cytoreductive hepatic surgery for neuroendocrine tumors. *Surgery.* 1990;108:1091–1096.
65. Solorzano CC, Lee JE, Pisters PWT, et al. Nonfunctioning islet cell carcinoma of the pancreas: survival results in a contemporary series of 163 patients. *Surgery.* 2000; 130:1078–1085.
66. Wiedenmann B, Jensen RT, Mignon M, et al. Preoperative diagnosis and surgical management of neuroendocrine gastroenteropancreatic tumors: general recommendations by a consensus workshop. *World J Surg.* 1998;22:309–18.
67. Bartsch DK, Langer P, Wild A, et al. Pancreaticoduodenal endocrine tumors in multiple endocrine neoplasia type 1: surgery or surveillance? *Surgery.* 2000;128:958–965.
68. Tyler DS, Evans DB. Reoperative pancreaticoduodenectomy. *Ann Surg.* 1994;219:211–221.
69. Baron PL, Aabakken LE, Cole DJ, et al. Differentiation of benign from malignant pancreatic masses by endoscopic ultrasound. *Ann Surg Oncol.* 1997;4:639–643.
70. Faigel DO, Ginsberg GG, Bentz JS, et al. Endoscopic ultrasound-guided real-time fine-needle aspiration biopsy of the pancreas in cancer patients with pancreatic lesions. *J Clin Oncol.* 1997;15:1439–1443.
71. Suits J, Frazee R, Erickson RA. Endoscopic ultrasound and fine needle aspiration for the evaluation of pancreatic masses. *Arch Surg.* 1999;134:639–642.
72. Takahashi H, Nakano K, Adachi Y, et al. Multiple nonfunctional pancreatic islet cell tumor in multiple endocrine neoplasia type I: a case report. *Acta Pathol Jpn.* 1988;38:667–682.
73. Thompson NW. Surgical treatment of the endocrine pancreas and Zollinger-Ellison syndrome in the MEN 1 syndrome. *Henry Ford Hosp Med J.* 1992;40:195–198.
74. Norton JA, Fraker DL, Alexander HR, et al. Surgery to cure the Zollinger-Ellison syndrome. *N Engl J Med.* 1999;341: 635–644.
75. Lowney JK, Frisella MM, Lairmore TC, Doherty GM. Pancreatic islet cell tumor metastasis in multiple endocrine neoplasia type 1: correlation with primary tumor size. *Surgery.* 124:1043–1048; discussion 1048–1049.
75a. Thompson NW. Management of pancreatic endocrine tumors in patients with multiple endocrine neoplasia type 1. *Surg Oncol Clin N Am.* 1998;7(4):881–891.
76. Slooter GD, Mearadji A, Breeman WA, et al. Somatostatin receptor imaging, therapy and new strategies in patients with neuroendocrine tumours. *Br J Surg.* 2001;88:31–40.
77. Bilchik AJ, Sarantou T, Foshag LJ, et al. Cryosurgical palliation of metastatic neuroendocrine tumors resistant to conventional therapy. *Surgery.* 1997;122:1040–1047.
78. Falconi M, Bassi C, Bonora A, et al. Role of chemoembolization in synchronous liver metastases from pancreatic endocrine tumours. *Dig Surg.* 1999;16:32–38.
79. Lehnert T. Liver transplantation for metastatic neuroendocrine carcinoma: an analysis of 103 patients. *Transplantation.* 1998;66:1307–1312.
80. Le Treut YP, Delpero JR, Dousset B, et al. Results of liver transplantation in the treatment of metastatic neuroendocrine tumors: a 31-case French multicentric report. *Ann Surg.* 1997;225:355–364.
81. Que FG, Nagorney DM, Batts KP, et al. Hepatic resection for metastatic neuroendocrine carcinomas. *Am J Surg.* 1995;169:36–42.
82. Evans DB, Abbruzzese JL, Willet CG. Cancer of the pancreas. In: DeVita VT, Jr, Hellman S, Rosenberg SA, eds. (6th ed.). Philadelphia: Lippincott; 2001:1126–1160.
83. Nagakawa T, Konishi I, Ueno K, et al. Extended radical pancreatectomy for carcinoma of the head of the pancreas. *Hepatogastroenterology.* 1998;45:849–854.
84. Nagakawa T, Konishi I, Ueno K, et al. Surgical treatment of pancreatic cancer: the Japanese experience. *Int J Pancreatol.* 1991;9:135–143.
85. Alessiani M, Tzakis A, Todo S, et al. Assessment of five-year experience with abdominal organ cluster transplantation. *J Am Coll Surg.* 1995;180:1–9.
86. Skogseid B. Nonsurgical treatment of advanced malignant neuroendocrine pancreatic tumors and midgut carcinoids. *World J Surg.* 2001;25:700–703.
87. Brentjens R, Saltz L. Islet cell tumors of the pancreas: the medical oncologist's perspective. *Surg Clin North Am.* 2001;81:527–542.
88. Tennvall J, Ljungberg O, Ahren B, et al. Radiotherapy for unresectable endocrine pancreatic carcinomas. *Eur J Surg Oncol.* 1992;18:73–76.
89. Bilchik AJ, Sarantou T, Foshag LJ, et al. Cryosurgical palliation of metastatic neuroendocrine tumors resistant to conventional therapy. *Surgery.* 1997;122:1040–1047.
90. Falconi M, Bassi C, Bonora A, et al. Role of chemoembolization in synchronous liver metastases from pancreatic endocrine tumours. *Dig Surg.* 1999;16:32–38.
91. Lehnert T. Liver transplantation for metastatic neuroendocrine carcinoma: an analysis of 103 patients. *Transplantation.* 1998;66:1307–1312.
92. Miller CA, Ellison EC. Therapeutic alternatives in metastatic neuroendocrine tumors. *Surg Oncol Clin N Am.* 1998;7:863–879.

93. Moertel CG, Hanley JA, Johnson LA. Streptozocin alone compared with streptozocin plus fluorouracil in the treatment of advanced islet-cell carcinoma. *N Engl J Med.* 1980;303:1189–1194.
94. Moertel CG, Lefkopoulo M, Lipsitz S, et al. Streptozocin-doxorubicin, streptozocin-fluorouracil or chlorozotocin in the treatment of advanced islet-cell carcinoma. *N Engl J Med.* 1992;326:519–523.
95. Chen H, Hardacre JM, Uzar A, et al. Isolated liver metastases from neuroendocrine tumors: does resection prolong survival? *J Am Coll Surg.* 1998;187:88–92; discussion 92–93.
96. Sarmiento JM, Que FG, Grant CS, et al. Concurrent resections of pancreatic islet cell cancers with synchronous hepatic metastases: outcomes of an aggressive approach. *Surgery.* 2002;132:976–982; discussion 982–983.
97. Chamberlain RS, Canes D, Brown KT, et al. Hepatic neuroendocrine metastases: does intervention alter outcomes? *J Am Coll Surg.* 2000;190:432–445.
98. Chung MH, Pisegna J, Spirt M, et al. Hepatic cytoreduction followed by a novel long-acting somatostatin analog: a paradigm for intractable neuroendocrine tumors metastatic to the liver. *Surgery.* 2001;130:954–962.
99. Siperstein AE, Berber E. Cryoablation, percutaneous alcohol injection, and radiofrequency ablation for treatment of neuroendocrine liver metastases. *World J Surg.* 2001;25:693–696.
100. Yao KA, Talamonti MS, Nemcek A, et al. Indications and results of liver resection and hepatic chemoembolization for metastatic gastrointestinal neuroendocrine tumors. *Surgery.* 2001;130:677–682; discussion 682–685.
101. Proye C. Natural history of liver metastasis of gastroenteropancreatic neuroendocrine tumors: place for chemoembolization. *World J Surg.* 2001;25:685–688.
102. Eriksson BK, Larsson EG, Skogseid BM, et al. Liver embolizations of patients with malignant neuroendocrine gastrointestinal tumors. *Cancer.* 1998;83:2293–2301.
103. Falconi M, Bassi C, Bonora A, et al. Role of chemoembolization in synchronous liver metastases from pancreatic endocrine tumours. *Dig Surg.* 1999;16:32–38.
104. Carroll NM, Alexander HR, Jr. Isolation perfusion of the liver. *Cancer J.* 2002;8:181–93.

CHAPTER 48

Management of Metastatic Islet Cell Carcinoma

James C. Yao, MD
Maria A. Kouvaraki, MD, PhD
Sanjay Gupta, MD

Islet cell carcinomas, which are relatively uncommon cancers of the pancreas, may have dramatic manifestations ranging from intractable diarrhea to variceal bleeding. Some patients present with bowel or biliary obstruction, whereas in others, tumors may be found incidentally during surgery for unrelated reasons.

The epidemiology of islet cell carcinoma has not been well described. In examining data of the Surveillance, Epidemiology, and End Results Program (SEER), we observed an incidence of 0.3 per 100,000 in 1999.[1] Sixty-seven percent of islet cell patients who were staged had developed a metastases at the time of diagnosis. Among the estimated population of 292 million, we can expect approximately 880 new cases of islet cell carcinoma in 2003; of these, 590 will have metastasized at diagnosis.

Although islet cell carcinoma is frequently indolent in its clinical behavior, it can also be aggressive and resistant to treatment. In the SEER database, the median survival of patients with metastatic islet cell carcinoma diagnosed from 1992 through 1999 was only 21 months (Fig. 48.1).[1] However, long-term survival beyond 8 years has also been reported among patients with metastatic disease.

Management of patients with metastatic islet cell carcinoma requires an understanding of the disease process and a multimodalities approach. Here we review the various strategies for treating patients who have metastatic islet cell carcinomas.

Chemotherapy

Systemic chemotherapy has been studied in a small number of phase II clinical trials. Because the disease is relatively rare, patients with carcinoid and pancreatic endocrine tumors were grouped together in many of these trials. Further complicating the interpretation of the data was the fact that earlier trials often counted as a response either a drop in biochemical markers or a shrinkage in tumor size. Since the introduction of somatostatin analogues for symptom control, we have advocated objective tumor shrinkage as the standard for judging therapeutic effectiveness.

Single-Agent Therapy

Streptozocin is the single agent that has been most widely studied in islet cell carcinoma. Its clinical benefit was first reported in 1973 by Broder and Carter.[2]

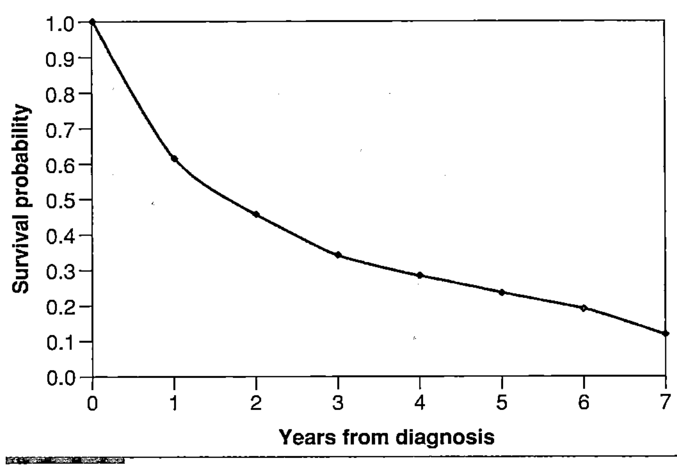

Figure 48.1
Survival of 375 patients with metastatic islet cell carcinoma in the SEER 11 database. Pancreatic primary and ICD-O-2 histology code 8150-8157 and 8240-8249 were used to select patients. The median survival was 21 months. Survival rates at 1, 2, 3, 4, and 5 years were 61%, 46%, 34%, 28%, and 24%, respectively.

The authors reported a response rate of 50% in 52 of the patients treated in that study. Subsequently, in one arm of a randomized trial, Moertel et al.[3] treated 42 patients with streptozocin alone and observed a response in 14 patients (36%). These investigators also studied doxorubicin in a single-arm phase II trial, finding evidence of a response in 4 of 20 patients (20%). Chlorozotocin demonstrated clinical activity in two single-agent clinical trials. In one small phase II trial, investigators demonstrated a response in 7 of 17 patients (42%).[4] Subsequently, chlorozotocin was studied as one arm of a randomized trial in which 10 of 33 patients (30%) receiving chlorozotocin responded to therapy.[5] Despite this evidence of therapeutic activity, chlorozotocin is not commercially available at this time.

Dacarbazine has also been studied in islet cell carcinoma. In a small trial with 11 islet cell patients, 1 patient (9%) had responded to the treatment.[6] However, in a subsequent phase II trial that included 42 patients with measurable disease, a 33% response rate was observed.[7]

5-Fluorouracil has often been included in combination chemotherapy regimens for islet cell carcinoma, yet its activity as a single agent has not been studied in clinical trials. An anecdotal report of complete response was published 15 years ago.[8] Other evidence of activity is inferred from a clinical trial that showed a higher response rate for the combination of 5-fluorouracil and streptozocin than for streptozocin alone.[3] Etoposide and carboplatin have also been studied as single agents in phase II settings, although clinical activity was not observed.[9,10]

Combination Chemotherapy

As several single agents showed moderate clinical activity, combination chemotherapy trials were conducted in hope of improving the outcome. Among the combinations, 5-fluorouracil plus streptozocin is the most thoroughly tested regimen. In four separate studies of 7, 43, 33, and 31 patients, respective response rates of 29%, 63%, 45%, and 54% were observed.[3,5,11,12]

This combination was then tested against the combination of streptozocin plus doxorubicin by the Eastern Cooperative Oncology Group.[5] The doxorubicin-containing regimen resulted in a higher response rate (69% vs 45%; $P = 0.05$) and longer time to disease progression (2.2 vs 1.4 years; $P = 0.004$). However, in a recent retrospective review of 16 cases at Memorial Sloan-Kettering Cancer Center, only 1 response (6%) was observed.[13] This 10-fold difference in response rates has aroused considerable controversy about the role of chemotherapy in treating islet cell carcinoma. Some differences may be accounted for by the fact that, in the earlier studies, either a decrease in biochemical parameters or a decrease in tumor measurement was counted as a response. For example, in a study by Eriksson et al.,[14] the response rates based on either decreased biochemical parameters or decreased tumor measurement were 36% for streptozocin plus doxorubicin and 58% for streptozocin plus 5-fluorouracil. When only radiologic response was counted, the response rates were 8% and 32%.[14]

Triple-combination chemotherapy consisting of 5-fluorouracil, streptozocin, and doxorubicin has been studied in two small trials with 10 and 12 patients whose response rates were 40% and 55%, respectively.[15,16] In light of the continuing controversy regarding the role of chemotherapy in the management of unresectable and metastatic islet cell carcinoma, we recently reviewed our experience with 84 patients treated with the 5-fluorouracil streptozocin and doxorubicin combination. Thirty-two patients (38%) had a radiologic response to treatment as determined by the Response Evaluation Criteria in Solid Tumors (RECIST) criteria.[17] A full multivariate analysis of the effect of tumor, patient, and treatment-related factors on response, time to progression, and survival is under way. We have also observed significant cytoreduction of locally advanced islet cell carcinoma that allowed some patients with otherwise unresectable tumors to undergo surgery (Fig. 48.2). Systemic chemotherapy is important in the management of patients with metastatic or unresectable islet cell carcinoma. We recommend combination chemotherapy for selected patients with symptomatic, bulky, or progressive disease. The regimens we recommend are summarized in Table 48.1.

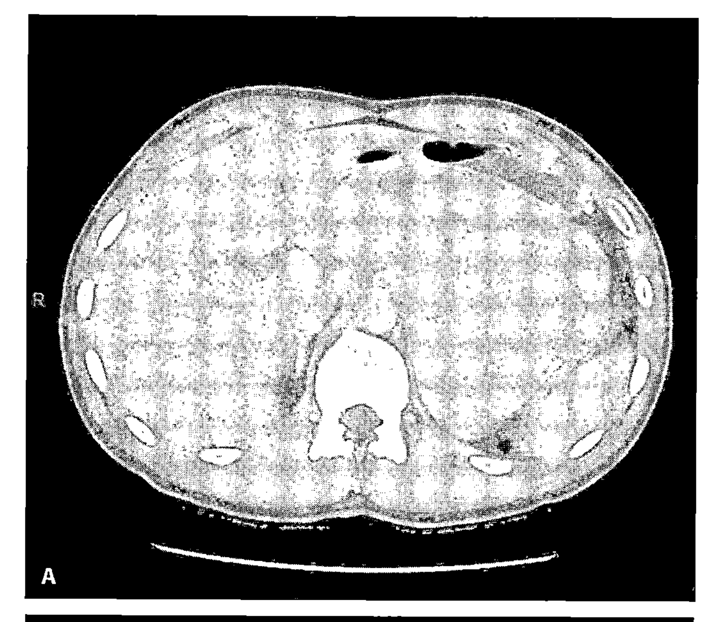

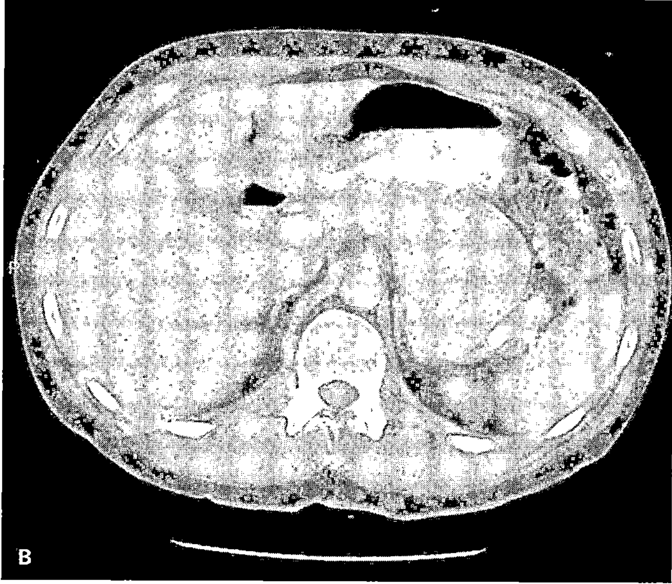

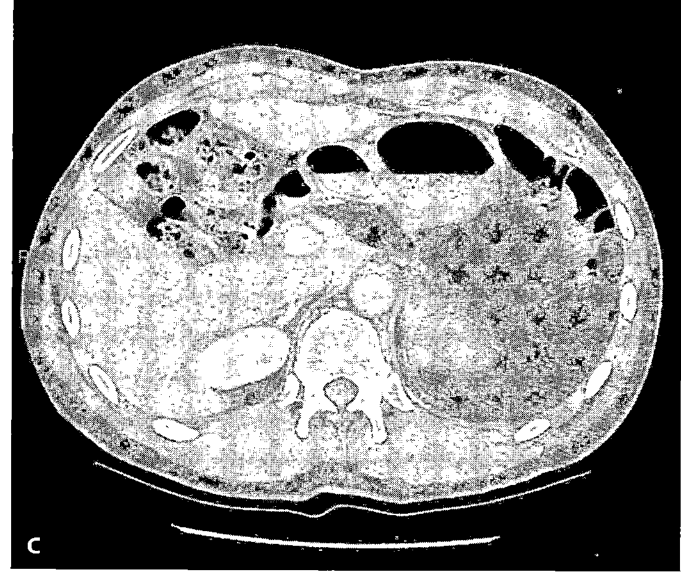

Figure 48.2
CAT Scan demonstrates a patient with locally advanced islet cell carcinoma whose response to 5-fluorouracil, streptozocin, and doxorubicin chemotherapy-enabled surgical resection. **(A)** Pretreatment. **(B)** After 10 courses of 5-fluorouracil, streptozocin, and doxorubicin. **(C)** After surgical resection.

Table 48.1 Selected Chemotherapy Regimens for Islet Cell Carcinoma

5-Fluorouracil, streptozocin, and doxorubicin—28-day cycle
5-Fluorouracil 400 mg/m^2/day intravenous bolus days 1–5
Streptozocin 400 mg/m^2/day intravenous days 1–5
Doxorubicin 40 mg/m^2 on day 1 only
5-Fluorouracil and streptozocin—42-day cycle
5-Fluorouracil 400 mg/m^2/day intravenous bolus days 1–5
Streptozocin 500 mg/m^2/day intravenous days 1–5
Streptozocin and doxorubicin—42-day cycle
Streptozocin 500 mg/m^2/day intravenous days 1–4
Doxorubicin 50 mg/m^2 on days 1 and 22

Biologic Therapy

Somatostatin Analogues

Somatostatin is a hormone that binds to specific high-affinity membrane receptors on target tissues, such as the brain, pancreas, pituitary, and gastrointestinal tract, and on neoplastic tissue.[18-20] To date, five subtypes of somatostatin receptors have been identified.[21] Studies have shown all five subtypes to bind to somatostatin with high affinity.[22] Synthetic analogues have differing binding profiles. With octreotide, a somatostatin analogue, high-affinity binding is observed for type 2 and type 5 receptors, low affinity for type 1 and type 4, and medium affinity for type 3.[22]

Somatostatin inhibits the release of a number of hormones, including growth hormone, insulin, glucagon, gastrin, and secretin. It also regulates exocrine secretions,[18,19,22] glandular secretions, neurotransmission, smooth-muscle contractility, and absorption of nutrients.[18,19,23]

Somatostatin is cytostatic to tumor cells.[24,25] Proposed mechanisms for this effect include indirect inhibition of autocrine, paracrine, or endocrine growth factors (growth hormone, insulin-like growth factor, or its related peptides); direct binding of somatostatin receptors; and antiangiogenetic properties.[26-28] Indeed, in one colon cancer study, octreotide was shown to reduce tissue and serum vascular endothelial growth factor levels.[29]

Clinically, the use of somatostatin is limited by its short half-life. Somatostatin analogues, with longer half-lives, are helpful in controlling hormone-related symptoms in a majority of patients. Octreotide, with a half-life of 90–120 minutes, is frequently given at 50–500 μg subcutaneously three times a day. Longer acting somatostatin analogues have obviated the need for multiple daily injections in most patients. Lanreotide, a long-acting somatostatin analogue given every 10–14 days, is effective against carcinoid syndrome.[30] Depot octreotide given as a 10- to 30-mg intramuscular injection has a longer half-life; it make take up to 12 weeks to reach steady state and may be given once a month.[31] Among symptomatic patients, the concurrent use of subcutaneous octreotide is advised for 14 days after the first injection of octreotide long-acting release (LAR) to allow the depot formulation to take effect. Higher doses have been used for which a clear benefit is yet to be demonstrated.

Anecdotal reports of tumor shrinkage with octreotide have been reported in carcinoid and islet cell carcinomas. In a larger series, tumor shrinkage was infrequently observed.[32,33] One exception was the case of a gastric carcinoid lesion arising in a patient with hypergastrinemia. Successful suppression of gastrin output with somatostatin analogues may result in the regression of primary gastric carcinoid in this setting.[34,35] Stabilization of growing neuroendocrine tumors has also been reported,[32,33] but definitive randomized trials are lacking.

Interferon

With interferon, also used in therapy of low-grade neuroendocrine carcinoma, a decrease in hormone production has been observed, although the mechanism of action is not well understood. Possible mechanisms include direct inhibition of cell proliferation, immune cell-mediated cytotoxicity, and induction of differentiation. Interferon may also block the cell cycle in the G0/G1 phase by dephosphorylation of the retinoblastoma gene.[36,37] Furthermore, interferon can downregulate the transcription factor Sp1 and inhibit angiogenesis.[38,39]

Interferon activity has been described by a number of investigators. However, many of the studies have included a mix of gastrointestinal carcinoids and a small number of islet cell carcinomas.[40-42] In one study, 57 patients with islet cell carcinoma were treated with interferon. Biochemical responses were observed in 27 patients (47%), whereas radiologic responses were observed in only 7 patients (12%). Currently, interferon is used infrequently to control hormonal symptoms because its toxic effects, fever, fatigue, anorexia, weight loss, and depression with chronic use. Newer pegylated formulations hold promise.

Ablative Therapy

Hepatic Artery Embolization

Despite the considerable activity that has been observed with front-line combination chemotherapy, patients are rarely cured of their disease. Second-line chemotherapy is far less effective. Because the liver is the most common site of metastasis, therapy has been directed to the liver region. Hepatic artery embolization takes advantage of the liver's dual blood supply. The normal liver derives only 25% of its blood supply from the hepatic artery, whereas metastases receive 95% of their blood supply from that artery. Thus, interruption of the hepatic artery supply preferentially causes ischemic necrosis of the metastases while sparing most of the normal liver.

Early studies of vascular occlusion involved surgical ligation of the common hepatic artery. Despite early successes, responses were usually short-lived because of rapid development of collateral vessel circulation.[43] Techniques of creating transient ischemia[44] and more selective embolization of the tumor vasculature[45] were developed to reduce reactive angiogenesis and collateral formation. Currently, most procedures follow a percutaneous approach. In hepatic artery chemoembolization before the vessels are blocked, cytotoxic agents are administered intra-arterially. This approach has the potential of delivering a higher dose of chemotherapy to liver metastases.

Trials of hepatic arterial vascular occlusion have produced biochemical responses of 13%–52% and tumor responses of 37%–38%.[44,46,47] From trials using chemoembolization or intra-arterial chemotherapy in addition to embolization, the reported biochemical response rates have ranged from 47%–91% and the tumor response rates from 8%–60%.[48-54] There are no data from randomized trials.

We recently reviewed the M. D. Anderson Cancer Center experience with hepatic artery embolization in patients with islet cell carcinomas. From 1992 through 2000, 54 patients with islet cell carcinoma underwent hepatic artery embolization (32 patients) or hepatic artery chemoembolization (22 patients). Most had bulky liver metastases. In 21 patients (39%), more than 50% of the liver was replaced by cancerous lesions. Objective tumor response as documented by computed tomography was observed in 37% of all treated patients, and a reduction of tumor-related symptoms was observed in 59%.

When the blend embolization group was compared with the chemoembolization group, an improved response rate (50% vs 28%, $P = 0.024$) was observed with the addition of chemotherapy.

Based on these findings, we recommend hepatic artery chemoembolization in selected patients. The procedures should be carried out in a hospital setting because treatment-related toxic effects are common and may be severe. A constellation of transient symptoms and laboratory abnormalities, sometimes referred to as "postembolization syndrome," occurs in most patients. This includes abdominal pain, nausea, fever, fatigue, and elevation of liver enzymes. Crises related to massive hormonal release may occur in the presence of functional tumors. Prophylactic administration of somatostatin analogues should be considered. Major complications (even deaths) have been reported in clinical trials; they include gastrointestinal bleeding, gastric and duodenal ulceration, hepatic abscesses, ischemic necrosis of the gallbladder and small bowel, sepsis, renal failure, hepatorenal syndrome, portal vein thrombosis, arterial thrombosis, and arrhythmia. To minimize the risk of hepatic insufficiency, embolization should be carried out in one liver lobe at a time. In patients with bulky disease or poor liver function, more limited embolization of liver segments should be considered.

Surgical Resection and Liver Transplantation

Because of the relatively indolent behavior of the disease, aggressive surgical resection has a role management of metastatic islet cell carcinoma. Que et al.[55] reported the results of a study of 74 patients undergoing hepatic resection for neuroendocrine tumors. Twenty-three patients had islet cell carcinoma, whereas the rest had the carcinoid type. An overall 4-year survival rate of 73% was reported for the entire group. However, even when resection with curative intent was possible, relapses were common. In this selected group of 74 patients, two perioperative deaths (2.7%) were reported, and major complications occurred in 18 patients (24%).

In the setting of metastatic disease, we encourage resection for patients with solitary metastasis. Among patients with more extensive but still resectable disease, we advocate resection for those with favorable biologic characteristics. Liver resection should be avoided in patients with intermediate and high-grade histologic subtypes. A period of systemic chemotherapy or trial of hepatic artery chemoembolization may be used as part of a test-of-time approach to selecting patients whose disease is less likely to progress rapidly and who are therefore more likely to benefit from aggressive surgical intervention.

Finally, hepatic transplantation has been explored as an option for patients with unresectable disease. Operative morbidity and mortality are substantial, and data on survival benefits are lacking. In one series,[56] the authors showed that survival duration after liver transplantation was inferior for patients with islet cell carcinoma compared with that of patients who had carcinoid tumors (3-year survival, 8% vs 80%). The role of hepatic transplantation in the management of metastatic islet cell tumors remains to be defined.

Approaches to Treatment for Metastatic Islet Cell Carcinoma

The combination of somewhat slow tumor growth and few established treatment options presents unique and challenging treatment decisions to the practicing oncologist. A general approach to the treatment of this disease is outlined in Table 48.2.

Localized disease should be surgically excised whenever possible. When metastases are present, treatments should be tailored to the volume and site of the tumor and the general condition of the patient. Treatment with long-acting somatostatin analogues such as depot octreotide or lanreotide should be considered whenever a patient has hormonal syndrome.

Patients with low-volume asymptomatic metastatic disease may remain under observation. Computed tomography using three-phase contrast enhancement, magnetic resonance imaging, and plasma chromogranin A level may be used to assess tumor biology and changes in tumor volume. Patients with bulky, symptomatic, or progressive disease should undergo streptozocin-based systemic chemotherapy. Hepatic artery chemoembolization may be an effective palliative strategy for patients in whom chemotherapy for hepatic dominant disease has

Table 48.2 Approaches to Treatment of Islet Cell Carcinoma

Disease State	Tumor Volume	Hormonal Syndrome	Recommendation
Localized primary tumor	Any	Any	Surgical resection if possible
Single liver metastasis	Low	Any	Surgical resection or other ablative approaches*
Advanced disease, any site	Low	No	Consider observation alone, chemotherapy, or clinical trials
Advanced disease, any site	Any	Yes	Long-acting somatostatin analogues; consider clinical trials or interferon-α
Advanced disease, any site	Low but progressive	Any	Chemotherapy, clinical trials, or interferon-α
Advanced disease, liver metastasis only	High (>50% liver involvement)	Any	Chemotherapy, clinical trial, hepatic arterial vascular occlusion therapy; long-acting somatostatin analogues for patients with syndrome
Advanced disease, extrahepatic	High	Any	Chemotherapy or clinical trial; long-acting somatostatin analogues for patients with syndrome

* Cryoablation, radiofrequency ablation, alcohol injection

failed. Enrollment of patients in clinical trials should be encouraged whenever possible.

In this disease, which has an often diverse but relatively long natural history, better clinical and biological predictors of prognosis are needed to initiate appropriate treatment at all stages. Investigations in tumor biology such as the roles of *p53*, *bcl-2*, *bax*, *MEN1*, *FGF*, *TGF*, *PDGF*, and *VEGF* expression need to be expanded. Clinical trials with newer agents that affect angiogenesis, epidermal growth factor receptor, and apoptosis hold promise for the future.

References

1. Surveillance, Epidemiology, and End Results (SEER) Program (1973–1999). National Cancer Institute, DCCPS, Surveillance Research Program. Cancer Statistic Branch; 2001.
2. Broder LE, Carter SK. Pancreatic islet cell carcinoma: II: results of therapy with streptozotocin in 52 patients. *Ann Intern Med.* 1973;79:108–118.
3. Moertel CG, Hanley JA, Johnson LA. Streptozocin alone compared with streptozocin plus fluorouracil in the treatment of advanced islet-cell carcinoma. *N Eng J Med.* 1980;303:1189–1194.
4. Bukowski RM, McCracken JD, Balcerzak SP, et al. Phase II study of chlorozotocin in islet cell carcinoma: a Southwest Oncology Group study. *Cancer Chemother Pharmacol.* 1983;11:48–50.
5. Moertel CG, Lefkopoulo M, Lipsitz S, et al. Streptozocin-doxorubicin, streptozocin-fluorouracil or chlorozotocin in the treatment of advanced islet-cell carcinoma. *N Engl J Med.* 1992;326:519–523.
6. Altimari AF, Badrinath K, Reisel HJ, et al. DTIC therapy in patients with malignant intra-abdominal neuroendocrine tumors. *Surgery.* 1987;102:1009–1017.
7. Ramanathan RK, Cnaan A, Hahn RG, et al. Phase II trial of dacarbazine (DTIC) in advanced pancreatic islet cell carcinoma: study of the Eastern Cooperative Oncology Group-E6282. *Ann Oncol.* 2001;12:1139–1143.
8. Hansen R, Helm J, Wilson JF, et al. Nonfunctioning islet cell carcinoma of the pancreas: complete response to continuous 5-fluorouracil infusion. *Cancer.* 1988;62:15–17.
9. Saltz L, Lauwers G, Wiseberg J, et al. A phase II trial of carboplatin in patients with advanced APUD tumors. *Cancer.* 1993;72:619–622.
10. Kelsen D, Fiore J, Heelan R, et al. Phase II trial of etoposide in APUD tumors. *Cancer Treat Rep.* 1987;71:305–307.
11. Chernicoff D, Bukowski RM, Groppe CW Jr, et al. Combination chemotherapy for islet cell carcinoma and metastatic carcinoid tumors with 5-fluorouracil and streptozotocin. *Cancer Treat Rep.* 1979;63:795–796.
12. Eriksson B, Oberg K. An update of the medical treatment of malignant endocrine pancreatic tumors. *Acta Oncol.* 1993;32:203–208.
13. Cheng PN, Saltz LB. Failure to confirm major objective antitumor activity for streptozocin and doxorubicin in the treatment of patients with advanced islet cell carcinoma. *Cancer.* 1999;86:944–948.
14. Eriksson B, Skogseid B, Lundqvist G, et al. Medical treatment and long-term survival in a prospective study of 84 patients with endocrine pancreatic tumors. *Cancer.* 1990;65:1883–1890.
15. von Schrenck T, Howard JM, Doppman JL, et al. Prospective study of chemotherapy in patients with metastatic gastrinoma. *Gastroenterology.* 1988;94:1326–1334.

16. Rivera E, Ajani JA. Doxorubicin, streptozocin, and 5-fluorouracil chemotherapy for patients with metastatic islet-cell carcinoma. *Am J Clin Oncol.* 1998;21:36–38.
17. Therasse P, Arbuck SG, Eisenhauer EA, et al. New guidelines to evaluate the response to treatment in solid tumors: European Organization for Research and Treatment of Cancer, National Cancer Institute of the United States, National Cancer Institute of Canada. *J Natl Cancer Inst.* 2000; 92:205–216.
18. Reichlin S. Somatostatin. *N Engl J Med.* 1983;309:1495–1501.
19. Reichlin S. Somatostatin (second of two parts). *N Engl J Med.* 1983;309:1556–1563.
20. Lamberts S, Krenning E, Reubi J. The role of somatostatin and its analogs in the diagnosis and treatment of tumors. *Endocr Rev.* 1991;12:450–482.
21. Adams S, Baum RP, Hertel A, et al. Metabolic (PET) and receptor (SPET) imaging of well- and less well-differentiated tumours: comparison with the expression of the Ki-67 antigen. *Nucl Med Commun.* 1998;19:641–647.
22. Bruns C, Weckbecker G, Raulf F, et al. Molecular pharmacology of somatostatin-receptor subtypes. *Ann NY Acad Sci.* 1994;733:138–146.
23. Lambert P, Minghini A, Pincus W, et al. Treatment and prognosis of primary malignant small bowel tumors. *Am Surg.* 1996;62:709–715.
24. Lamberts S, Uitterlinden P, Verschoor L, et al. Long term treatment of acromegaly with the somatosatin analogue SMS201–995. *N Engl J Med.* 1985;313:1576–1580.
25. Schally A. Oncological applications of somatostatin analogue. *Cancer Res.* 1988;48:6977–6985.
26. Hillman N, Herranz L, Alvarez C, et al. Efficacy of octreotide in the regression of a metastatic carcinoid tumour despite negative imaging with In-111-pentetreotide (Octreoscan). *Exp Clin Endocrinol Diabetes.* 1998;106: 226–230.
27. Kvols LK, Moertel CG, O'Connell MJ, et al. Treatment of the malignant carcinoid syndrome: evaluation of a long-acting somatostatin analogue. *N Engl J Med.* 1986;315:663–666.
28. Oberg K. Treatment of neuroendocrine tumors. *Cancer Treat Rev.* 1994;20:331–355.
29. Cascinu S, Del Ferro E, Ligi M, et al. Inhibition of vascular endothelial growth factor by octreotide in colorectal cancer patients. *Cancer Invest.* 2001;19:8–12.
30. Tomassetti P, Migliori M, Gullo L. Slow-release lanreotide treatment in endocrine gastrointestinal tumors. *Am J Gastroenterol.* 1998;93:1468–1471.
31. Rubin J, Ajani J, Schirmer W, et al. Octreotide acetate long-acting formulation versus open-label subcutaneous octreotide acetate in malignant carcinoid syndrome. *J Clin Oncol.* 1999;17:600–606.
32. Arnold R, Trautmann ME, Creutzfeldt W, et al. Somatostatin analogue octreotide and inhibition of tumour growth in metastatic endocrine gastroenteropancreatic tumours. *Gut.* 1996;38:430–438.
33. Saltz L, Trochanowski B, Buckley M, et al. Octreotide as an antineoplastic agent in the treatment of functional and nonfunctional neuroendocrine tumors. *Cancer.* 1993;72:244–248.
34. Tomassetti P, Migliori M, Caletti GC, et al. Treatment of type II gastric carcinoid tumors with somatostatin analogues. *N Engl J Med.* 2000;343:551–554.
35. Ferraro G, Annibale B, Marignani M, et al. Effectiveness of octreotide in controlling fasting hypergastrinemia and related enterochromaffin-like cell growth. *J Clin Endocrinol Metab.* 1996;81:677–683.
36. Hanssen LE, Schrumpf E, Kolbenstvedt AN, et al. Treatment of malignant metastatic midgut carcinoid tumours with recombinant human alpha2b interferon with or without prior hepatic artery embolization. *Scand J Gastroenterol.* 1989;24:787–795.
37. Oberg K. Chemotherapy and biotherapy in neuroendocrine tumors. *Curr Opin Oncol.* 1993;5:110–120.
38. von Marschall Z, Scholz A, Cramer T, et al. Effects of interferon alpha on vascular endothelial growth factor gene transcription and tumor angiogenesis. *J Natl Cancer Inst.* 2003;95:437–448.
39. Valimaki M, Jarvinen H, Salmela P, et al. Is the treatment of metastatic carcinoid tumor with interferon not as successful as suggested? *Cancer.* 1991;67:547–549.
40. Biesma B, Willemse PH, Mulder NH, et al. Recombinant interferon alpha-2b in patients with metastatic apudomas: effect on tumours and tumour markers. *Br J Cancer.* 1992;66:850–855.
41. Schober C, Schmoll E, Schmoll HJ, et al. Antitumour effect and symptomatic control with interferon alpha 2b in patients with endocrine active tumours. *Eur J Cancer.* 1992; 10:1664–1666.
42. Bajetta E, Zilembo N, Di Bartolomeo M, et al. Treatment of metastatic carcinoids and other neuroendocrine tumors with recombinant interferon-alpha-2a: a study by the Italian Trials in Medical Oncology Group. *Cancer.* 1993;72:3099–3105.
43. Ajani J, Humberto C, Wallace S. Neuroendocrine tumors metastatic to the liver: vascular occlusion therapy. *Ann NY Acad Sci.* 1994;733:479–487.
44. Nobin A, Mansson B, Lunderquist A. Evaluation of temporary liver dearterialization and embolization in patients with metastatic carcinoid tumour. *Acta Oncol.* 1989;28:419–424.
45. Chuang VP, Soo CS, Carrasco CH, et al. Superselective catheterization technique in hepatic angiography. *Am J Radiol.* 1983;141:803–811.
46. Carrasco CH, Charnsangavej C, Ajani J, et al. The carcinoid syndrome: palliation by hepatic artery embolization. *AJR Am J Roentgenol.* 1986;147:149–154.
47. Eriksson BK, Larsson EG, Skogseid BM, et al. Liver embolizations of patients with malignant neuroendocrine gastrointestinal tumors. *Cancer.* 1998;83:2293–2301.
48. Ruszniewski P, Rougier P, Roche A, et al. Hepatic arterial chemoembolization in patients with liver metastases of endocrine tumors: a prospective phase II study in 24 patients. *Cancer.* 1993;71:2624–2630.
49. Therasse E, Breittmayer F, Roche A, et al. Transcatheter chemoembolization of progressive carcinoid liver metastasis. *Radiology.* 1993;189:541–547.
50. Perry LJ, Stuart K, Stokes KR, et al. Hepatic arterial chemoembolization for metastatic neuroendocrine tumors. *Surgery.* 1994;116:1111–1116.

51. Diaco DS, Hajarizadeh H, Mueller CR, et al. Treatment of metastatic carcinoid tumors using multimodality therapy of octreotide acetate, intra-arterial chemotherapy, and hepatic arterial chemoembolization. *Am J Surg.* 1995;169:523–528.
52. Drougas JG, Anthony LB, Blair TK, et al. Hepatic artery chemoembolization for management of patients with advanced metastatic carcinoid tumors. *Am J Surg.* 1998;175: 408–412.
53. Diamandidou E, Ajani JA, Yang DJ, et al. Two-phase study of hepatic artery vascular occlusion with microencapsulated cisplatin in patients with liver metastases from neuroendocrine tumors. *AJR Am J Roentgenol.* 1998;170:339–344.
54. Kim YH, Ajani JA, Carrasco CH, et al. Selective hepatic arterial chemoembolization for liver metastases in patients with carcinoid tumor or islet cell carcinoma. *Cancer Invest.* 1999;17:474–478.
55. Que FG, Nagorney DM, Batts KP, et al. Hepatic resection for metastatic neuroendocrine carcinomas. *Am J Surg.* 1995;169:36–42; discussion 42–43.
56. Treut YP, Delpero J, Dousset B, et al. Results of liver transplantation in the treatment of metastatic neuroendocrine tumors. *Ann Surg.* 1997;225:355–364.

4

Periampullary Tumors

CHAPTER 49

Pathology of Periampullary Tumors

Mari Mino, MD
Gregory Y. Lauwers, MD

The ampulla of Vater is the small anatomic compartment formed by the junction of the common bile duct and the main pancreatic duct before they open into the duodenum. The ampulla is encircled by bundles of smooth muscle derived from the musculature of the duodenum that forms the sphincter of Oddi and is interspersed with numerous glands. However, in practice, the ampulla of Vater is more broadly defined as the junction of the biliary and pancreatic ducts with the duodenum.[1] Given this strategic location, neoplasms of the ampulla are of obvious clinical importance, and icterus is the presenting symptom in most patients.

The frequency of ampullary neoplasms is low compared with that of neoplasms arising in other segments of the gastrointestinal tract, with the reported incidence at autopsy varying between 0.04% and 0.12%.[2-4] Notably, a significant proportion (37%–95%) of epithelial neoplasms involving the ampulla of Vater are malignant.[4-6]

Benign Epithelial Neoplasms

Ampullary Adenoma, Intestinal Type

Small intestinal adenomas have a propensity to aggregate around the ampulla and, to a lesser degree, the duodenum.[7-10] Approximately 50% of small-intestinal adenomas involve the papilla, whereas another 25% are distributed throughout the duodenum.[9] Ampullary adenomas of the intestinal type are encountered in two distinct clinical scenarios, either sporadic or in the setting of *familial adenomatous polyposis* (FAP).

Although uncommon in the general population, sporadic ampullary adenomas are being recognized more frequently because of the increased use of upper endoscopy. The patients are usually in the 6th decade of life (range, 30–80 years of age), and the adenomas measure an average of about 2 cm.[11,12] Although some reports claim that women outnumber men by more than 2 to 1, this experience is not shared by all investigators.[3,4,9,12,13]

Ampullary and periampullary adenomas are present in 50%–85.7% of patients with FAP.[14] Males and females are equally represented, and the median age is between 30 and 40 years.[14] In these patients, the adenomas can be multiple and involve the mucosal surface and the ampullary channels simultaneously.[14,15] Notably, microscopic changes may be observed even when the ampulla appears endoscopically normal.[14] Adenomas in patients with FAP are diagnosed within a mean follow-up of 17 years after colectomies for polyposis were performed.[2] During an extended surveillance of more than 10 years, the follow-up of 18 pa-

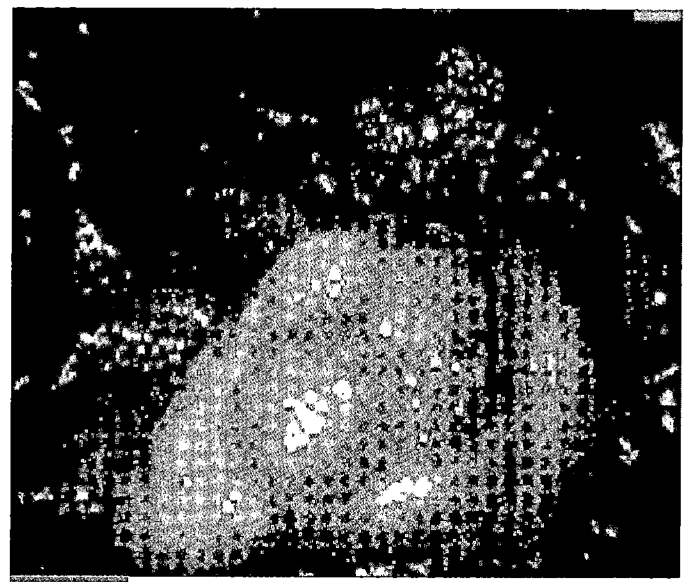

Figure 49.1
Endoscopic appearance of ampullary tubular adenoma. The papilla is covered by a reddish plaque of coarser mucosa.

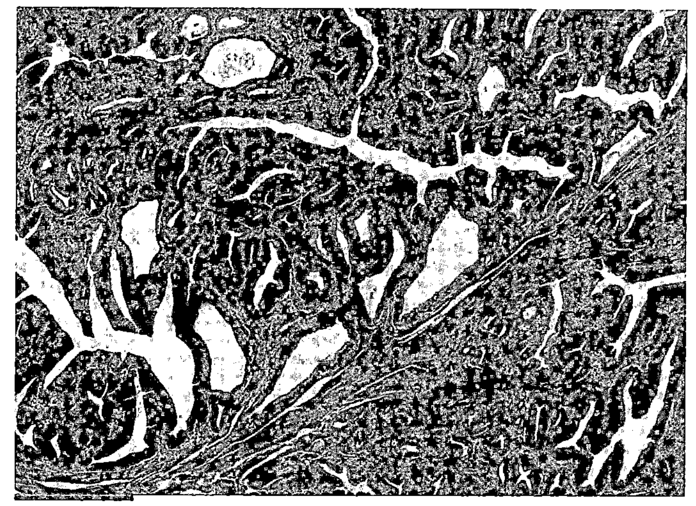

Figure 49.2
Tubular adenoma of the ampulla of Vater (intestinal type). The neoplastic epithelium covers the interconnecting ampullary channels.

tients with FAP showed that the histologic grade worsened in three of the 12 patients who initially had an adenoma, whereas adenomas developed in only two patients who had no previous adenomas.[16] Overall, the cumulative lifetime risk for developing adenomas is near 100%.[17] However, although patients with FAP have a 100- to 200-fold increased risk of adenocarcinomas, a multicenter analysis of 1262 patients with FAP demonstrated that periampullary adenocarcinomas occur in only approximately 4%.[18-20] Of interest, a group reported one case of ampullary carcinoma presenting as the first manifestation of attenuated FAP in a 38-year-old female.[21] Finally, a single report described the familial occurrence of ampullary adenomas in fraternal sisters with autosomal dominant polycystic kidney disease. The association of both disorders suggests a genetic alteration that remains unresolved.[22]

It is important to accurately diagnose ampullary adenomas because of the risk of malignant transformation. Evidence for an adenoma-carcinoma sequence similar to that encountered in colonic neoplasia has accumulated over the past 15 years. It includes the demonstration of residual adenomatous epithelium intermixed or at the immediate proximity of 44%–91% of resected ampullary adenocarcinomas.[23-25]

Clinical features Jaundice is the most frequent mode of presentation.[26] Fecal occult blood loss can also be detected. Weight loss, abdominal pain, and pancreatitis are less frequent.[2,8]

Endoscopic and gross appearances Ampullary adenomas can present as a plaque or a polypoid growth (Fig. 49.1). Ulceration is worrisome and could indicate the presence of adenocarcinoma. In surgical specimens, exophytic polypoid or plaque-like lesions composed of paler granular or papillary mucosa are usually observed.[11] Ampullary adenoma is typically solitary, but multiplicity is frequently described in patients with FAP, with the size of the polyps varying from 1 to 3 cm.[10,12]

Microscopic findings Tubular adenomas are composed of closely arranged glands lined by mucin-depleted columnar epithelium. The nuclei are prominent, hyperchromatic uniform, and usually cigar shaped. The dysplastic changes can involve only parts or the entirety of a single gland or villus. The adenomatous epithelium may not only involve the periampullary duodenal mucosal surface but also can extend along the ampullary channels (Fig. 49.2). The architecture may vary, but at least 25% of the neoplasm should be villous for a diagnosis of a tubulovillous adenoma to be achieved, and 50% should be villous for a diagnosis of papillary adenoma.[13] Overall, most adenomas are tubular (53.6%); less frequently, they are tubulovillous (36.3%) and villous (5.5%).[4] The latter are usually larger than tubular adenomas.[9,13] Low-grade dysplasia shows few mitotic figures and mild architectural changes (Fig. 49.3). Conversely, high-grade dysplasia is characterized by more complex architectural alterations with frequent back-to-back or small, abortive glands (Fig. 49.4). Also, instead of elongated basilar nuclei, worsening nuclear

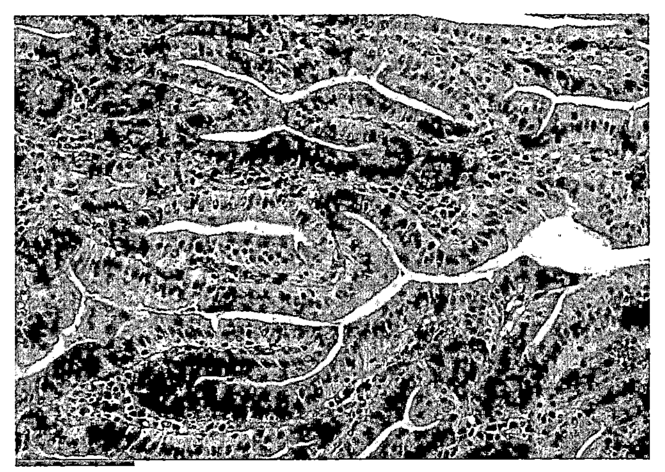

Figure 49.3
Tubular adenoma (intestinal type), low-grade dysplasia. The lining epithelium is composed of tall cells with elongated basilar nuclei. Mild architectural changes are seen.

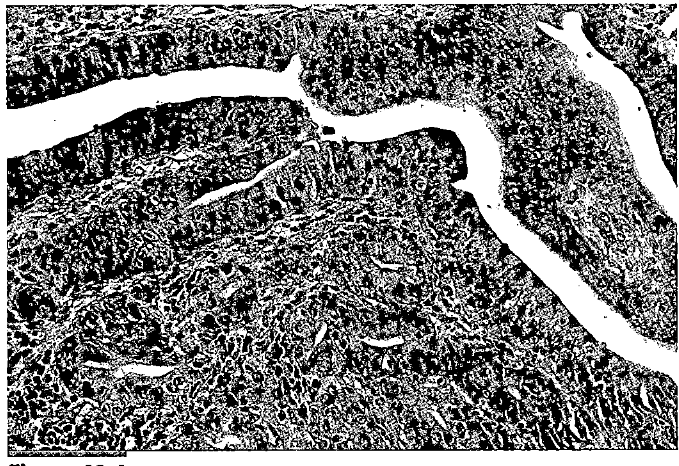

Figure 49.4
Tubular adenoma (intestinal type), high-grade dysplasia. The lining epithelium is characterized by more complex architectural alterations with frequent back-to-back and small, abortive glands. Larger, rounder nuclei with prominent nucleoli and significant stratification are identified.

atypia consisting of larger, rounded nuclei with prominent nucleoli and significant stratification can be identified. Perhaps because of their size, high-grade dysplasia and intramucosal carcinoma are more frequently observed in villous adenomas.[13] In one series, adenocarcinoma was present in 65% of villous adenomas.[27] When the nuclear atypia is particularly severe, a diagnosis of carcinoma in situ is sometimes made. We do not support this practice because of the potential for misunderstanding that may lead to pancreatoduodenectomy, whereas excellent results are achieved with local excision alone of these lesions.[2] Instead we prefer the term *high-grade dysplasia* over carcinoma in situ. Between the neoplastic epithelium, interspersed goblet cells, Paneth cells, and endocrine cells can be found (Fig. 49.5). Distinguishing between regenerative changes and dysplastic ampullary epithelium may be challenging. When attenuated epithelium is seen growing over an ulcerated surface, it can reasonably be assumed that the glands in the immediate vicinity of the ulceration are regenerative. In addition, regenerative epithelia usually display a gradual transition from normal epithelium to reactive epithelium. Also, the cells are usually uniform with basally oriented,

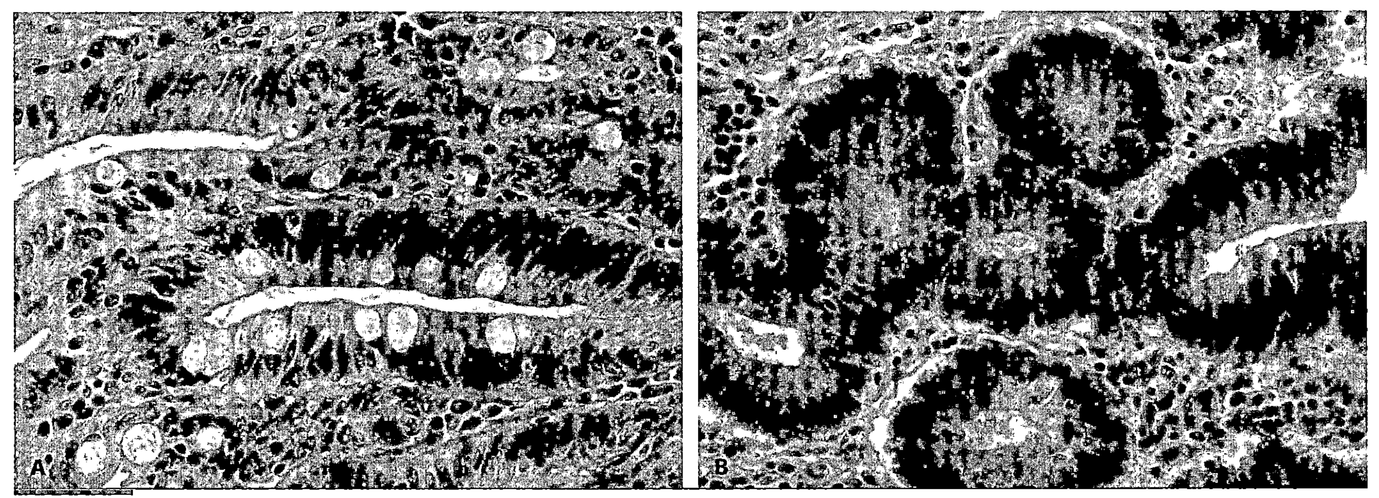

Figure 49.5
Tubular adenomas (intestinal type) with specialized cells. (A) Goblet cells and (B) Paneth cells are readily identified in these examples of low-grade tubular adenomas.

enlarged nuclei with homogeneous chromatin and multiple small nucleoli.

The accuracy of endoscopic biopsies in the diagnosis of ampullary adenomas is debated. Because the lesions may be large in comparison with the biopsy size and invasion may be focal, several surgical series have demonstrated that initial endoscopic evaluations of ampullary neoplasms frequently overlook malignant foci, and the reported false-negative rates range from 25% to 56%.[2,4,8,10,11,26] The accuracy of preoperative microscopic diagnosis is slightly improved when biopsies are performed after sphincterotomy, if multiple biopsies are obtained and step sections are examined.[28,29] Despite sampling problems, some workers have suggested that endoscopic treatment is satisfactory for the large majority of ampullary adenomas. In a series of 24 patients, complete endoscopic and microscopic remission were obtained in 67% of patients, and recurrence was observed in only one case (6%). After a mean follow-up of 81 months, no ampullary cancers were diagnosed, suggesting that the endoscopic analysis was satisfactory.[15]

Ampullary Adenoma, Biliary Type

Adenomatous lesions with architectural as well as cytologic features resembling neoplastic lesions of the pancreatic and biliary ductal systems are also observed. The readers are referred to the section Pancreaticobiliary-Type Adenocarcinoma in this chapter as well as Chapter 54 for a review of these lesions.

Ampullary Carcinomas

Ampullary carcinomas are uncommon and represent only 0.2% of gastrointestinal tract malignancies[30]; however, they account for up to half of the surgically operable pancreatoduodenal neoplasms.[31] The ampulla may also be overgrown by carcinomas that arise from adjacent structures, making it difficult, if not impossible, to determine in some cases whether the neoplasm originated in the periampullary duodenum, the distal common bile duct, the head of the pancreas, or the ampulla itself.[13] For those reasons, the nonspecific term *periampullary* has been used to refer to some neoplasms arising at the intersection of these four sites.[32-35] We believe that the designation "periampullary" should be avoided because it nonspecifically lumps clinically, grossly, microscopically, and genetically distinct neoplasms. Whenever possible, a specific organ of origin should be designated.

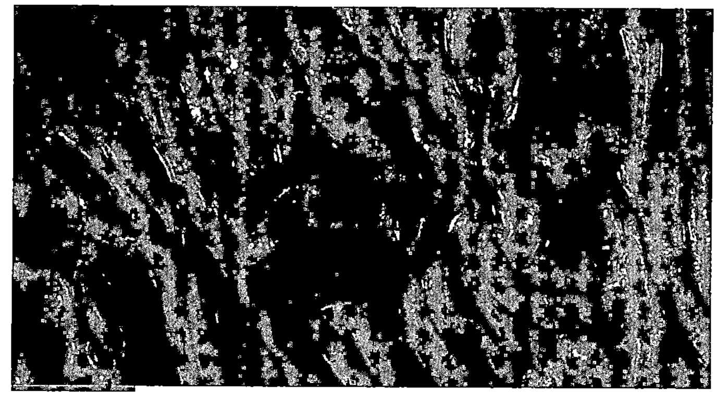

Figure 49.6
Macroscopic appearance of mixed exophytic adenocarcinoma.

Macroscopic features Ampullary carcinomas are often diagnosed at an early stage because of the precocity of symptoms that relate to its unique anatomic location. These patients tend to present at an early stage with persistent or intermittent jaundice, weight loss, abdominal pain, and less frequently, pancreatitis.[5,33] In one series of 149 cases, the mean greatest diameter of ampullary carcinoma was 2.7 cm, significantly smaller than carcinomas of the pancreatic head (3.5 cm).[31] In our practice, we use the modified classification of Cubilla and Fitzgerald.[13] This scheme combines the appearance of the duodenal lumen and the extent of the involvement of the ampulla and the periampullary duodenum. Four types are recognized: intra-ampullary, periampullary duodenal, mixed exophytic (Fig. 49.6) and mixed ulcerated[13] (Fig. 49.7). In a series of 116 cases, the mixed ulcerated type was the most common (39% of the cases), followed by the mixed exophytic (31%), intra-ampullary (24%), and periampullary duodenal (6%).[13] Intra-ampullary tumors tend to be smaller; they are less frequently associated with involvement of the pancreas, angiolymphatic invasion, and lymph node metastasis; and they have a better prognosis than the other types.[6]

Microscopic features Most ampullary adenocarcinomas show a tubular morphology and predominantly consist of simple or cribriformed glands. About 80% are well- or moderately differentiated, whereas about 20% are poorly differentiated.[5,24,36] Given the unique anatomic location, adenocarcinomas may display various histologic appearances and are further divided into intestinal type (Fig. 49.8) and pancreatobiliary type.

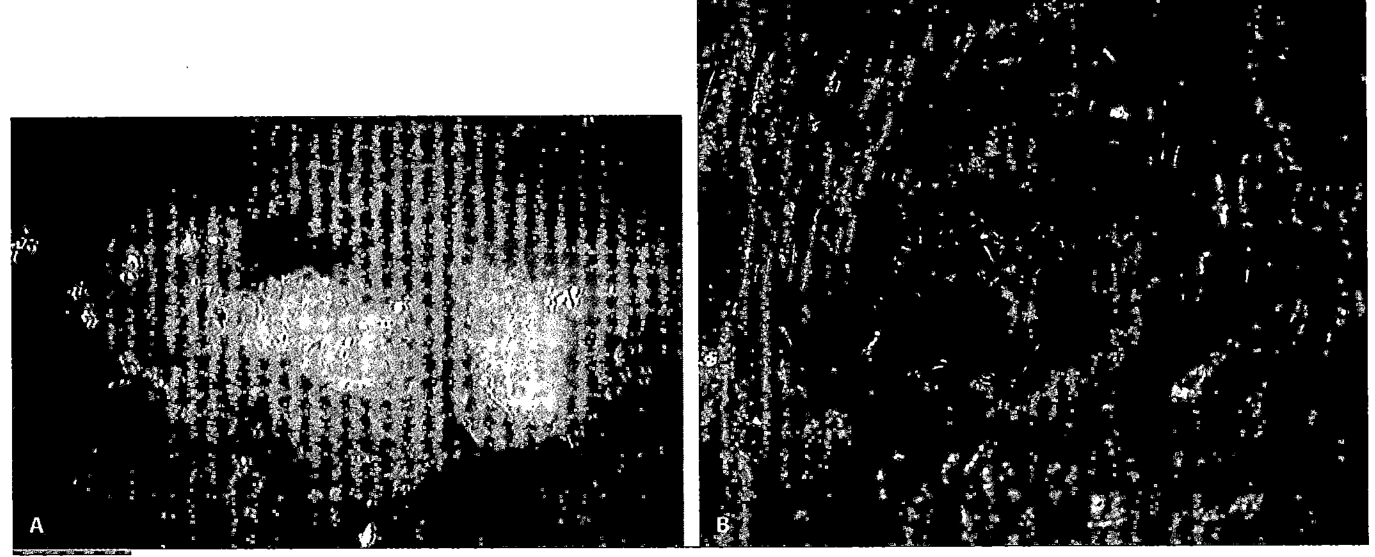

Figure 49.7
Macroscopic appearance of mixed ulcerated adenocarcinoma. (A) Endoscopic appearance. (Courtesy of Peter B. Kelsey, MD, Division of Gastroenterology, Massachusetts General Hospital, Boston, MA). (B) Surgical specimen. The papilla is replaced by an exophytic papillary and ulcerated tumor.

Intestinal-Type Adenocarcinoma

Intestinal-type adenocarcinomas are the most prevalent, representing approximately 50% of ampullary adenocarcinomas.[5,13] Intestinal-type adenocarcinomas closely resemble primary adenocarcinomas of the colon and are composed of simple or cribriformed glands lined by cells displaying pseudostratified and oval nuclei showing various degrees of atypia and variable numbers of mitoses (Fig. 49.9). Intraluminal central necrosis and inflammatory cells can be seen. Features suggestive of intestinal differentiation, such as a well-formed luminal brush border and goblet cells, may be present, but well-formed Paneth cells are rare in invasive adenocarcinomas. Instead, cells with small numbers of granules may be interspersed within the neoplastic epithelium, especially in well-differentiated cases.[7,37] Scattered endocrine cells can also be found more often in intestinal-type than in pancreatobiliary-type carcinomas.[13] As previously noted, residual adenoma (with or without high-grade dysplasia) can be detected in up to 90% of the cases).[24]

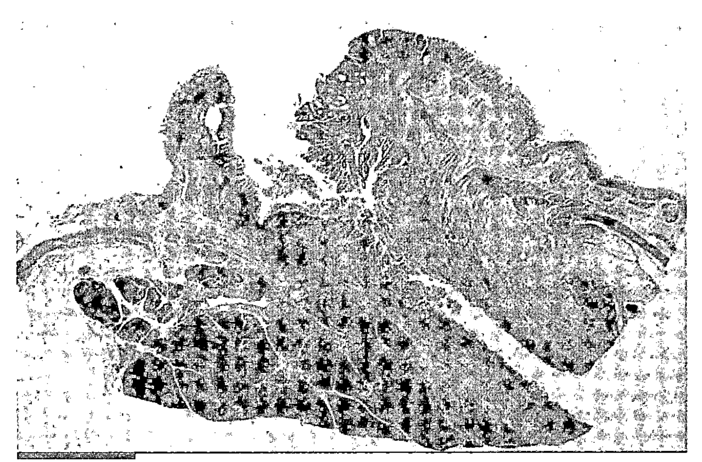

Figure 49.8
Adenocarcinoma, intestinal type. The neoplastic epithelium involves the ampullary ostium and channels and periampullary duodenal mucosa.

Pancreatobiliary-Type Adenocarcinoma

Approximately 20% of ampullary adenocarcinomas closely resemble adenocarcinomas of the pancreas and major bile ducts and are thus defined as the pancreatobiliary type. Simple or branching glands with a single layer of cuboidal cells with round and markedly atypical nuclei are often embedded in a prominent, hyalinized, desmoplastic stroma (Fig. 49.10). Focal papillary and/or micropapillary structures may be seen. Luminal necrotic debris is not common. A discrepancy between the degree of cytologic and architectural atypia is a characteristic of these neoplasms. In addition, poorly differentiated components, that is, single and/or small clusters of bizarre cells, are often intermingled. Perineural invasion is frequently observed in this type of carcinoma, but angiolymphatic invasion is seen less often than in the intestinal type.[13]

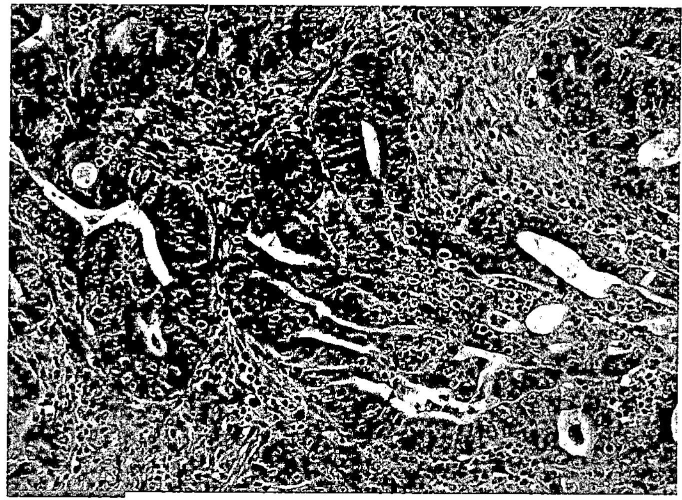

Figure 49.9
Adenocarcinoma, intestinal type. The tumor is composed of complexed glands lined by atypical cells. Note the typical luminal inflammation.

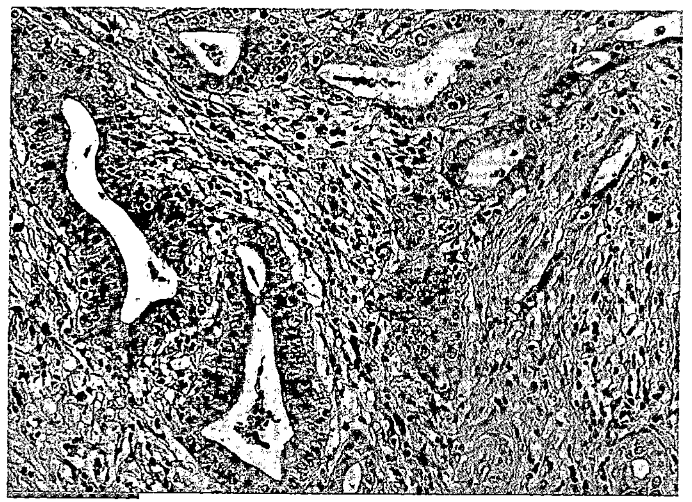

Figure 49.10
Adenocarcinoma, pancreatobiliary type. The tumor is composed of simple malignant glands lined by low columnar cells. Note the markedly atypical nuclei and the surrounding desmoplasia.

Some ampullary adenocarcinomas contain both intestinal and pancreatobiliary morphologies. It is recommended that these mixed neoplasms be classified as intestinal type unless pancreatobiliary morphology predominates.[38] However, some carcinomas are too poorly differentiated to be recognized as either type and should be reported as poorly differentiated adenocarcinomas, not otherwise specified.

The importance of the phenotype with regard to the prognosis is controversial; however, a trend toward improved survival for intestinal-type adenocarcinomas relative to the pancreatobiliary subtype was reported in a study of 101 resected cases (median survival, 59.6 versus 22.5 months).[5]

Unusual Histologic Subtypes of Ampullary Carcinomas

Papillary carcinoma This term has previously not been well defined and has often been used in the past without specific reference to invasion.[6,39] In one study, the term *papillary carcinoma* was applied to carcinomas without invasion in comparison with infiltrating carcinomas, a practice that is no longer followed.[13,40]

The diagnosis of invasive papillary carcinoma is contingent on the observation of invasive, complex, branching papillary structures with fibrovascular cores and/or micropapillary structures without fibrovascular cores (Fig. 49.11). The papillae can be lined by either intestinal-type or pancreatobiliary-type cells.

Noninvasive papillary carcinomas are, by definition, exophytic neoplasms arising in the intra-ampullary mucosa, and they are composed of pancreatobiliary-type epithelium.[13] Noninvasive papillary carcinomas are analogous to noninvasive intraductal papillary mucinous neoplasms of the pancreas[41] and noninvasive papillary carcinomas of the extrahepatic bile ducts.[42]

Papillary ampullary carcinomas are rare, representing 6% of the cases observed at the Massachusetts General Hospital (Mino M, Lauwers GY, personal experience).

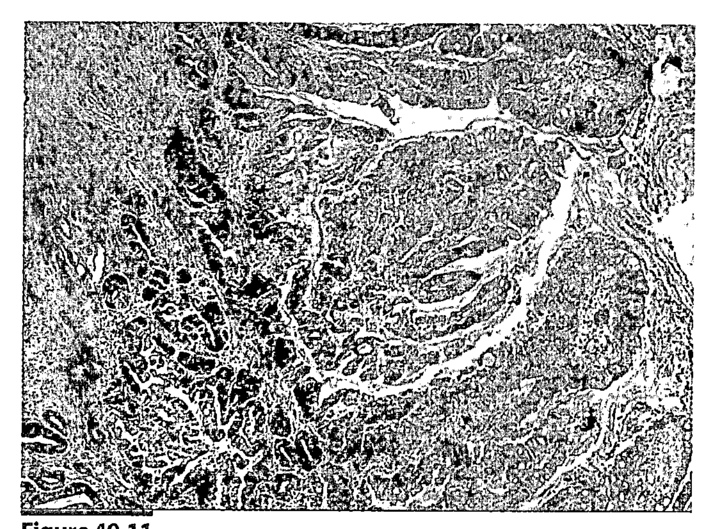

Figure 49.11
Papillary adenocarcinoma. Tall papillae are characteristic of this type. Note the subjacent invasion.

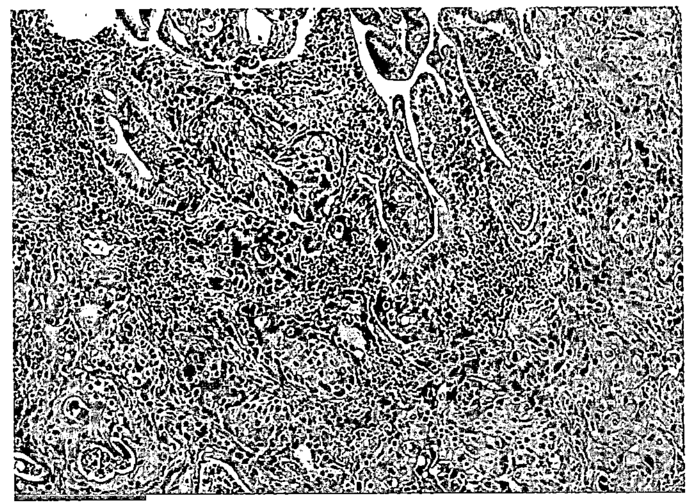

Figure 49.12
Adenosquamous carcinoma. Islands of squamous differentiation are intermixed with the glandular component.

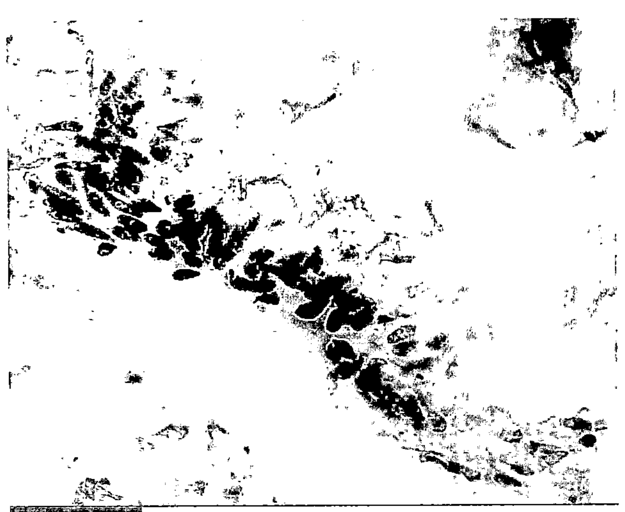

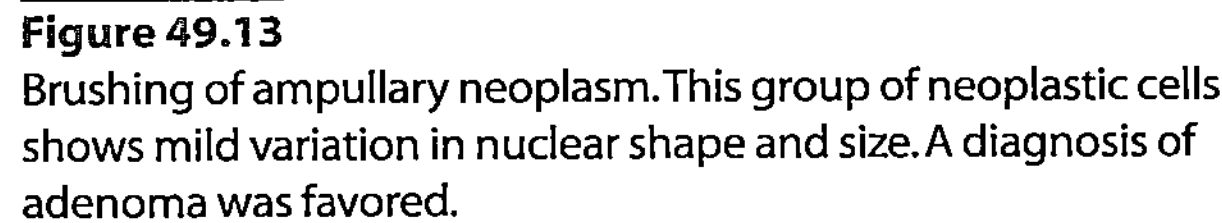

Figure 49.13
Brushing of ampullary neoplasm. This group of neoplastic cells shows mild variation in nuclear shape and size. A diagnosis of adenoma was favored.

Mucinous (colloid) carcinoma These carcinomas are grossly and microscopically similar to those arising in other segments of the gastrointestinal tract. By definition, more than 50% of the neoplasm should consist of pools of extracellular mucin, either lined by columnar epithelium displaying mild-to-moderate nuclear atypia or containing free-floating clusters of neoplastic cells. Some neoplasms show both growth patterns. Mucinous carcinomas are uncommon and represent only 4%–6.5% of ampullary carcinomas[39,43] (Mino M, Lauwers GY, MGH experience); however, focal mucinous differentiation is found in up to 20% of intestinal-type adenocarcinomas of the ampulla.[13]

Signet-ring cell carcinoma Pure signet-ring cell carcinoma of the ampulla is a rare neoplasm, with only rare examples being reported.[44,45] These carcinomas are composed of cells distended by abundant intracytoplasmic mucin that pushes the nuclei toward the periphery. A variable amount of extracellular mucin is also present. More than 50% of the neoplasm must consist of signet-ring cells with a diffuse growth pattern in order to classify. A signet-ring cell carcinoma primary to another organ, particularly the stomach, should be excluded before a diagnosis of a signet-ring cell carcinoma of the ampulla is established.

Unusual histologic subtypes Uncommonly diagnosed subtypes include intestinal-type adenocarcinoma with hepatoid features[46,47]; adenosquamous carcinoma (Fig. 49.12)[6,48]; squamous cell carcinoma; small cell carcinoma[49-51]; large-cell neuroendocrine carcinoma[52-54]; undifferentiated carcinoma, including one case with osteoclast-like giant cells[55]; and sarcomatoid carcinoma.[56-57] In addition, clear-cell carcinomas resembling the clear-cell carcinoma of the gallbladder and extrahepatic bile ducts have been reported.[58,59]

Cytology

Experience with brush cytology in the diagnosis of ampullary neoplasms is limited. In one series, a comparison of cytologic and biopsy diagnoses revealed a sensitivity and specificity of 100% for cytologic brushing.[60] The cytologic appearance of adenomas and adenocarcinomas is characterized by an increasing degree of cellular and architectural atypism ranging from cohesive clusters or small tubules to various numbers of single cells exhibiting a high nuclear-to-cytoplasmic ratio and a marked variation in nuclear size and contour, with or without prominent nucleoli (Fig. 49.13). Necrotic background may be seen.[60]

Ancillary Tests: Immunohistochemistry

Reactivity with monoclonal antibodies against carcinoembryonic antigen reveals moderate staining of the luminal membrane and faint cytoplasmic labeling of adenomas, whereas only minimal labeling of the luminal (glycocalyceal) borders of benign ampullary epithelium is observed in occasional cases. The intensity of the cytoplasmic labeling increases with increasing degree of atypia, and a diffuse and intense cytoplasmic carcinoembryonic antigen labeling is seen in 74%–100% of invasive carcinomas.[11,31,61,62] The difference in frequency and intensity of reactivity in relation to different histologic types and tumor grades is controversial.[11,13,31,63] Immunoreactivity with carbohydrate antigen 19-9 is also found in 60%–65% of ampullary carcinomas as well as in normal or benign epithelium of the ampulla.[31,61]

One study has demonstrated that a panel combining immunolabeling for keratin 7, keratin 20, and MUC2 can distinguish intestinal-type adenocarcinomas (keratin 7 negative, keratin 20 positive, MUC2 positive) from pancreatobiliary-type adenocarcinomas and papillary carcinomas (keratin 7 positive, keratin 20 negative, MUC 2 negative).[64] This immunohistochemical profiling may not only be helpful for diagnostic purposes but also supports the concept of a heterogeneous histogenesis for ampullary carcinomas.

Molecular Pathology

TP53 gene mutations have been demonstrated in 59%–94% of ampullary carcinomas.[65-69] Concomitantly, positive p53 immunolabeling is reported in 36%–40% of adenomas or adenomatous component of carcinomas[67,70]; thus, p53 accumulation appears to occur relatively late during the oncogenetic process. *KRAS2* oncogene mutations have been reported in 13%–75% of ampullary carcinomas.[65,70-77] *KRAS2* gene mutations are also found in up to 54% of adenomas, even in those with low-grade dysplasia, suggesting that *KRAS2* gene mutation is an early genetic event of the adenoma-carcinoma sequence.[31,74,77] Notably, the frequency and types of mutations are similar to those observed in colorectal carcinomas but differ from those seen in pancreatic cancer.[78,79] Other molecular abnormalities identified include the loss of *SMAD4/DPC4* tumor suppressor gene[70]; the overexpression of members of the type 1 growth factor receptor family, such as epidermal growth factor receptor, c-*erb*B-2, and c-*erb*B-3,[80,81] and ligands for the epidermal growth factor receptor (epidermal growth factor and transforming growth factor-α)[81,82]; and *APC* and *β-catenin* gene mutations.[77,83] High microsatellite instability, identified in 10%–15% of sporadic colorectal carcinomas, appears not to be involved in the development of ampullary carcinomas.[73,84]

Despite the better understanding of the molecular mechanisms, molecular markers have not yet entered the clinical diagnostic arena, and neither p53 expression abnormalities nor KRAS2 gene mutations correlate with prognosis.[66,73,74]

Staging

The current American Joint Committee on Cancer staging of ampullary carcinomas is listed in Table 49.1.[85] A major alteration from the previous staging consists of modifications of the T staging (between T3 and T4) to reflect the resectability of the tumors rather than the depth of pancreatic invasion. Modifications of the stages have also been implemented, in part, to retain consistency with the staging of neoplasms of the bile duct and the pancreas.

Table 49.1 TNM Tumor Staging*

Primary tumor (T)	
Tis	Carcinoma in situ
T1	Tumor limited to ampulla of Vater
T2	Tumor invades duodenum
T3	Tumor invades pancreatic parenchyma
T4	Tumor extends into pancreatic soft tissues or other adjacent structures
Regional lymph nodes (N)	
NX	Regional lymph nodes cannot be assessed
N0	Negative lymph node
N1	Lymph node metastasis present
Distant metastasis (M)	
MX	Distant metastasis cannot be assessed
M0	No metastasis
M1	Distant metastasis present

Stage Grouping			
Stage 0	Tis	N0	M0
Stage IA	T1	N0	M0
Stage IB	T2	N0	M0
Stage IIA	T3	N0	M0
Stage IIB	T1	N1	M0
	T2	N1	M0
	T3	N1	M0
Stage III	T4	Any N	M0
Stage IV	Any T	Any N	M1

*Modified from Geene et al.[85]

Prognostic Factors (see also Chapter 50)

The 5- and 10-year survival rates of invasive ampullary adenocarcinoma vary between 24% and 56%.[33,86-90] Over time, several histopathologic factors of prognostic relevance have been reported in different series. Strong indicators of prognosis, most demonstrated by multivariate analyses, include histologic type, with the biliary type associated with a worse prognosis[88]; tumor grade[86-88]; size of the carcinoma[86,87]; presence of lymphatic invasion and lymph node metastasis[88,89,91]; invasion of neighboring structures[87,91]; and presence of perineural invasion.[87]

MIB-1 labeling index of proliferation and DNA ploidy have also been reported to have some prognostic value.[92]

Endocrine Neoplasms

Carcinoid tumors are rare in the ampullary region, accounting only for about 2%–3% of periampullary neoplasms.[93] Most patients with ampullary endocrine neoplasms are male in their 5th or 6th decade of life.[93,94] The development of these neoplasms can be sporadic, for or associated with either Zollinger-Ellison syndrome or neurofibromatosis I, for which the association is particularly strong with African Americans.[93,95-97] Because of their infiltrative nature, they can present in a fashion similar to that of adenomas, with jaundice and obstructive pancreatitis.[93,98] They are less frequently associated with symptoms of hormonal secretion (i.e., gastrinoma) than other small-intestinal carcinoids.

Endoscopic/Gross Appearance

Ampullary carcinoids usually present as circumscribed, yellowish, submucosal nodules, with overlying mucosa being either intact (Fig. 49.14) or sometimes ulcerated. Their size may vary from a few millimeters to several centimeters (0.2–5.0 cm).[93] However, like most duodenal carcinoids, they usually measure less than 2 cm.[93,94]

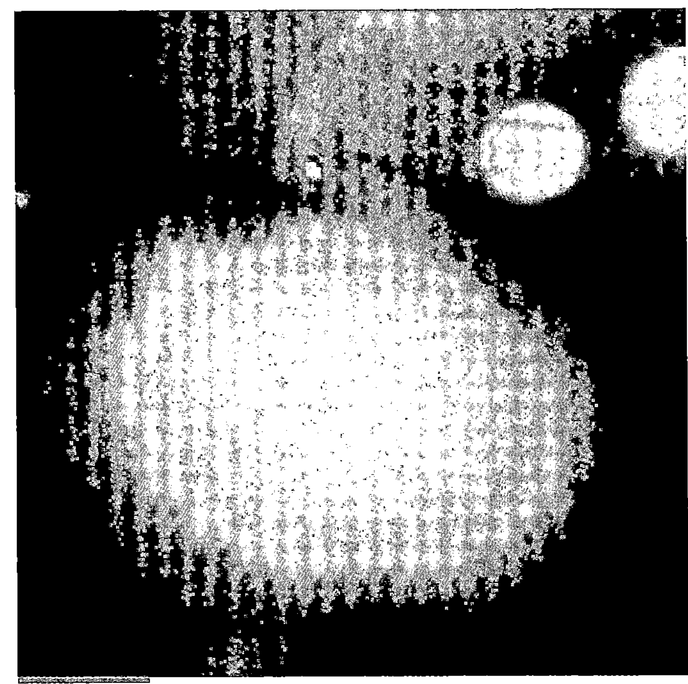

Figure 49.14
Endoscopic appearance of ampullary carcinoid. The bulging papilla has an intact mucosa, and the subjacent mass has a yellowish hue, characteristic of this neoplasm.

Microscopic Findings

The histologic appearance is similar to that of other carcinoid lesions of the duodenum, with cells forming solid islands or trabeculae infiltrating between the ducts and the smooth muscles of the ampulla (Fig. 49.15). The neoplastic cells are distinctly uniform, with a moderate amount of cytoplasm and round nuclei with the typical stippled chromatin. Mitoses are rare, and necrosis is usually absent. Given the frequent submucosal location of some of these neoplasms, large and deep biopsies may be necessary to secure a diagnosis. Cytologic fine-needle aspiration biopsy has been successful in confirming the diagnosis.[99]

As expected, most of these argyrophilic lesions label for generic endocrine markers, such as chromogranin A (92%) and synaptophysin (100%).[93] In most cases, this labeling is diffuse and strong, primarily for chromogranin, whereas about 10% of tumors are negative for all markers.[13,93] In these cases, ultrastructural analysis usually reveals neurosecretory granules. Carcinoembryonic antigen is expressed in 75% of the cases.[93]

Predicting the clinical behavior of ampullary carcinoids is difficult. Size (>2 cm), depth of penetration (involvement of muscularis propria), mitotic activity, and necrosis have all been associated with an unfavorable prognosis.[93] However, despite a high rate of nodal metastasis (between 33% and 50%), the clinical behavior of most of these neoplasms is generally relatively indolent, especially when they are submucosal and small in size.[93] A somatostatin-rich glandular carcinoid (somatostatinoma), variant of carcinoid tumors has been described. This type arises equally in both sexes and shows a stronger association with neurofibromatosis I.[95,100] In this group of patients, they represent the most common periampullary tumors.[93] Microscopically, they can present with a pre-

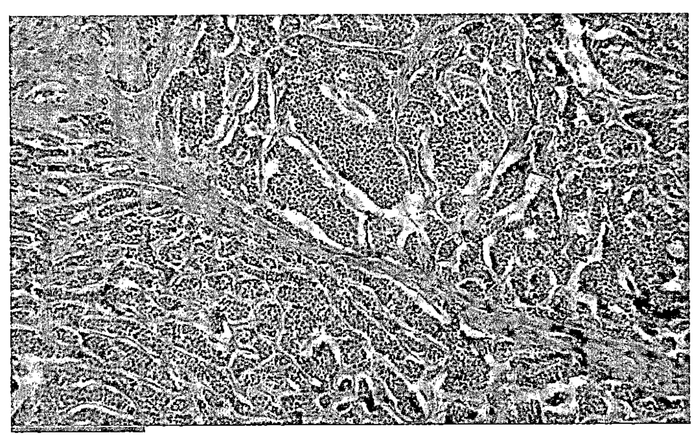

Figure 49.15
Ampullary carcinoid. Characteristic wide anastomosing trabeculae are set in a sclerotic stroma.

dominant tubuloglandular growth pattern that can be misdiagnosed as a well-differentiated adenocarcinoma. Solid or trabecular arrangements and intraglandular psammomatous calcifications both suggest the diagnosis of a somatostatinoma. Other lesions associated with neurofibromatosis (e.g., gastrointestinal stromal tumor and pheochromocytoma), should also raise the degree of suspicion for this diagnosis.[95,97,100] Although they are strongly immunoreactive to somatostatin antibody, about half of these tumors are negative for chromogranin A.[98] The rate of lymph node metastasis is between 25% and 50%; however, resection is usually curative.[96,97]

Gastrinomas, although frequently identified elsewhere in the duodenum, are relatively rare in the ampullary region. They can either be associated with multiple endocrine neoplasia type 1 or Zollinger-Ellison syndrome, or they may be sporadic. Despite their small size (most measuring <0.6 cm), gastrinoma have a higher tendency to behave aggressively, with lymph nodes and hepatic metastases (the latter seen in 45%–66% of the cases), particularly when they are associated with Zollinger-Ellison syndrome or Zollinger-Ellison/multiple endocrine neoplasia type 1 syndromes.[101]

Rare mixed endocrine/exocrine neoplasms have been reported.[102-104] They are usually small and composed of cells growing in small nests and tubules with interspersed signet-ring cells.[102,103] However, in one case, the signet-ring cells were not apparent.[104] Mucicarmine highlights the presence of mucin in the signet-ring cells as well as non–signet-ring cells, with a significant contingent of neoplastic cells also decorated by neuroendocrine markers, such as synaptophysin, chromogranin, and neuron-specific enolase. In practice, these tumors need to be differentiated from poorly differentiated adenocarcinomas with endocrine differentiation as well as signet-ring carcinomas. Although some report a clinical behavior intermediate between carcinoids and adenocarcinomas, one case was associated with a dismal prognosis.[13,104]

Gangliocytic Paraganglioma

Gangliocytic paragangliomas (GCPGs) are rare neoplasms of low malignant potential that predominantly affect adult men. Most cases are symptomatic, and the two most common modes of presentations are bleeding (68% of the cases) and abdominal discomfort (37% of the cases).[105-109] Common bile duct obstruction has also been reported.[107]

GCPGs can present as pedunculated or sessile, apparently arising in the submucosa and deforming the overlying mucosa (Fig. 49.16A). The morphology, immunocytochemistry, and ultrastructure suggest that GCPGs are neuroendocrine tumors with divergent differentiation.[105-108] Microscopically, they combine features of paraganglioma, carcinoid tumor, and ganglioneuroma. They are characteristically composed of epithelioid cell nests with transition to more spindle elements and well-developed ganglion cells (Fig. 49.16B).[105-109] The epithelioid cells frequently have a ribbon-like or trabecular arrangement and are nested by a delicate network of spindle cells. Although most GCPGs are not hormonally active, immunoreactivity for multiple polypeptides, including neuron-specific enolase, insulin, glucagon, pancreatic polypeptide, somatostatin, vasoactive intestinal peptide, and serotonin, may be revealed.[108,110-112] Chromogranin can be identified within the carcinoid-like areas of these neoplasms.[106,112] The ganglion cells express neuron-specific enolase, synaptophysin, and

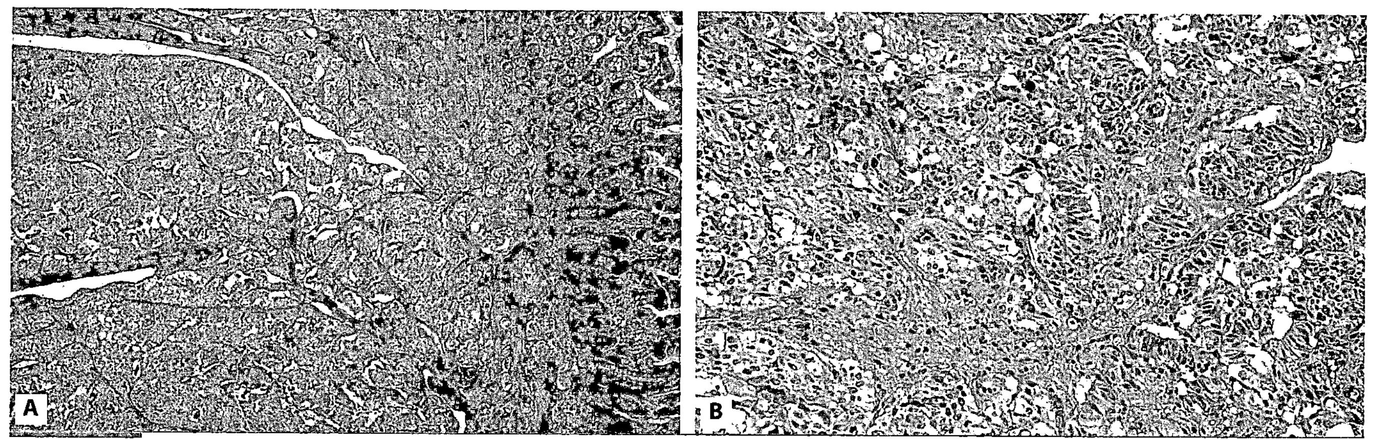

Figure 49.16
Gangliocytic paraganglioma. **(A)** Scanning view showing the lesion expending the ampullary submucosa. A nesting pattern is readily identified. **(B)** Higher magnification demonstrates the three cell types, with the epithelioid elements showing a ribbon-like arrangement separated by spindle cells and rare ganglion cells.

neurofilament protein, whereas immunolabeling for S-100 protein decorates the sustentacular network surrounding the epithelioid cells.[106,108,112] There is a single report of hormonally active, somatostatin-secreting GCPG, in which symptoms (e.g., diarrhea, steatorrhea) completely resolved after resection.[111] Rare cases of lymph node metastases have been reported, and those have always been exclusively composed of epithelioid cells.[105,113-117] Importantly, extranodal metastasis or death related to the disease has not been reported. Resection is curative, and long-term follow-up of most patients supports a benign behavior.

The nature of GCPG is a controversial issue. It has been postulated that GCPGs are hamartomatous proliferations that would arise from the ventral primordium of the pancreas and recapitulate, in an exaggerated fashion, the neuroinsular complexes described by Simard.[118] However, recent reports of GCPGs associated with neurofibromatosis and flow cytometric evidence of aneuploid and tetraploid populations, as well as the similarity with paragangliomas of the cauda equina, point to a true neoplasm.[107,119-121]

Benign and Malignant Mesenchymal Neoplasms

Primary mesenchymal neoplasms, both benign and malignant, are exceptionally rare in the ampulla. This may be explained by the fact that the ampulla contains minimal mesenchymal tissue and as a result, most ampullary mesenchymal tumors are likely to represent the extension of a duodenal neoplasm.

Benign Mesenchymal Neoplasms

Most benign periampullary mesenchymal neoplasms are either leiomyomas[122,123] or lipomas.[124] Other neoplasms include vascular tumors, such as hemangioma and lymphangioma,[125-127] and neurogenic tumors; neurofibroma[128]; and ganglioneuroma[129,130] likely to be diagnosed in a patient with neurofibromatosis 1. Granular cell tumors, which are benign neoplasms of Schwann cell origin, have been reported to occur in the biliary system, with one case involving the ampulla.[131]

Malignant Mesenchymal Neoplasms

Most malignant mesenchymal neoplasms arising in the periampullary duodenal wall are gastrointestinal stromal tumors.[13] Leiomyosarcomas involving the ampulla have also been reported.[33] These neoplasms are characterized by a cellular proliferation of plump spindle cells, often with mitotic activity; epithelioid types can occur. Because 39% of the gastrointestinal stromal tumors in the duodenum variably demonstrate immunoreactivity to smooth muscle actin,[132] the recent introduction of immunolabeling for the KIT protein, a marker for gastrointestinal stromal tumors, may lead to reclassification of some of the leiomyomas and leiomyosarcomas into gastrointestinal stromal tumors. Other reported malignant mesenchymal neoplasms include embryonal rhabdomyosarcoma[133,134] and Kaposi's sarcoma.[135]

Rare Periampullary Neoplasms

Lymphoma

Although primary non-Hodgkin's lymphomas of the gastrointestinal tract are the most frequent extranodal lymphomas, duodenal involvement occurs in less than 2% of lymphomas of the gastrointestinal tract, and only a few cases specifically involving the ampulla of Vater have been reported.[136] Endoscopy may reveal a mass, a slight enlargement of the papilla, or only granularity of the mucosa.[137,138] Dyspepsia, abdominal pain, and jaundice due to the infiltration of the sphincter of Oddi have been reported, and the overall clinical and radiologic appearance may mimic pancreatic carcinoma.[138-141] Most cases are high-grade B-cell lymphoma (Fig. 49.17) and extranodal marginal zone B-cell lymphoma (mucosa-associated lymphoid tissue lymphoma).[137,142-144] Noteworthy is an increase in the reports of follicular lymphoma in the ampulla.[141,145] Rare cases of T-cell lymphoma and lym-

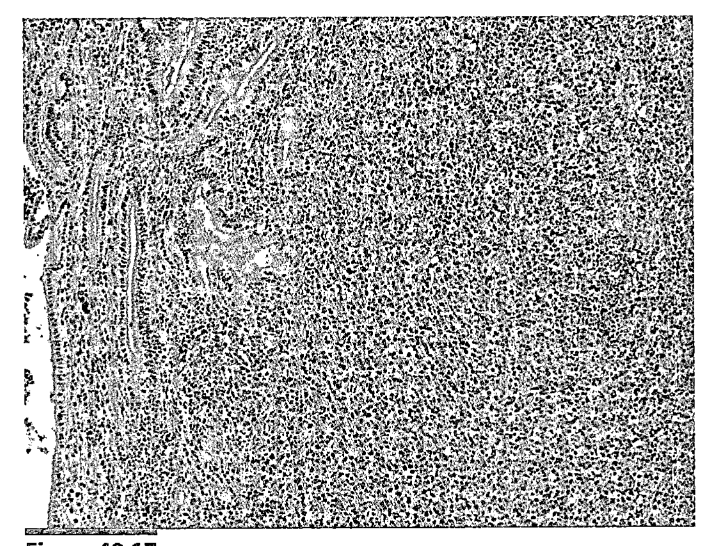

Figure 49.17
Ampullary lymphoma. This low-power view demonstrates the characteristic dense lymphoid infiltrate.

phoproliferative small intestinal disease have also been observed.[140,146]

Pseudotumors

Pseudotumors, whether inflammatory, hamartomatous, or hyperplastic, represent about 23% of the tumors identified in the ampullary region.[147] These lesions are important to recognize because they can either produce biliary obstruction or form masses that may easily be mistaken for a neoplastic process and may lead to unnecessary surgeries (in up to 18% of the cases) instead of being treated conservatively.[147]

Myoepithelial hamartoma (adenomyoma/adenomyomatous hamartoma) Ampullary adenomyomas are rare lesions believed by most to arise from ectopic pancreaticobilary-type ducts and ductules, although some favor a sequelae of chronic inflammation.[148,149] Most cases are asymptomatic, but few can present with obstructive jaundice and abdominal pain.[149] One report describes a case associated with severe weight loss, renal failure, and metabolic acidosis.[150]

Myoepithelial hamartomas take either the form of small nodules or ill-defined areas centered in the submucosa. They usually measure between 1 and 2 cm in their greatest dimension and are composed of an admixture of anastomosing and distended ducts lined by pancreaticobiliary-type cuboidal epithelium and surrounded by smooth muscle.[149] Inflammatory and regenerative cytologic atypia can be mistaken for adenomatous changes, but abnormal mitoses are not seen. Brunner glands and pancreatic acini can also be interspersed between the ducts.[7,151,152]

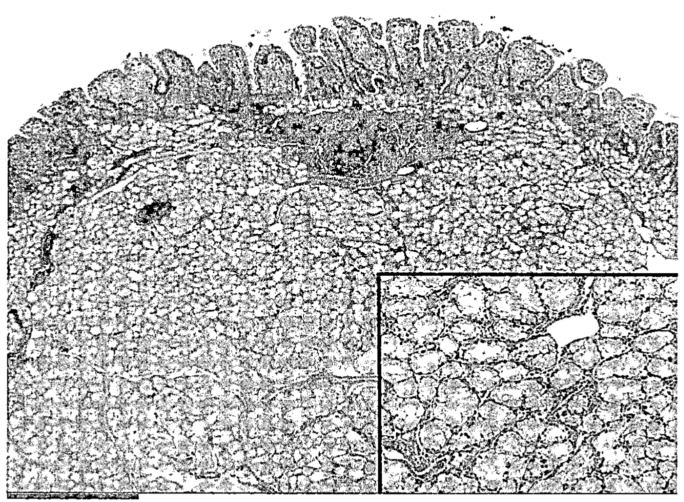

Figure 49.18
Brunner's gland hyperplasia. The hyperplastic lobules of Brunner's glands markedly expand the submucosa. The glandular elements are devoid of cytologic atypia (*inset*).

Rare cases of adenocarcinomas have been found in association with adenomyomatous hyperplasia, but these hypoproliferative lesions are not believed to be preneoplastic by most authors.[149,153,154]

The challenge presented by these lesions remains that despite advanced imaging techniques and preoperative endoscopic evaluation, the distinction from malignant tumors can be difficult, even at the time of frozen section, and can lead to unnecessary surgery.[149,152,155,156]

Brunner gland hyperplasia Brunner gland hyperplasia is an uncommon duodenal lesion that can be identified in the periampullary region. The hyperplasia of these submucosal glands has been attributed to increased secretin levels in patients with chronic renal failure and to hyperacidic gastric secretion.[157,158] Brunner gland hyperplasia usually presents as polypoid lesions that rarely exceed a few centimeters in size.[151,158] Most cases are asymptomatic, but hemorrhage and a rare example of obstructive jaundice have however been reported.[152,158] Histologically, these lesions are composed of densely packed lobules of benign Brunner glands that can distort the crypts and villi (Fig. 49.18). Cellular atypia and mitoses are usually absent, suggesting a hyperplastic process rather a neoplastic lesion.

Inflammatory pseudotumor Inflammatory pseudotumors composed of admixed inflammatory infiltrate encasing the ampullary epithelium have been described. They usually present in elderly patients and need to be distinguished from adenocarcinomas.[7] The distinction can be challenging because the epithelium can show varying degrees of reactive mucosal atypia. Endoscopic resection is curative.

Other rare inflammatory processes involving the ampulla of Vater have been observed. One case has been reported of eosinophilic gastroenteritis presenting with pancreaticobiliary obstruction and an ampullary mass mimicking an adenoma.[159] A very unusual case of xanthogranulomatous choledochitis resulting in ampullary stricture has also been published.[160]

Secondary Tumors of the Ampullary Region

Secondary involvement of the ampulla is most commonly direct extension from adjacent sites. Although rare, hematogenous metastases from distant organs have also been reported. The most common primary neoplasm is renal cell carcinoma.[161-164] The ampullary involvement may manifest many years after the initial diagnosis and/or resection of the primary neoplasm. Other neoplasms that metastasize to the ampulla include melanoma,[165] breast adenocarcinoma,[166] squamous cell carcinoma of the larynx,[167] endometrioid adenocarcinoma,[168] and osteosarcoma.[169]

References

1. Avisse C, Flament JB, Delattre JF. Ampulla of Vater: anatomic, embryologic, and surgical aspects. *Surg Clin North Am*. 2000;80:201–212.
2. Galandiuk S, Hermann RE, Jagelman DG, Fazio VW, Sivak MV. Villous tumors of the duodenum. *Ann Surg*. 1988;207:234–239.
3. Rosenberg J, Welch JP, Pyrtek LJ, Walker M, Trowbridge P. Benign villous adenomas of the ampulla of Vater. *Cancer*. 1986;58:1563–1568.
4. Stolte M, Pscherer C. Adenoma-carcinoma sequence in the papilla of Vater. *Scand J Gastroenterol*. 1996;31:376–382.
5. Howe JR, Klimstra DS, Moccia RD, Conlon KC, Brennan MF. Factors predictive of survival in ampullary carcinoma. *Ann Surg*. 1998;228:87–94.
6. Yamaguchi K, Enjoji M. Carcinoma of the ampulla of Vater: a clinicopathologic study and pathologic staging of 109 cases of carcinoma and 5 cases of adenoma. *Cancer*. 1987;59:506–515.
7. Attanoos R, Williams GT. Epithelial and neuroendocrine tumors of the duodenum. *Semin Diagn Pathol*. 1991;8: 149–162.
8. Ryan DP, Schapiro RH, Warshaw AL. Villous tumors of the duodenum. *Ann Surg*. 1986;203:301–306.
9. Perzin KH, Bridge MF. Adenomas of the small intestine: a clinicopathologic review of 51 cases and a study of their relationship to carcinoma. *Cancer*. 1981;48:799–819.
10. Bjork KJ, Davis CJ, Nagorney DM, Mucha P Jr. Duodenal villous tumors. *Arch Surg*. 1990;125:961–965.
11. Blackman E, Nash SV. Diagnosis of duodenal and ampullary epithelial neoplasms by endoscopic biopsy: a clinicopathologic and immunohistochemical study. *Hum Pathol*. 1985;16:901–910.
12. Yamaguchi K, Enjoji M. Adenoma of the ampulla of Vater: putative precancerous lesion. *Gut*. 1991;32:1558–1561.
13. Albores-Saavedra J, Henson DE, Klimstra DS. *Atlas of Tumors Pathology: Tumors of the Gallbladder, Extrahepatic Bile Ducts, and Ampulla of Vater.* Washington, DC: Armed Forces Institute of Pathology; 2000.
14. Noda Y, Watanabe H, Iida M, et al. Histologic follow-up of ampullary adenomas in patients with familial adenomatosis coli. *Cancer*. 1992;70:1847–1856.
15. Saurin JC, Chavaillon A, Napoleon B, et al. Long-term follow-up of patients with endoscopic treatment of sporadic adenomas of the papilla of Vater. *Endoscopy*. 2003;35:402–406.
16. Matsumoto T, Iida M, Nakamura S, et al. Natural history of ampullary adenoma in familial adenomatous polyposis: reconfirmation of benign nature during extended surveillance. *Am J Gastroenterol*. 2000;95:1557–1562.
17. Bjork J, Akerbrant H, Iselius L, et al. Periampullary adenomas and adenocarcinomas in familial adenomatous polyposis: cumulative risks and APC gene mutations. *Gastroenterology*. 2001;121:1127–1135.
18. Offerhaus GJ, Giardiello FM, Krush AJ, et al. The risk of upper gastrointestinal cancer in familial adenomatous polyposis. *Gastroenterology*. 1992;102:1980–1982.
19. Pauli RM, Pauli ME, Hall JG. Gardner syndrome and periampullary malignancy. *Am J Med Genet*. 1980;6:205–219.
20. Spigelman AD, Talbot IC, Penna C, et al. Evidence for adenoma-carcinoma sequence in the duodenum of patients with familial adenomatous polyposis. The Leeds Castle Polyposis Group (Upper Gastrointestinal Committee). *J Clin Pathol*. 1994;47:709–710.
21. Trimbath JD, Griffin C, Romans K, Giardiello FM. Attenuated familial adenomatous polyposis presenting as ampullary adenocarcinoma. *Gut*. 2003;52:903–904.
22. Norton ID, Pokorny CS, Painter DM, Johnson JR, Perkins KW. Fraternal sisters with adult polycystic kidney disease and adenoma of the ampulla of Vater. *Gastroenterology*. 1995;109:2007–2010.
23. Kozuka S, Tsubone M, Yamaguchi A, Hachisuka K. Adenomatous residue in cancerous papilla of Vater. *Gut*. 1981;22:1031–1034.
24. Baczako K, Buchler M, Beger HG, Kirkpatrick CJ, Haferkamp O. Morphogenesis and possible precursor lesions of invasive carcinoma of the papilla of Vater: epithelial dysplasia and adenoma. *Hum Pathol*. 1985;16:305–310.
25. Gertsch P, Preitner J, Fontolliet C. Carcinoma of Vater's ampulla and precursor states. *Schweiz Med Wochenschr*. 1987;117:1098–1100.
26. Komorowski RA, Cohen EB. Villous tumors of the duodenum: a clinicopathologic study. *Cancer*. 1981;47:1377–1386.
27. Jordan PH Jr, Ayala G, Rosenberg WR, Kinner BM. Treatment of ampullary villous adenomas that may harbor carcinoma. *J Gastrointest Surg*. 2002;6:770–775.
28. Menzel J, Poremba C, Dietl KH, Bocker W, Domschke W. Tumors of the papilla of Vater: inadequate diagnostic impact of endoscopic forceps biopsies taken prior to and following sphincterotomy. *Ann Oncol*. 1999;10:1227–1231.
29. Komorowski RA, Beggs BK, Geenan JE, Venu RP. Assessment of ampulla of Vater pathology: an endoscopic approach. *Am J Surg Pathol*. 1991;15:1188–1196.
30. Roder JD, Schneider PM, Stein HJ, Siewert JR. Number of lymph node metastases is significantly associated with survival in patients with radically resected carcinoma of the ampulla of Vater. *Br J Surg*. 1995;82:1693–1696.
31. Yamaguchi K, Enjoji M, Tsuneyoshi M. Pancreatoduodenal carcinoma: a clinicopathologic study of 304 patients and immunohistochemical observation for CEA and CA19-9. *J Surg Oncol*. 1991;47:148–154.
32. Martin FM, Rossi RL, Dorrucci V, Silverman ML, Braasch JW. Clinical and pathologic correlations in patients with periampullary tumors. *Arch Surg*. 1990;125:723–726.
33. Jones BA, Langer B, Taylor BR, Girotti M. Periampullary tumors: which ones should be resected? *Am J Surg*. 1985;149:46–52.

34. Sarmiento JM, Nagomey DM, Sarr MG, Farnell MB. Periampullary cancers: are there differences? *Surg Clin North Am.* 2001;81:543–555.
35. Kellum JM, Clark J, Miller HH. Pancreatoduodenectomy for resectable malignant periampullary tumors. *Surg Gynecol Obstet.* 1983;157:362–366.
36. Talbot IC, Neoptolemos JP, Shaw DE, Carr-Locke D. The histopathology and staging of carcinoma of the ampulla of Vater. *Histopathology.* 1988;12:155–165.
37. Ferrell LD, Beckstead JH. Paneth-like cells in an adenoma and adenocarcinoma in the ampulla of Vater. *Arch Pathol Lab Med.* 1991;115:956–958.
38. Chareton B, Coiffic J, Landen S, Bardaxoglou E, Campion JP, Launois B. Diagnosis and therapy for ampullary tumors: 63 cases. *World J Surg.* 1996;20:707–712.
39. Wise L, Pizzimbono C, Dehner LP. Periampullary cancer: a clinicopathologic study of sixty-two patients. *Am J Surg.* 1976;131:141–148.
40. Hayes DH, Bolton JS, Willis GW, Bowen JC. Carcinoma of the ampulla of Vater. *Ann Surg.* 1987;206:572–577.
41. Sessa F, Solcia E, Capella C, et al. Intraductal papillary-mucinous tumours represent a distinct group of pancreatic neoplasms: an investigation of tumour cell differentiation and K-ras, p53 and c-erbB-2 abnormalities in 26 patients. *Virchows Arch.* 1994;425:357–367.
42. Albores-Saavedra J, Murakata L, Krueger JE, Henson DE. Noninvasive and minimally invasive papillary carcinomas of the extrahepatic bile ducts. *Cancer.* 2000;89:508–515.
43. Seifert E, Schulte F, Stolte M. Adenoma and carcinoma of the duodenum and papilla of Vater: a clinicopathologic study. *Am J Gastroenterol.* 1992;87:37–42.
44. Gardner HA, Matthews J, Ciano PS. A signet-ring cell carcinoma of the ampulla of Vater. *Arch Pathol Lab Med.* 1990;114:1071–1072.
45. Eriguchi N, Aoyagi S, Jimi A. Signet-ring cell carcinoma of the ampulla of Vater: report of a case. *Surg Today.* 2003;33:467–469.
46. Gardiner GW, Lajoie G, Keith R. Hepatoid adenocarcinoma of the papilla of Vater. *Histopathology.* 1992;20:541–544.
47. Sato Y, Tominaga H, Tangoku A, Hamanaka Y, Yamashita Y, Suzuki T. Alpha-fetoprotein-producing cancer of the ampulla of Vater. *Hepatogastroenterology.* 1992;39:566–569.
48. Warren KW, Choe DS, Plaza J, Relihan M. Results of radical resection for periampullary cancer. *Ann Surg.* 1975;181:534–540.
49. Lee CS, Machet D, Rode J. Small cell carcinoma of the ampulla of Vater. *Cancer.* 1992;70:1502–1504.
50. Sarker AB, Hoshida Y, Akagi S, et al. An immunohistochemical and ultrastructural study of case of small-cell neuroendocrine carcinoma in the ampullary region of the duodenum. *Acta Pathol Jpn.* 1992;42:529–535.
51. Zamboni G, Franzin G, Bonetti F, et al. Small-cell neuroendocrine carcinoma of the ampullary region: a clinicopathologic, immunohistochemical, and ultrastructural study of three cases. *Am J Surg Pathol.* 1990;14:703–713.
52. Emory RE Jr, Emory TS, Goellner JR, Grant CS, Nagorney DM. Neuroendocrine ampullary tumors: spectrum of disease including the first report of a neuroendocrine carcinoma of non-small cell type. *Surgery.* 1994;115:762–766.
53. Mori K, Ikei S, Yamane T, et al. Pathological factors influencing survival of carcinoma of the ampulla of Vater. *Eur J Surg Oncol.* 1990;16:183–188.
54. Cavazza A, Gallo M, Valcavi R, De Marco L, Gardini G. Large cell neuroendocrine carcinoma of the ampulla of Vater. *Arch Pathol Lab Med.* 2003;127:221–223.
55. Molberg KH, Heffess C, Delgado R, Albores-Saavedra J. Undifferentiated carcinoma with osteoclast-like giant cells of the pancreas and periampullary region. *Cancer.* 1998;82:1279–1287.
56. Kench JG, Frommer DJ. Sarcomatoid carcinoma of the ampulla of Vater. *Pathology.* 1997;29:89–91.
57. Kijima H, Takeshita T, Suzuki H, et al. Carcinosarcoma of the ampulla of Vater: a case report with immunohistochemical and ultrastructural studies. *Am J Gastroenterol.* 1999;94:3055–3059.
58. Albores-Saavedra J, Molberg K, Henson DE. Unusual malignant epithelial tumors of the gallbladder. *Semin Diagn Pathol.* 1996;13:326–338.
59. Vardaman C, Albores-Saavedra J. Clear cell carcinomas of the gallbladder and extrahepatic bile ducts. *Am J Surg Pathol.* 1995;19:91–99.
60. Bardales RH, Stanley MW, Simpson DD, et al. Diagnostic value of brush cytology in the diagnosis of duodenal, biliary, and ampullary neoplasms. *Am J Clin Pathol.* 1998;109:540–548.
61. Kimura W, Ohtsubo K. Incidence, sites of origin, and immunohistochemical and histochemical characteristics of atypical epithelium and minute carcinoma of the papilla of Vater. *Cancer.* 1988;61:1394–1402.
62. Maxwell P, Davis RI, Sloan JM. Carcinoembryonic antigen (CEA) in benign and malignant epithelium of the gall bladder, extrahepatic bile ducts, and ampulla of Vater. *J Pathol.* 1993;170:73–76.
63. Batge B, Bosslet K, Sedlacek HH, Kern HF, Kloppel G. Monoclonal antibodies against CEA-related components discriminate between pancreatic duct type carcinomas and nonneoplastic duct lesions as well as nonduct type neoplasias. *Virchows Arch A Pathol Anat Histopathol.* 1986;408:361–374.
64. Fischer HP, Zhou H. [Pathogenesis and histomorphology of ampullary carcinomas and their precursor lesions: review and individual findings]. *Pathologe.* 2003;24:196–203.
65. Scarpa A, Capelli P, Zamboni G, et al. Neoplasia of the ampulla of Vater: K-ras and p53 mutations. *Am J Pathol.* 1993;142:1163–1172.
66. Takashima M, Ueki T, Nagai E, et al. Carcinoma of the ampulla of Vater associated with or without adenoma: a clinicopathologic analysis of 198 cases with reference to p53 and Ki-67 immunohistochemical expressions. *Mod Pathol.* 2000;13:1300–1307.
67. Younes M, Riley S, Genta RM, Mosharaf M, Mody DR. p53 protein accumulation in tumors of the ampulla of Vater. *Cancer.* 1995;76:1150–1154.
68. Teh M, Wee A, Raju GC. An immunohistochemical study of p53 protein in gallbladder and extrahepatic bile duct/ampullary carcinomas. *Cancer.* 1994;74:1542–1545.
69. Diamantis I, Karamitopoulou E, Perentes E, Zimmermann A. p53 protein immunoreactivity in extrahepatic bile duct and gallbladder cancer: correlation with tumor grade and survival. *Hepatology.* 1995;22:774–779.

70. McCarthy DM, Hruban RH, Argani P, et al. Role of the DPC4 tumor suppressor gene in adenocarcinoma of the ampulla of Vater: analysis of 140 cases. *Mod Pathol.* 2003;16:272–278.
71. Motojima K, Tsunoda T, Kanematsu T, Nagata Y, Urano T, Shiku H. Distinguishing pancreatic carcinoma from other periampullary carcinomas by analysis of mutations in the Kirsten-ras oncogene. *Ann Surg.* 1991;214:657–662.
72. Chung CH, Wilentz RE, Polak MM, et al. Clinical significance of K-ras oncogene activation in ampullary neoplasms. *J Clin Pathol.* 1996;49:460–464.
73. Rashid A, Ueki T, Gao YT, et al. K-ras mutation, p53 overexpression, and microsatellite instability in biliary tract cancers: a population-based study in China. *Clin Cancer Res.* 2002;8:3156–3163.
74. Howe JR, Klimstra DS, Cordon-Cardo C, Paty PB, Park PY, Brennan MF. K-ras mutation in adenomas and carcinomas of the ampulla of vater. *Clin Cancer Res.* 1997;3: 129–133.
75. Scarpa A, Zamboni G, Achille A, et al. ras-family gene mutations in neoplasia of the ampulla of Vater. *Int J Cancer.* 1994;59:39–42.
76. Stork P, Loda M, Bosari S, Wiley B, Poppenhusen K, Wolfe H. Detection of K-ras mutations in pancreatic and hepatic neoplasms by non-isotopic mismatched polymerase chain reaction. *Oncogene.* 1991;6:857–862.
77. Gallinger S, Vivona AA, Odze RD, et al. Somatic APC and K-ras codon 12 mutations in periampullary adenomas and carcinomas from familial adenomatous polyposis patients. *Oncogene.* 1995;10:1875–1878.
78. Smit VT, Boot AJ, Smits AM, Fleuren GJ, Cornelisse CJ, Bos JL. K-ras codon 12 mutations occur very frequently in pancreatic adenocarcinomas. *Nucleic Acids Res.* 1988;16:7773–7782.
79. Almoguera C, Shibata D, Forrester K, Martin J, Arnheim N, Perucho M. Most human carcinomas of the exocrine pancreas contain mutant c-K-ras genes. *Cell.* 1988;53:549–554.
80. Vaidya P, Kawarada Y, Higashiguchi T, Yoshida T, Sakakura T, Yatani R. Overexpression of different members of the type 1 growth factor receptor family and their association with cell proliferation in periampullary carcinoma. *J Pathol.* 1996;178:140–145.
81. Resnick MB, Gallinger S, Wang HH, Odze RD. Growth factor expression and proliferation kinetics in periampullary neoplasms in familial adenomatous polyposis. *Cancer.* 1995;76:187–194.
82. Bulow S, Skov Olsen P, Poulsen SS, Kirkegaard P. Is epidermal growth factor involved in development of duodenal polyps in familial polyposis coli? *Am J Gastroenterol.* 1988;83:404–406.
83. Rashid A, Gao YT, Bhakta S, et al. Beta-catenin mutations in biliary tract cancers: a population-based study in China. *Cancer Res.* 2001;61:3406–3409.
84. Park S, Kim SW, Kim SH, Darwish NS, Kim WH. Lack of microsatellite instability in neoplasms of ampulla of Vater. *Pathol Int.* 2003;53:667–670.
85. Geene FL, Page DL, Fleming ID, et al., eds. *AJCC Cancer Staging Manual.* 6th ed. New York: Springer; 2002.
86. Klempnauer J, Ridder GJ, Pichlmayr R. Prognostic factors after resection of ampullary carcinoma: multivariate survival analysis in comparison with ductal cancer of the pancreatic head. *Br J Surg.* 1995;82:1686–1691.
87. Nakai T, Koh K, Kawabe T, Son E, Yoshikawa H, Yasutomi M. Importance of microperineural invasion as a prognostic factor in ampullary carcinoma. *Br J Surg.* 1997;84:1399–1401.
88. Monson JR, Donohue JH, McEntee GP, et al. Radical resection for carcinoma of the ampulla of Vater. *Arch Surg.* 1991;126:353–357.
89. Talamini MA, Moesinger RC, Pitt HA, et al. Adenocarcinoma of the ampulla of Vater: a 28-year experience. *Ann Surg.* 1997;225:590–599; discussion 599–600.
90. Sperti C, Pasquali C, Piccoli A, Sernagiotto C, Pedrazzoli S. Radical resection for ampullary carcinoma: long-term results. *Br J Surg.* 1994;81:668–671.
91. Beger HG, Treitschke F, Gansauge F, Harada N, Hiki N, Mattfeldt T. Tumor of the ampulla of Vater: experience with local or radical resection in 171 consecutively treated patients. *Arch Surg.* 1999;134:526–532.
92. Shyr YM, Su CH, Wu LH, et al. Prognostic value of MIB-1 index and DNA ploidy in resectable ampulla of Vater carcinoma. *Ann Surg.* 1999;229:523–527.
93. Makhlouf HR, Burke AP, Sobin LH. Carcinoid tumors of the ampulla of Vater: a comparison with duodenal carcinoid tumors. *Cancer.* 1999;85:1241–1249.
94. Burke AP, Sobin LH, Federspiel BH, Shekitka KM, Helwig EB. Carcinoid tumors of the duodenum: a clinicopathologic study of 99 cases. *Arch Pathol Lab Med.* 1990;114:700–704.
95. Fuller CE, Williams GT. Gastrointestinal manifestations of type 1 neurofibromatosis (von Recklinghausen's disease). *Histopathology.* 1991;19:1–11.
96. Dayal Y, Tallberg KA, Nunnemacher G, DeLellis RA, Wolfe HJ. Duodenal carcinoids in patients with and without neurofibromatosis: a comparative study. *Am J Surg Pathol.* 1986;10:348–357.
97. Burke AP, Sobin LH, Shekitka KM, Federspiel BH, Helwig EB. Somatostatin-producing duodenal carcinoids in patients with von Recklinghausen's neurofibromatosis: a predilection for black patients. *Cancer.* 1990;65:1591–1595.
98. Bornstein-Quevedo L, Gamboa-Dominguez A. Carcinoid tumors of the duodenum and ampulla of vater: a clinicomorphologic, immunohistochemical, and cell kinetic comparison. *Hum Pathol.* 2001;32:1252–1256.
99. Guo M, Lemos LB, Bigler S, Baliga M. Duodenal somatostatinoma of the ampulla of Vater diagnosed by endoscopic fine needle aspiration biopsy: a case report. *Acta Cytol.* 2001;45:622–626.
100. Usui M, Matsuda S, Suzuki H, Hirata K, Ogura Y, Shiraishi T. Somatostatinoma of the papilla of Vater with multiple gastrointestinal stromal tumors in a patient with von Recklinghausen's disease. *J Gastroenterol.* 2002;37: 947–953.
101. Donow C, Pipeleers-Marichal M, Schroder S, Stamm B, Heitz PU, Kloppel G. Surgical pathology of gastrinoma. Site, size, multicentricity, association with multiple endocrine neoplasia type 1, and malignancy. *Cancer.* 1991;68:1329–1334.

102. Burke A, Lee YK. Adenocarcinoid (goblet cell carcinoid) of the duodenum presenting as gastric outlet obstruction. *Hum Pathol.* 1990;21:238–239.
103. Jones MA, Griffith LM, West AB. Adenocarcinoid tumor of the periampullary region: a novel duodenal neoplasm presenting as biliary tract obstruction. *Hum Pathol.* 1989;20:198–200.
104. Shah IA, Schlageter MO, Boehm N. Composite carcinoid-adenocarcinoma of ampulla of Vater. *Hum Pathol.* 1990;21:1188–1190.
105. Burke AP, Helwig EB. Gangliocytic paraganglioma. *Am J Clin Pathol.* 1989;92:1–9.
106. Hamid QA, Bishop AE, Rode J, et al. Duodenal gangliocytic paragangliomas: a study of 10 cases with immunocytochemical neuroendocrine markers. *Hum Pathol.* 1986;17:1151–1157.
107. Scheithauer BW, Nora FE, LeChago J, et al. Duodenal gangliocytic paraganglioma: clinicopathologic and immunocytochemical study of 11 cases. *Am J Clin Pathol.* 1986;86: 559–565.
108. Perrone T, Sibley RK, Rosai J. Duodenal gangliocytic paraganglioma: an immunohistochemical and ultrastructural study and a hypothesis concerning its origin. *Am J Surg Pathol.* 1985;9:31–41.
109. Reed RJ, Caroca PJ Jr, Harkin JC. Gangliocytic paraganglioma. *Am J Surg Pathol.* 1977;1:207–216.
110. Perrone T. Duodenal gangliocytic paraganglioma and carcinoid. *Am J Surg Pathol.* 1986;10:147–149.
111. Tomic S, Warner T. Pancreatic somatostatin-secreting gangliocytic paraganglioma with lymph node metastases. *Am J Gastroenterol.* 1996;91:607–608.
112. Collina G, Maiorana A, Trentini GP. Duodenal gangliocytic paraganglioma: case report with immunohistochemical study on the expression of keratin polypeptides. *Histopathology.* 1991;19:476–478.
113. Buchler M, Malfertheiner P, Baczako K, Krautzberger W, Beger HG. A metastatic endocrine-neurogenic tumor of the ampulla of Vater with multiple endocrineimmunoreaction–malignant paraganglioma? *Digestion.* 1985;31:54–59.
114. Korbi S, Kapanci Y, Widgren S. Malignant paraganglioma of the duodenum. Immunohistochemical and ultrastructural study of a case. *Ann Pathol.* 1987;7:47–55.
115. Inai K, Kobuke T, Yonehara S, Tokuoka S. Duodenal gangliocytic paraganglioma with lymph node metastasis in a 17- year-old boy. *Cancer.* 1989;63:2540–2545.
116. Hashimoto S, Kawasaki S, Matsuzawa K, Harada H, Makuuchi M. Gangliocytic paraganglioma of the papilla of Vater with regional lymph node metastasis. *Am J Gastroenterol.* 1992; 87:1216–1218.
117. Dookhan DB, Miettinen M, Finkel G, Gibas Z. Recurrent duodenal gangliocytic paraganglioma with lymph node metastases. *Histopathology.* 1993;22:399–401.
118. Simard L-C. Les complexes neuro-insulaires du pancreas humain. (Neurocrinie et fonction paraganglionnaire). *Arch D'Anat Microsc.* 1937;33:4–61.
119. Kheir SM, Halpern NB. Paraganglioma of the duodenum in association with congenital neurofibromatosis: possible relationship. *Cancer.* 1984;53:2491–2496.
120. Stephens M, Williams GT, Jasani B, Williams ED. Synchronous duodenal neuroendocrine tumours in von Recklinghausen's disease: a case report of co-existing gangliocytic paraganglioma and somatostatin-rich glandular carcinoid. *Histopathology.* 1987;11:1331–1340.
121. del Pino Porres FJ, Riesgo Suarez P, Boils Arroyo PL, et al. Nonchromaffin neurogenic tumors of the intestinal tract: a report of 2 cases and their relation to von Recklinghausen's neurofibromatosis. *Rev Esp Enferm Dig.* 1991;79:46–49.
122. Nemsmann B, Schroder D. [Juxtapapillary leiomyoma—a rare papillary tumor: presentation of an unusual disease picture]. *Fortschr Med.* 1984;102:565–566.
123. Culebras Fernandez JM, Gonzalez Bueno CM. [Leiomyoma of Vater's ampulla]. *Rev Esp Enferm Apar Dig.* 1974;42:165–172.
124. Koninger J, Butters M, Roos U, Bittner R. [Juxtapapillary intraduodenal lipoma as a rare cause of jaundice and acute pancreatitis]. *Z Gastroenterol.* 1994;32:157–159.
125. Sriram PV, Weise C, Seitz U, Brand B, Schroder S, Soehendra N. Lymphangioma of the major duodenal papilla presenting as acute pancreatitis: treatment by endoscopic snare papillectomy. *Gastrointest Endosc.* 2000;51:733–736.
126. Artaza T, Potenciano JM, Legaz M, Munoz C, Talavera A, Sanchez E. Lymphangioma of Vater's ampulla: a rare cause of obstructive jaundice: endoscopic therapy. *Scand J Gastroenterol.* 1995;30:804–806.
127. Friedrich HJ, Schramm H, Peckholz I. [Cavernous lymphangioma of Vater's papilla as a cause of occlusive icterus: case report]. *Zentralbl Chir.* 1985;110:1263–1265.
128. Klein A, Clemens J, Cameron J. Periampullary neoplasms in von Recklinghausen's disease. *Surgery.* 1989;106:815–819.
129. Gemer M, Feuchtwanger MM. Ganglioneuroma of the duodenum. *Gastroenterology.* 1966;51:689–693.
130. Goldman RL. Ganglioneuroma of the duodenum: relationship to nonchromaffin paraganglioma of the duodenum. *Am J Surg.* 1968;115:716–719.
131. Mackenzie DJ, Klapper E, Gordon LA, Silberman AW. Granular cell tumor of the biliary system. *Med Pediatr Oncol.* 1994;23:50–56.
132. Miettinen M, Kopczynski J, Makhlouf HR, et al. Gastrointestinal stromal tumors, intramural leiomyomas, and leiomyosarcomas in the duodenum: a clinicopathologic, immunohistochemical, and molecular genetic study of 167 cases. *Am J Surg Pathol.* 2003;27:625–641.
133. Caty MG, Oldham KT, Prochownik EV. Embryonal rhabdomyosarcoma of the ampulla of Vater with long-term survival following pancreaticoduodenectomy. *J Pediatr Surg.* 1990;25:1256–1258.
134. Isaacson C. Embryonal rhabdomyosarcoma of the ampulla of vater. *Cancer.* 1978;41:365–368.
135. Seitz JF, Giovannini M, Wartelle C, Monges G, Dhiver C, Gastaut JA. [Kaposi's sarcoma of Vater's ampulla associated with sclerosing cholangitis caused by Cryptosporidium in a patient with AIDS]. *Gastroenterol Clin Biol.* 1990;14:889–891.
136. Cirillo M, Federico M, Curci G, Tamborrino E, Piccinini L, Silingardi V. Primary gastrointestinal lymphoma: a clinicopathological study of 58 cases. *Haematologica.* 1992;77: 156–161.

137. Isomoto H, Kamihira S, Matsuo E, et al. A case of mucosa-associated lymphoid tissue lymphoma of the ampulla of Vater: successful treatment with radiation therapy. *Eur J Gastroenterol Hepatol.* 2003;15:1037–1041.
138. Nadal E, Martinez A, Jimenez M, et al. Primary follicular lymphoma arising in the ampulla of Vater. *Ann Hematol.* 2002;81:228–231.
139. Pawade J, Lee CS, Ellis DW, Vellar ID, Rode J. Primary lymphoma of the ampulla of Vater. *Cancer.* 1994;73:2083–2086.
140. Weinstock LB, Swanson PE, Bennett KJ, Van Amburg A, Wald SM, Shah NB. Jaundice caused by a clinically undetectable T-cell lymphoma infiltrating the sphincter of Oddi. *Am J Gastroenterol.* 2001;96:3186–3189.
141. Misdraji J, Fernandez del Castillo C, Ferry JA. Follicle center lymphoma of the ampulla of Vater presenting with jaundice: report of a case. *Am J Surg Pathol.* 1997;21:484–488.
142. Barek L, Orron D. Non-Hodgkin's lymphoma presenting as periampullary mass with obstructive jaundice. *J Comput Tomogr.* 1986;10:89–92.
143. Schoeppner HL, Wong DK, Bresalier RS. Primary small bowel lymphoma manifested as obstructive jaundice in a patient with AIDS. *South Med J.* 1995;88:583–585.
144. Ventrucci M, Gherlinzoni F, Sabattini E, Cipolla A, Ubalducci GM, Pileri S. Primary MALT-lymphoma of the papilla of Vater. *Dig Dis Sci.* 1998;43:214–216.
145. Yoshino T, Miyake K, Ichimura K, et al. Increased incidence of follicular lymphoma in the duodenum. *Am J Surg Pathol.* 2000;24:688–693.
146. Halline A, Lerios M, Melissas J, Segal I, Grieve TP. Primary lymphoma of the small bowel with obstructive jaundice and pancreatitis: a case report. *S Afr Med J.* 1987;72:61–62.
147. Leese T, Neoptolemos JP, West KP, Talbot IC, Carr-Locke DL. Tumours and pseudotumours of the region of the ampulla of Vater: an endoscopic, clinical and pathological study. *Gut.* 1986;27:1186–1192.
148. Narita T, Yokoyama M. Adenomyomatous hyperplasia of the papilla of Vater: a sequela of chronic papillitis? *Ann Diagn Pathol.* 1999;3:174–177.
149. Handra-Luca A, Terris B, Couvelard A, Bonte H, Flejou JF. Adenomyoma and adenomyomatous hyperplasia of the Vaterian system: clinical, pathological, and new immunohistochemical features of 13 cases. *Mod Pathol.* 2003;16:530–536.
150. Maran R, Gal R, Kyzer S, Feierman Z, Shapira G, Mittelman M. Severe weight loss, renal failure, and metabolic alkalosis due to duodenal adenomyoma. *Am J Gastroenterol.* 1993;88:472–473.
151. Fuller JW, Cruse CW, Williams JW. Hyperplasia of Brunner's glands of the duodenum. *Am Surg.* 1977;43:246–250.
152. Skellenger ME, Kinner BM, Jordan PH Jr. Brunner's gland hamartomas can mimic carcinoma of the head of the pancreas. *Surg Gynecol Obstet.* 1983;156:774–776.
153. Al Jitawi SA, Hiarat AM, Al-Majali SH. Diffuse myoepithelial hamartoma of the duodenum associated with adenocarcinoma. *Clin Oncol.* 1984;10:289–293.
154. Bergdahl L, Andersson A. Benign tumors of the papilla of Vater. *Am Surg.* 1980;46:563–566.
155. Kayahara M, Ohta T, Kitagawa H, Miwa K, Urabe T, Murata T. Adenomyomatosis of the papilla of Vater: a case illustrating diagnostic difficulties. *Dig Surg.* 2001;18:139–142.
156. Allgaier HP, Schwacha H, Kleinschmidt M, Thimme R, Schoffel U, Blum HE. Ampullary hamartoma: a rare cause of biliary obstruction. *Digestion.* 1999;60:497–500.
157. Pikielny SS, Bernheim J, Salomon A. Hyperplastic Brunner glands and chronic renal insufficiency (author's translation). *J Radiol Electrol Med Nucl.* 1978;59:493–495.
158. De Angelis G, Villanacci V, Lovotti D, et al. Hamartomatous polyps of Brunner's gland: presentation of 2 cases. Review of the literature. *Minerva Chir.* 1989;44:1761–1766.
159. Madhotra R, Eloubeidi MA, Cunningham JT, Lewin D, Hoffman B. Eosinophilic gastroenteritis masquerading as ampullary adenoma. *J Clin Gastroenterol.* 2002;34:240–242.
160. Goldar-Najafi A, Khettry U. Xanthogranulomatous choledochitis: a previously undescribed mass lesion of the hepatobiliary and ampullary region. *Semin Liver Dis.* 2003;23:101–106.
161. Leslie KA, Tsao JI, Rossi RL, Braasch JW. Metastatic renal cell carcinoma to ampulla of Vater: an unusual lesion amenable to surgical resection. *Surgery.* 1996;119:349–351.
162. Venu RP, Rolny P, Geenen JE, Hogan WJ, Komorowski RA, Ferstenberg R. Ampullary tumor caused by metastatic renal cell carcinoma. *Dig Dis Sci.* 1991;36:376–378.
163. Robertson GS, Gertler SL. Late presentation of metastatic renal cell carcinoma as a bleeding ampullary mass. *Gastrointest Endosc.* 1990;36:304–306.
164. McKenna JI, Kozarek RA. Metastatic hypernephroma to the ampulla of Vater: an unusual cause of malabsorption diagnosed at endoscopic sphincterotomy. *Am J Gastroenterol.* 1989;84:81–83.
165. Sans M, Llach J, Bordas JM, et al. Metastatic malignant melanoma of the papilla of Vater: an unusual case of obstructive cholestasis treated with biliary prostheses. *Endoscopy.* 1996;28:791–792.
166. Titus AS, Baron TH, Listinsky CM, Vickers SM. Solitary breast metastasis to the ampulla and distal common bile duct. *Am Surg.* 1997;63:512–515.
167. Buyukcelik A, Ensari A, Sarioglu M, Isikdogan A, Icli F. Squamous cell carcinoma of the larynx metastasized to the ampulla of Vater: report of a case. *Tumori.* 2003;89:199–201.
168. Silva R, Paiva ME, Santos CC. Obstructive jaundice caused by ampullary metastases of an endometrioid adenocarcinoma. *Gastrointest Endosc.* 1996;44:195–197.
169. Kadakia SC, Parker A, Canales L. Metastatic tumors to the upper gastrointestinal tract: endoscopic experience. *Am J Gastroenterol.* 1992;87:1418–1423.

50

Clinical Management of Ampullary Tumors

Rebekah R. White, MD
Bryan M. Clary, MD
Theodore N. Pappas, MD
Douglas S. Tyler, MD

Introduction

The ampulla of Vater is located at the confluence of the main pancreatic duct and the common bile duct, where they join to enter the major duodenal papilla, a prominence in the posteromedial wall of the second portion of the duodenum. Although initially described as a dilated common channel (thus, the name "ampulla"), this junction is anatomically quite variable, is rarely dilated, and is often not a common channel. The common bile duct and pancreatic duct may enter the duodenal papilla as a double-barreled opening or, occasionally, as separate openings.[1] Therefore, some anatomists consider a true ampulla to be absent in most people. Regardless, the functional entity that clinicians know as the ampulla of Vater is lined by an epithelial layer that transitions from pancreatic and biliary ductal epithelium to duodenal mucosal epithelium and is surrounded by the muscular sphincter of Oddi.

Because of their close proximity, tumors of the pancreatic head, distal common bile duct, second portion of the duodenum, and the ampulla of Vater are often discussed collectively as periampullary tumors. Tumors arising from the various tissues in this periampullary region can have similar clinical presentations and treatment approaches. Indeed, it is often difficult to determine the exact tissue of origin because tumors originating in the pancreas or common bile duct can extend to the ampulla and vice versa, and these tumors can possess similar histopathologic characteristics. However, these distinctions are not purely academic. As a result of the complex anatomy in this region, tumors of the ampulla of Vater can behave differently than other periampullary tumors and present unique management issues.

More than half of recognized ampullary neoplasms are adenomas, approximately 25% are carcinomas, and the rest are an assortment of benign and malignant tumor types, including lipomas, hemangiomas, leiomyofibromas, neuromas, neuroendocrine tumors, sarcomas (most commonly, gastrointestinal stromal tumors), and metastatic lesions. The spectrum of available treatment options for ampullary tumors ranges from endoscopic resection to pancreaticoduodenectomy, and the choice of treatment depends on both tumor and patient factors.

Presentation and Diagnosis

The clinical presentation of a periampullary tumor is not extremely helpful in determining its site of origin or whether it is benign or malignant. Common presenting symptoms include jaundice, abdominal pain, pancreatitis, and constitutional symptoms, such as weight loss. Jaundice is relatively more common in patients with adenocarcinoma (approximately 70% of patients) than in patients with benign lesions (20%–30% of patients),[2-6] whereas pancreatitis is relatively more common in patients with benign lesions.[5,6] Ampullary neoplasms are more likely than pancreatic or biliary tumors to present with anemia due to gastrointestinal bleeding from intraluminal growth. The timing of the onset of these symptoms with respect to the onset of constitutional symptoms may suggest a malignant etiology over a benign etiology, but none of these clinical presentations is prognostically very useful.

The diagnosis of an ampullary neoplasm is generally made after a diagnostic workup leads to an endoscopic examination. In patients with jaundice or abdominal pain, an initial abdominal ultrasound may demonstrate biliary ductal dilatation but rarely reveals an ampullary mass. Computed tomography (CT) may be performed early in a diagnostic workup, particularly if the suspicion for a malignant process is high. The presence of a periampullary mass on CT may render endoscopy unnecessary because in many treatment algorithms, a tissue diagnosis is not required before resection of a periampullary mass in which malignancy is suspected. However, the absence of a mass on CT obviously does not rule out a periampullary neoplasm. The presentation of obstructive jaundice without a mass lesion on CT warrants endoscopic retrograde cholangiopancreatography (ERCP), as does recurrent pancreatitis without clear etiology. It is during the approach to ERCP—or during duodenoscopy performed for the evaluation of abdominal pain or gastrointestinal bleeding—that ampullary masses are usually diagnosed. Endoscopic biopsy provides a histologic diagnosis, although the interpretation of this result should be tempered by the relatively low predictive value of a benign diagnosis. Depending on the diagnosis, ERCP and either endoscopic ultrasound (EUS) or intraductal ultrasound may provide additional information about the extent of local tumor invasion that influences subsequent management. CT, if not already performed, is recommended for the evaluation of both local tumor invasion and distant metastatic disease.

Benign Lesions

Although not true neoplasms, hamartomas (Brunner's gland hyperplasia), inflammatory pseudotumors, and adenomyomatosis are collectively much more common than adenomas. In addition, hamartomatous (Peutz-Jeghers) polyps, hemangiomas, neuromas, lipomas, and the polyps of the Cronkhite-Canada syndrome have essentially no malignant potential. If the patient is symptomatic, endoscopic resection—if technically feasible—is suitable for these benign lesions. Small, tubular adenomas might also be included in this category, given their relatively low likelihood of malignancy. Small, pedunculated lesions typically require only a single session for diathermy snare resection; larger lesions may require multiple sessions. Complications such as bleeding and pancreatitis are common but are usually minor and are able to be managed conservatively.[7] Relative contraindications to endoscopic resection include the presence of a duodenal diverticulum, Billroth II or Roux-en-Y anatomy, and large lesion size or circumference. Local surgical resection may be appropriate for lesions not amenable to endoscopic resection.

Malignant Tumors

At the other end of the spectrum, endoscopic biopsy may yield a malignant diagnosis. Adenocarcinoma is by far the most common ampullary malignancy and is the focus of this section, but neuroendocrine tumors, gastrointestinal stromal tumors, and metastatic lesions also occur in this region. Neuroendocrine tumors are discussed separately. Gastrointestinal stromal tumors, which should be presumed malignant, and certain isolated metastases to the ampulla, melanoma and renal cell carcinoma being the most common, may be treated with local ampullary resection or pancreaticoduodenectomy, as necessary to achieve complete resection.

Ampullary cancers represent less than 7% of malignant periampullary tumors[8] but because of their greater than 80% resectability rate, they are somewhat better represented (15%–25%) in series of resectable periampullary tumors.[9] Despite these sites being in such close proximity, ampullary adenocarcinoma has consistently been associated with survival superior to that of other periampullary tumors, with 5-year survival rates in recent series ranging from 33%–46%.[2-4,8,10,11] In the Johns Hopkins experience, patients undergoing resection for ampullary and duodenal cancers experienced the best 5-year survival rates (39% and 59%, respectively); cholangiocarcinoma was associated with intermediate survival (27%); and pancreatic cancer, the worst (15%).[9] In theory, even small tumors at the ampulla should lead to biliary obstruction, resulting in earlier clinical presentation. However, other incompletely understood biologic factors may also be involved. For instance, ampullary cancers are more likely to present with an expansive, intraluminal growth pattern than are pancreatic cancers, which typically present with an infiltrative growth pattern.[12] Ampullary cancers have also been associated with lower incidences of lymphatic, vascular, and perineural invasion, which may not be completely accounted for by earlier presentation.[13] Even when lymphatic involvement is present, the lymph nodes involved by ampullary carcinoma are usually limited to the posterior pancreatoduodenal nodes, unlike the more extensive lymph node involvement in pancreatic cancer.[14]

Numerous molecular differences have also been described. For instance, ampullary cancers are not associated with overexpression of EGFR as are pancreatic cancers.[15] Ampullary cancers have been associated with a lower incidence of p53 overexpression, which in turn correlates with lymph node metastasis and prognosis,[16] as well as a lower incidence of K-*ras* mutations.[17] Two histologic subtypes of ampullary carcinoma have been described: intestinal type and pancreaticobiliary type. The former is much more common, is more often associated with adenomatous changes, and has a more favorable outcome, similar to that of duodenal carcinoma.[8,18] In contrast, the pancreaticobiliary type appears to behave much more like a pancreatic and biliary primary. Because most ampullary cancers are of the intestinal type, they have a high incidence of microsatellite instability that is more similar to colon cancer than to pancreatic cancer,[19] and APC mutations are common in sporadic ampullary cancer (~50%), although they are rare in pancreatic cancer.[20] Arguably, ampullary carcinoma is actually a composite of two different diseases that should be considered to have biologic similarities to duodenal and pancreaticobiliary primaries.

In patients in whom the diagnosis of ampullary adenocarcinoma has been established by endoscopic biopsy, the most valuable staging study is a high-quality spiral CT with intravenous and oral contrast. CT is essential for the preoperative identification of distant metastatic disease, although one of its weaknesses remains its inability to identify small-volume hepatic and peritoneal metastases. CT also has a positive predictive value of approximately 80% in determining resectability and greater than 90% in predicting unresectability.[21,22] EUS has been touted as a supplement to CT in that it may provide superior assessment of T stage (Table 50.1), lymph node involvement, and portal vein invasion.[23-26] However, although EUS may be useful in staging selected high-risk surgical patients in whom local resection is being considered, we believe that its routine use is not necessary. EUS rarely alters the management of patients being offered radical resection, particularly because we do not consider lymph node involvement and portal vein invasion to be contraindications to resection for ampullary cancers. Similarly, ERCP should not automatically be performed in a patient in whom an ampullary malignancy has been diagnosed by other means, unless a delay in surgery is anticipated for a patient with jaundice, in which case the value of ERCP is the ability to palliate jaundice with endoscopic stenting.

Table 50.1 TNM Staging System* Ampullary Carcinoma

Tumor
- T1 Tumor limited to ampulla of Vater or sphincter of Oddie
- T2 Tumor invades duodenal wall
- T3 Tumor invades pancreas
- T4 Tumor invades peripancreatic soft tissues or other adjacent organs or structures

Nodes
- N0 No regional lymph node metastases
- N1 Regional lymph node metastases

Metastases
- M0 No distant metastases
- M1 Distant metastases

Stage	T	N	M
IA	T1	N0	M0
IB	T2	N0	M0
IIA	T3	N0	M0
IIB	T1-3	N1	M0
III	T4	Any N	M0
IV	Any T	Any N	M1

*Adapted from the 6th edition of the AJCC Cancer Staging Manual

There is general agreement that when a medically fit patient presents with a radiographically resectable ampullary adenocarcinoma, radical resection (Whipple pancreaticoduodenectomy) should be performed. Furthermore, a survival benefit for radical lymphadenectomy in combination with pancreaticoduodenectomy for ampullary cancer was demonstrated in a Japanese study,[27] suggesting that ampullary cancer may behave in a more Halstedian fashion than does pancreatic cancer, for which radical lymphadenectomy has not been shown to be beneficial. At the same time, others have used the relatively favorable prognosis of small ampullary cancers as an argument against radical resection. The presence of lymph node involvement in up to 20% of T1 tumors has led some to advocate local ampullary resection with limited regional lymph node dissection for such lesions.[4] No study has attempted to directly compare local ampullary resection with radical resection for small ampullary adenocarcinomas, but a few

Table 50.2 Results of Surgical Resection for T1 Ampullary Adenocarcinoma

Authors (year)	N	Positive Margins N (%)	Survival
Local resection			
Beger et al (1999)[4]	10	6 (60)	< 40% 5-year
Klein et al (1996)[29]	9	1 (11)	44% 5-year
Rattner et al (1996)[44]	2	0	NED at 15 and 56 months' follow-up
Branum et al (1996)[28]	8	NR	NR; recurrence in 75%
Pancreaticoduodenectomy			
Beger et al (1999)[4]	18	0	84% 5-year
Su et al (1999)[10]	19	0	181 months median
Roberts et al (1999)[11]	5	0	100% 5-year
Howe et al (1998)[8]	22	0	Median not reached (>59 months)
Klempnauer et al (1998)[3]	25	0	56% 5-year
Roder et al (1995)[53]	20	0	50% 5-year

Abbreviations: NED, no evidence of disease; NR, not reported.

studies of local ampullary resection have included small subsets of patients with adenocarcinomas[4,28,29] (Table 50.2). These patients, who were generally high-risk surgical candidates, experienced high rates of tumor recurrence and poor long-term survival. Although perhaps not comparable, patients with T1 tumors who underwent pancreaticoduodenectomy have generally enjoyed superior disease-free and overall survival rates that would seem to support this more aggressive approach (Table 50.2). The wide range of survival rates in these series is not surprising. The differences between dysplasia, carcinoma in situ, and invasive carcinoma can be subtle, even on permanent histology, and studies from different institutions may vary in their inclusion of patients with adenoma and carcinoma in situ.

Despite the probable long-term survival advantage for radical resection over local resection, there are still proponents of local ampullary resection for certain patients with small ampullary adenocarcinomas. However, the incidence of lymph node involvement increases with stage to greater than 20% for T2 tumors and greater than 50% for T3/4 tumors,[4] and, furthermore, local excision is not technically feasible for large tumors. Local resection is therefore a reasonable option only for patients with small malignant tumors who cannot tolerate radical resection. For patients with larger tumors or patients who cannot tolerate even a local resection, palliative endoscopic resection alone or in combination with endoscopic ablative therapies have been described with reasonable results.[30,31]

Negative prognostic factors after resection of ampullary adenocarcinoma generally have a lower incidence but are similar to those described for pancreatic adenocarcinoma, including advanced T stage, lymph node metastasis, positive surgical margins, neural invasion, and poor differentiation.[2,3,8,10] T stage and nodal status are the most consistently powerful predictors of survival but are clearly related to one another. A large drop-off between T2 and T3 tumors has been observed in some studies; in fact, pancreatic invasion (T3) has been associated with a high rate of lymph node metastasis and a prognosis similar to that of pancreatic primaries.[3,32]

Although ampullary cancers as a group have a favorable prognosis, clearly a subgoup exists that is at high risk for recurrence. However, as controversial as the roles of adjuvant and neoadjuvant therapy are for pancreatic cancer, there are less data and essentially no agreement on their roles for ampullary cancer. A few small series of patients receiving adjuvant therapy for "unfavorable" ampullary cancers have been reported. In one of the most recent series, 12 patients at Stanford University with lymph node metastasis, positive surgical margins, poorly differentiated tumors, tumor size greater than 2 cm, or neurovascular invasion received adjuvant chemoradiotherapy and had an 89% actuarial survival at 1 year.[33] Seventeen of 106 resected patients in the Johns Hopkins series received adjuvant therapy, without any apparent effect on survival.[2] Although no randomized, controlled trials specifically for ampullary cancer have been attempted, patients with ampullary cancer were included in the European Organization for Research and Treatment of Cancer study of adjuvant chemoradiotherapy for cancers of the periampullary region.[34] In this often-cited study, a trend toward a survival benefit was observed for pancreatic cancer, but no difference in survival was seen in the nonpancreatic periampullary cancer subgroup. However, this study did not specifically stratify for ampullary cancer, only a small percentage of nonpancreatic periampullary primaries were associated with lymph node metastases, and greater than 25% of patients did not receive the adjuvant therapy that they were randomly assigned to receive.

Several institutions, including our own, have adopted neoadjuvant (preoperative) treatment approaches to periampullary adenocarcinomas. Some of the theoretical advantages of preoperative chemoradiation include the assurance that chemoradiation is received by all patients eligible for resection, the delivery of chemoradiation to well-oxygenated tissues, and the potential to down-stage borderline or unresectable tumors. Most of the reported series have included only patients who had what were believed to be pancreatic adenocarcinomas.[35-37] In our own experience, at least eight patients with recognized ampullary primaries have received neoadjuvant chemoradiation followed by resection. All but one of these patients had at least a T2 primary tumor before treatment, and all underwent resection with negative margins, uninvolved lymph nodes, and significant histologic responses to chemoradiation. These anecdotal observations do not constitute proof of a beneficial effect, but they suggest that neoadjuvant therapy may be reasonably applied to patients with ampullary adenocarcinomas, particularly T3 and T4 tumors that appear to behave more like pancreatic adenocarcinomas.

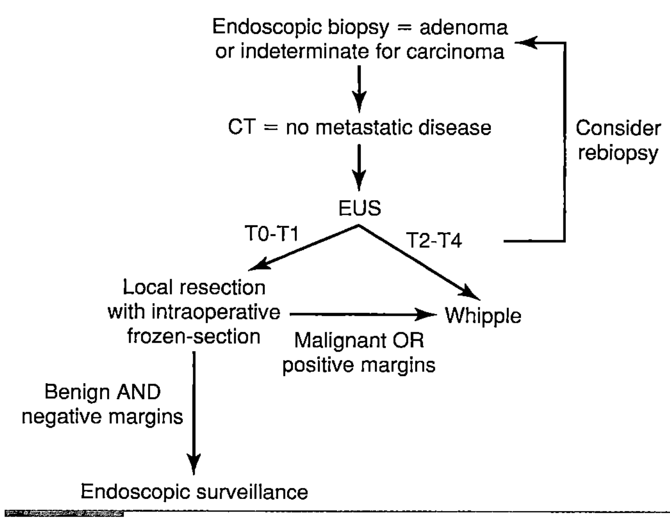

Figure 50.1
A proposed algorithm for the management of patients with an endoscopic diagnosis of adenoma.

Tumors with Malignant Potential

Adenomas are the most commonly diagnosed neoplasms of the ampulla. The duodenum is the least common location for adenomas in the gastrointestinal tract, but the ampulla is the most common within the duodenum, which suggests that their etiology may be related to biliary/pancreatic secretions. Unlike adenomas within the colon, villous and tubulovillous adenomas are much more common than tubular adenomas. Like adenomas within the colon, convincing evidence exists to support an adenoma-adenocarcinoma sequence. Adenocarcinoma is ultimately found in approximately 20% of tubular adenomas and in up to 60% of villous adenomas, and the likelihood of malignancy is related to the size of the lesion.[38] In addition, adenomatous changes are present in approximately 40% of adenocarcinomas.[39] Patients with adenomas tend to be younger than patients with adenocarcinoma,[5,40] and the degree of dysplasia present within the adenoma appears to be related to risk of invasive carcinoma.[41] Molecular changes associated with carcinoma, such as K-*ras* mutations, APC mutations, and loss of heterozygosity at chromosome 5q, have also been found in adenomas.[19,42,43] These provide indirect but compelling evidence that carcinogenesis is a multistep accumulation of mutations, but no specific marker has been identified that can differentiate between dysplasia and carcinoma. Although it is generally agreed that pancreaticoduodenectomy is the treatment of choice for invasive carcinoma, the management of adenomas is more controversial because of the desire to avoid pancreaticoduodenectomy in patients with benign disease.

Endoscopic biopsy is the mainstay of diagnosis (Fig. 50.1). However, the distinctions between hyperplasia, dysplasia, and carcinoma can sometimes be difficult to make, even for the most experienced pathologist. Furthermore, focal areas of malignancy may arise within deeper layers of the adenoma, and superficial biopsy using a simple forceps technique has been associated with false-negative rates of 25%–50% due to sampling error.[4,5,44-46] Gross findings characteristic of invasive carcinoma, such as firmness and ulceration, should make one question a benign biopsy result. More aggressive biopsy strategies, such as snare resection, may marginally improve the performance of endoscopic biopsy.[7,45] However, this technique is associated with a 10%–20% incidence of complications (e.g., hemorrhage, cholangitis, and pancreatitis) and should not be performed before EUS, because it prevents the accurate assessment of depth of invasion.[7] Ampullary snare resection is used only occasionally at our institution, in situations in which EUS yields results that are believed to be discordant with the endoscopic biopsy results. Snare resection may lead to over- or underestimation of histologic changes due to cautery effect[30] and should be combined with delayed superficial biopsies if not surgical resection. With or without these more aggressive biopsy strategies, the positive predictive value of endoscopic biopsy remains superior to that of the negative predictive value (Table 50.3).

Table 50.3 Endoscopic Biopsy of Ampullary Neoplasms

Authors (year)	*N*	% Carcinoma (Final Histology)	PPV (Malignant), %	NPV (Malignant), %
Rattner et al (1996)[44]	21	29	50	73
Sauvanet et al (1997)[45]	26	69	100	46
Cahen et al (1997)[46]	23	43	NA	70
Beger et al (1999)[4]	90	70	94	43
Clary et al (2000)[5]	34	50	100	78

Abbreviations: PPV, positive predictive value; NPV, negative predictive value; NA, not applicable.

Therefore, endoscopic biopsy is useful in that a definitive diagnosis of malignancy can reliably dictate a more aggressive approach (i.e., pancreaticoduodenectomy). However, if the biopsy is indeterminate for malignancy or even if the biopsy is clearly benign, malignancy within the adenoma cannot be excluded, and surgical resection is still recommended in medically fit patients.

The most valuable role of EUS in the management of ampullary neoplasms is in the evaluation of patients with an endoscopic diagnosis of adenoma. Although EUS alone does not provide histologic information and therefore cannot distinguish between adenoma and T1 adenocarcinoma, it provides information about local invasion into the duodenal wall (T2) and beyond. EUS is therefore useful in identifying tumors that are not amenable to local resection.[24-26,44,47] Patients with lesions confined to the ampulla by EUS and a histologic diagnosis of adenoma (Fig. 50.2) can be taken to the operating room without further workup for local ampullary resection with intraoperative frozen-section analysis. Clear evidence of pancreatic invasion by EUS (Fig. 50.3) is highly suggestive of malignancy, and these patients should be staged and treated accordingly. However, overestimation of T stage because of inflammation and edema from pancreatitis is an important limitation of this technique and has been reported to occur in 29% to 36% of lesions confined to the ampulla on final histology.[44-46,48] This distinction is obviously dependent on the skill and experience of the

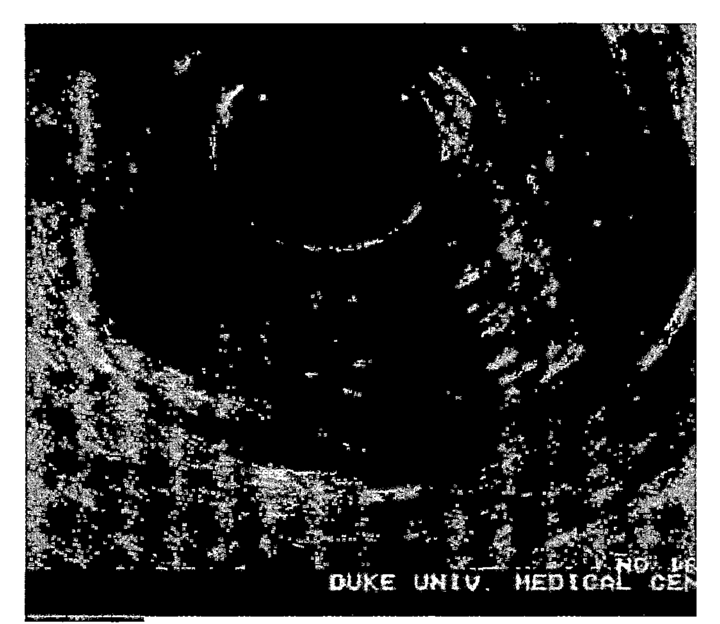

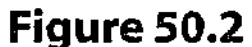

Figure 50.2
An image obtained by endoscopic ultrasound (EUS) of an ampullary adenoma. The intact muscularis propria (MP) indicates that the tumor is confined to the ampulla (T0 or T1).

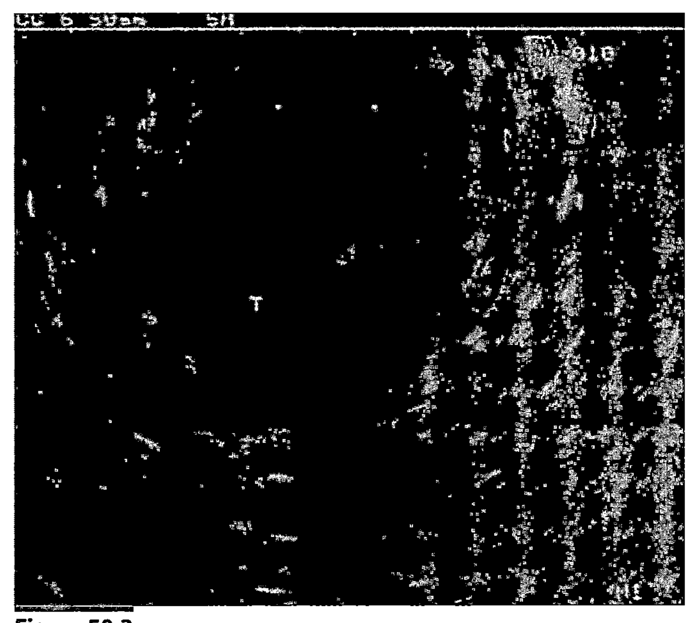

Figure 50.3
An image obtained by endoscopic ultrasound (EUS) of an ampullary adenocarcinoma with pancreatic invasion (T3 or T4).

endoscopist. When EUS suggests invasion beyond the ampulla in the setting of an endoscopic diagnosis of adenoma, we strongly consider a second endoscopic biopsy before the patient undergoes radical resection.

Ampullary neoplasms are often diagnosed in patients with jaundice during the performance of ERCP; therefore, ERCP is often performed before the results of endoscopic biopsy are available. Otherwise, similar to the patient with ampullary adenocarcinoma, ERCP is not routinely indicated in patients in whom the diagnosis of adenoma has been established by other means, unless a delay in surgery is anticipated. However, if ERCP is intended for endoscopic stent placement, EUS should, if possible, be performed before ERCP, because the presence of an endobiliary stent may result in tumor understaging.[25] When these two techniques are combined, intraductal ultrasound involves the use of a high-frequency probe that is small enough to be introduced into the pancreatic or common bile duct at the time of ERCP. This relatively new technique is reported to be more accurate than EUS for detecting invasion beyond the ampulla,[26,49] but it has not achieved widespread use.

Transduodenal ampullary resection was first described by Halsted in 1899,[50] but it was associated with high operative mortality and low long-term survival. Numerous variations on this operation have since been reported, but decreases in mortality and morbidity associated with pancreaticoduodenectomy over the years have resulted in the increased application of pancreaticoduodenectomy to periampullary neoplasms. With improvements in the accuracy of preoperative staging, there seems to have been a resurgence in the popularity of local ampullary resection or ampullectomy.

This technique has been used at Duke University Medical Center for several years, with good results.[5,28,51,52] The abdomen is explored through a right subcostal incision to rule out metastatic disease. An extended Kocher maneuver of the duodenum is performed. The lesion is usually palpable through the duodenal wall, and a generous longitudinal duodenotomy is performed over the junction of the second and third portion of the duodenum. Stay sutures are placed. This exposure allows identification of the ampulla and cannulation of the common bile duct (Fig. 50.4). If the common bile duct cannot be cannulated through the center of the mass, either the mass may be partially resected or the common bile duct may be cannulated through the cystic duct after cholecystectomy. With the use of needle-tip cautery, an outline of a resection margin to achieve a 0.5- to 1.0-cm margin of normal tissue is created on the mucosal surface. The mass is then excised, with the depth of dissection being in the submucosal plane, working in a lateral-to-medial direction so that the common bile duct is transected before the pancreatic duct (Fig. 50.5).

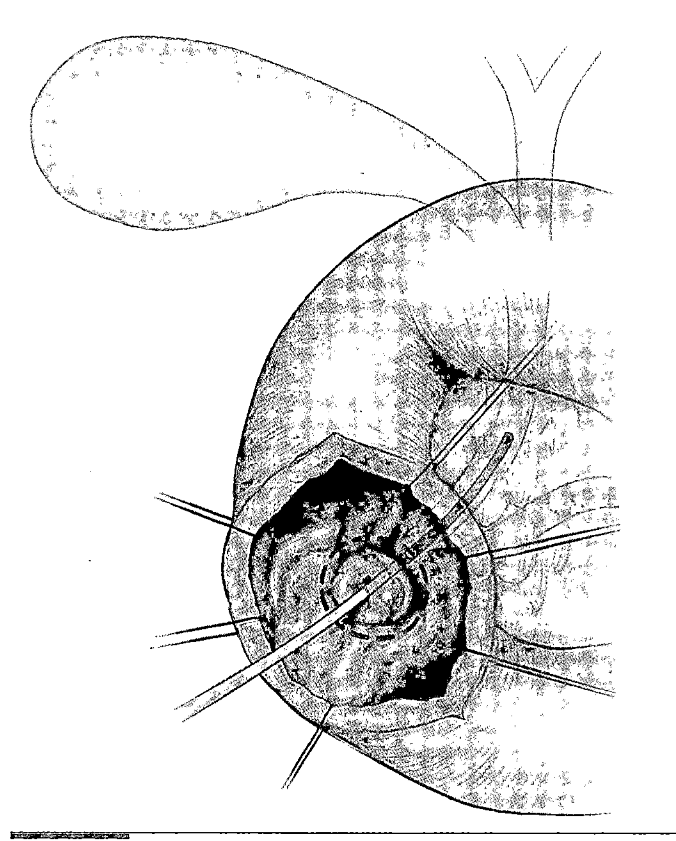

Figure 50.4
The ampulla is exposed via a longitudinal duodenotomy, and the common bile duct is cannulated. (Reprinted with permission from Clary et al.[52])

Once the specimen is excised, it is oriented for the pathologist and sent for frozen-section analysis to determine whether there is an invasive component and whether both the peripheral and the deep (common bile duct) margins are negative (Fig. 50.6). If an invasive component is identified or if a negative margin cannot be achieved, pancreaticoduodenectomy is performed. The success of this technique is therefore critically dependent on the accuracy of the frozen-section analysis. In a recent series of our patients in whom intraoperative frozen-section analysis was performed with careful step-sectioning, the final histology of adenoma was correctly predicted in all 16 patients. When all 39 of the patients undergoing ampullectomy by one senior author (T.N.P.) were reviewed, the negative predictive value of frozen-section analysis was 94%.[5]

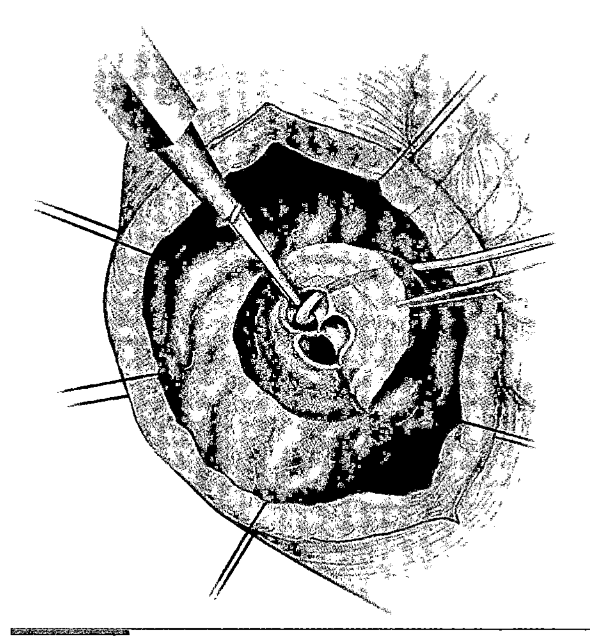

Figure 50.5
The ampulla is excised in the submucosal plane with a 0.5- to 1.0-cm cuff of normal duodenal mucosa. (Reprinted with permission from Clary et al.[52])

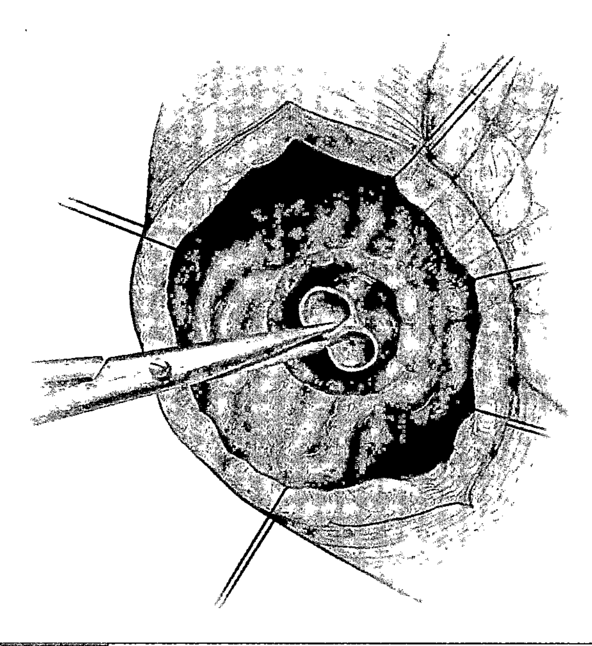

Figure 50.7
A common channel between the common bile duct and the pancreatic duct is created by incision of the intervening septum. (Reprinted with permission from Clary et al.[52])

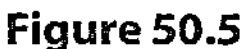

When a benign diagnosis and negative margins have been confirmed, reconstruction is begun by identifying the pancreatic duct and creating a common channel between the common bile duct and pancreatic duct by dividing the intervening septum with scissors (Fig. 50.7).

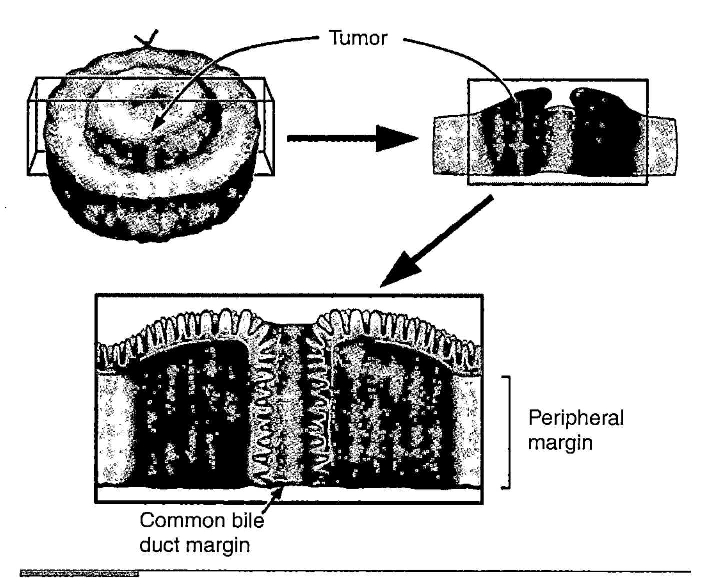

Figure 50.6
Intraoperative frozen-section analysis is used to assess for malignancy and margin status. Step-sectioning through the specimen is performed with identification of the inked peripheral and deep (common bile duct) margins. (Reprinted with permission from Clary et al.[52])

The duodenal mucosa is then circumferentially reapproximated to the common channel with the use of 5-0 Vicryl interrupted sutures, which are tied after the last suture is placed (Figs. 50.8 and 50.9). The duodenotomy is then closed in a transverse direction (Fig. 50.10).

Studies of ampullectomy for adenoma have been limited to small numbers of carefully selected patients but have generally reported acceptable rates of recurrence (Table 50.4). A notable exception is the Mayo Clinic series, which included patients (22%) with polyposis syndromes, who had a significantly higher rate of recurrence at 5 years (60%) than did patients with sporadic adenomas (24%). In this series, recurrences even after 10 years were observed, and almost 25% of recurrences were invasive cancers,[6] underscoring the importance of continued endoscopic surveillance after ampullectomy. In patients with sporadic adenomas, recurrence rates have ranged from zero to 26%, although longer follow-up may be necessary to truly assess the durability of this procedure for young patients. With surveillance, most but not all recurrences in these studies were amenable to endoscopic resection, local re-excision, or pancreaticoduodenectomy. After ampullectomy, complications occurred in 20%–25% of patients, including delayed gastric emptying, duodenal leak, pancreatitis, cholangitis, and common bile duct stricture. By comparison, the recurrence rate after pancreaticoduodenectomy for adenoma should

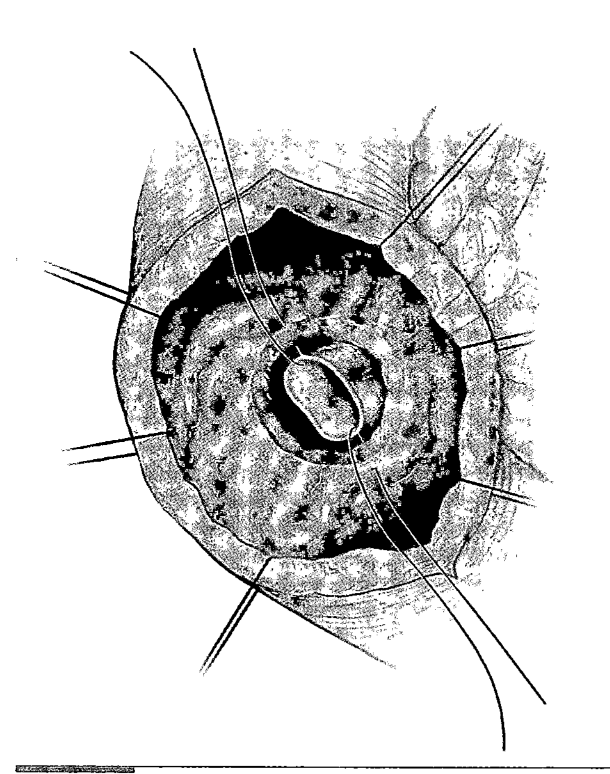

Figure 50.8
The common channel is approximated to the duodenal mucosa. (Reprinted with permission from Clary et al.[52])

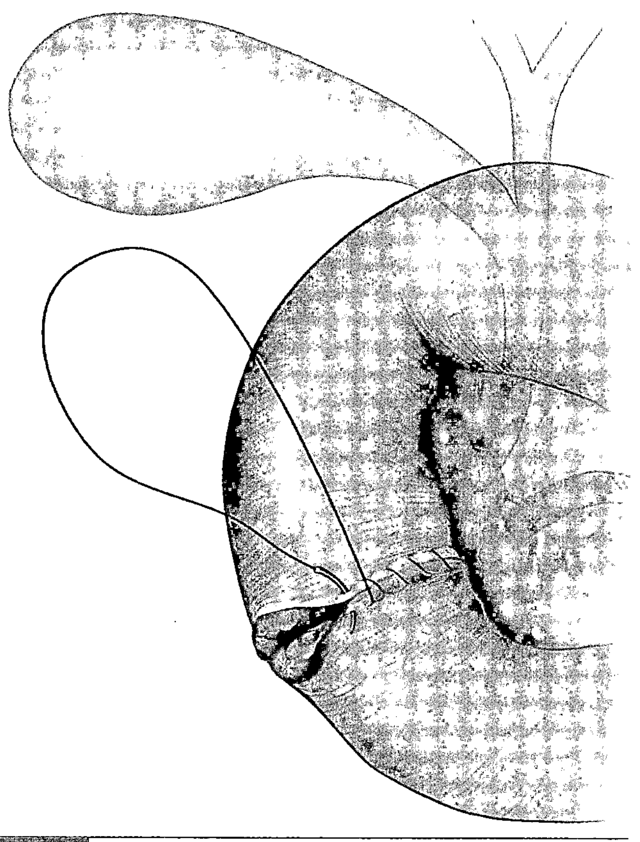

Figure 50.10
The duodenum is closed transversely after completion of the anastomosis. (Reprinted with permission from Clary et al.[52])

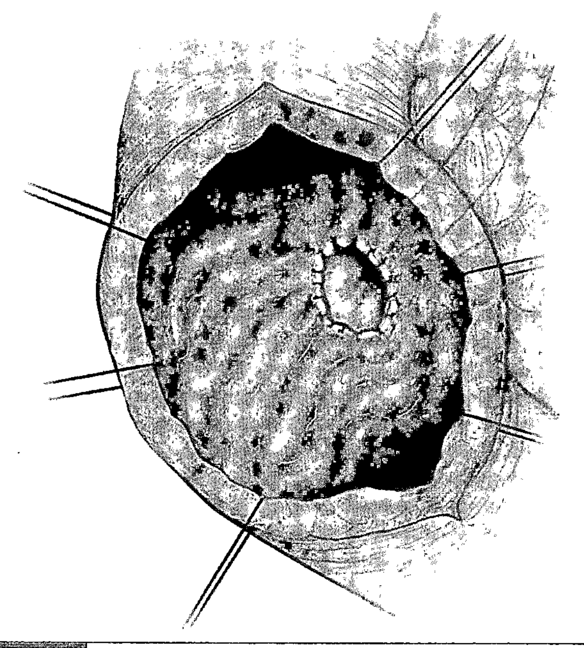

Figure 50.9
The completed anastomosis. (Reprinted with permission from Clary et al.[52])

Table 50.4 Results of Local Ampullary Resection for Adenoma

Authors (year)	*N*	Recurrences (%)	Median Follow-Up
Clary et al (2000)[5]	13	0	51 months
Farnell et al (2000)[6]	39*	10 (26%)	5.6 years
Posner et al (2000)[64]	18	2 (11%)	38 months (mean)
Beger et al (1999)[4]	37	0	43 months
Cahen et al (1997)[46]	8	2 (25%)	36 months

*Excluding 11 patients with polyposis syndrome.

approach zero,[4,6,46] but postoperative complications occur in 30%–50% of patients after pancreaticoduodenectomy for ampullary neoplasms, and postoperative mortality ranges from 3% to 5%.[2,4,8,53] We therefore advocate local ampullary resection with intraoperative frozen-section analysis for all patients with sporadic ampullary adenomas and recommend long-term endoscopic surveillance for early detection of local recurrence.

Familial Adenomatous Polyposis

Patients with ampullary adenomas in the setting of familial adenomatous polyposis (FAP) represent a unique situation. Duodenal adenomas are often multifocal, and with the increasing and earlier use of total abdominal proctocolectomy, periampullary adenocarcinoma is now the leading cause of death in these patients.[54] Because most patients with FAP develop duodenal adenomas, it is recommended that all patients with FAP undergo endoscopic surveillance at least every 3 years with biopsies of any abnormal tissue as well as the ampulla, even if no polyps are evident.[55] Patients with duodenal polyps greater than 10 mm, villous adenomas, adenomas with high-grade dysplasia, or any ampullary adenoma require further intervention because of the increased risk of malignancy. Due to the progressive nature of this disease, we recommend an attempt at endoscopic resection followed by repeat endoscopy within 6 months, reserving surgical intervention for patients with invasive care or diffuse disease for which endoscopic surveillance is not feasible. For patients with isolated ampullary adenomas, local resection has been described but has been plagued by high complication rates and high long-term recurrence rates of between 70% and 100%.[6,56,57] Pancreaticoduodenectomy is an option for patients requiring surgical intervention and is the only option for patients with ampullary cancer and FAP. However, for patients without evidence of malignancy, pancreas-sparing duodenectomy has been described as an alternative to radical pancreaticoduodenectomy that avoids the morbidity of pancreatic resection and anastamosis.[58-60] In this procedure, the duodenum is dissected off of the orifice of the common bile duct/pancreatic duct confluence. The duodenum is excised from just beyond the pylorus to the ligament of Treitz, and the proximal jejunum is brought up as a "neoduodenum" to which the common bile duct and pancreatic duct are anastomosed. Gastrointestinal continuity can be re-established either by a loop gastrojejunostomy, as it is performed at our institution,[60] or as an end-to-end duodenojejunostomy.[58,59] Complications—ampullary leak being most common—occurred in 33%–60% of patients in these three small series, but there were no postoperative deaths. Jejunal polyps, which were treated endoscopically, have been observed in several patients on follow-up endoscopy, and lifelong surveillance should be continued. Whether the development of drugs to prevent polyp formation, such as the cyclooxygenase inhibitors, will affect the indications for surgery or the need for endoscopic surveillance is not yet clear.

Neuroendocrine Tumors

Neuroendocrine tumors encompass a diverse array of histologies, all of which defy categorization as benign or malignant on the basis of the primary lesion alone. Carcinoids are the most common neuroendocrine tumor to involve the ampulla, but the ampulla is an uncommon location for carcinoids to occur.[61-63] Approximately 30% of ampullary carcinoids occur in patients with von Recklinghausen's neurofibromatosis; carcinoids in these patients are often somatostatin-rich and have been referred to as *somatostatinomas*.[63] However, ampullary neuroendocrine tumors of any type rarely produce clinically evident endocrine syndromes. Regional and/or distant metastases are present in 20%–45% of patients with ampullary carcinoids, but despite this, the prognosis is excellent, with 5-year survival rates of up to 90%.[61,63] The incidence of metastasis has correlated poorly with tumor size in the small numbers of patients studied. This observation is in contrast to other foregut carcinoids, and we believe that local ampullary resection is reasonable in patients with small (<1 cm) ampullary carcinoids and no apparent lymph node metastases. Patients with larger tumors or with obvious lymph node metastases appear to benefit from radical resection (pancreaticoduodenectomy) because some unresected patients die of local/regional disease progression without liver metastasis. Patients with liver metastases are unlikely to derive much therapeutic benefit from radical resection (unless the liver disease is resected as well), and local ampullary resection can provide palliation of obstructive symptoms with less morbidity.

Conclusion

The most common ampullary neoplasms are adenomas and adenocarcinomas, which appear to be related through an adenoma-adenocarcinoma sequence similar to that of colon polyps. Endoscopic biopsy is useful in making the diagnosis of an ampullary neoplasm but cannot reliably exclude the presence of invasive cancer. EUS can be helpful in identifying evidence of local invasion suggestive of invasive cancer. Malignant tumors are best treated with radical resection (pancreaticoduodenectomy), and ampullary adenocarcinomas have a much better prognosis than do pancreatic adenocarcinomas and cholangiocarcinomas. Local ampullary resection with intraoperative frozen-section analysis is less morbid than pancreaticoduodenectomy and is recommended for patients with benign ampullary adenomas.

References

1. Avisse C, Flament JB, Delattre JF. Ampulla of Vater: anatomic, embryologic, and surgical aspects. *Surg Clin North Am.* 2000;80:201–212.
2. Talamini MA, Moesinger RC, Pitt HA, et al. Adenocarcinoma of the ampulla of Vater: a 28-year experience. *Ann Surg.* 1997;225:590–599.
3. Klempnauer J, Ridder GJ, Maschek H, Pichlmayr R. Carcinoma of the ampulla of vater: determinants of long-term survival in 94 resected patients. *HPB Surg.* 1998;11:1–11.
4. Beger HG, Treitschke F, Gansauge F, et al. Tumor of the ampulla of Vater: experience with local or radical resection in 171 consecutively treated patients. *Arch Surg.* 1999;134: 526–532.
5. Clary BM, Tyler DS, Dematos P, et al. Local ampullary resection with careful intraoperative frozen section evaluation for presumed benign ampullary neoplasms. *Surgery.* 2000;127:628–633.
6. Farnell MB, Sakorafas GH, Sarr MG, et al. Villous tumors of the duodenum: reappraisal of local vs. extended resection. *J Gastrointest Surg.* 2000;4:13–21.
7. Binmoeller KF, Boaventura S, Ramsperger K, Soehendra N. Endoscopic snare excision of benign adenomas of the papilla of Vater. *Gastrointest Endosc.* 1993;39:127–131.
8. Howe JR, Klimstra DS, Moccia RD, et al. Factors predictive of survival in ampullary carcinoma. *Ann Surg.* 1998;228: 87–94.
9. Yeo CJ, Sohn TA, Cameron JL, et al. Periampullary adenocarcinoma: analysis of 5-year survivors. *Ann Surg.* 1998; 227:821–831.
10. Su CH, Shyr YM, Lui WY, P'Eng FK. Factors affecting morbidity, mortality and survival after pancreaticoduodenectomy for carcinoma of the ampulla of Vater. *Hepatogastroenterology.* 1999;46:1973–1979.
11. Roberts RH, Krige JE, Bornman PC, Terblanche J. Pancreaticoduodenectomy of ampullary carcinoma. *Am Surg.* 1999;65:1043–1048.
12. Yamaguchi K, Enjoji M. Carcinoma of the ampulla of Vater: a clinicopathologic study and pathologic staging of 109 cases of carcinoma and 5 cases of adenoma. *Cancer.* 1987;59:506–515.
13. Yamaguchi K, Enjoji M, Tsuneyoshi M. Pancreatoduodenal carcinoma: a clinicopathologic study of 304 patients and immunohistochemical observation for CEA and CA19-9. *J Surg Oncol.* 1991;47:148–154.
14. Shirai Y, Ohtani T, Tsukada K, Hatakeyama K. Patterns of lymphatic spread of carcinoma of the ampulla of Vater. *Br J Surg.* 1997;84:1012–1016.
15. Friess H, Wang L, Zhu Z, et al. Growth factor receptors are differentially expressed in cancers of the papilla of Vater and pancreas. *Ann Surg.* 1999;230:767–774.
16. Park SH, Kim YI, Park YH, et al. Clinicopathologic correlation of p53 protein overexpression in adenoma and carcinoma of the ampulla of Vater. *World J Surg.* 2000;24:54–59.
17. Howe JR, Klimstra DS, Cordon-Cardo C, et al. K-ras mutation in adenomas and carcinomas of the ampulla of vater. *Clin Cancer Res.* 1997;3:129–133.
18. Matsubayashi H, Watanabe H, Yamaguchi T, et al. Differences in mucus and K-ras mutation in relation to phenotypes of tumors of the papilla of Vater. *Cancer.* 1999;86:596–607.
19. Achille A, Biasi MO, Zamboni G, et al. Cancers of the papilla of Vater: mutator phenotype is associated with good prognosis. *Clin Cancer Res.* 1997;3:1841–1847.
20. Imai Y, Oda H, Tsurutani N, et al. Frequent somatic mutations of the APC and p53 genes in sporadic ampullary carcinomas. *Jpn J Cancer Res.* 1997;88:846–854.
21. Fuhrman G, Charnsangavej C, Abbruzzese J, et al. Thin-section contrast-enhanced computed tomography accurately predicts the resectability of malignant pancreatic neoplasms. *Am J Surg.* 1994;167:104–113.
22. Loyer EM, David CL, Dubrow RA, et al. Vascular involvement in pancreatic adenocarcinoma: reassessment by thin-section CT. *Abdom Imaging.* 1996;21:202–206.
23. Rosch T, Braig C, Gain T, et al. Staging of pancreatic and ampullary carcinoma by endoscopic ultrasonography: comparison with conventional sonography, computed tomography, and angiography. *Gastroenterology.* 1992;102:188–199.
24. Kubo H, Chijiiwa Y, Akahoshi K, et al. Pre-operative staging of ampullary tumours by endoscopic ultrasound. *Br J Radiol.* 1999;72:443–447.
25. Cannon ME, Carpenter SL, Elta GH, et al. EUS compared with CT, magnetic resonance imaging, and angiography and the influence of biliary stenting on staging accuracy of ampullary neoplasms. *Gastrointest Endosc.* 1999;50:27–33.
26. Menzel J, Hoepffner N, Sulkowski U, et al. Polypoid tumors of the major duodenal papilla: preoperative staging with intraductal US, EUS, and CT. A prospective, histopathologically controlled study. *Gastrointest Endosc.* 1999;49: 349–357.
27. Shirai Y, Tsukada K, Ohtani T, Hatakeyama K. Carcinoma of the ampulla of Vater: is radical lymphadenectomy beneficial to patients with nodal disease? *J Surg Oncol.* 1996;61:190–194.
28. Branum GD, Pappas TN, Meyers WC. The management of tumors of the ampulla of Vater by local resection. *Ann Surg.* 1996;224:621–627.
29. Klein P, Reingruber B, Kastl S, et al. Is local excision of pT1-ampullary carcinomas justified? *Eur J Surg Oncol.* 1996; 22:366–371.
30. Farrell RJ, Noonan N, Khan IM, et al. Carcinoma of the ampulla of Vater: a tumour with a poor prognosis? *Eur J Gastroenterol Hepatol.* 1996;8:139–144.
31. Fowler AL, Barham CP, Britton BJ, Barr H. Laser ablation of ampullary carcinoma. *Endoscopy.* 1999;31:745–747.
32. Willett CG, Warshaw AL, Convery K, Compton CC. Patterns of failure after pancreaticoduodenectomy for ampullary carcinoma. *Surg Gynecol Obstet.* 1993;176:33–38.

33. Mehta VK, Fisher GA, Ford JM, et al. Adjuvant chemoradiotherapy for "unfavorable" carcinoma of the ampulla of Vater: preliminary report. *Arch Surg*. 2001;136:65–69.
34. Klinkenbijl JH, Jeekel J, Sahmoud T, et al. Adjuvant radiotherapy and 5-fluorouracil after curative resection of cancer of the pancreas and periampullary region: phase III trial of the EORTC gastrointestinal tract cancer cooperative group. *Ann Surg*. 1999;230:776–782; discussion 782–784.
35. Spitz F, Abruzzese J, Lee J, et al. Preoperative and postoperative chemoradiation strategies in patients treated with pancreaticoduodenectomy for adenocarcinoma of the pancreas. *J Clin Oncol*. 1997;15:928–937.
36. Hoffman JP, Lipsitz S, Pisansky T, et al. Phase II trial of preoperative radiation therapy and chemotherapy for patients with localized, resectable adenocarcinoma of the pancreas: an Eastern Cooperative Oncology Group Study. *J Clin Oncol*. 1998;16:317–323.
37. White R, Hurwitz H, Lee C, et al. Neoadjuvant chemoradiation for localized adenocarcinoma of the pancreas. *Ann Surg Oncol*. 2001;8:758–765.
38. Wittekind C, Tannapfel A. Adenoma of the papilla and ampulla–premalignant lesions? *Langenbecks Arch Surg*. 2001;386:172–175.
39. Seifert E, Schulte F, Stolte M. Adenoma and carcinoma of the duodenum and papilla of Vater: a clinicopathologic study. *Am J Gastroenterol*. 1992;87:37–42.
40. Motton G, Veraldi GF, Fracastoro G, et al. Vater's papilla and periampullary area villous adenoma: personal experience about nine cases and review of the literature. *Hepatogastroenterology*. 1996;43:448–455.
41. Heidecke CD, Rosenberg R, Bauer M, et al. Impact of grade of dysplasia in villous adenomas of Vater's papilla. *World J Surg*. 2002;26:709–714.
42. Sato T, Konishi K, Kimura H, et al. Adenoma and tiny carcinoma in adenoma of the papilla of Vater–p53 and PCNA. *Hepatogastroenterology*. 1999;46:1959–1962.
43. Serafini FM, Carey LC. Adenoma of the ampulla of Vater: a genetic condition? *HPB Surg*. 1999;11:191–193.
44. Rattner DW, Fernandez-del Castillo C, Brugge WR, Warshaw AL. Defining the criteria for local resection of ampullary neoplasms. *Arch Surg*. 1996;131:366–371.
45. Sauvanet A, Chapuis O, Hammel P, et al. Are endoscopic procedures able to predict the benignity of ampullary tumors? *Am J Surg*. 1997;174:355–358.
46. Cahen DL, Fockens P, de Wit LT, et al. Local resection or pancreaticoduodenectomy for villous adenoma of the ampulla of Vater diagnosed before operation. *Br J Surg*. 1997;84:948–951.
47. Tio TL, Mulder CJ, Eggink WF. Endosonography in staging early carcinoma of the ampulla of vater. *Gastroenterology*. 1992;102:1392–1395.
48. Mukai H, Nakajima M, Yasuda K, et al. Evaluation of endoscopic ultrasonography in the pre-operative staging of carcinoma of the ampulla of Vater and common bile duct. *Gastrointest Endosc*. 1992;38:676–683.
49. Itoh A, Goto H, Hirooka Y, et al. Endoscopic diagnosis of pancreatic cancer using intraductal ultrasonography. *Hepatogastroenterology*. 2001;48:928–932.
50. Halsted W. Contributions to the surgery of the bile passages, especially the common bile duct. *Boston Med Surg J*. 1899;141:645–654.
51. Farouk M, Niotis M, Branum GD, et al. Indications for and the technique of local resection of tumors of the papilla of Vater. *Arch Surg*. 1991;126:650–652.
52. Clary BM, Pappas TN, Tyler DS. Transduodenal local resection for periampullary neoplasms. In: Evans DB, Abbruzzese JL, Pisters PW, eds. *Pancreatic Cancer: M.D. Anderson Solid Tumor Oncology Series*. New York: Springer-Verlag; 2001:181–191.
53. Roder JD, Schneider PM, Stein HJ, Siewert JR. Number of lymph node metastases is significantly associated with survival in patients with radically resected carcinoma of the ampulla of Vater. *Br J Surg*. 1995;82:1693–1696.
54. Belchetz LA, Berk T, Bapat BV, et al. Changing causes of mortality in patients with familial adenomatous polyposis. *Dis Colon Rectum*. 1996;39:384–387.
55. Wallace MH, Phillips RK. Preventative strategies for periampullary tumours in FAP. *Ann Oncol*. 1999;10:201–203.
56. Alarcon FJ, Burke CA, Church JM, van Stolk RU. Familial adenomatous polyposis: efficacy of endoscopic and surgical treatment for advanced duodenal adenomas. *Dis Colon Rectum*. 1999;42:1533–1536.
57. Penna C, Bataille N, Balladur P, et al. Surgical treatment of severe duodenal polyposis in familial adenomatous polyposis. *Br J Surg*. 1998;85:665–668.
58. Chung RS, Church JM, vanStolk R. Pancreas-sparing duodenectomy: indications, surgical technique, and results. *Surgery*. 1995;117:254–259.
59. Sarmiento JM, Thompson GB, Nagorney DM, et al. Pancreas-sparing duodenectomy for duodenal polyposis. *Arch Surg*. 2002;137:557–562.
60. Kalady MF, Clary BM, Tyler DS, Pappas TN. Pancreas-preserving duodenectomy in the management of duodenal familial adenomatous polyposis. *J Gastrointest Surg*. 2002;6:82–87.
61. Emory RE Jr, Emory TS, Goellner JR, et al. Neuroendocrine ampullary tumors: spectrum of disease including the first report of a neuroendocrine carcinoma of non-small cell type. *Surgery*. 1994;115:762–766.
62. Hatzitheoklitos E, Buchler MW, Friess H, et al. Carcinoid of the ampulla of Vater: clinical characteristics and morphologic features. *Cancer*. 1994;73:1580–1588.
63. Makhlouf HR, Burke AP, Sobin LH. Carcinoid tumors of the ampulla of Vater: a comparison with duodenal carcinoid tumors. *Cancer*. 1999;85:1241–1249.
64. Posner S, Colletti L, Knol J, et al. Safety and long-term efficacy of transduodenal excision for tumors of the ampulla of Vater. *Surgery*. 2000;128:694–701.

SECTION 5

Cystic Neoplasms

CHAPTER

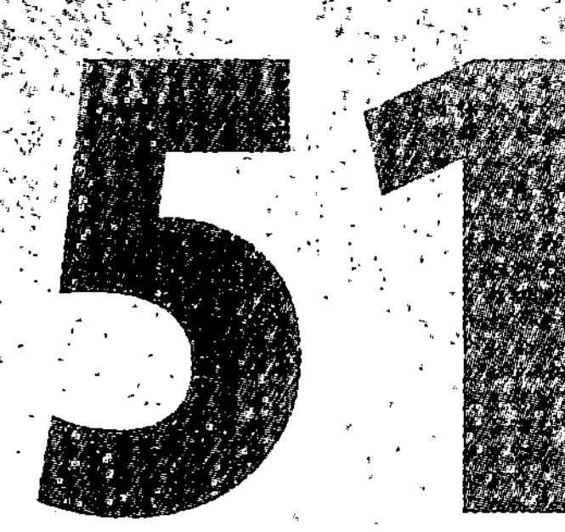

Pathological Classification of Cystic Neoplasms of the Pancreas

N. Volkan Adsay, MD

Dorland's Medical Illustrated Dictionary defines a cyst as "any closed cavity or sac, normal or abnormal, lined by epithelium, and especially one that contains a liquid or semisolid material."[1] In the pancreas, however, this term has been applied to a variety of lesions, ranging from radiologically low-attenuated tumors to any process that forms a cavity, in some cases, whether it has an epithelial lining or not. Therefore, the term *cyst* has become associated with some pancreatic lesions that do not fulfill the dictionary definition of the term.

In the ensuing text, we discuss the pathological classification and biology of pancreatic neoplasms that have been designated as cystic and review the lesions that should be considered in their differential diagnosis.

Importance of Cystic Lesions

As discussed in the previous chapters, the most common (>80%) and most important neoplasm of the pancreas is invasive ductal adenocarcinoma, and to an extent, ductal adenocarcinoma has become almost synonymous with "pancreatic cancer." Virtually all ductal adenocarcinomas are solid tumors; cystic transformation, either due to necrosis or to degeneration, is exceedingly uncommon in this neoplasm.

Cystic lesions constitute 5%–10% of the tumors of the pancreas. Interestingly, but perhaps not too surprisingly, most of these are either benign or indolent neoplasms with a prognosis that is significantly better than the dismal outcome of invasive ductal adenocarcinoma.[2-7] Conversely, most benign or indolent neoplasms of the pancreas are also cystic. This creates an important dichotomy in the differential diagnosis of pancreatic neoplasms: Whereas the vast majority of solid neoplasms are invasive ductal adenocarcinomas (and have a dismal prognosis), most cystic lesions are either benign, or at most, indolent.

Classification

There is no formal classification of cystic lesions of the pancreas; however, conceptually and practically, cystic lesions can be categorized on the basis of the following:

A. The mechanism of cyst formation and the nature of the cyst lining.

1. *Pseudocysts*. Pseudocysts are cavities containing fluid and necrotic debris rich in pancreatic exocrine enzymes. They lack an epithelial lining and are usually a complication of pancreatitis.[8] Technically, neoplasms that undergo degeneration or central necrosis that lead to a cavity formation

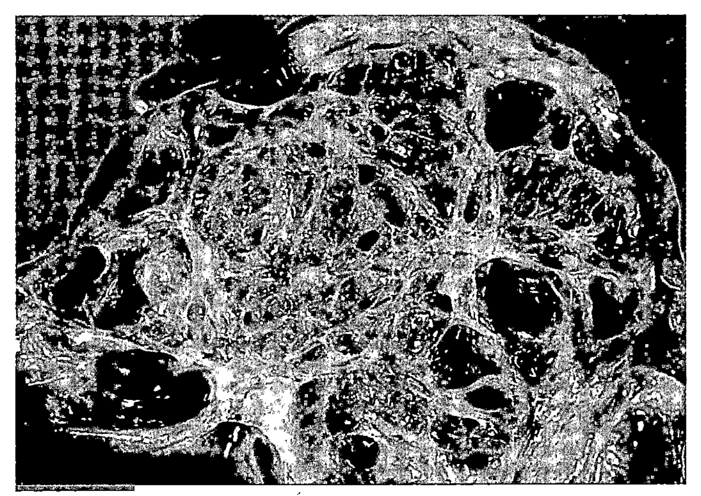

Figure 51.1
Microcystic type of cystic neoplasm in the pancreas. Numerous small cysts, most of which measure no more than several millimeters, form the microcystic pattern. Serous cystadenoma (microcystic, glycogen-rich adenoma) shown here is the prototypical and almost the sole example of microcystic neoplasia in the pancreas. This well-circumscribed appearance, along with spongelike microcystic pattern and stellate scar, is pathognomonic for serous cystadenoma.

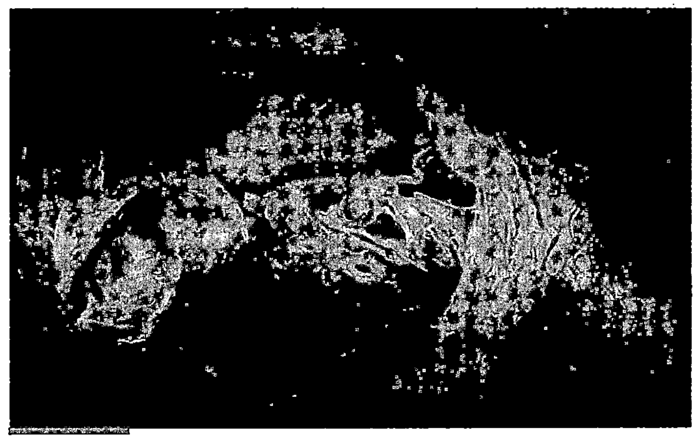

Figure 51.2
Megacystic (oligocystic) pattern. In contrast to the microcystic pattern, the loculi in this mucinous cystic neoplasm are fewer in number and larger in size, most measuring in the order of centimeters. It is difficult to predict the grade of this mucinous cystic neoplasm from the macroscopic findings alone. Although this lesion is of moderate complexity and devoid of papillary nodules, extensive sampling and thorough microscopic examination would be necessary to determine whether in situ or invasive carcinoma is present.

are also "pseudocystic," but neoplasms are excluded from the category of pseudocysts.[9-11]

2. *True cysts*. This category includes neoplasms such as mucinous cystic neoplasms[12] (MCNs) and serous cystadenomas,[13] which are composed of epithelium-lined cavities. These are true cysts because (1) they have an epithelial lining, and (2) they differ from the following group by their de novo nature.
3. *Cystic transformation of pre-existing normal tissue elements*. The typical examples of this phenomenon are cystic acinar transformation[14] and intraductal papillary mucinous neoplasm (IPMN),[15] in which the proliferation of neoplastic cells within the native ducts of the pancreas leads to cystic dilatation of normal tubular structures, culminating in a multilocular cystic mass.

B. Macroscopic configuration, pancreatic cystic lesions can also be classified in the following way:
   1. *Microcystic*. Microcystic lesions are composed of numerous small cysts with most measuring a few millimeters (Fig. 51.1). This configuration is quite specific for serous cystadenoma and therefore has become synonymous with this neoplasm (microcystic adenoma).[13,16]
   2. *Macro(oligo, mega)-cystic*. Cystic lesions containing a small number of loculi, usually less than 10, with each locule measuring several centimeters, are classified as megacystic (Fig. 51.2).[2] Most cystic lesions other than serous (microcystic) adenomas are in this category.

Pathology, Biology, and Differential Diagnosis of Pancreatic Cysts

Despite the potential usefulness of the aforementioned categorizations, the current pathological classification of pancreatic cysts reflects their differentiation (biology) and provides significant prognostic and therapeutic information. The remainder of this chapter therefore focuses on the current pathological classification of cystic lesions of the pancreas. Clinical features and management issues are included only as they relate to the pathological classification and are discussed in further detail in Chapters 52 and 53.

The relative frequencies of cystic lesions in the pancreas vary substantially from institution to institution, from primary versus tertiary care centers, and presumably even from region to region. The lesions are discussed herein in an order that reflects both the frequency and

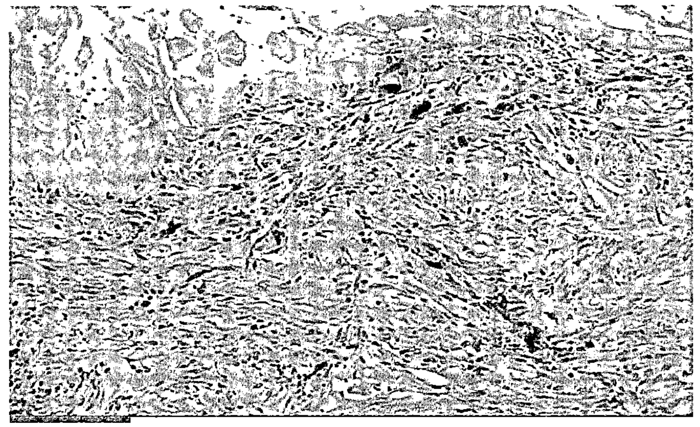

Figure 51.3
Pseudocyst. Pseudocyst is defined as a debris-filled cavity devoid of an epithelial lining. In the pancreas, the term *pseudocyst* is used specifically for a complication of pancreatitis that develops by post-necrotic resorption of peripancreatic fat. Often, as seen in this example, the contents *(upper)* are acidophilic amorphous material composed of acinar enzymes admixed with fat necrosis. Granulation tissue develops in the adjacent tissue *(lower)*, which may later transform into a fibrous pseudocapsule.

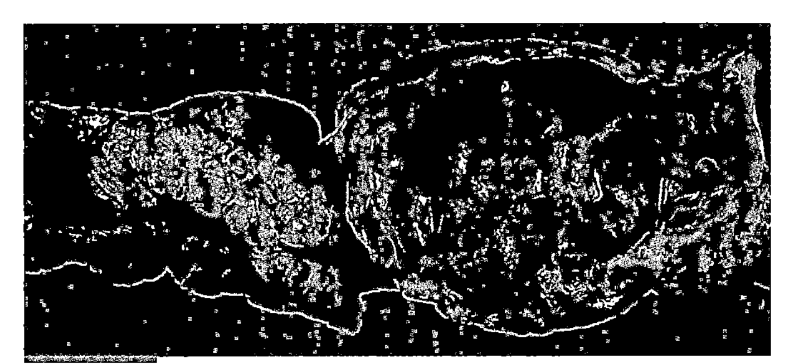

Figure 51.4
Solid-pseudopapillary neoplasm mimicking pancreatic pseudocyst. Solid-pseudopapillary neoplasm of the pancreas commonly undergoes cystic degeneration, which may be extensive in some cases and may clinically resemble a pseudocyst.

the clinical significance of different cystic lesions in this author's experience, based on a large surgical and autopsy database from an institution that serves both as a primary and a tertiary care center, as well as a consultation database.

Pseudocysts

Most cavity-forming lesions of the peripancreatic region are pseudocysts.[8,17,18] Pseudocysts are a nonneoplastic complication of pancreatitis. Pseudocysts develop when a focus of peripancreatic fat necrosis is resorbed, producing a debris-filled space rich in pancreatic exocrine enzymes (Fig. 51.3). Pseudocysts may measure up to several centimeters. The pathological findings vary, depending on the stage of the process. The cyst contents, originally necrotic fat, transform into a mixture of necrotic cells, enzymes, scavenger cells, hematoidin pigment, cholesterol clefts, and sometimes neutrophils. There is no epithelial lining. The tissue that surrounds the necrotic material first produces granulation tissue (Fig. 51.3) and eventually becomes a fibrotic pseudocapsule. Depending on the severity and the duration of the pancreatitis, the pseudocyst may resolve spontaneously or may achieve a size that is no longer self-resorbable and requires surgical intervention.

Pseudocysts do not present a risk of malignant degeneration, and the treatment of pseudocysts differs dramatically from that of cystic neoplasms of the pancreas. Fortunately, the clinical diagnosis of a pseudocyst is usually straightforward; however, neoplasms may mimic a pseudocyst. There are case reports of virtually every pancreatic neoplasm presenting like a pseudocyst.[19-24] For example, solid-pseudopapillary neoplasms can undergo massive cystic degeneration (Fig. 51.4), and MCNs[25] may become infected and exhibit suppurative contents. The ovarian stroma characteristic of the latter may be confused microscopically with the granulation tissue of pseudocysts and vice versa. Proper sampling is essential for the correct diagnosis in such cases. Ductal adenocarcinoma may rarely undergo central necrosis and may clinically mimic pseudocysts.[26-29]

Serous Cystic (Microcystic, Glycogen-Rich) Neoplasms

Serous cystadenoma is a benign neoplasm composed of uniform cuboidal glycogen-rich epithelial cells (Figs. 51.5 and 51.6) that form small cysts containing serous fluid. Serous cystadenomas are the prototypical and almost sole example of microcystic pancreatic neoplasms. In fact, the gross appearance of most serous cystadenomas—multiple small cysts and a stellate scar—can be almost diagnostic of the entity (Fig. 51.1). Serous cystadenomas usually present as relatively large masses measuring up to 25 cm, mostly in the body or tail of the pancreas, and are seen predominantly in females (female:male = 7:3). The mean age of the patients is 61 years.[7,13,16,30-33] Microscopically, these neoplasms have distinctive morphologic features. The cells lining the small cysts have clear cytoplasm, well-defined cytoplasmic borders, and small, round uniform nuclei (Fig. 51.6). A rare macrocystic variant of the serous cystadenoma has been reported,[34-36] as has a solid variant.[37]

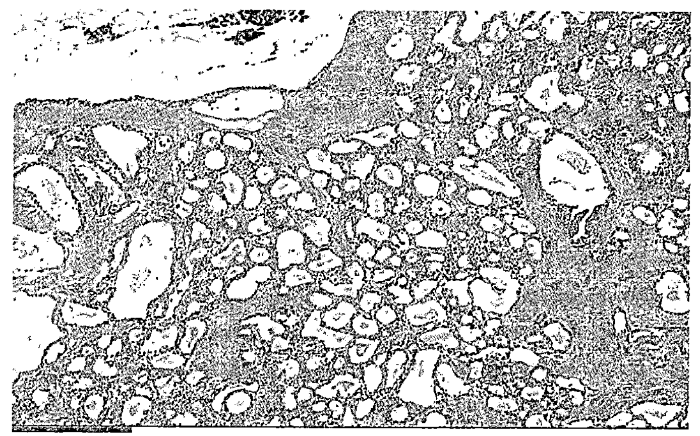

Figure 51.5
Serous cystadenoma, microscopic pattern. Serous cystadenoma of the pancreas typically exhibits tightly packed, small glandular elements, a few of which may become dilated. The cells are cytologically bland (see Fig. 51.6).

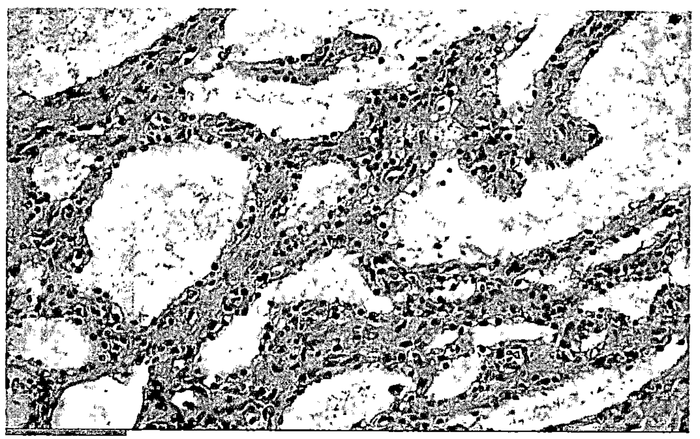

Figure 51.6
Serous cystadenoma, cytologic features. Serous cystadenomas are composed of uniform, cuboidal, and glycogen-rich epithelial cells. The nuclei are small and round and have dense homogenous chromatin.

Serous cystadenomas do not harbor the molecular genetic alterations that are characteristic of infiltrating ductal adenocarcinomas of the pancreas, such as mutations in the *KRAS2*, *SMADH4/DPC4*, *TP53*, and *p16* genes.[38,39] Instead, von Hippel-Lindau gene alterations have been implicated in the pathogenesis of serous cystadenomas.[40]

Of interest, serous cystadenomas are often reported to co-exist or "collide" with other pancreatic neoplasms[41-47] and with congenital pathological conditions.[48,49]

Oligocystic (macrocystic) variant of serous cystadenoma Although the vast majority of serous cystadenomas exhibit a microcystic growth pattern, rare examples are oligocystic (megacystic, macrocystic), that is, composed of fewer but larger loculi[34,36,50] (Fig. 51.7). The epithelial lining of these cysts may become denuded, and it may be difficult to distinguish oligocystic serous cystadenomas from mucinous neoplasms or pseudocysts[51] unless the lesion is extensively sampled and examined carefully to identify the characteristic glycogen-rich clear cells.

Serous cystadenocarcinoma Most serous cystic neoplasms of the pancreas are entirely benign, serous cystadenomas. A handful of malignant serous cystic neoplasms, serous cystadenocarcinomas, have been reported.[31,52-58] Most of these are microscopically identical to serous cystadenomas, and no morphologic findings, other than the presence of metastases, have been found to distinguish these malignant variants from their benign counterparts. The possibility that serous lesions in the liver represent a metachronous neoplasm rather than a metastasis is difficult to exclude and renders "serous cystadenocarcinoma" a dubious entity. Conversely, in two reported cases, an otherwise classical serous cystadenoma showed focal malignant-appearing morphologic features[54,57]; however, in these cases, the clinical and biologic significance of these morphologic changes could not be determined because of the lack of follow-up information. For practical purposes, although the vast majority of serous cystic neoplasms are benign, there are very rare examples of metastasis developing from these neoplasms.[31,53] We have seen examples of metastatic ovarian clear-cell adenocarcinoma and clear-cell renal cell carcinoma that were mistaken as serous cystadenocarcinomas.

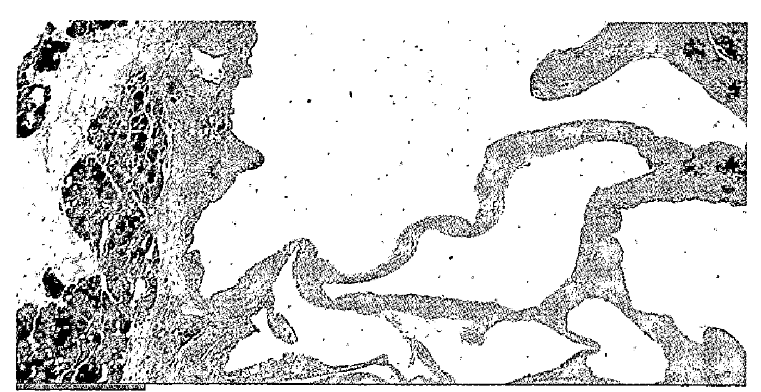

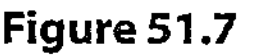

Figure 51.7
Oligocystic variant of serous cystadenoma. Although most serous cystadenomas are microcystic, some, as depicted in this micrograph, are composed of fewer and larger loculi. Such examples may be mistaken for mucinous cystic neoplasms or other megacystic (oligocystic) tumors.

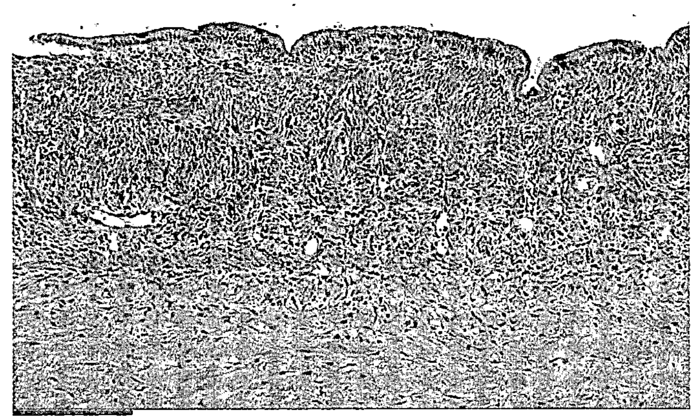

Figure 51.8
Mucinous cystadenoma. The cyst is lined by tall, columnar mucinous cells without cytologic atypia or architectural complexity. Therefore, the lesion would qualify as a mucinous cystadenoma, provided that the tumor has been thoroughly investigated. In the adjacent wall, a densely hypercellular spindle-cell stroma with cytomorphologic characteristics of ovarian stroma is seen.

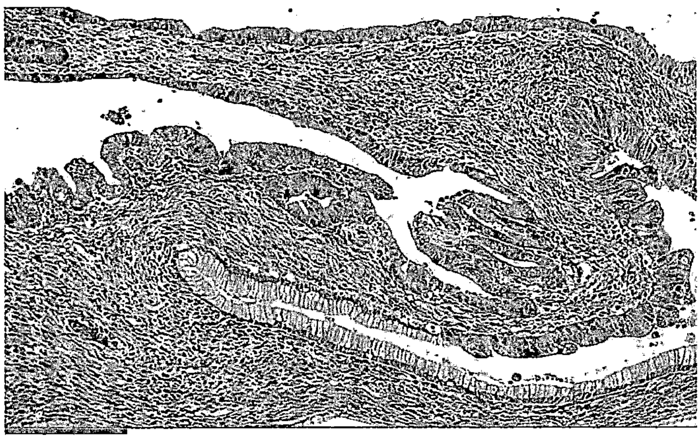

Figure 51.9
Mucinous cystic neoplasm with carcinoma in situ. Some parts of the cyst lining exhibit severe cytologic atypia, including high nuclear-to-cytoplasmic ratio, mucin depletion, hyperchromatism, pleomorphism, nuclear contour irregularities, and cellular disorganization. These areas qualify as carcinoma in situ. The abrupt transition from the low-grade areas (composed of simple columnar cells with abundant apical mucin) to those with carcinoma in situ is evident. The septae are composed of ovarian-like stroma pathognomonic of mucinous cystic neoplasms.

Mucinous Cystic Neoplasms (MCNs)

MCNs are epithelial neoplasms of the pancreas characterized by a mucinous epithelium and a distinctive ovarian type of stroma (Fig. 51.8). MCNs have distinctive clinicopathologic characteristics: they are seen almost exclusively in perimenopausal females (mean age, 48; male:female = 1:9) and the neoplasm is most often located in the tail of the pancreas.[12,59-63] Macroscopically, these neoplasms are composed of large, multilocular cysts ranging in size from one to several centimeters (Fig. 51.2). The cysts have thick, fibrotic walls. Unless fistula formation is present, the cysts do not communicate with the pancreatic ductal system. The wall of the cysts may have velvety papillations and may appear trabeculated and thickened. The cyst contents are often mucoid, but hemorrhage and a more watery consistency may also be noted. Solid areas within the neoplasm should be sampled extensively for microscopic examination because they may harbor an invasive component.

Morphologically, MCNs of the pancreas are similar to MCNs that occur in the retroperitoneum, ovary, and liver. This resemblance includes the presence of a distinctive cellular stroma (referred to as ovarian-like) (Fig. 51.8). This stroma is a very common and is an entity-defining feature of these neoplasms, to an extent that it has almost become a requirement for the diagnosis. There are two hypotheses about the origin of a neoplasm in the pancreas with ovarian-type stroma. The first hypothesis is that these neoplasms arise from rests of embryonic ovarian tissue deposited in the pancreas. This hypothesis is supported by the close proximity of the left ovarian primordium to the tail of the pancreatic anlage in fetal life. The second hypothesis proposed to account for these neoplasms is that the stroma represents a recapitulation of periductal fetal mesenchyme, the primitive mesenchyme present around the pancreatic and hepatic ducts in the developing fetus.[64] Regardless of its origin, it is clear that this stroma is hormone sensitive; it is often admixed with luteal-type cells, and it regularly expresses progesterone receptors. Moreover, some MCNs are reported to be associated with ovarian thecomas,[65] further suggesting a hormone influence in the pathogenesis of these neoplasms.

The cysts in MCNs are lined by tall, columnar, mucin-producing epithelium (Figs. 51.8 through 54.9), which may exhibit gastric foveolar-type intracellular mucin or intestinal-type features with goblet cells. Scattered neuroendocrine cells are present in most cases, and they can be demonstrated by immunohistochemical labeling for neuroendocrine markers, such as chromogranin and synaptophysin.

Some MCNs have purulent contents and these may be misdiagnosed as pseudocysts both during surgery and also histopathologically, especially if the epithelium is denuded, and the remaining ovarian stroma resembles the granulation tissue of pseudocysts. Inflammation may also impart a more complex architecture to an otherwise simple MCN and raise the suspicion for malignancy.[66]

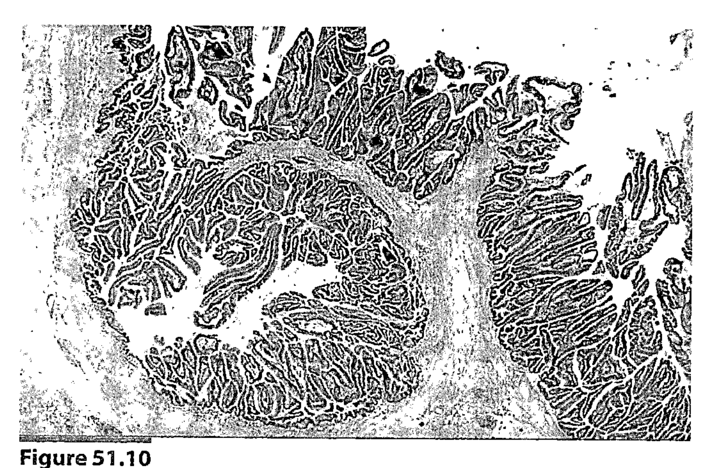

Figure 51.10
Intraductal papillary mucinous neoplasm of the pancreas. The pancreatic duct is filled and dilated by a papillary/villous proliferation.

MCNs can show a wide range of cytologic and architectural atypia; some are histologically bland, with uniform, basally oriented nuclei and minimal architectural atypia (Fig. 51.8), whereas others exhibit prominent papillary proliferations that form intraluminal polypoid masses with cribriform architecture and substantial cytologic atypia (Fig. 51.9). Epithelial atypia may be multifocal, and there is often an abrupt transition between histologically bland epithelium and epithelium with severe atypia (Fig. 51.9). Numerous sections may be required for the proper evaluation of these neoplasms. This may explain why the studies from the Armed Forces Institute of Pathology,[59,62] a referral center where the diagnosis is generally based on a few selected slides submitted for consultation, have failed to demonstrate that dysplasia and even the presence of an invasive cancer are prognostically relevant. For that reason, the authors from the Armed Forces Institute of Pathology regard all MCNs, regardless of their grade, as "low-grade malignant neoplasms," that is, cystadenocarcinoma.[59,62] However, more recently, studies from other authors who performed more complete examination and extensive sampling of the neoplasms concluded that the presence or absence of an associated invasive carcinoma does accurately predict the outcome.[12,61,63,67-69] It is also our experience that patients with completely resected MCNs without atypia (mucinous cystadenomas) are almost always cured. These MCNs tend to be small as well (<3 cm). MCNs with moderate atypia are classified as MCNs with moderate dysplasia, and those with significant architectural and cytologic atypia are classified as MCN with carcinoma in situ.[67,68] Patients with these last two grades of noninvasive MCNs are also almost always cured if their tumors are surgically resected.

If an invasive carcinoma is present, the neoplasm should be classified as a mucinous cystadenocarcinoma.[67,68] The invasive carcinomas that arise in association with MCNs are usually tubular/ductal type. These MCNs with an invasive carcinoma usually pursue a more indolent course than ordinary infiltrating ductal adenocarcinoma. It is difficult to determine whether this implies that the invasive carcinomas arising from MCNs are biologically different (although they may look morphologically identical to invasive ductal adenocarcinoma) or whether the presence of an MCN allows for earlier diagnosis of invasive carcinoma. The same concept is also true for IPMNs.

In addition to their association with invasive tubular adenocarcinomas, some MCNs may be associated with invasive colloid carcinoma, undifferentiated carcinoma with osteoclast-like giant cells,[70,71] or high-grade sarcoma.[72]

Intraductal Papillary Mucinous Neoplasms

IPMNs are epithelial neoplasms characterized by an intraductal proliferation of neoplastic mucin-producing cells, usually arranged in papillary patterns[15,73-84] (Figs. 51.10 through 51.17). The papillae may range from microscopic to large nodular masses. Mucin production by the neoplastic cells is usually associated with intraluminal mucin secretion, which leads to cystic dilatation of the ducts, and at times, to mucin extrusion from the ampulla of Vater, a finding that is virtually diagnostic of an IPMN. Depending on the location of the primary process and subsequent mechanical changes in the ducts, IPMNs may present as a spectrum of multilocular cystic masses (Fig. 51.11) or villous/papillary nodules (Fig. 51.12) or with mucin extrusion from the ampulla. This spectrum is reflected in the variety of designations that had been given to these neoplasms, including mucinous duct ectasia,[85] ductectatic mucinous cystadenoma,[86] mucin-producing tumor,[87,88] villous adenoma,[89] and papillary carcinoma.[90,91] The term *intraductal papillary mucinous neoplasm* is now widely accepted as the designation of these neoplasms. IPMNs are estimated to account for ~ 5% of pancreatic neoplasms; however, IPMNs are being reported in increasing numbers and may be more common than previously recognized.[74,78]

Clinically, patients with an IPMN usually present in the seventh to eighth decade of life with nonspecific abdominal symptoms, although in some, a history of pancreatitis is noted. Endoscopic findings, particularly mucin extrusion from the ampulla of Vater, and radiologic find-

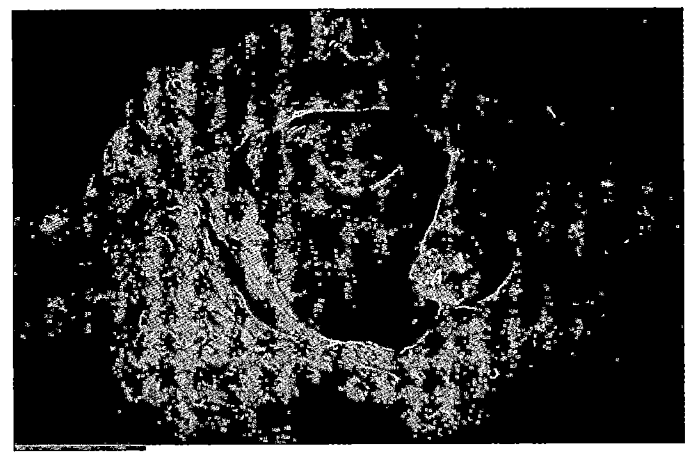
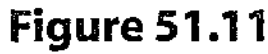

Figure 51.11
Intraductal papillary mucinous neoplasm with prominent cystic change in the ducts. In specimens such as this one, intraductal papillary mucinous neoplasm transforms the pancreatic ducts into a multilocular cystic mass resembling mucinous cystic neoplasms, hence the name "ductectatic mucinous cystadenoma/cystadenocarcinoma" previously applied to these tumors. This phenomenon appears to be more common in the branch duct type.

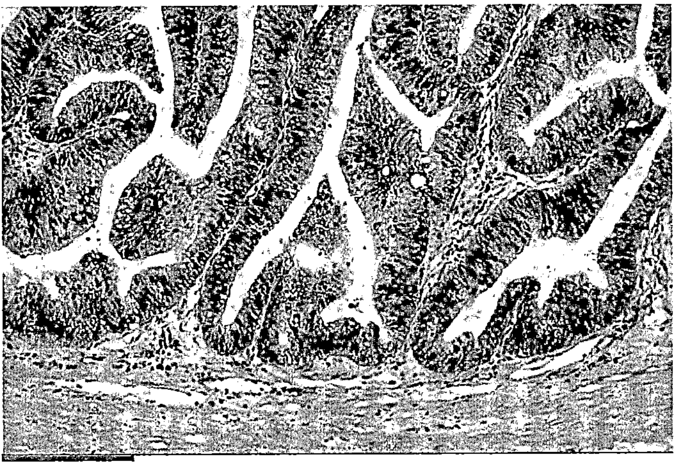

Figure 51.13
Intestinal type papillae in intraductal papillary mucinous neoplasms. The papillae are morphologically similar to those of colonic villous adenomas and exhibit cigar-shaped, pseudostratified nuclei. There is also immunophenotypic and molecular evidence that this pattern indeed represents intestinal differentiation.

ings, especially ectasia of the pancreatic ducts, are virtually diagnostic for these neoplasms. IPMNs occur predominantly in the head of the pancreas.

Macroscopic examination of IPMNs is imperative for documenting the involvement of the pancreatic ductal system and the distribution of the disease within the ductal system (Figs. 51.11 and 51.12). Some IPMNs primarily involve the main pancreatic duct, whereas others involve the branch ducts. The latter have been referred to as *branch duct–type IPMNs*, and branch-duct IPMNs have a predilection for the uncinate process. IPMNs may be localized or multicentric, or, rarely, the entire pancreatic duct may be involved. Careful examination and sampling of the specimen for an invasive carcinoma component are of vital importance.

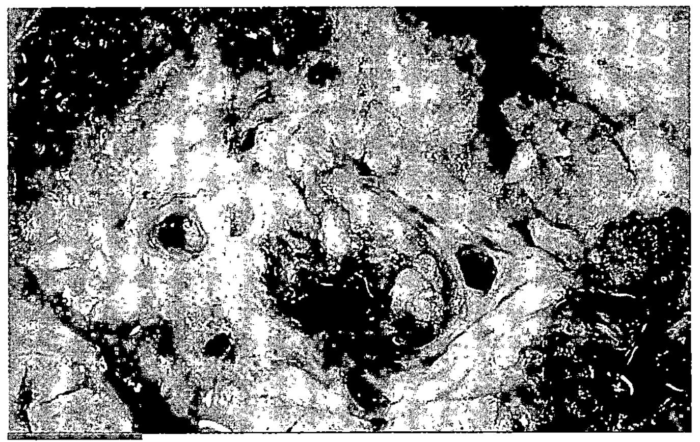

Figure 51.12
Intraductal papillary mucinous neoplasm, predominantly papillary. Some intraductal papillary mucinous neoplasms, especially the main-duct types, may exhibit ducts filled with prominent papillary nodules. In this example, tan, granular nodules are seen both in the main duct and in the branch duct *(at the center)*.

Microscopically, the cystically dilated ducts of IPMNs contain mucin-producing cells with various degrees of atypia. Papillae with two distinct morphologic patterns may be present.[73,92-96] The intestinal type of epithelium is morphologically similar to the epithelium of villous adenomas of the colon (Fig. 51.13). The pancreatobiliary type of epithelium is characterized by more complex papillae with cuboidal cells and prominent nucleoli (Fig. 51.14). The first type of epithelium does, in fact, show molecular characteristics of intestinal differentiation, as evidenced by MUC2 and CDX2 expression, which are regarded as key molecules in intestinal programming, in addition to their tumor-suppressor properties.[97] Papillae with the pancreatobiliary pattern, conversely, typically do not express CDX2 and MUC2 but may instead express MUC1, a "marker" of aggressive phenotype in the pancreas.[97]

Although IPMNs and MCNs have some features that overlap, the two can be distinguished by clinical, gross, and microscopic findings. MCNs occur predominantly in perimenopausal females and in the tail of the pancreas. IPMNs are seen predominantly in elderly males and in the head of the pancreas.[15,63,98] Whereas IPMNs involve the pancreatic ducts, MCNs typically do not communicate with the ductal system. MCNs often have thick cyst

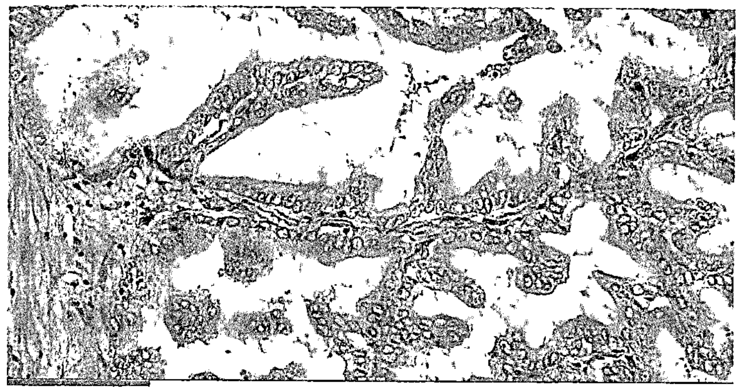

Figure 51.14
Pancreatobiliary type papilla in intraductal papillary mucinous neoplasm. In contrast with the intestinal type depicted in Fig. 51.13, pancreatobiliary-type papillae are more complex (arborizing), and the nuclei are more round.

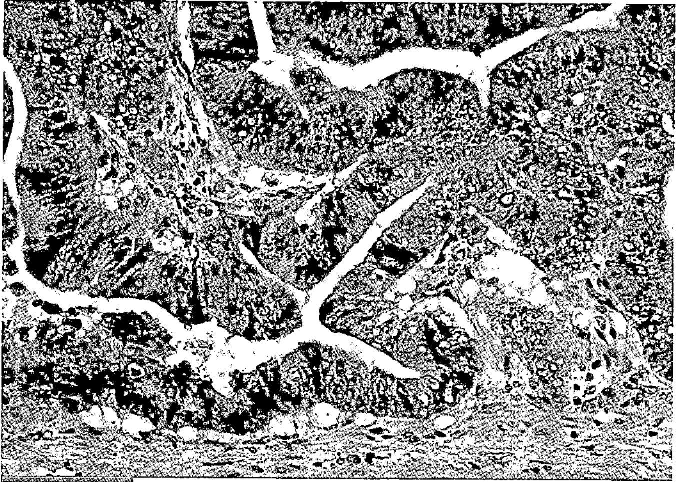

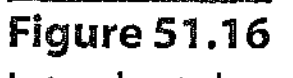

Figure 51.16
Intraductal papillary mucinous neoplasm with carcinoma in situ. In contrast to the adenoma shown in Fig. 51.15, this example exhibits multilayered epithelium with marked cellular disorganization and cytologic atypia, including high nuclear-to-cytoplasmic ratio, pleomorphism, and nuclear irregularities.

walls. The presence of ovarian stroma is diagnostic for MCNs and has almost become a requirement for the diagnosis of this tumor type. The differential diagnosis of IPMNs should also include ampullary adenomas that may extend intraluminally into the pancreatic ducts.

IPMNs also need to be distinguished both conceptually and practically from the smaller microscopic lesions of the pancreatic ducts known as *pancreatic intraepithelial neoplasia* (PanIN), and from nonneoplastic localized duct ectasia (Kimura lesions[99] and retention cysts). The distinction between IPMNs and PanIN is primarily based on size. IPMNs are larger (≥ 1 cm) and usually form a macroscopic and/or radiologic detectable mass.[100,101]

As advocated by the World Health Organization classification,[67,68] noninvasive IPMNs are graded as adenoma, borderline tumor, and carcinoma in situ (Figs. 51.15 and 51.16). Invasive adenocarcinoma, which occurs in ~35% of cases, is usually either of the colloid[102] (Fig. 51.17) or tubular (ordinary ductal) type.[15,73]

Overall 5-year survival for patients with an IPMN is > 70%.[15,73-84] This is not surprising, considering that most IPMNs are noninvasive. Interestingly, some patients with surgically resected noninvasive IPMNs later experience a recurrence and some even experience metastases. These cases most likely represent multifocal disease, a

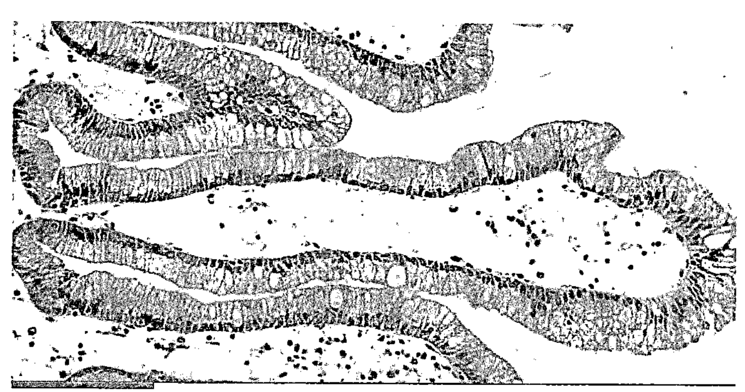

Figure 51.15
Intraductal papillary mucinous adenoma. The papillae are lined by a single layer of well-polarized, tall, columnar mucinous cells without any nuclear atypia. Cytomorphology, especially the pale color of the mucin, is reminiscent of gastric foveolar epithelium.

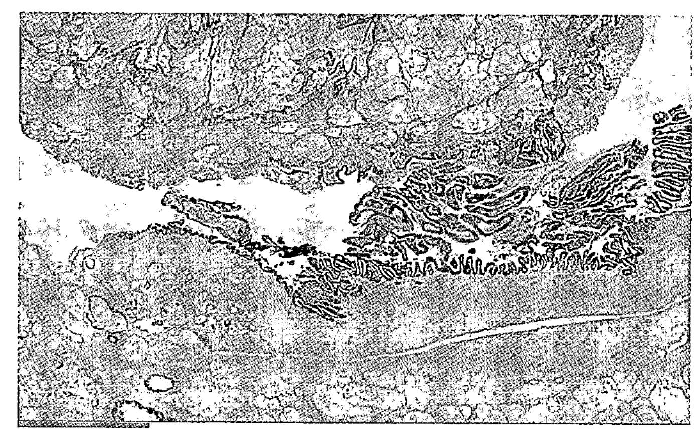

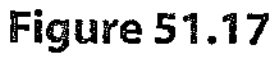

Figure 51.17
Invasive colloid carcinoma associated with intraductal papillary mucinous neoplasm. The main duct at the center is involved by the intraductal papillary mucinous neoplasm. In addition, the remainder of the pancreatic parenchyma is replaced by numerous pools of mucin, many of which are devoid of epithelial cells. This pattern is characteristic of invasive colloid carcinoma (also called mucinous noncystic carcinoma).

finding that is uncommon with MCNs. Multifocality of disease and of dysplasia in IPMNs necessitates the careful evaluation of these neoplasms, with complete removal, careful examination of the surgical margins, and thorough pathological examination.[73,77]

Multifocality and the potential for an associated invasive carcinoma to be present make the management of these tumors problematic. A multidisciplinary approach by experts familiar with this tumor type may be crucial. It seems that IPMNs that are of the branch-duct type (as determined by their location and radiologic findings), and those that are simple (small, predominantly cystic, and without complex nodularities) usually prove to be adenomas and are highly amenable to conservative approach. Conversely, main-duct type IPMNs, and those that are large, complex, and nodular often prove to be carcinomas and may require more aggressive therapy. Total pancreatectomy may be necessary if the disease is extensive[77] (discussed in further detail in Chapter 53).

Another problematic area in the management of IPMNs is the status of surgical resection margins.[77] In general, it is believed that the presence of carcinoma at the surgical margins bears too high a risk for the patient, and the resection of additional pancreatic parenchyma is probably warranted for these patients, if clinically feasible. On the other hand, the impact of adenomatous epithelium at the pancreatic parenchymal margin is probably negligible; however, the relative risk of later developing an invasive carcinoma in these patients is also difficult to determine.

IPMNs appear to be genetically much more stable than conventional infiltrating ductal adenocarcinomas and lack (or exhibit at much lower levels) the molecular/genetic alterations of the latter. Mutations in the *KRAS2*, *p16*, and *TP53* genes are significantly less common in IPMNs, and *SMADH4/DPC4* loss is not usually detected.[83,103-105] Also, IPMNs frequently express MUC2 and CDX2,[97] which have tumor-suppressor activity and encode for intestinal type mucin-related glycoproteins. Somatic mutations of the gene associated with Peutz-Jeghers syndrome, *STK11/LKB1*, are detectable in one third of IPMNs.[106] There are also differences between the molecular phenotype of IPMNs and that of PanINs as well. PanINs lack MUC2 expression, and high-grade PanINs may show MUC1 expression and *SMADH4/DPC4* loss. Whether some of these molecular alterations may have utility in the prognostication for and stratification of patients into different treatment categories is too soon to tell. Some studies have found MUC1 expression,[94,101,107] p53 overexpression,[108] and telomerase activity[109] to be associated with more aggressive clinical course. These and other potential markers ought to be studied further.

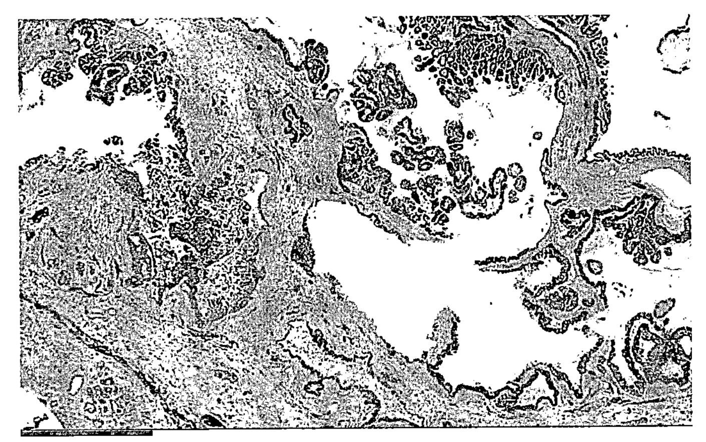

Figure 51.18
Intraductal oncocytic papillary neoplasm. As in intraductal papillary mucinous neoplasm, there are multiple intraductal papillary nodules associated with cystic dilatation of the ducts.

Intraductal Oncocytic Papillary Neoplasms

Intraductal oncocytic papillary neoplasm (IOPN) is a special subtype of IPMNs.[110] Grossly, these neoplasms exhibit cystic dilatation of the pancreatic ducts, many of which contain large, tan, and friable nodular proliferations (Fig. 51.18). The neoplasms are relatively large (mean size, 5.2 cm) at the time of diagnosis. The papillae of IOPNs are lined by eosinophilic cells with a "pancreaticobiliary" pattern of growth. These are exuberant, arborizing papillae lined by one- to five-cell layers of cuboidal cells. The nuclei in IOPNs contain single, prominent, and eccentric nucleoli. In addition to the oncocytic cytoplasm, a distinctive feature that appears to be relatively specific for these neoplasms is the presence of intraepithelial lumina (Fig. 51.19). These lumina are round, punched-out spaces within the epithelium that often give the proliferation a cribriform architecture, similar to that seen in oncocytic schneiderian papillomas of the sinonasal tract. These intraepithelial lumina often contain mucin. The cells of IOPNs are oncocytic (Fig. 51.19), as a result of the abundance of mitochondria and the paucity of other organelles, which is reflected histologically as abundant, granular, acidophilic cytoplasm. In most cases, the degree of cytoarchitectural atypia, the exuberance of the papillae, and the presence of mitoses qualify for the diagnosis of at least carcinoma in situ.

In other organs, oncocytic change (which is probably a degenerative phenomenon secondary to oxidative stress on the cells) is associated with a different biologic behavior than that occurring in the nononcocytic counterparts of these neoplasms. Whether this applies also to

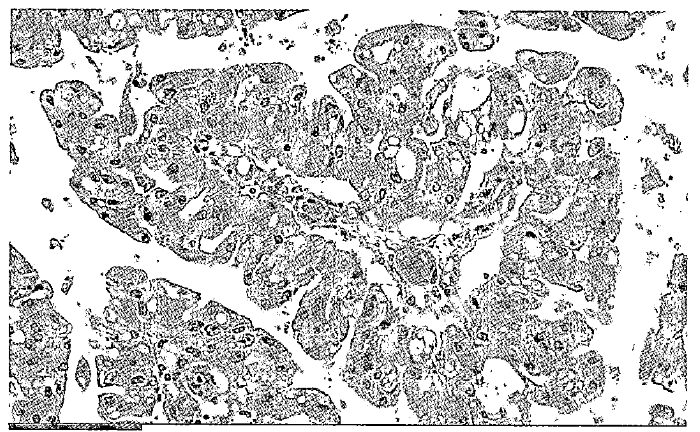

Figure 51.19
Intraductal oncocytic papillary neoplasm. The cells are oncocytic, i.e, they contain abundant granular acidophilic cytoplasm and round nuclei with a single prominent nucleolus. Punched-out spaces referred to as *intraepithelial lumina* are characteristic.

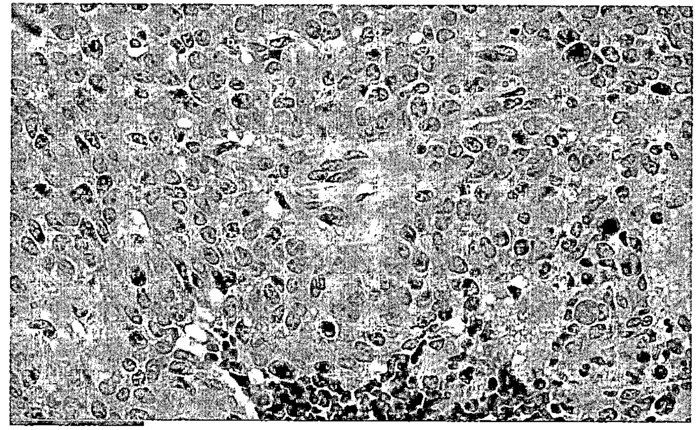

Figure 51.20
Solid-pseudopapillary tumor. This peculiar neoplasm of undetermined origin has distinctive morphologic characteristics. Often, the tumor has marked cystic degeneration, as demonstrated in Fig. 51.4. In well-preserved solid areas exemplified in this photomicrograph, it is a densely cellular neoplasm in which the nuclei are bland, are round to oval, and often exhibit nuclear grooves. Scattered hyaline globules are seen.

the pancreas remains to be seen. Preliminary molecular analyses have shown that IOPNs may differ from the conventional IPMNs, by the lack of *KRAS2* gene mutations and alternate MUC phenotypes (N.V. Adsay and D.S. Klimstra, unpublished observations, 2003).

The data on the clinical course of IOPNs are limited[110-114]; however, the course seems to be similar to that of other IPMNs but may be even more indolent.

Solid-Pseudopapillary Tumor

Solid-pseudopapillary tumor is the most recent name advocated by the World Health Organization[67,68] for a distinctive and enigmatic neoplasm in the pancreas that often presents as a cystic mass, and for this reason, it was previously (and is sometimes still) referred to as a "solid and cystic,"[115,116] "solid and papillary,"[117] "cystic and papillary," and "papillary-cystic"[118,119] tumor. The plethora of names used previously for solid-pseudopapillary tumor reflects the enigmatic nature of this neoplasm. It is now known that the cavities that form in solid-pseudopapillary tumors are not "true" cysts (there is no epithelial lining) but rather represent a necrotic/degenerative process[10,11] (Fig. 51.4). The cystic areas often contain blood, necrotic debris, and clusters of foamy macrophages. Viable neoplastic cells form pseudopapillae (creating an ependymoma-like appearance), hyaline globules, and cell clusters (Fig. 51.20). The nuclei are uniform, nuclear grooves may be present, and the cells usually have eosinophilic cytoplasm, but the cytoplasm can also be clear. The histologic appearance of these neoplasms can mimic neuroendocrine neoplasms, but solid-pseudopapillary tumors lack neuroendocrine chromatin and do not intensely label with markers of neuroendocrine differentiation, such as chromogranin.

Solid-pseudopapillary tumor is somewhat of an enigma. It is one of very few neoplasms in which the direction of differentiation of the neoplastic cells has yet to be established. Solid-pseudopapillary tumor is practically unique to the pancreas, with no close kindred in any other organ. Meanwhile, it does not show clear-cut pathogenetic relationship to any of the cells normally found in the pancreas; there is no evidence of uniform ductal, acinar, or endocrine differentiation.[10,11] Even the epithelial differentiation of this tumor type is incomplete and dubious. Immunohistochemically, the neoplastic cells express nonspecific markers, such as vimentin, CD56, α_1-antitrypsin and neuron-specific ("nonspecific") enolase; meanwhile, epithelial markers (keratins) are usually only focally or weakly expressed. Chromogranin, the most specific endocrine marker, is typically negative; solid-pseudopapillary tumors reported to be strongly chromogranin positive in the literature most likely represent pancreatic endocrine neoplasms with cystic degeneration. Similarly, the reports on high-grade pancreatic tumors that expressed CD99 (Ewing's marker) and t(11:22) translocation, in the author's opinion, may represent primitive neuroectodermal tumor of this organ.[120] Recently, CD10 expression and APC/β-catenin pathway and cyclin-D1 alterations were found to be almost uniformly present (> 90%) in solid-pseudopapillary tumors. This interesting finding is extremely helpful diagnostically

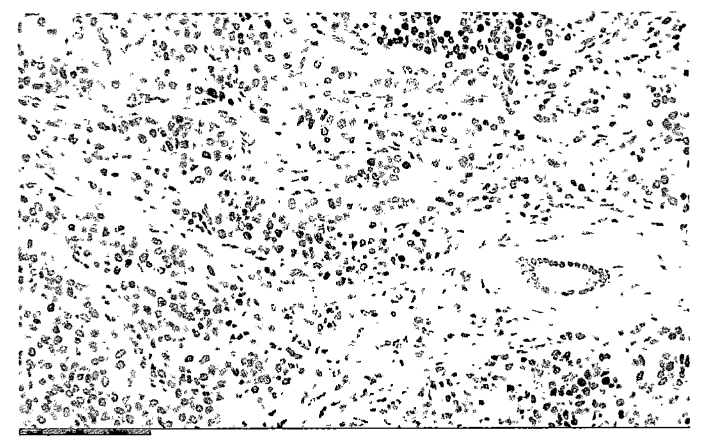

Figure 51.21
Progesterone receptor expression in solid-pseudopapillary tumor. Immunohistochemical expression of progesterone receptors in the nuclei is depicted. This, along with its much higher incidence in young females, suggest a role for hormones in the pathogenesis of this tumor.

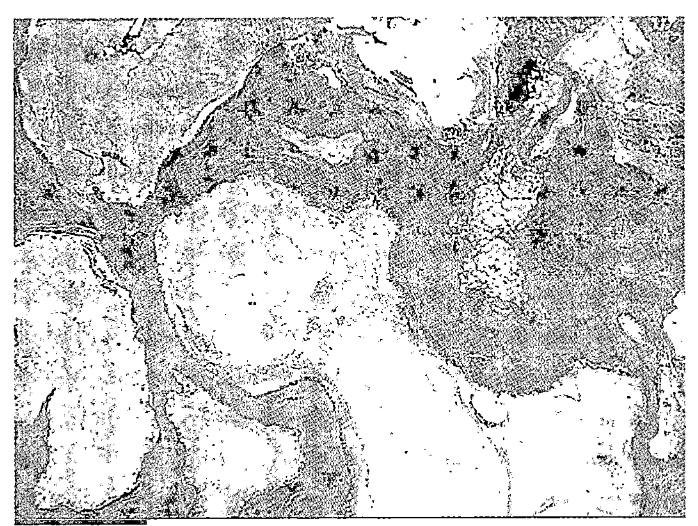

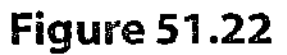

Figure 51.22
Large-duct pattern of invasive ductal adenocarcinoma. In some cases of ductal adenocarcinoma, the invasive tubular units may acquire a microcystic appearance. Microscopically, the invasive units may be difficult to distinguish from noninvasive ductal elements and therefore may be mistaken histologically as intraductal papillary mucinous neoplasm or mucinous cystic neoplasm.

and may prove to be important in unraveling the pathogenesis of this peculiar tumor.

Another puzzling aspect of solid-pseudopapillary tumors is that they almost exclusively occur in young females[10,116] (mean age, 25 years; male:female <1/9). Moreover, the neoplastic cells consistently express progesterone receptors[10] (Fig. 51.21) and also the β form of estrogen receptors,[121] suggesting a role for hormones in the evolution of these neoplasms.

More than 80% of solid-pseudopapillary tumors are cured by surgical resection.[10] Metastases (either to liver or peritoneum, but only seldom to lymph nodes)[10, 123] may occur in a small percentage of patients, but even some patients with metastases are cured after surgical resection of the metastases. Only a few deaths have been attributed to solid-pseudopapillary neoplasm. There do not appear to be any reliable histopathologic criteria to distinguish solid-pseudopapillary tumors that can metastasize from those that do not.[122]

Cystic Forms of Otherwise Typically Solid Pancreatic Tumors

Cystic change in ordinary ductal adenocarcinoma Rarely, conventional infiltrating ductal adenocarcinoma of the pancreas may undergo cystic change.[26-29] In our experience, this occurs in less than 1% of cases.[26] In some pancreatic cancers, a large, radiologically detectable cyst may form because of central necrosis. In these cases, what appears radiologically to be a cyst often proves microscopically to be solid, necrotic tissue surrounded by a cuff of viable neoplastic cells. Such cases can be misdiagnosed before surgery as "pseudocysts."[28] In other cases, infiltrating ductal adenocarcinoma can obstruct the pancreatic duct and lead to cystic dilatation of the upstream duct. The dilated upstream duct can show reactive epithelial changes, which may be indistinguishable from IPMNs. There is also a large-duct (microcystic) variant of ductal adenocarcinoma[124] (Fig. 51.22) in which the infiltrating tubular units are larger than those of ordinary ductal adenocarcinoma. This variant mimics IPMNs or MCNs at the microscopic level, but not at the clinical or macroscopic levels,[125] because the dilatation in the infiltrating tubules is of a minimal degree and creates a microcystic pattern at most.

Cystic change in other invasive carcinomas Other invasive malignant neoplasms of the pancreas, such as undifferentiated carcinoma with osteoclast-like giant cells[22] or squamous cell carcinomas[126] have also occasionally been reported to present as cystic masses.

Cystic pancreatic endocrine neoplasms (cystic islet cell tumors) Cystic pancreatic endocrine neoplasms are rare[9,127]; they constitute 5%–10% of pancreatic endocrine neoplasms.[9,128] In contrast to the cystic change in other solid tumors (especially those in ductal adenocarcinomas),

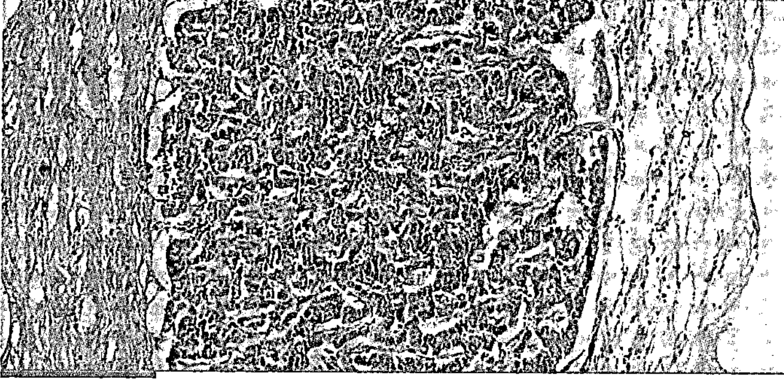

Figure 51.23
Cystic pancreatic endocrine neoplasm (islet cell tumor). A small percentage of pancreatic endocrine neoplasms present as a cystic mass. The cyst lumen (top) contains degenerated cells and granular material, whereas the lining of the cyst is composed of a thick band of pancreatic endocrine neoplasm with the typical thin, delicate vasculature and uniform round cells in nested and trabecular patterns.

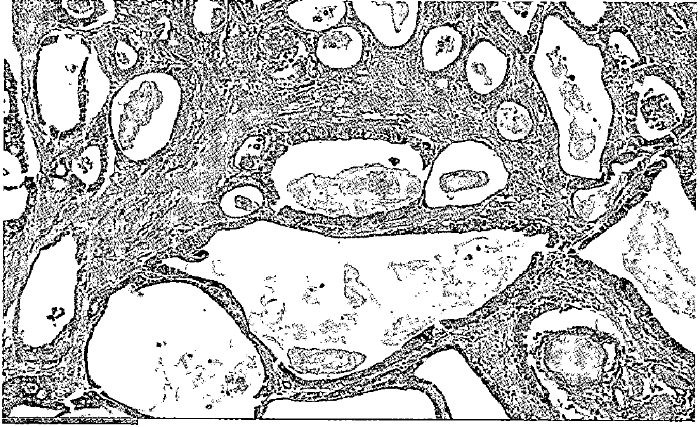

Figure 51.24
Acinar cell cystadenocarcinoma. Instead of the solid sheet-like growth pattern typical of conventional acinar cell carcinomas, the rare acinar cell cystadenocarcinoma is composed of glands, some of which show marked cystic dilatation. On closer inspection, characteristic features of acinar cell carcinomas, including basophilia of the basal cytoplasm, granular acidophilia of the apical cytoplasm, and prominence of nucleoli are evident.

the cyst formation in pancreatic endocrine neoplasms does not appear to be due to necrosis. Rather, the cysts are lined by a ragged cuff of well-preserved neoplastic endocrine cells (Fig. 51.23), and the cysts are filled with a clear serosanginous fluid instead of necrotic debris. The cyst formation is usually unilocular and at the center of the tumor. In some cases, however, the process is more microcystic and includes multiple small cysts.[129] Some cystic pancreatic endocrine neoplasms achieve significant sizes, up to 25 cm.[130] Most cystic pancreatic endocrine neoplasms are clinically nonfunctioning. The pathological diagnosis of these cystic pancreatic endocrine neoplasms is relatively simple if attention is paid to the cytologic features of the lesion. Microscopic examination of the solid areas of these neoplasms reveals characteristic cytomorphologic features of a well-differentiated pancreatic endocrine neoplasm, including round, monotonous cells with a moderate amount of cytoplasm and a distinctive nuclear chromatin pattern. Often, the neoplastic cells have a trabecular growth pattern.

"Mucinous Nonneoplastic Cysts," "Mucoceles," and "Retention Cysts"

In general, most "mucinous cysts" (cysts lined by mucinous epithelium) in the pancreas are neoplastic. However, obstruction and fibrosis may lead to cystic dilatation of the upstream ducts[8,131] (i.e., a retention cyst, or if mucus filled, a mucocele).[132,133] Mucinous nonneoplastic cyst is also possibly a related concept.[134] There is no precise definition for these lesions or specific criteria to distinguish them from IPMNs, MCNs, or, for those that are small, from PanINs. Our approach to these lesions is to accept them as nonneoplastic only if they are simple (unilocular), and lined by either low-cuboidal or attenuated cells. In these cases, finding an obstruction of the pancreatic duct helps establish the diagnosis. However, we classify those lesions lined by tall-columnar-mucinous cells, forming papillae, or are more complex (multilocular) as neoplastic (PanIN if they are smaller than 1 cm and IPMN if they are ≥ 1 cm). Admittedly, these criteria are arbitrary and may not have wide consensus.

Acinar Cell Cystadenocarcinoma

A cystic form of acinar cell carcinoma is well documented but is extremely uncommon; only a handful of cases have been documented in the literature.[135-138] However, that the term *cystic acinar cell carcinoma*[139-141] had also been erroneously applied during the 1980s to the neoplasm currently known as *solid-pseudopapillary neoplasm*, at which time solid-pseudopapillary tumors were mistaken to be of acinar origin. True acinar cell cystadenocarcinomas[135-138] are composed of neoplastic cells that form acini with prominent lumen formation (in contrast to ordinary acinar cell carcinomas, which have a more solid growth pattern[142]). Some of these cysts may measure up to several centimeters. The cysts in these neoplasms are true cysts with an epithelial lining composed of cells with acinar differentiation rather than a degenerative phenomenon (Fig. 51.24). The cells often contain abundant apical, acidophilic zymogen granules, and immunolabeling reveals the expression of pancreatic exocrine enzymes, including trypsin, amylase, and lipase. In the examples the author has seen, the cysts contained granular debris admixed with crystalline material, presumably composed of enzymatic secretions. One example contained an admixed endocrine component and also focal intraductal growth. Acinar cell cystadenocarcinomas are often large. Their biology seems not to be significantly different from that of their solid counterparts (see Chapter 2), with liver metastases developing early in the course of the disease.

Acinar Cell Cystadenoma

Until recently, the conventional thought was that all acinar neoplasms in the pancreas were malignant, albeit solid or cystic. In 2000, however, an entity referred to as *acinar cell cystadenoma* (also called *cystic acinar transformation*) was described.[8,14] This phenomenon is uncommon, often incidental, but may rarely produce a clinically detectable cystic mass (measuring up to several centimeters), in which the cysts are lined by cytologically bland acinar cells.[14,143-145] Immunohistochemical labeling for markers of acinar differentiation (trypsin, lipase, and amylase) are positive. Interestingly, they are also cytokeratin7 positive, whereas normal acinar cells are negative for this marker. Acinar cell cystadenoma occurs in young adults and children, and the consensus is that it is a benign process.

Lymphoepithelial Cysts

Lymphoepithelial cysts are benign cystic lesions occurring predominantly in males in the fifth to sixth decade of life.[146] They may be unilocular or multilocular. The cyst contents may vary from serous to cheesy/caseous appearing, depending on the degree of keratin formation present. The cyst walls are usually thin. Microscopically, the cysts are lined by well-differentiated stratified squamous epithelium, which may or may not have prominent keratinization. In some areas, the lining may appear more transitional, and in others, it may be flat, cuboidal, and focally denuded. Sebaceous elements and mucinous cells are uncommon and when present should suggest a diagnosis of dermoid cyst. The squamous epithelium is surrounded by a band of dense lymphoid tissue composed of mature T lymphocytes with intervening germinal centers formed by B cells, which may be abundant in some cases. In some examples, the lymphoid tissue has a thin capsule and a subcapsular sinus, suggesting that the process may have arisen in a peripancreatic lymph node. Solid lymphoepithelial islands (microscopic clusters of epithelial cells admixed with lymphocytes, akin to the so-called epimyoepithelial islands in the salivary gland lymphoepithelial cysts) may also be present. Some of these epithelial nests form microcysts. It is uncommon for lymphoepithelial cysts to become infected or acutely inflamed; however, the adjacent pancreas may contain granulomas, collections of foamy histiocytes, and fat necrosis and thereby mimic acute pancreatitis. Lymphoepithelial cysts of the pancreas do not appear to be associated with any autoimmune conditions, human immunodeficiency virus infection, lymphoma, or carcinoma, all of which have been documented to occur in their salivary gland counterparts.

Epidermoid Cysts within Intrapancreatic Accessory Spleen

Epidermoid cysts within intrapancreatic accessory spleen are rare. They occur almost exclusively in the tail of the pancreas,[147-149] where accessory spleens are not too uncommon. They are seen in younger patients (second–third decade). The cysts are lined by attenuated squamous cells and are usually nonstratified, surrounded by normal-appearing splenic tissue.

Dermoid Cysts

Dermoid cysts are also exceedingly rare tumors in the pancreas region.[147] They are reported in younger patients (second–third decade) and are morphologically similar to the teratomas occurring in other sites, although some examples are composed predominantly of epidermal elements, such that they are difficult to distinguish from lymphoepithelial cysts. The presence of sebaceous glands or hair follicles is more typical of dermoid cysts.

Lymphangioma

Lymphangiomas may also present as pancreatic and peripancreatic cystic masses[150,151] and may closely mimic lymphoepithelial cysts (especially those with denuded epithelium) because they also contain prominent lymphoid tissue. Lymphangiomas are lined by endothelial cells, as demonstrated by immunohistochemical labeling for endothelial markers (CD31, CD34, factor VIII, and Ulex) and the lack of staining for epithelial markers (cytokeratins). Lymphangiomas may become very large, measuring up to 25 centimeters.[152] They are benign.

Paraduodenal Wall Cyst (Cystic Dystrophy)

These cysts appear to occur as a consequence of chronic fibrosing inflammation in the periampullary region in which one or more of the accessory pancreatic ducts form a cyst on the duodenal wall and mimic duodenal duplication.[8,153,154] This phenomenon usually occurs in the background of microcystic trabeculation of the duodenal wall by myoadenomatosis type of changes that form a pseudotumor, which may also involve the adjacent pancreas in the groove area (the so-called groove pancreatitis[155]). The cyst wall may be lined partly by ductal epithelium and partly by inflammation, as well as granulation tissue.[156] In our experience,[153,154] this process is often located in the second portion of the duodenum, centered around the accessory ampulla, and may be associated with scarring of common bile duct, mimicking pancreatic cancer. We believe that paraduodenal wall cysts are closely related to the so-called cystic dystrophy.[157] In our experience, they occur predominantly in males, often with a history of alcohol abuse at age 40 to 50 years of age and in the context of severe abdominal symptoms (Dr. G. Zamboni, personal communication, Italy, 2003). Some were interpreted to be associated with pancreatic heterotopia in the duodenal wall.[158]

Secondary Neoplasms That Are Cystic

Rarely, neoplasms metastatic to the pancreas (or neoplasms that secondarily involve the pancreas) can exhibit cystic change.[159,160] We have seen examples of metastatic ovarian and renal cell carcinoma in the pancreas that presented as cystic masses. We have also seen a gastrointestinal stromal tumor with marked cystic degeneration that presented as a cystic mass in the pancreatic region. Cystic lesions of the common bile duct and duodenum may also mimic pancreatic cysts.[24,161,162]

Cystic Mesenchymal Neoplasms

Some mesenchymal neoplasms that occur in the pancreatic region may present as cystic lesions. Schwannomas in the pancreas especially tend to be cystic.[163-165] We have seen an example in which the spindle cells surrounding the cysts mimicked the ovarian-like stroma of the MCNs. Some sarcomas may also be cystic.[166]

Pancreatic Cysts Associated with Congenital, Developmental, and Hereditary Disorders

von Hippel-Lindau Syndrome A substantial number of patients with the von Hippel-Lindau syndrome develop pancreatic cysts. The cysts are usually multiple[40,167,168] and may involve the entire pancreas. Morphologically, the epithelial lining of these cysts is indistinguishable from the epithelium seen in serous cystadenomas, although some are mixed serous-endocrine neoplasms. Instead of forming a discreet mass, however, the cysts in patients with the von Hippel–Lindau syndrome may be scattered haphazardly throughout the pancreas.

Polycystic kidney disease and medullary cystic kidney Patients with polycystic kidney disease, both adult and infantile types, may have cystic lesions in the pancreas.[169] Rarely, patients with medullary cystic kidneys may also have pancreatic cysts.[170]

Congenital "enterogenous" (duplication) cysts and duodenal diverticula Congenital cysts of foregut derivation may also occur in the pancreas,[171-173] although very rarely. Essentially, these are regarded as gastrointestinal (enteric) duplications,[174] and some appear to be true diverticula.[162] They may have respiratory (bronchogenic) or ciliated epithelium.[175-177] We have seen two examples with ciliated epithelium; one of these contained inner and outer muscular coats typical of intestinal wall and had an associated high-grade papillary adenocarcinoma with pancreatobiliary type features. Although the carcinoma in this case appeared to be confined to the cyst wall, the patient experienced widespread metastases.

Cystic fibrosis In patients with cystic fibrosis, the genetic defect in the cystic fibrosis transmembrane conductance regulator protein increases the viscosity of pancreatic secretions, which in turn leads to the cystic dilatation of the pancreatic ducts[178,179] by causing intraluminal impaction, in addition to lobular atrophy and parenchymal fibrosis. However, this dilatation in the ducts is generally not clinically detectable.

Other congenital syndromes Cystic transformation of the pancreas has been described in a variety of congenital syndromes,[180] including Ivemark, trisomy 13 or 15, Meckel-Gruber, Elejalde, glutaric aciduria, chondrodysplasia, short rib polydactyly (Jeune and Saldino-Noonan),[181] a newly described syndrome (Balci et al.[182]), and others with no specific names.[183] A patient with choledochal cyst was also reported to have multiple pancreatic cysts.[184]

"Familial fibrocystic pancreatic atrophy" This is an interesting phenomenon described in a pancreatic cancer family from Seattle, Washington, and is characterized by a lobulocentric pancreatic atrophy associated with fibrocystic (microcystic) changes and endocrine cell proliferation.[185] These do not appear to form clinically detectable cysts. In the background of this peculiar fibrocystic process, PanINs and various invasive neoplasias, including anaplastic carcinoma as well as small-cell carcinoma, have developed in some members of this family.

Cysts associated with congenital infections Cytomegalovirus infection has also been implicated in cyst formation in the pancreas of newborns.

Miscellaneous Cysts

Other rare cysts that can occur in the pancreas include parasitic cysts, such as echinococcal cyst[186-188]; necrotic tuberculous infections[189,190]; cystic change in amyloidosis[191]; and endometriotic cysts,[192] some with massive hemorrhage.[193]

Unclassifiable Cysts

Some cysts cannot be classified into one of the well-documented entities. An example is the case reported by H.D. Friedman as a nonmucinous, glycogen-poor cystadenocarcinoma of the pancreas.[194] We have also seen cases that do not fit pathologically into any of the well-described categories. If such a case is encountered, an attempt ought to be made to determine the potential biologic nature of the lesion on the basis of the degree of cellularity, atypia, and architectural complexity of the process.

References

1. Dorland WAN. *Dorland's Illustrated Medical Dictionary*. Philadelphia: WB Saunders; 1988.
2. Adsay NV, Klimstra DS, Compton CC. Cystic lesions of the pancreas. *Semin Diagn Pathol.* 2000;17:1–6.
3. Fernandez-del Castillo C, Targarona J, Thayer SP, et al. Incidental pancreatic cysts: clinicopathologic characteristics and comparison with symptomatic patients. *Arch Surg.* 2003;138:427–423; discussion 433–434.
4. Sarr MG, Murr M, Smyrk TC, et al. Primary cystic neoplasms of the pancreas: neoplastic disorders of emerging importance current state-of-the-art and unanswered questions. *J Gastrointest Surg.* 2003;7:417–428.
5. Compton CC. Histology of cystic tumors of the pancreas. *Gastrointest Endosc Clin North Am.* 2002;12:673–696.
6. Klöppel G, Kosmahl M. Cystic lesions and neoplasms of the pancreas: the features are becoming clearer. *Pancreatology.* 2001;1:648–655.
7. Warshaw AL, Compton CC, Lewandrowski K, et al. Cystic tumors of the pancreas: new clinical, radiologic, and pathologic observations in 67 patients. *Ann Surg.* 1990;212:432–443; discussion 444–445.
8. Klöppel G. Pseudocysts and other non-neoplastic cysts of the pancreas. *Semin Diagn Pathol.* 2000;17:1–7.
9. Adsay NV, Klimstra DS. Cystic forms of typically solid pancreatic tumors. *Semin Diagn Pathol.* 2000;17:66–81.
10. Klimstra DS, Wenig BM, Heffess CS. Solid-pseudopapillary tumor of the pancreas: a typically cystic tumor of low malignant potential. *Semin Diagn Pathol.* 2000;17:66–81.
11. Solcia E, Capella C, Klöppel G. Tumors of the pancreas. Armed Forces Institute Pathology. *Atlas of Tumor Pathology*. vol. 20. Washington, DC: American Registry of Pathology; 1997:53–64.
12. Wilentz RE, Albores-Saavedra J, Hruban RH. Mucinous cystic neoplasms of the pancreas. *Semin Diagn Pathol.* 2000;17:31–43.
13. Compton CC. Serous cystic tumors of the pancreas. *Semin Diagn Pathol.* 2000;17:43–56.
14. Zamboni G, Terris B, Scarpa A, et al. Acinar cell cystadenoma of the pancreas: a new entity? *Am J Surg Pathol.* 2002;26:698–704.
15. Adsay NV, Longnecker DS, Klimstra DS. Pancreatic tumors with cystic dilatation of the ducts: intraductal papillary mucinous neoplasms and intraductal oncocytic papillary neoplasms. *Semin Diagn Pathol.* 2000;17:16–30.
16. Compagno J, Oertel JE. Microcystic adenomas of the pancreas (glycogen-rich cystadenomas): a clinicopathologic study of 34 cases. *Am J Clin Pathol.* 1978;69:289–298.
17. Kerr AA. Cysts and pseudocysts of the pancreas. *Surg Gynecol Obstet.* 1918;27:40.
18. Klöppel G, Maillet B. Pseudocysts in chronic pancreatitis: a morphological analysis of 57 resection specimens and 9 autopsy pancreata. *Pancreas.* 1991;6:266–274.
19. Jin YM, Yim H, Choi IJ. Pancreatic serous cystadenoma mimicking pseudocyst. *Yonsei Med J.* 1997;38:63–65.
20. Munoz NA, Takehara H, Komi N, et al. Papillary and cystic tumor of the pancreas possibly concealed within a pseudocyst. *Acta Paediatr Jpn.* 1992;34:316–323.
21. Machado MC, Montagnini AL, Machado MA, et al. Cystic neoplasm diagnosed as pancreatic pseudocyst: report of 5 cases and review of the literature. *Rev Hosp Clin Fac Med Sao Paulo.* 1994;49:246–249.
22. Oehler U, Jurs M, Klöppel G, et al. Osteoclast-like giant cell tumour of the pancreas presenting as a pseudocyst-like lesion. *Virchows Arch.* 1997;431:215–218.
23. Myung SJ, Kim MH, Lee SK, et al. Adenosquamous carcinoma of the pancreas: differentiation from pancreatic pseudocyst. *Gastrointest Endosc.* 1998;47:410–413.
24. Di Sena V, de Paulo GA, Macedo EP, et al. Choledochal cyst mimicking a pancreatic pseudocyst: case report and review. *Gastrointest Endosc.* 2003;58:620–624.
25. Kuba H, Yamaguchi K, Shimizu S, et al. Chronic asymptomatic pseudocyst with sludge aggregates masquerading as mucinous cystic neoplasm of the pancreas. *J Gastroenterol.* 1998;33:766–769.
26. Adsay NV, Andea A, Weaver D, et al. Centrally necrotic invasive ductal adenocarcinomas of the pancreas presenting clinically as macrocystic lesions [abstract]. *Mod Pathol.* 2001;13:1125A.
27. Lee LY, Hsu HL, Chen HM, et al. Ductal adenocarcinoma of the pancreas with huge cystic degeneration: a lesion to be distinguished from pseudocyst and mucinous cystadenocarcinoma. *Int J Surg Pathol.* 2003;11:235–239.

28. Kaplan JO, Isikoff MB, Barkin J, et al. Necrotic carcinoma of the pancreas: "the pseudo-pseudocyst." *J Comput Assist Tomogr*. 1980;4:166–167.
29. Otani T, Atomi Y, Hosoi Y, et al. Extensive invasion of a ductal adenocarcinoma into the wall of a pancreatic pseudocyst. *Pancreas*. 1996;12:416–419.
30. Hodgkinson DJ, ReMine WH, Weiland LH. Pancreatic cystadenoma: a clinicopathologic study of 45 cases. *Arch Surg*. 1978;113:512–519.
31. Strobel O, Z'Graggen K, Schmitz-Winnenthal FH, et al. Risk of malignancy in serous cystic neoplasms of the pancreas. *Digestion*. 2003;68:24–33.
32. Yasuhara Y, Sakaida N, Uemura Y, et al. Serous microcystic adenoma (glycogen-rich cystadenoma) of the pancreas: study of 11 cases showing clinicopathological and immunohistochemical correlations. *Pathol Int*. 2002;52:307–312.
33. Alpert LC, Truong LD, Bossart MI, et al. Microcystic adenoma (serous cystadenoma) of the pancreas: a study of 14 cases with immunohistochemical and electron-microscopic correlation. *Am J Surg Pathol*. 1988;12:251–263.
34. Casadei R, Santini D, Greco VM, et al. Macrocystic serous cystadenoma of the pancreas: diagnostic, therapeutic and pathological considerations of three cases. *Ital J Gastroenterol Hepatol*. 1997;29:54–57.
35. Lewandrowski K, Warshaw A, Compton C. Macrocystic serous cystadenoma of the pancreas: a morphologic variant differing from microcystic adenoma. *Hum Pathol*. 1992;23:871–875.
36. Sperti C, Pasquali C, Perasole A, et al. Macrocystic serous cystadenoma of the pancreas: clinicopathologic features in seven cases. *Int J Pancreatol*. 2000;28:1–7.
37. Perez-Ordonez B, Naseem A, Lieberman PH, et al. Solid serous adenoma of the pancreas: the solid variant of serous cystadenoma? *Am J Surg Pathol*. 1996;20:1401–1405.
38. Gerdes B, Wild A, Wittenberg J, et al. Tumor-suppressing pathways in cystic pancreatic tumors. *Pancreas*. 2003;26:42–48.
39. Kim SG, Wu TT, Lee JH, et al. Comparison of epigenetic and genetic alterations in mucinous cystic neoplasm and serous microcystic adenoma of pancreas. *Mod Pathol*. 2003;16:1086–1094.
40. Mohr VH, Vortmeyer AO, Zhuang Z, et al. Histopathology and molecular genetics of multiple cysts and microcystic (serous) adenomas of the pancreas in von Hippel-Lindau patients. *Am J Pathol*. 2000;157:1615–1621.
41. Quatresooz P, Honore P, Vivario M, et al. Multifocal serous cystadenoma of the pancreas synchronous with ampullary adenocarcinoma. *Ann Pathol*. 2002;22:317–320.
42. Baek SY, Kang BC, Choi HY, et al. Pancreatic serous cystadenoma associated with islet cell tumour. *Br J Radiol*. 2000;73:83–86.
43. Ustun MO, Tugyan N, Tunakan M. Coexistence of an endocrine tumour in a serous cystadenoma (microcystic adenoma) of the pancreas, an unusual association. *J Clin Pathol*. 2000;53:800–802.
44. Posniak HV, Olson MC, Demos TC. Coexistent adenocarcinoma and microcystic adenoma of the pancreas. *Clin Imaging*. 1991;15:220–222.
45. Keel SB, Zukerberg L, Graeme-Cook F, et al. A pancreatic endocrine tumor arising within a serous cystadenoma of the pancreas. *Am J Surg Pathol*. 1996;20:471–475.
46. Kim YW, Park YK, Lee S, et al. Pancreatic endocrine tumor admixed with a diffuse microcystic adenoma: a case report. *J Korean Med Sci*. 1997;12:469–472.
47. Montag AG, Fossati N, Michelassi F. Pancreatic microcystic adenoma coexistent with pancreatic ductal carcinoma: a report of two cases. *Am J Surg Pathol*. 1990;14:352–355.
48. Masatsugu T, Yamaguchi K, Chijiiwa K, et al. Serous cystadenoma of the pancreas associated with pancreas divisum. *J Gastroenterol*. 2002;37:669–673.
49. Inadome N, Yamaguchi K, Shimizu S, et al. Serous cystadenoma of the pancreas with hypoplasia of the dorsal pancreas: report of a case. *Nippon Shokakibyo Gakkai Zasshi*. 1998;95:455–459.
50. Egawa N, Maillet B, Schroder S, et al. Serous oligocystic and ill-demarcated adenoma of the pancreas: a variant of serous cystic adenoma. *Virchows Arch*. 1994;424:13–17.
51. Cohen-Scali F, Vilgrain V, Brancatelli G, et al. Discrimination of unilocular macrocystic serous cystadenoma from pancreatic pseudocyst and mucinous cystadenoma with CT: initial observations. *Radiology*. 2003;228:727–733.
52. Bassi C, Salvia R, Molinari E, et al. Management of 100 consecutive cases of pancreatic serous cystadenoma: wait for symptoms and see at imaging or vice versa? *World J Surg*. 2003;27:319–323.
53. Wu CM, Fishman EK, Hruban RK, et al. Serous cystic neoplasm involving the pancreas and liver: an unusual clinical entity. *Abdom Imaging*. 1999;24:75–77.
54. Abe H, Kubota K, Mori M, et al. Serous cystadenoma of the pancreas with invasive growth: benign or malignant? *Am J Gastroenterol*. 1998;93:1963–1966.
55. George DH, Murphy F, Michalski R, et al. Serous cystadenocarcinoma of the pancreas: a new entity? *Am J Surg Pathol*. 1989;13:61–66.
56. Haarmann W, Mittelkotter U, Smektala R. Monstrous recurrence of serous cystadenocarcinoma of the pancreas. *Zentralbl Chir*. 1997;122:122–125.
57. Kamei K, Funabiki T, Ochiai M, et al. Multifocal pancreatic serous cystadenoma with atypical cells and focal perineural invasion. *Int J Pancreatol*. 1991;10:161–172.
58. Eriguchi N, Aoyagi S, Nakayama T, et al. Serous cystadenocarcinoma of the pancreas with liver metastases. *J Hepatobiliary Pancreat Surg*. 1998;5:467–470.
59. Compagno J, Oertel JE. Mucinous cystic neoplasms of the pancreas with overt and latent malignancy (cystadenocarcinoma and cystadenoma): a clinicopathologic study of 41 cases. *Am J Clin Pathol*. 1978;69:573–580.
60. Albores-Saavedra J, Choux R, Gould EW, et al. Cystic tumors of the pancreas. *Pathol Annu*. 1994;2:19–51.
61. Wilentz RE, Talamani MA, Albores-Saavedra J, et al. Morphology accurately predicts behavior of mucinous cystic neoplasms of the pancreas. *Am J Surg Pathol*.1999;23:1320–1327.
62. Thompson LDR, Becker RC, Pryzgodski RM, et al. Mucinous cystic neoplasm (mucinous cystadenocarcinoma of low malignant potential) of the pancreas: a clinicopathologic study of 130 cases. *Am J Surg Pathol*. 1999;23:1–16.

63. Zamboni G, Scarpa A, Bogina G, et al. Mucinous cystic tumors of the pancreas: clinicopathological features, prognosis, and relationship to other mucinous cystic tumors. *Am J Surg Pathol*. 1999;23:410–422.
64. Khalife I, Qureshi F, Jacques S, et al. The nature of "ovarian-like" mesenchyme of pancreatic and hepatic mucinous cystic neoplasms: a recapitulation of the periductal fetal mesenchyme? [abstract]. *Mod Pathol*. 2004;17, 304A.
65. Colovic R, Barisic G, Colovic N, et al. Double mucinous cystadenoma of the pancreas associated with thecoma of the ovary. *Acta Chir Iugosl*. 2002;49:95–97.
66. Maire F, Hammel P, Terris B, et al. Benign inflammatory pancreatic mucinous cystadenomas mimicking locally advanced cystadenocarcinomas: presentation of 3 cases. *Pancreatology*. 2002;2:74–78.
67. Klöppel G, Lüttges J. WHO-classification 2000: exocrine pancreatic tumors. *Verh Dtsch Ges Pathol*. 2001;85:219–228.
68. Klöppel G, Hruban RH, Longnecker DS, et al. Pathology and genetics of tumours of the digestive system. In: Kleihues P, Sobin LH, Hamilton SR, et al., eds. *World Health Organization Classification of Tumours*. Lyon, France: IARC Press; 2000:219-252.
69. Sarr MG, Carpenter HA, Prabhakar LP, et al. Clinical and pathologic correlation of 84 mucinous cystic neoplasms of the pancreas: can one reliably differentiate benign from malignant (or premalignant) neoplasms? *Ann Surg*. 2000;231:205–212.
70. Sarnaik AA, Saad AG, Mutema GK, et al. Osteoclast-like giant cell tumor of the pancreas associated with a mucinous cystadenocarcinoma. *Surgery*. 2003;133:700–701.
71. Aoki Y, Tanimura H, Mori K, et al. Osteoclast-like giant cell tumor of the pancreas associated with cystadenocarcinoma. *Nippon Geka Hokan*. 1989;58:452–460.
72. van den Berg W, Tascilar M, Offerhaus GJ, et al. Pancreatic mucinous cystic neoplasms with sarcomatous stroma: molecular evidence for monoclonal origin with subsequent divergence of the epithelial and sarcomatous components. *Mod Pathol*. 2000;13:86–91.
73. Adsay NV, Conlon KC, Zee SY, et al. Intraductal papillary-mucinous neoplasms of the pancreas: an analysis of in situ and invasive carcinomas in 28 patients. *Cancer*. 2002;94:62–77.
74. Adsay NV. The "new kid on the block": Intraductal papillary mucinous neoplasms of the pancreas: current concepts and controversies. *Surgery*. 2003;133:459–463.
75. Klöppel G. Clinicopathologic view of intraductal papillary-mucinous tumor of the pancreas. *Hepatogastroenterology*. 1998;45:1981–1985.
76. Longnecker DS. Observations on the etiology and pathogenesis of intraductal papillary-mucinous neoplasms of the pancreas. *Hepatogastroenterology*. 1998;45:1973–1980.
77. Chari ST, Yadav D, Smyrk TC, et al. Study of recurrence after surgical resection of intraductal papillary mucinous neoplasm of the pancreas. *Gastroenterology*. 2002;123:1500–1507.
78. Tollefson MK, Libsch KD, Sarr MG, et al. Intraductal papillary mucinous neoplasm: did it exist prior to 1980? *Pancreas*. 2003;26:E55-E58.
79. Cellier C, Cuillerier E, Palazzo L, et al. Intraductal papillary and mucinous tumors of the pancreas: accuracy of preoperative computed tomography, endoscopic retrograde pancreatography and endoscopic ultrasonography, and long-term outcome in a large surgical series. *Gastrointest Endosc*. 1998;47:42–49.
80. Fukishima N, Mukai K, Kanai Y, et al. Intraductal papillary tumors and mucinous cystic tumors of the pancreas: clinicopathologic study of 38 cases. *Hum Pathol*. 1997;28:1010–1017.
81. Azar C, Van de Stadt J, Rickaert F, et al. Intraductal papillary mucinous tumours of the pancreas: clinical and therapeutic issues in 32 patients. *Gut*. 1996;39:457–464.
82. Loftus EV, Jr., Olivares-Pakzad BA, Batts KP, et al. Intraductal papillary-mucinous tumors of the pancreas: clinicopathologic features, outcome, and nomenclature. Members of the Pancreas Clinic, and Pancreatic Surgeons of Mayo Clinic. *Gastroenterology*. 1996;110:1909–1918.
83. Sessa F, Solcia E, Capella C, et al. Intraductal papillary-mucinous tumours represent a distinct group of pancreatic neoplasms: an investigation of tumour cell differentiation and K-ras, p53 and c-erbB-2 abnormalities in 26 patients. *Virchows Arch*. 1994;425:357–367.
84. Shimizu M, Manabe T. Mucin-producing pancreatic tumors: historical review of its nosological concept. *Zentralbl Pathol*. 1994;140:211–223.
85. Agostini S, Choux R, Payan MJ, et al. Mucinous pancreatic duct ectasia in the body of the pancreas. *Radiology*. 1989;170:815–816.
86. Yanagisawa A, Ohashi K, Hori M, et al. Ductectatic-type mucinous cystadenoma and cystadenocarcinoma of the human pancreas: a novel clinicopathological entity. *Jpn J Cancer Res*. 1993;84:474–479.
87. Yamada M, Kozuka S, Yamao K, et al. Mucin-producing tumor of the pancreas. *Cancer*. 1991;68:159–168.
88. Yamaguchi K, Tanaka M. Mucin-hypersecreting tumor of the pancreas with mucin extrusion through an enlarged papilla. *Am J Gastroenterol*. 1991;86:835–839.
89. Payan MJ, Xerri L, Moncada K, et al. Villous adenoma of the main pancreatic duct: a potentially malignant tumor? *Am J Gastroenterol*. 1990;85:459–463.
90. Milchgrub S, Campuzano M, Casillas J, et al. Intraductal carcinoma of the pancreas. *Cancer*. 1992;69:651–656.
91. Morohoshi T, Kanda M, Asanuma K, et al. Intraductal papillary neoplasms of the pancreas: a clinicopathologic study of six patients. *Cancer*. 1989;64:1329–1335.
92. Nakamura A, Horinouchi M, Goto M, et al. New classification of pancreatic intraductal papillary-mucinous tumour by mucin expression: its relationship with potential for malignancy. *J Pathol*. 2002;197:201–210.
93. Yonezawa S, Nakamura A, Horinouchi M, et al. The expression of several types of mucin is related to the biological behavior of pancreatic neoplasms. *J Hepatobiliary Pancreat Surg*. 2002;9:328–341.
94. Lüttges J, Brocker V, Kremer B, et al. Immunohistochemical mucin expression and DPC4 status in intraductal papillary mucinous tumors (IPMTs) of the pancreas [abstract]. *Pancreas*. 2000;21:459.

95. Lüttges J, Zamboni G, Longnecker D, et al. The immunohistochemical mucin expression pattern distinguishes different types of intraductal papillary mucinous neoplasms of the pancreas and determines their relationship to mucinous noncystic carcinoma and ductal adenocarcinoma. *Am J Surg Pathol.* 2001;25:942–948.
96. Lüttges J, Feyerabend B, Buchelt T, et al. The mucin profile of noninvasive and invasive mucinous cystic neoplasms of the pancreas. *Am J Surg Pathol.* 2002;26:466–471.
97. Adsay NV, Merati K, Basturk O, et al. Pathologically and biologically distinct types of epithelium in intraductal papillary mucinous neoplasms: delineation of an "intestinal" pathway of carcinogenesis in the pancreas [in press] *Am J Surg Pathol, June 2004.*
98. Yamaguchi K, Yokohata K, Noshiro H, et al. Mucinous cystic neoplasm of the pancreas or intraductal papillary-mucinous tumour of the pancreas. *Eur J Surg.* 2000;166:141–148.
99. Kimura W, Nagai H, Kuroda A, et al. Analysis of small cystic lesions of the pancreas. *Int J Pancreatol.* 1995;18: 197–206.
100. Hruban RH, Takaori K, Klimstra D, et al. An illustrated consensus on the classification of pancreatic intraepithelial neoplasia (PanIN) and intraductal papillary mucinous neoplasms (IPMNs). *Am J Surg Pathol.* 2004;28(8): 977–987.
101. Adsay NV, Merati K, Andea A, et al. The dichotomy in the preinvasive neoplasia to invasive carcinoma sequence in the pancreas: differential MUC1 and MUC2 expression supports the existence of two separate pathways of carcinogenesis. *Mod Pathol.* 2002;15:1087–1095.
102. Adsay NV, Pierson C, Sarkar F, et al. Colloid (mucinous noncystic) carcinoma of the pancreas. *Am J Surg Pathol.* 2001;25:26–42.
103. Iacobuzio-Donahue CA, Klimstra DS, Adsay NV, et al. Dpc-4 protein is expressed in virtually all human intraductal papillary mucinous neoplasms of the pancreas: comparison with conventional ductal adenocarcinomas. *Am J Pathol.* 2000;157:755–761.
104. Hruban RH, Iacobuzio-Donahue C, Wilentz RE, et al. Molecular pathology of pancreatic cancer. *Cancer J.* 2001;7:251–258.
105. Z'graggen K, Rivera JA, Compton CC, et al. Prevalence of activating K-ras mutations in the evolutionary stages of neoplasia in intraductal papillary mucinous tumors of the pancreas. *Ann Surg.* 1997;226:491–498; discussion 498–500.
106. Sato N, Rosty C, Jansen M, et al. STK11/LKB1 Peutz-Jeghers gene inactivation in intraductal papillary-mucinous neoplasms of the pancreas. *Am J Pathol.* 2001;159:2017–2022.
107. Yonezawa S, Taira M, Osako M, et al. MUC-1 mucin expression in invasive areas of intraductal papillary mucinous tumors of the pancreas. *Pathol Int.* 1998;48:319–322.
108. Kawahira H, Kobayashi S, Kaneko K, et al. p53 protein expression in intraductal papillary mucinous tumors (IPMT) of the pancreas as an indicator of tumor malignancy. *Hepatogastroenterology.* 2000;47:973–977.
109. Inoue H, Tsuchida A, Kawasaki Y, et al. Preoperative diagnosis of intraductal papillary-mucinous tumors of the pancreas with attention to telomerase activity. *Cancer.* 2001;91:35–41.
110. Adsay NV, Adair CF, Heffess CS, et al. Intraductal oncocytic papillary neoplasms of the pancreas. *Am J Surg Pathol.* 1996;20:980–994.
111. Jyotheeswaran S, Zotalis G, Penmetsa P, et al. A newly recognized entity: intraductal "oncocytic" papillary neoplasm of the pancreas. *Am J Gastroenterol.* 1998;93:2539–2543.
112. Noji T, Kondo S, Hirano S, et al. Intraductal oncocytic papillary neoplasm of the pancreas shows strong positivity on FDG-PET. *Int J Gastrointest Cancer.* 2002;32:43–46.
113. Patel SA, Adams R, Goldstein M, et al. Genetic analysis of invasive carcinoma arising in intraductal oncocytic papillary neoplasm of the pancreas. *Am J Surg Pathol.* 2002; 26:1071–1077.
114. Thompson K, Castelli MJ, Gattuso P. Metastatic papillary oncocytic carcinoma of the pancreas to the liver diagnosed by fine-needle aspiration. *Diagn Cytopathol.* 1998;18: 291–296.
115. Uchimi K, Fujita N, Noda Y, et al. Solid cystic tumor of the pancreas: report of six cases and a review of the Japanese literature. *J Gastroenterol.* 2002;37:972–980.
116. Zhu X, He L, Zeng J. Solid and cystic tumor of pancreas, analysis of 14 pediatric cases. *Zhonghua Yi Xue Za Zhi.* 2002;82:1180–1182.
117. Lieber MR, Lack EE, Roberts JR Jr, et al. Solid and papillary epithelial neoplasm of the pancreas: an ultrastructural and immunocytochemical study of six cases. *Am J Surg Pathol.* 1987;11:85–93.
118. Miettinen M, Partanen S, Fraki O, et al. Papillary cystic tumor of the pancreas. An analysis of cellular differentiation by electron microscopy and immunohistochemistry. *Am J Surg Pathol.* 1987;11:855–865.
119. Ladanyi M, Mulay S, Arseneau J, et al. Estrogen and progesterone receptor determination in the papillary cystic neoplasm of the pancreas: with immunohistochemical and ultrastructural observations. *Cancer.* 1987;60: 1604–1611.
120. Maitra A, Weinberg AG, Schneider N, et al. Detection of t(11;22)(q24;q12) translocation and EWS-FLI-1 fusion transcript in a case of solid pseudopapillary tumor of the pancreas. *Pediatr Dev Pathol.* 2000;3:603–605.
121. Morales A, Duarte-Rojo A, Angeles-Angeles A, et al. The beta form of the estrogen receptor is predominantly expressed in the papillary cystic neoplasm of the pancreas. *Pancreas.* 2003;26:258–263.
122. Nishihara K, Nagoshi M, Tsuneyoshi M, et al. Papillary cystic tumors of the pancreas: assessment of their malignant potential. *Cancer.* 1993;71:82–92.
123. Saiura A, Umekita N, Matsui Y, et al. Successful surgical resection of solid cystic tumor of the pancreas with multiple liver metastases and a tumor thrombus in the portal vein. *Hepatogastroenterology.* 2000;47:887–889.
124. Andea A, Lonardo F, Adsay V. Microscopically cystic and papillary "large-duct-type" invasive adenocarcinoma of the pancreas: a potential mimic of intraductal papillary mucinous and mucinous cystic neoplasms [abstract]. *Mod Pathol.* 1999, p179A.

125. Denis B, Claudel L, Marcellin L, et al. Presence of microcysts within a cystic tumor of the pancreas does not rule out malignancy: report of two cases. *Gastroenterol Clin Biol.* 2003;27:651–654.
126. Colarian J, Fowler D, Schor J, et al. Squamous cell carcinoma of the pancreas with cystic degeneration. *South Med J.* 2000;93:821–822.
127. Iacono C, Serio G, Fugazzola C, et al. Cystic islet cell tumors of the pancreas: a clinico-pathological report of two nonfunctioning cases and review of the literature. *Int J Pancreatol.* 1992;11:199–208.
128. Ahrendt SA, Komorowski RA, Demeure MJ, et al. Cystic pancreatic neuroendocrine tumors: is preoperative diagnosis possible? *J Gastrointest Surg.* 2002;6:66–74.
129. Ligneau B, Lombard-Bohas C, Partensky C, et al. Cystic endocrine tumors of the pancreas: clinical, radiologic, and histopathologic features in 13 cases. *Am J Surg Pathol.* 2001;25:752–760.
130. Kotoulas C, Panayiotides J, Antiochos C, et al. Huge nonfunctioning pancreatic cystic neuroendocrine tumour: a case report. *Eur J Surg Oncol.* 1998;24:74–76.
131. Toth IR, Lang JN. Giant pancreatic retention cyst in cystic fibrosis: a case report. *Pediatr Pathol.* 1986;6:103–110.
132. Iwase K, Takenaka H, Oshima S, et al. A case of pancreatic cyst containing gall sludge. *Gastroenterol Jpn.* 1992;27:550–553.
133. Morise Z, Yamafuji K, Tsuji T, et al. A giant retention cyst of the pancreas (cystic dilatation of dorsal pancreatic duct) associated with pancreas divisum. *J Gastroenterol.* 2002;37:1079–1082.
134. Kosmahl M, Egawa N, Schroder S, et al. Mucinous nonneoplastic cyst of the pancreas: a novel nonneoplastic cystic change? *Mod Pathol.* 2002;15:154–158.
135. Cantrell BB, Cubilla AL, Erlandson RA, et al. Acinar cell cystadenocarcinoma of human pancreas. *Cancer.* 1981;47:410–416.
136. Ishizaki A, Koito K, Namieno T, et al. Acinar cell carcinoma of the pancreas: a rare case of an alpha- fetoprotein-producing cystic tumor. *Eur J Radiol.* 1995;21:58–60.
137. Joubert M, Fiche M, Hamy A, et al. Extension of an acinar cell pancreatic carcinoma with cystic changes invading the Wirsung canal. *Gastroenterol Clin Biol.* 1998;22:465–468.
138. Stamm B, Burger H, Hollinger A. Acinar cell cystadenocarcinoma of the pancreas. *Cancer.* 1987;60:2542–2547.
139. Arai T, Kino I, Nakamura S, et al. Solid and cystic acinar cell tumors of the pancreas: a report of two cases with immunohistochemical and ultrastructural studies. *Acta Pathol Jpn.* 1986;36:1887–1896.
140. Learmonth GM, Price SK, Visser AE, et al. Papillary and cystic neoplasm of the pancreas: an acinar cell tumour? *Histopathology.* 1985;9:63–79.
141. Doppl W, Muhrer KH, Stambolis C. Acinar cell tumor of the pancreas: a solid cystic benign neoplasm of young females. *Med Welt.* 1983;34:480–483.
142. Klimstra DS, Heffess CS, Oertel JE, et al. Acinar cell carcinoma of the pancreas: a clinicopathologic study of 28 cases. *Am J Surg Pathol.* 1992;16:815–837.
143. Albores-Saavedra J. Acinar cystadenoma of the pancreas: a previously undescribed tumor. *Ann Diagn Pathol.* 2002;6:113–115.
144. Chatelain D, Paye F, Mourra N, et al. Unilocular acinar cell cystadenoma of the pancreas an unusual acinar cell tumor. *Am J Clin Pathol.* 2002;118:211–214.
145. Couvelard A, Terris B, Hammel P, et al. Acinar cystic transformation of the pancreas (or acinar cell cystadenoma), a rare and recently described entity. *Ann Pathol.* 2002;22:397–400.
146. Adsay NV, Hasteh F, Cheng JD, et al. Lymphoepithelial cysts of the pancreas: a report of 12 cases and a review of the literature. *Mod Pathol.* 2002;15:492–501.
147. Adsay NV, Hasteh F, Cheng JD, et al. Squamous-lined cysts of the pancreas: lymphoepithelial cysts, dermoid cysts (teratomas) and accessory-splenic epidermoid cysts. *Semin Diagn Pathol.* 2000;17:56–66.
148. Fink AM, Kulkarni S, Crowley P, et al. Epidermoid cyst in a pancreatic accessory spleen mimicking an infected abdominal cyst in a child. *AJR Am J Roentgenol.* 2002;179:206–208.
149. Yokomizo H, Hifumi M, Yamane T, et al. Epidermoid cyst of an accessory spleen at the pancreatic tail: diagnostic value of MRI. *Abdom Imaging.* 2002;27:557–559.
150. Bishop MD, Steer M. Pancreatic cystic lymphangioma in an adult. *Pancreas.* 2001;22:101–102.
151. Paal E, Thompson LD, Heffess CS. A clinicopathologic and immunohistochemical study of ten pancreatic lymphangiomas and a review of the literature. *Cancer.* 1998;82:2150–2158.
152. Igarashi A, Maruo Y, Ito T, et al. Huge cystic lymphangioma of the pancreas: report of a case. *Surg Today.* 2001;31:743–746.
153. Adsay NV, Tranchida P, Hasteh F, et al. Pseudotumoral pancreatitis: a clinicopathologic analysis of 33 patients with mass-forming pancreatitis with emphasis on the probable mechanisms [abstract]. *Mod Pathol.* 2000;13:179A.
154. Tranchida P, Taylor JP, Weaver D, et al. Paraduodenal pancreatitis: a clinically and pathologically distinct form of pseudotumoral chronic pancreatitis associated with abnormalities of accessory duct, accessory ampulla, or duodenal wall [abstract]. *Mod Pathol.* 2003;14:286A.
155. Stolte M, Weiss W, Volkholz H, et al. A special form of segmental pancreatitis: "groove pancreatitis." *Hepatogastroenterology.* 1982;29:198–208.
156. Liu TH, Consorti ET. Inflammatory pseudotumor presenting as a cystic tumor of the pancreas. *Am Surg.* 2000;66:993–997.
157. Procacci C, Graziani R, Zamboni G, et al. Cystic dystrophy of the duodenal wall: radiologic findings. *Radiology.* 1997;205:741–747.
158. Suda K, Takase M, Shiono S, et al. Duodenal wall cysts may be derived from a ductal component of ectopic pancreatic tissue. *Histopathology.* 2002;41:351–356.
159. Adsay V, Andea A, Kilinc N, et al. Secondary tumors of the pancreas: an analysis of a large surgical and autopsy database and review of the literature. *Virchows Arch.* 2004; in press.

160. Ramirez Plaza CP, Suarez Munoz MA, Santoyo Santoyo J, et al. Pancreatic cystic metastasis from pulmonary carcinoma: report of a case. *Ann Ital Chir.* 2001;72:95–99.
161. Vogel JD, Yeo CJ. Choledochal cyst or pancreatic (retention) cyst: a case report. *J Gastrointest Surg.* 2003;7:754–757.
162. Macari M, Lazarus D, Israel G, et al. Duodenal diverticula mimicking cystic neoplasms of the pancreas: CT and MR imaging findings in seven patients. *AJR Am J Roentgenol.* 2003;180:195–199.
163. Tan G, Vitellas K, Morrison C, et al. Cystic schwannoma of the pancreas. *Ann Diagn Pathol.* 2003;7:285–291.
164. Lee JS, Kim HS, Jung JJ, et al. Ancient schwannoma of the pancreas mimicking a cystic tumor. *Virchows Arch.* 2001; 439:697–699.
165. Hsiao WC, Lin PW, Chang KC. Benign retroperitoneal schwannoma mimicking a pancreatic cystic tumor: case report and literature review. *Hepatogastroenterology.* 1998;45:2418–2420.
166. Liu DM, Jeffrey RB, Jr., Mindelzun RE. Malignant fibrous histiocytoma presenting as cystic pancreatic mass. *Abdom Imaging.* 1999;24:299–300.
167. Girelli R, Bassi C, Falconi M, et al. Pancreatic cystic manifestations in von Hippel-Lindau disease. *Int J Pancreatol.* 1997;22:101–109.
168. Hough DM, Stephens DH, Johnson CD, et al. Pancreatic lesions in von Hippel-Lindau disease: prevalence, clinical significance, and CT findings. *AJR Am J Roentgenol.* 1994;162:1091–1094.
169. Silverman JF, Prichard J, Regueiro MD. Fine needle aspiration cytology of a pancreatic cyst in a patient with autosomal dominant polycystic kidney disease: a case report. *Acta Cytol.* 2001;45:415–419.
170. Valentini AL, Brizi MG, Mutignani M, et al. Adult medullary cystic disease of the kidney and pancreatic cystic disease: a new association. *Scand J Urol Nephrol.* 1999;33:423–425.
171. Andronikou S, Sinclair-Smith C, Millar AJ. An enteric duplication cyst of the pancreas causing abdominal pain and pancreatitis in a child. *Pediatr Surg Int.* 2002;18:190–192.
172. Dipaola G, Camoglio FS, Chironi C, et al. Congenital true pancreatic cyst in pediatric age: case report. *Pediatr Med Chir.* 2002;24:63–65.
173. Caillot JL, Rongieras F, Voiglio E, et al. A new case of congenital cyst of the pancreas. *Hepatogastroenterology.* 2000;47:916–918.
174. Keller MS, Weber TR, Sotelo-Avila C, et al. Duodenal duplication cysts: a rare cause of acute pancreatitis in children. *Surgery.* 2001;130:112–115.
175. Andersson R, Lindell G, Cwikiel W, et al. Retroperitoneal bronchogenic cyst as a differential diagnosis of pancreatic mucinous cystic tumor. *Dig Surg.* 2003;20:55–57.
176. Majeski J, Harmon J. Benign enterogenous cyst of the pancreas. *South Med J.* 2000;93:337–339.
177. Munshi IA, Parra-Davila E, Casillas VJ, et al. Ciliated foregut cyst of the pancreas. *HPB Surg.* 1998;11:117–119.
178. Monti L, Salerno T, Lucidi V, et al. Pancreatic cystosis in cystic fibrosis: case report. *Abdom Imaging.* 2001;26:648–650.
179. Toth IR, Lang JN. Giant pancreatic retention cyst in cystic fibrosis: a case report. *Pediatr Pathol.* 1986;6:103–110.
180. Boulanger SC, Borowitz DS, Fisher JF, et al. Congenital pancreatic cysts in children. *J Pediatr.* Surg 2003;38: 1080–1082.
181. Balci S, Altinok G, Teksen F, et al. A 34-week-old male fetus with short rib polydactyly syndrome (SRPS) type I (Saldino-Noonan) with pancreatic cysts. *Turk J Pediatr.* 2003;45:174–178.
182. Balci S, Bostanoglu S, Altinok G, et al. New syndrome? Three sibs diagnosed prenatally with situs inversus totalis, renal and pancreatic dysplasia, and cysts. *Am J Med Genet.* 2000;90:185–187.
183. Drut R, Drut M. Pancreatic cystic dysplasia (dysgenesis) presenting as a surgical pathology specimen in a patient with multiple malformations and familial ear pits. *Int J Surg Pathol.* 2002;10:303–308.
184. Xie XY, Strauch E, Sun CC. Choledochal cysts and multilocular cysts of the pancreas. *Hum Pathol.* 2003;34:99–101.
185. Meckler KA, Brentnall TA, Haggitt RC, et al. Familial fibrocystic pancreatic atrophy with endocrine cell hyperplasia and pancreatic carcinoma. *Am J Surg Pathol.* 2001; 25:1047–1053.
186. Haddad MC. Hydatid cyst of the pancreas as a cause of pancreatic cystic lesions. *AJR Am J Roentgenol.* 2003;181: 885–886; author reply 886.
187. Bolognese A, Barbarosos A, Muttillo IA, et al. Echinococcus cyst of the pancreas: description of a case and review of the literature. *G Chir.* 2000;21:389–393.
188. Yorganci K, Iret D, Sayek I. A case of primary hydatid disease of the pancreas simulating cystic neoplasm. *Pancreas.* 2000;21:104–105.
189. Echenique Elizondo M, Amondarain Arratibel JA, Liron de Robles Sanz C. Cystic neoplasms of the pancreas: a series. *Rev Esp Enferm Dig.* 2003;95:317–321, 311–316.
190. Liu Q, He Z, Bie P. Solitary pancreatic tuberculous abscess mimicking prancreatic cystadenocarcinoma: a case report. *BMC Gastroenterol.* 2003;3:1.
191. Matsuda M, Sakurai S, Suzuki A, et al. Fatal acute pancreatitis with cystic formation in reactive systemic AA amyloidosis secondary to rheumatoid arthritis. *Intern Med.* 2003;42:888–892.
192. Lee DS, Baek JT, Ahn BM, et al. A case of pancreatic endometrial cyst. *Korean J Intern Med.* 2002;17:266–269.
193. Sumiyoshi Y, Yamashita Y, Maekawa T, et al. A case of hemorrhagic cyst of the pancreas resembling the cystic endometriosis. *Int Surg.* 2000;85:67–70.
194. Friedman HD. Nonmucinous, glycogen-poor cystadenocarcinoma of the pancreas. *Arch Pathol Lab Med.* 1990; 114:888–891.

CHAPTER 52

Imaging of Cystic Pancreatic Tumors

Chuslip Charnsangavej, MD
Eric P. Tamm, MD

Cystic tumors of the pancreas are uncommon, accounting for 1%–2% of pancreatic tumors. Recent advances in imaging techniques and the common use of imaging studies for screening examination have increased the detection and diagnosis of cystic lesions in the pancreas. Some of these lesions are found in patients who are symptomatic, but many are purely incidental findings in those who have no symptoms or who have symptoms that are not related. The diagnosis and management of patients presenting with a pancreatic cystic mass depend on clinical information, laboratory findings, and more importantly, imaging characteristics of the cystic mass. In this chapter, we describe clinical findings and morphologic and imaging findings of common cystic tumors of the pancreas. We also discuss the approach to the diagnosis of cystic tumors when a cystic lesion is found on imaging studies as an incidental finding.

Cystic Neoplasms

Cystic tumors of the pancreas are rare tumors that originated from the ductal component of the gland, and they account for only 1%–2% of pancreatic neoplasms. Although many types of pancreatic tumors can have cystic appearances, the true cystic tumors originated from ductal epithelium are uncommon. The most common cystic tumors are serous microcystic and macrocystic cystadenoma, mucin-producing cystic tumors, intraductal papillary mucinous tumors (IPMTs), and solid papillary cystic tumors.[1-3]

Serous Microcystic and Macrocystic Cystadenoma

Clinical and pathologic features Serous cystadenoma is considered a benign tumor without malignant potential.[4,5] Although a malignant version has been reported, it is extremely rare, and some have been reported to be in association with the typical ductal adenocarcinoma. The tumor originates from ductal epithelium, and the fluid in the cyst contains serous fluid with glycogen-rich content. Morphologically, two types of serous cystadenoma have been described: a microcystic serous cystadenoma and a macrocystic or oligocystic serous cystadenoma. The majority of serous cystadenoma are the microcystic type, accounting for approximately 75% of the cases.[5]

Microcystic serous cystadenoma can be found as an incidental finding or in patients who present with symptoms associated with upper abdominal mass such as pain or pressure symptoms. Most microcystic serous

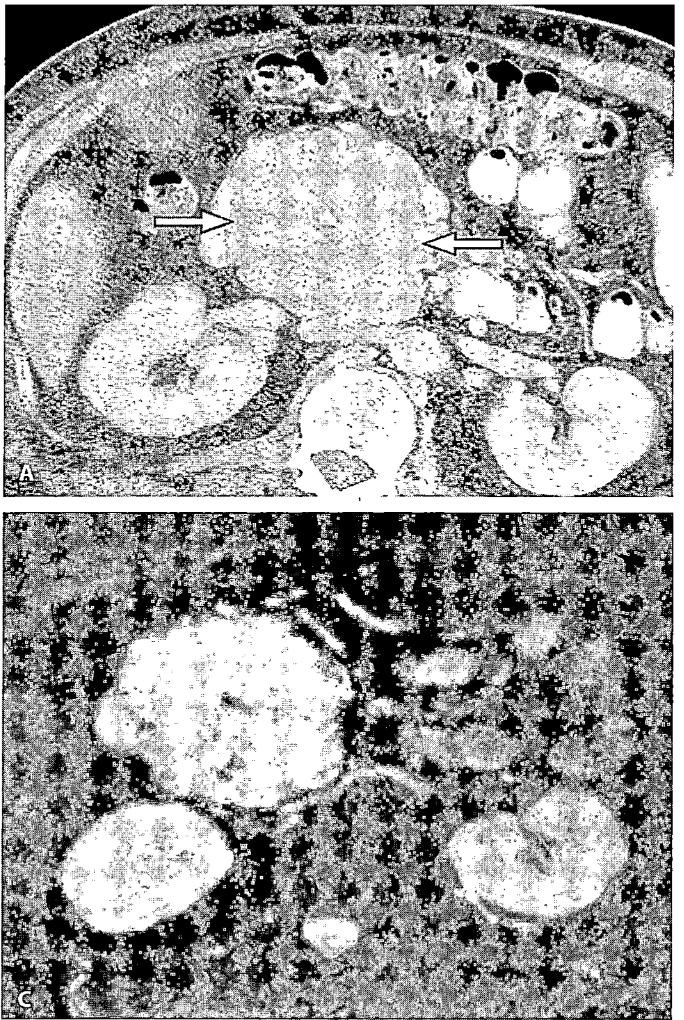

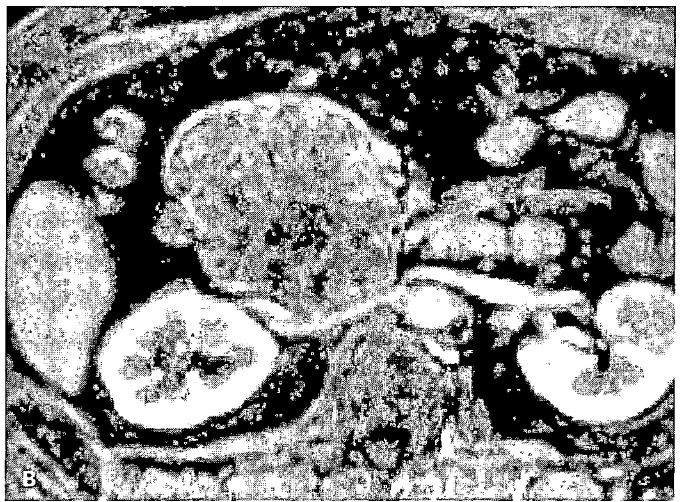

Figure 52.1
Microcystic serous cystadenoma, CT, and MR appearances. **(A)** The CT at the level of the head of the pancreas shows a well-circumscribed mass (*arrows*) containing numerous tiny cysts. A small calcification is seen in the fibrovascular septum. **(B)** After contrast, a T1-weighted MR image shows enhancement of the lesion with numerous cysts. **(C)** A T2-weighted MR image shows high signal intensity cysts in the mass with thin septum that have low signal intensity.

cystadenomas occur sporadically, and in 3%–5%, they may occur in association with a clinical syndrome such as von Hippel-Lindau disease and polycystic renal and hepatic disease.[6,7] The sporadic form is most frequently found in older females (older than 60 years old). Because this tumor is mostly benign and is found incidentally in older patients, a less aggressive approach in the management of this tumor will be most likely. Therefore, imaging characteristics of this lesion will be crucial for clinical decision making, whether surgical exploration or resection would be necessary. When the mass is large, it can produce pressure symptoms, dyspepsia, or weight loss. It may require surgical intervention.

Imaging features The gross morphologic appearance of microcystic cystadenoma is that of a well-circumscribed mass containing numerous small cysts with fibrovascular septum. The typical imaging characteristic of this tumor reflects the gross morphologic appearance. The mass is generally well circumscribed with a density measurement that is close to water density or that is slightly higher on the unenhanced computed tomography (CT). Individual tiny cysts may not be appreciable on unenhanced CT. After a bolus intravenous contrast injection, the tumor becomes hyperdense because of the enhancement of the septum. The tiny cysts, mostly smaller than 1 cm, within the mass can be easily recognized on CT and magnetic resonance (MR) (Figs. 52.1 and 52.2).[8-14] A central scar can be seen in 13–20%. Calcification in the central scar was reported in 11–38% of these tumors (Fig. 52.2).[8-11] The tumor is generally well circumscribed and is not invasive or metastatic. On rare occasion, obstruction of the bile duct may be observed. Obstruction of the pancreatic duct is also uncommon; however, large tumors can cause displacement and extrinsic compression of the duct. On ultrasonography (US), microcystic cystadenoma

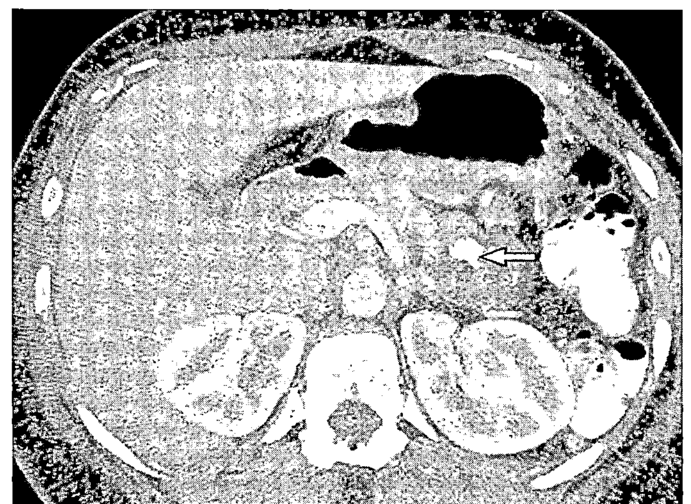

Figure 52.2
Microcystic serous cystadenoma with central calcification often described as "sunburst" appearance (*arrow*), shown on CT.

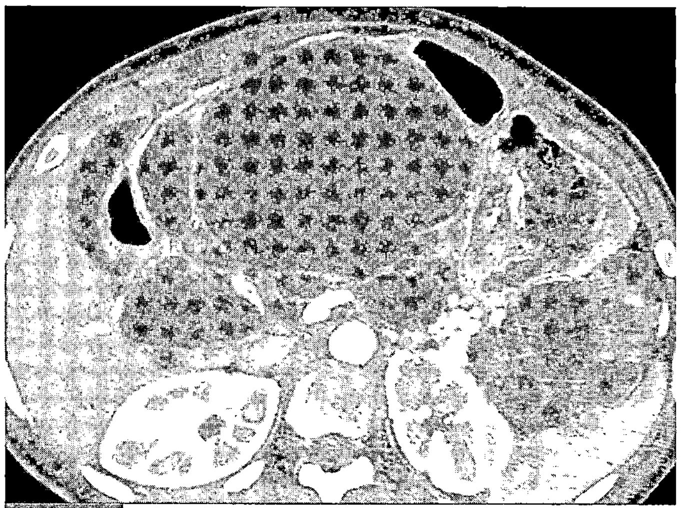

Figure 52.3
Macrocystic serous cystadenoma in a patient with von Hippel-Lindau disease. Note the large cystic locules in this type of serous cystadenoma.

have been shown to be irregular anechoic masses with central hyperechoic areas with possible acoustic shadowing if the lesions are calcified. Lesions with numerous tiny cysts may have a hypoechoic appearance without a well defined anechoic area. The reported diagnostic accuracy of serous cystadenoma is quite variable depending on the imaging techniques, criteria of interpretation, and gold standard.[11-14] Using the criteria of central scar, small cysts in a well-circumscribed cystic mass and the appearance of a honeycomb should result in a high positive predictive value. Common mistakes, such as misinterpretation of the lesion as a solid tumor or a neuroendocrine tumor, can occur when scanning techniques are not properly performed. Thin-section (2- to 5-mm slice thickness) and multiphasic contrast enhanced scanning will improve the detection of small cysts and enhancement of the fibrovascular septum. Without thin-section scanning, the tiny cysts may not be easily recognized, and the lesion can be mistaken as a solid tumor. Moreover, the hypervascularity of the fibrovascular septum could produce rapid enhancement of the lesion during the early phase of scanning. The lesion can be mistaken as a hypervascular tumor such as a neuroendocrine tumor.

On the other hand, in cases with a macrocystic serous cystadenoma, the positive predictive value could be low because of the inability to distinguish a serous cystadenoma from a pseudocyst or a mucin-producing cystic lesion.[1,5,13,14] In this case, aspiration of fluid in the cyst under US guidance via endoscopy to examine the characteristic of the fluid is the common diagnostic approach.[15-18]

Macrocystic Serous Cystadenoma

This is an uncommon variant of serous cystadenoma, with a reported incidence of approximately 10%–26% of serous cystadenoma.[4,5] This type of serous cystadenoma forms a unilocular or multilocular cystic mass, in which individual cysts are much larger than tiny cysts seen in the microcystic type (Fig. 52.3). The wall or septum of this cystic tumor does not contain fibrovascular tissue and is not hypervascular. The combination of these criteria, the lack of wall enhancement, the location of the tumor (in the pancreatic head), and contour lobulation are considered important signs for distinguishing this lesion from a mucin-producing cystic tumor.

Mucin-Producing Cystic Tumors

Clinical and pathologic features The mucin-producing cystic tumor is a group of tumors that may have various malignant potentials from a benign tumor such as a mucinous cystadenoma to a malignant tumor such as a cystadenocarcinoma that can be invasive and metastatic.[19-24] Many pathologists believe that a benign cystadenoma can transform to a cystadenocarcinoma over time. Clinical and pathologic studies during the past 2 decades have distinguished mucin-producing cystic tumors from IPMTs, which in the past were classified as a subtype of mucin-producing cystic tumors.[23,24]

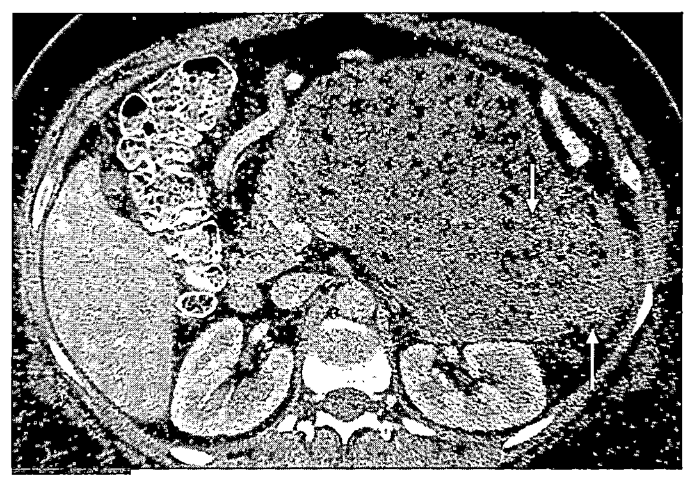

Figure 52.4
Mucin-producing cystic tumor, CT appearances. Note the large cystic mass arising from the body and tail of the pancreas with area of cystic nodules, septation, and solid nodule (*arrows*), known as the "daughter" nodule.

The tumor typically is a unilocular or multilocular cystic mass with a dense, thick fibrous wall that may contain tumor nodules or dystrophic calcification. The columnar epithelial cells lining the inner wall of the cyst produce mucin that accumulates in the cyst. The submucosal layer consists of highly cellular stroma of spindle cells with elongated nuclei similar to the "ovarian stroma." This is one of the most important pathologic features that distinguish mucin-producing cystic tumors from IPMTs. The tumor vascularity in mucin-producing cystic tumors is quite variable.

The tumor is more commonly seen in middle-aged females (between 40 to 50 years old). Approximately two thirds of this tumor occurs in the body and tail of the pancreas. It generally produces symptoms from pressure symptoms to weight loss. One of the most important clinical questions in dealing with cystic lesions in the pancreas is to distinguish mucin-producing cystic tumors from serous cystadenoma and other benign cystic lesions. This is because surgical resection is most likely the treatment of choice because of the malignant potential of mucin-producing cystic tumors.[2,3,22] Imaging studies and image-guided aspiration biopsy to evaluate the content of the cyst are currently used for this decision-making process.

Imaging features The CT appearance of a mucin-producing cystic tumor is that of a loculated, fluid-filled cystic mass with septation and nodules in the wall (Fig. 52.4).[8-10,25-29] The wall of the cystic mass is often thickened and can be identified. Curvilinear or peripheral calcification can be seen in the wall of the cystic mass in approximately 10%–20% of the cases. Similar morphologic features can be seen on US and MR imaging (MRI). Mucinous fluid in the cyst has T1 and T2 relaxation times similar to water (Fig. 52.5) or fluid in inflammatory pancreatic pseudocysts or serous cystadenoma and cannot distinguish one from the other. Enhancement of the wall, septum, and nodule may not be as intense as the fibrovascular septum of microcystic cystadenoma.

Imaging studies generally cannot distinguish cystadenoma from cystadenocarcinoma unless there are evidences of invasion of pancreatic parenchyma, vascular invasion, and metastasis.

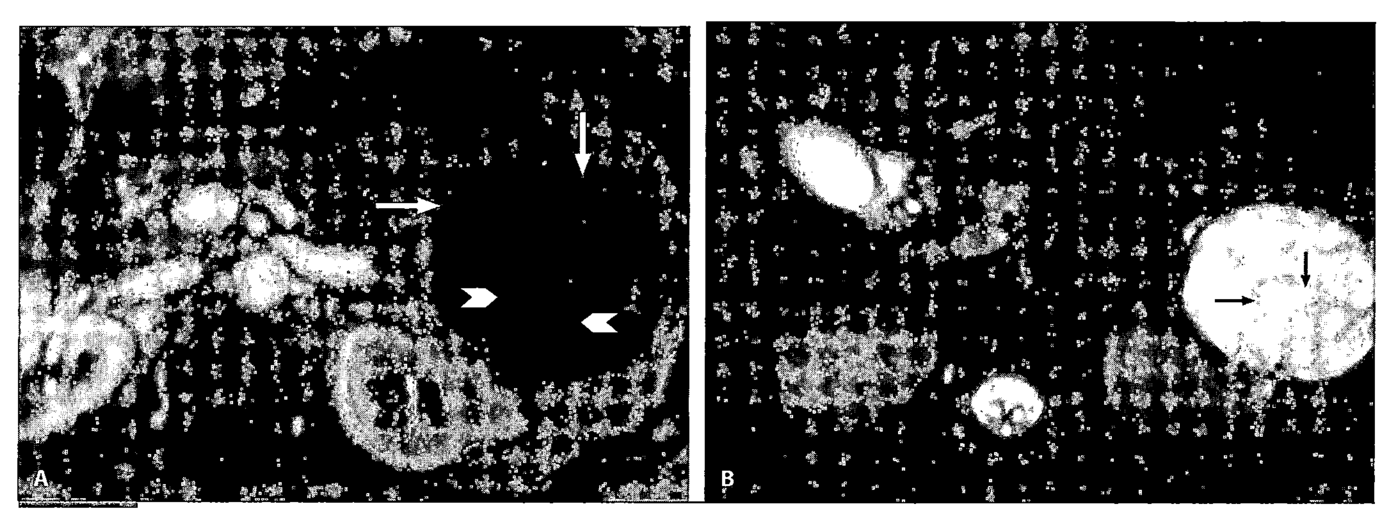

Figure 52.5
Mucin-producing cystic tumor, MR appearances. **(A)** After contrast, a T1-weighted MR image shows a cystic mass (*arrows*) arising from the tail of the pancreas with low signal intensity and septation (*arrowheads*). **(B)** A T2-weighted image shows septation (*arrows*) and a "daughter nodule" that have low signal intensity.

IPMTs

Clinical and pathologic features This type of tumor originates from ductal epithelium forming a papillary projection into the duct. The tumor produces mucin that accumulates in the pancreatic duct. The tumor by itself or its mucinous product can cause ductal obstruction and ductal stricture resulting in gross morphologic appearances of cystic lesions or diffuse dilation of the duct and atrophy of the pancreatic parenchyma. The epithelial cell of the primary tumor can have various degrees of cellular atypia and stromal invasion from a dysplastic, premalignant lesion to adenoma, carcinoma in situ, and invasive carcinoma.[23,24]

Previously, this group of tumors was classified as a subtype of mucin-producing cystic tumors, commonly known as ductectatic mucinous cystadenoma and cystadenocarcinoma, or mucinous ductectasia.[23-25] It was not until the past 2 decades that this type of tumor has been recognized and distinguished from mucin-producing cystic tumors because of the differences in their clinical and pathologic features. Clinically, IPMT is more frequently seen in males than in females (an approximate 2:1 ratio) and in an older age group (60–70 years old) than those patients with mucin-producing cystic tumors. The patients commonly present with signs and symptoms of obstruction of the pancreatic duct and bile duct, such as recurrent bouts of pancreatitis and obstructive jaundice. The course of progression and the malignant potential of IPMT can be variable depending on the phenotypes of the tumors.

The gross morphologic appearances of IPMT can be classified into two types: the main duct type and the side branch type. In the main duct type, there is diffuse dilation of the main pancreatic duct and the side branch. The ductal obstruction can be caused by the solid papillary growth of the tumors by itself or by the mucinous product of the benign dysplastic lesion in the ductal wall. The mucin in the pancreatic duct can accumulate, distend the duct, and protrude into the ampulla and the duodenum, causing the classic "fish mouth" appearance of the ampulla, as observed by endoscopic view or on CT. The main duct type is frequently associated with atrophy of the pancreatic parenchyma.

The branch duct type is frequently seen in the head of the pancreas but can be seen at any side branch of the main pancreatic duct. Obstruction of the secondary branch, by the primary tumor or mucin, at the site where it joins the main duct produces a morphologic feature of a multiseptated cystic mass or a cystic locule in that region of the pancreas.

IPMT has the classic histologic feature of columnar epithelial cells forming papillary projection into the ductal lumen. Unlike mucin-producing cystic tumors that have highly cellular, ovarian-type stromal cells, the submucosa layer of IPMT consists of inflammatory cells.

Imaging features The characteristic imaging features of the main duct type of IPMT is that of diffuse dilation of the main pancreatic duct and its side branch (Figs. 52.6 and 52.7).[30-34] The pancreatic parenchyma is atrophic because of chronic ductal obstruction. The classic features of chronic pancreatitis, including calcification of the pancreatic parenchyma and beaded appearance of pancreatic ductal dilation, are not present in IPMT, but atrophy of

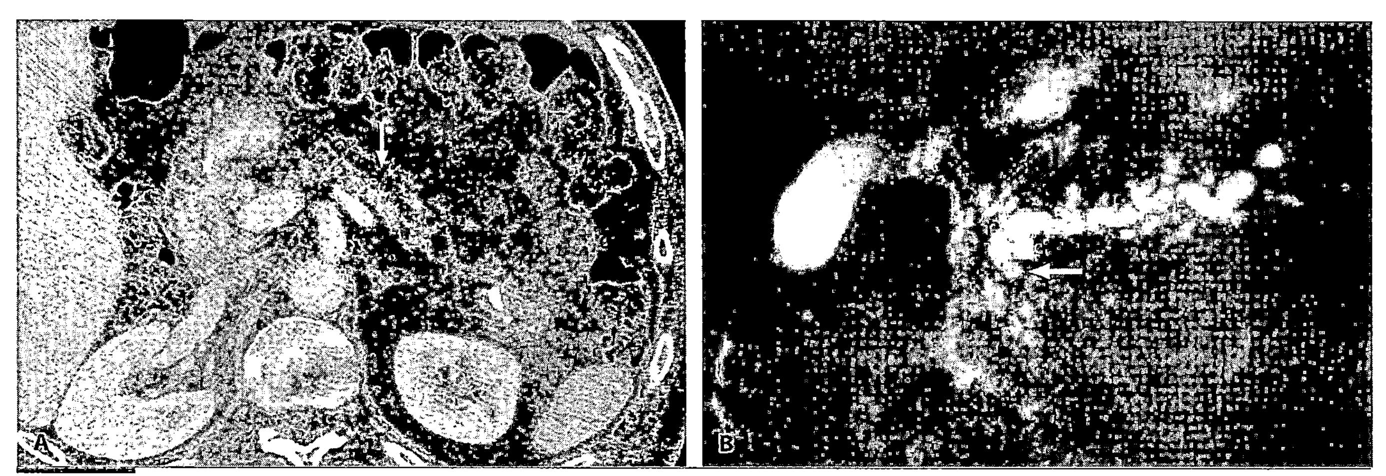

Figure 52.6
IPMT causing dilation of the main pancreatic duct in the body and tail simulating chronic pancreatitis. A pathologic specimen that showed mucin obstructing the duct and dysplastic lesions was found in the ductal epithelium without invasive carcinoma. **(A)** CT scan at the level of the body of the pancreas shows dilated pancreatic duct (*arrow*). **(B)** MR cholangiopancreatography shows diffuse pancreatic ductal dilation with stricture of the duct (*arrow*) at the pancreatic head.

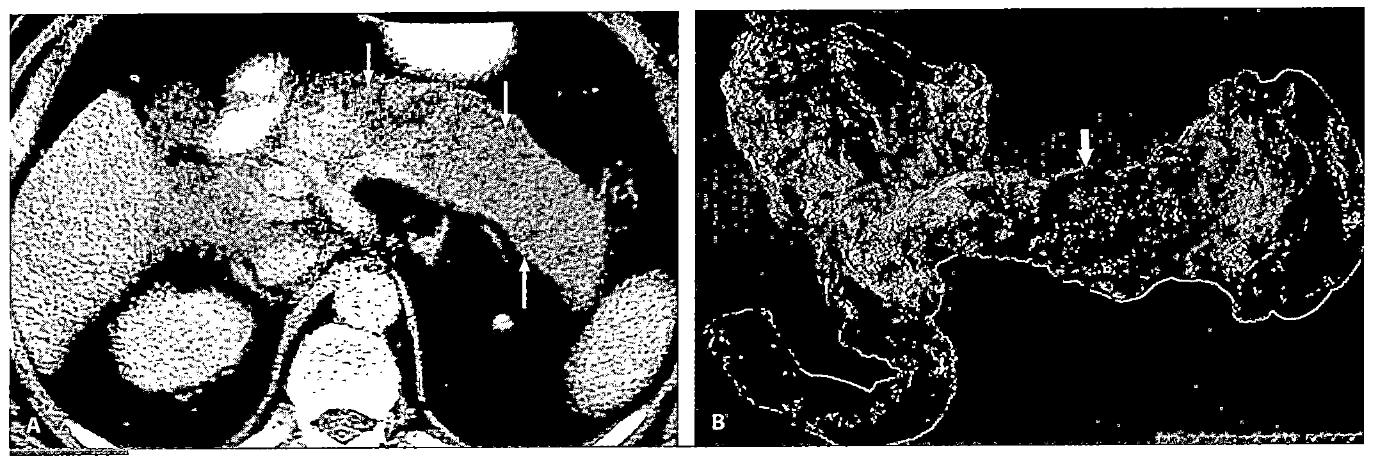

Figure 52.7
IPMT involving the entire body of the pancreas. This was a patient with lymphoma who had multiple episodes of pancreatitis. **(A)** CT at the level of the body of the pancreas shows diffuse low-density changes (*arrows*) throughout the body. This is due to a diffusely dilated pancreatic duct with pancreatic parenchyma atrophy. **(B)** A photograph of gross pathologic specimen shows diffuse dilation of pancreatic duct (*arrow*) in the body and tail of the pancreas, which was filled with mucin.

the pancreatic parenchyma may be similar. The key features that make the diagnosis of IPMT more likely are diffuse dilation of the duct without beaded appearances, protrusion of the dilated duct and ampulla into the duodenum (the fish mouth sign) (Fig. 52.8), and the lack of calcifications in the pancreatic duct or in the pancreatic parenchyma.

In patients who do not have ductal dilation down to the ampulla, the appearances of the site of ductal stricture should be carefully analyzed to determine the causes. The lack of mass at the stricture site could make it difficult to distinguish chronic pancreatitis from IPMT because it is not possible to define dysplastic or early lesions in IPMT using current imaging techniques (Fig. 52.6). The presence of intraductal lesion at the stricture site favors the diagnosis of IPMT, whereas the mass causing extrinsic compression to the duct would favor the diagnosis of pancreatic ductal adenocarcinoma.

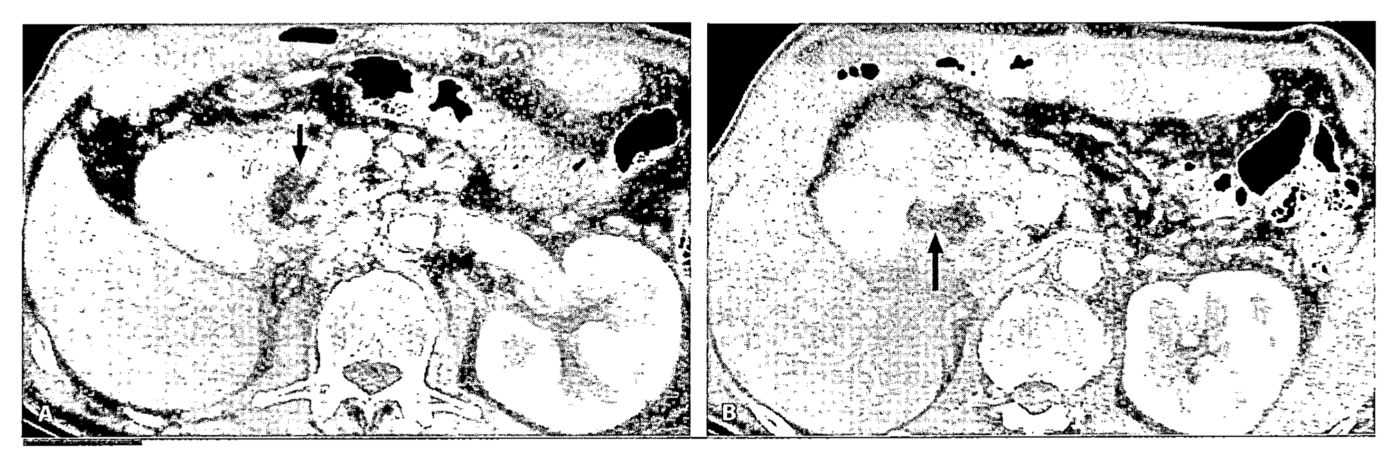

Figure 52.8
IPMT of the head of the pancreas with a "fish mouth" appearance of the ampulla. **(A)** A CT at the level of the head of the pancreas shows a cystic lesion (*arrow*) with tumor nodules in the head of the pancreas. **(B)** A CT at the level of the ampulla shows the dilated ampulla (*arrow*), which was filled with mucin, protruding into the duodenum producing a "fish mouth" appearance.

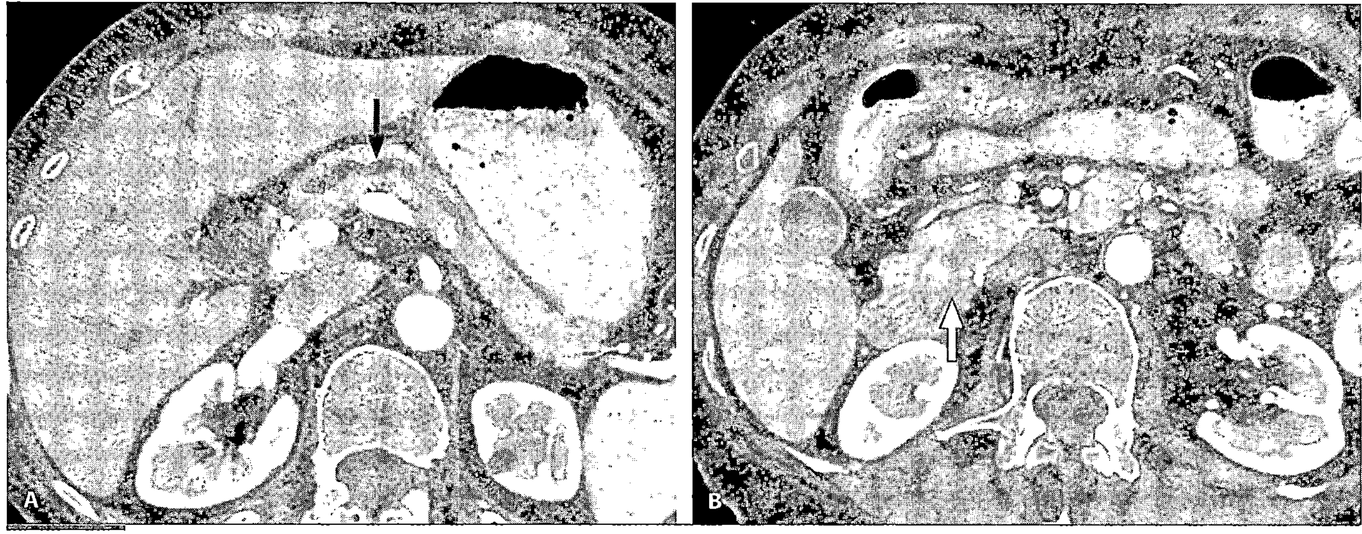

Figure 52.9
IPMT of the head of the pancreas presenting as a solid, enhancing, intraductal lesion. Histologic examination showed invasive papillary carcinoma. **(A)** A CT at the level of the body and tail shows dilation of the main pancreatic duct (*arrow*). **(B)** A CT at the level of the head of the pancreas shows a lesion (*arrow*) growing in the main pancreatic duct toward the ampulla.

The presence of a hyperdense-enhancing, intraductal mass is also another important sign for IPMTs. In our experience, 5%–10% of the main duct type of IPMT could present with intraductal mass causing obstruction of the pancreatic duct without a large amount of mucin accumulating in the duct (Fig. 52.9). This type of lesion could be diagnosed as an adenocarcinoma if the lesion was diagnosed by aspiration biopsy without surgical resection and examination of the entire specimen.

The imaging features of the side branch type of IPMT are quite different from the main duct type. Obstruction of the side branch of the pancreatic duct can cause segmental dilation of those secondary and tertiary branches or can form a cystic lesion. In the head of the pancreas and in the uncinate process, dilation of these secondary and tertiary ducts can form a tortuous, multiseptated cystic mass (Fig. 52.10), previously described as ductectasia. Further progression of this mass can obstruct the main pancreatic duct later. Obstruction of the secondary branch in the body and tail of the pancreas usually results in a cystic formation of variable size (Fig. 52.11). IPMTs of the side branch can be a single lesion or multiple lesions.

Currently, MR cholangiopancreatography has become the imaging technique of choice to demonstrate the extent of ductal involvement in IPMT (Fig. 52.6).[33,34] However, the accurate diagnosis of early lesions or dysplastic lesions and the ability to distinguish them from malignant lesions remain unresolved with the current technology. The positive predictive value for advanced disease may be high using the criteria of enhancing intraductal lesions and the presence of invasive tumors (hypodense mass) associated with cystic lesions in

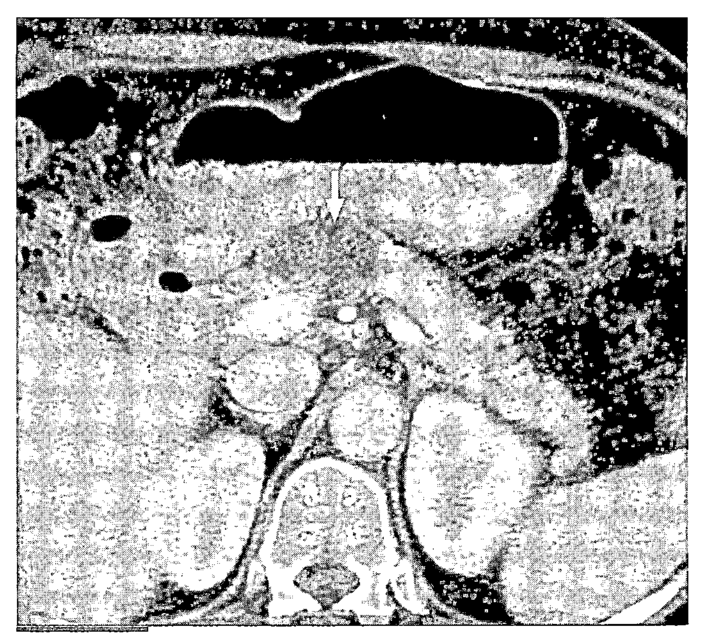

Figure 52.10
The branch duct type of IPMT. The CT shows cystic lesion (*arrow*) in the neck of the pancreas with septation. The main pancreatic duct is slightly dilated. The cystic lesion was due to mucin obstructing the branch duct and causing dilation of the branch duct.

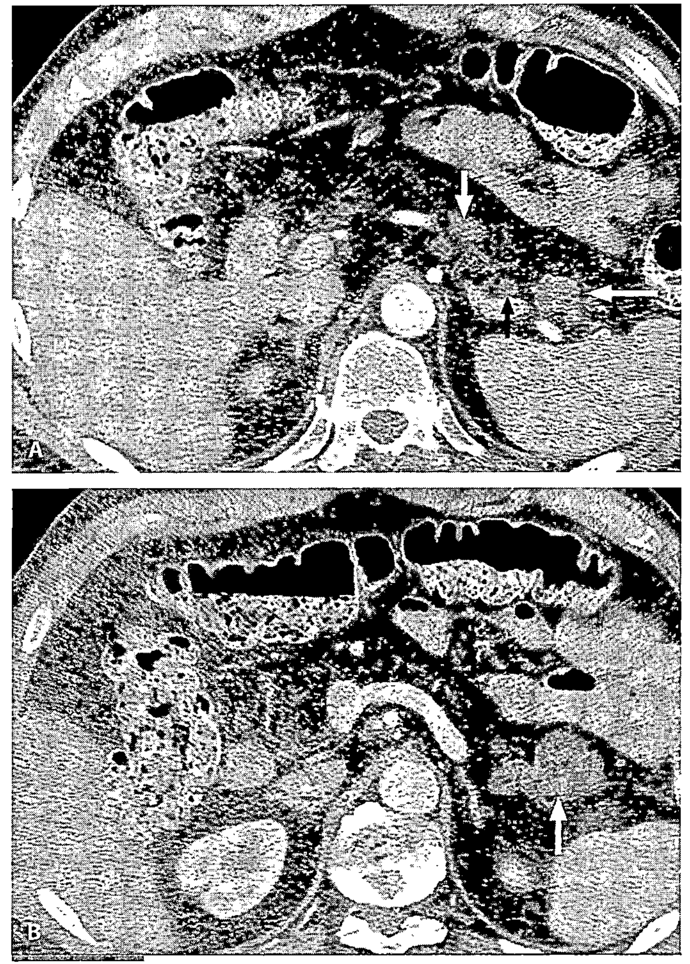

Figure 52.11
The branch duct type of IPMT in a patient with diffuse fatty replacement of pancreatic parenchyma. **(A)** A CT at the level of the body and tail of the pancreas shows multiple cystic locules (*arrows*) in the body and tail of the pancreas. Note the fatty changes of the pancreatic parenchyma. **(B)** Note the multiloculated cystic lesion (*arrow*) at the tail of the pancreas.

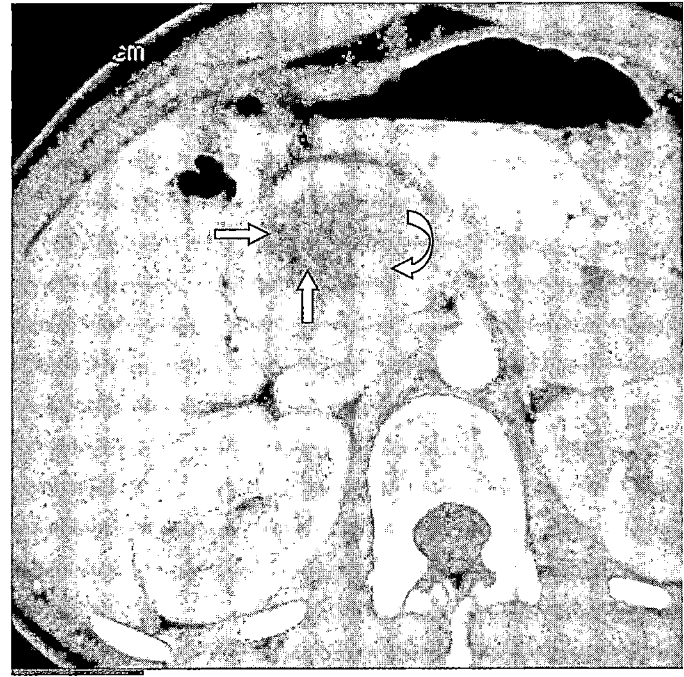

Figure 52.12
A solid papillary epithelial neoplasm at the head of the pancreas in a 14-year-old girl. A CT scan shows a mass in the head of the pancreas with an area of cystic change and old hemorrhage (*arrows*) in the center. The solid component (*curved arrow*) is still seen at the periphery of the tumor.

addition to vascular invasion and distant metastasis. This has become an important research focus that will make an impact in the management of patients with IPMT as to which tumors should be , which patients can be observed, and what extent surgery should be performed.

Solid Papillary Epithelial Neoplasms

Clinical and pathologic features This is another rare cystic tumor with low malignant potential. It is frequently seen in young females. The tumors usually have a well-defined margin and a thick capsule. However, the internal architecture of the tumor is rather complex because it may contain solid-component, hemorrhagic areas and cystic degeneration.[35,36] The patient may present because of pressure symptoms or mass effect or acute abdominal pain because of hemorrhage in the mass.

Imaging features CT of this tumor shows various features depending on the content of the tumor from cystic, hemorrhagic, and solid mass (Figs. 52.12 and 52.13). The key features to suggest the diagnosis are the patients' ages and the appearances of mixed solid and cystic masses in a well-circumscribed mass.

Other Cystic Lesions

Benign congenital cysts of the pancreas are rare. Some of the patients with benign pancreatic cysts may be associated with syndromes, which cysts are found in many organs, such as von Hippel-Lindau disease, and polycystic disease. Other types of benign cysts that may be acquired may also include lymphoepithelium cysts, posttraumatic cysts, and pseudocysts.

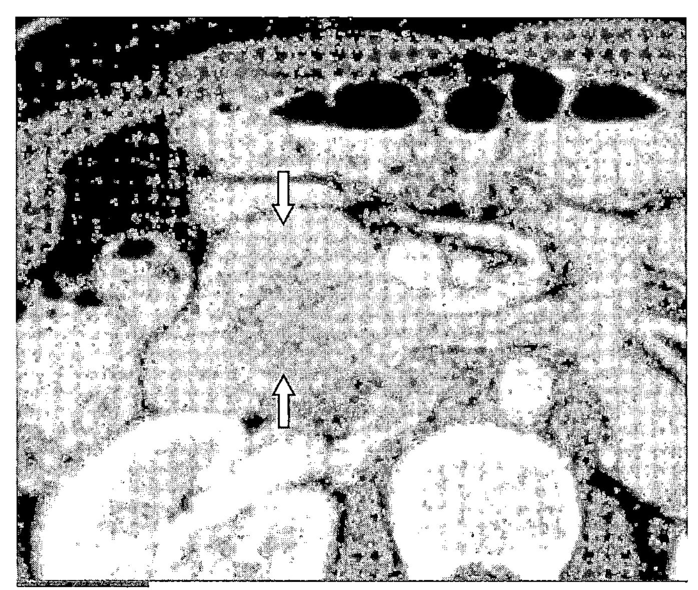

Figure 52.13
A solid papillary epithelial neoplasm at the head of the pancreas in a 17-year-old woman. CT scan shows a large solid tumor (*arrows*) in the head of the pancreas without cystic degeneration or hemorrhagic appearance.

Radiologic Imaging Approach to Cystic Lesions

In the imaging analysis of a cystic lesion based on CT and MRI, multiple factors should be taken into consideration in order to come up with an appropriate diagnosis, including the size of the lesion and its growth rate, the density and signal intensity of the lesion, the characteristic of the wall, the presence of septation or locules within the lesion, the presence of calcification and its characteristics, the enhancement of the lesion, and the relationship between the lesion and the pancreatic duct. These characteristics depend largely on the refinement of the scanning technique, particularly for the analysis of small lesions. Analysis of cystic lesions using screening CT examination at 7- to 10-mm slice thickness may be applicable for large cystic lesions but cannot be applied to lesions smaller than 2 cm or lesions containing small cysts because the screening technique cannot detect those tiny cysts of 2 to 5 mm or smaller, commonly present in microcystic cystadenoma. We prefer a specific CT imaging protocol using multiphasic scanning technique after a bolus intravenous contrast injection at 4 to 5 ml/sec and scanning at a 2- to 3-mm slice thickness. Similar scanning concept using fast, dynamic, multiphasic scanning at 3- to 5-mm slice thickness after a bolus of intravenous contrast enhancement is also applied in MRI.

Single-Locule Cyst

A cyst with single locule has many differential diagnoses. The specific diagnosis cannot be made on imaging findings alone. The following steps should be considered in the analysis of a single-locule cyst. CT density should be measured on both unenhanced CT and postcontrast CT. CT density measurement of a cystic lesion higher than water density should raise the possibility of a complicated cyst such as posttraumatic pseudocyst, hemorrhagic lesion, lesion with cystic degeneration such as a solid papillary epithelial neoplasm, cystic neuroendocrine tumor, and a possibility of microcystic cystadenoma. The thickness of the wall and presence of calcification in the wall are important to recognize. A cyst with water density with thickened wall should favor the diagnosis of a chronic inflammatory pseudocyst, posttraumatic cyst, or a mucin-producing cystic neoplasm. The presence of calcification also favors these diagnoses. The thin-walled cyst favors the diagnosis of acute or subacute pseudocyst, a serous cystadenoma (oligocystic or macrocystic type), a lymphoepithelial cyst, or a benign simple cyst.

Clinical management of this type of cyst depends largely on the size and clinical and laboratory findings. The diagnosis of pancreatic pseudocysts is favorable in patients who had history of alcohol abuse, gallstones, and previous trauma. Patients who have symptoms of chronic abdominal pain, weight loss, and elevation of serum CEA, CA 19-9 should be suspicious for having cystic neoplasm such as a mucin producing cystic tumors, and IPMT. The management of patients without symptoms will depend largely on the size of the lesion. Cystic lesions smaller than 2 cm found incidentally rarely have the diagnosis of malignancy. Fernandez–del Castillo et al.[2] found that only approximately 3% of cystic lesions smaller than 2 cm in patients who have no symptoms are malignant. Therefore, cystic lesions smaller than 2 cm can be followed at a regular 6 to 12-month interval to document the growth rate of the lesion.[2,37] Cystic lesions between 2 and 5 cm may need to be aspirated to determine the characteristics of fluid content. Imaging findings alone are not specific to characterize these lesions. We currently use endoscopic ultrasonography and aspiration of fluid under US guidance to obtain the diagnosis of these lesions. Cystic lesions larger than 5 cm often require surgical intervention or drainage depending on the most likely diagnosis based on clinical, laboratory findings, and endoscopic ultrasonography–guided aspiration.

Cyst with Multiple Large Locules and Septations

Three major differential diagnoses for cysts with multiple septations and multiple locules are mucin-producing cystic tumor, side branch type of IPMT, and macrocystic serous cystadenoma. Cysts with thick wall, calcification, and nodule in the septation and wall favor the diagnosis of mucin-producing cystic tumor, particularly if the patient is female and between 30 to 60 years old. A hydatid cyst may have the appearance similar to a mucin-producing cystic tumor, but the lesion is rare outside of the endemic area. Lesions with a thin wall, that are well circumscribed, and that lack of a nodule favor the diagnosis of macrocystic or oligocystic cystadenoma. Pseudocyst and lymphangioma may be considered in the differential diagnosis. Cystic lesions with multiple septations associated with pancreatic ductal dilation and communication with pancreatic duct favor the diagnosis of IPMT. The presence of enhancing tumor nodule and infiltration into the surrounding parenchyma should raise the concern of the malignant version of IPMT.

The role of positron emission tomography using F-18 FDG has been explored to determine whether increased uptake in the cystic lesion could be used to predict malignancy.[38] An early study suggested that it was highly accurate in predicting malignancy. However, it may not be sensitive enough to predict whether the lesion should be resected because many premalignant lesions did not have a high uptake of glucose.

Cyst with Tiny Cystic Locules and with Enhancement Simulating Solid Lesion

This is the lesion that is often mistaken as a hypervascular neoplasm. The key findings are the presence of tiny cystic locules in the well-circumscribed mass with early enhancement of the septa. The lesion is typical for a microcystic serous cystadenoma. Aspiration of this lesion often yields nondiagnostic tissue.

Conclusion

Current imaging techniques allow excellent morphologic assessment of cystic tumors of the pancreas. Careful analysis of a cystic lesion should include the density of cystic fluid, the enhancement of the lesion, the appearance of the wall, and the internal architecture of the cyst. Proper analysis can provide initial guidelines for clinical management of patients with a cystic lesion of the pancreas. Future research should focus on the development of imaging techniques and interpretation criteria that have the ability to distinguish the types of cystic fluid (mucinous vs serous) and the ability to characterize and distinguish a premalignant lesion from a malignant lesion.

References

1. Le Borgne J, de Calan L, Partensky C. Cystadenomas and cystadenocarcinomas of the pancreas: a multiinstitutional retrospective study of 398 cases: French Surgical Association. *Ann Surg.* 1999;230:152–161.
2. Fernandez-del Castillo C, Targarona J, Thayer SP, Rattner DW, Brugge WR, Warshaw AL. Incidental pancreatic cysts: clinicopathologic characteristics and comparison with symptomatic patients. *Arch Surg.* 2003;138:427–433; discussion 433–434.
3. Box JC, Douglas HO. Management of cystic neoplasms of the pancreas. *Am Surg.* 2000;66:495–501.
4. Compton C. Serous cystic tumors of the pancreas. *Semin Diagn Pathol.* 2000;17:43–55.
5. Bassi C, Salvia R, Molinari E, Biasutti C, Falconi M, Pederzoli P. Management of 100 consecutive cases of pancreatic serous cystadenoma: wait for symptoms and see at imaging or vice versa? *World J Surg.* 2003;27:319–323.
6. Hough DM, Stephens DH, Johnson CD, Binkovitz LA. Pancreatic lesions in von Hippel-Lindau disease: prevalence, clinical significance, and CT findings. *AJR Am J Roentgenol.* 1994;162:1091–1094.
7. Girelli R, Bassi C, Falconi M, et al. Pancreatic cystic manifestations in von Hippel-Lindau disease. *Int J Pancreatol.* 1997;22:101–109.
8. Friedman AC, Lichtenstein JE, Dachman AH. Cystic neoplasms of the pancreas radiological-pathological correlation. *Radiology.* 1983;149:45–50.
9. Johnson CD, Stephens DH, Charboneau JW, Carpenter HA, Welch TJ. Cystic pancreatic tumor: CT and sonographic assessment. *AJR Am J Roentgenol.* 1988;151:1133–1138.
10. Minami M, Itai Y, Ohtomo K, Yoshida H, Yoshikawa K, Iio M. Cystic neoplasms of the pancreas: comparison of MR imaging with CT. *Radiology.* 1989;171:53–56.
11. Procacci C, Graziani R, Bicego E, et al. Serous cystadenoma of the pancreas: report of 30 cases with emphasis on imaging findings. *J Comput Assist Tomogr.* 1997;21:373–382.
12. Cohen-Scali F, Vilgrain V, Brancatelli G, et al. Discrimination of unilocular macrocystic serous cystadenoma from pancreatic pseudocyst and mucinous cystadenoma with CT: initial observations. *Radiology.* 2003;228: 727–733.
13. Curry CA, Eng J, Horton KM, et al. CT of primary cystic pancreatic neoplasms: can CT be used for patient triage and treatment? *AJR Am J Roentgenol.* 2000;175:99–103.
14. Procacci C, Biastitutti C, Carbognin G, et al. Characterization of cystic tumors of the pancreas: CT accuracy. *J Comput Assist Tomogr.* 1999;23:906–912.
15. Lewandrowski KB, Southern JF, Pins MR, Compton CC, Warshaw AL. Cystic fluid analysis in the differential diagnosis of pancreatic cysts: a comparison of pseudocysts, serous cystadenomas, mucinous cystic neoplasms and mucinous cystadenoma. *Am Surg.* 1993;217:41–47.

16. Carlson SK, Johnson CD, Brandt KR, Batts KP, Salomao DR. Pancreatic cystic neoplasms: the role and sensitivity of needle aspiration biopsy. *Abdom Imaging.* 1998;23:387–393.
17. Sperti C, Pasquali C, Guolo P. Serum tumor markers and cystic fluid analysis are useful for the diagnosis of pancreatic cystic tumors. *Cancer.* 1996;78:237–243.
18. Frossard JL, Amouyal P, Amouyal G, et al. Performance of endosonography-guided fine needle aspiration and biopsy in the diagnosis of pancreatic cystic lesions. *Am J Gastroenterol.* 2003;98:1516–1524.
19. Demos TC, Posniak HV, Harmath C, Olson MC, Aranha G. Cystic lesions of the pancreas. *AJR Am J Roentgenol.* 2002;179:1375–1388.
20. Whang EE, Danial T, Dunn JC, et al. The spectrum of mucin-producing adenocarcinoma of the pancreas. *Pancreas.* 2000;21:147–151.
21. Wilentz RE, Albores-Saavedra J, Hruban R. Mucinous neoplasms of the pancreas. *Semin Diagn Pathol.* 2000;17:31–42.
22. Sarr MG, Carpenter HA, Prabhakar L, et al. Clinical and pathologic correlation of 84 mucinous cystic neoplasms of the pancreas. *Ann Surg.* 2000;231:205–212.
23. Fukushima N, Mukai K. Differential diagnosis between intraductal papillary-mucinous tumors and mucinous cystic tumors of the pancreas. *Int J Surg Pathol.* 2000;8:271–278.
24. Yamaguchi K, Tanaka M. Intraductal papillary-mucinous tumor of the pancreas: a historical review of the nomenclature and recent controversy. *Pancreas.* 2001;23:12–19.
25. Itai Y, Moss AA, Ohtomo K. Computed tomography of cystadenoma and cystadenocarcinoma of the pancreas. *Radiology.* 1982;145:419–425.
26. Lima JE, Javitt MC, Mathur SC. Mucinous cystic neoplasm of the pancreas. *RadioGraphics.* 1999;19:807–811.
27. Buetow PC, Rao P, Thompson LD. Mucinous cystic neoplasms of the pancreas: radiologic-pathologic correlation. *RadioGraphics.* 1998;18:433–449.
28. Grogan JR, Saeian K, Taylor AJ, Quiroz F, Demeure MJ, Komorowski RA. Making sense of mucin-producing pancreatic tumors. *AJR Am J Roentgenol.* 2001;176:921–929.
29. Scott J, Martin I, Redhead D, Hammond P, Garden OJ. Mucinous cystic neoplasms of the pancreas: imaging features and diagnostic difficulties. *Clin Radiol.* 2000;55:187–192.
30. Itai Y, Ohashi K, Nagai H, et al. Ductectatic mucinous cystadenoma and cystadenoma of the pancreas. *Radiology.* 1986;161:697–700.
31. Fukukura Y, Fujiyoshi F, Sasaki M, Inoue H, Yonezawa S, Nakajo M. Intraductal papillary mucinous tumors of the pancreas: thin-section helical CT findings. *AJR Am J Roentgenol.* 2000;174:441–447.
32. Taouli B, Vilgrain V, Vullierme MP, et al. Intraductal papillary mucinous tumors of the pancreas: helical CT with histopathologic correlation. *Radiology.* 2000;217:757–764.
33. Silas AM, Morin MM, Raptopoulos V, Keogan MT. Intraductal papillary mucinous tumors of the pancreas. *AJR Am J Roentgenol.* 2001;176:179–185.
34. Lim JH, Lee G, Oh YL. Radiologic spectrum of intraductal papillary mucinous tumors of the pancreas. *RadioGraphics.* 2001;21:323–337.
35. Klimstra D, Wenig B, Heffness C. Solid-pseudopapillary tumor of the pancreas: a typically cystic carcinoma of low malignant potential. *Semin Diagn Pathol.* 2000;17:66–80.
36. Buetow PC, Buck JL, Pantongrag-Brown L, et al. Solid papillary epithelial neoplasm of the pancreas: imaging-pathologic correlation in 56 cases. *Radiology.* 1996;199:707–711.
37. Megibow AJ, Lombardo FP, Guarise A, et al. Cystic pancreatic masses: cross-sectional imaging observations and serial follow-up. *Abdom Imaging.* 2001;26:640–647.
38. Sperti C, Pasquali C, Chierichetti F, Liessi G, Ferlin G, Pedrazzoli S. Value of 18-fluorodeoxyglucose positron emission tomography in the management of patients with cystic tumors of the pancreas. *Ann Surg.* 2001;234:675–680.

CHAPTER

53

Surgical Treatment of Cystic Neoplasms

Carlos Fernández-del Castillo, MD

The current management of cystic neoplasms of the pancreas is the result of important advances in this field over the past 25 years. The landmark publications by Compagno and Oertel[1,2] set the basis for the pathological differential diagnosis of this heterogeneous group of lesions, previously referred to only as pancreatic cystadenomas and cystadenocarcinomas and described only in isolated case reports. Simultaneously, the use of computed tomography (CT) and ultrasound became widespread, and this contributed by disclosing increasing numbers of cases in asymptomatic or minimally symptomatic patients and by providing clinicians with both objective parameters for follow-up and morphologic features useful in the differential diagnosis. Endoscopic retrograde cholangiopancreatography, and more recently, endoscopic ultrasound, magnetic resonance imaging, and magnetic resonance cholangiopancreatography have also played a role by providing additional parameters that not only help differentiate pseudocysts from cystic tumors but also distinguish the many varieties of neoplastic cysts. Finally, refinements in pancreatic surgery have made resection of these lesions increasingly safe and justify the diagnostic effort by providing reasonable expectations for cure. The mortality for pancreatic resection in specialized centers is currently less than 2%,[3,4] which has resulted in expanded indications for pancreatectomy; in contrast to previous decades in which pancreatic resection was confined to proven malignancy given the high morbidity and mortality rates associated with surgery. Before 1990, cystic neoplasms were the indication for less than 10% of pancreatic resections at the Massachusetts General Hospital, whereas in the past 5 years, they accounted for 23%.[5]

As described in Chapter 51, there are many varieties of cystic tumors of the pancreas. This chapter addresses only serous cystadenomas, mucinous cystic neoplasms, and intraductal papillary mucinous neoplasms (IPMNs), which together make up approximately 95% of the cystic neoplasms of the pancreas.

Surgical Treatment of Serous Cystadenomas

Most serous cystadenomas of the pancreas are firm, well-circumscribed, multinodular tumors. Approximately half are located in the head or uncinate process of the pancreas, and the rest in the neck, body, or tail of the gland.[2,6-8] These tumors can be large (mean size, 7 cm; range, 1–25 cm) and can occasionally encompass the entire pancreas (Fig. 53.1). When cut, they typically have numerous small cysts filled

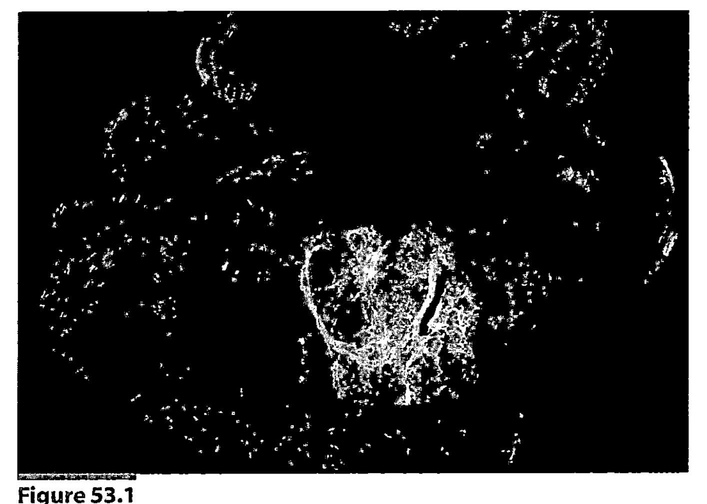

Figure 53.1
Total pancreatectomy specimen of a serous cystadenoma involving the entire pancreas.

with clear liquid and ranging in size from less than a millimeter to about 2 cm, giving them a spongy or honeycomb appearance. Lewandrowski et al.[9] have described unilocular serous cystadenomas, ranging in size from 2.5 to 8 cm, and which had been previously described as congenital or dysgenetic simple cysts of the pancreas. Whether these "macrocystic" serous cystadenomas represent a distinct entity or the end of a spectrum of cystadenomas is unclear, but they seem to have the same benign clinical course and histologic appearance. In the recent series by Bassi et al.[10] describing 100 cases of serous cystadenoma, 26% corresponded to this unilocular or macrocystic type, which is also referred to as *oligomacrocystic variant*.

Serous cystadenomas are more common in females. Most patients present with vague symptoms, usually mild upper abdominal pain or discomfort, epigastric fullness, or moderate weight loss. Because of increased detection by CT, a larger proportion of serous cystadenomas (perhaps more than 50%) are now asymptomatic.[10,11] Occasionally, they present as a palpable mass or with more specific symptoms, such as jaundice, pancreatitis, or even acute hemoperitoneum, and rarely may be associated with the von Hippel-Lindau syndrome.[12]

For symptomatic patients with serous cystadenoma, surgical resection is the best treatment. This consists of a Whipple procedure for tumors in the head of the pancreas, or a distal pancreatectomy for tumors in the body and tail. A splenectomy is not necessary if a distal pancreatectomy is performed for a serous cystadenoma, given the benign nature of this tumor, and the spleen can often be preserved, relying on the short gastric vessels alone.[13] For cases located in the neck or proximal body of the pancreas, a middle pancreatectomy is an option that spares the distal pancreas, thereby lessening the risk of diabetes[14] (Fig. 53.2). Pyke et al.[6] described enucleation in eight cases, but the high morbidity and mortality in those patients indicate that this is not an appropriate technique for removing a serous cystadenoma from the pancreas, unless the tumor is very small. A recent paper described cystojejunostomy as an option for patients with high surgical risk and serous cystadenomas.[10] We strongly believe that this is an inappropriate treatment for any cystic neoplasm of the pancreas, even if it is performed only with palliative intent.

Serous cystadenomas are indolent, slow-growing tumors, and only a handful of malignant cases have been reported. A recent review compiled 16 well-documented cases of malignant serous cystadenoma, although in six patients the pancreatic tumor was histologically benign, and the diagnosis of cancer was made on the basis of synchronous or metachronous lesions in other organs, mostly liver, raising the possibility of multifocal disease, rather than metastatic spread.[15] Based on their review of the literature, these authors concluded that malignant serous cystadenomas make up 3% of all serous tumors of the pancreas. Because there is unequivocal bias toward reporting an extremely rare lesion such as a serous cystadenocarcinoma rather than benign tumors, the prevalence must be lower than that, and most authors agree that the risk of malignancy in a serous cystadenoma is less than 1%.[16] Therefore, malignant potential is not to be used as an argument for surgical resection.

Because many patients with serous cystadenomas are elderly (average age at diagnosis, 65 years), it is reasonable to manage asymptomatic patients expectantly. When patients are identified at a younger age, the decision not to operate may not be as straightforward, because the tumors do increase in size and may eventually become symptomatic. In our own unpublished experience, the likelihood of symptoms increases with the size of the tumor (43% with tumors less than 4 cm vs 77% in larger tumors), and the average rate of growth is about 0.45 cm/year. If a conservative management is adopted, it is important to fully ascertain that the lesion that is to be observed is truly a serous cystadenoma and not a mucinous cyst or other potentially malignant lesion. Except in the most typical cases, in which the radiologic appearance is pathognomonic (i.e., central sunburst calcification), sampling of the tumor for markers and cytology should be performed. Aspiration of a serous cystadenoma should yield nonviscous fluid with low carcinoembryonic antigen and amylase levels, and if

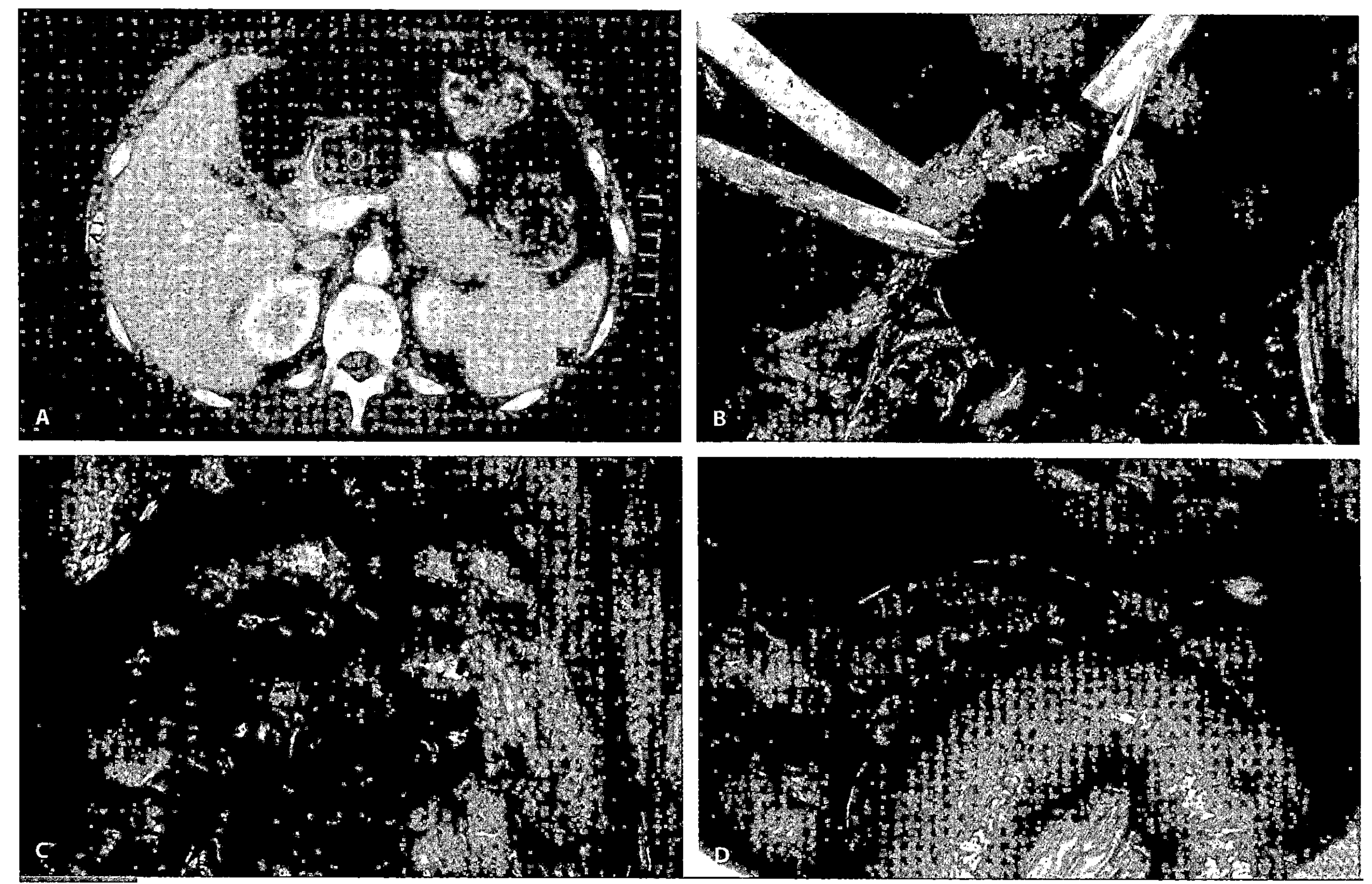

Figure 53.2
Unilocular serous cystadenoma involving the neck of the pancreas treated with a middle pancreatectomy. **(A)** Top left: computed tomographic scan. **(B)** Top right: the tumor and adjacent pancreas are dissected from the portosplenic confluence. **(C)** Bottom left: the tumor has been removed and the cut end of the proximal pancreas has been oversewn. **(D)** Bottom right: a Roux-en-Y loop of jejunum is anastomosed to the distal pancreas.

cells are obtained (which is rare), they are cuboidal and have a clear cytoplasm.[11]

Mucinous Cystic Neoplasm

Mucinous cystic neoplasms are the most frequently encountered cystic tumors of the pancreas. At the Massachusetts General Hospital, they constituted 40% of 300 cystic neoplasms seen over a 22-year period, and in the French Surgical Association series, they constituted 44% of 522 cases.[17] In contrast to serous cystadenomas, which are almost exclusively benign, it is well recognized that mucinous cystic neoplasms encompass a spectrum that ranges from benign but potentially malignant lesions to carcinomas with a very aggressive behavior.[18,19] One of the prominent features of mucinous cystadenocarcinoma is its histologic heterogeneity, with coexistence of benign-appearing and malignant epithelia being seen in nearly all tumors. From a surgical perspective, this is a very important characteristic because one cannot exclude malignancy with a needle or an incisional biopsy. In fact, very extensive pathological sampling of these lesions is required to be certain that a tumor is benign, and frequently, the entire specimen needs to be processed for that purpose.[20,21] In four recent series, carcinoma, either in situ or invasive, has been found in 34%–48% of mucinous cystic neoplasms.[17,19,21,22]

Macroscopically, most mucinous cystic neoplasms appear as multilocular tumors with smooth, glistening surfaces. The cysts are filled with thick, mucoid material or hemorrhagic fluid, and the walls are dense and fibrous and are calcified in about 10% of cases. Some neoplasms are unilocular, and some contain large whitish nodules projecting into the cyst lumen (Fig. 53.3). The average size is

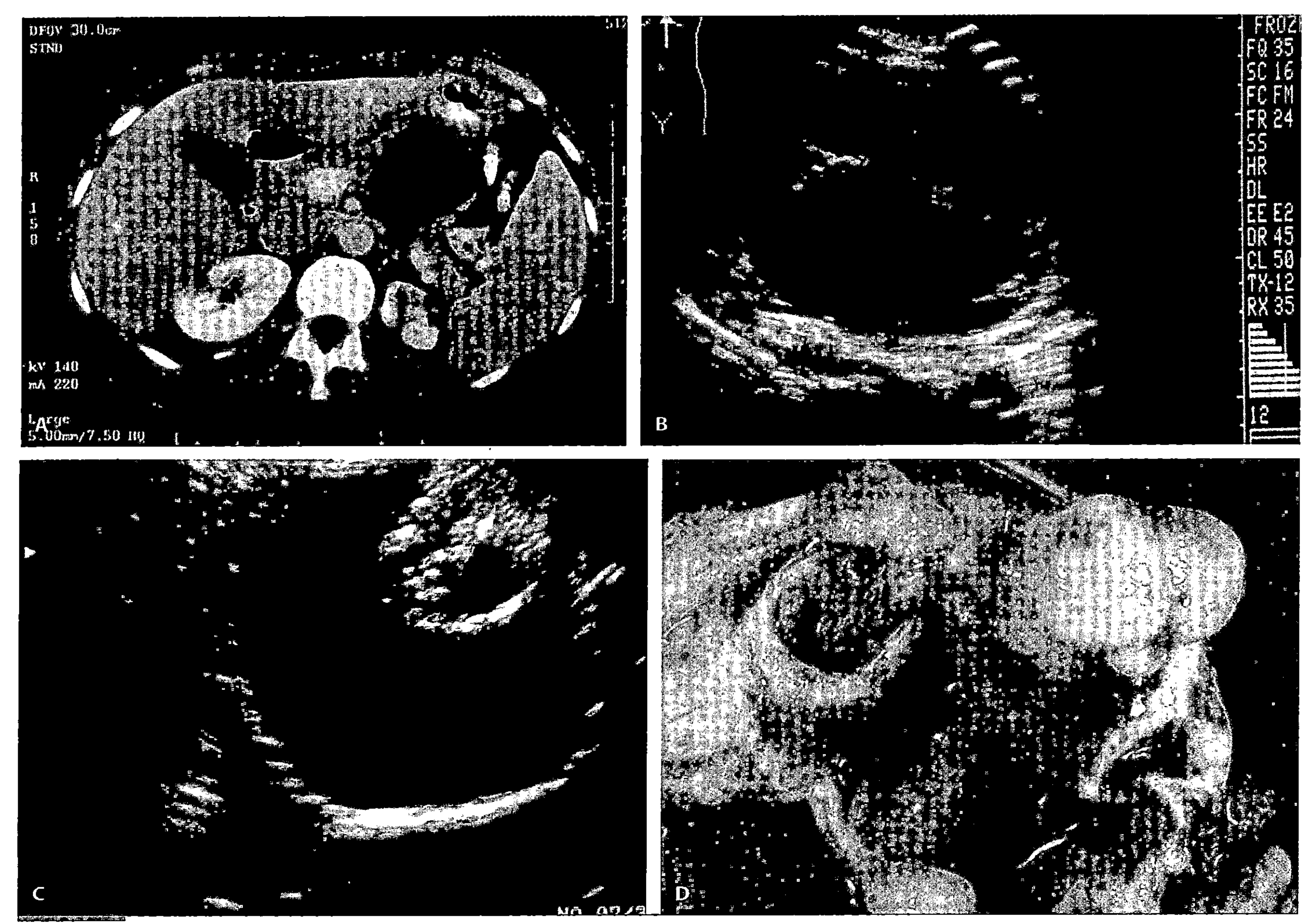

Figure 53.3
Mucinous cystadenoma of the tail of the pancreas. **(A)** Top left: computed tomographic scan. **(B)** Top right and **(C)** bottom left: images from endoscopic ultrasound showing septation and nodular projections. **(D)** Bottom right: cut gross specimen showing mural nodules.

8.1 cm (range, 1.5–36 cm), with malignant tumors being significantly larger than benign ones.[19,21-23] Between 65% and 95% are located in the body and tail of the pancreas.

More than 80% of mucinous cystic neoplasms occur in females, most of them in the fifth and sixth decades of life, with an age range of 18–85 years. Symptoms are very nonspecific and include upper abdominal discomfort or pain, weight loss, postprandial fullness, and less commonly, jaundice or a palpable mass. As with serous cystadenomas, most mucinous cystic neoplasms are incidental findings identified during imaging performed for other reasons.[11]

Surgical excision is indicated for all mucinous cystic neoplasms because extensive histologic sampling (to confirm it is benign) cannot be achieved until the tumor is excised, and because the current thinking is that most, if not all, of these tumors will evolve into cancer if left untreated. This concept is based on epidemiologic data showing that patients with invasive cancer within a mucinous cystic neoplasm are older and have larger tumors.[19,21,22] Studies of the molecular pathology of these lesions indicate a stepwise increase in the frequency of K-*ras* and *p53* mutations, in a manner similar to that seen in the adenoma-carcinoma sequence of colon cancer.[24] In one study, a significant age difference of 9.5 years was found between patients with cystadenocarcinoma (invasive or in situ) and those with mucinous cystadenomas or borderline tumors.[21] In another study, there was a stepwise age increase between patients with mucinous cystadenomas, borderline and in situ tumors and those with invasive carcinoma (48, 53, and 64 years, respectively).[22]

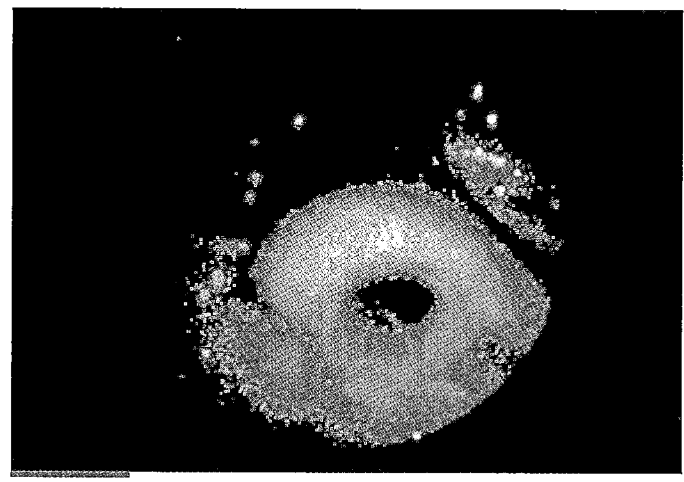

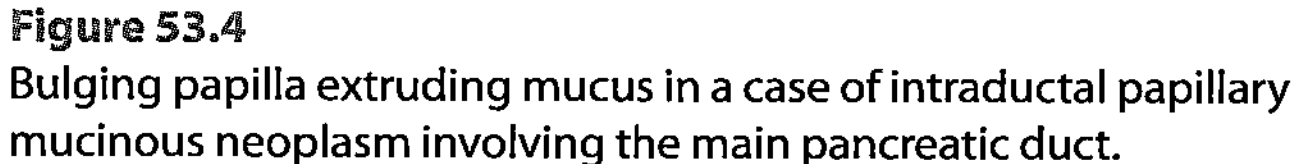

Figure 53.4
Bulging papilla extruding mucus in a case of intraductal papillary mucinous neoplasm involving the main pancreatic duct.

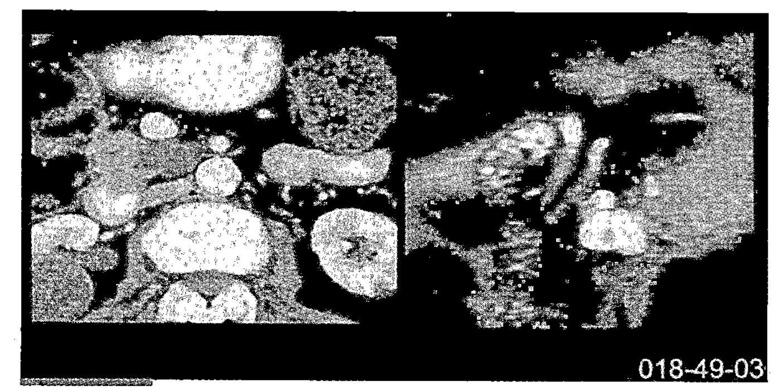

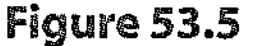

Figure 53.5
Side-branch intraductal papillary mucinous neoplasm. Left panel, computed tomography showing a multicystic lesion in the uncinate process of the pancreas. Right panel: magnetic resonance cholangiopancreatography showing that the lesion originates in a side branch that communicates with the main pancreatic duct.

Because most mucinous cystic neoplasms are located in the body and tail of the pancreas, they require a distal pancreatectomy. It may be appropriate to preserve the spleen in small lesions, but in larger ones, or whenever there is a higher suspicion of an established carcinoma, a splenectomy should also be carried out in order to remove the lymph node basin that can potentially be involved. A laparoscopic approach is certainly feasible for small or even medium-sized mucinous cystic neoplasms located in the tail of the pancreas,[25] but it is very important not to rupture the cyst during the procedure because spillage of contents could potentially lead to tumor spread. In addition, the cyst should be removed intact (i.e., not morselized) so that the pathologist can perform an appropriate gross and microscopic examination. For tumors in the head of the gland, a Whipple procedure is indicated. An occasional small tumor in the neck or proximal body of the pancreas can be treated with a middle-segment pancreatectomy.

Although enucleation has been described as an alternative for the surgical management of these tumors,[26] the high complication rate as well as the need to provide the pathologist with adequate surrounding pancreatic parenchyma in order to assess for invasion, makes it a very unattractive option. Furthermore, there is evidence that suggests that the pancreatic ducts in direct proximity to mucinous cystic neoplasms harbor K-*ras* mutations.[24]

Results of surgical treatment are excellent. Three recent large series show that even if carcinoma is present within the specimen, as long as it is not invasive (high grade dysplasia or carcinoma in-situ), the cure rate is 100%, thus avoiding the need for long-term surveillance.[19,21,22] For patients with invasive mucinous cystadenocarcinoma, the 5-year survival is only 30%–40%, which is still better than that of the more common ductal adenocarcinoma of the pancreas. There are no data on adjuvant treatment for these lesions.

Intraductal Papillary Mucinous Neoplasms (IPMNs)

In the 20 years that have elapsed since its initial description by Ohashi and coworkers,[27] IPMN has become one of the most common diagnoses in the field of pancreatology. Its epidemiology, natural history and proper management remain in a state of flux, and therefore, surgical treatment is not standarized.

In its classic form, which was formerly referred to as *mucinous ductal ectasia*, IPMN presents as a dilated pancreatic duct full of mucus that extrudes through a bulging ampulla (Fig. 53.4). Patients have recurrent episodes of pancreatitis-like pain, with or without hyperamylasemia, and not infrequently have steatorrhea, diabetes, and weight loss. Not surprisingly, this clinical picture has led to the diagnosis of chronic pancreatitis in many of these patients. In this form of IPMN, the tumor originates in the main pancreatic duct, more commonly in the cephalic portion, and from there spreads to the rest of the duct.

It is now well-recognized that IPMNs can also originate in the side branches of the pancreatic ductal system. These occur mostly in the uncinate process of the pancreas, but they can be seen in the neck and distal pancreas as well (Fig. 53.5). A large proportion of these patients are asymptomatic and are detected by CT or ultrasound performed for other reasons, but others may present

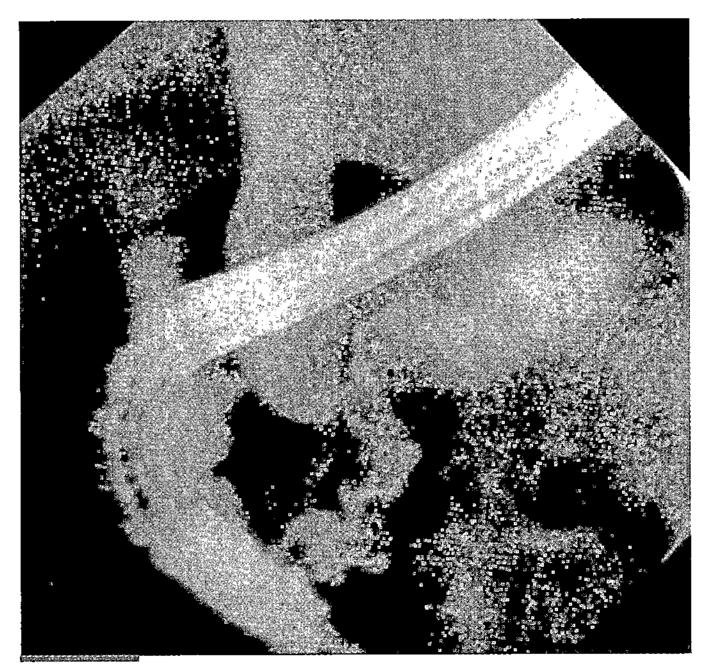

Figure 53.6
Endoscopic retrograde cholangiopancreatography from a patient with carcinoma arising in an intraductal papillary mucinous neoplasm presenting with recent-onset jaundice and a history of recurrent abdominal pain for many years. Note the bile duct obstruction (stented) and the multiple filling defects in the main pancreatic duct.

with abdominal pain or pancreatitis. It is unclear whether this variant represents an entity that remains localized or one that will inevitably spread into the main ductal system, but studies do show that the side-branch IPMNs have smaller tumors and may have a lower likelihood of being malignant.[28-31]

Both main- and branch-duct IPMNs occur typically in the seventh and eighth decades of life. Initial reports suggested a strong male predominance, but more recent series indicate an equal distribution. In a recent experience with 140 patients, more than 25% were asymptomatic, and the most common symptoms were abdominal pain (65%), weight loss (44%), acute pancreatitis (23%), jaundice (17%), diabetes (12%), and steatorrhea (6.5%).[32]

Histopathologically, IPMNs encompass a spectrum of epithelial changes ranging from adenoma to invasive adenocarcinoma, with borderline tumors and carcinoma in situ in between. Like in mucinous cystic neoplasms, extensive sampling of the specimen is required to rule out cancer. In our experience, 42% of patients had invasive carcinoma and 18% had in situ tumors.[32] Patients with malignant IPMN tended to have larger tumors, a larger proportion of solid component, and a higher incidence of jaundice or recent-onset diabetes[33] (Fig. 53.6). The average age of patients with main-duct IPMN and malignant tumors is 6.4 years older than that of patients with adenomas or borderline lesions. This supports the current view that most if not all IPMNs eventually become malignant.

The surgical management of IPMNs is different than that of serous cystadenomas and mucinous cystic neoplasms. Whereas in the latter two, the surgeon can accurately locate the tumor from the preoperative studies and plan a segmental pancreatic resection (either a Whipple or a distal or a middle pancreatectomy), that is not always the case in IPMN. In IPMN, preoperative studies show a dilated pancreatic duct in the main-duct variety, but not necessarily the intraductal mass, which is often small. Because of the overproduction of mucus, dilation can occur both proximally and distal to the tumor, making location problematic. This difficulty is compounded by the propensity of the tumor to spread microscopically along the duct.

At the Massachusetts General Hospital, it is our policy to obtain a spiral CT and an endoscopic retrograde cholangiopancreatography or a magnetic resonance cholangiopancreatography in all patients with suspected IPMN. Furthermore, we often perform endoscopic ultrasound to better define the presence or absence of intraductal mass and to sample both the fluid and the solid components. With this information, we plan the surgical intervention (be it a Whipple procedure or a distal, total, or middle pancreatectomy, with or without splenic preservation), but we are prepared to change this plan, depending on the intraoperative findings. We have not found that intraoperative ultrasound adds much more to preoperative imaging, but we rely heavily on the frozen-section diagnosis of the transection margin of the pancreas. Because IPMN extends along the pancreatic duct and can do so without obvious macroscopic tumor, it is important to rule out the presence of tumor at the margin so that tumor is not left behind. A denuded epithelium within the duct is not uncommon in IPMN, and de-epithelialization should not be erroneously interpreted as a "negative" margin, because recurrence has often occurred in this setting.[33] We are also using intraoperative pancreatoscopy to inspect the ductal system of the remaining pancreas. This can potentially identify "skip" lesions if they are macroscopic. The presence of these skip lesions has been proposed on the basis of recurrence of IPMT in the remaining pancreas in the setting of a truly negative transection margin.[34,35]

Because of the potential to modify or extend the surgical resection at the time of surgery, it is important that the surgeon discuss and evaluate the risks and consequences of a total pancreatectomy with the patient before surgery. This process obviously needs to be carefully individualized. Whereas a total pancreatectomy may be appropriate in a young, fit patient who has an IPMN with carcinoma in the head of the pancreas that is extending into the body and tail, it may not be the right operation for an elderly or frail patient with an IPMN that is only an adenoma or a borderline tumor, even if it is present at the transection margin. In our experience, 63% of patients have required a Whipple procedure (not infrequently extended to the left of the mesenteric vessels), 17% a distal pancreatectomy, and 19% a total pancreatectomy.[32] In 29/140 cases, results of the frozen section transection margin altered the surgical plan, underscoring the importance of this information throughout the surgery.

The survival of patients with IPMN, even when malignant and invasive, can be quite good. In our recent experience with follow-up of 137 resected patients, 5- and 10-year disease-specific survival for 80 patients with adenoma, borderline tumors, or carcinoma in-situ was 100%, and the comparable statistics for the 57 patients with invasive carcinoma were 60% and 50%, respectively.[32] Forty-one percent of patients with invasive cancer had positive lymph node metastases, and remarkably, their 5-year survival was 45%, which is markedly better than that of the usual ductal pancreatic adenocarcinoma, wherein long-term survival of resected patients with positive lymph nodes is rare.[36,37] If recurrence occurs in the remaining pancreas, further resection is warranted, because several series have shown that some of these cases are salvageable.[32,34,38] This may indeed be one of the most curable forms of pancreatic cancer.

References

1. Compagno J, Oertel JE. Mucinous cystic neoplasms of the pancreas with overt and latent malignancy (cystadenocarcinoma and cystadenoma). *Am J Clin Pathol.* 1978;69:573-580.
2. Compagno J, Oertel JE. Microcystic adenomas of the pancreas (glycogen-rich cystadenomas). *Am J Clin Pathol.* 1978;69:289–298.
3. Fernández-del Castillo C, Rattner DW, Warshaw AL. Standards for pancreatic resection in the 1990s. *Arch Surg.* 1995;130:295–300.
4. Yeo CJ, Cameron JL, Sohn TA, Lillemoe KD, Pitt HA, Talamini MA, et al. Six hundred fifty consecutive pancreaticoduodenectomies in the 1990s. *Ann Surg.* 1997;226:248–260.
5. Balcom JH, Rattner DW, Warshaw AL, Chang Y, Fernández-del Castillo C. Ten-year experience with 733 pancreatic resections: changing indications, older patients, and decreasing length of hospitalization. *Arch Surg.* 2001;136:391–398.
6. Pyke CM, van Heerden JA, Colby TV, Sarr MG, Weaver AL. The spectrum of serous cystadenoma of the pancreas. *Ann Surg.* 1992;215:132–139.
7. Torres-Barrera G, Fernández-del Castillo C, Reyes E, Robles-Diaz G, Campuzano M. Microcystic adenoma of the pancreas. *Dig Dis Sci.* 1987;32:454–458.
8. Warshaw AL, Compton CC, Lewandrowski K, Cardenosa G, Mueller PR. Cystic tumors of the pancreas: new clinical, radiologic, and pathologic observations in 67 patients. *Ann Surg.* 1990;212:432–445.
9. Lewandrowski K, Warshaw AL, Compton CC. Macrocystic serous cystadenoma of the pancreas: a morphologic variant differing from microcystic adenoma. *Hum Pathol.* 1992;23:871–875.
10. Bassi C, Salvia R, Molinari E, Biasutti C, Falconi M, Pederzoli P. Management of 100 consecutive cases of pancreatic serous cystadenoma: wait for symptoms and see at imaging or vice versa? *World J Surg.* 2003;27:319–323.
11. Fernández-del Castillo C, Targarona J, Thayer SP, Rattner DW, Brugge WR, Warshaw AL. Incidental pancreatic cysts: clinico-pathologic characteristics and comparison to symptomatic patients. *Arch Surg.* 2003;138:427–434.
12. Hammel P, Vilgrain V, Terris B, Penfornis A, Sauvanet A, Correas JM, et al. Pancreatic involvement in von Hippel-Lindau disease. *Gastroenterology.* 2000;119:1087–1095.
13. Warshaw AL. Conservation of the spleen with distal pancreatectomy. *Arch Surg.* 1988;123:550–553.
14. Warshaw AL, Rattner DW, Fernández-del Castillo C, Z'Graggen K. Middle segment pancreatectomy: a novel technique for conserving pancreatic tissue. *Arch Surg.* 1998;133:327–331.
15. Strobel O, Z'Graggen K, Schmitz-Winnenthal FH, Friess H, Kappeler A, Zimmermann A, et al. Risk of malignancy in serous cystic neoplasms of the pancreas. *Digestion.* 2003;68:24–33.
16. Abe H, Kubota K, Mori M, et al. Serous cystadenoma of the pancreas with invasive growth: benign or malignant? *Am J Gastroenterol.* 1998;93:1963–1966.
17. Le Borgne J, de Calan L, Partensky C, and the French Surgical Association. Cystadenomas and cystadenocarcinomas of the pancreas: a multiinstitutional retrospective study of 398 cases. *Ann Surg.* 1999;230:152–161.
18. Albores-Saavedra J, Angeles-Angeles A, Nadji M, Henson DE, Alvarez L. Mucinous cystadenocarcinoma of the pancreas: morphologic and immunocytochemical observations. *Am J Surg Pathol.* 1987;11:11–20.
19. Wilentz RE, Albores-Saavedra J, Zahurak M, Talamini MA, Yeo CJ, Cameron JL, et al. Pathologic examination accurately predicts prognosis in mucinous cystic neoplasms of the pancreas. *Am J Surg Pathol.* 1999;23:1320–1327.
20. Albores-Saavedra J, Gould EW, Angeles-Angeles A, Henson DE. Cystic tumors of the pancreas. *Pathol Annu.* 1990;25: 19–50.
21. Zamboni G, Scarpa A, Bogina G, Iacono C, Bassi C, Talamini G, et al. Mucinous cystic tumors of the pancreas: clinicopathological features, prognosis, and relationship to other mucinous cystic tumors. *Am J Surg Pathol.* 1999;23:410–422.
22. Sarr MG, Carpenter HA, Prabhakar LP, Orchard TF, Hughes S, van Heerden JA, et al. Clinical and pathologic correlation of 84 mucinous cystic neoplasms of the pancreas. *Ann Surg.* 2000;231:205–212.

23. Thompson LDR, Becker RC, Prygodzki RM, Adair CF, Heffess CS. Mucinous cystic neoplasm (mucinous cystadenocarcinoma of low-grade malignant potential) of the pancreas: a clinicopathological study of 130 cases. *Am J Surg Pathol.* 1999;23:1–16.
24. Jimenez RE, Warshaw AL, Z'Graggen K, Hartwig W, Taylor DZ, Compton CC, et al. Sequential accumulation of *K-ras* mutations and *p53* overexpression in the progression of pancreatic mucinous cystic neoplasms to malignancy. *Ann Surg.* 1999;230:501–511.
25. Park AE, Heniford BT. Therapeutic laparoscopy of the pancreas. *Ann Surg.* 2002;236:149–158.
26. Talamini MA, Moesinger R, Yeo CJ, Poulose B, Hruban RH, Cameron JL, et al. Cystadenomas of the pancreas: is enucleation an adequate operation? *Ann Surg.* 1998;227:896–903.
27. Ohashi K, Murakami Y, Maruyama M. Four cases of mucin-producing cancer of the pancreas on specific findings of the papilla of Vater [in Japanese]. *Prog Dig Endosc.* 1982;20:348–351.
28. Kobari M, Egawa S, Shibuya K, Shimamura H, Sunamura M, Takeda K, et al. Intraductal papillary mucinous tumors of the pancreas comprise 2 clinical subtypes: differences in clinical characteristics and surgical management. *Arch Surg.* 1999;134:1131–1136.
29. Nakagohri T, Kenmochi T, Kainuma O, Tokoro Y, Asano T. Intraductal papillary mucinous tumors of the pancreas. *Am J Surg.* 1999;178:344–347.
30. Sugiyama M, Atomi Y, Kuroda A. Two types of mucin-producing cystic tumors of the pancreas: diagnosis and treatment. *Surgery.* 1997;122:617–625.
31. Terris B, Ponsot P, Paye F, Hammel P, Sauvanet A, Molas G, et al. Intraductal papillary mucinous tumors of the pancreas confined to secondary ducts show less aggressive pathologic features as compared with those involving the main pancreatic duct. *Am J Surg Pathol.* 2000;24:1372–1377.
32. Salvia R, Fernández-del Castillo C, Bassi C, Thayer SP, Falconi M, Mantovani W, et al. Main duct intraductal papillary mucinous neoplasms of the pancreas: clinical predictors of malignancy and long-term survival following resection. *Ann Surg.* 2004; in press.
33. Falconi M, Salvia R, Bassi C, Zamboni G, Talamini G, Pederzoli P. Clinicopathological features and treatment of intraductal papillary mucinous tumor of the pancreas. *Br J Surg.* 2001;88:376–381.
34. Sohn TA, Yeo CJ, Cameron JL, Iacobuzio-Donahue CA, Hruban RH, Lillemoe KD. Intraductal papillary mucinous neoplasms of the pancreas: an increasingly recognized clinicopathologic entity. *Ann Surg.* 2001;234:313–322.
35. Traverso LW, Peralta EA, Ryan JA, Kozareck RA. Intraductal neoplasms of the pancreas. *Am J Surg.* 1998;175:426–432.
36. Delcore R, Rodriguez FJ, Forster J, Hermreck AS, Thomas JH. Significance of lymph node metastases in patients with pancreatic cancer undergoing curative resection. *Am J Surg.* 1996;172:463–469.
37. Yeo CJ, Cameron JL, Lillemoe KD, Sohn TA, Campbell KA, Sauter PK, et al. Pancreaticoduodenectomy with or without distal gastrectomy and extended retroperitoneal lymphadenectomy for periampullary adenocarcinoma, part 2. *Ann Surg.* 2002;236:355–368.
38. Chari ST, Yadav D, Smyrk T, DiMagno EP, Miller LJ, Raimondo M, et al. Study of recurrence after surgical resection of intraductal papillary mucinous neoplasm of the pancreas. *Gastroenterology.* 2002;123:1500–1507.

COMMENTARY—CHAPTERS 51–53

Ralph H. Hruban, MD

One of the most exciting developments in the war against pancreatic cancer has been the dramatic advances made in our understanding of cystic neoplasms. Cystic neoplasms are particularly exciting because they provide an opportunity for a cure—noninvasive neoplastic cysts are often large enough to be detected and removed before they give rise to an invasive carcinoma. The surgical resection of noninvasive intraductal papillary mucinous neoplasms (IPMNs) and mucinous cystic neoplasms (MCNs) prevent these lesions from progressing to invasive, potentially incurable, cancer. Chapters 51–53 by Drs. Volkan Adsay, Chulsip Charnsangavej, and Carlos Fernández-del Castillo provide excellent reviews of the pathology, radiology, and surgical management of these important neoplasms. The authors of these chapters raise seven questions that deserve emphasis:

1. How can a small IPMN be distinguished from a large focus of pancreatic intraepithelial neoplasia (PanIN)?
2. Are IPMNs and MCNs localized neoplasms, or do they represent a field defect?
3. How can we explain metastases arising in patients with apparently benign MCNs?
4. Should well-demarcated, mucin-producing cystic lesions without obvious ductal involvement and lacking ovarian-type stroma be classified as IPMNs or MCNs?
5. Does the existing World Health Organization (WHO) nomenclature for in situ and infiltrating carcinomas in IPMNs and MCNs accurately reflect the current state of knowledge of these entities?
6. How can we explain solid-pseudopapillary tumors when there doesn't appear to be a normal cell type in the pancreas with a corresponding direction of differentiation?
7. Should all small cystic lesions detected radiologically be surgically resected?

This commentary briefly addresses each of these questions with the use of the framework of knowledge established in Chapters 51–53.

How Can a Small IPMN Be Distinguished from a Large Pancreatic Intrepithelial Neoplasia?

Twenty years ago, life was simple—cystic neoplasms were either serous or mucinous. All serous cystic neoplasms were benign, and a third of MCNs progressed to an invasive cancer.[1,2] Then, in 1982, Ohhashi et al.[3] described a type of mucin-producing cystic neoplasm called *mucous secreting pancreatic cancer* and emphasized the distinction of this neoplasm from the MCN and ductal adenocarcinoma. These neoplasms were subsequently described by surgeons, gastroenterologists, pathologists, and radiologists, leading to a confusing array of terminology. The name *intraductal papillary mucinous neoplasm* was eventually agreed on, and criteria for the diagnosis and grading of IPMNs were accepted.[4] As described in Chapters 51–53, IPMNs are papillary mucin-producing neoplasms that arise in the larger pancreatic ducts. A third of IPMNs are associated with an invasive cancer.[5] The invasive cancers associated with IPMNs are often colloid carcinomas,[6] and it is generally agreed that the complete surgical resection of a noninvasive IPMN greatly reduces the risk of a subsequent invasive cancer.[7] The recognition that IPMNs are a distinct entity with a distinct treatment has been a significant advance in the battle against pancreatic cancer.

Advances in our understanding of the biology and clinical behavior of IPMNs have been paralleled by advances in our understanding of the biology and clinical behavior of noninvasive precursor lesions in the smaller pancreatic ducts, known as *pancreatic intraepithelial neoplasia* (PanINs).[8,9] PanINs are small microscopic lesions that can give rise to conventional infiltrating ductal adenocarcinoma of the pancreas. The recognition that PanINs can give rise to invasive pancreatic cancer has formed the basis for studies aimed at advancing our understanding of the earliest events responsible for the development of pancreatic cancer, and it has opened the door to the development of screening tests for early, potentially curable, pancreatic neoplasia.

The distinction between IPMNs and PanINs has been made primarily on the basis of size. Lesions <1 cm have been designated PanINs, whereas those ≥ 1 cm have been designated IPMNs. As our experience with these neoplasms has grown, however, it has become clear that there can be overlap in the size of these lesions. Some IPMNs are <1 cm, and some PanINs involve larger ducts (>1 cm).[10] An international meeting of experts on precursor lesions of pancreatic cancer was therefore held at The Johns Hopkins Hospital from August 18 to 19, 2003.[11] The purpose of this meeting was to define an internationally acceptable set of diagnostic criteria for PanINs and IPMNs, and to address ambiguities that exist in the previously reported classification systems for these neoplasms.[11] The definitions of PanINs and IPMNs agreed on at this meeting include the following:

> *Pancreatic intraepithelial neoplasia* (PanIN) is a microscopic papillary or flat noninvasive epithelial neoplasm arising in the pancreatic ducts. PanINs are characterized by columnar to cuboidal cells with varying amounts of mucin and degrees of cytological and architectural atypia. PanINs usually involve ducts <5 mm in diameter.[11]
>
> The *intraductal papillary mucinous neoplasm* (IPMN) is a grossly visible, noninvasive mucin producing, predominantly papillary or rarely, flat epithelial neoplasm arising from the main pancreatic duct or branch ducts, with varying degrees of ductal dilatation. IPMNs usually produce a lesion greater than 1 cm in diameter, and include a variety of cell types with a spectrum of cytological and architectural atypia.[11]

It is hoped that these internationally agreed on definitions will provide a uniform standard for the study of these important precursors to invasive pancreatic cancer.

Are IPMNs and MCNs Localized Lesions, or Do They Represent a Field Defect?

As described in Chapters 51–53, IPMNs can be distinguished from MCNs by the presence of a characteristic ovarian stroma in MCNs and by the extensive involvement of the pancreatic ducts in IPMNs.[4,12-14] Based on these distinctions, numerous other differences have been found between MCNs and IPMNs. For example, IPMNs occur slightly more often in men than in women (male:female ratio of 6:4), whereas MCNs are much more common in women than in men (male:female ratio of 1:9).

Recent follow-up studies of several large series of patients with IPMNs have shown that patients with surgically resected IPMNs have a small but significant risk of subsequently developing a second IPMN or even an invasive carcinoma. For example, Chari et al.[7] reported that five of 60 noninvasive IPMNs recurred after partial pancreatectomy. The recurrence of a noninvasive IPMN likely represents a second primary because none of the 13 patients with a noninvasive IPMN who underwent total pancreatectomy recurred. This suggests a field defect—the development of a second IPMN in apparently uninvolved portions of the pancreatic duct distant from the original surgically resected IPMN. Although the jury is still out on field defects in pancreata with MCNs, most studies to date suggest that patients with a surgically resected noninvasive MCN are cured. The remainder of their duct system does not appear to be at increased risk. This difference between IPMNs and MCNs is a critical one and has profound implications for patient treatment and follow-up. Patients with an IPMN need to be monitored carefully after surgery, and patients with a surgically resected noninvasive MCN are likely to be cured.

How Can We Explain Metastases Arising in Patients with Apparently Benign MCNs?

If MCNs are localized neoplasms and the remainder of their duct system does not appear to be at risk, how then do we explain the reports of metastases arising in patients with surgically resected, apparently benign MCNs?[15] For example, the group from the Armed Forces Institute of Pathology has suggested that completely resected noninvasive MCNs can metastasize.[15] Rather than suggesting something very peculiar about the biology of MCNs, it is more likely that reports of metastases arising in patients with apparently benign MCNs simply represent gross undersampling of the lesions for histopathologic examination.[16] Small, invasive carcinomas can arise in an otherwise benign-appearing, large MCN. If this small focus is not sampled and the patient later develops metastatic disease, the situation might give the erroneous appearance of a metastasis from a benign neoplasm.[16]

The focality of carcinomas and the frequent abrupt transition from completely bland epithelium to epithelium with significant dysplasia dictate that MCNs should be entirely resected and entirely submitted for histologic examination before a carcinoma can be excluded.[14,16] A benign diagnosis cannot be established on biopsy alone, nor can it be established in an inadequately examined specimen.

Should Well-Demarcated, Mucin-Producing Cystic Lesions without Obvious Ductal Involvement and Lacking Ovarian-Type Stroma Be Classified as IPMNs or MCNs?

Although the distinction between MCNs and IPMNs is clinically important, the recent description of a "branch duct type" of IPMN has led to some confusion as to how MCNs can be distinguished from branch duct type IPMNs. In contrast to main duct type IPMNs, the branch duct type, as their name suggests, involve the side branches of the main pancreatic duct.[17,18] It can be very difficult to grossly and microscopically distinguish between branch duct type IPMNs and MCNs. Well-demarcated, mucin-producing cystic lesions without obvious ductal involvement and lacking ovarian-type stroma are sometimes encountered, yet they do not appear to fit nicely within the definitions of either entity.

The associated features of these neoplasms can help distinguish between branch duct type IPMNs and MCNs. For example, IPMNs tend to involve the head of the gland and arise in men and women at close to the same frequency, whereas MCNs tend to involve the tail of the gland and occur primarily in women.[4,12] However, these features cannot be the only criteria used to distinguish between branch duct IPMNs and MCNs. Some MCNs arise in men, and some IPMNs arise in the tail of the gland. Better criteria need to be established to distinguish between branch duct type IPMNs and MCNs.

While we wait for the classification of these "intermediate" lesions to be resolved, several approaches are possible. At one extreme, and this is the position held by the author of this commentary, the presence or absence of ovarian-type stroma should be used to distinguish between an IPMN and an MCN. If ovarian-type stroma is present, the lesion should be considered an MCN. If ovarian-type stroma is not present, then the lesion should be designated an IPMN. Alternatively, an intermediate group could be established. This would foster the detailed study of these lesions, with the eventual goal of identifying histologic, immunohistochemical, or molecular markers to classify these lesions, and, importantly, to guide therapy.

Does the Existing World Health Organization Nomenclature for In Situ and Infiltrating Carcinomas in IPMNs and MCNs Accurately Reflect the Current State of Knowledge of These Entities?

The current WHO nomenclature lumps IPMNs with in situ carcinoma together with IPMNs with an invasive carcinoma under the single designation "intraductal papillary mucinous carcinoma."[4] Similarly, the current WHO nomenclature lumps MCNs with in situ carcinoma together with MCNs with an invasive carcinoma under the single designation "mucinous cystadenocarcinoma."[12] This classification scheme is unfortunate for several reasons. First, the presence or absence of an invasive carcinoma is by far the single most important predictor of prognosis for patients with IPMNs and MCNs.[7,16,19] This important prognostic information is lost if noninvasive and invasive neoplasms are lumped. Second, the extent of invasion is also a very important predictor of prognosis. For example, Zamboni et al.[19] have shown that the size of the associated invasive carcinoma is a significant prognosticator in patients with MCNs.

This author believes that the invasive and noninvasive components should be separately designated when an invasive carcinoma arises in association with an IPMN or an MCN. Compare, for example, the amount of information conveyed in these two pathology reports on the same resected cancer: "well-differentiated intraductal papillary mucinous carcinoma (10 cm)" versus "infiltrating well-differentiated colloid carcinoma (1 cm) arising in association with an intraductal papillary mucinous neoplasm with carcinoma in situ (9 cm)."

How Can We Explain the Existence of Solid Pseudopapillary Tumors When There Doesn't Appear to Be a Normal Cell Type in the Pancreas with a Corresponding Direction of Differentiation?

Solid pseudopapillary tumors are a real enigma. They are clinically, grossly, and microscopically distinctive neoplasms, and yet, despite extensive study, the direction of differentiation (cell type) of these tumors has not been defined.[20] These low-grade malignant neoplasms arise primarily in women in their twenties.[21] They are grossly solid and cystic and are microscopically composed of noncohesive polygonal cells that surround delicate blood vessels and form solid masses with frequent cystic degeneration and intracystic hemorrhage. Numerous attempts have been made to define the direction of differentiation of these cells. At the ultrastructural level, they show evidence of epithelial differentiation, including an incomplete basal lamina, poorly defined intercellular junctions, and scattered desmosomes.[21] The neoplastic cells usually contain numerous mitochondria and some annulate lamellae, but the findings are otherwise nonspecific. Similarly, immunohistochemical labeling demonstrates the expression of cytokeratin, but immunolabeling for chromogranin, insulin, glucagon, somatostatin, amylase, lipase, calretinin, α-inhibin, and estrogen receptors is usually negative.[21] This pattern of immunolabeling does not correspond to any known normal cell type in the pancreas.

Although the direction of differentiation of solid pseudopapillary tumors remains a mystery, two reports have advanced our ability to diagnose these neoplasms, and they provide insight into how solid pseudopapillary tumors arise. First, it has

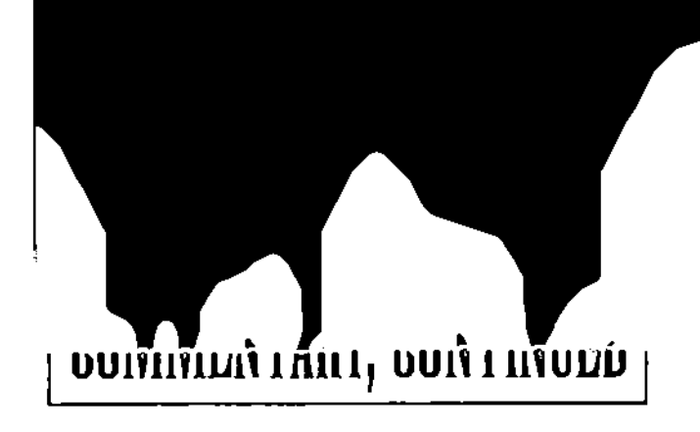

been demonstrated that almost all solid pseudopapillary tumors express CD10.[22] CD10, also known as neutral endopeptidase 24.11 or neprilysin, is a zinc metalloproteinase that functions as part of a regulatory loop to control concentrations of certain peptide substrates and associated peptide-mediated signal transduction.[22] The role of CD10 differs from tissue to tissue, depending on the substrates available.[22] The almost ubiquitous expression of CD10 by solid pseudopapillary tumors provides an immunohistochemical marker that can be used to distinguish solid pseudopapillary tumors from other neoplasms of the pancreas.

Second, Abraham et al.[23] have shown that >90% of solid pseudopapillary tumors harbor *β-catenin* gene mutations and that these mutations result in the abnormal nuclear accumulation of the *β-catenin* gene product. *β-catenin* gene mutations do not occur in infiltrating ductal adenocarcinomas of the pancreas. *β-catenin* gene mutations therefore represent a fundamental genetic difference between these two neoplasms. In addition, immunolabeling for the *β-catenin* gene product can be used to aid in the interpretation of difficult biopsies of the pancreas. A nuclear pattern of labeling for the *β-catenin* gene product and positive labeling for CD10 strongly support the diagnosis of a solid pseudopapillary tumor.

Should All Small Cystic Lesions Detected Radiologically Be Surgically Resected?

Increased abdominal imaging, including increased numbers of "virtual physical examinations," combined with improved resolution, has resulted in a dramatic increase in the number of cystic pancreatic lesions that are found in asymptomatic patients. The challenge is to determine which of these lesions should be surgically resected and which should not. Although it is generally agreed that larger MCNs and IPMNs should be surgically resected, not all cysts in the pancreas are neoplastic, and the benefit of removing small, 1- to 2-cm MCNs and branch duct type IPMNs in patients in their 70s and 80s is debatable. Nonneoplastic cystic spaces in the pancreas include retention cysts, congenital cysts, and simple variations in anatomy. Unless they cause symptoms, there is probably little to be gained by the removal of such cysts. Similarly, our current understanding of the natural history of small MCNs and branch duct type IPMNs is so poor that it is difficult to judge if the benefits of their removal justify the significant risks associated with pancreatic surgery.

There is no easy answer to this problem, and the challenge is certain to grow. This author believes that further studies on at least two levels are needed. First, detailed studies carefully correlating radiologic findings with gross and microscopic pathology are needed to define criteria that can reliably distinguish between neoplastic and nonneoplastic cysts. This approach helped advance high-resolution computed tomographic scanning of the lung,[24] and it needs to be systematically applied to cystic lesions in the pancreas. Second, studies are needed to identify and characterize the natural history and molecular alterations specific for neoplastic pancreatic cysts.[25] For example, if a panel of methylation markers can be identified that are specific for neoplastic cysts with a significant likelihood of progressing, then these markers could be applied to aspirated cyst fluid to distinguish between cysts that should be resected and those that can be watched. Parenthetically, serous cystadenomas present a similar challenge. Shortcomings in our knowledge of the natural history of these neoplasms make it difficult to evaluate the benefit of surgically removing asymptomatic serous cystadenomas.

The first significant strides in the war against cancer of the pancreas are likely to be made by scientists, pathologists, radiologists, gastroenterologists, and surgeons studying cystic neoplasms of the pancreas. Chapters 51–53 by Drs. Volkan Adsay, Chulsip Charnsangavej, and Carlos Fernández-del Castillo set the framework for the excitement to come.

References

1. Compagno J, Oertel JE. Mucinous cystic neoplasms of the pancreas with overt and latent malignancy (cystadenocarcinoma and cystadenoma): a clinicopathologic study of 41 cases. *Am J Clin Pathol*. 1978;69:573–580.
2. Compagno J, Oertel JE. Microcystic adenomas of the pancreas (glycogen-rich cystadenomas): a clinicopathologic study of 34 cases. *Am J Clin Pathol*. 1978;69:289–298.
3. Ohhashi K, Murakami Y, Maruyama M, et al. "Ductectatic" mucinous cystadenoma and cystadenocarcinoma of the pancreas. *Radiology*. 1986;161:697–700.
4. Longnecker DS, Adler G, Hruban RH, Klöppel G. Intraductal papillary-mucinous neoplasms of the pancreas. In: Hamilton SR, Aaltonen LA, eds. *World Health Organization Classification of Tumours. Pathology and Genetics of Tumours of the Digestive System*. Lyon: IARC Press; 2000:237–240.
5. Sohn TA, Yeo CJ, Cameron JL, et al. Intraductal papillary mucinous neoplasms of the pancreas: an increasingly recognized clinicopathologic entity. *Ann Surg*. 2001;234:313–321.
6. Seidel G, Zahurak M, Iacobuzio-Donahue C, et al. Almost all infiltrating colloid carcinomas of the pancreas and periampullary region arise from in situ papillary neoplasms: a study of 39 cases. *Am J Surg Pathol*. 2002;26:56–63.
7. Chari ST, Yadav D, Smyrk TC, et al. Study of recurrence after surgical resection of intraductal papillary mucinous neoplasm of the pancreas. *Gastroenterology*. 2002;123:1500–1507.
8. Hruban RH, Adsay NV, Albores-Saavedra J, et al. Pancreatic intraepithelial neoplasia (PanIN): a new nomenclature and classification system for pancreatic duct lesions. *Am J Surg Pathol*. 2001;25:579–586.
9. Hruban RH, Goggins M, Parsons JL, Kern SE. Progression model for pancreatic cancer. *Clin Cancer Res*. 2000;6:2969–2972.

10. Takaori K. Dilemma in classifications of possible precursors of pancreatic cancer involving the main pancreatic duct: PanIN or IPMN? *J Gastroenterol*. 2003;38:311–313.
11. Hruban RH, Takaori K, Klimstra DS, Adsay NV, Albores-Saavedra J, Biankin AW, Biankin SA, Compton C, Fukushima N, Furukawa T, Goggins M, Kato Y, Klöpper G, Longnecker D, Lüttges J, Maitra A, Offerhaus GJA, Shimizu M, Yonezawa S. An illustrated consensus on the classification of pancreatic intraepithelial neoplasia (PanIN) and intraductal papillary mucinous neoplasms (IPMNs). *Am J Surg Pathol*. 2004;28:977–987.
12. Zamboni G, Klöppel G, Hruban RH, et al. Mucinous cystic neoplasms of the pancreas. In: Hamilton SR, Aaltonen LA, eds. *World Health Organization Classification of Tumours. Pathology and Genetics of Tumours of the Digestive System*. Lyon: IARC Press; 2000:234–236.
13. Adsay NV, Longnecker DS, Klimstra DS. Pancreatic tumors with cystic dilatation of the ducts: intraductal papillary mucinous neoplasms and intraductal oncocytic papillary neoplasms. *Semin Diagn Pathol*. 2000;17:16–30.
14. Wilentz RE, Albores-Saavedra J, Hruban RH. Mucinous cystic neoplasms of the pancreas. *Semin Diagn Pathol*. 2000;17:31–42.
15. Thompson LDR, Becker RC, Przygodzki RM, et al. Mucinous cystic neoplasm (mucinous cystadenocarcinoma of low-grade malignant potential) of the pancreas: a clinicopathologic study of the pancreas. *Am J Surg Pathol*. 1999;23:1–16.
16. Wilentz RE, Albores-Saavedra J, Zahurak M, et al. Pathologic examination accurately predicts prognosis in mucinous cystic neoplasms of the pancreas. *Am J Surg Pathol*. 1999;23:1320–1327.
17. Kobari M, Egawa S, Shibuya K, et al. Intraductal papillary mucinous tumors of the pancreas comprise 2 clinical subtypes: differences in clinical characteristics and surgical management. *Arch Surg*. 1999;134:1131–1136.
18. Kuroda A. Recent progress in clinicopathology of pancreatic tumors: Tan to Sui. *Biliary Tract Pancreas*. 1988;9:1459–1472.
19. Zamboni G, Scarpa A, Bogina G, et al. Mucinous cystic tumors of the pancreas: clinicopathological features, prognosis, and relationship to other mucinous cystic tumors. *Am J Surg Pathol*. 1999;23:410–422.
20. Klöppel G, Lüttges J, Klimstra DS, et al. Solid-pseudopapillary neoplasm. In: Hamilton SR, Aaltonen LA, eds. *World Health Organization Classification of Tumours: Pathology and Genetics of Tumours of the Digestive System*. Lyon: IARC Press; 2000:246–248.
21. Klimstra DS, Wenig BM, Heffess CS. Solid-pseudopapillary tumor of the pancreas: a typically cystic carcinoma of low malignant potential. *Semin Diagn Pathol*. 2000;17:66–80.
22. Notohara K, Hamazaki S, Tsukayama C, et al. Solid-pseudopapillary tumor of the pancreas: immunohistochemical localization of neuroendocrine markers and CD10. *Am J Surg Pathol*. 2000;24:1361–1371.
23. Abraham SC, Klimstra DS, Wilentz RE, et al. Solid-pseudopapillary tumors of the pancreas are genetically distinct from pancreatic ductal adenocarcinomas and almost always harbor beta-catenin mutations. *Am J Pathol*. 2002;160:1361–1369.
24. Hruban RH, Meziane MA, Zerhouni EA, et al. High resolution computed tomography of inflation fixed lungs. *Am Rev Respir Dis*. 1987;136:935–940.
25. Sato N, Ueki T, Fukushima N, et al. Aberrant methylation of CpG islands in intraductal papillary mucinous neoplasms of the pancreas. *Gastroenterology*. 2002;123:365–372.

SECTION

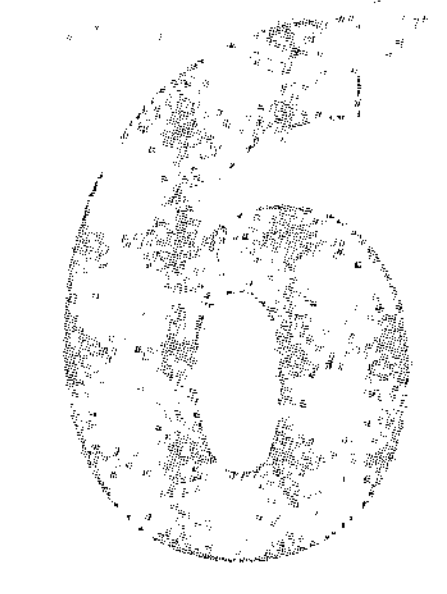

Other Rare Tumors

CHAPTER 54

Tumors of the Distal Common Bile Duct

Jorge Albores-Saavedra, MD

For diagnostic, prognostic, and therapeutic purposes, it has been useful to divide the extrahepatic biliary tree into three parts: upper, middle, and lower thirds. The common bile duct, which constitutes the lower third of the extrahepatic biliary tree, is in turn divided into four parts in relation to the duodenum and the pancreas: (1) supraduodenal (the longest part), (2) retroduodenal, (3) intrapancreatic, and (4) intraduodenal.[1] The latter two parts are considered to be the distal portion of the common bile duct. This chapter deals with both benign and malignant tumors that arise from the intrapancreatic and intraduodenal portions of the common bile duct. Histologically, these tumors are similar to those that originate in the proximal portions of the common bile duct as well as in the upper and middle thirds of the extrahepatic bile ducts.[1,2] Therefore, the same terminology and classifications are used, regardless of the location of the tumor. Frequently malignant tumors that originate in the distal portion of the common bile duct extend into the pancreas and simulate primary malignancies of this organ, a feature that justifies their inclusion in a book dedicated primarily to pancreatic cancer.

Benign Epithelial Tumors

Adenoma

Adenomas of the common bile duct are exceedingly rare benign epithelial neoplasms with an intestinal phenotype.[3-7] To our knowledge, the pyloric and biliary types of adenoma, which are the most common and the rarest forms of adenoma of the gallbladder, respectively, have not been described in the common bile duct.[1] We believe that biliary papillomatosis and cystadenomas of the common bile duct should not be included in the adenoma category, because they differ in clinical presentation and morphologic features. It should also be kept in mind that ampullary adenomas of intestinal type may extend into the common bile duct and simulate primary tumors at this site. It is therefore not surprising that most of the available information on adenomas of the common bile duct is based on case reports. We have summarized our experience with six cases elsewhere.[1]

Less common than carcinomas, adenomas are usually small, well-circumscribed, polypoid nodules. They are often single, may be pedunculated or sessile, and fre-

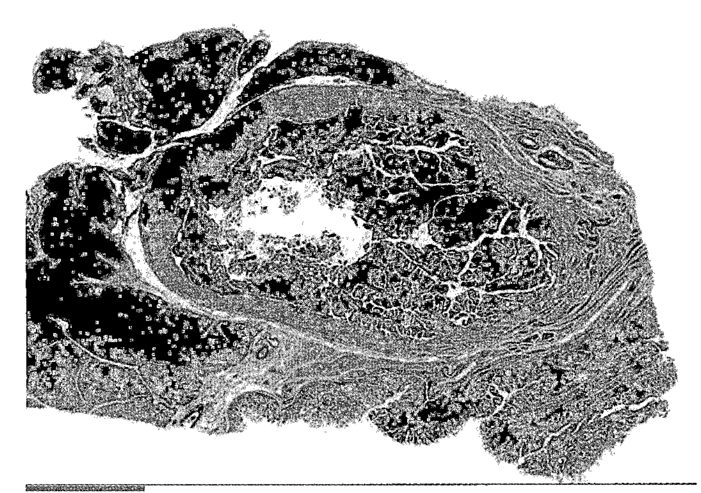

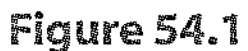

Figure 54.1
This tubulovillous adenoma fills most of the lumen of the common bile duct, which is distended and has a thickened wall. Inspissated bile is also seen.

quently obstruct the common bile duct, leading to jaundice. The jaundice often has an insidious onset and can be intermittent or persistent. Occasionally, patients present with symptoms of ascending cholangitis or relapsing acute pancreatitis.[8-10] Distinction of adenomas from malignant tumors is difficult before biopsy. However, the correct diagnosis can sometimes be suspected on the basis of cholangiography, endoscopic ultrasonography, or selective angiography. Adenomas of the distal common bile duct have been reported in patients with familial adenomatous polyposis/Gardner's syndrome.[9,11,12] Patients with Peutz-Jeghers syndrome rarely develop hamartomatous polyps in the distal common bile duct.[8] The simultaneous occurrence of adenomas of the distal common bile duct and high-grade pancreatic intraepithelial neoplasia or adenocarcinoma of the duodenum has been documented.[12]

Adenomas of the distal common bile duct have an intestinal phenotype and therefore are classified like colonic adenomas, according to their growth patterns. Tubular (composed of more than 80% tubular glands), villous (more than 80% villous components), and tubulovillous (each component comprising more than 20% of the adenoma) adenomas have been reported[1,3-5] (Figs. 54.1 and 54.2). The glands and papillary structures of tubular and villous adenomas, respectively, are lined by columnar pseudostratified cells showing variable degrees of dysplasia (Figs. 54.3 and 54.4). Some of the adenomas contain goblet, Paneth, and endocrine cells. The endocrine cells show immunoreactivity for

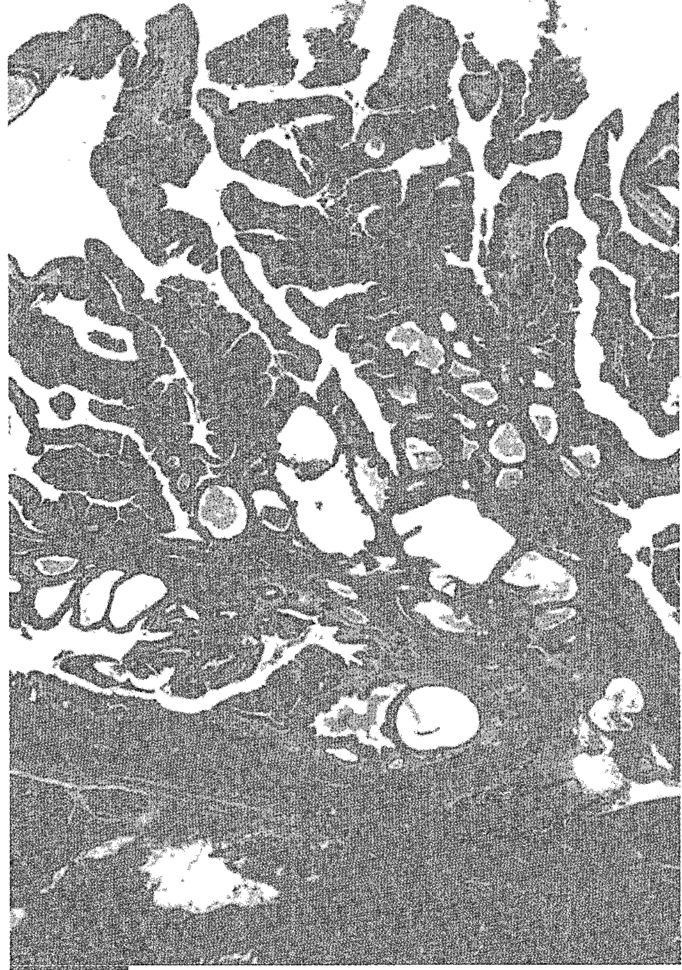

Figure 54.2
Low-power view of a villous adenoma that arose in the distal common bile duct. Part of the pancreas is shown (*bottom*).

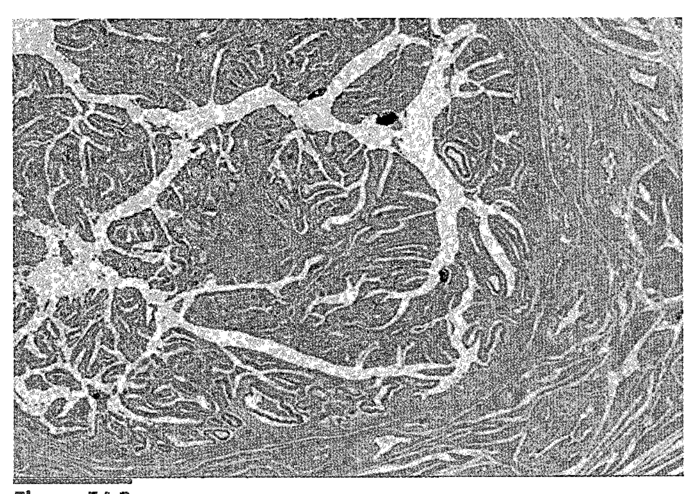

Figure 54.3
Higher magnification of the adenoma shown in Fig. 54.1. Both villous and tubular components are depicted.

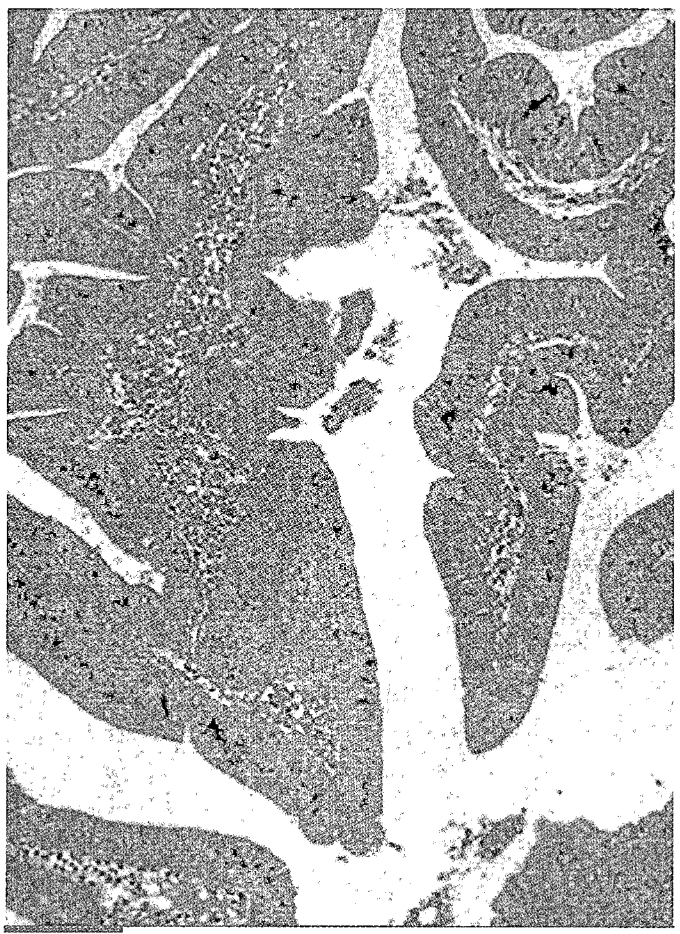

Figure 54.4
Higher magnification of the tumor shown in Fig. 54.2. The papillary structures are lined by dysplastic, columnar, pseudostratified cells with an intestinal phenotype.

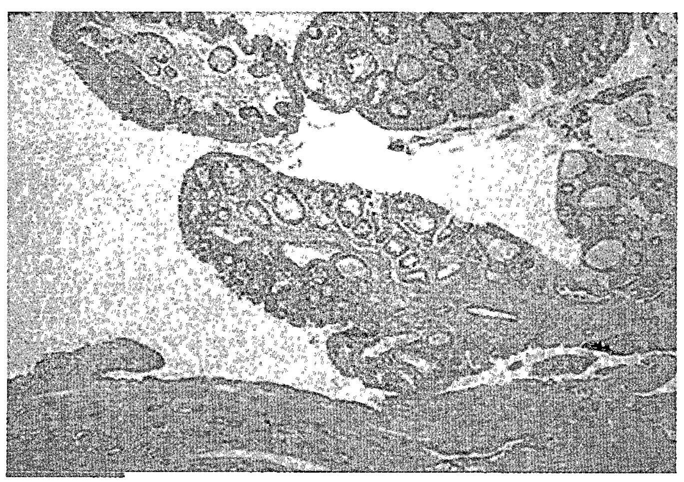

Figure 54.5
Tubular adenoma of the ampulla of Vater that extended into the common bile duct simulating a primary tumor at this site.

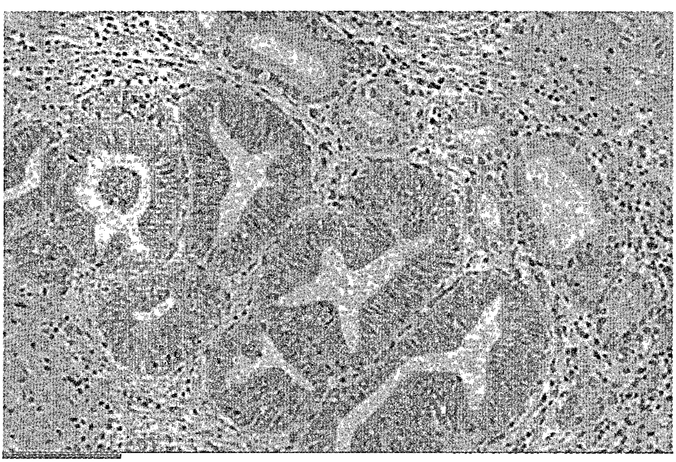

Figure 54.6
Tubular adenoma of distal common bile duct that extended into intramural glands. The lobular architecture of the glands is maintained. Glands lined by nonadenomatous epithelium are also present.

chromogranin, serotonin, and peptide hormones.[1,2] The clinical significance of the endocrine cells and their hormones is unknown. High-grade dysplasia and in situ and invasive carcinoma usually occur in larger adenomas. Adenomas of the distal common bile duct should be distinguished from adenomas of the ampulla of Vater that extend into the distal common bile duct, a common occurrence in tumors greater than 1.5 cm. (Fig. 54.5). Conversely, adenomas may extend into the intramural glands of the distal common bile duct and simulate stromal invasion (Fig. 54.6). When pedunculated and small, adenomas of the distal common bile duct can be resected endoscopically.[10] Large and sessile adenomas usually require a Whipple procedure.

Cystadenoma

Cystadenoma is a distinctive benign neoplasm belonging to a family of mucinous cystic tumors that can arise in the pancreas, liver, extrahepatic bile ducts, gallbladder, and retroperitoneum unattached to any organ.[13] The pancreas liver and extrahepatic biliary tree are the most common sites. Cystadenomas of the extrahepatic bile ducts occur almost exclusively in middle-aged females, and the most common location is the common bile duct.[14] Usually larger than noncystic adenomas, some cystadenomas are palpable on physical examination, and they are occasionally painful. They may reach up to 20 cm in greatest dimension.[14,15] Most cystadenomas lead to obstructive jaundice. Elevated serum levels of carcinoembryonic antigen (CEA) and CA19-9 have been reported in patients with these tumors.[16-18]

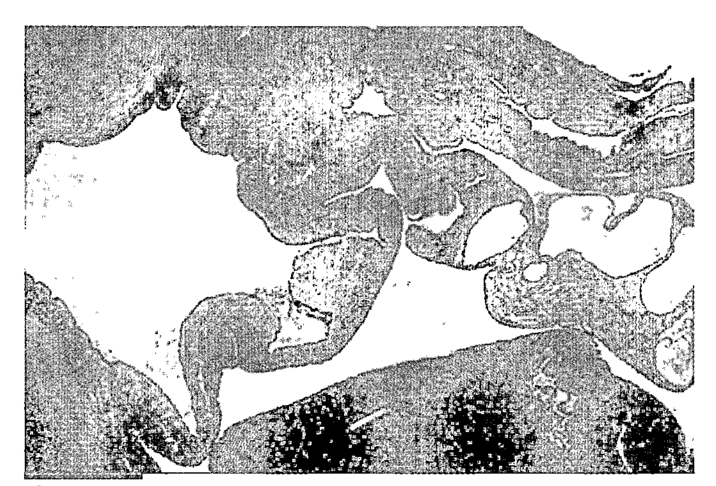

Figure 54.7
Low-power view of a multiloculated biliary cystadenoma. The locules are of different sizes and contain a cellular stroma and areas of fibrosis.

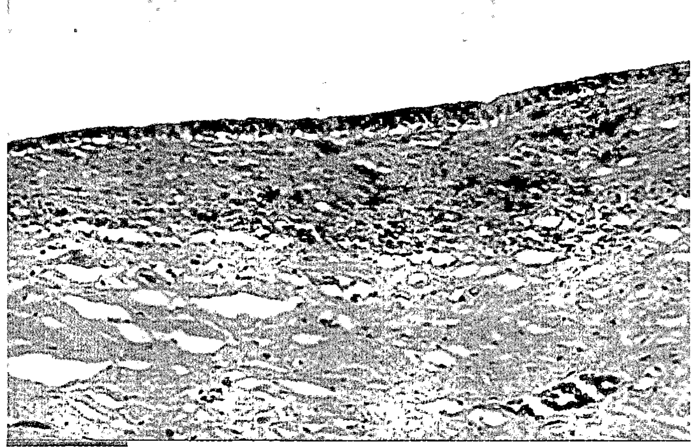

Figure 54.8
The characteristic three-layer architecture of biliary cystadenoma is shown. The inner layer is composed of cuboidal cells of biliary type, the subepithelial band of cellular stroma resembles ovarian stroma, and the outer layer consists of hyalinized connective tissue.

Cystadenomas are multilocular or unilocular, well-demarcated cystic masses that contain serous or mucinous fluid rich in CEA. Only rarely, the cyst content is hemorrhagic. The inner surface can be smooth, granular, or trabeculated. Frequently, small polypoid excrescences project into the lumens of the locules.

The locules of most cystadenomas have a characteristic three-layer structure: a cuboidal or columnar lining epithelium, a cellular ovarian-like stroma, and an outer layer of hyalinized fibrous tissue (Figs. 54.7 and 54.8). The surface lining epithelial cells are either cuboidal, resembling biliary cells, or columnar and mucin-secreting, similar to gastric foveolar cells. Goblet and Paneth cells are present in 20% of the tumors. One third of cystadenomas contain scattered chromogranin-positive endocrine cells.[14,19] These three cell types reflect intestinal differentiation. The lining epithelium shows immunoreactivity for cytokeratin, epithelial membrane antigen, CEA, and the carbohydrate antigen CA19-9. Approximately 13% of the tumors show dysplastic changes, suggesting that some cystadenomas may progress to carcinoma.[14] The ovarian-like stroma is composed of spindle-shaped cells that are focally immunoreactive for smooth muscle actin, desmin, and inhibin. The spindle cells also show immunoreactivity for estrogen and progesterone receptors.[17,20,21] By electron microscopy, the spindle cells are heterogeneous and have been identified as undifferentiated mesenchymal cells, fibroblasts, and myofibroblasts.[13] Secondary changes are often seen in the stroma including hemorrhage, cholesterol clefts, and pigmented or foamy macrophages. Cystadenomas of the distal portion of the common bile duct usually recur after incomplete excision. Despite the foci of dysplasia present in 13% of the tumors, malignant transformation has rarely been reported only in cystadenomas of the common bile duct.[15]

Papillomatosis

Biliary papillomatosis is a rare clinicopathologic entity characterized by multicentric complex papillary neoplasms that often involve extensive areas of the biliary tract, including the gallbladder and the intrahepatic bile ducts.[22-31] Extension into pancreatic ducts has even been observed.[24] The papillary lesions usually lead to obstruction and dilatation of the extrahepatic and intrahepatic bile ducts, which may result in ascending cholangitis and death. Because of frequent multifocality and extensive involvement of the bile ducts, it is difficult to accomplish complete surgical excision. Local recurrence is therefore common. Curettage and drainage may relieve symptoms temporarily, but cure can be achieved only by total hepatectomy and liver transplantation. The disease affects both sexes equally. Most patients who present with biliary obstruction are between 50 and 60 years of age. Percutaneous transhepatic cholangiography usually reveals multiple filling defects and mural irregularities along the dilated and distorted biliary tree.[25]

Histologically, multiple and complex papillary lesions as well as glandlike structures project into the lumen of the bile ducts (Fig. 54.9). The lining epithelial cells are cuboidal or columnar and contain a variable amount of mucin (Fig. 54.10). The nuclei are round, ovoid, or elongated with small nucleoli. Cytologic atypia and mitotic figures are uncommon, although obvious carcinomatous changes occur in some cases.[32] Examples of biliary

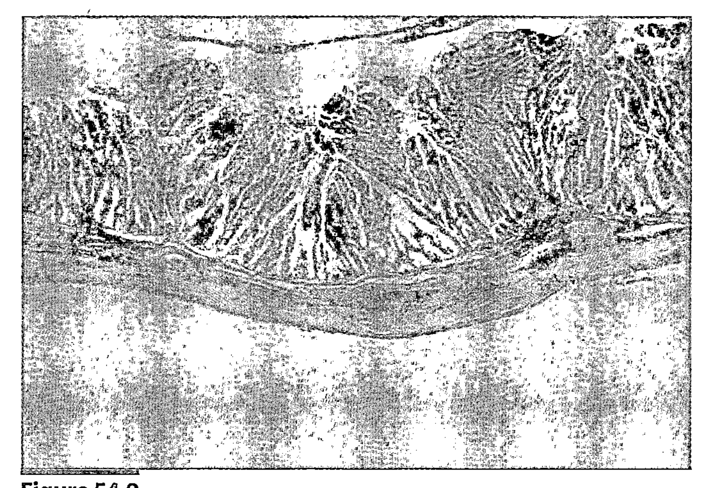

Figure 54.9
Papillomatosis. Multiple long papillary structures project into the lumen of the common bile duct. There is no invasion of the ductal wall.

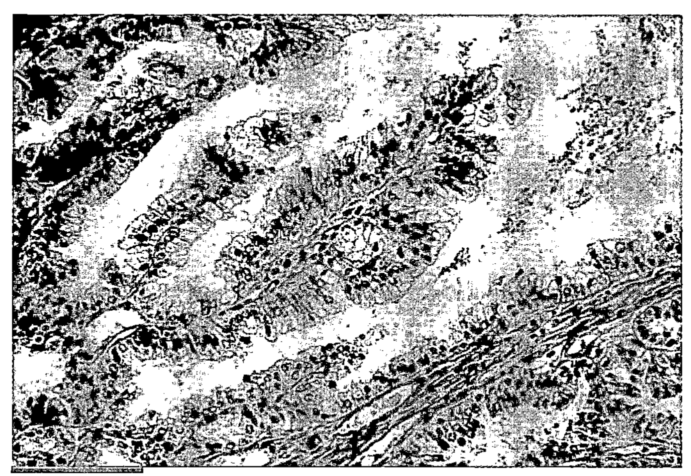

Figure 54.10
Higher magnification of Fig. 54.9. The papillary structures are lined by columnar mucin-producing cells with basal nuclei.

papillomatosis with abundant extracellular mucin closely resemble intraductal papillary mucinous neoplasms of the pancreas.[33] Some investigators believe that biliary papillomatosis should be regarded as a form of intraductal papillary carcinoma that may invade the ductal wall and metastasize.[1,24]

Little is known about the molecular pathogenesis of biliary papillomatosis. A point mutation at codon 12 of the *KRAS2* gene was detected in a case of biliary papillomatosis that arose in a congenital choledochal cyst.[26] Whereas *KRAS2* gene mutations and allelic losses on chromosomes 5q and 18q appear to be infrequent events in biliary papillomatosis, microsatellite instability is relatively common and appears to play a role in the pathogenesis of some of these tumors.[34] The prognosis of patients with biliary papillomatosis is poor. The mean survival period in 13 patients for whom adequate follow-up was available was 3 years.[24] Five patients (38%) survived for more than 5 years. Two patients lived for 6 years after curettage and external drainage. However, almost half of the patients died within 3 years of diagnosis.[24]

Malignant Epithelial Neoplasms of the Distal Common Bile Duct

Malignant epithelial neoplasms can arise in any segment of the extrahepatic biliary tree, but most seem to arise in the upper third, near the hilar area (49%). Approximately 19% of carcinomas of the extrahepatic bile ducts originate in the distal portion of the common bile duct. In the United States, the incidence of carcinoma of the extrahepatic bile ducts is 0.54 cases per 100,000 population.[1]

These neoplasms characteristically occur in older people. In our series, the age range varied from 34 to 87 years, with a mean of 66 years for men and 70 years for women.[1] Although these neoplasms are slightly more common in men, the rates for carcinomas of the distal common bile duct are essentially the same in blacks and whites.

The etiology of extrahepatic bile duct cancer is unknown. However, numerous risk factors have been documented. The association of extrahepatic bile duct carcinoma with ulcerative colitis and sclerosing cholangitis has long been established.[35,36] Patients with a history of long-standing ulcerative colitis and sclerosing cholangitis have a relative risk of developing bile duct carcinoma of 31.2%.[1] As a group, patients who develop extrahepatic bile duct carcinoma as a complication of ulcerative colitis and sclerosing cholangitis are younger (mean, 42 years) than those who have carcinoma of the extrahepatic bile ducts unassociated with these two inflammatory diseases.

Studies, largely from Japan, indicate that a congenitally abnormal choledochopancreatic junction predisposes to carcinoma of the gallbladder and the common bile duct.[37] As result of the congenital anomaly, the common channel (i.e., the pancreatobiliary duct) is usually abnormally long and is no longer under the control of the sphincter of Oddi. Cancer may be the result of reflux of pancreatic juice into the common bile duct or into choledochal cysts. The pancreatic juice is able to induce metaplastic changes in the mucosa that may progress to dysplasia, in situ carcinoma, and invasive carcinoma.[37] Rarely, carcinomas of the bile duct have been described in association with certain congenital anomalies, including congenital absence of the gallbladder.[1]

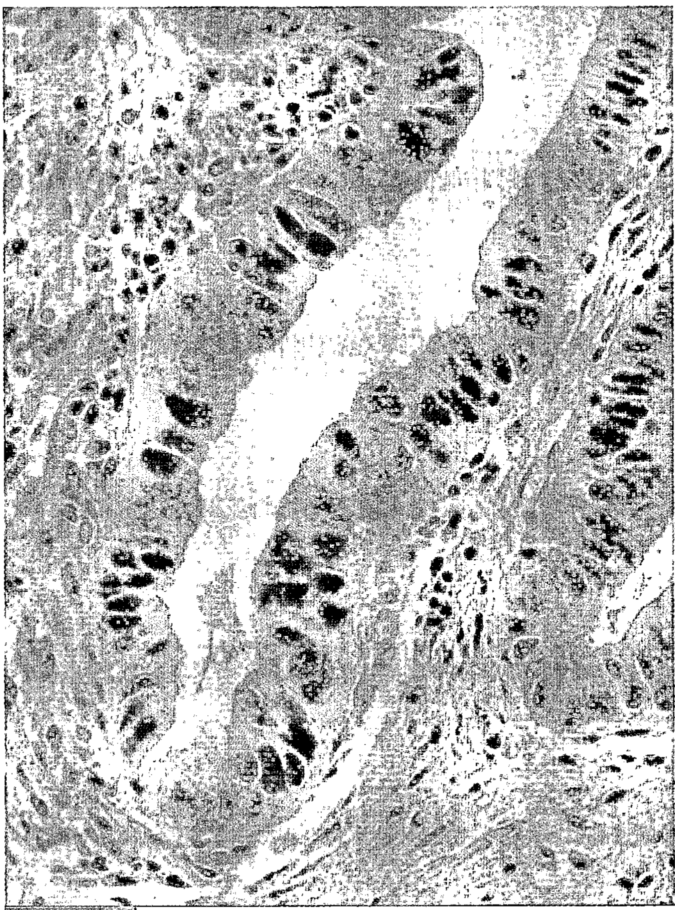

Figure 54.11
High-grade dysplasia of the common bile duct. The lining epithelial cells show large, pseudostratified, hyperchromatic nuclei.

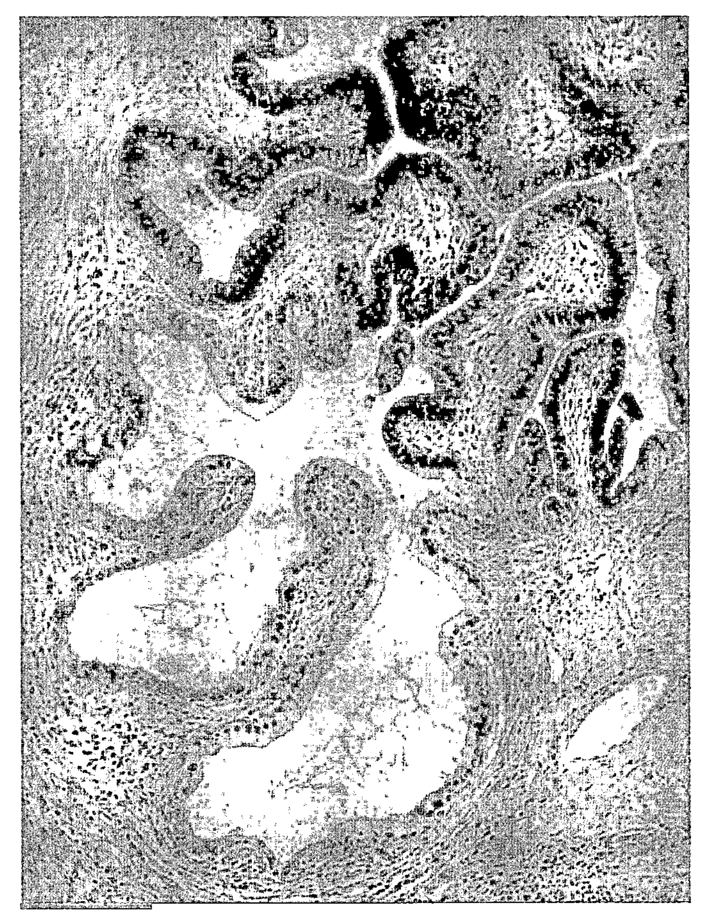

Figure 54.12
Dysplastic cells extend into the sacculi of Beale, mimicking invasion.

Patients with familial adenomatous polyposis coli occasionally develop carcinoma of the common bile duct. The bile duct carcinoma in these patients is probably an expression of the underlying genetic abnormality that occurs in familial adenomatous polyposis coli.[11,38]

In the Orient, infestation with the liver flukes *Clonorchis sinensis* or *Opisthorchis viverrini* has long been associated with carcinoma of both the intrahepatic and the extrahepatic biliary tree.[39,40] With persistent infection, the mucosa becomes hyperplastic. Later, adenomatous changes develop that can progress to dysplasia and carcinoma.

Choledocholithiasis does not appear to play a role in the etiology of carcinoma of the common bile duct, although cholelithiasis has been proposed as a risk factor.[1]

Twenty percent to 30% of patients with carcinoma of the extrahepatic bile ducts have gallstones.[1] Cholecystectomy for cholelithiasis appears to reduce the risk of extrahepatic bile duct carcinoma beginning 10 years after surgery.[1] Less than 20% of carcinomas of the common bile duct are associated with choledocholithiasis.

Dysplasia and Carcinoma in situ

During the past two decades, numerous studies have shown that flat dysplasia and carcinoma in situ occur commonly in the mucosa adjacent to invasive carcinomas of the extrahepatic bile ducts.[1,41] Moreover, foci of bile duct dysplasia have been described in association with primary sclerosing cholangitis, ulcerative colitis, infestation with *C. sinensis* or *O. viverrini*, abnormal choledochopancreatic junction, and choledochal cysts.[1] As a result, it is now generally accepted that the dysplasia-carcinoma sequence is the usual pathway for the development of invasive carcinoma of the extrahepatic bile ducts. Only a very small proportion of bile duct carcinomas arise from preexisting adenomas of intestinal type.

Morphologically, dysplasia is characterized by large cuboidal or columnar atypical cells that show pseudostratification, loss of polarity, and increased mitotic activity (Figs. 54.11 and 54.12). Dysplasia is graded as mild, moderate, or severe, depending on the severity of nuclear atypia. The terms low- and high-grade dysplasia are also used. In carcinoma in situ, the cells are indistinguishable from those of invasive carcinoma but are confined to the surface epithelium. Both dysplasia and in situ carcinoma may extend into the sacculi of Beale and intramural glands and simulate invasion.

Dysplasia and carcinoma in situ should be distinguished from epithelial reactive atypia, which occurs in association with nonspecific chronic inflammation. For instance, if a stent has been left in the common bile duct for longer than 2 weeks, atypical reactive changes can be very prominent and may simulate high-grade dysplasia or carcinoma in situ.[1] In contrast to dysplasia and carcinoma in situ, atypical reactive cells are heterogeneous. They may be cuboidal or columnar and have clear or basophilic cytoplasm. The nuclei are either hyperchromatic or vesicular with prominent nucleoli. Pseudostratification and even formation of pseudocribriform structures may occur. A variable number of mitotic figures are present. Intraepithelial inflammatory cells are common. Like neoplastic cells, atypical reactive cells may extend into the intramural glands and simulate invasion. It is advisable to avoid a diagnosis of dysplasia or in situ carcinoma in areas with extensive inflammation. In small endoscopic biopsies, the distinction between reactive atypia and dysplasia or carcinoma in situ may be impossible.

Invasive Carcinoma

Clinical features Carcinomas of the distal common bile duct usually cause early obstruction that results in jaundice, which can rapidly progress or fluctuate. Jaundice often appears while the neoplasm is relatively small before lymphatic dissemination has occurred. Other symptoms include right upper quadrant pain, malaise, anorexia, nausea, vomiting, and weight loss. If ascending cholangitis develops, chills and fever appear. The gallbladder may be dilated and palpable. A palpable mass or ascites indicates advanced disease, which precludes complete resection of the carcinoma. The liver is enlarged and may become nodular because of metastasis or secondary biliary cirrhosis. Laboratory findings reflect extrahepatic bile duct obstruction. They include hyperbilirubinemia, bilirubinuria, and an increase in serum alkaline phosphatase and glutamic oxaloacetic transaminase levels. Elevated serum levels of CEA and the carbohydrate antigen CA19-9 can be detected in most patients with these tumors. However, these serum markers lack specificity and may increase with extrahepatic obstruction from any cause.

Transhepatic or endoscopic retrograde cholangiopancreatography is essential to determine the site of obstruction and sometimes the extent of the lesion. Endoscopic ultrasonography is also a reliable procedure in the diagnosis and staging of these tumors. Cytologic examination of endoscopic retrograde cholangiopancreatographic brushings is a useful procedure for the diagnosis of carcinoma of the common bile duct.[42,43] According to different series, the sensitivity of cytologic brushings varies from 40% to 70%, and its specificity between 70% and 100%. Malignant cells are often arranged in disordered cords or sheets and show enlarged nuclei with irregular contours, an increased nuclear:cytoplasmic ratio, chromatin clumping, nuclear molding, prominent nucleoli, and cytoplasmic vacuoles.[43] *KRAS2* mutational analysis of endoscopic retrograde cholangiopancreatographic brushings has been considered a valuable diagnostic adjunct to conventional light microscopy.[44] However, *KRAS2* gene mutations are not specific for malignancy and can be detected in hyperplastic ductal epithelial lesions from both bile ducts and pancreas.[1,44]

Gross pathology Carcinomas of the common bile duct usually appear as nodular, polypoid, or diffusely infiltrating lesions. A combination of these gross patterns is often seen. Occasionally, there is minimal thickening or induration of the bile duct wall, which when opened longitudinally reveals only a roughened and granular mucosa. These subtle changes can be overlooked on gross examination, even by experienced surgeons and pathologists.

Most common bile duct carcinomas are firm, gray-white, and ill defined. A few are friable and show necrosis, especially spindle and giant cell carcinomas. Mucinous carcinomas have a gelatinous appearance. When carcinoma of the distal common bile duct coexists with carcinoma of the ampulla, the carcinomas appear as two distinct nodules separated by normal mucosa. Some tumors spread along the entire biliary ductal system, and their site of origin is impossible to determine with certainty.

Microscopic features The microscopic features of carcinoma of the common bile duct do not differ from those arising in the upper portion of the extrahepatic bile ducts. The vast majority (> 85%) are well- to moderately differentiated adenocarcinomas with an abundant desmoplastic stroma.[1,45] Small, medium-sized, and long tubular glands are identified in most of these neoplasms (Figs. 54.13 and 54.14). The lining epithelial cells vary from low cuboidal to tall columnar, mucin-secreting cells resembling gastric foveolar cells. Well-differentiated adenocarcinomas lined by cuboidal or columnar cells with minimal atypia, basal nuclei, and inconspicuous nucleoli may have a deceptively benign appearance and are difficult to recognize on small biopsy samples. The infiltrative pattern and the lack of a lobular arrangement of the glands are helpful features in

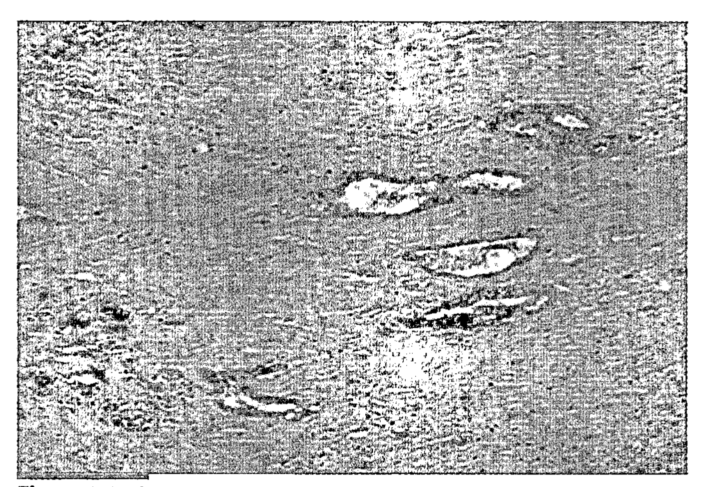

Figure 54.13
Well-differentiated adenocarcinoma. Several small tubular glands that contain mucin lie in an abundant desmoplastic stroma.

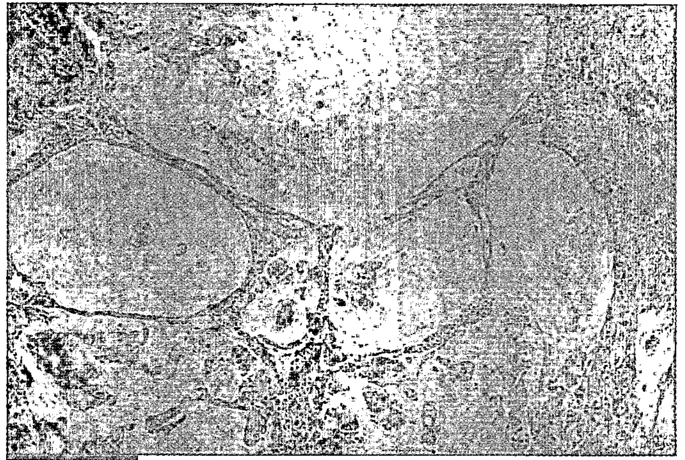

Figure 54.15
Mucinous carcinoma of common bile duct. Pools of mucin contain small clusters and strands of neoplastic cells.

the diagnosis of carcinoma. Moderately differentiated adenocarcinomas may show cribriform or pseudoangiomatous patterns.[1] Mucinous, signet-ring, and small-cell carcinomas are exceedingly rare and are similar to those that occur in other organs[1] (Fig. 54.15). Intestinal-type adenocarcinomas have a close resemblance to colonic adenocarcinomas[1] (Fig. 54.16). Clear-cell carcinomas usually contain foci of conventional bile duct adenocarcinoma, often secrete mucin, and are immunoreactive for CEA, features that allow distinction from metastatic renal cell carcinoma.[46] For prognostic reasons, papillary carcinomas should be classified into noninvasive (Fig. 54.17) or minimally invasive (<1 mm) and invasive types. Noninvasive and minimally invasive carcinomas behave as in situ carcinomas, whereas invasive papillary carcinomas

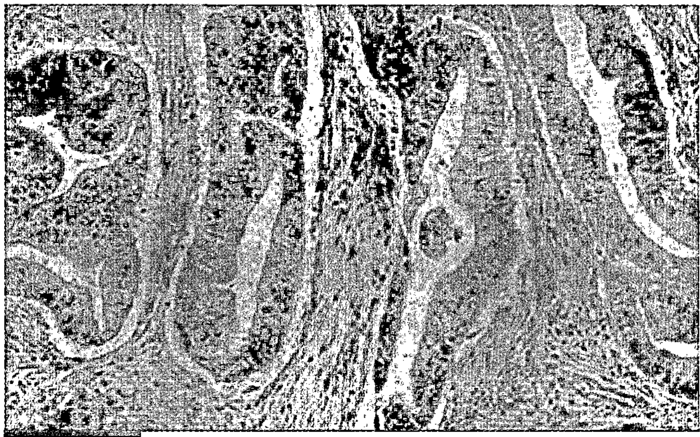

Figure 54.16
Intestinal-type adenocarcinoma. The tubular glands are lined by columnar neoplastic cells with intestinal phenotype.

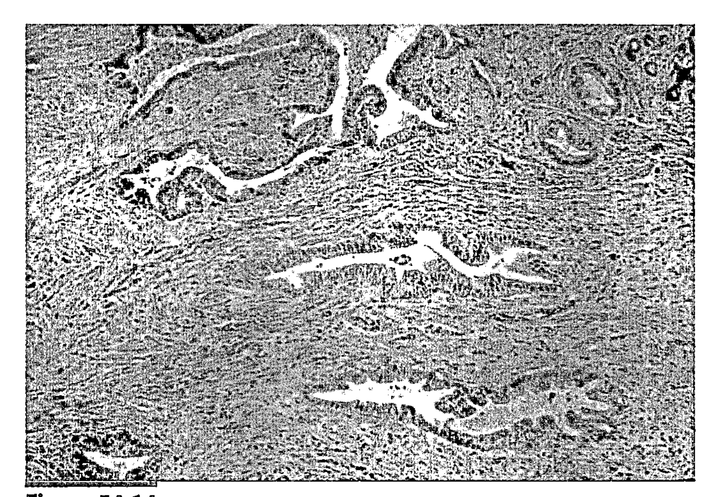

Figure 54.14
Well-differentiated adenocarcinoma. Long, branching, tubular glands are surrounded by abundant fibrous stroma.

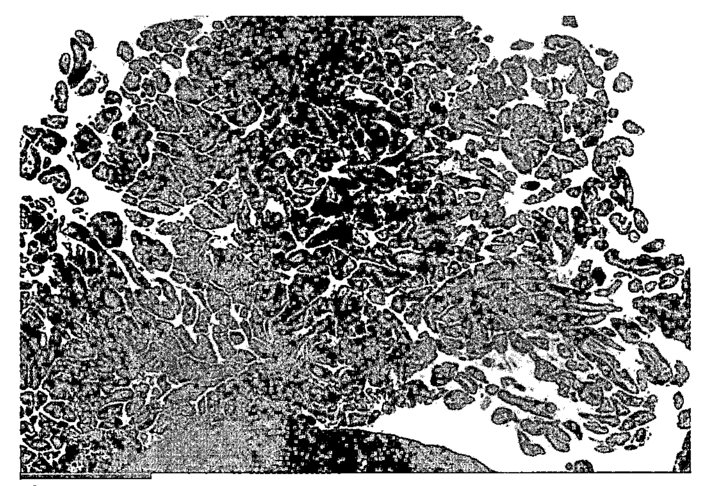

Figure 54.17
Noninvasive papillary carcinoma. Innumerable complex papillary structures project into the lumen but do not invade the wall of the common bile duct.

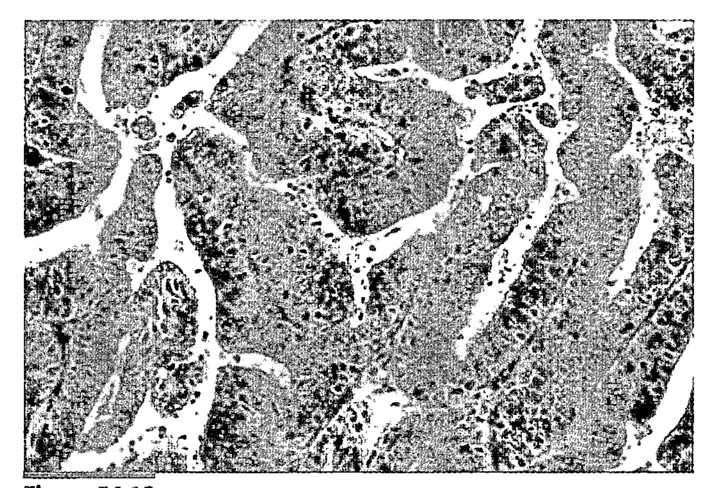

Figure 54.18
Invasive papillary carcinoma. The pseudostratified neoplastic cells are cuboidal or columnar and show biliary phenotype.

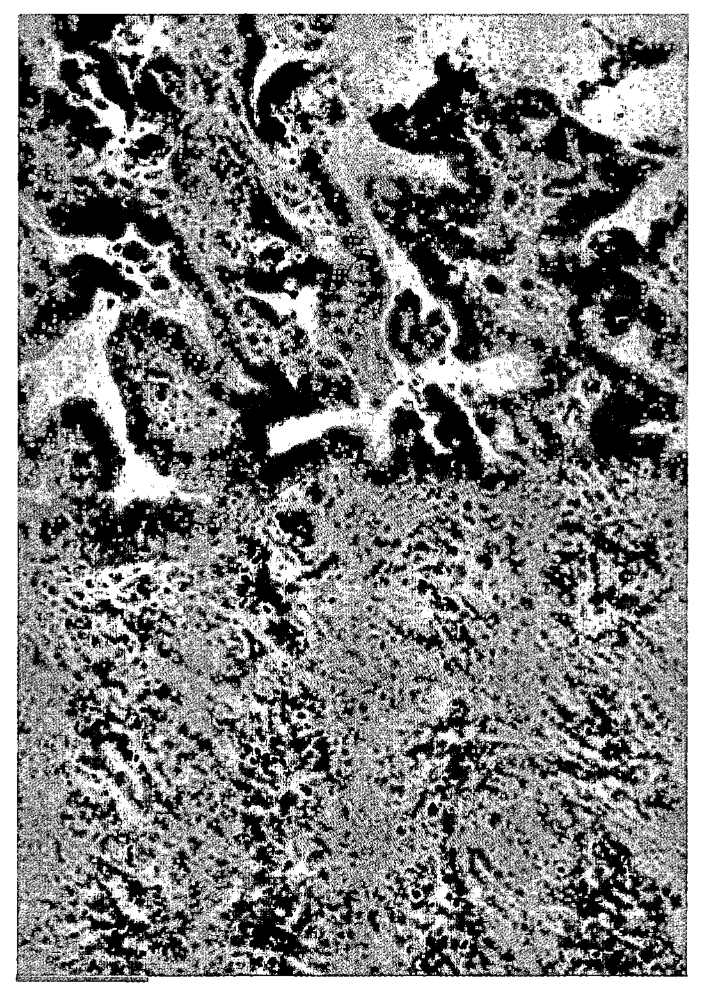

Figure 54.19
Noninvasive papillary carcinoma with invasive small (oat) cell carcinoma.

are associated with a poor prognosis (10-year survival rate, 21%). Microscopically, these papillary carcinomas are well to moderately differentiated and are characterized by complex papillary structures with or without gland formation that project into the lumen of the bile duct.[47,48] Most papillary neoplasms show a biliary phenotype (Fig. 54.18), but a minority exhibit an intestinal phenotype. The invasive component can be papillary, glandular, or both. Some of these carcinomas may dedifferentiate into small (oat)cell carcinoma (Fig. 54.19), giant-cell carcinoma or undifferentiated non-small (non-oat) cell carcinoma.[48] Adenosquamous carcinomas show glandular and squamous components with variable degrees of differentiation. Pure squamous cell carcinomas are usually moderately differentiated and are similar to those that occur in the gallbladder. Adenocarcinomas or undifferentiated carcinomas containing spindle cells and numerous osteoclast-like giant cells resembling giant-cell tumor of bone have been described in the common bile duct.[1] The mononuclear cells are epithelial membrane antigen positive, and the nonneoplastic osteoclast-like giant cells are CD-68 reactive. Undifferentiated carcinomas composed entirely of cytokeratin-positive spindle cells have also been reported.[49] Adenocarcinomas with gastric foveolar cell phenotype are extremely well-differentiated tumors that have been confused with adenomas because of their focally well-defined lobular pattern[45] (Figs. 54.20 and 54.21). The predominant neoplastic cells are tall, slender, columnar, and mucin-secreting, resembling gastric foveolar cells. Perineural invasion and foci of less-differentiated adenocarcinoma in the deep portions of the tumor facilitate recognition. Despite their deceptively benign microscopic appearance, these tumors behave as conventional adenocarcinomas of the common bile duct.

Immunohistochemistry Most well- to moderately differentiated adenocarcinomas of the common bile duct are diffusely immunoreactive to cytokeratins 7 and 19; most are negative or at the most focally reactive for cytokeratin 20[50,51] (Fig. 54.22). These neoplasms show both cytoplasmic and membrane reactivity for CEA.[52] In our experience, the great majority of carcinomas of the common bile duct abnormally express p53 protein.[48,53,54] In fact, in small biopsy samples, immunolabeling for CEA and p53 can help separate neoplastic glands from normal intramural glands, which are negative for these markers (Figs. 54.23 through 54.25). Approximately one third of well- to moderately differentiated adenocarcinomas of

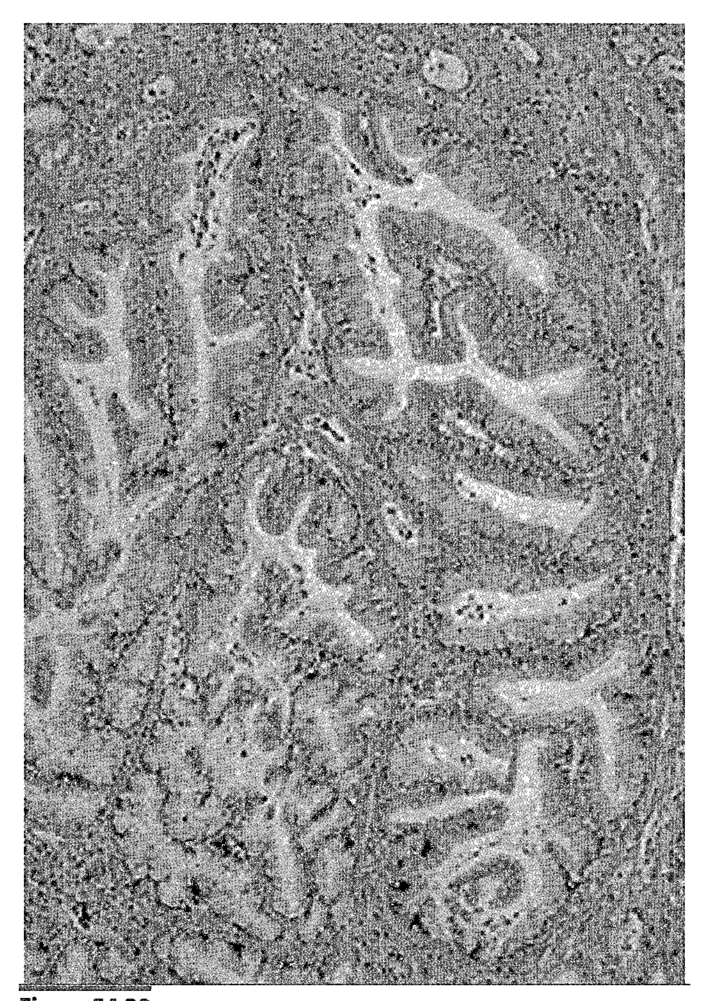

Figure 54.20
Adenocarcinoma of gastric foveolar type. Lobules of neoplastic glands like this simulate an adenoma.

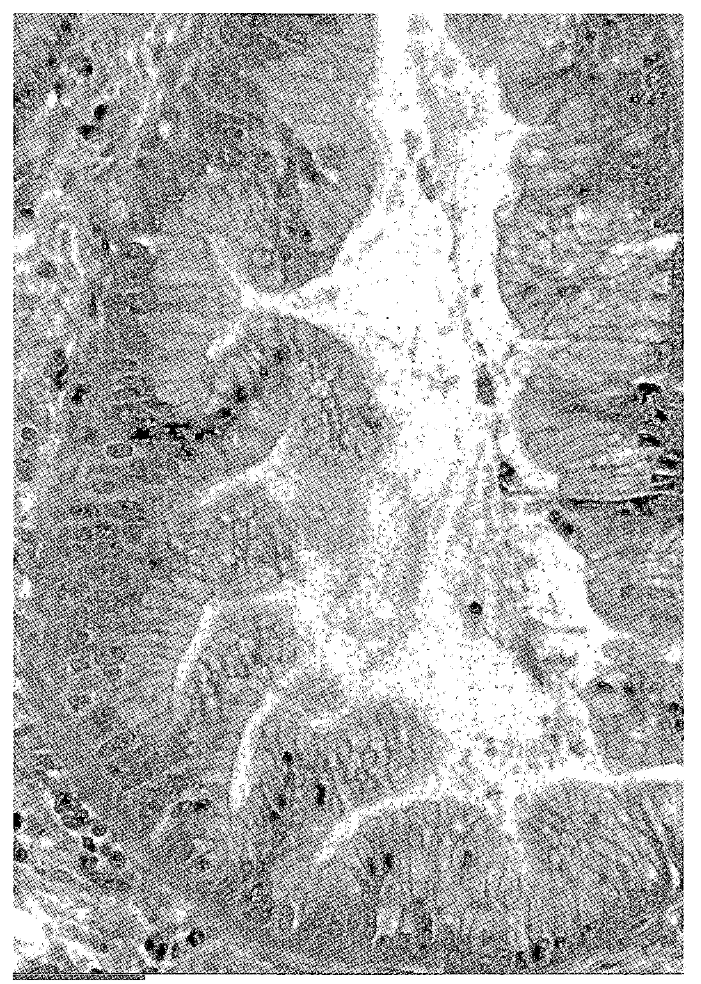

Figure 54.21
Adenocarcinoma of gastric foveolar type. A neoplastic gland is lined by tall, slender, columnar cells with basal nuclei and abundant mucin-containing cytoplasm.

the common bile duct contain chromogranin-positive endocrine cells.[1,55] These endocrine cells are more abundant in the intestinal type of adenocarcinoma. Loss of Dpc4 protein expression has been noted in 55%–62% of adenocarcinomas of the common bile duct, including invasive papillary carcinomas.[48,56]

Carcinomas of the common bile duct express MUC1 and MUC2 mucins, which are high-molecular-weight glycoproteins with different functions. In one study, MUC1, an anti-adhesion molecule, was highly expressed by poorly differentiated carcinomas, whereas MUC2, a cell differentiation molecule, was frequently expressed by well-differentiated carcinomas.[57] Likewise, well-differentiated carcinomas of the common bile duct show higher immunohistochemical expression of E-cadherin, a transmembrane glycoprotein that mediates calcium-dependent adhesion of cells, than that appearing in poorly differentiated carcinomas.[58] Similar immunohistochemical findings have been reported with α-catenin, a cell-to-cell adhesion molecule.[58] In addition, well-differentiated adenocarcinomas of the common bile duct show immunoreactivity for CD44 standard form and its variants v3 and v6 (a transmembrane glycoprotein involved in cell-to-cell and cell-to-matrix interactions).[58]

Molecular pathology Numerous studies have shown that codon 12 *KRAS2* gene mutations are common and appear to be an early event in the molecular pathogenesis of invasive adenocarcinoma of the extrahepatic bile ducts.[59-61] The reported incidence of these mutations has varied from zero to 100%, but the true figure probably lies between 55% and 65%. *KRAS2* gene mutations have been detected in hyperplastic bile duct lesions, providing support for an early event in the

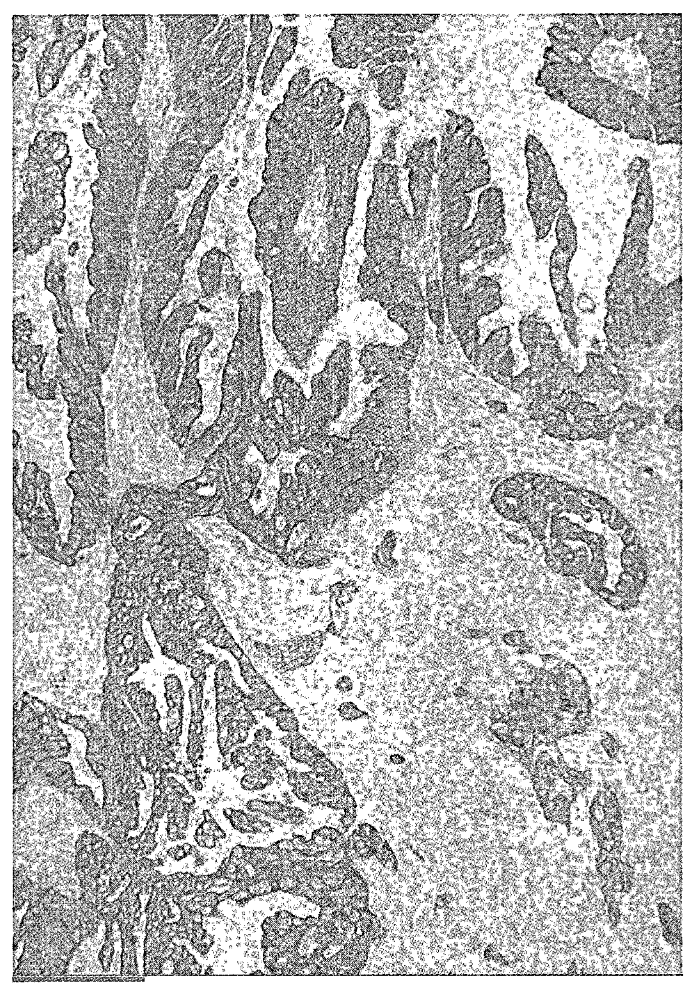

Figure 54.22
Invasive papillary adenocarcinoma. Both the papillary noninvasive and the invasive glandular components show strong immunoreactivity for cytokeratin 7.

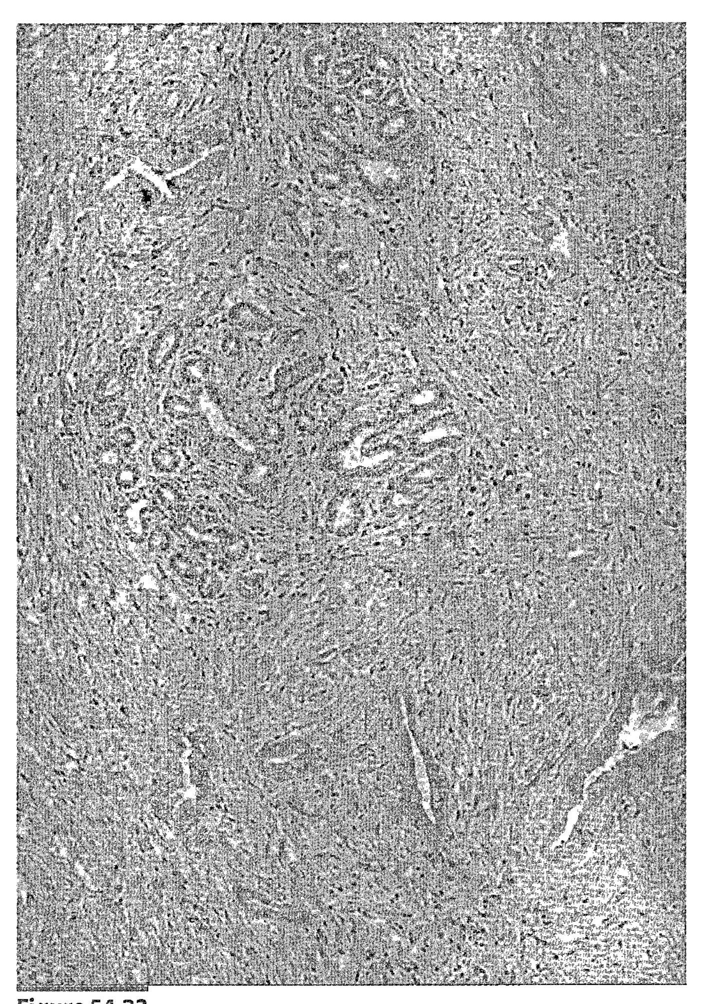

Figure 54.23
Well-differentiated adenocarcinoma. Intramural glands maintain their lobular architecture, whereas the neoplastic glands are distributed at random and lie in an abundant fibrous stroma.

molecular pathway of these tumors. Most adenocarcinomas of the extrahepatic bile ducts abnormally express p53 protein. P53 expression probably correlates with genetic mutation because a significant proportion of intrahepatic cholangiocarcinomas (essentially the same neoplasm in a different location) harbor mutations of the *TP53* gene.[62-64] Common bile duct carcinomas also harbor mutations of the *SMAD4/DPC4* tumor suppressor gene.[65] In one series of 32 extrahepatic bile duct carcinomas, 16% had point mutations in the *SMAD4/DPC4* gene[65] by single-strand conformational analysis.[65] Rijken et al.[66] studied 14 distal common bile duct carcinomas by comparative genomic hybridization and found that the most frequent site of loss was the long arm of chromosome 18, which houses the *SMAD4/DPC4* locus.

Prognosis In patients with carcinoma of the extrahepatic bile duct, those with neoplasms located in the distal common bile duct appear to have a better prognosis, both due to relatively early diagnosis and the higher resectability rate of these tumors. The 5-year survival rate for this group of patients with all stages combined is 28%.[67] Stage of disease, histologic type, and perineural and lymphovascular invasion are the most important prognostic factors.[68] The 5-year survival rate of patients without nodal metastases is better than that of patients with nodal metastases.[69] In one series, the 5-year survival rate for radically resected, node-negative tumors was 54%.[70] Noninvasive and minimally invasive papillary carcinomas behave as in situ carcinomas. None of the nine patients with these types of papillary carcinomas reported on by Albores-Saavedra et al.[47] died as a

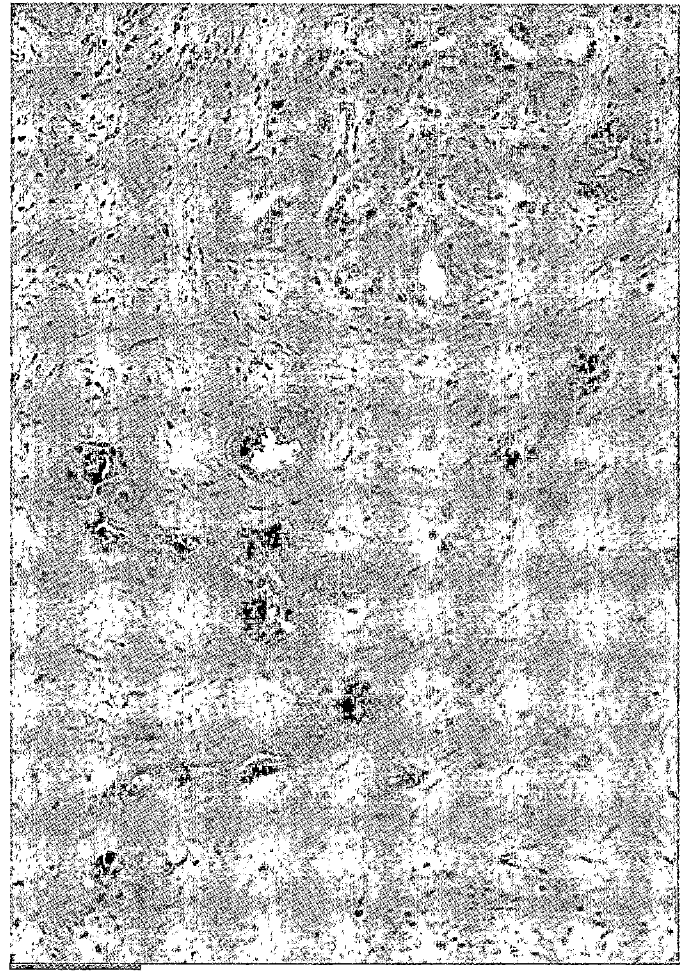

Figure 54.24
Well-differentiated adenocarcinoma shown in Figure 54.23. The neoplastic glands are positive for carcinoembryonic antigen, whereas the normal intramural glands are negative.

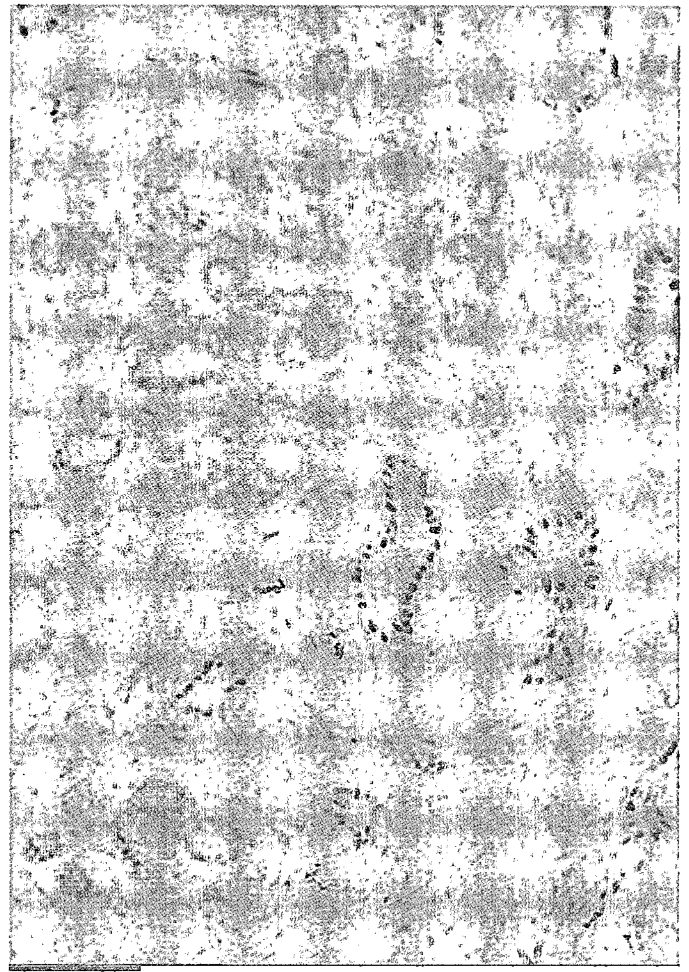

Figure 54.25
Well-differentiated adenocarcinoma shown in Figures 54.23 and 54.24. The neoplastic glands are p53 positive, whereas the intramural glands are unreactive.

direct result of the neoplasm, whereas six of 10 patients with invasive papillary carcinoma reported on by the same group died because of local recurrence or metastasis.[48] Of 174 invasive papillary carcinomas compiled by the Surveillance, Epidemiology, and End Results program of the National Cancer Institute, 71 were confined to the ductal wall, and 61 had regional node metastasis. Papillary carcinomas confined to the ductal wall had better 10-year relative survival rates than conventional adenocarcinoma limited to the wall (21% vs 12%).[48] Likewise, papillary carcinomas with lymph node metastasis had a better prognosis than conventional adenocarcinomas with nodal metastasis (10-year relative survival rate of 12% vs 5 %).[48] In our experience, there is no correlation between p53, ki67, and Dpc4 expression in these neoplasms and patient survival.

Endocrine Tumors

Carcinoid Tumors

Carcinoid tumors of the extrahepatic biliary tree are exceedingly rare endocrine neoplasms that represent 0.1% of all carcinoids of the gastrointestinal tract.[1] The most common location in the biliary tree is the common bile duct.[71-79] Recognition of these tumors is important because they differ clinically and morphologically from carcinomas of the common bile duct. Although both carcinoids and carcinomas can have similar presenting clinical features, including painless jaundice with or without pruritus, carcinoid tumors are more common in young adult females, whereas carcinomas show a slight male predominance and typically present in the 6th or 7th decade of life. Carcinoid tumors have been reported in

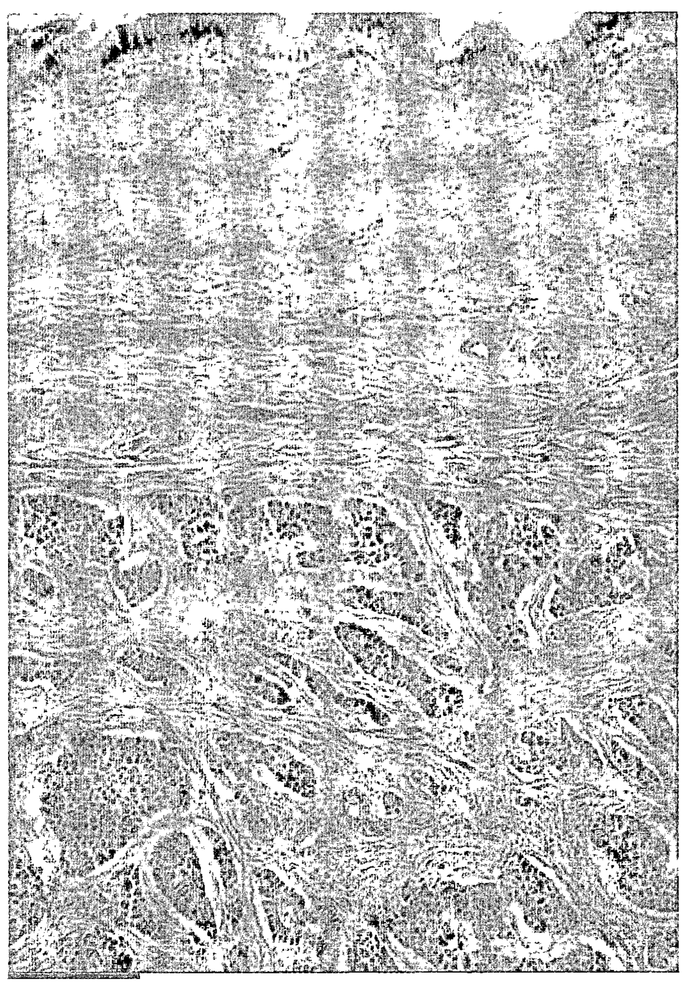

Figure 54.26
Carcinoid tumor of common bile duct. Between the tumor and the normal surface biliary epithelium, there is a band of dense fibrous tissue.

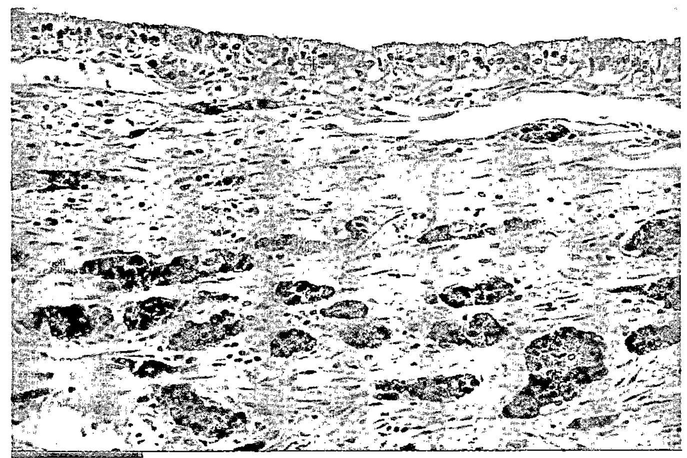

Figure 54.27
Carcinoid tumor of common bile duct. The neoplastic cells show immunoreactivity for serotonin.

association with multiple endocrine neoplasia type 1 and the von Hippel-Lindau syndrome,[1,71] whereas the incidence of carcinomas is increased in patients with ulcerative colitis and primary sclerosing cholangitis. Perhaps more importantly, the prognosis of these two tumors is markedly different. Whereas carcinomas are aggressive neoplasms with a high mortality rate, carcinoid tumors are far more indolent.[79] In fact, patients with carcinoid tumors have reasonable long-term life expectancy, even in the presence of hepatic metastases.[9]

Carcinoid tumors are usually small, firm, and poorly demarcated submucosal nodules. Occasionally, they appear as polypoid lesions that project into the lumen of the common bile duct. On sectioning, they are firm and gray-white or yellow. Carcinoid tumors are composed of small, uniform cells arranged in nests, cords, or trabeculae with an intervening fibrous, often hyalinized, stroma (Fig. 54.26). Tubular structures are occasionally present. The nuclei are round or ovoid with finely granular chromatin and small inconspicuous nucleoli. The cytoplasm is granular, eosinophilic, or clear. Although submuscosal, these neoplasms often ulcerate the overlying epithelium and may also extend into the periductal soft tissues and pancreas. Carcinoid tumors of the common bile duct probably arise from the endocrine cells normally present in the intramural glands. We have not seen the tubular or goblet cell variants of carcinoid tumors in the common bile duct. Most carcinoid tumors of the common bile duct are argyrophilic, and some are argentaffin. They are usually diffusely positive for chromogranin and synaptophysin. Most are immunoreactive for serotonin, and some are also reactive for peptide hormones, such as somatostatin, gastrin, and pancreatic polypeptide[71,76] (Fig. 54.27). The immunoreactivity for Dpc4 in two tumors suggests that Dpc4 abnormalities may not be critical in the pathogenesis of common bile duct carcinoids.[79] These tumors lack reactivity for p53 protein and do not show *TP53* gene mutations. In our series of seven carcinoids, a mutation in codon 12 of the *KRAS2* gene was detected in one tumor.[79]

Paragangliomas are exceedingly rare benign neoplasms that can occur in the common bile duct. Although usually small (<1 cm in greatest dimension), they appear as well-to-poorly demarcated nodules that can lead to bile duct obstruction.[80] Microscopically, the neoplasm is composed of chief and sustentacular cells. The chief cells are arranged in nests ("zellballen") separated by thin fibrous septa that contain capillaries. The sustentacular cells, highlighted by immunolabeling for the S100 protein, are seen around the nests of chief cells, which are chromogranin positive. Peptide hormones have not been detected in paragangliomas of the extrahepatic biliary tree.

Benign Nonepithelial Tumors

Granular Cell Tumor

Granular cell tumors of the extrahepatic bile ducts are histologically distinctive neoplasms of uncertain histogeneses that usually lead to obstruction and are often confused with carcinoma both clinically and by imaging techniques.[81-86] They are more common in the common bile duct than in other segments of the biliary tree. Ninety percent of the patients are young women (mean age, 34 years), and 65% are black. Children and adolescents are rarely affected, with only a few cases having been reported.

Jaundice and abdominal pain are the characteristic manifestations of common bile duct tumors. Cholangiography and ultrasound reveal the site of obstruction. Because the symptoms and radiologic findings lack specificity, it is impossible to diagnose granular cell tumors before biopsy or surgical excision.

Occasionally, granular cell tumors are multicentric and may arise in different sites synchronically or asynchronically.[81,85] As a result, patients with granular cell tumor of the common bile duct may have similar neoplasms in the gallbladder, skin, omentum, esophagus, and stomach.[1,85] These multicentric lesions should not be confused with metastases. Granular cell tumors of the common bile duct appear as poorly demarcated, firm, yellow-tan submucosal nodules that usually protrude into the lumen and are no greater than 2 cm.

Microscopically, the submucosal neoplasms are composed of clusters, cords, or sheets of large polygonal, ovoid, round, or spindle-shaped granular cells that infiltrate the wall of the common bile duct, eventually obliterating the lumen. The cells have abundant, eosinophilic, and granular periodic acid–Schiff positive cytoplasm. Large cytoplasmic hyaline globules are seen in most tumors. Nuclei are small, round, centrally placed, and hyperchromatic. A mild degree of nuclear pleomorphism occurs in a few cases, but mitotic figures are not seen. Granular cell tumors of the common bile duct may extend into the periductal connective tissue or pancreas. Rarely, perineural invasion and direct extension into lymph nodes occurs. These changes should not be interpreted as evidence of malignancy.[1] In fact, malignant granular cell tumors have not been described in the common bile duct. Hyperplasia of the overlying surface epithelium and reactive atypia of intramural glands occur in association with some of these neoplasms, findings that have been confused with carcinoma[86] (Fig. 54.28).

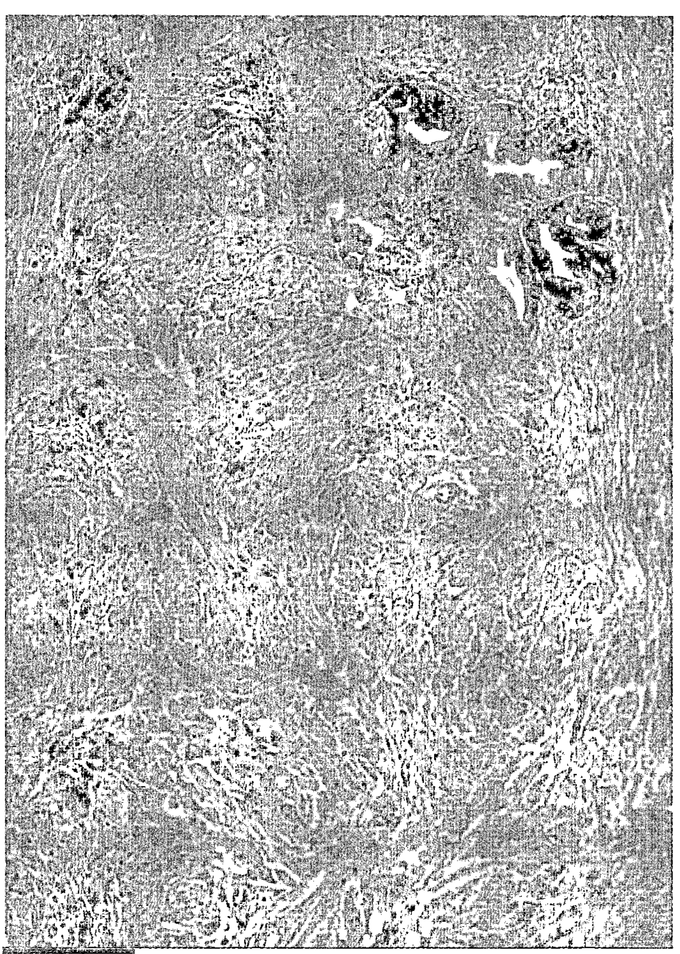

Figure 54.28
These reactive intramural glands, which are embedded in the granular cell tumor, have been misinterpreted as adenocarcinoma.

Granular cell tumors of the common bile duct show immunoreactivity for vimentin, S100 protein, myelin basic protein, and inhibin.[87] By electron microscopy, the cells contain numerous autophagic lysosomes, myelin-like figures, and degenerated mitochondria.[1]

Neurofibromas, lipomas, and leiomyomas have rarely been described in the common bile duct.[1] Some of these neoplasms are symptomatic, whereas others constitute autopsy findings. Histologically, they do not differ from those that occur in the soft tissues. In contrast to the gallbladder, pancreas, and liver, single or multiple leiomyomas associated with acquired or congenital immunodeficiencies have not been reported in the common bile duct.[88]

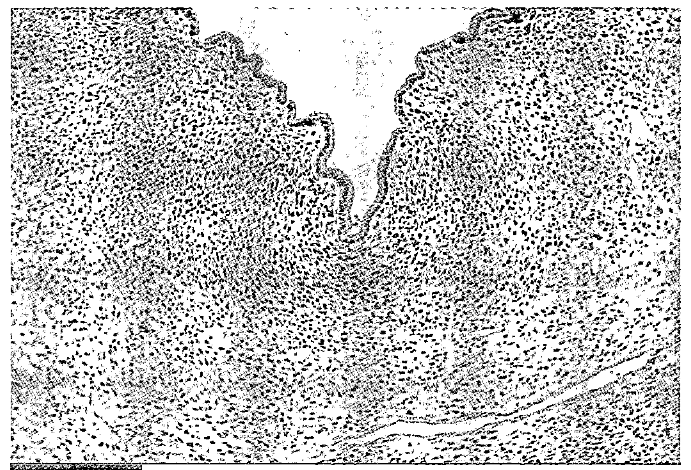

Figure 54.29
Embryonal rhabdomyosarcoma covered by normal biliary epithelium. The tumor is densely cellular and composed of small, round cells.

Malignant Mesenchymal Neoplasms

Embryonal Rhabdomyosarcoma (Sarcoma Botryoides)

The common bile duct is the most common location of embryonal rhabdomyosarcoma of the extrahepatic biliary tree. Although exceedingly rare, embryonal rhabdomyosarcoma is the most common biliary tract malignancy in children.[89,90] Intermittent jaundice, with or without abdominal distention, fever, and loss of appetite is the typical clinical presentation. These symptoms are often attributed to hepatitis, which results in delayed treatment.

Grossly, these neoplasms can be sessile or pedunculated. They often have a gelatinous appearance and form polypoid structures with a characteristic grape-like appearance. The malignant cells are located immediately beneath a single layer of normal-appearing biliary epithelium (Fig. 54.29). The neoplastic cells are small, round or ovoid, contain scant cytoplasm, and are admixed with globoid or strap rhabdomyoblasts that have abundant eosinophilic cytoplasm. These two types of cells form the cambium layer. Stellate cells loosely arranged in a myxomatous stroma are also seen. In our experience, muscle-specific actin, desmin, and MYOD1 are the best immunohistochemical markers for rhabdomyosarcoma of the common bile duct (Fig. 54.30). Myoglobin stains only the better-differentiated tumors that are easy to identify with conventional stains. The prognosis of embryonal rhabdomyosarcoma of the biliary tree has greatly improved with multidrug chemotherapy and irradiation, and it correlates with stage of disease.[91,92]

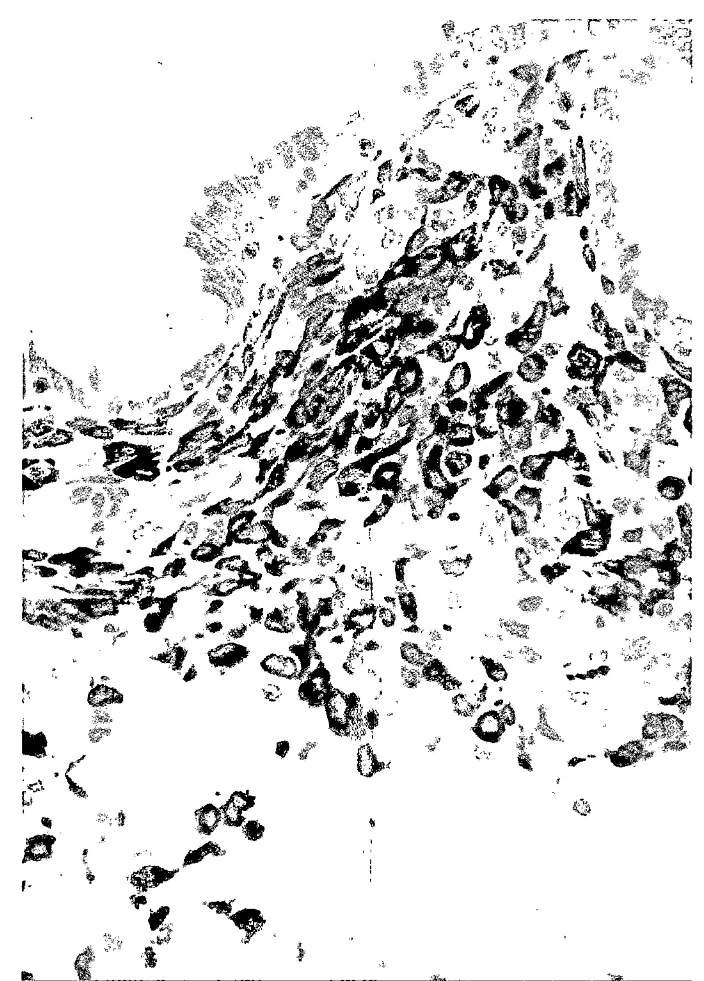

Figure 54.30
Embryonal rhabdomyosarcoma. Most neoplastic cells are desmin positive. The overlying biliary epithelium is unreactive.

Leiomyosarcoma is an exceeding rare neoplasm of the common bile duct—only a few cases have been reported. We described a case of malignant fibrous histiocytoma of the common bile duct, which appears to be the first and only case reported so far.[1]

Malignant Lymphoma

Malignant lymphomas of any type may infiltrate the wall of the common bile duct as part of a systemic process. Some may lead to obstruction and are symptomatic, whereas others are incidental autopsy findings. Primary large B-cell and small lymphocytic lymphomas of the common bile duct have occasionally been reported.[93,94] Patients present with obstructive jaundice, and a clinical diagnosis of sclerosing cholangitis or carcinoma is usually made before biopsy. Most of the patients experience systemic disease months or years after diagnosis.

Tumor-like Lesions

A number of tumor-like lesions occur in the distal common bile duct. Some of these, such as choledochal cyst and ectopic pancreas, most likely represent congenital anomalies. Others, including pyloric and intestinal metaplasia, are associated with, and are probably induced by, inflammatory changes or associated with benign and malignant tumors. The pathogenesis of primary papillary hyperplasia remains unknown.[95] Although some of these tumor-like lesions, especially pyloric, intestinal, and squamous metaplasia, are asymptomatic, others can give rise to symptoms and may be mistaken for neoplasms; still others are considered cancer precursors.

Choledochal Cysts

Congenital cysts and fusiform dilatations of the extrahepatic bile ducts involve predominantly the common bile duct (choledochal cyst). Choledochal cysts are classified according to their shape and location.[96-98] Diagnosis is based primarily on the appearance of the bile ducts, as assessed by imaging studies or by gross inspection, because these lesions have no distinctive histologic features. Choledochal cysts are found in all age groups and have a female predominance. Most cases are recognized in the first two decades of life, usually as a result of an abdominal mass and common bile duct obstruction. In children, jaundice is the most common presentation. Some of the cysts are quite large and can reach up to 15 cm in diameter. Biliary tract anomalies have occasionally been reported in association with choledochal cysts, including double common bile duct, double gallbladder, absent gallbladder, and stenosis of the intrahepatic bile ducts.[99] An anomalous pancreatobiliary junction is reported in 64%–97% of patients with choledochal cysts.[99] It has been postulated that reflux of pancreatic enzymes into the bile duct weakens the wall by damaging intercellular junctions of the surface epithelium. In addition, reflux of pancreatic enzymes can cause chronic inflammation with fibrosis and surface erosion. Histologically, the cyst wall is composed of dense fibrous tissue, which usually lacks an epithelial lining, although islands of intact mucosa may be seen. Over time, metaplastic changes, dysplasia, and carcinoma may develop.[100] *KRAS2* gene mutations have been detected in normal, dysplastic, and neoplastic biliary epithelium.[101] Up to 15% of patients with choledochal cysts may develop carcinoma; however, the incidence of carcinoma varies with age. It is estimated to be less than 0.1% in children younger than 10 years, 6.8% in people between 10 and 20 years of age, and 15% in patients older that 20 years.[102] Adenocarcinoma is the most common malignant neoplasm in choledochal cysts, but adenosquamous carcinomas, carcinoid tumors, and rhabdomyosarcomas have also been reported[1] (Fig. 54.31).

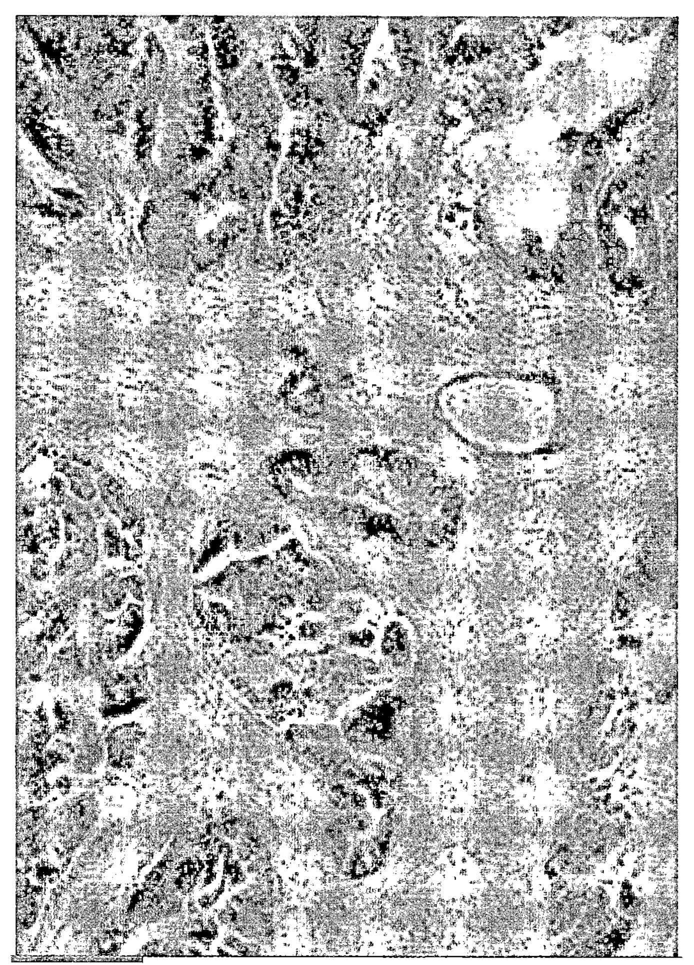

Figure 54.31
Invasive adenocarcinoma infiltrating the wall of a choledochal cyst. An in situ component not seen here was also identified.

Amputation or traumatic neuroma is a tumor-like nodular lesion that develops months or years after biliary tract surgery. Abdominal pain is the usual presenting symptom. Most traumatic neuromas involve the duct wall and periductal connective tissue. Rarely, however, they grow into the lumen of the common bile duct and lead to obstruction.[103,104] Microscopically, traumatic neuroma is composed of distorted nerve fibers separated by variable amounts of fibrous tissue.

Heterotopic tissue, including gastric mucosa and pancreas, has been reported in the common bile duct. Ectopic

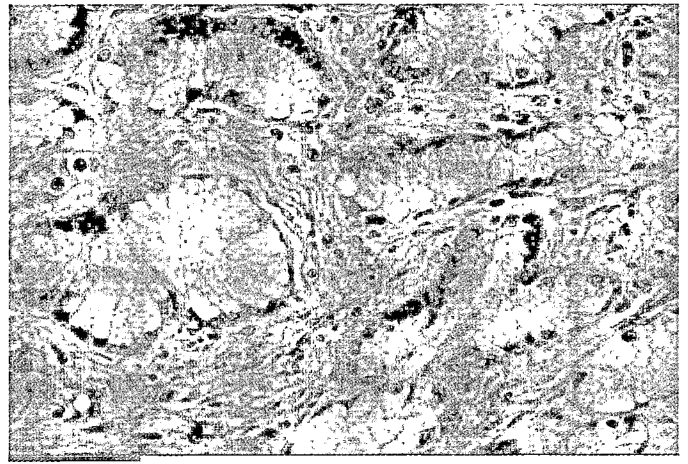

Figure 54.32
Pyloric gland metaplasia of intramural glands. The columnar cells that line the glands have abundant mucin-containing cytoplasm and small basal nuclei.

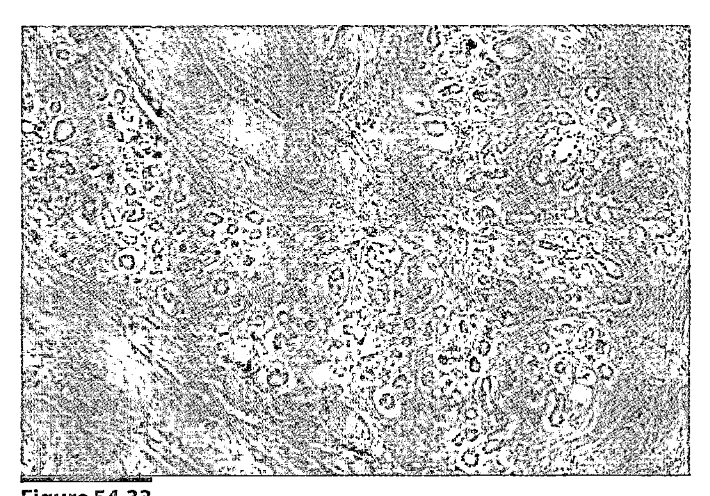

Figure 54.33
Hyperplasia of intramural glands. Lobules of intramural glands have extended beyond the ductal wall. Fibrosis and marked nerve proliferation are seen around the gland lobules.

gastric mucosa is commonly an incidental microscopic finding, whereas ectopic pancreas often leads to obstruction and jaundice and may mimic carcinoma clinically.[1]

Pyloric Gland, Intestinal, and Squamous Metaplasia

Pyloric gland metaplasia is the most common metaplastic lesion of the common bile duct and involves primarily the intramural glands (Fig. 54.32). It arises in a background of chronic inflammation or in association with benign and malignant tumors. Intestinal and squamous metaplasia usually coexist with pyloric gland metaplasia and are also incidental microscopic findings.[105]

Hyperplasia of Intramural Glands

In contrast to pyloric, intestinal, and squamous metaplasia, which are usually incidental microscopic findings, hyperplasia of intramural glands can be symptomatic and can simulate carcinoma both clinically and histologically.[106] It is usually seen in association with chronic inflammation, including primary sclerosing cholangitis and benign and malignant epithelial neoplasms. We have seen one case not associated with chronic inflammation or tumor. The florid type of intramural gland hyperplasia, which extends beyond the ductal wall and is accompanied by extensive fibrosis and marked nerve proliferation, may lead to bile duct obstruction. The intramural glands maintain their lobular pattern and show no cytologic atypia (Fig. 54.33). Rarely, however, the glands may invade nerves and can closely simulate carcinoma. The hyperplastic glands show low proliferative activity, as measured by the MIB-1 labeling index, and lack reactivity for P53 and monoclonal CEA, whereas carcinoma nearly always shows reactivity for these markers.[106]

In our experience, most lesions known as adenomyomatous hyperplasia, adenomyoma, or hamartoma of the ampulla of Vater are examples of florid hyperplasia of intramural glands of the terminal portion of the common bile duct rather than heterotopic pancreatic tissue lacking acinar elements and islets of Langerhans.[107] Hyperplasia of intramural glands of the terminal portion of the common bile duct may form a nodule or have a diffuse growth pattern. It is usually symptomatic and gives rise to abdominal pain and obstructive jaundice. The occasional coexistence of hyperplasia of intramural glands with carcinoma should not be misinterpreted as malignant transformation but rather as a reactive process induced by the tumor, as occurs in other segments of the biliary tree.

References

1. Albores-Saavedra J, Henson DE, Klimstra DS. Tumors of the gallbladder, extrahepatic bile ducts, and ampulla of Vater. *Atlas of Tumor Pathology*. 3rd series, Fascicle 27. Washington, DC: Armed Forces Institute of Pathology; 2000.
2. Albores-Saavedra J, Henson DE, Sobin LH. *World Health Organization International Histological Classification of Tumors of the Gallbladder and Extrahepatic Bile Ducts*. 2nd ed. Berlin, Germany: Springer-Verlag; 1991.
3. Hanafy M, McDonald P. Villous adenoma of the common bile duct. *J Roy Soc Med*. 1993;86:603–604.
4. Jao Y, Tseng LJ, Wu CJ, et al. Villous adenoma of the common bile duct. *Gastrointest Endosc*. 2003;57:561–562.

5. Buckley JG, Salimi Z. Villous adenoma of the common bile duct. *Abdom Imaging*. 1993;18:245–246.
6. Erwald R. Gardner's syndrome with adenoma of the common bile duct, a case report. *Acta Chir Scand*. 1984;520:63–68.
7. Jarvinen HJ, Nyberg M, Peltokallio P. Biliary involvement in familial adenomatosis coli. *Dis Colon Rectum*. 1983;26:525–528.
8. Parke MC, Knight M. Peutz-Jeghers syndrome causing obstructive jaundice due to polyp in common bile duct. *J Roy Soc Med*. 1983;76:701–703.
9. Futami H, Furuta T, Hanai H, et al. Adenoma of the common bile duct in Gardner's syndrome may cause relapsing acute pancreatitis. *J Gastroenterol*. 1997;32:558–561.
10. Sturgis TM, Fromkes JJ, Marsh W. Adenoma of the common bile duct: endoscopic diagnosis and resection. *Gastrointest Endosc*. 1992;38:504–505.
11. Komorowski RA, Tresp MG, Wilson SD. Pancreatobiliary involvement in familial polyposis coli/Gardner's syndrome. *Dis Colon Rectum*. 1986;29:55–58.
12. Spigelman AD, Farmer KC, James M, et al. Tumours of the liver, bile ducts pancreas and duodenum in a single patient with familial adenomatous polyposis. *Br J Surg*. 1991;78:979–980.
13. Albores-Saavedra J, Vardaman C, Vuitch F. Non-neoplastic polypoid lesions and adenomas of the gallbladder. *Pathol Annu*. 1993;28:145–177.
14. Devaney K, Goodman ZD, Ishak KG. Hepatobiliary cystadenoma and cystadenocarcinoma: a light microscopic and immunohistochemical study of 70 patients. *Am J Surg Pathol*. 1994;18:1078–1091.
15. O'Shea JS, Shah D, Cooperman AM. Biliary cystadenocarcinoma of extrahepatic duct origin arising in previously benign cystadenoma. *Am J Gastroenterol*. 1987;82:1306–1310.
16. Thomas JA, Scriven MW, Puntis MC, et al. Elevated CA19-9 levels in hepatobiliary cystadenoma with mesenchymal stroma: two case reports with immunohistochemical confirmation. *Cancer*. 1992;70:1841–1847.
17. Vuitch F, Battifora H, Albores-Saavedra J. Demonstration of steroid hormone receptors in pancreato-biliary mucinous cystic neoplasms [abstract]. *Lab Invest*. 1983;68:114A.
18. Lee JH, Chen DR, Pang SC, et al. Mucinous biliary cystadenoma with mesenchymal stroma: expression of CA19-9 and carcinoembryonic antigen in serum and cystic fluid. *J Gastroenterol*. 1996;31:732–736.
19. Terada T, Kitamura Y, Ohta T, et al. Endocrine cells in hepatobiliary cystadenomas and cystadenocarcinomas. *Virchows Arch*. 1997;430:37–40.
20. Scott FR, More L, Dhillon AP. Hepatobiliary cystadenoma with mesenchymal stroma: expression of oestrogen receptors in formalin-fixed tissue. *Histopathology*. 1995; 26:555–558.
21. Grayson W, Teare J, Myburgh JA, et al. Immunohistochemical demonstration of progesterone receptors in hepatobiliary cystadenoma with mesenchymal stroma. *Histopathology*. 1996;29:461–463.
22. Bronnimann S, Zimmermann A, Baer HU. Diffuse bile duct papillomatosis: high rate of recurrence and risk of malignant transformation. *Chirurgie*. 1996;67:93–97.
23. Cheng MS, AhChong AK, Mak KL, et al. Case report: two cases of biliary papillomatosis with unusual associations. *J Gastroenterol Hepatol*. 1999;14:464–467.
24. Hubens G, Delvaux G, Willems G, et al. Papillomatosis of the intra-and extrahepatic bile ducts with involvement of the pancreatic duct. *Hepatogastroenterology*. 1991;38:413–418.
25. Kim YS, Myung SJ, Kim SY, et al. Biliary papillomatosis: clinical, cholangiographic and cholangioscopic findings. *Endoscopy*. 1998;30:763–767.
26. Ohita H, Yamaguchi Y, Yamakawa O, et al. Biliary papillomatosis with the point mutation of K-ras gene arising in congenital choledochal cyst. *Gastroenterology*. 1993; 105:1209–1212.
27. Sagar PM, Omar M, Macrie J. Extrahepatic biliary papillomatosis occurring after removal of a dysplastic gallbladder. *HPB Surg*. 1993;6:219–221.
28. Seo DW, Lee SK, Kim MH. Biliary papillomatosis. *Gastrointest Endosc*. 2000;51:67.
29. Taguchi J, Yasunaga M, Kojiro M, et al. Intrahepatic and extrahepatic biliary papillomatosis. *Arch Pathol Lab Med*. 1993;117:944–947.
30. Terada T, Mitsui T, Nakanuma Y, et al. Intrahepatic biliary papillomatosis arising in nonobstructive intrahepatic biliary dilatations confined to the hepatic left lobe. *Am J Gastroenterol*. 1991;86:1523–1526.
31. Tireli M, Uslu A. Multiple biliary papillomatosis. *HPB Surg*. 1992;26:125–127.
32. Neumann RD, LiVolsi VA, Rosenthal NS, et al. Adenocarcinoma in biliary papillomatosis. *Gastroenterology*. 1976; 70:779–782.
33. Kim HJ, Kim MH, Lee, SK, et al. Mucin-hypersecreting bile duct tumor characterized by a striking homology with an intraductal papillary mucinous tumor (IMPT) of the pancreas. *Endoscopy*. 2002;32:389–393.
34. Abraham SC, Lee JH, Boitnott JK, et al. Microsatellite instability in intraductal papillary neoplasms of the biliary tract. *Mod Pathol*. 2002;15:1309–1317.
35. Mir-Madjlessi SH, Farmer RG, Sivak MV, Jr. Bile duct carcinoma in patients with ulcerative colitis. Relationship to sclerosing cholangitis: report of six cases and review of the literature. *Dig Dis Sci*. 1987;32:145–154.
36. Bergquist A, Ekbom AH, Olsson R, et al. Hepatic and extrahepatic malignancies in primary sclerosing cholangitis. *J Hepatol*. 2002;36:321–327.
37. Aoki H, Sugaya H, Shimazu M. A clinical study on cancer of the bile duct associated with anomalous arrangements of the pancreaticobiliary ductal system: analysis of 569 cases collected in Japan. *J Biliary Tract Pancreatol*. 1987; 40:880–883.
38. Jarvinen HJ, Nyberg M, Peltokallio P. Biliary involvement in familial adenomatosis coli. *Dis Colon Rectum*. 1983;26: 525–528.
39. Sher L, Iwatsuki S, Lebeau G, et al. Hilar cholangiocarcinoma associated with clonorchiasis. *Dig Dis Sci*. 1989;34:1121–1123.
40. Haswel-Elkins MR, Statarug S, Elkins DB. Opisthorchis viverrini infection in Northeast Thailand and its relationship to cholangiocarcinoma. *J Gastroenterol Hepatol*. 1992;7: 538–548.

41. Suzuki M, Takahashi T, Ouchi K, et al. The development and extension of hepatohilar bile duct carcinoma: a three-dimensional tumor mapping in the intrahepatic biliary tree visualized with the aid of a graphics computer system. *Cancer*. 1989;64:658–666.
42. Ryan ME. Cytologic brushings of ductal lesion during ERCP. *Gastrointest Endosc*. 1991;37:139–142.
43. Cohen MB, Wittchow RJ, Johlin FC, et al. Brush cytology of the extrahepatic biliary tract: comparison of cytologic features of adenocarcinoma and benign biliary strictures. *Modern Pathol*. 1995;8:498–502.
44. Sturm PD, Rauws EA, Hruban RH, et al. Clinical value of K-ras codon 12 analysis and endobiliary brush cytology for the diagnosis of malignant extrahepatic biliary stenosis. *Clin Cancer Res*. 1999;5:629–635.
45. Albores-Saavedra J, Delgado R, Henson DE. Well differentiated adenocarcinoma, gastric foveolar type of the extrahepatic bile ducts: a previously unrecognized and distinctive variant of bile duct carcinoma. *Ann Diagn Pathol*. 1999;3:75–80.
46. Vardaman C, Albores-Saavedra J. Clear cell carcinoma of the gallbladder and extrahepatic bile ducts. *Am J Surg Pathol*. 1995;19:91–99.
47. Albores-Saavedra J, Murakata LA, Krueger JE, et al. Noninvasive and minimally invasive papillary carcinomas of the extrahepatic bile ducts. *Cancer*. 2000;89:508–515.
48. Hoang MP, Murakata LA, Katabi N, et al. Invasive papillary carcinoma of the extrahepatic bile ducts: a clinicopathologic and immunohistochemical study of 13 cases. *Mod Pathol*. 2002;15:1251–1258.
49. Nagai E, Shinohara M, Yonemasu H, et al. Undifferentiated carcinoma of the common bile duct: case report and review of the literature. *HBP Surg*. 2002;9:627–631.
50. Rullier A, LeBail B, Fawaz R, et al. Cytokeratin 7 and 20 expression in cholangiocarcinomas varies along the biliary tract but still differs from that in colorectal carcinoma metastasis. *Am J Surg Pathol*. 2000;42:870–876.
51. Duval JV, Savas, L, Banner BF. Expression of cytokeratins 7 and 20 in carcinoma of the extrahepatic biliary tract, pancreas and gallbladder. *Arch Pathol Lab Med*. 2000;124:1196–2000.
52. Yamaguchi K, Enjoji M, Nakayama F. Cancer of the extrahepatic bile duct: a clinicopathologic study of immunohistochemistry for CEA, CA 19-9, and p21. *World J Surg*. 1988;12:11–17.
53. Diamantis I, Karamitopoulou E, Perentes E, et al. p53 protein immunoreactivity in extrahepatic bile duct and gallbladder cancer: correlation with tumor grade and survival. *Hepatology*. 1995;22:774–779.
54. Suto T, Sugai T, Nakamura S, et al. Assessment of p53, MIB (Ki-67 antigen) and argyrophilic organizer regions in carcinoma of the extrahepatic bile duct. *Cancer*. 1998;82:86–95.
55. Yamamoto M, Takahashi I, Iwamoto T, et al. Endocrine cells in extrahepatic bile duct carcinoma. *J Cancer Res Clin Oncol*. 1984;108:331–335.
56. Argani P, Shaukat A, Kaushal M, et al. Differing rates of loss of DPC4 expression and of p53 overexpression among carcinoma of the proximal and distal bile duct: evidence for biologic distinction. *Cancer*. 2001;91:1332–1341.
57. Tamada S, Goto M, Nomoto M, et al. Expression of MUC1 and MUC2 mucins in extrahepatic bile duct carcinomas: its relationship with tumor progression and prognosis. *Pathol Int*. 2002;52:713–723.
58. Mikami T, Saegusa M, Mitomi H, et al. Significant correlations of E-cadherin, catenin and CD44 variant form expression with carcinoma cell differentiation and prognosis of extrahepatic bile duct carcinomas. *Am J Clin Pathol*. 2001;116:369–376.
59. Watanabe M, Asaka M, Tanaka J, et al. Point mutation of K-ras gene codon 12 in biliary tract tumors. *Gastroenterology*. 1994;107:1147–1153.
60. Imai M, Hoshi T, Ogawa K. K-ras codon 12 mutations in biliary tract tumors detected by polymerase chain reaction denaturing gradient gel electrophoresis. *Cancer*. 1994;73:2727–2733.
61. Matsubara T, Sakurai Y, Sasayama Y, et al. K-ras point mutations in cancerous and noncancerous biliary epithelium in patients with pancreaticobiliary maljunction. *Cancer*. 1996;77:1752–1757.
62. Kiba T, Tsuda H, Pairojkul C, et al. Mutations of the p53 tumor suppressor gene and the ras gene family in intrahepatic cholangiocellular carcinomas in Japan and Thailand. *Mol Carcinog*. 1993;8:312–318.
63. Kang YK, Kim WH, Lee HW, et al. Mutation of p53 and K-ras, and loss of heterozygosity of APC in intrahepatic cholangiocarcinoma. *Lab Invest*. 1999;79:477–483.
64. Hahn SA, Bartsch D, Schroers A, et al. Mutations of DPC4/SMAD4 gene in biliary tract carcinoma. *Cancer Res*. 1998;58:1124–1126.
65. Rijken AM, Hu J, Perlman EJ, et al. Genomic alterations in distal bile duct carcinoma by comparative genomic hybridization and karyotype analysis. *Genes Chromosomes Cancer*. 1999;26:185–191.
66. Tompkins RK, Thomas D, Wile A, et al. Prognostic factors in bile duct carcinoma: analysis of 96 cases. *Ann Surg*. 1981;194:447–455.
67. Henson DE, Albores-Saavedra J, Corle D. Carcinoma of the extrahepatic bile ducts: histologic types, stage of disease, grade, and survival rates. *Cancer*. 2000;70:1498–1501.
68. Wade TP, Prasad CN, Virgo KS, et al. Experience with distal bile duct cancers in U.S. Veterans Affairs hospitals: 1987-1991. *J Surg Oncol*. 1997;64:242–245.
69. Fong Y, Blumgart LH, Lin E, et al. Outcome of treatment for distal bile duct cancer. *Br J Surg*. 1996;83:1712–1715.
70. Fellows IW, Leach IH, Smith PG, et al. Carcinoid tumor of the common bile duct: a novel complication of von Hippel-Lindau syndrome. *Gut*. 1990;31:728–729.
71. Alexander IA, Thomson KK, Klune GA. Primary common bile duct carcinoid: demonstration by computed tomography, ultrasonography and angiography. *Aust Radiol*. 1986;30:34–37.
72. Angeles-Angeles A, Quintanilla-Martinez L, Larriva-Sahd J. Primary carcinoid of the common bile duct: immunohistochemical characterization of a case and review of the literature. *Am J Clin Pathol*. 1991;96:341–344.

73. Barron-Rodriguez LP, Manivel JC, Mendez-Sanchez N, et al. Carcinoid tumor of the common bile duct: evidence for its origin in metaplastic endocrine cells. *Am J Gastroenterol.* 1991;8:1073–1076.
74. Kopelman D, Schein M, Kerner H, et al. Carcinoid tumor of the common bile duct. *HPBS Surg.* 1996;10:41–43.
75. Hao L, Friedman AL, Navarro VJ, et al. Carcinoid tumor of the common bile duct producing gastrin and serotonin. *J Clin Gastroenterol.* 1996;23:63–65.
76. Nahas SC, Lourencao JL, Gazoni E, et al. Carcinoid tumor of the common bile duct: report of a case. *Rev Hosp Clin Fac Med Univ Sao Paulo.* 1998;53:26–28.
77. Ross AC, Hurley JB, Hay WB, et al. Carcinoid of the common bile duct: a report and literature review. *Can J Surg.* 1999;42:59–63.
78. Mandujano-Vera G, Angeles-Angeles A, de la Cruz-Hernandez J, et al. Gastrinoma of the common bile duct: immunohistochemical and ultrastructural study of a case. *J Clin Gastroenterol.* 1995;20:321–324.
79. Maitra A, Krueger JE, Tascilar M, et al. Carcinoid tumors of the extrahepatic bile ducts: a study of seven cases. *Am J Surg Pathol.* 2000;24:1501–1510.
80. Caceres M, Mosquera LF, Shih JA, et al. Paraganglioma of the bile duct. *South Med J.* 2001;94:515–518.
81. Aisner SC, Khaneja S, Ramirez O. Multiple granular cell tumors of the gallbladder and biliary tree: report of a case. *Arch Pathol Lab Med.* 1982;106:470–471.
82. Lindberg G, Saborian H, Housini I, et al. The clinicopathologic spectrum of granular cell tumors [abstract]. *Lab Invest.* 1996;74:9A.
83. Lafreniere R, Demetrick DJ, Benediktsson H. Granular cell neoplasm of the extrahepatic biliary tree: morphological, ultrastructural and immunohistochemical study of review of the literature. *J Surg Oncol.* 1991;46:60–66.
84. Mackenzie DJ, Klapper E, Gordon LA, et al. Granular cell tumor of the biliary system. *Med Pediatr Oncol.* 1994;23:50–56.
85. Mauro MA, Jaques PF. Granular cell tumors of the esophagus and common bile duct. *J Can Assoc Radiol.* 1981;32:254–256.
86. Eisen RN, Kirby WM, O'Quinn JL. Granular cell tumors of the biliary tree: a report of two cases and review of the literature. *Am J Surg Pathol.* 1991;15:460–465.
87. Murakata LA, Ishak KG. Expression of inhibin-alpha by granular cell tumors of the gallbladder and extrahepatic bile ducts. *Am J Surg Pathol.* 2000;42:895.
88. Monforte-Munoz H, Kapoor N, Albores-Saavedra J. Epstein-Barr virus-associated leiomyomatosis and post-transplant lymphoproliferative disorder in a child with severe combined immunodeficiency: case report and review of the literature. *Ped Dev Pathol.* 2003;6:449–457.
89. Davis GL, Kissane JM, Ishak KG. Embryonal rhabdomyosarcoma (sarcoma botryoides) of the biliary tree: report of five cases and a review of the literature. *Cancer* 1969;24:333–342.
90. Lack EE, Perez-Atayde AR, Schuster SR. Botryoid rhabdomyosarcoma of the biliary tract. *Am J Surg Pathol.* 1981;5:643–652.
91. Ruymann FB, Raney RB, Crist WM, et al. Rhabdomyosarcoma of the biliary tree in childhood: a report from the Intergroup Rhabdomyosarcoma Study. *Cancer.* 1985;56:575–581.
92. Maurer HM, Gehan EA, Beltangady M, et al. The Intergroup Rhabdomyosarcoma Study-II. *Cancer.* 1993;71:1904–1922.
93. Brouland JP, Molimard JP, Nemeth J, et al. Primary T-cell rich B-cell lymphoma of the common bile duct. *Virchows Arch (A).* 1993;423:513–517.
94. Chiu KW, Changchien CS, Chen L, et al. Primary malignant lymphoma of common bile duct presenting as acute obstructive jaundice. *J Clin Gastroenterol.* 1995;20:259–261.
95. Albores-Saavedra J, Defortuna SM, Smothermon WE. Primary papillary hyperplasia of the gallbladder and cystic and common bile ducts. *Hum Pathol.* 1990;21:228–231.
96. Katyal D, Lees GM. Choledochal cysts: a retrospective review of 28 patients and a review of the literature. *Can J Surg.* 1992;35:584–588.
97. O'Neill JA Jr: Choledochal cyst. *Curr Probl Surg.* 1992;29:361–410.
98. Todani T, Watanabe Y, Narusue M, et al. Congenital bile duct cysts: classification, operative procedures and review of thirty-seven cases, including cancer arising from choledochal cyst. *Am J Surg.* 1997;134:263–269.
99. Komi N, Tamura T, Miyoshi Y, et al. Nationwide survey of cases of choledochal cyst: analysis of coexistent anomalies, complications and surgical treatment in 645 cases. *Surg Gastroenterol.* 1984;3:69–72.
100. Komi N, Tamura T, Miyoshi Y, et al. Histochemical and immunohistochemical studies on development of biliary carcinoma in forty-seven patients with choledochal cyst-special reference to intestinal metaplasia in the biliary duct. *Jpn J Surg.* 1985;15:273–278.
101. Matsubara T, Sakurai Y, Sasayama Y, et al. K-ras point mutations in cancerous and noncancerous biliary epithelium in patients with pancreaticobiliary maljunction. 1996;77:1752–1757.
102. Voyles CR, Smadja WC, Shands C, et al. Carcinoma in choledochal cysts: age-related incidence. *Arch Surg.* 1983;118:986–988.
103. Arai A. A case of obstructive jaundice by neuromas in the common bile duct. *Acta Hepatol Jpn.* 1984;25:813–817.
104. Larson DM, Storsteen KA. Traumatic neuroma of the bile ducts with intrahepatic extension causing obstructive jaundice. *Hum Pathol.* 1984;15:287–209.
105. Hoang MP, Murakata LA, Padilla-Rodriguez AL, et al. Metaplastic lesions of the extrahepatic bile ducts: a morphologic and immunohistochemical study. *Mod Pathol.* 2001;14:1119–1125.
106. Katabi N, Albores-Saavedra J. The extrahepatic bile duct lesions in end-stage primary sclerosing cholangitis. *Am J Surg Pathol.* 2003;27:349–355.
107. Handra-Luca A, Teris B, Couvelard A, et al. Adenomyoma and adenomyomatous hyperplasia of the Vaterian system: clinical pathological and new immunohistochemical features of 13 cases. *Mod Pathol.* 2003;16:530–536.

Italicized page locators denote photographs/figures; t denotes a table.

A

B

C

E

G

H

N

O

Q

R

S

U